W9-APU-698

CLINICAL ONCOLOGY

∎∎∎

RAYMOND E. LENHARD, JR., MD

ROBERT T. OSTEEN, MD

TED GANSLER, MD

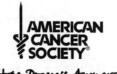

AMERICAN CANCER SOCIETY

Hope. Progress. Answers.

Managing Editor: Lois F. Hall
Copyeditor: Marius Broekhuizen
Production Manager: Candace Magee
Production Editor: Tom Gryczan
Production Coordinators: Suzy Crawford and Shange Amani
Graphic Designer/Figures: Dana Wagner
Design/Composition: Graphic Composition, Inc., Athens, GA
CD-ROM Developer: Snider Publishing Services, Franklin, NY
Publisher: Emily Pualwan

The American Cancer Society, Inc., Atlanta, Georgia 30329

03 02 01 00   5 4 3 2 1

Library of Congress Cataloging-in-Publication Data

Clinical oncology / [edited by] Raymond E. Lenhard, Jr.,
Robert T. Osteen, Ted Gansler.—1st ed.
    p. ; cm.
  Includes bibliographic references and index.
  ISBN 0-944235-15-8
    1. Cancer. I. Lenhard, R. E. (Raymond E.) II. Osteen,
Robert T., 1941– III. Gansler, Ted S. IV. American Cancer
Society.
   [DNLM: 1. Neoplasms. QZ 200 C6407 2000]
RC261 .C6513 2000
616.99′44—dc21
                                  00-032290
                                     CIP

Book and CD-ROM sold as a package only (ISBN 0-944235-15-8)

Institutional and international orders distributed through
Blackwell Science, Inc.

In the US: **Blackwell Science, Inc.**
              350 Main Street
              Malden, MA 02148
              Phone: 781-388-8250
              Toll Free Phone: 1-800-215-1000
              Fax: 781-388-8270

Order by telephone
in the US 1-800-215-1000
in Canada 800-665-1148
in Australia 03-9347-0300
outside North America and Australia 44-01235-465500

Contents

Preface

CLINICAL ONCOLOGY, THE AMERICAN CANCER Society's textbook of cancer, was conceived and produced as a source of information on the wide range of issues in cancer. We hope that it will help health care providers adopt practices to encourage prevention and early detection and to offer state-of-the-art diagnosis and treatment. The textbook was designed as a resource for medical and nursing students and for primary-care physicians, nurses, and others responsible for creating medical care plans, the goal of which is to return the cancer patient to as productive and healthy a life as possible. It offers practical and immediate information and clinical approaches and serves as a bridge to more specialized and comprehensive textbooks and the literature. Although it is directed primarily to generalists in the health professions, it also will serve as a ready resource for those with special interest in oncology.

Many changes have been made in this edition of *Clinical Oncology*. The most apparent is the format: It has been reorganized to address in more logical order the full scope of cancer. We have incorporated elements from our *Textbook of Clinical Oncology*, 2nd Edition and our *Cancer Manual*, 9th Edition, which was developed by the American Cancer Society Massachusetts Division. The production of a CD-ROM version of this text containing hundreds of images has given us the opportunity to enhance with color art and graphics the presentation of some subjects, which was not possible using a print medium alone. In addition, this new edition places an emphasis on directing the reader to reliable electronic databases, where the next step in inquiry can be taken. Medical information in general, and cancer information in particular, is experiencing an ever-climbing growth rate. We believe that the printed page is one of many routes that can be taken and that while printed textbook chapters are a fundamental guide to strategic thinking and medical approaches, up-to-the-minute data can be presented in a more timely fashion in the dynamic world of electronic web sites.

The reader will note a further shift in our approach to the topic of cancer control, particularly the importance of primary prevention and early detection. Increasing importance is placed on our new knowledge of genetics and other biological factors and their use as a guide to prognosis and selection of treatment. Genetic subclasses of histologic diagnosis are emerging, and the various histologic types are associated with very different responses to treatment and outcome. This is illustrated especially well by acute leukemia and non-Hodgkin's lymphomas. Nowhere has more change occurred than in cancer treatment. Systemic therapy has expanded greatly, with the introduction of entirely new classes of systemic drugs that demonstrate new mechanisms of action, driven by current information based on fundamental biochemical characteristics of cancer cells that differentiate them from normal cells.

The trend currently is toward multidisciplinary management of cancer and the use of treatment strategies to cure the disease while preserving intact the primary site of the cancer and that organ's function. For many types of cancer, the integration of medical and psychological support has been realized, and the return of the patient to normal employment and activities of daily living has emerged as an achievable goal. Health care providers are exhibiting a growing emphasis on consideration of all facets of patients' well-being, including financial, occupational, legal, and socio-cultural issues.

Clinical Oncology is the outcome of the collaborative efforts of a team of American Cancer Society volunteers who donated their time and talent to this project. Their commitment and dedication made this new edition possible. For both editorial board members and chapter authors, this was a volunteer effort for which they receive no payment or honoraria.

It is equally important to note individuals' generous financial contributions to the American Cancer Society, which have made possible the production and distribution of this book. These contributions enabled the Society to render this service to the education of health care providers and, ultimately, to the primary beneficiaries of this effort—cancer patients and their families.

Raymond E. Lenhard, Jr., MD
Robert T. Osteen, MD
Ted Gansler, MD

Introduction

THE AMERICAN CANCER SOCIETY

The American Cancer Society is the nationwide community-based voluntary health organization dedicated to eliminating cancer as a major health problem by preventing cancer, saving lives from cancer, and diminishing suffering from cancer through research, education, and service. The Society originated in 1913 with a group of 10 physicians and 5 laypersons who met in New York City to found the American Society for the Control of Cancer. Its stated purpose at that time was to "disseminate knowledge concerning the symptoms, treatment, and prevention of cancer; to investigate conditions under which cancer is found; and to compile statistics in regard thereto." This organization later was renamed the *American Cancer Society* and today is one of the oldest and largest voluntary health agencies in the United States.

Today's Society includes more than 2 million volunteers and is governed by an elected board of directors from throughout the United States, half of whom are members of the medical and scientific professions and half of whom are lay members. The Society is a community-based organization made up of thousands of local volunteer leaders who form the connection between the community and the Society's national programs in cancer prevention, early cancer detection, and service to cancer patients and their families.

Editorial Board

Contributors

Steven A. Ahrendt, MD
Medical College of Wisconsin
Department of Surgery
Milwaukee, Wisconsin

Barbara L. Andersen, PhD
Ohio State University
Department of Psychology
Columbus, Ohio

Kenneth C. Anderson, MD
Harvard Medical School
Dana-Farber Cancer Institute
Boston, Massachusetts

Noreen Aziz, MD, PhD
National Cancer Institute
Division of Cancer Control and
    Population Sciences
Bethesda, Maryland

Dileep Bal, MD, MS, MPH
California Department of Health
Cancer Control Branch
Sacramento, California

David G. Bostwick, MD
Bostwick Laboratories
Richmond, Virginia

Luther W. Brady, MD
Hahnemann University Hospital
Department of Radiation Oncology
Philadelphia, Pennsylvania

John A. Carucci, MD, PhD
New York University School of
    Medicine
Department of Dermatology
New York, New York

Barrie R. Cassileth, PhD
Memorial Sloan-Kettering Cancer
    Center
New York, New York

Bruce D. Cheson, MD
National Cancer Institute
Division of Cancer Treatment and
    Diagnosis
Bethesda, Maryland

Orlo H. Clark, MD, FACS
University of California at San Francisco
Mt. Zion Medical Center
Department of Surgery
San Francisco, California

Reiner Class, PhD
Medical College of Pennsylvania-
    Hahnemann University
Department of Radiation Oncology
Philadelphia, Pennsylvania

Charles S. Cleeland, PhD
University of Texas MD Anderson
    Cancer Center
Pain Research Group
Houston, Texas

Everardo Cobos, MD
Texas Tech University Health Sciences
    Center
Department of Internal Medicine
Lubbock, Texas

Michael R. Cooper, MD
Duke University Comprehensive Cancer
    Center
Durham, North Carolina

M. Robert Cooper, MD
Wake Forest University Baptist Medical
    Center
Comprehensive Cancer Center
Winston-Salem, North Carolina

Mary E. Costanza, MD
University of Massachusetts Medical
    School
Division of Hematology and Oncology
Worcester, Massachusetts

Lisa M. DeAngelis, MD
Memorial Sloan-Kettering Cancer
    Center
New York, New York

Angela DeMichele, MD
University of Pennsylvania
Division of Hematology and Oncology
Philadelphia, Pennsylvania

Colin P. N. Dinney, MD
University of Texas MD Anderson
    Cancer Center
Division of Urology
Houston, Texas

Paul M. Dodd, MD
Memorial Sloan-Kettering Cancer
    Center
Division of Medical Oncology
New York, New York

Paul F. Engstrom, MD
Fox Chase Cancer Center
Temple University Medical School
Philadelphia, Pennsylvania

Harmon J. Eyre, MD
American Cancer Society
Medical Affairs and Research
Atlanta, Georgia

Abbie L. Fields, MD
Albert Einstein College of Medicine
Montefiore Medical Center
Division of Gynecologic Oncology
Bronx, New York

Leonard M. Finn, MD
University of Massachusetts Medical
    School
Boston University School of Medicine
Tufts University School of Medicine
Boston, Massachusetts

Irvin D. Fleming, MD, FACS
University of Tennessee Center for
    Health Sciences
Department of Surgery
Methodist Healthcare Cancer Center
Memphis, Tennessee

**Elizabeth T. H. Fontham, MPH,
DrPH**
Louisiana State University School of
    Medicine
Department of Public Health and
    Preventive Medicine
New Orleans, Louisiana

Arlene A. Forastiere, MD
Johns Hopkins University
Johns Hopkins Oncology Center
Baltimore, Maryland

Leslie G. Ford, MD
National Cancer Institute
Division of Cancer Prevention
Bethesda, Maryland

Jorge E. Freire, MD
Thomas Jefferson University
Department of Radiation Oncology
Philadelphia, Pennsylvania

Robert J. Friedman, MD, MSc
New York University School of
  Medicine
Department of Dermatology
New York, New York

John H. Glick, MD
University of Pennsylvania Cancer
  Center
Department of Medicine
Philadelphia, Pennsylvania

**John L. Gollan, MD, PhD, FRACP,
  FRCP**
Brigham and Women's Hospital
Gastroenterology Division
Harvard Medical School
Boston, Massachusetts

Daniel M. Green, MD
Roswell Park Cancer Institute
State University of New York at Buffalo
School of Medicine and Biomedical
  Sciences
Buffalo, New York

Howard M. Grodman, MD
Floating Hospital for Children
New England Medical Center
Boston, Massachusetts

Howard B. Gutstein, MD
University of Texas MD Anderson
  Cancer Center
Research Division
Houston, Texas

**Rohan J. H. Hammett, MBBS,
  FRACP**
Royal North Shore Hospital
Division of Medicine
St. Leonard's, New South Wales,
  Australia

Louis B. Harrison, MD
Beth Israel Medical Center
Department of Radiation Oncology
New York, New York

Clark W. Heath, Jr., MD
American Cancer Society (emeritus)
Department of Epidemiology and
  Surveillance Research
Atlanta, Georgia

Elisabeth I. Heath, MD
Johns Hopkins University
Johns Hopkins Oncology Center
Baltimore, Maryland

Richard F. Heitmiller, MD
Johns Hopkins University
Baltimore, Maryland

Ronald B. Herberman, MD
Pittsburgh Cancer Center
Pittsburgh, Pennsylvania

Martin J. Heslin, MD
University of Alabama at Birmingham
Birmingham, Alabama

C. Stratton Hill, Jr., MD
University of Texas MD Anderson
  Cancer Center
Houston, Texas

Scott A. Hundahl, MD, FACS
Queen's Cancer Institute
The Queen's Medical Center
Honolulu, Hawaii
Commission on Cancer
Chicago, Illinois

Joan G. Jones, MD
Albert Einstein College of Medicine
Weiler Hospital
Bronx, New York

William K. Kelly, DO
Cornell University Medical College
Memorial Sloan-Kettering Cancer
  Center
Department of Medicine
New York, New York

Leroy J. Korb, MD
Northwest Prostate Institute
Department of Radiation Oncology
Seattle, Washington

John E. Lahaniatis, MD
Medical College of Pennsylvania-
  Hahnemann University
Philadelphia, Pennsylvania

Donald L. Lamm, MD
West Virginia University
Robert C. Byrd Health Sciences Center
Department of Urology
Morgantown, West Virginia

Walter Lawrence, Jr., MD
Massey Cancer Center (emeritus)
Medical College of Virginia of Virginia
  Commonwealth University
Division of Surgical Oncology
Richmond, Virginia

Raymond E. Lenhard, Jr., MD
Johns Hopkins Oncology Center
  (emeritus)
Johns Hopkins University School
  of Medicine
Baltimore, Maryland

Frederick P. Li, MD
Dana-Farber Cancer Institute
Harvard Medical School
Harvard School of Public Health
Boston, Massachusetts

Marvin J. Lopez, MD, FACS, FRCSC
St. Elizabeth's Medical Center
Department of Surgery
Boston, Massachusetts

Karen C. Marcus, MD
Children's Hospital
Department of Radiation Oncology
Joint Center for Radiation Therapy
Harvard Medical School
Boston, Massachusetts

Patricia Marks, RN, MSN
University of Massachusetts Medical
  Center
Department of Family Medicine
Worcester, Massachusetts

Mary Jane Massie, MD
Barbara White Fishman Center for
  Psychological Counseling
Memorial Sloan-Kettering Cancer
  Center
Department of Psychiatry and
  Behavioral Sciences
New York, New York

Ronald P. McCaffrey, MD
The Cancer Center
Lowell General Hospital
Lowell, Massachusetts

Curtis J. Mettlin, PhD
Roswell Park Cancer Institute
Buffalo, New York

Glenn B. Mieszkalski, MD
Holy Name Regional Cancer Center
Holy Name Hospital
Teaneck, New Jersey

Donald M. Miller, MD, PhD
University of Alabama at Birmingham
Birmingham, Alabama

Kenneth B. Miller, MD
New England Medical Center Hospital
Boston, Massachusetts

Gerald P. Murphy, MD, DSc
Pacific Northwest Cancer Foundation
Northwest Hospital
Cancer Research Division
Seattle, Washington

Robert T. Osteen, MD
Brigham and Women's Hospital
Department of Surgery
Harvard Medical School
Boston, Massachusetts

Rose Mary Padberg, RN, MA, OCN
National Cancer Institute
Division of Cancer Prevention
Rockville, Maryland

Donald Maxwell Parkin, MD
International Agency for Research on
Cancer
Lyon, France

Shreyaskumar Patel, MD
University of Texas MD Anderson
Cancer Center
Houston, Texas

Snehal R. Patel, MD, FRCS
Memorial Sloan-Kettering Cancer
Center
Head and Neck Service
New York, New York

Curtis A. Pettaway, MD
University of Texas MD Anderson
Cancer Center
Department of Urology
Houston, Texas

John D. Pfeifer, MD, PhD
Washington University School of
Medicine
Department of Pathology
St. Louis, Missouri

Henry A. Pitt, MD
Medical College of Wisconsin
Department of Surgery
Milwaukee, Wisconsin

Alan Pollack, MD
University of Texas MD Anderson
Cancer Center
Houston, Texas

Raphael E. Pollock, MD, PhD
University of Texas MD Anderson
Cancer Center
Department of General Surgery
Houston, Texas

Jerome B. Posner, MD
Memorial Sloan-Kettering Cancer
Center
Department of Neurology
New York, New York

Marianne N. Prout, MD, MPH
Boston University School of Medicine
Department of Surgery
Boston, Massachusetts

Sridhar Ramaswamy, MD
Dana-Farber Cancer Institute
Division of Hematology and Oncology
Boston, Massachusetts

Philip N. Redlich, MD, PhD
Medical College of Wisconsin
Department of Surgery
Milwaukee, Wisconsin

Darrell S. Rigel, MD
New York University Medical Center
Ronald O. Perelman Department of
Dermatology
New York, New York

David P. Ringer, PhD, MPH
American Cancer Society
Extramural Grants
Atlanta, Georgia

David S. Rosenthal, MD
Harvard University Health Services
Harvard Medical School
Cambridge, Massachusetts

Paul E. Rosenthal, MD
North Adams Regional Hospital
Eileen Barrett Oncology Center
North Adams, Massachusetts

Andrew J. Roth, MD
Memorial Sloan-Kettering Cancer
Center
Cornell University Medical College
Department of Psychiatry
New York, New York

Carolyn D. Runowicz, MD
Albert Einstein College of Medicine
Montefiore Medical Center
Division of Gynecologic Oncology
Bronx, New York

Lowell E. Schnipper, MD
Beth Israel Deaconess Medical Center
Oncology Division
Boston, Massachusetts

Mary Ann Sens, MD, PhD
West Virginia University
Robert C. Byrd Health Sciences Center
Department of Pathology
Morgantown, Virginia

Ashok R. Shaha, MD, FACS
Memorial Sloan-Kettering Cancer
Center
Head and Neck Service
New York, New York

Daniel Shasha, MD
Beth Israel Medical Center
New York, New York

Carol L. Shields, MD
Wills Eye Hospital
Department of Ocular Oncology
Philadelphia, Pennsylvania

Jerry A. Shields, MD
Wills Eye Hospital
Department of Ocular Oncology
Philadelphia, Pennsylvania

Lawrence N. Shulman, MD
Dana-Farber Cancer Institute
Department of Adult Oncology
Boston, Massachusetts

Robert A. Smith, PhD
American Cancer Society
Cancer Control
Atlanta, Georgia

Hassan Y. Tehrani, MB, ChB
St. Elizabeth's Medical Center
Department of Surgery
Boston, Massachusetts

Charles R. Thomas, Jr., MD
Medical University of South Carolina
Department of Radiation Oncology
Charleston, South Carolina

Gillian M. Thomas, MD, FRCPC
Toronto Sunnybrook Regional Cancer
Centre
University of Toronto
Departments of Radiation Oncology and
Obstetrics and Gynecology
Toronto, Ontario, Canada

Andrew T. Turrisi, III, MD
Medical University of South Carolina
Department of Radiation Oncology
Charleston, South Carolina

Marshall M. Urist, MD
University of Alabama at Birmingham
Division of General Surgery
Birmingham, Alabama

**Claudette G. Varricchio, DSN, RN,
FAAN**
National Cancer Institute
Division of Cancer Prevention
Bethesda, Maryland

Mark R. Wick, MD
Washington University School of
    Medicine
Department of Pathology
St. Louis, Missouri

Todd E. Williams, MD
Medical University of South Carolina
Department of Radiation Oncology
Charleston, South Carolina

Phyllis A. Wingo, PhD, MS
American Cancer Society
Epidemiology and Surveillance
Atlanta, Georgia

Theodore E. Yaeger, MD
University of Florida
Halifax Medical Center
Department of Radiation Oncology
Daytona Beach, Florida

Alan W. Yasko, MD
University of Texas MD Anderson
    Cancer Center
Houston, Texas

CD-ROM IMAGE CONTRIBUTORS

Eugene Battles, MD
Emory University School of Medicine
Divisions of Cytopathology and Surgical
    Pathology
Department of Pathology and
    Laboratory Medicine
Atlanta, Georgia

Harry S. Clarke, Jr., MD, PhD
Emory University School of Medicine
Department of Urology
Atlanta, Georgia

Cynthia Cohen, MD
Emory University School of Medicine
Division of Surgical Pathology
Department of Pathology and
    Laboratory Medicine
Atlanta, Georgia

Robert Eckstein, MB, BS
Royal North Shore Hospital
Department of Anatomical Pathology
University of Sydney
St. Leonard's, New South Wales,
    Australia

Diane C. Farhi, MD
Quest Diagnostics
Tucker, Georgia

Anthony A. Gal, MD
Emory University School of Medicine
Division of Surgical Pathology
Department of Pathology and
    Laboratory Medicine
Atlanta, Georgia

Ted Gansler, MD
American Cancer Society
Health Content Products
Atlanta, Georgia

Hans E. Grossniklaus, MD
Emory University School of Medicine
Division of Ocular Pathology
Department of Ophthalmology and
    Department of Pathology and
    Laboratory Medicine
Atlanta, Georgia

Raghu Halkar, MD
Emory University School of Medicine
Division of Nuclear Medicine
Department of Radiology
Atlanta, Georgia

Hunter T. Hardy, MD
Emory University School of Medicine
Division of Pathology Informatics
Department of Pathology and
    Laboratory Medicine
Atlanta, Georgia

Jeannine T. Holden, MD
Emory University School of Medicine
Division of Hematopathology
Department of Pathology and
    Laboratory Medicine
Atlanta, Georgia

Stephen B. Hunter, MD
Emory University School of Medicine
Division of Neuropathology
Department of Pathology and
    Laboratory Medicine
Atlanta, Georgia

Karen P. Mann, MD, PhD
Emory University School of Medicine
Division of Hematopathology
Department of Pathology and
    Laboratory Medicine
Atlanta, Georgia

Debra Monticciolo, MD
St. Peter's Hospital
Department of Medical Imaging
Albany, New York

Susan Muller, DMD
Emory University School of Medicine
Division of Oral Pathology
Department of Pathology and
    Laboratory Medicine
Atlanta, Georgia

Patricia A. O'Shea, MD
Emory University School of Medicine
Division of Pediatric Pathology
Department of Pathology and
    Laboratory Medicine
Atlanta, Georgia

Douglas C. B. Redd, MD
Emory University School of Medicine
Division of Interventional Radiology
Department of Radiology
Atlanta, Georgia

C. Whitaker Sewell, MD
Emory University School of Medicine
Division of Surgical Pathology
Department of Pathology and
    Laboratory Medicine
Atlanta, Georgia

Shobha Sharma, MD
Emory University School of Medicine
Divisions of Gastrointestinal and
    Surgical Pathology
Department of Pathology and
    Laboratory Medicine
Atlanta, Georgia

Robin Warshawsky, MD
North Shore University Hospital
Department of Radiology
Manhasset, New York

Carl Washington, MD
Emory University School of Medicine
Department of Dermatology
Atlanta, Georgia

1

Measuring the Occurrence of Cancer: Impact and Statistics

■ ■ ■

Phyllis A. Wingo
Donald Maxwell Parkin
Harmon J. Eyre

IMPACT OF CANCER ON FAMILIES, SURVIVORS, AND THE UNDERSERVED

Cancer has been present throughout human history. Egyptian and Incan mummies show evidence of the disorder. Greek physicians described it, and Hippocrates provided its name. However, accurate information regarding the occurrence of cancer has been captured only within the last century. In the United States in 1900, cancer was the eighth leading cause of death after pneumonia, tuberculosis, heart disease, stroke, and assorted other conditions. In the last half of the twentieth century, cancer has been the second leading cause of death in the United States after heart disease, accounting for approximately one in every four deaths in America. Throughout this time, the quality of cancer statistics has improved greatly .

Cancer has an impact on individuals, families, and our society as a whole. This impact can be measured in multiple ways. At current rates, approximately one in two men and one in three women will develop cancer in their lifetimes [1]. Cancer affects two of every three families in America. The annual costs of cancer are estimated at approximately $107 billion: $37 billion for direct medical costs, $11 billion for indirect morbidity costs (cost of lost productivity), and $59 billion for indirect mortality costs [2]. Treatment of breast, lung, and prostate cancers account for more than one-half of these direct medical costs.

The National Cancer Institute (NCI) estimates that more than 8 million cancer survivors are alive in the United States today [1]. Some have been treated, are cured, and have fully adopted a normal lifestyle, whereas others live with chronic pain or other permanent disability (or both) related to the disease or its treatment. As interest in evaluating health-related quality of life of cancer patients and survivors continues to grow, so does the importance of the existence of a scientifically sound basis for measuring, monitoring, and analyzing the health-related quality of life in specific populations. Despite a number of methodological issues that continue to challenge researchers in this field, reasonable scientific consensus maintains that health-related quality of life is a multidimensional construct that must include, at a minimum, the following four domains: physical, psychological, spiritual, and social functioning. The Behavioral Research Center of the American Cancer Society (ACS) is undertaking several population-based approaches to understanding better the health-related quality of life in cancer patients throughout their cancer experience, from diagnosis and treatment to the end of life.

Cancer affects various racial and ethnic populations in different ways. In the United States, black men have the highest incidence of cancer and the highest death rate. Other subpopulations have specific cancer problems that differ from the majority population. The excess cancer mortality in the socioeconomically disadvantaged and medically underserved populations is a result of the complex array of social forces and individual behaviors. Central to these social forces is access to health care, including prevention, information, early detection capability, and quality treatment. Importantly, we must continue to collect statistics of these problems with the hope that doing so will lead to solutions.

COLLECTING AND REPORTING US CANCER STATISTICS

Statistics are used for measuring the occurrence of cancer in the population and for monitoring trends in incidence, mortality, survival, and patterns of care. They are used also for planning and evaluating cancer control programs and for prioritizing the allocation of scarce health care resources (e.g., screening, diagnosis, treatment, patient services). Additionally, they are used for advancing population-based epidemiologic and health services research and for serving as the foundation for a national comprehensive cancer control strategy [3]. Statistics can delineate variations in cancer occurrence in specific populations or geographic regions and can identify areas in need of increased attention and research. In recent years, for example, analyses of breast cancer incidence and 5-year survival rates by stage of disease at diagnosis provided insights into the results of increased cancer control efforts in mammography screening and afforded advances in diagnostic and treatment protocols for breast cancer. Generally, significant decreases in breast cancer mortality during 1990 through 1996 in the United States have been attributed to the increased use of adjuvant therapies and mam-

mography screening in the late 1980s [1, 4, 5]. The significant increase in prostate cancer incidence during the late 1980s and early 1990s, followed by a decrease after 1993, may be related to the following sequence of events: (1) the dissemination of prostate-specific antigen (PSA) screening into a previously unscreened population, (2) the resultant diagnoses of previously undetected prevalent cancer cases in the community, and (3) the consequent deficit of prevalent cases that occurs after widespread screening [4].

The collection of data related to cancer in the United States has evolved under several systems of tumor registries [6]. In general, the data derive from hospital registries, which may be part of an individual hospital's cancer program, and from population-based registries, which usually are associated with state health departments or the institutions to which they delegate authority. Hospital registries furnish complex data for the evaluation of care within the hospital, such as the annual reports provided to hospitals that participate in the Approvals Program of the American College of Surgeons. Hospital registries also serve as the primary source of data for the state population-based registries. Population-based registries record and consolidate information from all reports of new cancer cases diagnosed within a specific geographic area and thus provide data for determining incidence rates.

The cancer registrar carries the major responsibility for data collection and other day-to-day registry operations [7, 8]. The registrar seeks out the sources of patient information, abstracts and integrates the data into a comprehensive format, resolves discrepancies, and protects patient confidentiality [6]. The registrar also regularly reports data to hospital tumor boards, state cancer registries, national registry programs, and the Joint Commission on Accreditation of Healthcare Organizations. Registry operations and the quality of the data collected by the registrar are guided by standards established by the Commission on Cancer of the American College of Surgeons, which has a long history of registry oversight through its Approvals Program, and the Surveillance, Epidemiology, and End Results (SEER) Program of the NCI [9, 10]. The organizations that collect and report population-based statistics pertaining to cancer in the United States are described briefly here.

Surveillance, Epidemiology, and End Results Program

The NCI SEER program evolved from the National Cancer Act of 1971, which included a mandate to collect, analyze, and disseminate data to aid in the prevention, treatment, and diagnosis of cancer in the United States [1, 6]. Although the 10 registries in the current program cover only approximately 14% of the US population, SEER cancer statistics frequently are used as the national data for the United States. Cases are coded according to the second edition of the *International Classification for Diseases for Oncology* groupings for the specific cancer sites and are followed up annually to determine survival [1, 11]. Cancer incidence and survival rates from SEER and cancer mortality from the National Center for Health Statistics are published annually in the *SEER Cancer Statistics Review, 1973–1996* [1], and are available on the Internet at www.seer.ims.nci.nih.gov.

National Program of Cancer Registries

In 1992, Congress enacted the Cancer Registries Amendment Act (Public Law 102–515) to establish the National Program of Cancer Registries at the Centers for Disease Control and Prevention (CDC) [12]. In 1990, 10 states had no cancer registry, and 40 states had registries operating at different levels, usually constrained by financial and personnel resources necessary to achieve the minimum reporting standards. By 1997, 45 states, the District of Columbia, Puerto Rico, the Virgin Islands, and Palau were receiving appropriations from the CDC to support their cancer registries [6]. The National Program of Cancer Registries expects to cover 97% of the US population when all funded states achieve full compliance with the reporting standards [6]. State-specific cancer incidence and mortality data are available through the North American Association of Central Cancer Registries (NAACCR).

North American Association of Central Cancer Registries

The NAACCR was established in 1987 as an umbrella organization to provide support to cancer registries and tumor registrars in hospitals and population-based settings. The NAACCR sets reporting standards for cancer registries and works collaboratively with government agencies, professional associations, private organizations, and cancer registrars toward the compatibility of data collection methods [6]. For cancer cases diagnosed from 1991 through 1995, *Cancer Incidence in North America* included cancer incidence data from 36 state cancer registries in the United States, six metropolitan areas that participate in the SEER program, and 12 cen-

tral cancer registries in Canada [13]. *Cancer Incidence in North America* also combines cancer incidence statistics from the highest-quality registries to estimate rates for the total United States [13]. For 1991 through 1995, the combined incidence rates for the entire United States were based on cases reported by 19 state cancer registries and two metropolitan areas and are estimated to cover approximately 45% of the US population. For cancer deaths that occurred from 1991 through 1995, *Cancer Incidence in North America* included cancer mortality data from 50 states, the District of Columbia, six metropolitan areas that participate in SEER, and 12 Canadian territories and provinces [14]. These data are available on the Internet at www.naaccr.org. As data quality in the state cancer registries continues to improve, the *Cancer Incidence in North America* data are likely to be cited as the national data for the United States.

National Center for Health Statistics

As part of the CDC, the National Center for Health Statistics serves as the principal repository for vital and health statistics in the United States [15, 16]. State legislation requires that death certificates be completed for all deaths, and federal legislation requires national collection and reporting of deaths. Causes of death are reported by certifying physicians on standard death certificates filed in the states. The information is processed and consolidated into a national database by the National Center for Health Statistics. For cancer mortality statistics, the underlying cause of death is selected for tabulation according to the procedures specified by the World Health Organization (WHO) in the relevant *Manual of the International Classifications of Disease, Injuries, and Causes of Death* (ICD codes).

STATISTICS FOR MEASURING CANCER OCCURRENCE
Population-Based Versus Hospital-Based Data

Kleinbaum et al. [17] noted that "the use of populations distinguishes epidemiology from clinical medicine and other biomedical sciences, which typically involve a small number of individuals, tissues, or organs" (p. 20). Epidemiologists collect data from many individuals and use statistical methods to make inferences about the general population. Hospital-based or clinic-based data are important for describing patterns of disease and care for patients, individual hospitals, and groups of hospitals and for generating hypotheses that require additional investigation. However, physician or patient referral patterns may influence the characteristics of the patients admitted to hospitals such that the data are not representative of the general population or the population of all cancer cases. Population-based data, as collected by the aforementioned registry programs, are needed to be able to describe the occurrence of cancer in specific populations in which age structures, racial and ethnic makeup, access to screening and treatment, and exposure to environmental and behavioral risk factors vary.

Definitions of Cancer Statistics

The key measures for describing the occurrence of cancer are prevalence, incidence, mortality, and survival. *Prevalence* refers to the number of individuals who have cancer at a specific time; *incidence* refers to the number of individuals who have a new diagnosis of cancer in a specific period; and *mortality* refers to the number of cancer deaths that occur in a specific period. The estimated new cancer cases and cancer deaths for the United States in 2000 that are presented in this report are estimated by the ACS, and the methods have been described previously [18]. Survival is described later.

The most basic function of a cancer registry is providing cancer incidence statistics. The *cancer incidence rate* refers to the rate at which new cancer cases occur in the population. The numerator is the number of new cancer cases that occur during a specific period, whereas the denominator is the population at risk of having cancer diagnosed during the same period [19]. The incidence rates presented in this report derive from SEER for the United States [1] and from the International Agency for Research on Cancer (IARC) and the International Association of Cancer Registries for other countries around the world [20].

Cancer registries do not provide cancer prevalence statistics routinely. The estimation of prevalence requires the registry to have been operating for many years (so that cases diagnosed in earlier years may be counted) and to be able to determine which cancer patients have died and which have moved out of the registration area. Determining vital status and residency is possible only when the cancer registry has appropriate resources for conducting follow-up and has access to motor vehicle or voter registration files, city directories, and regional telephone directories (as used by the SEER

Program) [21] or population registers (as used in Nordic countries) [22].

The *cancer prevalence rate* refers to the total number of individuals who have cancer at a specific time, divided by the population at risk of having cancer at the same time [19]. Agreement is lacking as to what is meant by "having" the disease. Some researchers, for example, define it to mean ever having had cancer diagnosed, even if that diagnosis occurred many years ago and the patient's disease has since been cured. Other researchers define it to mean currently being treated for cancer or at least still being followed up medically. A useful compromise is to estimate the prevalence of cancer as the number of living individuals in whom cancer has been diagnosed in the last 5 years [23].

Information regarding deaths from cancer may be obtained from registries. However, the usual source of such data is vital statistics derived from the registration of deaths, which is a statutory requirement in many countries. Usually, death registration requires that both the fact and cause of death be recorded and, in many countries, that the cause of death be specified by a medical practitioner. The accuracy of death certificate data depends on the disease under study (e.g., rapidly fatal diseases are recorded more accurately) and on the physician who records the cause of death (e.g., attending physician versus the coroner) [24]. The *cancer death rate* refers to the proportion of a population that dies from cancer during a specific period. The numerator is the number of persons dying from cancer during the specific period; the denominator is the size of the population [19]. The cancer death rates presented in this report are from SEER for the United States [1] and from WHO for other countries around the world [25].

ADJUSTED RATES AND STANDARD POPULATIONS

The foregoing rates refer to "crude" or unadjusted rates. Crude rates for populations that differ from one another by age, race, or some other factor cannot be compared without considering these differences. For example, crude cancer death rates for Florida in the United States cannot be compared to crude cancer death rates for Georgia because Florida has an older population and, therefore, has crude cancer death rates higher than those in Georgia.

Crude rates can be adjusted or standardized to remove the effects of the differences. Adjustment by age, race, or any other factor requires selecting a standard population. The standard population may be one of the populations being compared, a different population altogether, or a theoretic population [26]. Usually, cancer incidence and death rates are expressed per 100,000 population for a specific period and usually are age-adjusted by the direct method to the 1970 US standard population or to the world standard population [27, 28]. The new 2000 US standard population will be used for the first time for cases and deaths occurring in 1999 (Dr. Harry Rosenberg, National Center for Health Statistics, personal communication, September 1998) and will result in rates of higher magnitude.

The cancer incidence and death rates for the United States are age-adjusted to the 1970 standard; the cancer incidence and death rates for other countries are age-adjusted to the world standard. Therefore, the international cancer rates cannot be compared directly to the US cancer rates. However, the US cancer rates that are included in tables with international data are age-adjusted to the world standard and may be compared with those data.

RELATIVE SURVIVAL

Monitoring survival after cancer diagnosis is rather more difficult than monitoring incidence and mortality rates, because it requires follow-up of registered cases to determine outcome. The observed survival rate represents overall survival as opposed to disease-specific survival and estimates the proportion of cancer patients who survived through the specified year. The observed survival rate is needed for calculating the relative survival rate and generally is computed using actuarial methods and 1-year intervals [29, 30].

The relative survival rate for cancer is the observed survival rate for a group of cancer patients compared with the survival rate for those persons in the general population who are similar to those in the patient group with respect to age, gender, race, and calendar year of observation [30]. Relative survival provides an adjustment for deaths due to causes other than cancer and usually is expressed as a 5-year rate. A relative survival rate of 100 indicates that survival for the specific group of cancer patients was the same as survival in the subgroup of the general population with the same characteristics as the cancer patients; a relative survival rate of less than 100 indicates that survival in the specific group of cancer patients was lower than survival for similar persons in the general population; a relative survival rate greater than 100 indicates better survival in cancer patients than in similar persons in the general population [30]. The relative survival rates presented in this report are from the SEER program [31] and several European and developing countries [32, 33]. Survival rates should be interpreted with caution because 5-year relative survival rates are based on data from patients who received their diagnosis and were treated at least 8 years ago and do not reflect completely the most recent advances in treatment.

RELATIVE AND ATTRIBUTABLE RISK

Epidemiologists use the word *risk* in several ways. *Lifetime* risk refers to the probability that individuals, over the course of their entire lifetimes, will receive a diagnosis of or will die from cancer. In the United States, the lifetime risk of developing cancer is approximately 1 in 2 for men and 1 in 3 for women [1].

Relative risk in cancer studies measures the strength of the relationship between a specific risk factor and cancer by comparing risk among persons with a trait or exposure to risk among persons without the trait or exposure. For example, women who have a family history of breast cancer have approximately twice the risk of developing breast cancer as do women who do not have such a history (i.e., the relative risk is 2.0).

Attributable risk refers to the risk difference in cancer incidence or mortality between individuals with an exposure or trait and individuals without such an exposure or trait. For example, in an analysis of death rates for smokers and those who never smoked in the United States during 1990, 418,690 deaths were attributed to smoking [34].

Consider the following example. Women who have used hormone replacement therapy (HRT) for 5 to 9 years have a relative risk of 1.19 for developing breast cancer [35]. This figure means that they are 19% more likely to develop breast cancer than are women who have never used HRT. Among 1,000 women who started HRT at age 50 and used it for 10 years, an estimated 83 breast cancers may be diagnosed during the next 25 years. For women of the same ages who never used HRT, an estimated 77 breast cancers may be diagnosed over the same period. This estimate means that an excess of six breast cancers (the difference between 83 and 77) may be attributed to HRT use for every 1,000 users.

PATTERNS AND TRENDS IN US CANCER STATISTICS
All Sites Combined

In 2000 in the United States, approximately 1,220,100 persons are expected to receive new diagnoses of cancer, and 552,200 persons are expected to die from this disease (Table 1.1) [36]. Cancers of the lung and bronchus, prostate, female breast, and colon or rectum together account for more than 50% of all new cancer diagnoses and cancer deaths in the United States.

The occurrence of cancer varies significantly by demographic characteristics. Cancer rates increase with age; in 2000, more than 60% of new cancer cases and more than 70% of cancer deaths are expected to occur after age 65. The occurrence of cancer also varies significantly by race and ethnicity (Table 1.2). In the United States during 1990 through 1996, black men had the highest overall cancer incidence rate [1]. Among women, incidence rates are highest among whites, followed by blacks. For both men and women, incidence rates for Asians and Pacific Islanders and Hispanics are similar and are lower than for blacks and whites. Incidence rates for American Indians and Alaskan Natives are significantly lower than for other racial and ethnic populations.

For all cancer sites combined, cancer death rates among blacks in the United States are higher than for other racial or ethnic populations during the years 1990 through 1996 (see Table 1.2) [1]. For both men and women, whites have the second highest cancer death rates. Asians and Pacific Islanders, American Indians and Alaskan Natives, and Hispanics have cancer death rates significantly lower than those for blacks and whites, and the rates among these three racial and ethnic populations are similar in magnitude.

In 2000, the ACS, NCI, NAACCR, and CDC reported to the nation on progress related to cancer prevention and control in the United States [5]. For all sites combined, cancer incidence rates decreased on average −0.8% per year from 1990 through 1997 [5] after significantly increasing by +1.2% per year from 1973 through 1990 [4]. The trend for the most recent period was not statistically significant. However, the change in direction of the trends between the two periods did achieve statistical significance [4]. Declines were greater for persons who were 65 years and older than for younger persons: −1.1% per year for persons 65 to 74 years ($p > .05$); −2.2% per year for persons aged 75 to 84 years ($p < .05$); and −2.4% per year for persons 85 years and older ($p < .05$) [5]. Although most age groups demonstrated significant annual increases during 1973 through 1990 [4], all ages showed declines or slight increases during 1990 through 1997 [5].

Similarly, a reversal in cancer mortality trends occurred during the 1990s. After significantly increasing on average +0.4% per year from 1973 through 1990 [4], cancer death rates for all sites combined decreased

significantly an average of −0.8% per year from 1990 through 1997 [5]. The change in direction and the difference in trends between the two periods were statistically significant [4]. Declines were greater for men than for women and primarily were confined to persons who were younger than age 65 at the time of death.

Five Leading Incidence and Mortality Sites in Men and Women

Lung cancer is the second leading cause of cancer and the leading cause of cancer death in both men and women in the United States [36]. In 2000, some 89,500 men (14%) and 74,600 women (12%) are expected to receive a new diagnosis of lung cancer (see Table 1.1). Deaths from this cancer are expected to number 89,300 (31%) in men and 67,600 (25%) in women (see Table 1.1).

The patterns of lung cancer incidence and mortality are very different for men and women in the United States (Figs. 1.1–1.4) [1]. Lung cancer incidence and mortality rates are declining significantly in men (see Figs. 1.1, 1.3). Incidence rates in men have declined from a high of 86.5 per 100,000 in 1984 to 70.0 per 100,000 in 1996; and death rates have declined from 75.2 per 100,000 in 1990 to 68.2 per 100,000 in 1996. Conversely, lung cancer incidence rates in women increased perhaps 4% per year through 1991 to 43.2 per 100,000 and now may be leveling off (see Fig. 1.2). The slowing increase in rates in women may be due to decreasing rates among women 40 to 59 years of age and among black and Hispanic women [5]. Lung cancer death rates continue to increase significantly in US women (on average, +1.4% per year from 1990 through 1996) [5]; since 1987, lung cancer death rates in women have exceeded breast cancer death rates (see Fig. 1.4) [1].

In the United States, prostate cancer is expected to be the most common cancer in men (180,400 cases in 2000) and the second leading cause of cancer death in men (31,900 in 2000; see Table 1.1). Prostate cancer accounts for approximately 29% of new cancer cases in men and 11% of cancer deaths. Prostate cancer incidence rates in the United States increased dramatically during the late 1980s and early 1990s to a high of 190.8 per 100,000 in 1992 [1], probably due to the increased use of PSA screening (Fig. 1.1). In the years 1993 through 1996, prostate cancer incidence rates declined. Not known is whether incidence rates will continue to decline, level off, or resume the pattern of increase apparent before PSA testing. Prostate cancer mortality de-

Table 1.1 Estimated New Cancer Cases* and Deaths by Sex for All Sites, United States, 2000

Site	Estimated New Cases			Estimated Deaths		
	Both Sexes	**Male**	**Female**	**Both Sexes**	**Male**	**Female**
All sites	1,220,100	619,700	600,400	552,200	284,100	268,100
Oral cavity and pharynx	30,200	20,200	10,000	7,800	5,100	2,700
Tongue	6,900	4,500	2,400	1,700	1,100	600
Mouth	10,900	6,500	4,400	2,300	1,300	1,000
Pharynx	8,200	5,900	2,300	2,100	1,500	600
Other oral cavity	4,200	3,300	900	1,700	1,200	500
Digestive system	226,600	117,600	109,000	129,800	69,300	60,500
Esophagus	12,300	9,200	3,100	12,100	9,200	2,900
Stomach	21,500	13,400	8,100	13,000	7,600	5,400
Small intestine	4,700	2,300	2,400	1,200	600	600
Colon	93,800	43,400	50,400	47,700	23,100	24,600
Rectum	36,400	20,200	16,200	8,600	4,700	3,900
Anus, anal canal, and anorectum	3,400	1,400	2,000	500	200	300
Liver and intrahepatic bile duct	15,300	10,000	5,300	13,800	8,500	5,300
Gallbladder and other biliary organs	6,900	2,900	4,000	3,400	1,200	2,200
Pancreas	28,300	13,700	14,600	28,200	13,700	14,500
Other digestive organs	4,000	1,100	2,900	1,300	500	800
Respiratory system	179,400	101,500	77,900	161,900	93,100	68,800
Larynx	10,100	8,100	2,000	3,900	3,100	800
Lung and bronchus	164,100	89,500	74,600	156,900	89,300	67,600
Other respiratory organs	5,200	3,900	1,300	1,100	700	400
Bones and joints	2,500	1,500	1,000	1,400	800	600
Soft tissue (including heart)	8,100	4,300	3,800	4,600	2,200	2,400
Skin (excluding basal and squamous)	56,900	34,100	22,800	9,600	6,000	3,600
Melanoma-skin	47,700	27,300	20,400	7,700	4,800	2,900
Other non-epithelial skin	9,200	6,800	2,400	1,900	1,200	700
Breast	184,200	1,400	182,800	41,200	400	40,800
Genital system	265,900	188,400	77,500	59,000	32,500	26,500
Uterine cervix	12,800		12,800	4,600		4,600
Uterine corpus	36,100		36,100	6,500		6,500
Ovary	23,100		23,100	14,000		14,000
Vulva	3,300		3,400	800		800
Vagina and other genital, female	2,100		2,100	600		600
Prostate	180,400	180,400		31,900	31,900	
Testis	6,900	6,900		300	300	
Penis and other genital, male	1,100	1,100		300	300	
Urinary system	86,700	58,600	28,100	24,600	15,700	8,900
Urinary bladder	53,200	38,300	14,900	12,200	8,100	4,100
Kidney and renal pelvis	31,200	18,800	12,400	11,900	7,300	4,600
Ureter and other urinary organs	2,300	1,500	800	500	300	200
Eye and orbit	2,200	1,200	1,000	200	100	100
Brain and other nervous system	16,500	9,500	7,000	13,000	7,100	5,900
Endocrine system	20,200	5,600	14,600	2,100	1,000	1,100
Thyroid	18,400	4,700	13,700	1,200	500	700
Other endocrine	1,800	900	900	900	500	400
Lymphoma	62,300	35,900	26,400	27,500	14,400	13,100
Hodgkin's disease	7,400	4,200	3,200	1,400	700	700
Non-Hodgkin's lymphoma	54,900	31,700	23,200	26,100	13,700	12,400

Table 1.1   Estimated New Cancer Cases and Deaths by Sex for All Sites, United States, 2000 (*continued*)

Site	Estimated New Cases			Estimated Deaths		
	Both Sexes	Male	Female	Both Sexes	Male	Female
Multiple myeloma	13,600	7,300	6,300	11,200	5,800	5,400
Leukemia	30,800	16,900	13,900	21,700	12,100	9,600
Acute lymphocytic leukemia	3,200	1,800	1,400	1,300	700	600
Chronic lymphocytic leukemia	8,100	4,600	3,500	4,800	2,800	2,000
Acute myeloid leukemia	9,700	4,800	4,900	7,100	3,900	3,200
Chronic myeloid leukemia	4,400	2,600	1,800	2,300	1,300	1,000
Other leukemia	5,400	3,100	2,300	6,200	3,400	2,800
Other and unspecified primary sites	34,000	15,700	18,300	36,600	18,500	18,100

*Excludes basal and squamous cell skin cancers and in situ carcinomas except urinary bladder. Carcinoma in situ of the breast accounts for about 42,600 new cases annually, and melanoma carcinoma in situ accounts for about 28,600 new cases annually. Estimates of new cases are based on incidence rates from the National Cancer Institute Surveillance, Epidemiology, and End Results (NCI SEER) program 1979–1996. American Cancer Society, Surveillance Research, 2000.

creased significantly (on average, –2.2% per year) from 1990 through 1997 [5], after significantly increasing between 1973 and 1990 (+1.0% per year; Fig. 1.3) [4].

Breast cancer is expected to be the most common cancer (184,200 in 2000) and the second leading cause of cancer death (41,200 in 2000) in US women (see Table 1.1) [36]. After increasing approximately 4% per year in the middle to late 1980s, probably due to increased use of mammography screening, breast cancer incidence rates have leveled off in recent years (Fig. 1.2) [1]. Breast cancer death rates in 1990 through 1996 are higher in black women (31.4 per 100,000) than in white women (25.7 per 100,000). During 1990 through 1997, US breast cancer death rates decreased significantly (on average, –2.1% per year) [5]; this decline was a significant reversal from the significantly increasing death rates during 1973 through 1990 (+0.2% per year; Fig. 1.4) [4].

Colorectal cancers are the third most common cause of cancer and cancer death in men and women in the United States [36]. In 2000, approximately 93,800 men and women are expected to receive new diagnoses of colon cancer, and some 36,400 were expected to develop rectal cancer; deaths from colon and rectal cancer are expected to be 47,700 and 8,600, respectively (see Table 1.1) [36]. Incidence rates during 1990 through 1996 range from 16.4 per 100,000 among American Indians and Alaskan Natives to 50.4 per 100,000 among blacks. The incidence of colorectal cancer peaked in the mid-1980s in the United States for men and women; since then, incidence rates have declined (see Figs. 1.1, 1.2) [1]. During the years 1990 through 1996, incidence rates declined significantly in all racial and ethnic groups except American Indians and Alaskan Natives [1].

Mortality from colorectal cancer also has been declining in the United States (see Figs. 1.3, 1.4) [1]. After declining an average 0.9% per year from 1973 through 1990 [4], colorectal cancer mortality declined at an even greater rate between 1990 and 1997 (–1.8% annually) [5]. During this time, colorectal death rates declined for men and women in all racial and ethnic groups except Alaskan Natives and American Indian men and women, and Asian and Pacific Islander women.

Cancer of the urinary bladder is the fourth leading cause of cancer in men and the eighth leading cause in women [36]. In 2000, an estimated 38,300 new cases are expected to occur in men, and 14,900 cases are expected to occur in women; deaths from this cancer are expected to number 8,100 and 4,100 in men and women, respectively (see Table 1.1). Incidence rates for 1992 through 1996 were nearly four times higher in men (28.9 per 100,000) than in women (7.7 per 100,000) and were nearly two times higher in whites (18.1 per 100,000) than in blacks (9.8 per 100,000) [1]. Among the 10 leading cancer incidence sites, the reversal in trends—from an increase between 1973 and 1990 [4] to a decrease between 1990 and 1997 [5]—observed for all sites combined and for cancers of the lung, prostate, and colon and rectum was also observed for urinary bladder cancer. The difference in the average annual percentage change between the two periods was significant for urinary bladder cancer, and urinary bladder cancer incidence rates decreased on average –1.0% per year between 1990 and 1997 [5]. Bladder cancer death rates declined throughout 1973 through 1996 [1].

Cancer of the uterine corpus ranks fourth in the top 10 cancer incidence sites for women in the United

Table 1.2 Cancer Incidence and Mortality Rates by Site, Gender, and Race or Ethnicity, United States, 1990–1996

Race, ethnicity	All Sites M	All Sites F	Lung M	Lung F	Female Breast	Prostate	Colon-Rectum M	Colon-Rectum F	Non-Hodgkin's Lymphoma M	Non-Hodgkin's Lymphoma F	Stomach M	Stomach F	Urinary Bladder M	Urinary Bladder F	Melanoma M	Melanoma F	Ovary	Uterine Corpus	Liver M	Liver F	Leukemia M	Leukemia F	Kidney M	Kidney F	Esophagus M	Esophagus F
SEER Incidence																										
All races	482.8	342.9	74.5	41.7	109.1	151.9	53.4	37.3	19.4	12.1	11.2	5.0	28.6	7.4	15.0	10.0	14.8	21.1	6.0	2.3	13.3	8.0	12.3	6.1	6.3	1.8
White	480.2	351.6	73.1	43.3	113.2	147.3	53.2	36.8	20.2	12.7	9.7	4.2	31.2	7.9	17.0	11.5	15.7	22.5	4.7	1.8	14.0	8.3	12.6	6.3	5.7	1.6
African-American	598.0	335.6	112.3	46.2	99.3	222.9	58.1	44.9	15.4	8.2	17.1	7.5	15.6	6.0	1.1	0.7	10.3	14.9	7.8	2.7	10.7	6.9	14.5	6.9	13.5	4.2
Asian, Pacific Islander	325.5	244.9	52.4	22.5	72.6	81.5	47.5	31.4	13.4	8.6	20.3	11.0	12.5	3.4	1.2	0.9	10.6	13.6	16.6	6.1	8.5	5.8	7.0	3.0	4.5	0.8
American Indian, Alaska Native	177.8	136.8	25.3	13.5	33.9	46.5	21.5	12.4	4.3	4.0	6.3	4.4	4.3	1.1	0.8	1.1	9.1	7.4	7.4	4.1	3.6	3.1	11.0	5.9	2.5	0.4
Hispanic*	326.9	243.2	38.8	19.6	69.4	102.8	35.7	24.0	15.0	9.8	14.5	7.6	14.1	3.8	2.8	2.8	11.7	13.3	8.8	3.1	9.7	6.5	10.6	5.8	4.4	—
US mortality																										
All races	215.1	141.2	71.9	33.2	25.9	25.9	21.9	14.9	8.2	5.4	6.3	2.9	5.6	1.7	3.2	1.5	7.7	3.4	4.7	2.1	8.4	4.9	5.0	2.3	6.2	1.5
White	208.8	139.8	70.1	33.8	25.7	23.7	21.5	14.5	8.5	5.6	5.6	2.6	5.8	1.7	3.5	1.7	7.9	3.2	4.3	2.0	8.5	4.9	5.1	2.4	5.6	1.3
African-American	308.8	168.1	100.8	32.8	31.4	54.8	27.8	20.0	6.1	3.7	12.5	5.5	4.5	2.3	0.4	0.4	6.4	5.8	7.0	2.9	7.9	4.7	5.1	2.3	13.4	3.5
Asian, Pacific Islander	129.2	83.5	34.9	14.9	11.4	10.7	13.4	9.0	5.1	3.1	11.1	6.3	1.9	0.8	—	—	4.1	1.8	13.6	5.1	4.6	2.9	2.1	0.9	3.4	0.7
American Indian, Alaska Native	123.3	90.2	40.5	19.8	12.3	14.3	11.0	8.9	3.5	2.7	5.9	3.0	—	—	—	—	4.3	2.0	5.1	2.7	3.8	2.9	5.0	2.9	3.3	—
Hispanic*	131.8	86.3	32.0	11.0	15.3	16.7	13.2	8.4	6.0	3.8	8.0	4.3	2.8	0.8	0.8	0.5	4.9	2.5	6.9	3.1	5.2	3.6	4.0	1.8	3.5	0.7

*Hispanic is not mutually exclusive from whites, African-Americans, Asian Pacific Islanders, and American Indians.

—Statistic not shown; rate is based on fewer than 25 cases for the time interval.

Note: Rates are per 100,000 and are age-adjusted to the 1970 US standard population.

Source: Data adapted from the LAG Ries, CL Kosary, BF Hankey et al. (eds); SEER Cancer Statistics Review, 1973–1996. Bethesda, MD: National Cancer Institute, 1999.

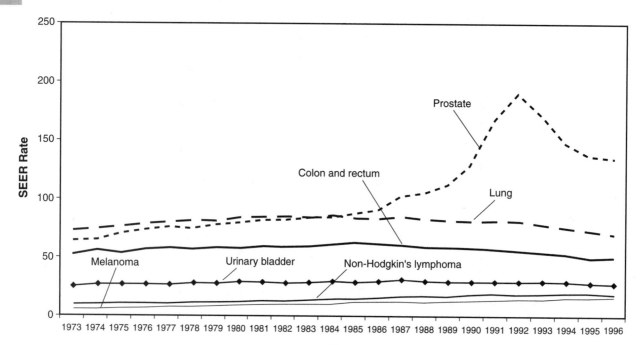

Figure 1.1   Age-adjusted cancer incidence rates for men by site, United States, 1973–1996. Rates are per 100,000 and are age-adjusted to the 1970 US standard population. (Data adapted from the LAG Ries, CL Kosary, BF Hankey, et al. [eds], *SEER Cancer Statistics Review, 1973–1996*. Bethesda, MD: National Cancer Institute, 1999.)

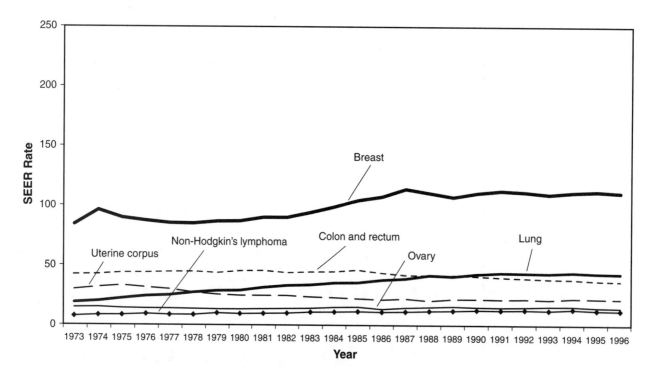

Figure 1.2   Age-adjusted cancer incidence rates for women by site, United States, 1973–1996. Rates are per 100,000 and are age-adjusted to the 1970 US standard population. (Data adapted from the LAG Ries, CL Kosary, BF Hankey, et al. [eds], *SEER Cancer Statistics Review, 1973–1996*. Bethesda, MD: National Cancer Institute, 1999.)

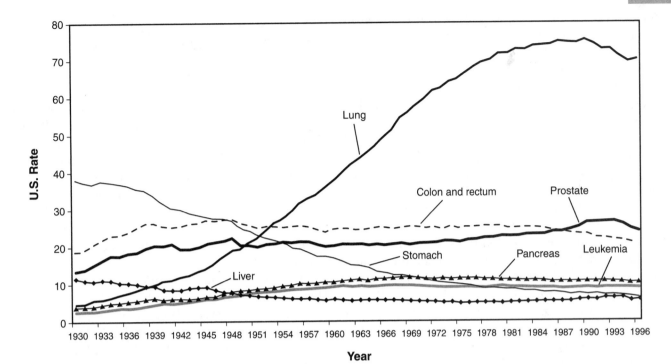

Figure 1.3 Age-adjusted cancer mortality for men by site, United States, 1930–1996. Rates are per 100,000 and are age-adjusted to the 1970 US standard population. (Data adapted from the National Center for Health Statistics, *Vital Statistics of the United States, 1930–1959: Vol 2: Mortality, parts A and B.* Washington, DC: Public Health Service, 1930–1997; and from the National Center for Health Statistics, *Vital Statistics of the United States* [public use data file documentation: mortality detail for ICD-7 1960–67, ICD-8A 1968–78, ICD-9 1979–95]. Hyattsville, MD: Public Health Service, 1998.)

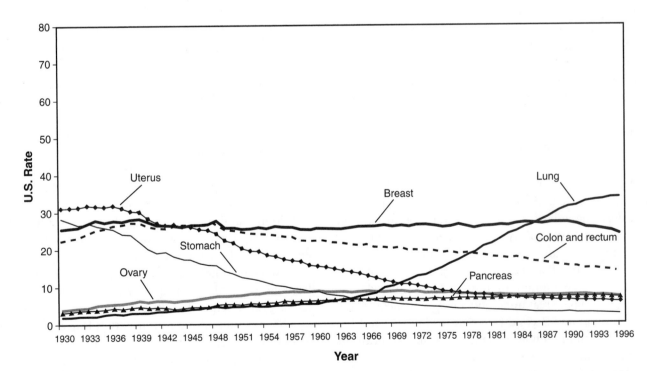

Figure 1.4 Age-adjusted cancer mortality for women by site, United States, 1930–1996. Rates are per 100,000 and are age-adjusted to the 1970 US standard population. (Data adapted from the National Center for Health Statistics, *Vital Statistics of the United States, 1930–1959: Vol 2: Mortality, parts A and B.* Washington, DC: Public Health Service, 1930–1997; and from the National Center for Health Statistics, *Vital Statistics of the United States* [public use data file documentation: mortality detail for ICD-7 1960–67, ICD-8A 1968–78, ICD-9 1979–95]. Hyattsville, MD: Public Health Service, 1998.)

States, with an estimated 36,100 women expected to receive a new diagnosis in 2000 (see Table 1.1) [36]. From 1992 through 1996, incidence rates were 21.5 per 100,000, and death rates were 3.3 per 100,000 [1]. Trends in the incidence of cancer of the corpus uteri and uterus, not otherwise specified, decreased significantly during 1973 through 1990 (–2.5% per year), due primarily to changes in prescribing practices for unopposed noncontraceptive estrogens [4]; incidence rates have been approximately level between 1990 and 1996 (see Fig. 1.2) Death rates for cancer of the corpus uteri and uterus, not otherwise specified, decreased over both periods [4].

Pancreatic cancer ranks fourth as the leading cause of cancer death in men and women in the United States; in 2000, 13,700 men and 14,500 women are expected to die from this disease (see Table 1.1) [36]. This cancer ranks among the leading causes of cancer death because only 7% of pancreatic cancers are diagnosed at the local stage [1].

Ovarian cancer is the sixth leading cause of cancer and fifth leading cause of cancer death in US women; in 2000, an estimated 23,100 women are expected to receive new diagnoses of this cancer, and 14,000 are expected to die from this disease (see Table 1.1) [36]. Most ovarian cancers (60%) are diagnosed when the tumor has spread to distant sites; thus, only 50% of women in whom this cancer is diagnosed survive 5 years [1].

Non-Hodgkin's lymphoma is the fifth leading cause of cancer and cancer death in US men and the fifth leading cause of cancer and the sixth leading cause of cancer death in US women (see Table 1.1) [36]. Incidence rates for non-Hodgkin's lymphoma nearly doubled throughout the years 1973 through 1995 (8.6 per 100,000 in 1973 and 15.5 per 100,000 in 1996) [1]. Interestingly, the average annual percentage change for non-Hodgkin's lymphoma in the 1990s was significantly lower than in 1973 to 1990, suggesting a slowing in the annual increase in incidence rates for this disease [4, 5]. Non-Hodgkin's lymphoma death rates were increasing significantly throughout this time.

The leading 10 cancer incidence sites in men also include skin (melanoma), oral cavity, kidney, blood (leukemia), and pancreas and, in women, they include skin (melanoma) and thyroid [36]. The leading 10 causes of cancer death in men also include leukemia and cancers of the esophagus, liver, and stomach and, in women, cancers of the blood (leukemia), brain, and stomach and multiple myeloma.

COLLECTING AND REPORTING INTERNATIONAL CANCER STATISTICS
World Health Organization

The numbers and rates of cancer deaths according to cause are published by government statistics offices in many countries and are compiled by the WHO. The WHO makes data available both as printed tables in the *World Health Statistics Annuals* and also, in more detail, in the WHO mortality database on computer tapes or diskettes [25]. In recent years, the IARC has collaborated closely with the WHO to make cancer mortality data available via the Internet at www.dep.iarc.fr through the CancerMondial site.

The great advantages of mortality data are comprehensive coverage and availability via the aforementioned mechanisms. In 1990, mortality statistics were available from 65 countries, covering 28% of the world population. In the 1996 *World Health Statistics Annual,* mortality data for 83 countries were presented, although not all were of the same quality [25]. For some countries, mortality data are very incomplete because not all sections of the population are subject to death registration. Sometimes (though not always) this exception is stated explicitly, and death rates that are implausibly low may be published. In recent years, both the Pan American Health Organization [37] and the WHO [25] have published tables with quantitative estimates of the coverage of death registration in the countries for which mortality statistics are provided. In addition, the quality of information about the cause of death is variable and may be related to the completion of certificates by nonmedical personnel. Again, the WHO recently provided tabulations of the relevant percentages, at least for some countries. Otherwise, the quality of the data must be judged from such indicators as the proportion of cancer deaths coded to "senility and ill-defined conditions" and the proportion of cancer deaths without specification of the primary site or with only vague descriptions of site specification (ICD-9 codes 195–199).

Besides national vital statistics, other sources of information regarding cancer mortality can be useful for making international comparisons. China presents a notable example, in that information is available from at least two different sample surveys of deaths [38]. One of these sources concerns the continuous collection of information on cause of death in a relatively small but random sample (0.8%) of the Chinese population. This information supplements data published from the vital statistics program that, although much larger (a population of 100–120 million), is confined to relatively affluent areas of the country (the eastern coastal provinces in particular).

International Agency for Research on Cancer and International Association of Cancer Registries

INCIDENCE

No one knows how many cancer registries exist and, regardless, the distinction between registries that provide accurate, bona fide data about incidence in a well-defined population and those achieving only partial, incomplete coverage is not clear-cut. More than 300 population-based registries are members of the International Association of Cancer Registries, which provides a professional forum for registries worldwide. The IARC collaborates with the Association to make data available to the scientific and public health communities. The best-known source is *Cancer Incidence in Five Continents*, which brings together registry data of good quality and hence provides information for valid international comparisons of incidence. The latest volume (VII), covering mainly the period from 1988 through 1992, was published in 1997 [20] and was made available also on a computer diskette with special software for extraction and analysis of the data [39].

Some registries are excluded because of questions about completeness or validity of the data. Nevertheless, for many parts of the world, partial or incomplete data may provide vital clues about contemporary patterns of cancer.

SURVIVAL

Until recently, little interest has been evinced in international comparative statistics regarding cancer survival. Individual cancer registries published results in their annual reports, but whether they used methodology that was sufficiently similar to permit comparisons among them was unclear. This situation has changed recently with the publication of relative survival data from 11 European countries in the EUROCARE project [32] and from several developing countries [33].

Methods and Data Limitations

The foregoing data sources may be used to develop a comprehensive set of estimates of cancer incidence, mortality, and survival throughout the world. The inci-

dence and mortality data for 167 countries, 25 cancer sites, both genders, and 5 broad age groups are now available in the GLOBOCAN package, available as a compact disk (with software for analysis and presentation of the results) [40] or via the Internet at www.dep.iarc.fr.

The methods used to produce these estimates have been described previously [41, 42]. National incidence data and national mortality data were used whenever they were available and were judged to be sufficiently accurate. Sometimes, correction factors were applied to published mortality data in light of documented and quantified underregistration of deaths for a country. When only one of the pair was available, the other was estimated from it. Using regression models, incidence can be estimated from mortality, given sufficient information from cancer registries in the same or similar countries about the relationship of mortality to incidence by age, gender, and site. Conversely, mortality can be derived from incidence with data about survival in similar populations.

Without national-level information regarding incidence or mortality, disease patterns must be inferred from samples. The sample survey of deaths in China, a random sample, was taken to represent the national cancer mortality profile. The national incidence figures were obtained by using mortality-to-incidence ratios from Chinese cancer registries. More often, the national pattern of cancer incidence must be inferred from the results of one or several cancer registries. Incidence rates for India were developed from seven registries in that country, for example. The populations covered by these registries may not be representative of the country, and they are more likely to be urban. Death rates then can be estimated using the survival data from the same registries.

Failing other sources of information, a "best guess" of the cancer profile was made from whatever data could be obtained about the relative frequency of different cancers (using data sets that were as representative as possible) and partitioning a national incidence for "all cancers" by the relevant proportions. Mortality then was derived using the best available estimate of survival in the same population.

PATTERNS AND TRENDS IN INTERNATIONAL CANCER STATISTICS

For 30 countries in different regions of the world, Table 1.3 shows selected results for cancer incidence, and Table 1.4 illustrates cancer mortality. The incidence and

Table 1.3 Estimated Worldwide Cancer Incidence Rates and Number of Cases, by Site and Gender, 1990

	Lung		Stomach		Breast	Colon-Rectum		Liver		Prostate	Cervix	Esophagus		Bladder		Leukemia	
	M	F	M	F	F	M	F	M	F	M	F	M	F	M	F	M	F
Africa																	
Algeria[a]	2.8	6.2	3.2	18.4	7.2	6.1	1.5	1.0	3.4	13.6	0.5	0.9	8.9	2.2	2.7	1.6	
Mali[a]	5.1	1.5	18.9	10.6	9.8	5.5	2.1	48.0	17.0	5.3	24.4	1.6	0.6	10.2	2.1	0.9	2.0
South Africa[b]	8.2	12.1	4.6	33.2	11.9	9.1	20.5	6.7	32.4	40.8	33.7	12.4	12.5	3.2	5.6	3.6	
Uganda[a]	3.9	0.4	4.9	3.2	17.7	6.9	5.1	9.2	3.4	26.8	34.2	17.0	8.3	2.5	0.5	0.7	1.3
North America																	
USA[c]	70.0	33.4	8.1	3.9	87.1	44.4	32.8	3.3	1.4	95.1	9.1	5.3	1.4	24.3	5.4	10.5	6.2
Central America and Caribbean																	
Cuba[d]	17.7	9.6	5.2	34.3	15.1	17.5	5.1	4.3	31.3	23.8	4.9	1.8	10.4	2.9	6.1	4.8	
Costa Rica[d]	15.5	5.4	51.8	23.6	28.3	10.8	10.8	6.6	3.8	27.5	25.0	4.0	1.5	6.6	1.7	7.8	6.3
Trinidad and Tobago[c]	16.5	4.9	15.6	8.2	53.5	18.4	15.0	4.6	3.2	66.1	22.4	5.1	0.7	5.5	2.4	5.3	5.2
South America																	
Argentina[c]	57.0	7.7	20.7	7.6	74.1	28.0	24.6	3.3	1.8	21.9	27.6	11.0	4.0	13.5	2.8	6.0	4.4
Brazil[d]	28.2	6.8	31.3	13.7	45.2	17.5	15.5	3.1	1.8	29.7	30.6	9.3	1.9	11.9	2.8	6.3	4.7
Colombia[c]	19.1	10.0	38.3	24.3	28.7	11.2	11.5	3.1	2.4	25.4	31.6	6.1	3.2	5.9	2.2	6.7	5.7
Asia																	
China[c]	34.7	13.4	43.6	19.0	11.8	13.3	10.2	35.8	11.5	1.1	5.0	21.6	9.9	3.3	1.0	4.5	3.5
Israel[d]	27.5	9.0	13.2	6.4	72.2	38.8	30.9	3.2	1.7	24.8	5.2	1.7	1.1	24.9	5.1	7.5	5.1
India[a]	9.6	2.2	6.2	3.3	21.2	5.4	3.8	2.6	1.2	5.2	26.9	8.0	5.4	3.7	0.9	3.5	2.3
Japan[c]	38.9	11.2	77.9	33.3	28.6	39.5	24.6	27.6	6.9	8.5	9.7	9.5	1.6	8.9	2.0	5.7	3.7
Kuwait[d]	22.8	9.8	5.5	3.8	33.0	8.9	5.5	6.6	3.0	8.1	6.8	1.7	1.8	9.1	3.1	5.8	4.9
Kyrgyzstan[c]	43.6	7.3	35.0	18.4	19.9	11.3	8.1	12.4	5.4	12.2	16.2	12.3	6.3	9.6	0.8	5.5	3.4
Philippines[a]	52.7	14.9	9.7	5.8	41.5	16.3	12.8	20.7	7.1	16.5	22.3	2.6	1.4	4.3	1.3	5.4	5.1
Thailand[a]	24.9	11.9	5.8	2.9	13.2	8.8	6.0	39.9	16.0	3.9	23.0	4.1	1.4	4.9	1.3	3.7	3.1
Europe																	
Czech Republic[d]	78.2	10.4	19.9	10.1	47.3	49.1	28.9	6.7	2.8	25.0	17.7	4.3	0.6	15.6	3.4	9.3	5.9
Denmark[d]	52.4	24.8	9.4	5.3	76.2	39.3	32.8	3.8	2.2	33.5	16.2	4.9	1.5	28.8	8.0	9.8	6.3
Finland[d]	54.8	8.5	17.2	10.3	68.7	24.0	19.9	4.9	3.0	43.4	3.9	3.5	1.9	15.7	3.4	7.1	5.2
France[c]	50.3	5.7	11.8	4.9	61.0	35.6	23.0	8.0	1.7	39.2	10.0	11.0	1.1	16.7	2.4	8.7	5.8
Germany[c]	50.8	8.5	19.8	10.3	67.5	43.6	32.8	3.4	1.6	37.5	12.6	5.0	0.9	16.3	3.2	8.5	5.6
Italy[c]	63.7	8.4	21.6	10.5	55.0	31.3	21.7	10.8	3.7	16.3	8.9	4.4	0.4	25.3	3.5	9.5	6.2
Netherlands[d]	74.2	12.9	15.9	6.9	82.0	37.7	29.7	1.6	0.7	41.8	7.6	5.3	2.1	15.6	3.3	7.8	5.0
Russian Federation[c]	82.2	10.0	45.5	20.9	34.7	24.8	18.7	5.2	2.7	12.7	11.3	7.9	1.3	12.8	2.1	7.4	5.0
Spain[c]	51.7	4.1	17.9	8.5	46.6	28.6	20.3	7.4	2.9	18.3	8.6	6.1	0.4	24.2	3.1	7.9	5.4
United Kingdom[d]	66.3	24.5	16.9	7.4	71.7	35.5	26.7	2.2	1.1	30.1	13.4	8.0	4.1	21.2	6.4	8.5	5.7
Oceania																	
Australia[c]	47.1	15.2	10.5	4.7	70.5	44.7	33.3	2.6	1.0	51.6	10.8	4.4	2.4	14.5	4.5	10.7	6.3
World	37.5	10.8	24.5	11.6	33.0	19.4	15.3	14.7	4.9	19.8	15.4	10.2	4.2	9.9	2.3	5.6	4.0
Cases (× 1,000)	772	265	511	287	796	402	381	316	121	396	371	213	103	203	58	130	101

[a]Estimate from regional incidence data.

[b]Estimate from frequency data (corrected for under reporting).

[c]Estimate from national mortality data and cancer registry data.

[d]National incidence data.

[e]Estimate from sample mortality data.

Note: Rates are per 100,000 and are age-adjusted to the world standard population.

Source: Data adapted from Ferley J, Parkin DM, Pisani P. GLOBOCAN: Cancer Incidence and Mortality Worldwide in 1990. [IARC CancerBase No. 3.] Lyon, France: International Agency for Research on Cancer, 1998.

death rates have been age-adjusted to the world population so that they can be compared directly, without the confounding effect of the very different age structures of the populations in these countries. The cancers selected represent the 10 with the highest annual number of cases in the world and the leading 10 in terms of deaths. The age-adjusted rates for the world are shown, as are the estimated numbers of cases and deaths.

Table 1.5 shows relative survival rates for these cancers in the SEER registries for cases diagnosed in 1986

Table 1.4 Estimated Worldwide Cancer Mortality Rates and Number of Deaths, by Site and Gender, 1990

	Lung		Stomach		Colon-Rectum		Liver		Breast	Esophagus		Cervix	Leukemia		Pancreas		Prostate
	M	F	M	F	M	F	M	F	F	M	F	F	M	F	M	F	M
Africa																	
Algeria[a]	17.0	2.6	5.4	2.7	4.6	3.9	1.5	0.9	8.3	0.4	0.8	7.4	2.3	1.3	0.5	0.4	2.1
Mali[a]	4.7	1.4	16.0	9.1	3.5	1.4	45.1	16.0	4.5	1.4	0.5	12.9	0.7	1.7	2.2	0.8	3.3
South Africa[a]	28.3	7.5	10.4	3.9	7.8	5.9	19.4	6.4	15.1	29.9	10.8	21.6	4.8	3.1	2.9	1.9	19.6
Uganda[a]	3.6	0.3	4.1	2.7	4.5	3.2	8.7	3.2	8.1	14.8	7.3	17.9	0.5	1.1	1.1	0.6	16.2
North America																	
USA[b]	58.3	25.2	5.4	2.6	17.4	12.9	3.3	1.6	23.4	4.8	1.2	3.5	6.6	4.3	7.7	5.8	18.6
Central America and Caribbean																	
Cuba[b]	42.8	15.6	8.4	4.3	11.4	12.4	4.4	3.7	15.6	4.4	1.6	10.6	4.8	3.6	4.9	3.9	22.1
Costa Rica[b]	15.1	5.6	45.4	19.7	6.9	7.3	8.1	5.0	11.7	4.2	1.2	12.1	5.8	4.6	6.6	5.3	16.0
Trinidad and Tobago[b]	14.5	3.9	11.1	5.8	11.0	9.2	4.6	3.4	19.4	3.8	0.6	13.9	3.9	3.7	5.8	4.1	34.4
South America																	
Argentina[b]	38.8	6.2	12.3	5.3	13.9	9.8	5.9	3.7	21.5	8.3	2.4	9.5	5.1	3.5	8.1	5.3	13.7
Brazil[a]	26.1	6.3	27.0	11.8	11.4	10.1	2.9	1.7	20.7	8.2	1.7	16.4	5.3	4.0	4.7	3.6	17.9
Colombia[b]	17.1	8.2	28.1	17.7	5.3	5.9	5.4	6.9	9.9	4.5	2.5	16.1	5.1	4.1	7.0	5.2	13.1
Asia																	
China[c]	32.0	12.4	35.3	15.5	8.7	6.7	34.7	11.1	4.3	19.8	9.1	2.8	4.1	3.1	2.3	1.2	0.7
Israel[b]	28.3	8.9	9.2	5.0	16.7	13.2	3.0	1.8	25.0	2.0	1.1	2.7	6.9	5.0	7.9	6.3	10.3
India[a]	9.0	2.0	5.5	3.1	3.5	2.4	2.5	1.1	11.0	7.5	5.1	15.3	2.7	1.8	1.5	1.0	3.2
Japan[b]	31.7	8.8	35.9	16.7	15.9	10.6	21.0	5.6	6.7	7.1	1.1	3.4	4.4	2.8	8.8	5.2	4.2
Kuwait[b]	21.1	9.0	4.7	3.3	5.9	3.6	6.3	2.8	14.9	1.5	1.6	3.7	5.0	4.2	5.1	3.1	4.9
Kyrgyzstan[b]	37.0	5.4	30.1	12.4	7.6	6.9	18.4	5.1	8.7	9.1	3.3	6.4	3.2	2.3	4.3	2.9	3.7
Philippines[a]	48.7	13.8	8.4	5.0	10.6	8.3	19.5	6.7	18.9	2.3	1.3	12.1	4.5	4.3	4.0	3.1	9.9
Thailand[a]	22.9	11.0	5.0	2.5	5.7	3.8	37.8	15.2	6.0	3.6	1.2	12.1	3.1	2.6	1.8	1.2	2.3
Europe																	
Czech Republic[b]	76.8	10.0	18.9	9.5	35.0	19.9	7.7	3.7	22.4	4.3	0.6	7.0	7.7	5.0	11.6	6.9	15.5
Denmark[b]	52.5	23.7	8.0	4.8	23.9	19.6	2.2	1.3	29.5	5.3	1.5	6.2	7.0	4.5	8.8	7.3	20.8
Finland[b]	49.4	7.0	13.4	8.0	12.7	9.9	3.2	2.0	18.0	3.1	1.7	1.9	4.3	2.8	9.4	7.3	18.3
France[b]	47.7	5.4	9.4	4.6	18.6	12.6	10.2	2.2	21.2	11.3	1.3	3.9	6.5	4.3	7.6	4.4	20.3
Germany[b]	49.6	8.1	15.9	9.0	22.5	17.5	4.4	2.0	23.1	5.0	0.9	4.8	6.2	4.0	8.4	5.6	18.5
Italy[b]	57.8	7.7	18.1	9.3	16.3	11.4	13.4	5.6	21.6	4.3	0.7	3.5	6.6	4.3	7.7	4.9	13.0
Netherlands[b]	70.3	11.0	12.9	5.8	18.7	15.0	1.8	0.9	28.7	5.5	1.9	3.0	5.8	3.9	8.2	6.2	19.8
Russian Federation[b]	74.6	7.6	42.8	18.8	17.7	12.9	5.9	2.9	14.7	8.9	1.9	6.3	5.6	3.7	8.0	3.7	6.8
Spain[b]	46.6	3.7	14.8	7.4	15.0	10.2	8.6	4.5	17.8	5.7	0.7	3.2	5.2	3.8	5.9	3.5	14.4
United Kingdom[b]	61.4	21.8	13.4	6.2	21.2	15.9	2.2	1.2	30.4	8.0	3.8	5.2	5.3	3.6	7.5	5.7	17.5
Oceania																	
Australia[b]	41.9	13.0	7.2	3.6	20.3	14.8	2.7	1.0	21.2	4.7	1.8	3.2	6.0	3.9	6.6	4.9	17.9
World	33.7	9.2	19.1	9.2	10.7	8.6	14.2	4.9	12.9	9.3	3.8	8.0	4.4	3.2	4.4	3.1	8.2
Number (× 1,000)	693	228	397	230	222	215	306	121	314	194	93	190	103	81	96	78	165

[a]Estimate from incidence and survival data.

[b]National mortality data.

[c]Estimate from sample mortality data.

Note: Rates are per 100,000 and are age-adjusted to the world standard population.

Source: Data adapted from Ferley J, Parkin DM, Pisani P. GLOBOCAN: Cancer Incidence and Mortality Worldwide in 1990. [IARC CancerBase No. 3] Lyon, France: International Agency for Research on Cancer, 1998.

through 1993 and followed up through 1994 [31], in European registries participating in the EUROCARE project [32], and in selected developing countries [33].

Lung cancer was the most common cancer in 1990, in terms of both incidence and mortality. Worldwide, it is by far the most common cancer among men, with the highest rates observed in North America and Europe (especially eastern Europe). Moderately high rates also are seen in Argentina, Australia, and the Philippines (see Table 1.3). In women, incidence rates are lower (an overall rate of 10.8 per 100,000 women, as compared with 37.5 per 100,000 men). The highest rates are in the United States of America and northern Europe. Notably, the incidence in China is rather high (13.4 per

Table 1.5   Five-Year Relative Survival (%) from Population-Based Cancer Registries Around the World

Site	SEER Program [31]	EUROCARE [32]	India [33]	China [33]	Developing Countries [33]
Lung	15.5	8	7	8	8
Stomach	21	18	7	18	14
Breast	84	67	49	60	55
Colon-rectum	61.5	41	42	32	35
Liver	6	N/A	N/A	3	6
Prostate	88	N/A	40	40	40
Cervix	69	59	48	49	49
Esophagus	11	5	6	9	12
Bladder	81	N/A	18	47	42
Blood	42	27	20	10	16
Pancreas	4	4	2	5	5

SEER = Surveillance, Epidemiology, and End Results; N/A = not available.

100,000), similar to that in, for example, Australia and New Zealand (16.1 per 100,000).

Lung cancer remains a highly lethal disease. Relative survival at 5 years as measured by the SEER program in the United States is 14%, whereas average relative survival in Europe is 8%, not much better than the 7% in developing countries (see Table 1.5).

The number of cases worldwide has increased by 16% since 1985 (+4% in men and +21% in women), which represents a 2.5% increase in the actual risk in men and a 9.5% increase in women (with the remainder due to population growth and aging). The trends, however, are very different among countries and between the genders. In men, several populations have passed the peak of the tobacco-related epidemic, and incidence rates are declining (e.g., United States and the countries of northern and western Europe). In contrast, incidence and mortality are increasing rapidly in southern and eastern European countries. In women, the epidemic is less advanced. Most Western countries still are showing a rising trend in incidence and mortality. In many countries, evidence of an increasing trend is not apparent thus far; however, for a few countries (e.g., United Kingdom), the peak of risk already may have been reached.

Stomach cancer is the second most frequent cancer, with 798,000 new cases and 627,000 deaths in 1990, although it is relatively less common in women (see Table 1.3). Age-adjusted incidence rates are highest in Japan (77.9 per 100,000 in men, 33.3 in women) and China. High rates also are present for both genders in eastern Europe and in some parts of Central and South America. The rates are low in East and North Africa, North and South America, and Southeast Asia (5.9–9.0 per 100,000 in men and 2.6–5.3 per 100,000 in women). Relative survival from stomach cancer is mod-

est: 21% based on the SEER data and 18% on average in European registries.

A steady decline has been recorded in the risk of gastric cancer incidence and mortality in most countries. In 1990, the estimated number of cases worldwide was just 6% greater than in 1985; given the population increase and aging, this figure represents a decline of some 4% to 5% in age-adjusted risk.

Breast cancer is the third most frequent cancer in the world (796,000 cases in 1990) and by far the most common malignancy of women (21% of all new cases; see Table 1.3). It is the fifth cause of death from cancer overall, although still the leading cause of cancer mortality in women. The 314,000 annual deaths represent 14.1% of female cancer deaths (see Table 1.4). Breast cancer incidence rates are high in all of the "developed" areas (except for Japan, where it is third after stomach and colorectal cancer), with the highest age-adjusted incidence in the United States (87.1 per 100,000; see Table 1.3). The rates are low (< 30 per 100,000) in most of sub-Saharan Africa (with the exception of South Africa) and in most of Asia (the Philippines being a notable exception). The lowest incidence is in China (11.8 per 100,000).

Generally, the prognosis in breast cancer is rather good, as illustrated by the relative survival figures in Table 1.5. Relative survival in the SEER program is 84% and in the EUROCARE project was 67%. Even in developing countries, more than 50% of women can expect to survive for more than 5 years.

Incidence rates of breast cancer are increasing in most countries, and usually the changes are greatest where rates previously were low. Since 1985, the annual increase in incidence rates has been approximately +0.5%, but the rate of increase is considerably higher than this in east Asia, including China.

Colorectal cancers accounted for 783,000 new cancer cases and caused 437,000 deaths in 1990 (see Tables 1.3, 1.4). Unlike that for most sites, the incidence is not very different in men and women. Relative survival at 5 years is 62% in the SEER program, 41% in European and Indian cancer registries, and slightly lower in China and developing countries (32% and 35%, respectively). Incidence of colorectal cancer is higher in developed countries than in developing countries, with the highest rates in the United States, Australia, and northern and western Europe, and moderately high incidence rates in south and east Europe and in Argentina. Incidence rates are low in Africa and Asia, except for Japan, which now has an incidence similar to that in western Europe. The incidence rates of colon cancer are increasing in most areas, especially in men, although (as noted) this no longer is evident in the United States.

Liver cancer is the fifth most frequent cancer worldwide in terms of numbers of cases (437,000; see Table 1.3) and fourth in terms of mortality (427,000 deaths; see Table 1.4). This finding reflects the extremely poor prognosis for this cancer; relative survival rates are 3% to 6% in the United States and developing countries. The areas of high incidence are western and southern Africa and eastern and Southeast Asia. The incidence is low in Europe (with any substantial risk only in southern Europe), in the Americas, and in southern and western Asia.

Prostate cancer is the sixth most common cancer in the world (in terms of number of new cases) and is fourth in frequency in men (see Table 1.3). The total annual number of cases is 396,000. It is predominantly a cancer of the elderly, with 81% of cases in the world occurring after age 65. Incidence rates are influenced by the diagnosis of latent cancers that results from the screening of asymptomatic individuals. Thus, where this practice of screening is common, the "incidence" may be very high (e.g., 95.1 per 100,000 in the United States). Incidence is high also in northern and western Europe and in Australia. The age-adjusted rates show that several developing areas also have a relatively high occurrence of disease—parts of sub-Saharan Africa, Latin America, and the Caribbean in particular. In contrast, the incidence rates in Asia (and particularly in China) are low.

Prostate cancer mortality is considerably lower than incidence (165,000 deaths in 1990), and the rates show less diversity than incidence (see Table 1.4). Relative survival is significantly greater in high-risk countries (88% in SEER versus 40% in developing countries). This more favorable prognosis well could be due to detection of more latent cancer by screening procedures,

which also explains the absence of any change in mortality in the presence of the large increase in incidence. Nevertheless, a fairly marked gradient in mortality still exists, with age-adjusted death rates ranging from 0.7 per 100,000 in China to 34.4 per 100,000 in Trinidad and Tobago. Recently, prostate cancer mortality declined significantly in the United States between 1990 and 1996 [5].

The incidence of prostate cancer has risen briskly over the last 5 years—a nearly 3.7% annual increase worldwide. Much of this increase was due to the huge surge in the United States (a 9.5% average annual increase between 1985 and 1990), a change that has been reversed since 1992.

Cervical cancer is the seventh most common cancer overall and the third most common in women, in whom it reflects 9.8% of all cancers (371,000 new cases per year; see Table 1.3). It is much more common in developing countries, with the highest incidence rates recorded in Latin America and the Caribbean, sub-Saharan Africa, and southern and Southeast Asia. In developed countries, the incidence rates generally are low, with age-adjusted rates less than 14 per 100,000. Very low rates are observed also in China and the Middle East.

Cervical cancer death rates are substantially lower than is incidence (see Table 1.4). Relative survival rates vary among regions, with fairly good prognosis in low-risk regions (69% in SEER and 59% in the European registries; see Table 1.5). Even in developing countries, where many cases present at an advanced stage, relative survival rates are fair (49% on average).

Cervical cancer incidence and mortality have declined rather substantially, a decrease observed most clearly in western countries having well-developed screening programs (e.g., in Finland). Declines are evident also in some developing countries, most notably in China, where current incidence and death rates are very low.

Esophageal cancer is the eighth most common cancer worldwide, responsible for 316,000 new cases in 1990 (see Table 1.3), and it is sixth most common cause of death from cancer, with 286,000 deaths (see Table 1.4). Cancer of the esophagus is the fourth site characterized by very poor survival, the other three being the liver, pancreas, and lung. Eleven percent of affected patients survive at least 5 years in the United States, and 5% do so in Europe. Geographic variation in incidence is very striking. High-risk areas include South and eastern Africa, China, central Asia (Kyrgyzstan), Argentina, Brazil, and (in men only) France. Incidence in women is also relatively high in India.

Some 261,000 annual new cases of bladder cancer are estimated worldwide (see Table 1.3). Only one-fifth of the cases (58,000) occur in women. The areas of high risk are those where the effects of long-term exposure to tobacco smoking still are evident: Europe, North America, and Israel. The estimated relative survival from bladder cancer varies substantially worldwide. It is very good in North America (81% from SEER) and only 42% in developing countries (see Table 1.5). No measure is available for Europe. Part of this inconsistency is an artifact due to different practices adopted by cancer registries with respect to the inclusion of in situ and even benign tumors.

Leukemias account for some 231,000 new cases each year (see Table 1.3), and 184,000 deaths (see Table 1.4). This rather high ratio of deaths to cases (80%) reflects the poor prognosis of this cancer in many parts of the world. The lowest incidence rates are observed in sub-Saharan Africa (probably representing failure of diagnosis to some extent), and the highest are seen in North America and Australia–New Zealand. Variations in mortality are somewhat less, owing to better survival (and hence lower mortality) in developed countries.

Pancreas cancer enters into the top 10 causes of cancer deaths in the world (168,000 per year; see Table 1.4) because of the very poor prognosis (relative survival < 5%; see Table 1.5). The death rates are highest in Europe, the United States, and Japan, where incidence and death rates are 6 to 12 per 100,000 in men and 4 to 7 per 100,000 in women. The only developing countries with rates in this range are in Latin America.

SUMMARY

Population research contributes to our understanding of cancer at many levels. Certain fundamental concepts such as individual risk, survival, and population attributable risk are measurable only in populations, not in individuals. Population-based statistics regarding cancer incidence, mortality, and survival are essential for identifying high-risk populations, monitoring progress against disease, developing cancer control programs, and assessing program needs for patient services.

REFERENCES

1. Ries LAG, Kosary CL, Hankey BF, et al. (eds). *SEER Cancer Statistics Review, 1973–1996.* Bethesda, MD: National Cancer Institute, 1999.
2. Thom TJ. Economic costs of neoplasms, arteriosclerosis, and diabetes in the United States. *In Vivo* 10:255–260, 1996.
3. Centers for Disease Control and Prevention. *The National Program of Cancer Registries: At-A-Glance, 1998.* Atlanta: Centers for Disease Control and Prevention, 1998.
4. Wingo PA, Ries LAG, Rosenberg HM, et al. Cancer incidence and mortality, 1973–1995: a report card for the U.S. *Cancer* 82:1197–1207, 1998.
5. Ries LAG, Wingo PA, Miller DS, et al. Annual report to the nation on the status of Cancer, 1973–1997, with a special section on colorectal cancer. *Cancer* 88:2398–2424, 2000.
6. Swan J, Wingo P, Clive R, et al. Cancer surveillance in the U.S.: can we have a national system? *Cancer* 83:1282–1291, 1998.
7. Menck H, Smart C (eds). *Central Cancer Registries: Design, Management, and Use.* Chur, Switzerland: Harwood Academic, 1994.
8. Jensen OM, Parkin DM, Maclennan R, et al. *Cancer Registration: Principles and Methods.* Lyon, France: International Agency for Research on Cancer, 1991.
9. *Standards of the Commission on Cancer: Vol II. Registry Operations and Data Standards (ROADS).* Chicago: American College of Surgeons, 1996.
10. *SEER Extent of Disease—1998, Codes and Coding Instructions* (3rd ed). Washington, DC: National Cancer Institute, Public Health Service, National Institutes of Health, January 1998.
11. Percy C, Van Holten V, Muir C (eds). *International Classification of Diseases for Oncology* (2nd ed). Geneva: World Health Organization, 1990.
12. State cancer registries: status of authorizing legislation and enabling regulations—United States, October 1993. *MMWR* 43:71–75, 1994.
13. Chen VW, Wu XC, Andrews PA (eds). *Cancer in North America, 1990–1995: Vol 1. Incidence.* Sacramento, CA: North American Association of Central Cancer Registries, 1999.
14. Chen VW, Wu XC (eds). *Cancer in North America, 1990–1995: Vol 2: Mortality.* Sacramento, CA: North American Association of Central Cancer Registries, 1999.
15. National Center for Health Statistics. *Vital Statistics of the United States, 1930–1959: Vol II: Mortality, parts A and B.* Washington, DC: Public Health Service, 1930–1997.
16. National Center for Health Statistics. *Vital Statistics of the United States.* [Public use data file documentation: mortality detail for ICD-7 1960–67, ICD-8A 1968–78, ICD-9 1979–95.] Hyattsville, MD: Public Health Service, 1998.
17. Kleinbaum DG, Kupper LL, Morgenstern H. *Epidemiologic Research.* Belmont, CA: Lifetime Learning Publications, 1982.
18. Wingo PA, Landis S, Parker S, et al. Using cancer registry and vital statistics data to estimate the number of new cancer cases and deaths in the United States for the upcoming year. *Registry Manage* 25:43–51, 1998.
19. Last JM (ed). *A Dictionary of Epidemiology.* New York: Oxford University Press, 1988.
20. Parkin DM, Whelan SL, Ferlay J, et al. (eds). *Cancer Incidence in Five Continents,* vol VII. [IARC Sci. Pub. No. 143.] Lyon, France: International Agency for Research on Cancer, 1997:1028–1029.
21. Gloeckler Ries LA, Pollack ES, Young JL. Cancer patient

survival: surveillance, epidemiology, and end results program, 1973–1979. *J Natl Cancer Inst* 70:693–707, 1983.

22. Tulinius H, Storm HH, Pukkala E, et al. Cancer in the Nordic countries 1981–1986. *Acta Pathol Microbiol Immunol Scand* 100(suppl):31, 1992.

23. Pisani P, Ferlay J. Prevalence data. In Ferlay J, Black RJ, Pisani P, et al. (eds), *EUCAN90: Cancer in the European Union*. [IARC CancerBase No. 1.] Lyon, France: International Agency for Research on Cancer, 1996.

24. Kelsey JL, Thompson WD, Evans AS. *Methods in Observational Epidemiology*. New York: Oxford University Press, 1986.

25. World Health Organization. *World Health Statistics Annual, 1996*. Geneva: World Health Organization, 1998.

26. Becerra J, Eaker ED. Measures of disease frequency in reproductive health. In Wingo PA, Higgins JE, Rubin GL, Zahniser SC (eds), *An Epidemiologic Approach to Reproductive Health*. Geneva: World Health Organization, 1992.

27. Fleiss JL. *Statistical Methods for Rates and Proportions* (2nd ed). New York: Wiley, 1981.

28. Waterhouse J, Muir C, Correa P, Powell J (eds). *Cancer Incidence in Five Continents*, vol III. [IARC Sci. Pub. No. 15.] Lyon, France: International Agency for Research on Cancer, 1976.

29. Wingo PA, Gloekler-Ries LA, Parker SL, Heath CW. Long-term cancer patient survival in the United States. *Cancer Epidemiol Biomarkers Prev* 7:271–282, 1998.

30. Ederer F, Axtell LM, Cutler SJ. The relative survival rate: a statistical methodology. *Monogr Natl Cancer Inst* 6:101–121, 1961.

31. Ries LAG, Kosary CL, Hankey BF, et al. (eds). *SEER Cancer Statistics Review, 1973–1994*. [NIH Pub. No. 97–2789.] Bethesda, MD: National Cancer Institute, 1997.

32. Berrino F, Sant M, Verdecchia A, et al. (eds). *Survival of Cancer Patients in Europe: The EUROCARE Study*. [IARC Sci. Pub. No. 132.] Lyon, France: International Agency for Research on Cancer, 1995.

33. Sankaranarayanan R, Black RJ, Parkin DM (eds). *Cancer Survival in Developing Countries*. [IARC Sci. Pub. No. 145.] Lyon, France: International Agency for Research on Cancer, 1998.

34. Cigarette smoking–attributable mortality and years of potential life lost—United States, 1990. *MMWR* 42:645–648, 1993.

35. Collaborative Group on Hormonal Factors in Breast Cancer. Breast cancer and hormone replacement therapy: collaborative reanalysis of data from 51 epidemiological studies of 52,702 women with breast cancer and 108,411 women without breast cancer. *Lancet* 350:1047–1059, 1997.

36. Greenlee RT, Murray T, Bolden S, Wingo PA. Cancer statistics, 2000. *CA Cancer J Clin* 50:7–33, 2000.

37. Pan American Health Organization. *Health Statistics from the Americas* (1995 ed). Washington, DC: Pan American Health Association, 1995.

38. World Health Organization. *World Health Statistics Annual*. Geneva: World Health Organization, 1993.

39. Ferlay J, Black R, Whelan SL, Parkin DM. *CI5VII: Cancer Incidence in Five Continents*, vol VII. [IARC CancerBase No. 2.] Lyon, France: International Agency for Research on Cancer, 1997.

40. Ferlay J, Parkin DM, Pisani P. *GLOBOCAN: Cancer Incidence and Mortality Worldwide*. [IARC CancerBase No. 3.] Lyon, France: International Agency for Research on Cancer, 1998.

41. Parkin DM, Pisani P, Ferlay J. Estimates of the worldwide incidence of twenty-five major cancers in 1990. *Int J Cancer* 80:827–841, 1999.

42. Pisani P, Parkin DM, Bray FI, Ferlay J. Estimates of the worldwide mortality from twenty-five major cancers in 1990. *Int J Cancer* 80:18–29, 1999.

2

Principles of Cancer Biology

■ ■ ■

David P. Ringer
Lowell E. Schnipper

As we enter a new millennium, we also embark on a new era in the battle against cancer. The tools and approaches available to medical science for treatment of patients with diagnosed cancer have moved beyond those predominantly developed through empiric processes of observation and experience. Dramatic technical advances in the areas of molecular biology, eukaryotic cell biochemistry, cellular immunology, virology, cytogenetics, cell culture, and animal models of multistage carcinogenesis have provided significant new insights into the molecular basis of cancer biology. This understanding already has opened new doors to the treatment of cancer.

One such advance is a novel treatment based on the construction of a monoclonal antibody targeted against a specific cancer cell gene product (e.g., an aberrant cell growth factor receptor) to treat certain forms of aggressive breast cancer. Other advances include progress in the use of steroid hormone antagonists, such as tamoxifen, not only to treat existing breast cancer but also to prevent the emergence of new breast cancers in high-risk women. Powerful new cancer-arresting antiangiogenesis compounds capable of reversing the growth of new blood vessels in a wide variety of solid cancer tumors now await testing in well-designed clinical trials. Furthermore, the future will bring another significant paradigm shift in cancer biology. Completion of the federally funded Human Genome Project within the next five years will permit expansion of our understanding of the molecular basis of cancer founded on a full structural description of the human genome.

HISTORIC PHENOTYPIC ALTERATIONS IN CANCER CELL BIOLOGY

Past investigations based on the use of in vitro cultures of transformed cells from animal and human tumors and on the use of normal cells transformed in vitro by viruses, irradiation, or chemical carcinogens have allowed the identification of cellular features that distinguish the cell biology of cancer cells from that of normal cells. These hallmarks of cancer cell biology have, in turn, provided researchers with important intermediate end points in experimental assays and have provided key entry points for the investigation of the cellular and molecular mechanisms of carcinogenesis. These historic phenotypic characteristics provide a useful context for understanding key molecular events in carcinogenesis.

Cell Structure

Cancer cells in histologically fixed and stained tissue sections and cancer cells in cell cultures show an increased nucleus-to-cytoplasm ratio characterized by increased nuclear size, enlarged nucleoli, and irregular chromatin distributions. Cancer cells in cell culture also appear to be more rounded in overall shape in contrast to noncancerous cells, which appear flattened along the growth surface. The rounded appearance is linked to changes in the structural organization of actin polymers in the cell cytoskeleton.

Contact Inhibition During Cell Proliferation

Typically, cancer cells fail to stop proliferating when cell density reaches that of a monolayer of cells in contact with one another (i.e., loss of contact inhibition). The loss of contact inhibition is correlated with the loss of signaling between cells by small-molecule movement through gap junctions between adjacent cells. As a result, cancer cells overgrow and form multicell layers called *foci*.

Alterations in Anchorage-Dependent Growth

Normal, noncancerous cells grown in cell culture require direct contact and anchorage to a solid surface for proliferative growth. Cancer cells fail to show anchorage dependence and typically will proliferate on semisolids, such as soft agar, or in solutions. Notably, cancer cells in culture produce less fibronectin, a protein used by cells for adhesion to a growth surface.

Growth Factor Requirements

Normal human cells in cell culture require the presence of high levels (5%) of fetal calf serum for optimal proliferative growth. In the presence of low levels of sera (< 1%), cells remain viable but do not proliferate readily. The lessened dependence on exogenously supplied growth factors corresponds with cancer cell ability to display autonomous growth characteristics. Malignant cells can produce growth factors and can express receptors for these same growth factors and, thus, lose their dependence on exogenously supplied growth factors. The hypothesis that cancer cells may stimulate their own proliferation independent of normal external regulatory controls has been termed the *autocrine stimulatory hypothesis* of cancer.

Cell Population–Doubling Capacity (Immortalization)

Typically, normal human cells grown in culture display a finite number of population doublings or passages in cell culture before they stop growing and die. Often, this process is termed *in vitro aging* or *senescence*. Cancer cells in culture show no restriction in their number of proliferative generations. This unlimited capacity for proliferative growth is termed *immortalization*. Cancer cell reexpression of telomerase—a telomere-lengthening activity (a telomere being the distal end of a chromosome) absent in most normal cells—plays a key role in enabling cancer cells to have an unlimited capacity for proliferation in cell culture.

GENETIC AND EPIGENETIC MECHANISMS FOR ALTERED GENOTYPE IN CANCER CELLS
Genetic Mechanisms

Several decades of research were required to establish what now is taken to be axiomatic: that the phenotypic changes associated with cancer cell biology are the result of changes to the cell genome. The basis for defining cancer as a disease of the genome came from voluminous data showing that agents strongly associated with increased risk for cancer (e.g., x-rays and certain chemicals) also caused mutations in DNA. This association led to development of the somatic cell mutation theory for cancer causation, wherein mutated genes in somatic cells of a target organ initiate carcinogenesis that culmi-

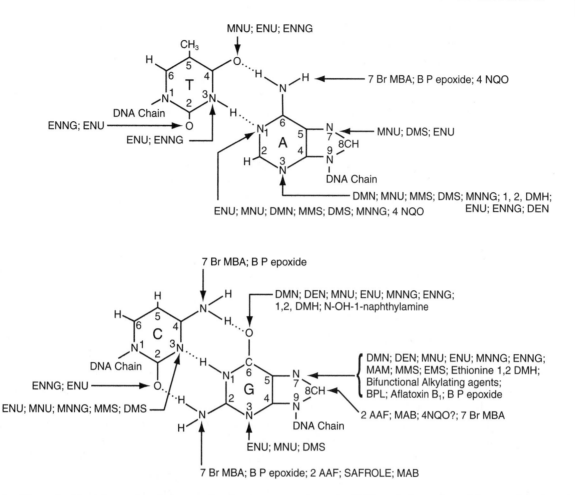

Figure 2.1 Sites of adduct formation between the four common bases in DNA and the activated forms of various known chemical carcinogens. (Reprinted with permission from E Farber, Chemical carcinogens: a biological perspective. *Am J Pathol* 106[2]:271–296, 1982.) *MNU* = *N*-methyl-*N*-nitrosourea; *ENU* = *N*-ethyl-*N*-nitrosourea; *ENNG* = *N*-ethyl-*N'*-nitro-*N*-nitroso-guanidine; *7 Br MBA* = 7-bromomethylbenz[a]anthracene; *BP epoxide* = benzo[a]pyrene epoxide; *4NQO* = 4-nitroquinoline-*N*-oxide; *DMS* = dimethyl methanesulfonate; *DMN* = dimethylnitrosamine; *MMS* = methyl methanesulfonate; *MNNG* = *N*-methyl-*N'*-nitro-*N*-nitrosoguanidine; *DMH* = dimethylhydrazine; *DEN* = diethylnitrosamine; *MAM* = methylazoxymethanol; *EMS* = ethyl methanesulfonate; *BPL* = β-propiolactone; *AAF* = acetylaminofluorene; *MAB* = methylaminoazobenzene.

nates in a primary tumor in that organ. Generally, DNA-damaging events leading to the initiation of cancer were found to comprise two general classes: point mutations and chromosomal changes.

POINT MUTATIONS

Point mutations result from unrepaired irradiation or chemical damage to DNA purine and pyrimidine bases, resulting in single-base changes within gene sequences. A summary representative of the types of chemical agents and their points of attack on DNA purines and pyrimidines is shown in Figure 2.1. The mutational damage to a gene sequence takes the form of DNA base

substitutions, deletions, or insertions and results in altered protein expression, half-life, or functional properties in the cell. However, mutating agents generate a large array of DNA damage, not all of which is linked to the development of cancer. Thus, localization of damage to a key cancer-related gene generally is not possible.

CHROMOSOMAL REARRANGEMENTS

Cancer-related genomic alterations have been found also to result from chromosomal translocations and gene copy-number amplification. Such early chromosomal alterations as the Philadelphia chromosome in chronic myelogenous leukemia and the 13q deletion of retinoblastoma initially were identified through association with rare and/or early-onset cancers. Recent advances in chromosomal banding techniques have permitted greater visualization of specific regions within chromosomes and have revealed the presence of a broad range of nonrandom chromosomal changes related to specific cancers. This approach has been particularly successful when applied to the study of oncogene activation, because once the normal genomic location of a protooncogene is identified, an association can be established between the activation of particular oncogenes and the chromosomal rearrangements, deletions, and amplifications observed at closely linked chromosomal sites. Specific examples of chromosomal changes involving oncogenes and associated human cancers are presented in Table 2.1.

Other evidence demonstrating the requirement for an altered cellular genotype in cancer has come from research of cancer-causing viruses. The investigation of cells transformed by such DNA viruses as SV40 and polyomavirus revealed that cancer cells had retained several viral genes in the cellular genome. Subsequent studies showed both that these viral genes were responsible for the cancerlike transformation of cells and that their continued presence was required for maintaining the transformed state. Several distinct classes of tumor viruses have been revealed to play key roles in the inception of cancer in both animals and humans.

RETROVIRUSES

Retroviruses have an RNA genome. They are composed of several genes with such shorthand designations as *gag* (encoding for viral core proteins), *pol* (encoding for the enzyme reverse transcriptase, which allows these viruses to make DNA copies of themselves and therefore to integrate their genetic material into the genome of the cell they infect), and *env* (encoding for a virion glycoprotein). In addition, the acute transforming retroviruses include nucleic acid sequences transduced from the genetic information of the host cell; such cellular gene sequences are necessary to the transforming activity of the acutely acting retroviruses and have been termed *viral oncogenes*. To date, oncogene-bearing retroviruses have been shown to arise only in certain animal species (notably chickens, mice, rats, and monkeys).

Another group of retroviruses that are found in humans lack their own oncogenes and cause cancer by integrating into the host genome and controlling the expression of cellular genes. The human T-cell lymphotropic virus is an example of this second type of transforming retrovirus and is associated with a cancer of T

lymphocytes. Furthermore, the human T-cell lymphotropic virus may be transmitted horizontally in the manner of classic infectious diseases or may persist in an asymptomatic carrier state in susceptible populations and, after a long latency, can result in a cancer of T lymphocytes of the mature-differentiation phenotype. It is endemic in southern Japan, the Caribbean, Africa, Central America, parts of South America, and the southeastern United States.

HUMAN PAPILLOMAVIRUSES

Human papillomaviruses (HPVs) are small DNA viruses that infect epithelial cells and often are associated with mucosal and cutaneous lesions (e.g., benign genital warts and low grades of cervical intraepithelial neoplasia that regress spontaneously). The papillomavirus subtypes associated with benign cutaneous warts (e.g., HPV-1) are not associated with cervical cancer, whereas those implicated in the genesis of cervical cancer do not cause skin warts. HPV serotypes 16 and 18 are found in the majority of cervical cancers and are implicated in the pathogenesis of this type of cancer. Its transforming gene, *E7*, can immortalize rodent cells and cooperate with other oncogenes to transform cells into a neoplastic phenotype. An interesting effect associated with the E7 protein is its ability to interact with the retinoblastoma gene product and to impair this protein's cell-cycle regulatory function. Another gene product of the HPV, *E6*, can cause degradation of the cell's *p53* gene product. The *p53* and retinoblastoma gene products are cell-cycle regulatory proteins that function as tumor suppressors. Another viral protein, E5, can complex with several types of human peptide hormone receptors and can cause sustained signaling of receptor kinases. Thus, the virus's abilities to inactivate two of the cell's key tumor suppressor proteins and to mimic growth hormone activity would appear to facilitate its promotion of unconstrained proliferation of the infected cell.

HEPATITIS B AND C VIRUSES

The hepatitis B virus (HBV) and the hepatitis C virus (HCV) pose major public health problems. Approximately 300 million chronic HBV carriers exist worldwide and are at greatly increased risk for hepatocellular carcinoma. Genetic sequences belonging to the HBV have been identified in most samples of hepatocellular carcinoma in many Asian countries where HBV is endemic and hepatocellular carcinoma is one of the most common cancers. DNA and serologic evidence of HBV infection is less common in North American and Euro-

Table 2.1   Oncogenes and Their Mechanisms of Activation, Functional Properties, and Associated Cancers

Oncogene	Activation Mechanism	Functional Properties	Associated Cancers
bcr-abl	Chromosomal translocation t(9;22)(q34;q11)*	Chimeric nonreceptor tyrosine kinase	Acute lymphocytic leukemia, chronic myelogenous leukemia
b-Cat	Point mutation	Transcriptional coactivator (linking E-cadherin and cytoskeleton)	Melanoma, colorectal cancer
bcl-2	Chromosomal translocation t(14;18)(q32;q21)	Antiapoptosis	B-cell lymphoma, colorectal cancer
cdk4	Amplification, point mutation	Cyclin-dependent kinase	Sarcoma
erb-B1	Amplification	Growth factor receptor	Squamous cell carcinoma, glioblastoma, astrocytoma
erb-B2/neu	Amplification	Growth factor receptor	Breast, gastric, ovarian cancer
gli	Amplification	Transcription factor	Sarcoma, glioma
hst	Amplification	Growth factor-like	—
met	Point mutation	Receptor tyrosine kinase	Carcinomas; sarcomas of lung, breast, cervix
mdm-2	Amplification	*p53*-Binding protein	Gastric sarcomas
myc family (C-, L-, N-)	Amplifications; C-, chromosomal translocation t(8;14)(q24;q32)	Transcription factor	C-: Burkitt's lymphoma, small-cell lung carcinoma, acute T-cell lymphoma; L-: small-cell lung carcinoma; N-: neuroblastoma, small-cell lung carcinoma
plm-RARa	Chromosomal translocation	Chimeric transcription factor	Acute promyelocytic leukemia
ras family (H-, K-, N-)	Point mutations	p21 GTPase	H-: bladder cancer; K-: pancreatic cancer, colorectal cancer, lung adenocarcinoma, endometrial cancer; N-: myeloid leukemia
ret	Chromosomal translocation, point mutation	Receptor tyrosine kinase	Thyroid cancer (papillary, medullary), sarcoma
smo	Point mutations	Transmembrane signaling	Skin (basal cell) cancer
trk	Chromosomal translocation	Receptor tyrosine kinase	Thyroid carcinoma, colorectal carcinoma
ttg	Chromosomal translocation t(11;14)(p15;q11)	Transcription factor	T-cell acute lymphocytic leukemia
w2a-pbx1	Chromosomal translocation	Chimeric transcription factor	Pre-B-cell acute lymphocytic leukemia

*Chromosomal sites involved in translocation.
Source: Adapted from J Cortner, S Vande Woude, GF Vande Woude, Genes involved in oncogenesis. *Adv Vet Med* 40:51–102, 1997; TL Goodrow, One decade of comparative molecular carcinogenesis. *Prog Clin Biol Res* 395:57–80, 1996; and DA Haber, ER Fearon, The promise of cancer genetics. *Lancet* 351(suppl 2):S111–S118, 1998.

pean hepatocellular carcinoma cases. Although the association between the DNA of HBV and liver cancer is clear, a causative relationship has not been established. Nonetheless, some investigators have suggested that the mechanism involves the ability of HBV to cause chronic tissue damage. This action, in turn, leads to chronic compensatory hyperplasia of the surviving cells, a pro-

cess that acts effectively as a tumor-promoting stimulus. Activation of oncogenes and inactivation of tumor suppressor genes resulting from integration of HBV sequences is another mechanism believed to contribute hepatocarcinogenesis.

More recently, HCV has become recognized as the major causative factor responsible for non-A, non-B hepatitis. With the advent of serologic and molecular techniques to identify HCV or humoral responses to it, epidemiologic studies have provided strong evidence for an association between HCV infection and hepatocellular carcinoma. The mechanisms underlying this association are not yet understood.

EPSTEIN-BARR VIRUS

The Epstein-Barr virus (EBV) is a prevalent virus widely known for causing infectious mononucleosis. Early studies showed an association of EBV with Burkitt's lymphoma, and EBV became the first human virus that could be linked with leading to cancer in humans. EBV genes can immortalize previously uninfected B lymphocytes in tissue culture through the actions of nine specific viral genes, of which the genes for latent membrane protein 1 and the nuclear antigens 1, 2, 3A, and 3C appear to be required for constitutive expression. In the absence of a normally functioning immune system (as in the X-linked lymphoproliferative syndrome) or in the state of profound immunosuppression after organ transplantation, malignant lymphoproliferative disorders can arise more readily and are composed of cells that contain EBV genes.

Epigenetic Mechanisms

Besides the genetic mechanisms for altering the cellular genome, nongenetic or epigenetic mechanisms exist. Epigenetic mechanisms exert their effect on the genome by acting through cellular regulatory circuits without causing a change in gene sequence. The primary (if not only) example of an epigenetic mechanism operating in vertebrates is that involving the methylation of DNA cytosines. Methylation at the C-5 position of DNA cytosines by DNA cytosine-5-methlyltransferase results in the formation of 5-methylcytosines along the DNA sequence, primarily at CpG dinucleotide sites. The regions in the genome in which the CpG sites cluster together are called *CpG islands,* and much evidence indicates that the state of cytosine C-5 methylation in these islands alters the rate of gene transcription, thereby altering the levels of proteins that govern cellular function.

Although the exact molecular mechanisms are not known, in general, hypermethylation of DNA cytosines in CpG islands has been found to be associated with the downregulation of gene transcription and hypomethylation at these sites with the upregulation gene transcription. Hypermethylation plays an important role

in normal embryonic development through the functional silencing of genes. A mechanism in somatic cells through which alterations in DNA cytosine methylation may support tumor development involves changing the normal functional status of cell-cycle regulatory genes that control the proliferative state of the cell. Transcriptional silencing of several cell-cycle suppressor genes through hypermethylation of CpG islands in the gene promoter regions has been associated with a number of cancer types. For example, studies have reported the hypermethylation-related silencing of the *RB* gene in retinoblastoma tumors, the von Hippel-Lindau gene in renal cancers, and the *H19* gene in Wilms' tumor.

PRIMARY MOLECULAR TARGETS OF ALTERED GENE EXPRESSION IN CANCER CELLS

Understanding cancer at the molecular level has advanced rapidly because of expanded knowledge about how select sets of regulatory genes control cell proliferation and cell differentiation. Now accepted is that human tumors arise largely through a sequence of multiple alterations in specific families of cell regulatory genes. Generally, the gene families have been classified either as altered genes (termed *oncogenes*) in which functional activation in the cell was tied strongly to cancer causation or as altered genes (termed *tumor suppressor genes*) in which functional loss in the cell strongly supported cancer development. Characteristically, activation of oncogenes increases cell proliferation, whereas inactivation of tumor suppressor genes increases cell proliferation by abrogation of their normal function of blocking cell proliferation.

Oncogenes

Initial insights into the identity of important gene families associated with cancer development came from research involving tumor viruses. Studies demonstrated that a small number of viral genes, or viral oncogenes, incorporated into the cellular genome could act to create cancerlike changes in cellular phenotype and could lead to cell transformation. Subsequent discoveries that some viral oncogenes could be shown to have arisen from genes normally present in the cellular genome led to the realization that certain normal genes could be converted by viruses into cancer-causing oncogenes. This concept was extended to an examination of the possibility that a small number of mutated cellular genes in cells without tumor viruses could act also as oncogenes.

A now-well-documented concept for many human cancers is that oncogenes arise from normal, wild-type cellular genes (termed *protooncogenes*) after an alteration in DNA structure resulting in inappropriate functional activation of that gene. Much evidence suggests that the protein products of protooncogenes typically have roles in regulating normal cell processes (e.g., cell growth and cell differentiation). Furthermore, as mutant forms of alleles, oncogenes characteristically are functionally dominant to the wild-type form of the alleles when both are present in the same cell.

As can be seen in Table 2.1, oncogenes are composed of genes involved in the control of cell proliferation, differentiation, and apoptosis (programmed cell death). Discussion of several of these oncogenes in greater detail illustrates their functional diversity and the mechanisms for their activation.

v-sis

The *v-sis* oncogene, originally isolated from a transforming retrovirus known to cause sarcomas in monkeys, codes for a protein with an amino-acid sequence virtually identical to that of the hormone platelet-derived growth factor (PDGF), a protein with mitogenic characteristics. PDGF is capable of causing the growth of such connective-tissue cells as fibroblasts.

erb-B2

The *erb-B2* oncogene, also known as *HER2/neu,* is a member of the same gene family as the cell-surface receptors for epidermal growth factor. Like PDGF, it is responsible for stimulating cell proliferation. Similar to other members of this family, *erb-B2* exhibits tyrosine kinase activity, an enzyme activity characteristic of many proteins that play regulatory roles within cells. Gene amplification and protein overexpression of *erb-B2* in human breast cancer and is associated with an adverse prognosis. In clinical trials employing adjuvant chemotherapy to treat breast cancer effectively, a marked improvement in both progression-free and overall survival was observed after the use of a specific type of chemotherapy for the systemic treatment of tumors that overexpress *erb-B2*. More recently, a monoclonal antibody to the erb-B2 protein, called *trastuzumab (Herceptin),* has been therapeutically useful in women whose breast cancer is characterized by erb-B2 overexpression and has progressed after standard chemotherapy.

ras

The *ras* family of oncogenes encodes a protein, p21, with a cellular location at the inner surface of the cytoplasmic membrane and guanosine triphosphatase (GTPase) activity that modulates cellular growth. The GTPase activity enables p21 to shut off its own growth-promoting functions. The mutated, oncogenic form of *ras* proteins has greatly reduced GTPase activity and presumably leads to a loss of normal regulatory ability. Studies comparing nucleotide sequences of transforming *H-ras* genes obtained from human and animal tumors with sequences of normal *H-ras* genes revealed that the oncogene carries nucleotide changes in either the twelfth or the sixty-first codon of the gene. The single-nucleotide base pair changes each lead to a single amino acid substitution in the 189–amino acid sequence of the p21 protein for *H-ras*. Mutations at these "hot-spot" regions are found also to lead to the activation of *K-ras* and *N-ras,* two genes homologous to *H-ras*. Commonly, *ras* is altered in polyps and in carcinomas of the colon.

Other studies of humans with lung cancer or myeloid leukemia have revealed the presence of mutated *ras* genes in the malignant cells but structurally normal *ras* genes in corresponding normal tissue. Furthermore, animal studies have shown that in animals exposed to chemical carcinogens (e.g., nitrosomethylurea), tumors that develop carry mutated *ras* genes, whereas adjacent normal tissues exhibit a normal *ras* gene structure. In this manner, single-gene mutations by environmental carcinogens have been implicated directly in carcinogenesis.

myc

In Burkitt's lymphoma, a reciprocal translocation including the *c-myc* gene on the distal segment of the long arm of chromosome 8 and the long arm of chromosome 14 or chromosome 2 results in abnormal expression of the *c-myc* gene. Because the *myc* protein has been associated with cellular proliferation, abnormal *myc* expression is hypothesized to be related to abnormal growth. The *myc* protein is located in the nucleus, where it acts as a transcription factor controlling the expression of cell growth–promoting genes.

The *c-myc* oncogene has been found also to be amplified in cell lines obtained from small-cell lung cancer. Characteristically, these cells express high levels of *c-myc* RNA and proliferate more rapidly than do cells without the *c-myc* amplification. Other forms of the *myc* oncogene that have been found to be amplified in small-cell lung cancers and neuroblastomas are *L-myc* and *N-myc*, respectively. In neuroblastoma, *N-myc* amplification is an unfavorable and clinically significant prognostic factor.

abl

The Philadelphia chromosome, observed in malignant cells of patients with chronic myelogenous leukemia, was the first example of a specific chromosomal rearrangement to be associated with cancer. This reciprocal translocation between chromosomes 9 and 22 has been shown to result in the translocation of the *abl* protooncogene from its normal site on chromosome 9 to a characteristic region on chromosome 22 (termed *bcr*). Consequently, the protein encoded by the new *bcr-abl* gene displays a new terminus with a novel function, a chimeric, nonreceptor tyrosine kinase. The fact that the *bcr* region on chromosome 22—to which the gene is translocated—is highly invariant suggests that this particular region may play an important role in the biology of this form of leukemia.

bcl-2

Apoptosis (programmed cell death), a process highly conserved throughout evolution, enables cells to cause their self-destruction by activating a cellular suicide pathway. The pathway is characterized by the condensation and fragmentation of nuclear and cytoplasmic components. The process is recognized as having important biological roles in mediating both the development and the homeostasis of animal cells in tissues. It also provides organisms with a means for destroying cells that have been seriously damaged. Numerous observations have linked specific neoplasms (e.g., non-Hodgkin's lymphoma) to a gene named *bcl-2* that is important in the regulation of apoptosis. *Bcl-1* normally functions to block apoptosis, and its cellular levels are regulated carefully in normal cells. In certain low-grade lymphomas, characterized by a nonrandom translocation between chromosomes 14 and 18, the *bcl-2* gene is translocated, dysregulated, and overexpressed. Cells demonstrating this genetic defect do not undergo programmed cell death normally, and this limitation is believed to be a key factor contributing to the massive accumulation of neoplastic lymphocytes seen in low-grade B-cell lymphomas. Generally, the induction of cell death through activation of apoptosis now is held also to be the central mechanism used by most chemotherapeutic drugs (e.g., 5-fluorouracil; taxol and bleomycin; dexamethasone; and cisplatin) to exert their cytotoxic effects on cancer cells. Overexpression of *bcl-2* has been found to correlate with resistance to chemotherapy. Consequently, the monitoring of *bcl-2* levels could have diagnostic, prognostic, and therapeutic relevance.

Tumor Suppressor Genes

Unlike oncogenes, tumor suppressor genes require the loss of both functional alleles to support an increase in cancer. Investigations of such cancers as familial retinoblastoma led to the initial studies showing that the inactivation of certain genes could lead to an increase in cancer causation. In this example, cancer is triggered when an individual inherits one defective retinoblastoma (*RB*) gene allele from one parent at birth, followed by loss of the function of the second allele at some point after birth through a somatic mutation.

Table 2.2 summarizes the currently identified tumor suppressor genes, their functional characteristics, and associated human cancers. Tumor suppressor genes, like oncogenes, also involve a variety of functional categories, including growth regulation, differentiation, and apoptosis. Two examples of tumor suppressor genes studied most frequently are the *RB* and *p53* genes.

RB

Because both *RB* genes are lost or inactivated in retinoblastoma, logical inferences are that no functional copy of this gene is present and that its influence as an essential regulator of cellular proliferation is lost. The heterozygous state of normal and abnormal *RB* alleles has been observed not to be associated with neoplasia, indicating that either one of the functioning alleles effectively can control cell proliferation. Further insight into the mechanism by which inactivation of the *RB* gene contributes to neoplasia has come from the study of several different oncogenic DNA viruses. Structurally distinct proteins critical to the development of neoplasia by a human adenovirus (the *Ela* gene and its protein); *SV40* (the large T-antigen gene and its protein); and HPV-16 (the *E7* gene and its protein) have been shown to act by binding and sequestering the protein product of the *RB* gene. Inactivation of this important regulator of cell proliferation appears to be of central importance to the cancer-causing capacity of these viruses. Either the loss of *RB* alleles or the inactivation of RB1 protein product would appear to allow the cell to downregulate *RB* growth-inhibitory pathways and thereby contribute to a state of autonomous cell proliferation.

Table 2.2   Tumor Suppressor Genes and Their Corresponding Functions, Associated Cancers, and Syndrome Name

Tumor Supressor	Functional Properties	Syndrome Name	Associated Cancers
APC	Cytoplasmic, cytoskeletal	Familial adenomatous polyposis	Colorectal cancer
BRCA1, BRCA2	Transcription factor	Familial breast cancer	Breast, ovarian cancer
DNA ligase 1	DNA repair enzyme	46BR	Lymphoma
		Bloom syndrome	Carcinoma
		Ataxic telangiectasia	Lymphoma
ERCC	DNA repair enzyme	Xeroderma pigmentosum	Skin cancer
FACC	DNA repair enzyme	Fanconi's anemia	Leukemia
HMLH1, HMLH2	DNA repair enzyme	Lynch syndrome	Nonpolyposis colon
Merlin	Cytoplasm, cytoskeleton	Neurofibromatosis type 2	Acoustic neuroma, meningioma, glioma, schwannoma
NF1	Cytoplasm, cytoskeleton	Neurofibromatosis type 1	Neurofibroma, neurofibrosarcoma
RB	Transcription factor	Familial retinoblastoma	Retinoblastoma, osteosarcoma, breast carcinoma, small-cell lung carcinoma
VHL	Unknown	von Hippel-Lindau	Kidney (clear-cell) carcinoma, hemangioblastoma
WT1	Transcription	Familial Wilms' tumor	Wilms' kidney tumor, hepatoblastoma

Source: Adapted from J Cortner, S Vande Woude, GF Vande Woude, Genes involved in oncogenesis. *Adv Vet Med* 40:51–102, 1997; TL Goodrow, One decade of comparative molecular carcinogenesis. *Prog Clin Biol Res* 395:57–80, 1996; and DA Haber, ER Fearon, The promise of cancer genetics. *Lancet* 351(suppl 2):S111–S118, 1998.

p53

Another important negative regulator of cell proliferation, the inactivation of which is associated with cancer causation, is the gene for *p53*. This gene encodes for a transcription factor involved with both control of cell proliferation and apoptosis. Mutant forms of *p53* have been detected in as many as 50% of all human tumor DNA samples analyzed. Inactivation of *p53* appears to facilitate unlimited proliferative potential and proliferation in the face of damage to their genomes. Often, tumor cells that have normal *p53* alleles respond to chemotherapy-induced DNA damage by entering into apoptosis; cells carrying mutant *p53* resist this response. A striking demonstration of the importance of tumor suppressor genes in the genesis of common human cancers is seen in families in which affected individuals have inherited one mutant *p53* allele from one parent and a normal allele from the other. Acquisition of a somatic mutation after birth in the previously normal *p53* allele is associated with the development of cancer in the tissue in which the cells have acquired this second mutation. This syndrome, known as the *Li-Fraumeni syndrome*, is a well-characterized condition in which members of affected families are at increased risk for breast cancer, leukemia, brain tumors, and sarcomas. The malignant tumors are characterized by homozygous deletion of *p53*.

DNA Repair Genes

Recently, the tumor suppressor gene category included a new class of genes: the DNA repair genes. This large family of genes is responsible for maintaining genomic integrity in the cell by repairing the DNA damage caused by such agents as irradiation and mutagenic chemicals. Though the effect of functionally inactivating DNA repair genes is somewhat indirect (i.e., the loss of their activities functions to increase the rate of mutations in genes related more directly to cancer, such as oncogenes and other tumor suppressor genes), they have been classified as tumor suppressors because a loss of their function significantly contributes to an increase in cancer. Recent examples of the loss of the DNA repair function acting as tumor suppressors come from investigations of colon and breast cancers. A form of hereditary human colon cancer (called *hereditary nonpolyposis colon cancer*) is associated with mutations in the DNA of one of the two alleles belonging to one of a number of mismatch repair genes, including *PMS1, PMS2, MLH1, MSH2,* and *MSH6.* Similarly, in familial breast cancer, a

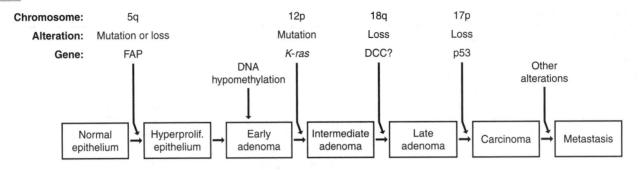

Figure 2.2   A genetic model for colorectal tumorigenesis. Tumorigenesis proceeds through a series of genetic alterations involving oncogenes (*ras*) and tumor suppressor genes (particularly those on chromosomes 5q, 17p, and 18q). The three stages of adenomas, in general, represent tumors of increasing size, dysplasia, and villous content. In patients with familial adenomatous polyposis, a mutation on chromosome 5q is inherited. This alteration may be responsible for the hyperproliferative (Hyperprolif.) epithelium present in such patients. In tumors arising in patients without polyposis, the same region also may be lost or mutated (or both) at a relatively early stage of tumorigenesis. Hypomethylation is present in very small adenomas in patients with or without polyposis, and this alteration may lead to aneuploidy, resulting in the loss of suppressor gene alleles. *Ras* gene mutation (usually *K-ras*) appears to occur in one cell of a preexisting small adenoma and, through clonal expansion, produces a larger and more dysplastic tumor. The chromosomes deleted most frequently include 5q, 17p, and 18q; the putative target of the loss event (i.e., the tumor suppressor gene) on each chromosome is indicated, as is the relative timing of the chromosome loss event. Usually, allelic deletions of chromosome 17p and 18q occur at a later stage of tumorigenesis than do deletions of chromosome 5q or *ras* gene mutations. However, the order of these changes is not invariant, and accumulation of these changes, rather than their order with respect to one another, seems most important. Tumors continue to progress once carcinomas have formed, and the accumulated loss of suppressor genes on additional chromosomes correlates with the ability of the carcinomas to metastasize and cause death. (Reprinted with permission from ER Fearon, B Vogelstein, A genetic model of colorectal tumorigenesis. *Cell* 61:759–767, 1990.)

mutation in one allele of the *BRCA1* or *BRCA2* gene is associated highly with a strong predisposition to human breast cancer. These genes have been associated with cellular response to DNA damage.

MULTISTAGE CARCINOGENESIS AND ASSOCIATED CLINICAL IMPLICATIONS

The investigation of transformed cells and their altered genotypes and phenotypes and the subsequent elucidation of the cellular mechanisms that they influence have generated a vast selection of possible biomarkers for early detection of cancer and have created future avenues for the design of new treatments. However, much important work remains in fitting the new information of cancer cell biology into the in vivo context of tissue biology. Within tissues, the multistage process of cancer initiation, promotion, and progression leads to the development of invasive primary tumors and the subsequent development of metastatic capacity. Also in this context, new, more effective diagnostic and therapeutic approaches to cancer will be developed.

One of the best-known examples of how cancer cell and molecular biology can be incorporated into the context of tissue biology is the pathogenesis of human colon cancer (Fig. 2.2). As shown, specific alterations in colon cell oncogenes and tumor suppressor genes are associated with specific stages in the stepwise development of cancer. Though the figure is neither a depiction of the only neoplastic pathway for colon cancer nor a complete list of somatic cell genes associated with colon cancer development, it does illustrate a new understanding of cancer cell biology. This knowledge is key to the design of molecular diagnostic tests capable of detecting cancer prior to its clinical appearance, of staging cancer, and of identifying important therapeutic targets for possibly arresting and reversing carcinogenesis.

A number of additional characteristics are important to understanding the development of a cancer. They include heterogeneity, tumor angiogenesis, and tumor-host interactions.

Tumor Cell Heterogeneity

Cancer arises through a multistep process estimated to involve from three to eight mutations. These changes result in a normal cell's evolution into a clinically identifiable malignant cell. The multistage model of cancer development is supported by morphologic observations of the multistage premalignant-to-malignant tumor transition and of experimental carcinogenesis involving the direct introduction of oncogenes into normal cells. In an important recent example of the latter, experiments by Hahn et al. [1] at the Whitehead Institute for Biomedical Research have demonstrated that several independent steps are needed to create a human tumor. These experiments showed that normal human cells could be transformed into cancer cells capable of tumor growth in immunologically defective nude mice when three genes were introduced into the normal cells. The artificially introduced genes were telomerase, to overcome telomerase shortening; the *ras* oncogene; and the *SV40* large T-cell antigen to inactivate tumor suppressor genes *p53* and *RB*. The simultaneous presence of all three genes was required for cell transformation.

Thus, though cancers may begin as monoclonal expansions of a cell with a single cancer-related mutation, subsequent mutations are required to drive the multistage development of cancer. This process gives rise to new clonal outgrowths. Frequently, this process of divergent subclonal evolution is associated with the appearance of increasing aneuploidy and new marker chromosomes in individual subclones. Also, the expression of specific cell-surface antigens frequently varies among the different subclones of a single tumor.

This developing tumor cell heterogeneity has clinical importance, because the emerging biological diversity creates cells that differ in such clinically relevant biological behavior as growth rate, metastatic potential, and susceptibility to chemotherapy. Hence, combination chemotherapy has been found usually to be more successful than is treatment with a single drug. Similarly, tumor cell heterogeneity might be expected also to explain the difficulty observed in therapy using a monoclonal antiidiotypic antibody to kill specific B-cell lymphomas; often, they exhibit a subsequent appearance of subpopulations of malignant lymphocytes that have an altered idiotype and escape killing by the antibody treatment.

Tumor Angiogenesis

The ability of a solid tumor to grow beyond a mass with a diameter of 1 to 2 mm depends on its ability to gain access to an increased supply of blood and to allow essential nutrients and metabolic waste exchange. This blood supply is provided by growth of new capillaries and larger vessels into the tumor mass from adjacent normal tissues; they are recruited by tumor-derived proteins termed *angiogenesis factors*. The production of tumor angiogenesis factors by malignant tumors permits continuous cycles of cell proliferation to further tumor growth.

Once malignant transformation has occurred, the clinical importance of the resulting cancer is determined not only by the proliferative ability of the primary tumor cells but by the propensity of these cells to invade adjacent tissues and to establish metastases. Increased contact with the circulatory system also provides tumor cells with an expanding portal through which they can enter the general circulation and colonize at distant sites in the body, forming metastases. Tumor invasion and metastasis has been correlated in some studies with tumor cell motility and the production by the malignant cells of tissue-destructive enzymes (e.g., collagenases, cathepsin B, and lysosomal hydrolases). These enzymes may permit tumor cells to destroy cell basement membranes and thereby directly to penetrate blood vessels and lymphatics. Only a small fraction of tumor cells entering the bloodstream actually lead to formation of metastases at distant sites. Numerous studies have demonstrated the presence of wide ranges of metastatic potential within a given population of tumor cells. This differential ability of tumor subclones to establish metastases represents yet another manifestation of tumor cell heterogeneity. The biological basis of this varying metastatic ability still is unclear, although experiments demonstrate that subclones having different metastatic potential may differ in both their oncogene biology and their expression of cell-surface membrane antigens.

A very active area of experimental antitumor therapy involves translating to the treatment of human cancers the research in animals that shows that such antiangiogenesis factors as angiostatin and endostatin can dramatically inhibit the growth and even reverse the size of primary tumors. The potential importance of such therapy is that it may be applicable to a wide variety of solid tumors, because the treatment focuses on blocking the general process of tumor angiogenesis rather than on destroying a heterogeneous population of tumor cells.

Tumor Cell–Host Interactions

Considerable evidence suggests that immune response plays an important role in regulating the development and growth of spontaneous tumors and their ability to metastasize. Support for this concept comes from documented instances of spontaneous tumor regressions, the dramatically increased incidence of cancer in immunodeficient or immunosuppressed patients, and a wealth of experimental evidence from studies in animal models. These observations have stimulated efforts to treat cancer with immunotherapy using such non-specific immunostimulatory substances as bacillus Calmette-Guérin and *Corynebacterium parvum*. However, these approaches have been unsuccessful, perhaps a not surprising outcome in view of the complexity of the immune response as it has been defined over the last several years.

An area of intense study involves the enumeration and characterization of the immunoeffector cells involved in the immune response to cancer. This inquiry includes investigations of the properties of cytotoxic T lymphocytes, macrophages, and natural killer and helper cells; the regulatory interaction of these cells; and the identity of the cell-surface structures recognized on cancer cells. Biological response modification, such as the stimulation of immune mechanisms against cancer, is an area of cancer therapeutics now under very active study.

The cloning of genes for such immunoregulatory substances as the interferons, the interleukins, and tumor necrosis factor has permitted studies of the biological effects of these substances. Often, tumor cells have been observed to fail to present at the cell surface the immunomodulatory proteins needed to facilitate antigen recognition by cells of the immune system. A dramatic demonstration of the importance of these molecules comes from several independently performed experiments showing that the introduction into a neoplastic cell of a gene that encodes a costimulatory immune molecule (i.e., B7) causes that cell to be recognized by the host animal's immune system. As a result, the host acquires the ability to reject the tumor. This observation has stimulated research into the possible therapeutic value of introducing costimulatory molecules into tumor cells and then using these cells as vaccines.

The use of monoclonal antibodies to characterize tumor cell-surface antigens has led to therapeutic trials using antibodies against cellular differentiation antigens. The first examples of such antibody-directed therapy in humans have used antibodies against B- and T-lymphocyte-related tumors in patients with refractory lymphocytic cancer. More highly targeted immunotherapy remains the goal of cancer immunologists. The availability of monoclonal antibodies with defined specificity, with in vitro cloned cytotoxic effector cell populations, and with purified immunoregulatory proteins produced by recombinant DNA techniques renders possible the testing of novel immunotherapeutic strategies.

NEW PARADIGMS AND FUTURE DIRECTIONS

Knowledge of the cellular and molecular basis of cancer has contributed to marked advances in the diagnosis and treatment of this disease. These advances, together with more successful and widespread use of more concentrated methods of early detection and treatment, have significantly improved the overall five-year US cancer survival rates. For example, the relative five-year survival rate among white Americans for all cancers between 1960 and 1963 (as compared to that between 1989 and 1994) is up significantly from 39% to 62% [2, 3].

The impact of a molecular understanding of cancer biology has been especially apparent in the diagnosis of lymphoid cancer. It has allowed the distinction between benign polyclonal and malignant monoclonal lymphoproliferations, for example, by characterizing these by cell type of origin. Defining the specific molecular alterations in solid tumors with regard to tumor lineage and subtype and predicting its likely biological behavior for use in diagnosis and prognosis also has begun.

Advances in understanding the molecular characteristics of cancer have led to a number of new strategies for cancer treatment that offer the advantages of being more specific in impeding the growth and development of cancer without general toxicity. Chimeric toxins that have been described contain part of the growth factor that binds to the cell receptor, which then is linked to a toxin molecule. When administered, this molecule gains entry to the cancer cell by binding to the normal receptor, with a single toxin molecule capable of killing a malignant cell. Another approach involves the use of the antisense molecules. These nucleic acids are complementary and therefore can bind to a messenger RNA (mRNA) sequence transcribed from a gene targeted for downregulation in the cell (e.g., a growth factor or growth factor receptor). By binding to this mRNA, the encoded gene cannot be translated into protein, and the cell will be damaged or killed by the loss of the specific gene's function. Some of these approaches already are being tested in clinical trials.

The increase in knowledge of cancer molecular biology also has caused a series of reconceptualizations of cancer, producing new paradigms to drive and direct future research and cancer control efforts. Medical science is on the threshold of entering a new era of knowledge that involves access to a complete description of the human genome. This will be provided by the human genome project and by the more focused cancer genome anatomy project. A primary result will be a new paradigm in which, for the first time, building a fully systematic approach to cancer investigations will be possible. Knowledge of the identity of all relevant components in the human genome and the ability to organize this information systematically with respect to biological systems, processes, and phenomena will permit an unprecedented level of rigor in scientific investigations. The promise of this new paradigm to cancer biology will be to provide an ability fully to interpret the effects of genetic changes that determine the nature of cancer. It will also allow the development of cancer interventions, including an understanding of all the complex networks and pathways associated with the pathways targeted for therapy.

A specific area of cancer biology likely to benefit from a full knowledge of the human genome will be the ability to move beyond the current limitations of familial genetic linkage studies in the investigation of cancer susceptibility genes. Normally, the genome of individuals other than identical twins has a genetic variability rate of approximately 1 different DNA base for every 900 DNA bases. A portion of this normal genetic variability is attributed to the polymorphic nature of many genes. The presence of different forms of polymorphic genes can play an important role in understanding an individual's capacity to respond to either exogenous or endogenous stimuli, because subtle differences in gene sequence can translate into important differences in biochemical function. For example, understanding which cigarette smokers actually will develop lung cancer likely will require a more intimate knowledge of individual differences in the polymorphic forms of various genes involved in the activation or detoxification metabolism of the chemical carcinogens in cigarette smoke. Ultimately, new knowledge based on the description of the human genome will permit the identification and classification of individuals with specific genetic dispositions into populations with defined cancer risks for different environmental exposures. Identification of highly susceptible populations by the more subtle characteristics of their individual genetic variability will provide key information for new public health policy and for clinical strategies in both treating and preventing cancer.

New areas of technologic development will be required also to translate into new treatments and interventions the expected flood of knowledge in cancer biology. New high-throughput approaches and techniques now constituting the field of combinatorial chemistry will be used. They will permit rapid screening of new varieties of synthetic molecules that selectively can mimic specific inhibitory and stimulatory properties of biological regulatory molecules found to be key control points in pathways regulating the development of cancer. A great increase in the volume of biological information will be generated by new molecular biology techniques that permit examining the expression of vast numbers of genes in a single assay (e.g., DNA chip array, mRNA differential displays, and protein fingerprint displays). The vast aggregations of new data that will be generated will require the field of informatics to provide new methods of computational analysis and communication of results that are not currently available.

REFERENCES

1. Hahn WC, Counter CM, Lundberg AS, et al. Creation of human tumour cells with defined genetic elements. *Nature* 400:464–468, 1999.
2. Landis SH, Taylor M, Bolden S, Wingo PA. Cancer statistics 1998. *CA Cancer J Clin* 48:6–30,1998.
3. Landis SH, Taylor M, Bolden S, Wingo PA. Cancer statistics 1999. *CA Cancer J Clin* 49:8–31, 1999.

SELECTED READINGS
Angiogenesis and Tumors

Fidler IJ, Kumar R, Bielenberg, DR, Ellis LM. Molecular determinants of angiogenesis in cancer metastasis. *Cancer J Sci Am* 4(suppl 1):S58–S66, 1998.

Kerbel, RS, Viloria-Petit A, Okada F, Rak J. Establishing a link between oncogenes and tumor angiogenesis. *Mol Med* 4:286–292, 1998.

McNamara DA, Harmey JH, Walsh TN, et al. Significance of angiogenesis in cancer therapy. *Br J Surg* 85:1044–1055, 1998

Rabbani SA, Metalloproteases and urokinase in angiogenesis and tumor progression. *In Vivo* 12:135–142, 1998.

Tobi M. Polyps as biomarkers for colorectal neoplasia. *Front Biosci* 15:D329–D338, 1999.

Winlaw DS. Angiogenesis in the pathobiology and treatment of vascular and malignant diseases. *Ann Thorac Surg* 64: 1204–1211, 1997.

Zetter BR. Angiogenesis and tumor metastasis. *Annu Rev Med* 49:407–424, 1998.

Apoptosis and Cancer

Albright CD, Liu R, Mar M, et al. Diet, apoptosis, and carcinogenesis. *Adv Exp Med Biol* 422:97–107, 1997.

Bold RJ, Termuhlen PM, McConkey DJ. Apoptosis, cancer and cancer therapy. *Surg Oncol* 6:133–142, 1997.

Ding HF, Fisher DE. Mechanisms of *p53*-mediated apoptosis. *Crit Rev Oncog* 9:83–98, 1998.

Glinsky GV. Apoptosis in metastatic cancer cells. *Crit Rev Oncol Hematol* 25:175–186, 1997.

Haq R, Zanke B. Inhibition of apoptotic signaling pathways in cancer cells as a mechanism of chemotherapy resistance. *Cancer Metastasis Rev* 17:233–239, 1998.

James SJ, Muskhelishvili L, Gaylor DW, et al. Upregulation of apoptosis with dietary restriction: implications for carcinogenesis and aging. *Environ Health Perspect* 106(suppl 1): 307–312, 1998.

LaCasse EC, Baird S, Korneluk RG, MacKenzie AE. The inhibitors of apoptosis (IAPs) and their emerging role in cancer. *Oncogene* 17:3247–3259, 1998.

Lyons SK, Clarke AR. Apoptosis and carcinogenesis. *Br Med Bull* 53:554–569, 1997.

Wyllie AH. Apoptosis and carcinogenesis. *Eur J Cell Biol* 73: 189–197, 1997.

Cancer Biology

Gonzalgo ML, Jones PA. Mutagenic and epigenetic effects of DNA methylation. *Mutat Res* 386:107–118, 1997.

Indulski JA, Lutz W. Molecular epidemiology: cancer risk assessment using biomarkers for detecting early health effects in individuals exposed to occupational and environmental carcinogens. *Rev Environ Health* 12:179–190, 1997.

Lee TC, Mukai S. Molecular events in tumor formation. *Int Ophthalmol Clin* 37:215–232, 1997.

Tsongalis GJ, Coleman WB. Molecular oncology: diagnostic and prognostic assessment of human cancers in the clinical laboratory. *Cancer Invest* 16:485–502, 1998.

Warren AJ, Shields PG. Molecular epidemiology: carcinogen-DNA adducts and genetic susceptibility. *Proc Soc Exp Biol Med* 216:172–180, 1997.

Chemoprevention and Cancer

Einspahr JG, Alberts DS, Gapstur SM, et al. Surrogate endpoint biomarkers as measures of colon cancer risk and their use in cancer chemoprevention trials. *Cancer Epidemiol Biomarkers Prev* 6:37–48, 1997.

El-Bayoumy K, Chung F, Richie J, et al. Dietary control of cancer. *Proc Soc Exp Biol Med* 216:211–223, 1997.

Rock CL. Nutritional factors in cancer prevention. *Hematol Oncol Clin North Am* 12:975–991, 1998.

Wattenberg LW. An overview of chemoprevention: current status and future prospects. *Proc Soc Exp Biol Med* 216: 133–141, 1997.

Oncogenes and Cancer

Beaupre DM, Kurzrock R. *Ras* and leukemia: from basic mechanisms to gene-directed therapy. *J Clin Oncol* 17: 1071–1079, 1999.

Buzard GS. Studies of oncogene activation and tumor sup-

pressor gene inactivation in normal and neoplastic rodent tissue. *Mutat Res* 365:43–58, 1996.

Cortner J, Vande Woude S, Vande Woude GF. Genes involved in oncogenesis. *Adv Vet* 40:51–102, 1997.

Dang CV, Lewis BC, Dolde C, et al. Oncogenes in tumor metabolism, tumorigenesis, and apoptosis. *J Bioenerg Biomembr* 29:345–354, 1997.

Goodrow TL. One decade of comparative molecular carcinogenesis. *Prog Clin Biol Res* 395:57–80, 1996.

Haber DA, Fearon ER. The promise of cancer genetics. *Lancet* 351(suppl 2):S111–S118, 1998.

Leong AS, Leong FJW. What we need to know about cancer genes. *Diagn Cytopathol* 18:33–40, 1998.

Rowley H. The molecular genetics of head and neck cancer. *J Laryngol Otol* 112:607–612, 1998.

Schwab M. Amplification of oncogenes in human cancer cells. *Bioessays* 20:473–479, 1998.

Tumor Invasion

Bryne M, Boysen M, Alfsen CG, et al. The invasive from of carcinomas. The most important area for tumour prognosis. *Anticancer Res* 18:4757–4764, 1998.

Noel A, Gilles C, Bajou K, et al. Emerging roles for proteinases in cancer. *Invasion Metastasis* 17:221–239, 1997.

Rabbani SA, Xing RH. Role of urokinase (uPA) and its receptor (uPAR) in invasion and metastasis of hormone-dependent malignancies. *Int J Oncol* 12:911–920, 1998.

Yan S, Sameni M, Sloane BF. Cathepsin B and human tumor progression. *Biol Chem* 379:113–123, 1998.

Tumor Metastasis

Woodhouse EC, Chuaqui RF, Liotta LA. General mechanisms of metastasis. *Cancer* 80(suppl 8):1529–1537, 1997.

Tumor Suppressors and Cancer

Ambs S, Hussain SP, Harris CC. Interactive effects of nitric oxide and the *p53* tumor suppressor gene in carcinogenesis and tumor progression. *FASEB J* 11:443–448, 1997.

Blackwood MA, Weber BL. *BRCA1* and *BRCA2:* from molecular genetics to clinical medicine. *J Clin Oncol* 16:1969–1977, 1998.

Dean M. Towards a unified model of tumor suppression: lessons learned from the human patched gene. *Biochim Biophys Acta* 1332:M43–M52, 1997.

Grander D. How do mutated oncogenes and tumor suppressor genes cause cancer? *Med Oncol* 15:20–26, 1998.

Ilyas M, Tomlinson IPM. The interactions of APC, E-cadherin and beta-catenin in tumour development and progression. *J Pathol* 182:128–137, 1997.

Palapattu GS, Bao S, Kumar TR, Matzuk MM. Transgenic mouse models for tumor suppressor genes. *Cancer Detect Prev* 22:75–86, 1998.

Semb H, Christofori G. The tumor-suppressor function of E-cadherin. *Am J Hum Genet* 63:1588–1593, 1998.

Steele RJC, Thompson PA, Lane DP. The p53 tumour suppressor gene. *Br J Surg* 85:1460–1467, 1998.

Weber BL. Update on breast cancer susceptibility genes. *Recent Results Cancer Res* 152:49–59, 1998.

Weisberg E, Sattler M, Ewaniuk DS, Salgia R. Role of focal adhesion proteins in signal transduction and oncogenesis. *Crit Rev Oncog* 8:343–358, 1997.

White RL. Tumor suppressing pathways. *Cell* 92:591–592, 1998.

Viruses and Cancer

Alani RM, Munger K. Human papillomaviruses and associated malignancies. *J Clin Oncol* 16:330–337, 1998.

Ambinder RF, Leman VM, Moore S, et al. Epstein-Barr virus and lymphoma. In Tallmean MS, Bordon LI (eds), *Diagnostic and Therapeutic Advances in Hematologic Malignances.* Boston: Kluwer Academic, 1999.

Buendia MA. Hepatitis B viruses and cancerogenesis. *Biomed Pharmacother* 52:34–43, 1998.

Campo MS. HPV and cancer: the story unfolds. *Trends Microbiol* 6:424–426, 1998.

Griffin BE, Xue S. Epstein-Barr virus infections and their association with human malignancies: some key questions. *Ann Med* 30:249–259, 1998.

Idilman R, De Maria N, Colantoni A, Van Thiel DH. Pathogenesis of hepatitis B- and C-induced hepatocellular carcinoma. *J Viral Hepat* 5:285–299, 1998.

Klein E. The complexity of the Epstein-Barr virus infection in humans. *Pathol Oncol Res* 4:3–7, 1998.

Knecht H, Berger C, Al-Homsi SA, et al. Epstein-Barr virus oncogenesis. *Crit Rev Oncol Hematol* 26:117–135, 1997.

Lyons SF, Liebowitz DN. The roles of human viruses in the pathogenesis of lymphoma. *Semin Oncol* 25:461–475, 1998.

McKaig RG, Baric RS, Olshan AF. Human papillomavirus and head and neck cancer: epidemiology and molecular biology. *Head Neck* 20:250–265, 1998.

Zur Hausen H. Yohei Ito Memorial Lecture: papillomaviruses in human cancers. *Leukemia* 13:1–5, 1999.

3

Cancer Etiology

∎ ∎ ∎

Clark W. Heath, Jr.
Elizabeth T. H. Fontham

OVERVIEW

The etiology of cancer can be viewed from two perspectives: its molecular origins within individual cells and its external causes in terms of personal and community risks. Either viewpoint is complex. Together, these perspectives form a multidimensional web of causation by which cancers arise from the interplay of causal events occurring in tandem over time.

Chapter 2 deals at length with the molecular and cellular nature of cancer biology. Those aspects of cancer etiology are, therefore, reviewed here only to the extent necessary for understanding the biological impact of host attributes and environmental exposures (what commonly are termed *nature* and *nurture* [1]). For the purposes of this chapter, environmental causes encompass the full spectrum of chemicals, radiation, infectious agents, and lifestyle factors, whereas host-related causes include not only heritable genetic events but immune mechanisms and endogenous hormones [2]. In this list of causal categories, the role of chance in relation to genetic mutations also should be included. Though the main focus here is on DNA damage arising from environmental exposures or transmitted by inheritance, DNA aberrations also can result from chance errors in the normal processes of cell division and repair.

Molecular Mechanisms

Fundamentally, cancer is a genetic disease resulting from mutations affecting genes that control normal cell function (proto-oncogenes and tumor suppressor genes) or from polymorphic gene activity governing enzyme systems that either activate or detoxify environmental carcinogens (phase I and phase II enzyme reactions). Therefore, carcinogenic mutations can arise in several different ways: genotoxic environmental exposures (e.g., chemicals, radiation), spontaneous DNA aberrations occurring during normal cell turnover, or inherited germline mutations, such as *BRCA1*.

Because cancers develop from initial mutations in a single cell, they are by nature monoclonal. The growth of clinically apparent cancer from that single mutated cell is a slow process, typically involving a latency of 20 to 30 years in adult-onset cancers. During that time, a succession of genetic and epigenetic events is required for cancer to develop [3]. The entire process involves two stages: *initiation*, the primary genetic mutation in a single cell, and *promotion*, those successive carcinogenic events that complete the neoplastic transformation of the initial mutated cell and facilitate its multiplication to form a diagnosable tumor. The later course of the cancer—its continued growth and, often, metastatic spread—represents a further stage called *progression*. In that phase, or in the later stages of promotion, new subclones commonly arise from the primary cell line as a result of continuing gene mutations. Often, those new mutations are marked by distinctive chromosomal changes (e.g., deletions, rearrangements, aneuploidy). Similar changes often are observed in primary cancer cell lines as well. A prime example is the Ph[1] chromosome (a 9/22 translocation) seen in most cases of chronic granulocytic leukemia. Such cytogenetic aberrations can provide clues regarding the chromosomal location of genes critical for carcinogenesis.

Criteria for Causation

Proving that a given molecular event or environmental exposure is an actual cause of cancer is not a simple matter. For causes in the realm of molecular or cellular metabolism (e.g., genetic changes, enzyme reactions), questions of causation can be approached experimentally. Limitations relate to the strength of observations, the reliability of available laboratory techniques, the ability of independent investigators to confirm the findings of others, and the extent to which observations ultimately fit with existing biological knowledge. For studies of human patients and epidemiologic research in human populations, areas in which ethical concerns greatly constrain experimental approaches, proof of causation rests mostly with careful interpretation of observational studies. Because bias and misleading or distorted data relationships are of constant concern, deciphering the causal implications of associations between putative risk factors and cancer occurrence often is difficult, especially when relative risk levels are low and observations are scanty.

In the face of such difficulties, much attention has been given over the last several decades to considerations that warrant particular attention in judging the causal implications of observed associations between risk factors and disease [4, 5]. The principal considerations are as follows:

1. Strength of the observed association
2. Consistency of the association in findings from various research studies
3. Presence of a biological gradient or dose-response relationship
4. Biological plausibility of the association in relation to existing scientific knowledge
5. Specificity of the association for particular discrete disease entities
6. Temporality of the association: confirmation that exposure precedes disease occurrence

Evidence that the association grows stronger as levels of exposure or dose rise is particularly important (dose-response), as is the extent to which the association makes biological sense and fits with existing scientific knowledge. Associations that are specific for particular diseases (as opposed to a wide range of loosely related disorders) also may be considered more likely to be causal, although for many associations between risk factors and chronic disease, this consideration is not met. (For example, tobacco use is associated causally not only with many different forms of cancer but with heart disease, chronic obstructive pulmonary disease, and other adverse health outcomes.) Lastly, in assessing causal associations, exposure to a putative causal agent clearly must be seen to precede disease occurrence, a judgment not always easily made in chronic disease settings in which latent periods can be long and uncertain.

In this context, a clear distinction must be drawn between truly causal associations and those risk and disease associations in which the factor under consideration is not itself causal but correlates closely with one that is. Both factors, in common epidemiologic parlance, are often termed *risk factors,* yet the distinction is most important. For example, age and socioeconomic status commonly are called *risk factors* for particular cancers, though neither is truly carcinogenic in its own right. Instead, both describe conditions in which cancer frequencies increase (with advancing age or lower socioeconomic class) as a reflection of accumulated carcinogenic exposures over time (in the case of age) or of increased opportunities for exposure or heightened dose (in poorer economic settings).

For much of what we know about environmental causes of cancer, especially chemical carcinogenesis, interpretation of epidemiologic data depends greatly on pertinent toxicologic research. In fact, most carcinogen risk assessments conducted by regulatory or science advisory agencies depend heavily on this dual source of information. Demonstration of carcinogenicity in animal models, of course, cannot be easily extrapolated to the human situation without considerable support from epidemiologic or clinical studies. Given those difficulties and the frequent need to extrapolate high-dose toxicologic data to low-dose human exposure settings, often the process of risk assessment must settle for tentative judgments regarding the human carcinogenicity of given chemical or physical risks (thus, such official designations as *possible* or *probable* human carcinogens).

In comparing chronic diseases, such as cancer, with acute diseases, such as bacterial or viral infections, drawing conclusions about causation, either in populations or in individual patients, clearly is considerably more difficult in the chronic disease setting. That is so for several reasons. First is the fact of long and variable latency in such chronic diseases as cancer. When disease appears within a few days or weeks after an acute toxic or infectious exposure, the task of linking cause to effect is considerably simpler than when the interval spans several years or even decades. Also, for most infectious diseases, existing laboratory methods identify specific causal agents in individual cases. At present, obviously this is not possible for cancers, although increased understanding of molecular mechanisms may permit more specific etiologic case diagnoses in the future. The low frequency of even the more common cancers at any one time contributes further to difficulties in exploring causation, especially in epidemiologic studies. The same can be said, of course, for uncertainties about the identification of environmental exposures to carcinogens, proving their occurrence, linking their exposure to at-risk populations, and assessing dose levels, especially when presumed exposures occurred in the remote past.

HOST FACTORS

Though considering cancer causation in terms of intrinsic and extrinsic factors (i.e., host and environment) is common, drawing the distinction is not always easy. Taken in their entirety, host risk factors may be considered conveniently within three major categories: inherited genes, hormones, and immunologic mechanisms. Each instance, however, allows ample opportunity for interplay with environmental forces. Therefore, frequent consideration must be given to the potential mutagenic effects of environmental chemicals and radia-

tion, or to the cellular impact of infectious agents and exogenous hormones, when host-oriented etiologic judgments are being formed.

Heredity

Cancer overall is not strongly heritable. For virtually all tumors, however, the incidence of same-site cancer, but not other cancers, is increased modestly (twofold to threefold) in close relatives of persons with cancer [2]. Hereditary cancer arises when carcinogenic mutations affect germ cells. Although rare, such oncogenes can raise the lifetime risk of cancer in affected persons to 80% or greater. Such a high risk renders heritable mutations of this sort among the strongest of all personal cancer causes, although their rarity makes their overall impact on total population cancer frequencies small. Still, the role of heritable risk in cancer etiology is of great importance because, in addition to dominant and recessive germ-cell mutations, numerous polymorphic genes play significant roles in the metabolism of environmental carcinogens and influence the occurrence of somatic mutations [6, 7].

More than 30 familial cancer syndromes have been documented, and the responsible genes have been identified [8]. The major classes of heritable genes affecting cancer risk are shown in Table 3.1. Future research well may expand this list. *Oncogenes* are included in the table, although this class of genes has not been found to underlie the inherited nature of familial cancer. They are critically important, however, in the fundamental processes of carcinogenesis, disrupting normal functions of cell metabolism and arising from proto-oncogenes that control those basic functions in most, if not all, species [9]. Oncogenes were initially discovered through studies of oncogenic RNA viruses in animals. During their life cycle within cells, such viruses form oncogenes from cellular proto-oncogenes.

The role of genetic factors in determining the risk of cancer long has been recognized through the heightened risk of skin cancers in persons of fair complexion. Such cancers represent the interaction of a person's genetic makeup with exposure to an environmental carcinogen, in this instance ultraviolet B (UVB) radiation. Family cancer syndromes now linked to inherited mutations in *tumor suppressor genes* were the first in which underlying gene defects were discovered. Initial work focused on familial retinoblastoma (the *RB1* gene), preceded in that instance by Knudsen's two-hit hypothesis, which postulated the need for two mutations in a cell before cancer could result [10]. In familial cases, the

Table 3.1 Genes Involved in Cancer Etiology

Category of Genes	Examples	Cancers Involved
Oncogenes (mutated proto-oncogenes)	*K-ras*	Adenocarcinoma (lung, pancreas, colon)
	myc	Small-cell lung cancer, Burkitt's tumor, other
	erb-B2	Breast, lung
	cyclin D1	Breast, lung, liver
	abl	All sites
	androgen receptor	Prostate
Tumor suppressor genes	*RB1*	Retinoblastoma, osteosarcoma
	WT1	Wilms' tumor
	APC	Familial adenomatous polyposis: colon
	p53	Li-Fraumeni syndrome: sarcoma, breast, brain, other
	BRCA1	Breast, ovary, colon, prostate
	BRCA2	Breast, pancreas (?)
	DCC	Colon
	p16	Melanoma, esophagus, pancreas, non-small-cell lung
DNA mismatch repair genes	*MLH1, MSH2* *PMS1, PMS2*	Hereditary nonpolyposis colon cancer: colon, rectum, endometrium, genitourinary tract, other gastrointestinal sites, ovary, pancreas, breast (?)
Genomic instability genes	*ATM*	Ataxia telangiectasia: leukemia, lymphoma, brain, ovary, stomach, breast (?)
	BLM	Bloom's syndrome: leukemia, lymphoma, skin, gastrointestinal tract
	FA-A, C	Fanconi's anemia: leukemia, liver, cervix, esophagus
Dominant transforming genes	*MEN1,* *MEN2A*	Multiple endocrine neoplasia
	MEN2B	Familial medullary thyroid cancer
Polymorphic carcinogen-metabolizing genes		Cytochrome P450s (CYP): phase I oxidative activation of genotoxic compounds to form DNA adducts
		Glutathione-S-transferases, *N*-acetyl transferases, UDP-glucuronosyltransferases, sulfotransferases, GSH-S-transferases, cyclooxygenases, epoxide hydrolases, NAD(P)H quinone reductases: phase II metabolic detoxification of carcinogens

first hit was visualized as affecting a germ cell (hence the heritable risk), whereas in the rarer instance of sporadic cases, a somatic cell was the site of both hits. Subsequent genetic studies in other clinical syndromes of familial cancer have identified other tumor suppressor gene mutations: the *APC* gene in familial adenomatous polyposis and the *p53* gene in the Li-Fraumeni syndrome. Discovery of the *BRCA1* and *BRCA2* genes in breast cancer families appears to account for the majority of such families [11, 12], although studies select for families with young-onset cases [13]. Only perhaps 7% of all breast cancer cases occur in multiple-case family settings.

Several other types of inherited gene mutations (see Table 3.1) have been linked to other familial cancer risk settings: DNA mismatch repair genes in the case of the familial colon cancer syndrome (hereditary nonpolyposis colon cancer or Lynch syndrome); genomic instability genes in ataxia telangiectasia, Bloom's syndrome, and Fanconi's anemia; and dominant transforming genes in multiple endocrine neoplasia and familial medullary thyroid cancer. Undoubtedly, further familial gene defects will be found as research continues. However, because such defects in heritable settings are rare, they are unlikely to account for more than a small portion of total cancer incidence. In contrast, polymorphic carcinogen-metabolizing genes well may prove to have considerable impact in shaping individual genetic cancer risks. By influencing enzyme systems that either activate environmental carcinogens (phase I) or detoxify them (phase II), such genes have the potential for determining a large portion of total cancer risk. Hence, a person at high risk for a particular carcinogen would show high phase I activity and low phase II activity for a relevant enzyme system, and a person at low risk would exhibit the reverse. Given the likelihood that most cancers result from environmental causes, the influence of such genetically determined processes of carcinogen metabolism well may be substantial.

Hormones

Endogenous hormones have received considerable research attention with respect to cancers of breast, ovary, and endometrium in women and those of prostate and testis in men [2]. No clear relationships have been seen for the male cancer sites, notably regarding serum levels of endogenous testosterone, although seemingly, androgen metabolism likely influences prostate cancer etiology [14]. Female cancer sites, however, demonstrate a clear etiologic role for endogenous estrogen (estradiol) in both breast and endometrial cancers and a probable role for gonadotropin in ovarian cancer. In breast cancer, much of the evidence relates to the well-known association of increased cancer risk with low parity, late age at first birth, early menarche, late menopause, and breast density, all conditions in which heightened exposure to endogenous estrogen may be expected [15, 16]. Those epidemiologic risk observations receive considerable support from animal experiments and from measurements of hormone levels in women. Findings regarding the possible influence of other hormones in breast cancer (prolactin, progesterone) have been largely inconclusive. In endometrial cancer, the etiologic role of estrogen is supported strongly by the fact that postmenopausal risk is increased greatly by estrogen replacement therapy in the absence of progesterone replacement. For ovarian cancer, estrogens do not appear to increase risk, although increased risk with nulliparity and decreased risk with oral contraceptive use [17] suggest a role for gonadotropin. It is well-known, of course, that the synthetic hormone diethylstilbestrol, once widely prescribed during pregnancy to prevent spontaneous abortion and premature birth, can cause clear-cell carcinoma of the vagina and cervix in women exposed in utero [18].

Immune Mechanisms

The occurrence of particular types of cancer under various conditions of immunologic impairment supports the general concept that normal mechanisms of immunosurveillance are important for control of carcinogenesis [2]. Evidence comes from a variety of sources, including such indirect evidence as the potential link between chronic mental depression and cancer, medi-

ated perhaps through impaired immunity [19]. Certain cancers, especially non-Hodgkin's lymphoma (NHL), occur with increased frequency in persons treated with immunosuppression for tissue transplantation or other medical reasons [20–22]. Less striking increases also occur for Kaposi's sarcoma and for cancers of skin, cervix, vulva, and anus. Similar excess incidence (again, NHL especially) is seen in certain rare hereditary syndromes characterized by immunodeficiency (e.g., Wiscott-Aldrich syndrome, ataxia telangiectasia). The acquired immunodeficiency syndrome (AIDS) is accompanied by this same spectrum of cancers (NHL, Kaposi's sarcoma, cancers of cervix, anus, etc.), and the frequency of NHL is increased in such immune-related disorders as rheumatoid arthritis and Sjögren's syndrome. Finally, certain illnesses characterized by excessive immunostimulation are accompanied by increased incidence of unusual lymphomas: Burkitt's tumor in children subject to intense malarial infection in Africa and New Guinea and jejunal B-cell lymphoma in young persons afflicted with immunoproliferative small-intestine disease in the Middle East (so-called Mediterranean lymphoma). The selective nature of cancer occurrence in these various disease conditions strongly suggests that immune mechanisms play an important etiologic role in cancers arising in cells related to the immune system itself and in cancers initiated by infectious agents.

ENVIRONMENTAL CAUSES

Estimates support that 75% or more of cancers are the result of environmental exposures. This conclusion arises from rate comparisons based on the recognition that site-specific cancer rates differ very widely from place to place in the world and that persons migrating from one country to another tend to develop rates similar to those in their new country [23]. Environmental exposures, of course, encompass all influences arising outside the host; therefore, they include the many carcinogenic exposures associated with personal lifestyle and behavior (e.g., diet, tobacco use) in addition to those arising in the general community and in workplace environments [2]. For some cancer sites, such as lung, larynx, and bladder, environmental factors clearly dominate the etiologic picture, whereas for others, such as breast, they seem unlikely to play a major role [24]. Because the actual carcinogenicity of environmental exposures depends on interactions between environmental agents and metabolic processes within the host, and because those processes involve cellular enzyme systems

Table 3.2 Proportions of Cancer Mortality Attributable to Different Categories of Environmental Causes: United States and Other Western Countries

Categories of Environmental Causes	Percentage of All Cancer Deaths	
	Most Reliable Estimate	Approximate Range of Variability in Estimates
Lifestyle exposures		
Constituents of diet	35	20–60
Use of tobacco	30	25–40
Patterns of reproduction	7	1–13
Consumption of alcohol	3	2–4
Community-based exposures		
Infectious agents	10 (?)	(?)
Workplace exposures	4	2–8
Natural physical exposures	3	2–4
Human-made pollution (air, water)	2	1–5
Medicines and medical procedures	1	0.5–3
Consumer products (food additives)	1	0.5–2

that, in turn, are under genetic control, all cancers can be argued to have a genetic origin, including the great majority in which environmental factors play a role.

Table 3.2 shows the relative contributions to cancer mortality of different sources of environmental carcinogens. Dietary habits and tobacco use are by far the most important sources, accounting for some 35% and 30%, respectively, of all cancer deaths in the United States [25]. These estimates are based on numerous epidemiologic studies, and their precision depends greatly on the ability of such studies to measure exposures accurately. Because such exposure measurement is particularly difficult in the case of dietary habits, the variability of diet risk estimates is substantial. Compared with lifestyle exposures, the total population cancer risks of non-lifestyle or community-based exposures are relatively small. Infectious agents, mostly oncogenic viruses, are likely to play the largest role, although their full impact is uncertain.

The risk percentages shown in Table 3.2 are not strictly additive, because many of the risks involved may overlap or interact. Also, in some categories, such as diet or food additives, exposures may involve substances that reduce cancer risks in addition to those that increase risk. Workplace or occupational exposures can, in many instances, represent large risks for the particular worker groups involved but quite small risks for the much larger general population. The overall risk estimate for occupational exposures contained in Table 3.2 is relatively small (4%) because its point of reference is the general population. The same can be said for medical exposures, for which therapeutic doses of radiation or certain chemotherapeutic agents can carry relatively high carcinogenic risk for individual patients but have no great impact on general population risks because of the limited number of such patients.

Chemicals

A wide variety of chemicals have carcinogenic potential [2]. For some, sufficient human and animal (toxicologic) evidence exists to establish carcinogenicity with certainty. For a larger number, however, evidence is incomplete, particularly with respect to human data. Inorganic arsenic is the only chemical to date in which human evidence is convincing but in which animal data are sparse [26]. Examples of chemicals or chemical mixtures for which further studies are needed include diesel exhaust fumes [27], various organic pesticides [28], and materials with estrogenic activity [29–31]. Because many new chemicals from human-made sources are introduced each year and, because the process of carcinogenicity testing is difficult, achieving a truly complete and current listing of actual chemical carcinogens is virtually impossible.

Classification systems in place at the US Environmental Protection Agency and the International Agency for Cancer Research group chemicals as *proved, probable,* and *possible* human carcinogens on the basis of the extent of available human and animal evidence. Table 3.3 lists chemicals in the proved category, together with the major cancer sites affected and the general exposure settings in which they have been observed.

Table 3.3 Proved Human Carcinogenic Chemicals (Excluding Pharmaceuticals)

Chemical	Exposure Settings	Major Cancer Sites
Arsenic	Air, water, workplace, diet	Liver, lung, skin
Asbestos	Air, workplace, water	Lung, pleura, gastrointestinal tract (?)
Benzene	Air, workplace, tobacco	Leukemia
Benzidine	Workplace	Bladder
Beryllium	Workplace	Lung
Cadmium	Workplace	Lung, prostate (?)
Chloroethers	Workplace	Lung
Chromium	Workplace, water	Lung
Mustard gas	Workplace	Lung, larynx, nasal cavity
Nickel	Workplace	Lung, nasal cavity
Vinyl chloride monomer	Workplace, air	Liver, brain (?), lung (?)
Radium	Workplace	Lung, bone
Radon	Workplace, air	Lung

The preponderance in Table 3.3 of proved carcinogens related to occupational exposures reflects the high exposure conditions under which human risks have occurred in workplace conditions in the past and, hence, the relative ease with which firm evidence of human carcinogenicity could be established. At the much-lower-exposure conditions generally seen in non-workplace settings (and today in most workplaces), establishing epidemiologic data confirming carcinogenicity is more difficult. Among probable carcinogens for which human data are strongly suggestive (if not convincing) are such airborne compounds as formaldehyde and 1,3-butadiene, such solvents as trichloroethylene, such pesticides as chlorophenoxy herbicides, and a wide variety of other chemicals (e.g., polychlorinated biphenyls, ethylene dibromide, 2,4,7,8-tetrachlorodibenzodioxin [TCDD or dioxin]).

Consideration of carcinogenic chemicals is complicated further by the fact that most exposures are to mixtures of compounds. Examples include (1) products of incomplete combustion, such as coke oven emissions and coal tar pitch (the carcinogenic substance responsible for the scrotal cancers in chimney sweeps described by Percival Pott in 1775); (2) the large number of carcinogens present in tobacco smoke (e.g., benzene, tars, such polycyclic aromatic hydrocarbons as benzo[a]pyrene, such aromatic amines as naphthylamine); and (3) the presence in chlorinated drinking water of potentially carcinogenic chemicals (albeit in low concentrations) arising from reactions between chlorine and organic residues (e.g., chloroform and various trihalomethanes). Also important are compounds that themselves may not be carcinogenic but that, after absorption, can give rise to carcinogens. Both nicotine in tobacco and nitrates in drinking water can be metabolized to form nitrosamines in the body.

Though chemicals in diet undoubtedly contribute greatly to overall cancer risk, their individual identification is difficult. Not only are the mixtures complex; by diverse mechanisms, the chemical constituents of food may influence carcinogenesis, including the likelihood that, in many instances, cancer development may be inhibited (anticarcinogens). Despite the constant concern that human-made additives or contaminants may present a major dietary cancer risk, such substances rarely are present in greater than trace amounts. Instead, the preponderance of dietary chemicals arise from natural sources, representing a wide range of biologically active compounds useful to plants and animals for protection against predators in natural settings.

Radiation

Ionizing radiation and the higher frequencies of ultraviolet (UV) light are the only forms of radiation known to cause cancer [2]. Only such high-frequency radiation has sufficient energy to damage tissue or, in the case of ionizing radiation, to disrupt molecular structure (i.e., ionize atoms by dislodging electrons) and hence cause cell mutations [32]. Although much research has focused on the possible ability of electromagnetic energy at lower frequencies (e.g., microwaves, radio waves, power frequency fields) to promote cancer, no firm associations have been made [33, 34].

Forms of ionizing radiation include cosmic rays, x-rays, gamma rays, and alpha and beta particles. Evidence of carcinogenicity comes from studies of medical exposures, workplace exposures, survivors of nuclear explosions, and various exposures to background terrestrial radiation, radon emissions [35], and nuclear fallout [36, 37]. Overall, ionizing radiation accounts for only approximately 4% to 5% of all human cancers. Although nearly all tissue sites can be affected, bone marrow, thyroid, and breast are the most sensitive. Varieties of cancer not clearly involved are prostate and cervix cancer, Hodgkin's disease, and chronic lymphocytic leukemia. Increased cancer frequencies have been seen at single-dose levels as low as 0.1 to 0.2 Sv in Japanese atom bomb survivors [38].

Total average exposure to ionizing radiation is estimated at approximately 3.6 mSv/yr. Most comes from natural sources: approximately 0.3 mSv each from the sun's cosmic rays and from the radioactive decay of terrestrial radionuclides; approximately 0.4 mSv from radionuclides within the human body (^{40}K in particular); and approximately 2 mSv from radon gases (lung dose mostly). Remaining sources consist of approximately 0.5 mSv from medical and dental radiation and approximately 0.1 mSv from nuclear fallout, nuclear power, and various consumer products.

Several uncertainties affect estimates of cancer risk from ionizing radiation. As direct measurement of low-dose risks (below approximately 0.1 Sv) are not feasible, estimates of such risks continue to be made using various extrapolation models. The most common approach uses a straight-line extrapolation to zero dose. This method well may exaggerate risks, as cellular repair of radiation damage may operate more effectively at lower doses. The effect of age on risk also must be considered, because younger persons may have greater sensitivities at given doses. A further uncertainty involves the effect of dose fractionation on eventual risks of cancer. Likely, a given dose received in a single exposure will be more carcinogenic than the same dose received in multiple exposures over time, given the greater opportunity for cell repair when exposures are intermittent.

Solar UV radiation contains three frequency ranges: UVA, UVB, and UVC. Though radiation at faster frequencies (UVC and much of UVB) is absorbed by the atmosphere's ozone layer, slower frequencies with longer wavelengths (UVA and a portion of UVB) reach the earth's surface. Only that UVB portion (and perhaps a small fraction of higher-frequency UVA) has sufficient energy to be carcinogenic, though only for skin and not for deeper organs [39]. The integrity of the ozone layer, therefore, is critical for controlling UVB exposure levels in particular and, hence, the occurrence of skin cancers. All forms of skin cancer are involved, melanoma as well as squamous and basal cell carcinomas. Incidence is higher in whites than in populations with greater melanin content in skin (blacks, Hispanics, Asians). Risk is particularly great in persons with blond complexions

and with certain hereditary conditions prone to radiation sensitivity (e.g., xeroderma pigmentosum). Cases are more common at warmer latitudes where solar radiation is more intense and in persons who work outdoors and who have frequent exposure to the sun. Persons whose sun exposure is heavy but intermittent or who have suffered severe sunburn in their youth may be at particular risk for melanoma.

Infectious Agents

The viral etiology of cancer has been studied since the early years of the twentieth century and now has been demonstrated clearly in many different species, including humans [2, 40]. Both DNA and RNA viruses are involved. After early discoveries regarding the viral causes of chicken leukosis, chicken sarcoma, and rabbit fibrosarcoma, attention focused on the RNA retrovirus origins of leukemia in mice and other species. From the mouse studies in particular came understanding of the reverse DNA transcriptase capacity of retroviruses, followed by the initial description of cellular oncogenes. Subsequent studies regarding similar RNA viruses in cats, cows, monkeys, and woodchucks and regarding the herpesvirus responsible for Marek's disease (lymphoma) in chickens have shown the importance of cellular immunity and long latency in the process of viral carcinogenicity. Such animal research has been important for understanding the biology of human viral oncogenesis.

Several viruses of different types are now known to cause human cancer or to play critical roles in human cancer development (Table 3.4). They include both RNA and DNA forms of virus, and they affect several different tissues and organs (lymphoid cells, liver, cervix uteri), although by no means the majority of cancer sites.

From time to time, various human herpesviruses (e.g., herpes simplex, cytomegalovirus) have been thought to be potentially oncogenic because of their capacity for latent cellular infection and apparent associations with particular cancers. To date, however, only Epstein-Barr virus (EBV), which infects B lymphocytes and is the causal agent for infectious mononucleosis, has been proved to be oncogenic. The cancer it causes—Burkitt's tumor—arises from B-lymphocytes but is extraordinarily rare outside of tropical Africa and New Guinea, where it is a common form of childhood cancer [41]. Disturbed cellular immune mechanisms resulting from hyperendemic malaria are postulated to play a major role in tumor development. The carcinogenic role of EBV infection is worldwide, however, recognized as causing naso-

Table 3.4 Viruses That Play a Role in the Etiology of Human Cancers

Virus Types	Specific Viruses	Cancers
DNA	Epstein-Barr herpesvirus (EBV)	Burkitt's tumor, Hodgkin's disease (?), nasopharyngeal cancer
	Human papillomavirus (HPV)	Cervix uteri carcinoma, anal carcinoma
	Hepatitis B virus (HBV)	Hepatocellular carcinoma
RNA	Hepatitis C virus (HCV)	Hepatocellular carcinoma
	Human T-cell leukemia virus type 1 (HTLV-1)	Adult T-cell leukemia
	Human immunodeficiency virus (HIV)	Kaposi's sarcoma, non-Hodgkin's lymphoma, cervix uteri carcinoma, anal carcinoma

pharyngeal carcinoma [42] and possibly some forms of lymphoma, including Hodgkin's disease [43].

Human papillomaviruses (HPVs), especially HPV types 16 and 18, are responsible for most cases of cervical cancer and hence are very important for total cancer incidence [44]. The same is true for the hepatitis viruses, given the high frequency of liver cancers in much of the world [45, 46]. Hepatocellular carcinoma develops when hepatitis B virus (HBV) infection is chronic. Such circumstances are not infrequent in developing countries in which perinatal infection often overwhelms the immature immune capacity of newborn infants. The great frequency of these two cancers (cervical and liver cancers) in many countries makes viral infection a truly major cause of cancer worldwide, substantially greater than the estimate of 10% (see Table 3.2) for Western countries. Both HPV and HBV are spread by sexual contact, and HBV (like the human immunodeficiency virus [HIV]) is spread through blood and blood products as well.

Adult T-cell leukemia, although a rare form of cancer, represents the only example to date of retrovirus oncogenicity in humans, with the possible exception of the several cancers associated with AIDS and HIV infection [47]. The malignancy is characterized by depressed cellular immunity and is seen largely in southern Japan [48] and in parts of the Caribbean, South America, West Africa, and the Pacific region. The origins of human T-cell leukemia virus type 1 (HTLV-1) are unclear, although its appears to be spread by sexual transmission and blood contact.

Although HIV is related closely to HTLV-1, it has not been shown clearly to cause cancers directly [49]. Instead, the increased occurrence of various tumors as part of the clinical complex of AIDS appears to be the result of HIV-induced cellular immunosuppression acting to facilitate infection by a variety of other oncogenic viruses [50]. For Kaposi's sarcoma, the cancer associated most closely with AIDS, the viral agent is not known, although growing evidence suggests herpesvirus activity [51–54]. The EBV virus is suspected in instances of NHL, and HPV is the likely agent for both cervical and anal cancers [44, 55].

Although viruses are the principal infectious agents involved in carcinogenesis, certain bacterial and parasitic infections also may play a role. Infection with *Helicobacter pylori* has been associated causally with a threefold to sixfold increased risk of gastric cancer [56]. *H. pylori* causes multifocal atrophic gastritis (a premalignant lesion), diffuse antral gastritis, and peptic ulcer disease. Although the exact mechanism of *H. pylori* carcinogenesis has not been established, the following mechanism may be involved: increased epithelial cell proliferation, impaired mucus secretion, and damaged foveolar cells; enhanced synthesis and delivery of carcinogens in situ, especially *N*-nitroso compounds, and inhibition of antioxidant activity in the stomach, especially *L*-ascorbic acid; and increased mutations resulting from the local inflammatory response to infection. Infection with the parasite *Schistosoma hematobium* has been linked causally to bladder cancer, and similar observations have been made with respect to liver cancers and other schistosomal illnesses. Infestation with the liver fluke *Opisthorchis viverrini* has been shown to cause hepatic cholangiocarcinoma.

LIFESTYLE ENVIRONMENT

As suggested, individual chemicals, genes, or physical agents do not by themselves provide a full picture of cancer causation. Single causes do not act alone. Instead, our experience with them occurs in settings in which many causal elements are present and interact. This condition is particularly true of the two most important areas of environmental cancer causation—tobacco use and dietary habits—each of which involves many different agents that can influence the process of carcinogenesis (see Table 3.2). For all categories of environmental risk, however, whether related to lifestyle or to community or workplace environments, epidemiologic research, our chief source of human evidence, regularly weighs the impact of selected risks against a wide array of competing or modifying variables [2].

Tobacco Use

Any mode of tobacco or tobacco smoke consumption—active smoking (cigarettes, cigars, pipes), passive inhalation of environmental tobacco smoke (ETS), and smokeless tobacco use (chewing tobacco, snuff)—carries risk of cancer. Continuous, active cigarette smoking, with inhalation of mainstream smoke, involves the greatest risk by far. For cancers of lung and larynx, wherein the risk is greatest, mortality rates are roughly 10 times greater for smokers than for nonsmokers (relative risk, 10.0) and can be as high as 30 times greater when cigarette consumption is especially heavy (two or more packs per day) [57, 58]. Increased cancer risk clearly is present for other sites but at lower levels. Such sites include the oropharynx, esophagus, pancreas, and bladder and include renal cell carcinoma and acute myelocytic leukemia. Suggestive (though not conclusive) evidence links active smoking with hepatocellular cancer, squamous cell carcinoma of the uterine cervix and, possibly, breast cancer [59, 60], whereas for other sites (prostate, colon and rectum, ovary, skin, lymphoid tissue, and central nervous system) no causal relationships are apparent. For one tissue site, uterine endometrium, risk is lower in smokers than in nonsmokers. The reason for this protective effect is not clear, but it may relate to the association of smoking with weight loss or with its apparent antiestrogen properties, obesity and estrogen sensitivity being associated with increased risk of endometrial cancer.

Because it usually does not involve regular inhalation of smoke, tobacco smoked by means other than cigarettes (cigars, pipes) is linked mostly to cancers of the mouth and nasopharynx and perhaps, to some extent, esophagus. The same is true for smokeless tobacco use, which most often gives rise to cancers at specific sites within the mouth where tobacco is habitually inserted or held. Snuff tobacco, being more finely ground, may have greater carcinogenic potential than do coarser chewing tobaccos.

Repeated epidemiologic studies have demonstrated a clear causal link between ETS and lung cancer, childhood respiratory disease, and (probably) cardiovascular disease [61, 62]. The increased cancer risk (approximately 20% or a relative risk of 1.2) is, of course, much weaker than for active smoking, as the inhaled smoke, a mixture of sidestream smoke and exhaled mainstream smoke, is greatly diluted. Epidemiologic evidence comes mainly from comparing lung cancer rates (mostly for women) in nonsmokers married to smokers to rates in nonsmokers married to nonsmokers.

Exposure to tobacco-related carcinogens is related closely to nicotine addiction. Because addiction almost always is acquired in adolescence or in early adulthood, and because nicotine addiction is not reversed easily, cancer risks reflect years of steady exposure. Latent periods of 20 or more years are usual between onset of addiction and cancer appearance. In some settings in which other carcinogen exposures are present, the lung cancer risk associated with cigarette smoking can be magnified in a multiplicative manner. This appears true for occupational exposures to asbestos fibers and ionizing radiation and (to some degree) for heavy alcohol use. Successful smoking cessation can reduce cancer risks 50% or more after 10 years, with diminished risk first appearing in perhaps 5 years. Risks appear to decline more steeply when cessation is achieved before age 50. Risk reductions for cardiovascular disease occur more promptly after cessation.

The exact carcinogenic roles of the many hazardous substances present in tobacco smoke are not entirely clear, although now considerable evidence suggests the many molecular mechanisms involved. The nicotine naturally contained in tobacco leaf is converted readily to oncogenic nitrosamines during curing of the leaf or by smoking. Tobacco smoke contains more than 40 carcinogenic chemicals (e.g., polycyclic aromatic hydrocarbons, aromatic amines, benzene, phenols, free radicals), many of which are genotoxic and thus can initiate the carcinogenic process by causing mutations in such genes as *p53* or *ras*. Others may promote cancer development by induction of genetically controlled enzyme systems capable of activating environmental carcinogens [63]. With efforts over time to reduce the tar and nicotine content of cigarette smoke and with the introduction of filter tips, patterns of smoking and the mix of carcinogens present in smoke have changed. Smaller tar particle size and deeper inhalation of smoke to satisfy nicotine craving appear to have resulted from these changes and may be responsible for an increasing frequency of adenocarcinomas arising deep within lung parenchyma.

Dietary Intake

The major role of diet and nutrition in influencing cancer risk is well established. As suggested in Table 3.2, approximately one-third of cancer mortality in developed countries may result from dietary causes. That estimate, however, is by no means as precise as the comparable estimate for mortality resulting from tobacco use, largely because of the complex composition of diet, the interrelated nature of its many constituents, and the difficulties involved in obtaining valid and precise measurements of specific dietary intakes for use in epidemiologic research [64]. Because the foods we eat contain both substances that can protect against cancer and substances with carcinogenic potential, evidence regarding the effects of diet on cancer frequency comes as much from observations regarding diet patterns associated with reduced risk as from observations regarding increased risk [2]. Table 3.5 illustrates the many components of diet that can influence susceptibility or resistance to carcinogenicity.

Of the various diet categories listed in Table 3.5, natural food substances (and perhaps chemicals formed in cooking and food preparation) account for the great majority of substances affecting cancer risk. Although synthetic contaminants and additives can contribute, they constitute only a tiny proportion of total diet bulk, when present at all. Given the vast number of substances present in diet and the potential for interaction among them, knowing the precise biological impact for any single substance is difficult. Most of our knowledge comes instead from epidemiologic studies using broader definitions of dietary subgroups or from toxicologic observations in which the effects of single dietary substances in animals are used to postulate effects in humans.

Table 3.5 Components of Diet with Carcinogenic or Anticarcinogenic Properties

Source and Nature	Examples
Natural food constituents	
Basic sources of energy	Carbohydrates, fats, proteins
Micronutrients	Vitamins, amino acids, minerals (e.g., beta-carotene, vitamin E, selenium)
Natural toxins	Hydrazines, urethane, psoralens, fungal metabolites (aflatoxins)
Other constituents	Fiber, alcohol, cholesterol
Synthetic or artificial constituents	
Industrial contaminants	Polychlorinated biphenyls (PCBs), cadmium, lead
Agricultural contaminants	Pesticides, growth hormones
Cooking, food processing	Heterocyclic amines, salt
Additives	Colors, flavors, preservatives, packaging

The earliest epidemiologic evidence came from population-wide comparisons in which site-specific cancer frequencies in different countries or particular population groups were correlated with local dietary or food consumption patterns. Such studies have given strong indications that high dietary content of saturated fat may be linked to high risk for various cancers, especially breast and colorectal cancers. Subsequent case-control and cohort studies, data based on individual-specific rather than population-wide dietary information, have failed to confirm such correlations in the case of breast cancer. For colorectal cancers, however, the association seems firm, supplemented by the additional finding of increased risk linked to increased consumption of red meat. Epidemiologic data also suggest links between fat intake and prostate and ovarian cancers, although not all findings are consistent [65, 66].

Regular consumption of alcohol (closely controlled for tobacco use) has been confirmed widely to increase cancer frequency at various organ sites: oral cavity, pharynx, esophagus, and liver in particular [67, 68]. Evidence is suggestive (but not yet convincing) with respect to cancers of colon and pancreas, whereas some (but not all) studies [69] report a modest increase in breast cancer risk associated with moderate alcohol intake [70–72]. The potential mechanism for the latter association is not clear, although for other alcohol-related cancers, direct contact between alcohol and tissue surfaces (e.g., mouth, esophagus) may facilitate carcinogenesis.

Considerable toxicologic and epidemiologic information suggests that total caloric energy intake, especially early in life, may increase cancer risks. Several human studies have reported that increased body height and weight, perhaps reflecting growth patterns in youth, is accompanied by increased risk of breast cancer in women [73]. Obesity is associated strongly with risk of endometrial and biliary cancers and is linked moderately with male colon cancer, renal cell cancer, postmenopausal breast cancer, and pancreatic cancer [74]. Other evidence of increased risk concerns specific chemical substances formed in food during cooking, notably heterocyclic amines during the broiling of meats. The extent of this potential risk has yet to be explored fully. In contrast, firm evidence demonstrates that preservation of foods by salting increases risk of gastric cancer. That risk has diminished greatly, however, in developed countries through the use of refrigeration and through increased availability of fruits and vegetables as dietary staples.

Reduction of cancer risks for most epithelial tumors, and especially colorectal cancer, has been demonstrated repeatedly in the presence of increased dietary intake of fresh fruits and vegetables. Evidence also suggests that phytoestrogens and other plant materials in the diet, such as tofu or soy products, may lead to reduced incidence of breast cancer [75, 76]. Although the exact nature of this dietary defense against cancer is not clear, suggested mechanisms focus on the chemical activity of various vitamins and minerals [77–79]. Fruit and vegetable sources of vitamin A and other micronutrients have been associated with lowered risks of lung and gastric cancers, but the evidence is not entirely consistent [80]. Because of its antioxidant properties, vitamin C has been studied widely, and reduced risks have been reported (though not always confirmed) for several cancer sites, including mouth, stomach, esophagus, and larynx. Similarly, vitamin E has been associated with lowered risks of lung and prostate cancers (though this has not been fully confirmed). Likewise, epidemiologic research concerning selenium has suggested reduced risk at particular cancer sites, especially prostate [81, 82] but also colon and breast. Though fiber in food has been postulated possibly to reduce colon cancer risk by speeding the transit time of exogenous carcinogens through the gastrointestinal tract, the evidence is not consistent [83].

Sexual and Reproductive Lifestyle

A prominent epidemiologic feature of uterine cervical cancer is its increasing frequency in relation to the number of sexual contacts. This lifestyle characteristic reflects the tumor's infectious viral etiology (HPV), and it holds true for each of the other various cancers related to infectious agents transmitted by sexual contact (HBV, HIV, HTLV-1) [2]. Because each of these latter viruses also are prone to transmission through intimate blood contact, sexual practices that facilitate such contact represent additional lifestyle risk factors.

Lifestyle patterns related to childbearing are well-known determinants of risk for female breast cancer [84]. The increased risk of breast cancer in single and nulliparous women first was noted in the mid–eighteenth century when Ramazzini in Italy remarked on its relative frequency in nuns. That risk pattern largely reflects the strong protective effect of an early full-term pregnancy, supplemented by some additional increased risk associated with a late first-term pregnancy and perhaps some protective influence from exceptionally high parity. Prolonged lactation also may have significant impact on breast cancer risk by delaying ovulatory cycles, thereby reducing cumulative estrogen exposure to breast tissue. Physical exercise well may

have a similar effect by delaying menarche, inducing anovular cycles, and reducing obesity (the latter being a significant risk factor for postmenopausal breast cancer) [85–87].

Finally, use of oral contraceptives represents a further aspect of reproductive lifestyle that may affect risk of cancer. Incidence of benign hepatoma is increased, as are perhaps risks of thyroid and cervix uteri cancer. Incidence of ovarian cancer, however, is decreased, whereas effects on breast cancer frequency appear to be minimal, limited perhaps to prolonged contraceptive use begun at an early age [88]. Risk of endometrial cancer, although increased by use of sequential oral contraceptives in years past, now is reduced in the presence of current combined formulations [89].

GENERAL ENVIRONMENT

Although well more than one-half of all environmental cancer risks arise from lifestyle sources, public concern long has focused more closely on exposures not primarily governed by lifestyle choices but determined mainly by place of residence and occupation. The reasons for this disproportionate emphasis are complex, but they have much to do with peoples' natural fear of what is unknown or unfamiliar to them and their sense of alarm and outrage concerning perceived hazards that are beyond their own control. Regarding exposure pathways and environmental concentrations that can result in high tissue dosage, concerns are well placed. Clearly, this reaction has been true of many workplace exposures in past years and, to some extent, remains true today. It also pertains to many forms of high-dose medical therapies. High-dose exposures, however, tend to focus on relatively small population groups (specific worker cohorts or patients receiving chemotherapy or radiotherapy), so their overall population impact is limited. Though the potential certainly exists for widespread high-dose residential exposures from pollution of air or water and, hence, major population impact—possibilities to which communities must always remain alert—actual exposure levels remain low in most developed countries. Less well understood is the added impact, if any, of low-dose exposures to complex mixtures of chemicals in the environment.

Occupational Exposures

Most of our early knowledge about occupational carcinogens comes from purely clinical observations, coupled

Table 3.6 Occupational Exposures and Cancer Sites for Which Carcinogenicity Is Clearly Established

Cancer	Carcinogen or Industrial Process
Bladder	Benzidine, 2-naphthylamine, 4-aminobiphenyl, dye manufacture
Bone	Mesothorium, radium
Hepatic angiosarcoma	Vinyl chloride monomer
Larynx	Mustard gas, sulfuric acid mist
Leukemia	Benzene
Lung	Arsenic, asbestos, beryllium, bis(chloromethyl)ether, cadmium, chromium, mustard gas, nickel, ionizing radiation, coal tar pitch, coal carbonization, painting, iron ore mining, foundry work
Nasal cavity	Nickel, mustard gas, radium, woodworking, shoe manufacture
Peritoneum, pleura	Asbestos
Skin	Arsenic, coal tar, mineral oils, ionizing and ultraviolet radiation

with information about personal workplace exposures [2]. Scrotal skin cancer in chimney sweeps, as recorded in 1775 by Sir Percival Potts, is the classic example of such an etiologic observation. Other instances include skin cancers in various occupations that involve contact with mineral oils (e.g., cutting oils) and lung cancers in miners and in occupations with exposure to such lung carcinogens as arsenic, asbestos, nickel, and chromium (Table 3.6). For occupational lung cancers, most conclusive clinical observations were made in the years prior to widespread cigarette smoking (approximately 1950 and before). Since then, definitive studies of potential workplace lung carcinogens have required more sophisticated epidemiologic analyses that control carefully for smoking histories, because tobacco use and occupational exposures often interact in a multiplicative fashion. Though astute clinical observations continue to be important in discovering occupational cancer hazards (witness the relationship of hepatic angiosarcomas to exposure to vinyl chloride monomer, first described in 1974), most work today relies on formal epidemiologic analyses coupled ideally with ongoing surveillance of workplace conditions [28, 90, 91]. Table 3.6 lists organ sites affected by occupational carcinogens and the principal chemical and physical agents or workplace processes for which carcinogenicity is fully established.

Proof of carcinogenicity, especially in the past, often has been possible mostly because of the existence of heavy exposure and high-dose conditions in many workplace settings. Also, it has been assisted greatly by industrial hygiene and worker assignment records

maintained by businesses and industries. Most workplace carcinogenicity studies, however, tend to be reactive, to be conducted only after health concerns have arisen among worker groups. Ideally, and perhaps increasingly in the future, such research should best grow from ongoing programs of occupational health surveillance and from advances in knowledge regarding particular human cancer risks under particular exposure conditions. One example of such research is a prospective study now under way in the United States regarding potential cancer risks related to pesticide exposures in agricultural work [92].

Health Care Exposures

Various uses of ionizing radiation and chemical medications in health care practice can contribute to carcinogenicity [2]. Although the cancer risks they pose can be substantial, they must of course be balanced against the underlying health risks involved in the diseases under treatment.

Much of our fundamental information about the cancer-producing potential of ionizing radiation comes directly from observations made in patients receiving high-dose radiotherapy for different health conditions [93]. In the past, many of these conditions were nonmalignant in nature: ankylosing spondylitis, thymic or tonsillar enlargement in childhood, ringworm dermatitis of the scalp, acute postpartum mastitis. Other evidence comes from increased risks of second cancers in cancer patients treated with x-ray therapy or radionuclides. Because such treatment often is given in combination with chemotherapeutic agents, deciphering specific risks resulting from specific treatment modalities often is difficult. Clearly, however, dosage levels at given tissue sites are critically important in determining risk, as well as site, of secondary cancer occurrence. In general, the radiation doses involved in the diagnostic uses of ionizing radiation are far below the levels at which excess cancer frequencies might be expected. Exceptions to this generalization include increased breast cancer frequency in women who in the past received repeated chest fluoroscopies when under care for tuberculosis [94] and a modest increase in childhood cancers after exposure to prenatal diagnostic irradiation.

Table 3.7 lists pharmaceutical medications that either clearly affect risk of cancer or have, to some extent, been suspected of having carcinogenic potential. Many different classes of drugs are involved, including cytotoxic compounds, immunosuppressants, antibacterials, analgesics, and sedatives. Not included are hormonal

Table 3.7 Medications with Potential for Human Carcinogenicity According to Certainty of Evidence

Evidence for Carcinogenicity	Medications
Sufficient	Azathioprine, busulfan, chloramphenicol, cyclophosphamide, cyclosporine, inorganic arsenic, melphalan, nitrogen mustard, phenacetin-containing analgesics, thiotepa
Probable	Adriamycin, chloramphenicol, cisplatin, epipodophyllotoxin, methoxsalen
Possible	Coal tar, calcium channel blockers, dacarbazine, diphenylhydantoin, iron dextran, isoniazid, methoxalen, metronidazole, phenazopyridine, phenobarbital, propylthiouracil, various diuretics
Decreased risk (protective)	Nonsteroidal antiinflammatory drugs (colorectal cancers)

drugs (discussed earlier). Evidence of carcinogenicity or of anticancer activity comes from both animal toxicologic investigations and human studies. For drugs in which cancer effects are established firmly, human data are generally consistent and well documented.

Determining the carcinogenicity of individual compounds often is a complex task in which the combined effects of cumulative dose, latency, and companion treatments require consideration. Where dose levels are relatively low, although exposure may be continuous, large numbers of patients need to be followed for health outcomes over long periods. Only in the instance of cancers arising after immunosuppressive therapy (e.g., azathioprine, cyclosporine) does it appear that latent periods may be short (often a matter of only months) [95]. NHLs and Kaposi's sarcomas are the most common cancers encountered in such settings, as opposed to the predominance of acute nonlymphocytic leukemias as the most common secondary cancers seen after cancer chemotherapy using various combinations of cytotoxic drugs (e.g., cyclophosphamide, chlorambucil, melphalan) [96–98]. In health care settings where such drugs are administered, some carcinogenic risk may exist also for nurses and other health care workers.

In some instances, on the other hand, use of medications may reduce rather than increase cancer risk. Chronic use of aspirin and other nonsteroidal antiinflammatory drugs now has been shown clearly to have such an effect with regard to colon cancers [99, 100] and perhaps to certain other organ sites as well [101]. Recent research regarding the antiestrogen drug tamoxifen suggests similar risk reductions in breast cancer occurrence [102].

Air, Water, and Soil Exposures

Though a wide variety of known cancer-causing agents can be conveyed in air, water, and soil, their concentrations are rarely at levels where any major impact on population cancer rates can be expected. Measuring such impact, however, is difficult. Concentrations can vary widely from place to place and time to time; quantitating individual or population exposure levels with any precision is difficult; and latent periods between exposure and cancer diagnosis are long and variable.

A possible carcinogenic role for air contaminants is suggested largely by differences in cancer rates between urban and rural environments, correlated to some degree with measured pollutant levels and supported somewhat by data suggesting increased risk for persons living near point sources of pollution [103–105]. In recent years, however, the historical aggregation of high lung cancer rates in urban areas of the United States has been replaced by elevated risks in the generally rural southeast. However exposure occurs, it seems unlikely to account for more than 0.1% to 0.2% of total cancer occurrence in the United States (approximately 2,000 cases per year), much of it perhaps related to airborne products of incomplete combustion. In other countries, of course, where regulations controlling air pollution may be lax, the population impact may be greater.

As with air, contamination of water can involve a wide range of pollutants, human-made or natural: organic compounds, inorganic solutes, particulate substances, radionuclides, and microbiological agents. Chlorinated organics resulting from water chlorination have been linked fairly consistently with modest increases in cancer risk, especially bladder cancer [106]. Inorganic arsenic in drinking water has been associated with the occurrence of skin, bladder, and lung cancers [26]. Nitrates from natural sources or traced to agricultural uses of nitrogen-containing fertilizers are metabolized to potentially carcinogenic nitroso compounds and have been associated with increased occurrence of gastric cancers. Other possible carcinogenic substances in water include asbestos fibers, chromium, and nickel.

Much of what may contaminate air and drinking water arises from substances contained in soil, either naturally or by way of industrial or agricultural pollution. In particular, various natural radionuclides, such as radon and its daughter elements, can contaminate indoor air or well-water from underground sources. Where uranium mining has occurred, mine tailings used in later home construction can pose potential cancer risks. Other human-made pollutants, such as dioxins, polychlorinated biphenyls, and various organic solvents, can represent possible sources of cancer risk when discarded in soil as a result of industrial accidents or in the course of improper waste disposal [29].

Unproved or Uncertain Risks

As indicated, the scientific identification of cancer causes is an exacting task. Often, differentiating true causes from noncausal associations is difficult, a difficulty especially common in public concerns about potential but unproved environmental hazards. In some situations, as in the case of water fluoridation [107] or of electrical and magnetic fields [33, 34], human, animal, and laboratory data linking exposures to cancer risk are either negative or weak and inconsistent. In others, such as residence near nuclear power plants [108] or consumption of very low-dose pesticide residues in food or water [109], potential exposures to known carcinogenic influences are below levels at which increased cancer risk might be expected. Whatever the setting, public concern can develop rapidly, despite the absence of any clear scientific evidence of true cancer risk. Similar concerns, equally severe, can arise in other situations as well: Witness recent controversies regarding suggested but unproved cancer risks related to induced abortion [110–112] and breast implants [113].

Finally, serious public concerns can arise also in the context of perceived cancer case "clusters" within small residential communities or particular workplaces in which the occurrence of several cases of cancer close in time can raise questions about suspected local carcinogenic exposures [114]. Frequently, such cancer clusters require serious and extensive public health attention, even though evidence of meaningful exposures may be doubtful and despite the fact that such small time-space case groupings are common reflections of random disease distribution. Our ability to conduct meaningful etiologic studies in settings of this sort is limited severely by the small number of cases involved, their long latencies, and the difficulties involved in identifying specific personal exposures retrospectively. Coupled to those restrictions is the likelihood that, whatever kind of investigation is undertaken, chance aggregation is the true cause of the case cluster under study. Though particular features of any given cluster may, in fact, suggest that it might be more than merely a chance event (and thus

demonstrate sound reasons for conducting some degree of scientific investigation), community residents, workplace employees, and health care professionals need to understand the severe limitations that will hamper any meaningful study, however well intentioned.

CONCLUSION

As our knowledge grows regarding the etiology of cancer, new opportunities may arise by which we can develop new or improved methods for its effective prevention or control (see Chapters 4, 5). Newly discovered cancer genes suggest selective screening approaches and possible new therapies. Enzyme systems that govern the metabolism and life cycle of cells or interact with environmental carcinogens lead to revised concepts of chemoprevention [115] or fresh approaches for controlling environmental exposures [116].

Though such research knowledge increases at a steady pace, its translation into effective programs of cancer control and prevention often is a slow and faltering process, depending less on the firmness of scientific evidence than on the readiness of society and its political will to take appropriate action. Tobacco control is the prime example of this difficulty: It is especially striking because not only has the scientific knowledge and the proof of causation needed for curbing tobacco use been at hand for more than 30 years, but tobacco use alone accounts for nearly one-third of all cancer cases in developed countries.

Though dietary factors probably are responsible for an even greater proportion of cases, translation of etiologic knowledge into preventive approaches is more difficult. The complexity of dietary ingredients, both carcinogens and anticarcinogens, and their probable interactive nature make difficult the prediction of the long-range effectiveness of particular dietary interventions.

For other environmental causes of cancer, regulatory controls in the United States have achieved a considerable degree of preventive control in terms of occupational exposures, medical uses of ionizing radiation and pharmaceuticals, and pollution of food, air, water, and soil. Such controls, of course, require constant updating and sufficient resources for their enforcement, tasks that are not always performed easily. All such measures are dose-dependent and are designed to reduce exposures to levels sufficiently low so that risks of cancer are virtually negligible.

At any time, though some aspects of cancer causation are established firmly, others are not. It is of great importance that this distinction be understood clearly and that preventive actions not be premature or inappropriate. Avoiding misguided preventive action is not easy, especially when incompletely informed public perceptions bring legal or political pressures to bear on the scientific process. Both the public and the scientific community must have a thorough understanding of the complexities involved in cancer causation and of the patience required in the process of identifying true causal factors.

References

1. Doll R. Nature and nurture: possibilities for cancer control. *Carcinogenesis* 17:177–184, 1996.
2. Schottenfeld D, Fraumeni JF Jr (eds). *Cancer Epidemiology and Prevention* (2nd ed). New York: Oxford University Press, 1996.
3. Pitot HC. The molecular biology of carcinogenesis. *Cancer* 72:962–970, 1993.
4. Hill AB. The environment and disease: association or causation? *Proc R Soc Med* 58:295–300, 1965.
5. Weed DL, Hursting SD. Biologic plausibility in causal inference: current method and practice. *Am J Epidemiol* 147:415–425, 1998.
6. Li FP. Phenotypes, genotypes, and interventions for hereditary cancers. *Cancer Epidemiol Biomarkers Prev* 4:579–582, 1995.
7. Hussain SP, Harris CC. Molecular epidemiology of human cancer: contribution of mutation spectra studies of tumor suppressor genes. *Cancer Res* 58:4023–4037, 1998.
8. Lindor NM, Greene MH. The concise handbook of family cancer syndromes. *J Natl Cancer Inst* 90:1039–1071, 1998.
9. Krontiris TG. Oncogenes. *N Engl J Med* 333:303–306, 1995.
10. Knudson AG Jr. Hereditary cancer, oncogenes, and anti-oncogenes. *Cancer Res* 45:1437–1443, 1985.
11. Struewing JP, Hartge P, Wacholder S, et al. The risk of cancer associated with specific mutations of *BRCA1* and *BRCA2* among Ashkenazi Jews. *N Engl J Med* 336:1401–1408, 1997.
12. Shattuck–Eidens D, Oliphant A, McClure M, et al. *BRCA1* sequence analysis in women at high risk for susceptibility mutations. *JAMA* 278:1242–1250, 1997.
13. Newman B, Mu H, Butler LM, et al. Frequency of breast cancer attributable to *BRCA1* in a population-based series of American women. *JAMA* 279:915–921, 1998.
14. Ross RK, Pike MC, Coetzee GA, et al. Androgen metabolism and prostate cancer: establishing a model of genetic susceptibility. *Cancer Res* 58:4497–4504, 1998.
15. Colditz GA. Relationship between estrogen levels, use of hormone replacement therapy, and breast cancer. *J Natl Cancer Inst* 90:814–823, 1998.
16. Boyd NF, Lockwood GA, Byng JW, et al. Mammographic densities and breast cancer risk. *Cancer Epidemiol Biomarkers Prev* 7:1133–1144, 1998.
17. Narod SA, Risch H, Moslehi R, et al. Oral contraceptives and the risk of hereditary ovarian cancer. *N Engl J Med* 339:424–428, 1998.
18. Hatch EE, Palmer JR, Titus-Ernstoff L, et al. Cancer risk in women exposed to diethylstilbestrol in utero. *JAMA* 280:630–634, 1998.
19. Penninx BWJH, Guralnik JM, Pahor M, et al. Chronically depressed mood and cancer risk in older persons. *J Natl Cancer Inst* 90:1888–1893, 1998.
20. Kinlen LJ. Incidence of cancer in rheumatoid arthritis and other disorders after immunosuppressive treatment. *Am J Med* 78(suppl 1A):44–49, 1985.
21. Curtis RE, Rowlings PA, Deeg HJ, et al. Solid cancers after bone marrow transplantations. *N Engl J Med* 336:897–904, 1997.
22. Dantal J, Hourmant M, Cantoravich D, et al. Effect of long-term immunosuppression in kidney-graft recipients on cancer incidence: randomized comparison of two cyclosporin regimens. *Lancet* 351:623–628, 1998.
23. Shimizu H, Mack TM, Ross RK, et al. Cancer of the gastrointestinal tract among Japanese and white immigrants in Los Angeles County. *J Natl Cancer Inst* 78:223–228, 1987.
24. Laden F, Hunter DJ. Environmental risk factors and female breast cancer. *Annu Rev Public Health* 19:101–123, 1998.
25. Doll R. The lessons of life: keynote address to the Nutrition and Cancer Conference. *Cancer Res* 52(suppl):2024–2029, 1992.
26. Smith AH, Goycolea M, Haque R, Biggs ML. Marked increase in bladder and lung cancer mortality in a region of northern Chile due to arsenic in drinking water. *Am J Epidemiol* 147:660–669, 1998.
27. Bhatia R, Lopipero P, Smith AH. Diesel exhaust exposure and lung cancer. *Epidemiology* 9:84–91, 1998.
28. Hooiveld M, Heederik DJJ, Kogevinas M, et al. Second follow-up of a Dutch cohort occupationally exposed to phenoxy herbicides, chlorophenols, and contaminants. *Am J Epidemiol* 147:891–901, 1998.
29. Hunter DJ, Hankinson SE, Laden F, et al. Plasma organochlorine levels and the risk of breast cancer. *N Engl J Med* 337:1253–1258, 1997.
30. Moysich KB, Ambrosone CB, Vena JE, et al. Environmental organochlorine exposure and postmenopausal breast cancer risk. *Cancer Epidemiol Biomarkers Prev* 7:181–188, 1998.
31. Hoyer AP, Grandjean P, Jorgensen T, et al. Organochlorine exposure and risk of breast cancer. *Lancet* 352:1816–1820, 1998.
32. Shore RE. Electromagnetic radiations and cancer: cause and prevention. *Cancer* 62:1747–1754, 1988.
33. Linet MS, Hatch EE, Kleinerman RA, et al. Residential exposure to magnetic fields and acute lymphoblastic leukemia in children. *N Engl J Med* 337:1–7, 1997.
34. Wartenberg D. Residential magnetic fields and childhood leukemia: a meta-analysis. *Am J Public Health* 88:1787–1794, 1998.
35. Lubin JH, Boice JD Jr. Lung cancer risk from residential radon: meta-analysis of eight epidemiologic studies. *J Natl Cancer Inst* 89:49–57, 1997.
36. Gilbert ES, Tarone R, Bouville A, Ron E. Thyroid cancer

rates and ^{131}I doses from Nevada atmospheric nuclear bomb tests. *J Natl Cancer Inst* 90:1654–1660, 1998.

37. Astakhova LN, Anspaugh LR, Beebe GW, et al. Chernobyl-related thyroid cancer in children of Belarus: a case-control study. *Radiat Res* 150:349–356, 1998.

38. Pierce DA, Shimizu Y, Preston DL, et al. Studies of the mortality of atomic bomb survivors. [Report 12, part 1: Cancer 1950–1990.] *Radiat Res* 146:1–27, 1996.

39. Council on Scientific Affairs. Harmful effects of ultraviolet radiation. *JAMA* 262:380 384, 1989.

40. Morris JDH, Eddleston ALWF, Crook T. Viral infection and cancer. *Lancet* 346:754 758, 1995.

41. de The G, The epidemiology of Burkitt's lymphoma: evidence for causal association with Epstein-Barr virus. *Epidemiol Rev* 1:32–54, 1979.

42. Zeng Y. Sero-epidemiological studies on nasopharyngeal carcinoma in China. *Adv Cancer Res* 44:121–138, 1985.

43. Sleckman BG, Mauch PM, Ambinder RF, et al. Epstein-Barr virus in Hodgkin's disease: correlation of risk factors and disease characteristics with molecular evidence of viral infection. *Cancer Epidemiol Biomarkers Prev* 7:1117–1121, 1998.

44. Ho GYF, Bierman R, Beardsley L, et al. Natural history of cervicovaginal papillomavirus infection in young women. *N Engl J Med* 338:423–428, 1998.

45. Lee WM. Hepatitis B virus infection. *N Engl J Med* 337:1733–1743, 1997.

46. Di Bisceglie AM. Hepatitis C. *Lancet* 351:351–355, 1998.

47. Sarma PS, Gruber J. Human T-cell lymphocytic viruses in human diseases. *J Natl Cancer Inst* 82:1100–1106, 1990.

48. Yamaguchi K. Human T-lymphotrophic virus type 1 in Japan. *Lancet* 343:213–216, 1994.

49. Schultz TF, Boshoff CH, Weiss RA. HIV infection and neoplasia. *Lancet* 348:587–591, 1996.

50. Selik RM, Rabkin CS. Cancer death rates associated with human immunodeficiency virus infection in the United States. *J Natl Cancer Inst* 90:1300–1302, 1998.

51. Gao S-J, Kingsley L, Hoover DR, et al. Seroconversion to antibodies against Kaposi's sarcoma–associated herpes-related latent nuclear antigens before the development of Kaposi's sarcoma. *N Engl J Med* 335:233–241, 1996.

52. Levy JA. Three new herpesviruses (HHV-6, -7, and -8). *Lancet* 349:558–562, 1997.

53. Regamey N, Tamm M, Wernli M, et al. Transmission of human herpesvirus 8 infection from renal-transplant donors to recipients. *N Engl J Med* 339:1358–1363, 1998.

54. Martin JN, Ganem DE, Osmond DH, et al. Sexual transmission and the natural history of human herpesvirus 8 infection. *N Engl J Med* 338:948–954, 1998.

55. Frisch M, Glimelius B, van den Brule AJC, et al. Sexually transmitted infection as a cause of anal cancer. *N Engl J Med* 337:1350–1358, 1997.

56. Correa P. *Helicobacter pylori* and the cell cycle. *J Natl Cancer Inst* 89:836–837, 1997.

57. Wynder EL. The past, present, and future of the prevention of lung cancer. *Cancer Epidemiol Biomarkers Prev* 7:735–748, 1998.

58. Doll R, Peto R, Wheatley K, et al. Mortality in relation to smoking: 40 years' observations of male British doctors. *Br Med J* 309:901–911, 1994.

59. Morabia A, Bernstein M, Heritier S, Khatchatrian N. Relation of breast cancer with passive and active exposure to tobacco smoke. *Am J Epidemiol* 143:918–928, 1996.

60. Lash TL, Aschengrau A. Active and passive cigarette smoking and the occurrence of breast cancer. *Am J Epidemiol* 149:5–12, 1999.

61. Fontham ETH, Correa P, Reynolds P, et al. Environmental tobacco smoke and lung cancer in non-smoking women: a multicenter study. *JAMA* 271:1752–1759, 1994.

62. Hackshaw AK, Law MR, Wald NJ. The accumulated evidence on lung cancer and environmental tobacco smoke. *Br Med J* 315:980–988, 1997.

63. Ishibe N, Hankinson SE, Colditz GA, et al. Cigarette smoking, cytochrome *P450 1A1* polymorphisms, and breast cancer risk in the Nurses' Health Study. *Cancer Res* 58:667–671, 1998.

64. Willett WC. Diet and health: what should we eat? *Science* 264:532–537, 1994.

65. Hebert JR, Hurley TG, Olendski BC, et al. Nutritional and socioeconomic factors in relation to prostate cancer mortality: a cross-national study. *J Natl Cancer Inst* 90:1637–1647, 1998.

66. Kushi LH, Mink PJ, Folsom AR, et al. Prospective study of diet and ovarian cancer. *Am J Epidemiol* 149:21–31, 1999.

67. Thun MJ, Peto R, Lopez AD, et al. Alcohol consumption and mortality among middle-aged and elderly U.S. adults. *N Engl J Med* 337:1705–1714, 1997.

68. Talamini R, La Vecchia C, Levi F, et al. Cancer of the oral cavity and pharynx in smokers who drink alcohol and in nondrinkers who smoke tobacco. *J Natl Cancer Inst* 90:1901–1903, 1998.

69. Zhang Y, Kreger BE, Dorgan JF, et al. Alcohol consumption and risk of breast cancer: the Framingham Study revisited. *Am J Epidemiol* 149:93–101, 1999.

70. Holmberg L, Baron JA, Byers T, et al. Alcohol intake and breast cancer risk: effect of exposure from 15 years of age. *Cancer Epidemiol Biomarkers Prev* 4:843–847, 1995.

71. Bowlin SJ, Leske MC, Varma A, et al. Breast cancer risk and alcohol consumption: results from a large case-control study. *Int J Epidemiol* 26:915–923, 1997.

72. Smith-Warner SA, Speigelman D, Yaun S-S, et al. Alcohol and breast cancer in women: a pooled analysis of cohort studies. *JAMA* 279:535–540, 1998.

73. Trentham-Dietz A, Newcomb PA, Storer BE, et al. Body size and risk of breast cancer. *Am J Epidemiol* 145:1011–1019, 1997.

74. Silverman DT, Swanson CA, Gridley G, et al. Dietary and nutritional factors and pancreatic cancer: a case-control study based on direct interviews. *J Natl Cancer Inst* 90:1710–1719, 1998.

75. Wu AH, Ziegler RG, Horn-Ross PL, et al. Tofu and risk of breast cancer in Asian-Americans. *Cancer Epidemiol Biomarkers Prev* 5:901–906, 1996.

76. Ingram D, Sanders K, Kolybaba M, Lopez D. Case-control study of phyto-oestrogens and breast cancer. *Lancet* 350:990–994, 1997.

77. Giovannucci E, Rimm EB, Wolk A, et al. Calcium and fructose intake in relation to risk of prostate cancer. *Cancer Res* 58:442–447, 1998.

78. Heinonen OP, Albanes D, Virtamo J, et al. Prostate can-

cer and supplementation with alpha-tocopherol and beta-carotene: incidence and mortality in a controlled trial. *J Natl Cancer Inst* 90:440–446, 1998.

79. Baron JA, Beach M, Mandel JS, et al. Calcium supplements for the prevention of colorectal adenomas. *N Engl J Med* 340:101–107, 1999.

80. Hennekens CH, Buring JE, Manson JE, et al. Lack of effect of long-term supplementation with beta carotene on the incidence of malignant neoplasms and cardiovascular disease. *N Engl J Med* 334:1145–1149, 1996.

81. Clark LC, Dalkin B, Krongrad A, et al. Decreased incidence of prostate cancer with selenium supplementation: results of a double-blind cancer prevention trial. *Br J Urol* 81:730–734, 1998.

82. Yoshizawa K, Willett WC, Morris SJ, et al. Study of prediagnostic selenium level in toenails and the risk of advanced prostate cancer. *J Natl Cancer Inst* 90:1219–1224, 1998.

83. Fuchs CS, Giovannucci EL, Colditz GA, et al. Dietary fiber and the risk of colorectal cancer and adenoma in women. *N Engl J Med* 340:169–176, 1999.

84. Kelsey JL, Gammon MD, John EM. Reproductive factors and breast cancer. *Epidemiol Rev* 15:36–47, 1993.

85. Mittendorf R, Longnecker MP, Newcomb PA, et al. Strenuous physical activity in young adulthood and risk of breast cancer (United States). *Cancer Causes Control* 6:347–353, 1995.

86. Thune I, Brenn T, Lund E, Gaard M. Physical activity and the risk of breast cancer. *N Engl J Med* 336:1269–1275, 1997.

87. Rockhill B, Willett WC, Hunter DJ, et al. Physical activity and breast cancer risk in a cohort of young women. *J Natl Cancer Inst* 90:1155–1160, 1998.

88. Collaborative Group on Hormonal Factors in Breast Cancer. Breast cancer and hormonal contraceptives: collaborative reanalysis of individual data on 53,297 women with breast cancer and 100,239 women without breast cancer from 54 epidemiological studies. *Lancet* 347:1713–1727, 1996.

89. Stanford JL, Brinton LA, Berman ML, et al. Oral contraceptives and endometrial cancer: do other risk factors modify the association? *Int J Cancer* 54:243–248, 1993.

90. Rinsky RA, Smith AB, Hornung R, et al. Benzene and leukemia: an epidemiologic risk assessment. *N Engl J Med* 316:1044–1050, 1987.

91. Stayner LT, Dankovic DA, Lemen RA. Occupational exposure to chrysotile asbestos and cancer risk: a review of the amphibole hypothesis. *Am J Public Health* 86:179–186, 1996.

92. Alavanja MRC, Sandler DP, McMaster SB, et al. The Agricultural Health Study. *Environ Health Perspect* 104:362–369, 1996.

93. Weiss HA, Darby SC, Doll R. Cancer mortality following x-ray treatment for ankylosing spondylitis. *Int J Cancer* 59:327–338, 1994.

94. Boice JD Jr, Preston D, Davis FG, et al. Frequent chest x-ray fluoroscopy and breast cancer incidence among tuberculosis patients in Massachusetts. *Radiat Res* 125:214–222, 1991.

95. Kripke ML. Immunoregulation of carcinogenesis: past, present, and future. *J Natl Cancer Inst* 80:722–727, 1988.

96. Boivin J-F, Hutchison GB, Zauber AG, et al. Incidence of second cancers in patients treated for Hodgkin's disease. *J Natl Cancer Inst* 87:732–741, 1995.

97. Smith MA, McCaffrey RP, Karp JE. The secondary leukemias: challenges and research directions. *J Natl Cancer Inst* 88:407–418, 1996.

98. Travis LB, Holowaty EJ, Bergfeldt K, et al. Risk of leukemia after platinum-based chemotherapy for ovarian cancer. *N Engl J Med* 340:351–357, 1999.

99. Thun MJ, Namboodiri MM, Heath CW Jr. Aspirin use and reduced risk of fatal colon cancer. *N Engl J Med* 325:1593–1596, 1991.

100. Berkel HJ, Holcombe RF, Middlebrooks M, Kannan K. Nonsteroidal antiinflammatory drugs and colorectal cancer. *Epidemiol Rev* 18:205–217, 1996.

101. Cramer DW, Harlow BL, Titus-Ernstoff L, et al. Over-the-counter analgesics and risk of ovarian cancer. *Lancet* 351:104–107, 1998.

102. Fisher B, Costantino JP, Wickerham L, et al. Tamoxifen for prevention of breast cancer: report of the National Surgical Adjuvant Breast and Bowel Project P-1 Study. *J Natl Cancer Inst* 90:1371–1388, 1998.

103. Archer VE. Air pollution and fatal lung disease in three Utah counties. *Arch Environ Health* 45:325–334, 1990.

104. Camus M, Siemiatycki J, Meek B. Nonoccupational exposure to chrysotile asbestos and the risk of lung cancer. *N Engl J Med* 338:1565–1571, 1998.

105. Landrigan PJ. Asbestos—still a carcinogen [editorial]. *N Engl J Med* 338:1618–1619, 1998.

106. Cantor KP, Lynch CF, Hildesheim ME, et al. Drinking water source and chlorination byproducts: I. Risk of bladder cancer. *Epidemiology* 9:21–28, 1998.

107. Chilvers C. Cancer mortality and fluoridation of water supplies in 35 US cities. *Int J Epidemiol* 12:397–404, 1983.

108. Jablon S, Hrubec Z, Boice JD Jr. Cancer in populations living near nuclear facilities. *JAMA* 265:1403–1408, 1991.

109. Ritter L. Report of a panel on the relationship between public exposure to pesticides and cancer. *Cancer* 80:2019–2033, 1997.

110. Daling JR, Brinton LA, Voigt LF, et al. Risk of breast cancer among white women following induced abortion. *Am J Epidemiol* 144:373–380, 1996.

111. Melbye M, Wohlfahrt J, Olsen JH, et al. Induced abortion and the risk of breast cancer. *N Engl J Med* 336:81–85, 1997.

112. Palmer JR, Rosenberg L, Rao RS, et al. Induced and spontaneous abortion in relation to risk of breast cancer (United States). *Cancer Causes Control* 8:841–849, 1997.

113. Brinton LA, Brown SL. Breast implants and cancer. *J Natl Cancer Inst* 89:1341–1349, 1997.

114. Heath CW Jr. Investigating causation in cancer clusters. *Radiat Environ Biophys* 35:133–136, 1996.

115. Lippman SM, Lee JJ, Sabichi AL. Cancer chemoprevention: progress and promise. *J Natl Cancer Inst* 90:1514–1528, 1998.

116. Perera FP. Molecular epidemiology: insights into cancer susceptibility, risk assessment, and prevention. *J Natl Cancer Inst* 88:496–509, 1996.

4

Cancer Prevention: Strategies for Practice

▪ ▪ ▪

Mary E. Costanza
Frederick P. Li
Leonard M. Finn
Marianne N. Prout
Patricia Marks
Dileep Bal

Cancer will develop in almost half of all persons now living in the United States; nearly one in four will die of the disease. Over the last 30 years, the number of cancer deaths has doubled, surpassed only by the number of deaths from cardiovascular disease. Cancer deaths now exceed 550,000 per year. This dramatic increase can be attributed to the increase in the size and average age of the population and to the rapid rise in the number of deaths from lung cancer. Excess deaths are also related to poverty, an important component of the susceptibility to developing cancer. For example, cancers of the lung, stomach, uterus, and cervix are more common among the poor.

Cancer is a preventable disease. Perhaps two-thirds of cancer deaths in the United States could be prevented by lifestyle changes. Two-thirds of all cancers can be linked to tobacco use, diet, obesity, and lack of exercise, all of which can be modified through action at both the individual and the societal level. This chapter summarizes ways in which physicians can help patients to reduce their risk for disease. In addition, it describes some of the public and professional resources available to aid physicians, nurses, and other health care professionals in this task.

EPIDEMIOLOGIC PROFILE: RISK FACTORS

At the cellular level, the development of cancer is a rare event. Of the many billions of cells in an organ, one cell may undergo transformation to a malignant state. Through clonal growth, that single transformed cell eventually may produce clinical disease. Carcinogenesis appears to be a multistep process that involves both initiating and promoting factors: An initiator transforms a normal cell into a malignant cell, whereas a promoter gives the transformed cell advantages that favor its growth. Carcinogenic influences may be of environ-

Table 4.1 Heritable Cancer Susceptibility Genes

Gene	Locus	Year Identified	Tumor Type	Gene Class
RB	13q	1986	Retinoblastoma and others	Suppressor
p53	17p	1990 (1986)	Sarcoma and others	Suppressor
NF1	17q	1990	Brain and others	Suppressor
WT1	11p	1990	Wilms' and others	Suppressor
APC	5q	1991	Colon and others	Suppressor
NF2	22q	1993	Brain and others	Suppressor
VHL	3p	1993	Renal and others	Suppressor
RET	10q	1993	Multiple endocrine neoplasia and others	Oncogene
MLH1	2p	1993–1994	Colon and others	Mismatch repair
MSH2	3p	1993–1994	Colon and others	Mismatch repair
MSH6	2p	1997	Colon and others	Mismatch repair
PMS1	2q; 7p	1994–1995	Colon and others	Mismatch repair
MTSI (p16)	9p	1994	Melanoma	Suppressor
BRCA1	17q	1994	Breast and others	Suppressor
BRCA2	13q	1995	Breast and others	Suppressor
PTC	9q	1996	Basal cell carcinoma	Suppressor
E-cadherin	16q	1998	Stomach	Suppressor

Source: Data adapted from DM Gertig, DJ Hunter, Genes and environment in the etiology of colorectal cancer. *Semin Cancer Biol* 8:285–298, 1998; A de la Chapelle, P Peltomaki, The genetics of hereditary common cancers. *Curr Opin Genet Dev* 8:298–303, 1998; and AG Knudson, Hereditary predisposition to cancer. *Ann NY Acad Sci* 833:58–67, 1997.

mental origin (non-host factors) or genetic origin (host factors). Prevention strategies focus on one or both of these. (It is worth noting that the epidemiologic–public health definition of *environmental* origin refers to all nongenetic factors, whereas the general public tends to view the term more specifically as referring to water and air pollution and the like. This difference in viewpoint sometimes produces an inaccurate perception of cancer etiology among lay people.) On the basis of analyses of variations in the incidence of cancer among communities and of changes in incidence over time or after the immigration of certain racial and ethnic groups, estimates project that up to 80% of cancers in the United States may be due in part to environmental factors, most of which are related to lifestyles.

Genetics

In the last decade, increasing numbers of inherited cancer susceptibility genes have been identified (Table 4.1). Although most of these genes are tumor suppressor genes, some are DNA mismatch repair genes, often also classified as tumor suppressor genes or oncogenes. The initial discoveries involved genes for rare cancers such as retinoblastoma and Wilms' tumor. More recently, several genes for hereditary nonpolyposis colon cancer were discovered, as were the *BRCA1* and *BRCA2* genes

for breast cancer. Data suggest that thousands of Americans carry a susceptibility gene for colon cancer and that these carriers have a greater than 50% lifetime probability of developing the disease. Likewise, other Americans carry a susceptibility gene for breast cancer. Of this total, approximately half have an inherited *BRCA1* mutation, and the remainder have other susceptibility genes. Women with a *BRCA1* mutation have a 50% to 80% lifetime probability of developing breast or ovarian cancers.

Environment

LIFESTYLE

Tobacco

Tobacco is a major cause of potentially preventable cancer deaths in the United States. The number of recorded deaths from lung cancer now approaches 200,000 per year. Yet, if no one in this country smoked, this figure would be only roughly 12,000. The risk for lung cancer increases with both the amount and the duration of smoking. Cessation of smoking gradually lowers this risk, but more than a decade must pass before the rate of lung cancer in ex-smokers approaches the low rate of this disease among nonsmokers. Mortality associated with lung cancer has risen sharply for several decades among men, and this disease has overtaken breast cancer as the leading cause of cancer deaths among American women. For both men and women, this increase in risk was preceded by substantial increases in tobacco use 20 years earlier. In addition to lung cancer, exposure to tobacco can cause cancer at other sites, including the oral cavity, larynx, pharynx, bladder, kidneys, esophagus, and (possibly) the pancreas, and substantially increases the risk for heart attack and stroke.

In an attempt to lower their risk for cancer and cardiovascular events, some cigarette smokers have switched to pipes and cigars. However, former cigarette smokers are much more likely to inhale than are other pipe and cigar smokers, so this switch may have little effect in reducing risk. Clearly, total cessation of smoking is the best advice. Ironically, this precaution has increased the popularity of chewing tobacco, particularly among young men who are influenced by seductive advertising that does not mention the risks of oral cancer posed by this form of tobacco use. Tobacco is carcinogenic, regardless of whether it is burned. The attributable risk of chewing tobacco use can be fairly striking: 90% in oral cancer and 65% in bladder cancer.

Alcohol

Excess consumption of alcohol is associated with cancers of the mouth, pharynx, larynx, and esophagus. Epidemiologic research suggests that approximately 5% of US cancer deaths are related to alcohol consumption. Alcoholism also can produce cirrhosis of the liver, which increases the risk for liver cancer. The relative harm associated with various alcoholic beverages and with pure alcohol is not well defined; possibly, additives and contaminants in these beverages are deleterious factors. Alcohol consumption is particularly harmful among cigarette smokers, because the two agents apparently act synergistically to increase the degree of cancer risk, particularly for cancers of the oral cavity, pharynx, and esophagus. Most reports have cited increased breast cancer incidence associated with daily consumption of one or more alcoholic beverages, but these findings are not universal.

Sunlight Exposure

The incidence of skin cancer is rising, with exposure to sunlight being the major factor in the development of such tumors. Until recently, the need to prevent skin cancer has not been given high priority, because most of such lesions can be cured by simple excision. However, the increasing incidence of melanoma is cause for concern. Sunburn during the teenage years is a major risk factor for melanoma. Tanning booths expose users to the same damaging light waves as those in natural sunlight, and although we still do not know the long-term effects of exposure to such rays, tanning booths should not be considered risk-free.

Diet and Obesity

Diet appears to play a role in the development of many cancers, particularly those of the digestive and reproductive organs. Although these cancers are potentially preventable, efforts at prevention have been hindered because our knowledge about specific carcinogenic factors is insufficient. Dietary carcinogens may exist within natural foodstuffs, may be produced as a result of cooking or improper storage, or may be generated through the activity of bile acids and intestinal flora. Moreover, inert dietary substances may influence bowel transit time and thus alter the duration of physical contact between gastrointestinal tract tissue and carcinogenic substances.

The evidence suggests that approximately one-third of the nearly 500,000 annual US cancer deaths are due to dietary factors. Another one-third are due to smoking. For those who do not smoke, diet and physical activity are the most modifiable determinants of cancer risk. Researchers have found extraordinarily consistent scientific evidence that the dietary intake of fruits and vegetables is related inversely to the risk of cancer at various sites. In terms of the abundance and consistency of data, the evidence supporting this diet-related reduction in cancer risk is second only to the evidence linking smoking with elevated cancer risk.

Much research is attempting to identify in plant foods the specific phytochemicals that lower the risk of cancer and to identify the mechanisms by which these substances work. Phytochemicals are substances found naturally in fruits, vegetables, and grains. Such substances as beta-carotene, lycopene, and isoflavones show powerful disease-fighting properties. Test results indicate that phytochemicals, vitamins, and minerals interact in various foods and act differently under various circumstances. More research and clinical trials with human subjects will be necessary to determine the effectiveness, safety, and dosage of these substances.

Few data are available regarding the effects of specific dietary changes on cancer risk. Recently, researchers became interested in the effects of dietary "anticarcinogens" that might serve to deactivate harmful substances. The relative importance of these and other dietary factors in cancer of the gastrointestinal tract and other sites is unknown. However, excess calories and consequent obesity appear to constitute risk factors for many gastrointestinal tract neoplasms.

Strong evidence from population studies indicates

Table 4.2 Occupational Exposures and Cancer

Associated Industry or Material	Carcinogen Involved	Site of Cancer
Asbestos	Asbestos	Lung
Brewing	Alcohol	Liver
Commercial fishing	Ultraviolet light	Skin
Demolition	Asbestos	Lung, pleura
Furniture manufacturing	Wood dusts	Nasal passages
Glue manufacturing	Benzene	Leukemia
Insulation	Asbestos	Lung, pleura
Ion-exchange resin production	Bischloro-methyl ether	Lung
Isopropyl alcohol manufacturing	Isopropyl alcohol	Nasal passages
Mineral oil	Polycyclic hydrocarbons	Lung, skin
Nickel refining	Nickel	Lung, nasal passages
Ore manufacturing	Chromium	Lung
Outdoor occupations	Ultraviolet light	Skin
Pesticides	Arsenic	Lung, skin
Petroleum production	Polycyclic hydrocarbons	Lung
Pigment manufacturing	Chromium	Lung
Rubber manufacturing	Aromatic amines	Bladder
Shipyards	Asbestos	Lung, skin
Smelting	Arsenic	Lung, skin
Uranium mining	Ionizing irradiation	Multiple sites
Varnish	Benzene	Leukemia
Vinyl chloride	Vinyl chloride	Liver

Note: Industry-related lung cancers are associated synergistically with tobacco use. Exposure to tobacco, alcohol, and certain dietary factors is far more important in the etiology of lung cancer than are any of the exposures listed in this table.
Source: Reprinted with permission from D Schottenfeld, JF Fraumeni (eds), *Cancer Epidemiology and Prevention* (2nd ed), New York: Oxford University Press, 1996.

that the incidence of breast, endometrial, colon, rectal, and prostate cancer is significantly higher among Asian individuals who have immigrated to the United States than it is in those who have remained in their native countries. Although many researchers believe that this increase is due to a profound increase in dietary fat consumption among immigrants, this hypothesis remains controversial. Epidemiologic studies suggest that high dietary fiber consumption may have a protective effect against cancer of the large bowel. In addition, foods rich in certain naturally occurring substances (vitamins A, C, and E and such trace elements as selenium) appear to be protective. Other studies have shown that certain population groups are at relatively low risk for cancer. Mormons and Seventh-Day Adventists, who are largely nonsmokers and teetotalers and, in the case of Seventh-Day Adventists, vegetarians, have substantially lower rates of cancer, primarily of the lungs and digestive tract, as compared with the general population.

Physical Activity

The lack of physical activity has been demonstrated consistently to be related to an increased incidence of colon cancer. The relationship includes recreational, oc- cupational, and total activity. Less consistent relationships have been found with breast and other cancers.

Occupational Exposures

Some human cancers are caused by occupational exposures to chemicals and irradiation (Table 4.2). Although estimates differ, some experts suggest that perhaps 20,000 cancer deaths annually may be attributed to occupational exposures. Of particular concern in recent years is asbestos, which can induce mesothelioma and lung cancer and may be involved also in colon cancer. Asbestos exposure may occur not only during the mining and manufacture of asbestos materials but from contact with such materials in the home, school, or workplace. Demolition or construction workers who rehabilitate old buildings also may be exposed unknowingly to this carcinogen. The risk for lung cancer is particularly high among asbestos workers who smoke (approximately 60 times greater than that among nonsmokers). Indeed, the risks for lung and bladder cancers are increased in most occupationally exposed individuals who also smoke.

National legislation now mandates that workers be informed when they are exposed to any known toxic agents in the workplace. Such information allows workers to avoid carcinogens, to exercise greater care, or to wear protective clothing when handling such substances. Concerned workers can obtain relevant information from their employers and can consult with a physician about the level of risk. Whether this public health measure eventually will reduce the risk of cancer is not yet clear.

Infectious Agents

Certain viruses have been implicated in a variety of human cancers. Follow-up studies of patients with chronic hepatitis B and/or C virus infections have shown that they are at a risk substantially higher than normal for primary liver cancer, one of the most common neoplasms in some parts of Asia and Africa. The Epstein-Barr virus is associated with nasopharyngeal carcinoma and Burkitt's lymphoma, particularly in immunodeficient individuals. Papillomaviruses have been studied extensively and, as a result, certain types have been implicated strongly in cervical cancer. The newest and one of the most dangerous infectious agents to emerge in this century is the human immunodeficiency virus, the likely cause of the acquired immunodeficiency syndrome. By late 1995, more than 500,000 cases of acquired immunodeficiency syndrome had been recorded in the United States. This syndrome may include Kaposi's sarcoma, lymphomas, and anorectal cancers. Another newly identified infectious agent implicated in stomach cancer development is *Helicobacter pylori,* which can be treated with antibiotics.

Pharmaceuticals and Other Forms of Medical Therapy

Medical treatments can have carcinogenic effects. Approximately 2,000 cancer cases per year may be due to prior irradiation exposure. In some instances, exposure consisted of therapy for cancer or other diseases. Postmenopausal estrogen therapy and antiestrogen (tamoxifen) therapy have been linked to the development of endometrial cancer; however, because estrogen-associated endometrial cancer carries a favorable prognosis, the drug has had a greater effect on the incidence of cancer than on mortality. Studies now indicate that low-dose progesterone reduces the incidence of uterine cancer associated with estrogen use. The risk for breast cancer may increase by as much as 40% with long-term estrogen therapy (i.e., longer than 15 years; note that a 40% increase might be the difference between cancer √tes of 10% and 14%). Daughters of women exposed to diethylstilbestrol during pregnancy are at greater risk for clear-cell adenocarcinoma of the vagina. Other drugs

with carcinogenic potential include alkylating agents (e.g., cyclophosphamide) that are associated with the development of acute nonlymphocytic leukemia. Chronic abuse of phenacetin increases the risk for cancers of the renal pelvis.

COMMUNITY EXPOSURES

Although such environmental factors as solid-waste contamination and air and water pollutants may be involved in cancer causation, definition of their precise role is not likely in the near future. Because our society is highly mobile, people often spend time in a variety of environments. The problem of identifying multiple exposures is compounded by the long latency period between the time of exposure to a carcinogen and the clinical manifestation of cancer. In addition, the impact of nonenvironmental cancer risk factors further obscures low-level environmental risks. The scientific basis for attributing a specific cancer in a specific individual to environmental exposure remains tenuous, even in areas where exposure to carcinogens has been documented and cancer incidence is unusually high. Nonetheless, physicians often are asked to assess environmental cancer risk in their communities; therefore, they should be aware of resources available to help them in this task (see Chapter 3).

PREVENTIVE STRATEGIES

To prevent cancer, health professionals can and should take an active role in teaching and counseling to raise public awareness about cancer risks and preventive measures. For example, people working in hazardous occupations could be counseled about the risks and can be encouraged to use safety equipment. Practicing physicians can help patients to eliminate carcinogenic exposures, especially through cessation of smoking. Other areas of intervention include counseling about alcohol use, physical activity, and dietary changes. Practitioners also can be a valuable source of information about cancer prevention clinical trials and can provide support for patients interested in participating in these critical investigations.

Tobacco-Related Cancers

Tobacco use causes at least 30% of all deaths from cancer. Children and adolescents are particularly important target groups for antismoking campaigns because people who start smoking at an early age have a cancer risk much greater than that of those who begin later in life. Teenage girls are the fastest-growing segment of the smoking population. Parents should be reminded that their smoking habits often are models for their children.

Communities may offer smoking cessation clinics staffed by volunteer, commercial, religious, or medical groups or by committed physicians, nurses, or other health professionals. By displaying antismoking materials and by forbidding tobacco use in their offices, physicians can contribute to the antismoking campaign. In the past, only half of all patients surveyed reported that their physicians advised them to stop smoking. Few formal behavior modification training programs were offered in medical schools, and most physicians thought they could do relatively little to aid patients who wanted to stop smoking. However, a critical reminder is that 74% of the patients who successfully quit smoking were advised by their physicians to stop.

APPROACHES TO SMOKING CESSATION

Most smoking cessation approaches employ three basic techniques: quitting outright, reducing tobacco use, and postponing the first cigarette of each day. Approximately 95% of the patients who successfully quit do so simply by going "cold turkey." Though some patients respond well to information and advice from a knowledgeable source, others may require additional support from their families or other people who are trying to quit smoking. Health professionals should assess a person's learning styles and behavioral histories to help in making this lifestyle change and other important health-related changes. The key to success is patient-centered counseling that tailors a particular program to an individual. If, for example, a medical history reveals that a patient is concerned about weight gain that occurred during previous attempts to quit smoking, referral to a weight-control program may improve the chance of success. Independent, goal-oriented patients may respond to the challenge and commitment of entering into a "no-smoking contract" with a health professional. Often, referral to a smoking-cessation program is an effective adjunct to physicians' counseling and also can be an effective alternative when physicians have advised patients to stop smoking but have not had time to counsel them about approaches for quitting.

Physicians' principal role in smoking cessation is to present data about the risks posed by smoking; these include an increase in cancer and in cardiovascular and respiratory disease. One educational technique involves asking patients what they know about the dangers of smoking and offering supplemental information. The next important step is to help patients decide to stop smoking and to establish a date and time to quit. Compliance is enhanced by an actual written contract to be signed by both physician and patient. An important aspect in planning a program is to note whether patients have tried to quit previously and to identify the optimal approach to stopping. Options include quitting cold turkey, tapering, postponing the first cigarette each day, or using tobacco substitutes (e.g., the nicotine patch, nicotine nasal spray, nicotine gum, nicotine inhaler). Sustained-release Bupropion may be used as an aid for smoking cessation and may be particularly helpful in smokers with significant negative mood during the cessation period or with a history of depression. In some cases, such techniques as hypnosis, aversion therapy, and acupuncture also are helpful. Most recently, cessation programs have become available on the Internet. Quitnet is one such Web-based counseling and support program.

A recent placebo-controlled study found that an 8-week treatment program involving the use of a 22-mg nicotine patch combined with physician intervention, nurse counseling, follow-up, and relapse prevention yielded a statistically significant improvement in smoking cessation rates among the treated participants. The most important factor in the successful cessation of smoking is total abstinence during the first 2 weeks. Clinicians should emphasize this fact to patients who are preparing to stop smoking. Counseling and support should be "front-loaded" (i.e., the help should be most intensive during the crucial first 2 weeks). Follow-up by phone or in the office should be performed during the second week to assess patients' smoking status. Patients who have remained abstinent should be congratulated on their success and should be encouraged to continue their efforts. For patients who have been unable to abstain completely but remain motivated, increased pharmacotherapy or enrollment in a formal smoking cessation program may be recommended. Patients who lack motivation may be asked to consider setting a new cessation date and completing appropriate activities to prepare for quitting.

ADDICTION AND DEPENDENCY

A critical factor is to take the time to help patients to understand why they began smoking and to identify reasons for their persistence in the behavior. By asking patients to answer the questions listed in Figure 4.1, physicians should be able to convince patients that nic-

1. Is it extremely difficult for you to refrain from smoking for a half-day? Yes ☐ No ☐

2. Do you have an intense, recurring craving for cigarettes? Yes ☐ No ☐

3. Do you feel a need to smoke a certain minimum number of cigarettes each day? Yes ☐ No ☐

4. Do you often find yourself smoking a cigarette and being unaware of when you lit it up? Yes ☐ No ☐

5. Do you link your smoking with other behavior, such as drinking coffee or talking on the telephone? Yes ☐ No ☐

6. Does it seem unlikely that you might unintentionally refrain from smoking for a whole day? Yes ☐ No ☐

7. Do you smoke more after having an argument with someone? Yes ☐ No ☐

8. Is smoking one of your greatest pleasures in life? Yes ☐ No ☐

9. Does the thought of never smoking make you feel unhappy? Yes ☐ No ☐

Figure 4.1 Questionnaire for assessing a patient's reasons for smoking and for convincing a patient of the addictive nature of nicotine.

otine is an addictive substance. Affirmative patient answers to all or most of these questions clearly demonstrates that smoking has become an addiction.

Health professionals should stress the role of habituation in smoking. Often, sharing a simple example with patients is useful. For example, many people smoke whenever they drink coffee. At first, such people may have had a cigarette with coffee because it was a convenient time (such as a coffee break) or because they drank coffee in a particular social situation in which others were smoking. With repetition, the association between drinking coffee and smoking became a habit. After a while, they wanted a cigarette whenever they had coffee, even if it was not a convenient time or an appropriate social setting. Other examples can be given: smoking while drinking a cocktail, talking on the telephone, writing reports, watching television, or relaxing.

Another aspect of this dependency is psychological. The most common example is the use of cigarette smoking to help to manage stress. Cigarettes may have become associated with relaxation because they were consumed at times of leisure during the habituation period. Over time, cigarettes became a crutch to help to relieve tension and to manage stress. In a similar fashion, cigarettes may be used as entertainment or as a defense against loneliness. Some people use cigarettes as stimulants and smoke when they are drowsy or need to increase productivity.

Frequently, patients feel ambivalent about stopping smoking; thus, an important factor is to acknowledge such feelings. Health professionals should stress that the desire to stop smoking and to avoid its health risks eventually will overpower the desire to continue smoking but that this reversal usually occurs only after a period of abstinence. Making a chart that lists both the reasons to quit and the forces at work to continue smoking can help patients to understand their ambivalence better.

WITHDRAWAL SYMPTOMS

Patients should be told about the possibility of withdrawal symptoms and how to cope with them. Advisers should emphasize the fact that no physical pain accompanies quitting and that the majority of withdrawal symptoms abate within 2 weeks. Common symptoms include craving, tension, lightheadedness, dizziness, coughing, and weight gain. Craving dissipates in minutes if ignored; when craving occurs, affected people should divert their attention with another activity, such as eating a carrot stick, making a telephone call, engaging in a relaxing exercise, or sucking on a cinnamon stick. Tension can be relieved by practicing a stress reduction technique (e.g., deep breathing) or increasing physical exercise. Coughing occurs as the lungs clean out accumulated secretions, so drinking extra glasses of water between meals can help to relieve this problem. Weight gain can be prevented by such tactics as eating carrot sticks or sucking on a cinnamon stick or artificially sweetened candy. While quitting, smokers should give themselves noncaloric rewards, such as going to a movie, engaging in physical activity, or selecting low-calorie snacks, especially vegetables.

COUNSELING

Because slips or relapses are common, counseling should include cautions about the temptation to resume smoking. Ex-smokers sometimes relapse during crises (e.g., death of a loved one, loss of a job) or as result of ordinary stress, fatigue, enticement by other smokers, or lowered resistance (e.g., during or after drinking alcohol). Therefore, patients should be encouraged to develop constructive coping mechanisms in place of smoking. Most successful quitters use relapses to plan more intelligent and effective strategies.

The American Cancer Society periodically conducts FreshStart group sessions to help people to stop smoking. Health professionals can refer their patients to such programs, or patients can contact the American Cancer Society Call Center at 1-800-ACS-2345.

Skin Cancer

Limiting exposure to sunlight (avoiding midday sun exposure, wearing a wide-brimmed hat, covering extremities during the brightest hours of the day, etc.) can help to prevent all types of skin cancer, including malignant melanoma. For people who have fair complexions, do not tan easily, and have suffered from sunburns at an early age, the risk is greatest. Everyone should use sunscreens and should avoid excessive exposure to the sun (see Chapter 24). Similar precautions should be taken by patients who have had skin cancer, by members of melanoma patients' families, and by people with dysplastic nevus syndrome, xeroderma pigmentosum, or nevoid basal cell carcinoma. Health professionals can play an important role in counseling patients.

Hepatoma

The hepatitis B and C viruses causes hepatitis in hundreds of thousands of people each year in North America alone. Some patients die of fulminant hepatitis, others develop chronic active hepatitis and cirrhosis. Some cirrhotic patients eventually develop hepatocellular cancer. A currently available vaccine can prevent hepatitis B and should be used in high-risk groups. Although a reduction in the incidence of hepatocellular cancer among vaccinated populations is expected, longer followup is needed before studies will be able to verify this hypothesis. Recent data from Taiwan have already detected a reduction in the incidence of hepatocellular carcinoma in vaccinated children. [1]

Chemoprevention

Chemoprevention of cancer is emerging as a clinical option and as an ongoing focus for clinical trials as the results of several large clinical trials of selected agents are published. *Chemoprevention* refers to the use of specific chemical agents to reverse or suppress either the processes of carcinogenesis or in situ cancer progression to invasive disease. Agents are selected for further evaluation on the basis of epidemiologic studies that have identified many factors that appear to increase or decrease the risk of developing specific cancers. As the mechanisms of carcinogenesis have been elucidated in the laboratory, agents with the capacity to enhance or inhibit specific mechanisms can be identified for clinical trials in humans. Chemoprevention agents are evaluated in an approach analogous to that taken in chemotherapy trials: Phase I, phase II, and phase III clinical trials are conducted to study dose-toxicity relationships, to assess the spectrum of antitumor activities, and to quantify the effects of promising drugs.

Chemoprevention trials differ both from other types of cancer prevention studies and from therapeutic studies in several important ways. Screening or risk factor modification studies may focus on either the individual or community, but chemoprevention trials are focused on individuals and are conducted through health care facilities. These constraints may result in difficulties in defining, reaching, and accruing participants, and the differences between the study participants and the general population must be kept in mind. The reference population denotes the general group to whom results should be applicable; the experimental population refers to the actual population among whom the trial is conducted; the study population is composed of the experimental population members who participate.

Chemoprevention trials are large, their size determined by the number of end points—usually cancers—needed for a statistically significant outcome to be ensured. Generally, such trials are restrictive, with strict enrollment criteria that reflect both substantive issues (the group of interest) and logistic issues (who is accessible, compliant, feasible for follow-up). In addition, participants reflect the characteristics of volunteers, of-

Table 4.3 Differences Between Cancer Prevention and Treatment Trials

Factors	Prevention Trials	Treatment Trials
Participants	Healthy volunteers	Patients
Disease end points	Multiple	Single
Morbidity, mortality	Low, increasing with time	High, decreasing with time
Interventions	Long-term	Short-term
Important late effects	Higher chance	Lower chance

ten introducing a "healthy volunteer" bias. Because noncompliance diminishes study power, selection for and maintenance and assessment of compliance are critical in long-term chemoprevention studies. Likewise, ascertaining outcomes is critical and requires both high follow-up rates and uniform methods; otherwise bias is introduced.

Chemoprevention trials are long and expensive. They incorporate all the dilemmas of therapeutic trials and raise additional ethical issues in dealing with healthy individuals. Because of the length of prevention trials, secular changes may occur in any of the outcomes or methods, in disease outcomes, assessment methods, and therapeutic options.

Primary-care practitioners must, therefore, become familiar with the strengths and the limitations of clinical trials of chemoprevention agents so as to assist their patients in making informed choices about participation in a chemoprevention trial or the initiation of therapy with a chemoprevention agent outside of the trial. Table 4.3 defines important differences between cancer prevention and treatment trials.

Several large-scale chemoprevention trials have been conducted in the United States. Table 4.4 updates the status of five large trials. Important variations in clinical chemoprevention trials may affect results; critical study decisions include design, inclusion and exclusion criteria for participants, recruitment and retention, and selection of outcomes. The use of factorial and more complex designs may result in stopping the testing of some of the agents. For example, in the Physicians' Health Study, aspirin was unblinded and recommended for prevention of cardiovascular events, whereas beta-carotene was continued for evaluation of effects on cancers. Selection of participants may be based on risk factors for cancer and risk factors for anticipated adverse effects; in the United States, Britain, and Italy, discordant results among three randomized studies of tamoxifen versus placebo to prevent breast cancer have been

attributed to variations in risk factors for breast cancer among the participants. The Breast Cancer Prevention Trial has published its results, noting a 49% decrease in risk of invasive breast cancer in the women who received tamoxifen as compared to placebo through 69 months of study. In contrast, the much smaller British and Italian studies reported no difference in their randomized controlled studies of tamoxifen versus placebo. Women in the British study were determined to be at higher risk for breast cancer, owing to the inclusion of a high number of women presumed to have BRCA1 or BRCA2. In both the British and Italian studies, hormonal therapy with estrogen or other agents was not precluded.

Recruitment can determine how applicable the results are to the general population. Failure to enroll sufficient numbers of minorities in the Breast Cancer Prevention Trial limited the knowledge of both beneficial and adverse effects in diverse populations. Failure to retain study participants can reduce markedly the statistical power of the study to demonstrate effects. Indeed, the failure to retain women in the European studies of tamoxifen has been cited to explain the discordant results.

Finally, rules for ending these studies may limit assessments of all outcomes and adverse effects. Large-scale prevention trials require external and expert monitoring of results so that adverse effects are identified quickly and statistically significant benefits are noted appropriately. Participation in prevention studies is conditional on ethical assessment of the results and prompt notification of participants about results that may affect their health. Such judgments about chronic disease end points always are difficult, especially when both beneficial and adverse effects are occurring.

Three of the studies listed in Table 4.4 had been unblinded earlier than initially planned. The Beta-Carotene and Retinol Efficacy Trial (CARET) trial was halted 21 months early because of an increase in lung cancer incidence and mortality in the intervention arm. The Physicians' Health Study stopped the aspirin component of the study and notified all participants that they should consider taking aspirin because of a 44% reduction of risk of myocardial infarction associated with taking 325 mg aspirin every other day. The subsequent analyses of cancer risks related to aspirin use are complex, as they incorporate data from both a randomized trial period and an observational period when participants chose whether to take aspirin.

Follow-up of all participants in the trials listed in Table 4.4 continues and is required to evaluate long-term changes in cancer rates. The results for these stud-

Table 4.4 Summary of Five Large US Chemoprevention Trials

Trial	Participants	Number	Intervention	End Points and Results
BCPT	High-risk women	13,388	Tamoxifen vs placebo	Breast cancer, 49%↓; bone fracture, 19%↓; cardiovascular disease, NC
CARET	US smokers and asbestos workers	18,314	Beta-carotene, retinyl palmitate	Lung cancer (incidence, 28%↑; mortality, 17%↑)
Physicians' Health Study	Male physicians	22,000	Aspirin, beta-carotene	Myocardial infarction, 44%↓; cancers, NC
PCPT	Men ages 55	18,000	Finasteride	Prostate cancer
Women's Health Initiative	Women ages 50–79	64,500	Two arms: hormone replacement therapy vs placebo; dietary modification (low-fat vs usual)	Breast cancer, colorectal cancer, cardiovascular disease, bone fractures

BCPT = Breast Cancer Prevention Trial; NC = no change; CARET = Beta-Carotene and Retinol Efficacy Trial; PCPT = Prostate Cancer Prevention Trial.

Source: Data adapted from B Fisher, JP Constantion, DL Wickerham, et al., Tamoxifen for prevention of breast cancer: report of the National Surgical Adjuvant Breast and Bowel Project P-l study. *J Natl Cancer Inst* 90:1371–1388, 1998; TJ Powles, R Eeles, S Ashley, et al., Interim analysis of the incidence of breast cancer in the Royal Marsden Hospital tamoxifen randomised chemoprevention trial. *Lancet* 352:98–101, 1998; U Veronesi, P Maisonneuve, A Costa, et al., Prevention of breast cancer with tamoxifen: preliminary findings from the Italian randomized trial among hysterectomized women. *Lancet* 352:93–97, 1998; GS Omenn, GE Goodman, MD Thornquist, et al., Risk factors for lung cancer and for intervention effects in CARET, the Beta-Carotene and Retinol Efficacy Trial. *J Natl Cancer Inst* 88:1550–1559, 1996; and T Sturmer, RJ Glynn, IM Lee, et al., Aspirin use and colorectal cancer: post-trial follow-up data from the Physicians' Health Study. *Ann Intern Med* 128:713–720, 1998.

ies will require many updates, not only of the cancer and cardiovascular outcomes but of long-term potential adverse effects of the drugs. The high cost of these trials is believed to be justified because of the potential to improve the health and longevity of many adults. New trials certainly merit serious attention and support by primary-care clinicians and their patients, because the partial answers available today require confirmation and elaboration and because new agents designed to retain effectiveness while minimizing adverse effects are being readied for clinical studies.

Dietary Considerations

In 1982, the US National Academy of Sciences' landmark report, "Diet, Nutrition and Cancer," was the first multidisciplinary, scientifically based report to suggest dietary recommendations to reduce the risk of cancer. Since then, the American Cancer Society, the US National Cancer Institute, the American Institute for Cancer Research, and many other national and international organizations have continued to review the research and make recommendations for public policy and personal dietary modifications.

The American Cancer Society's 1996 nutrition guidelines advise the public about dietary practices to reduce cancer risk (Table 4.5). These broad guidelines, intended to apply to persons of age 2 and older, are a useful tool to promote understanding among health professionals and to help them make appropriate recommendations to the public. These guidelines are consistent with the recommendations of other agencies promoting health and prevention of other diseases (e.g., the 1992 US Department of Agriculture Food Pyramid). The pyramid uses the concept of "building from the bottom" to show the relative proportions and numbers of servings of the various food groups in the recommended diet. For example, people should consume three to five servings of vegetables and two to four servings of fruit per day; this recommendation is consistent with the National Cancer Institute's recommendation that people consume a total of at last five servings of fruits and vegetables daily.

The American Institute for Cancer Research and the World Cancer Research Fund have reviewed diet and cancer findings from more than 4,500 studies. Their 1997 report was the first analysis of food and cancer prevention from a global perspective. It focuses on foods and whole diets rather than on compounds within foods. Of the 202 studies of the association between vegetables and fruit and cancer examined by a panel of the American Institute for Cancer Research, 78% show those foods to be cancer-preventive. The recommenda-

Table 4.5 American Cancer Society Guidelines on Diet, Nutrition, and Cancer Prevention

---

Choose most of the foods you eat from plant sources.
  Eat five or more servings of fruits and vegetables each day.
  Eat other foods from plant sources, such as breads, cereals, grain products, rice, pasta, or beans several times each day.

Limit your intake of high-fat foods, particularly from animal sources.
  Chose foods low in fat.
  Limit consumption of meats, especially high-fat meats.

Be physically active: achieve and maintain a healthy weight.
  Be at least moderately active for 30 min or more on most days of the week.
  Stay within your healthy weight range.

Limit consumption of alcoholic beverages if you drink at all.

Source: Reprinted with permission from the American Cancer Society 1996 Advisory Committee on Diet, Nutrition and Cancer Prevention. Guidelines on diet, nutrition and cancer prevention: reducing the risk of cancer with healthy food choices and physical activity. *Cancer* 46:325, 1996.

tions are similar to those of the American Cancer Society but add specifics about salt, food preparation, and storage. The most important message is that cancer often is a preventable disease.

Thus far, our limited knowledge about the nature of phytochemicals and how they work prevents prescribing particular foods or supplements. A number of dietary constituents have been proposed as being responsible for reducing cancer risk, including antioxidants, fiber, folic acid, and other nutritive and nonnutritive factors. Although specific agents and their mechanisms of action have not been determined, the compelling evidence of reduced cancer risk warrants appropriate action by the health care community. Primary-care providers should support public education about the role of diet in preventing cancer and should counsel their patients about dietary approaches for reducing cancer risk. The best advice to give patients is to eat a predominantly plant-based diet rich in vegetables (particularly legumes), fruits, and whole grains.

Physical Activity

Increasing physical activity can have important effects on decreasing the risk of developing colon cancer. Studies demonstrate that individuals with the highest activity levels have the lowest incidence of colon cancer. An added benefit of physical activity is weight reduction, also associated independently with a lower incidence of some cancers, including that of the colon, breast, and prostate.

Identifying High-Risk Patients for Prevention

Cancer risk factors tend to be site-specific (i.e., chemical carcinogens produce their effects in specific vulnerable sites). For example, irradiation-induced cancers develop only in exposed tissues. Cancer genes predispose a person to one type or several types of cancers rather than to cancers in general. Thus, the identification of risk factors serves as a guide to those organs and tissues likely to be affected. One important purpose of identifying such high-risk persons is to provide them with the opportunity to prevent the clinical development of cancer.

CARCINOGENS

In some cases, risk for cancer can be identified during a routine recording of medical history by questioning patients about their personal habits, particularly their use of tobacco and alcohol. Information about prior illnesses and treatments may reveal whether such patients have been exposed to potentially carcinogenic medications and irradiation treatments. An occupational history of exposure to carcinogens, particularly asbestos, is associated with a high risk for lung cancer and mesothelioma. Obesity, nulliparity, and infertility are risk factors for cancers of the female reproductive tract.

Although environmental factors may be associated with a high relative risk of cancer, the absolute risk to exposed individuals may be low. Thus, approximately one of six cigarette smokers who smoke 25 or more cigarettes per day dies of lung cancer. Chemoprevention studies in the heavy-smoker population, therefore, are not only practical but imperative. The risk is much smaller for most other environmental carcinogens. For example, exposure to 1 Gy (100 rads) of irradiation may be associated with approximately one instance of cancer per 1,000 exposed persons each year. Of every 1,000 daughters of women who took diethylstilbestrol during pregnancy, one woman will develop vaginal adenocarcinoma in early adulthood.

GENETICS

By contrast, cancer genes are much more potent carcinogenic factors than are many environmental carcinogens. Fewer than 5% of all cancers result from inherited genetic susceptibility or defects. However, for carriers of certain cancer genes (e.g., those for familial polyposis coli and hereditary retinoblastoma), the risk for cancer approaches 100%. Thus, the yield from surveillance of these patients will be high. When the certainty of future cancer in individual family members can be established, active preventive intervention may be justified.

To date, researchers have identified more than 200 inherited diseases that predispose to neoplasia. The identification of an increasing number of inherited cancer susceptibility genes, including genes for such common neoplasms as breast and colon cancer, will create new opportunities for intervention to reduce cancer morbidity and mortality. Intervention strategies include dietary modification; chemoprevention with such agents as aspirin and nonsteroidal antiinflammatory agents for colon cancer; and screening to detect precancerous lesions of the breast, colon, and other sites. Studies now under way are seeking to determine the effect of tamoxifen on carriers of *BRCA1*. In addition, some carriers of the breast cancer susceptibility gene may elect prophylactic mastectomy and prophylactic oophorectomy.

The availability of techniques to identify persons with a genetic susceptibility to cancer raises a number of legal, social, and ethical issues. The benefits of cancer predisposition testing must be weighed carefully against its potential drawbacks. Any genetic testing should be coupled with professional genetic counseling. Persons identified as gene carriers may suffer from discrimination and may have difficulty in gaining or keeping a job or in obtaining insurance. The National Advisory Council for the Human Genome Program recently recommended that cancer predisposition testing be regarded as a research activity. For various reasons, testing should be offered initially only to individuals and families at high risk and not to the general population. Because so many issues are involved in genetic testing, referral of interested patients to a center specializing in genetic counseling should precede any such testing. Recognition of the possibility of genetic cause of cancer in affected patients' families will be facilitated by remembering that genetic cancers tend to affect one or only a few different organs, occur at a relatively early age, and affect multiple generations.

PERSONAL HISTORY OF CANCER AND OTHER DISEASES

Patients cured of one cancer may be at high risk for the development of other cancers. Genetic susceptibility may be one important factor, or exposure of several organs to the same carcinogen also may be involved. In addition, such anticancer treatments as radiotherapy combined with chemotherapy may have a carcinogenic effect. As cancer therapy becomes more effective and more patients survive for long periods after treatment, more of these associated cancers may be seen.

GENERAL ADVICE FOR HIGH-RISK PATIENTS

In patients at higher-than-normal risk, rigorous intervention may be indicated. For example, the small number of patients identified as being at high risk for occupational cancers should be advised to avoid additional exposure to carcinogens. Among patients who are exposed to asbestos and who also smoke, the risk for lung cancer is multiplied dramatically. For patients with polyposis coli, Gardner's syndrome, or chronic ulcerative colitis of long duration, standard medical practice involves excision of those areas of the colon at risk before cancer appears. This procedure may be accomplished variously by total colostomy and ileorectal anastomosis, with periodic examinations of the residual rectum; by total proctocolectomy and permanent ileostomy; or by total colectomy, mucosal proctectomy, and ileoanal anastomosis. The presence of a dysplastic nevus is associated with an increased risk for malignant melanoma. Periodic surveillance and removal of such nevi appear to prevent the progression to melanoma.

Physicians' responsibility for early intervention in such situations extends not only to affected patients themselves but to their families. High-risk patients may be screened more often and in greater detail than are low-risk patients. For example, periodic physical examination might be performed more frequently and colonoscopy could be started at an earlier age in persons at high risk for colon cancer.

IMPLEMENTING PREVENTIVE SERVICES IN THE OFFICE SETTING

Although primary-care facilities usually have well-established procedures, recording systems, and clinical equipment for providing high-quality care to patients with acute medical problems, many still do not have similar systems for prevention of disease. Although involved physicians have a strong commitment to providing preventive services [2, 3]—already an accepted activity within their practice [4]—many studies document less than 50% compliance with such basic prevention service recommendations as Papanicolaou tests, mammograms, fecal blood testing, and sigmoidoscopy [5–7]. The barriers to preventive service performance by primary-care physicians has been well described: lack of time, the urgent demands of patients, physician uncertainty about conflicting guidelines, uncertainty about the value of screening tests, disorganized medical records, lack of direct gratification from screening, lack of reminders to physicians regarding overdue tests, lack of staff support, lack of organized office systems, and the lack of insurance coverage [8–12].

Many controlled studies have demonstrated that a team approach to preventive services improves the prevention and early detection of cancer [13–15]. To be effective, such an approach should make use of a carefully described prevention protocol combined with well-designed paper-based or computerized tools for tracking and reminding physicians and patients when screening should be performed [16–18]. The American Cancer Society's Advisory Group on Preventive Health Care Reminder Systems has documented five steps for preventive care. Every primary-care provider should be familiar with these steps:

1. *Perform a risk evaluation:* Identify which procedures and what type of counseling are due when patients come to the office. (This step may be accomplished by the office nurse.) Both acute-care visits and comprehensive physical examinations offer excellent opportunities for prevention.
2. *Recommend preventive procedures:* Document this in the medical record or on the flow sheet.
3. *Perform or order the appropriate procedures or counseling:* Document these procedures or other activities.
4. *Implement and document appropriate follow-up:* This is based on the results of the preventive procedures or activities.
5. *Determine patients' next preventive care needs:* Arrange for another office visit at that time.

Primary-care providers should create a personal written policy for preventive care, including screening and counseling activities, after reviewing guidelines from such national organizations as the American Cancer Society. After developing such policy, providers should audit 50 patient charts to establish baseline performance rates for their practice. After the new policies have been implemented for 6 to 12 months, a repeat audit should be performed to measure any improvement (or lack thereof). Staff members should be informed of and encouraged with the results, whether positive or negative. The following important tasks should be delegated to the office staff, with one person acting as coordinator: (1) reviewing when services were last provided to each patient; (2) recording results of preventive activities on a flow sheet or computer; (3) following up on these results; and (4) informing patients of when the next preventive services should be performed.

The US Department of Health and Human Services has developed "Put Prevention Into Practice" (PPIP) to increase the appropriate use of clinical preventive services [19]. These materials were based on research-tested interventions for improving the delivery of preventive services in primary-care settings. They have been revised and updated on the basis of new scientific information and evaluation of the users. The basic tool is a flow sheet for a patient's chart (Fig. 4.2). A prevention prescription pad also has been designed to enable providers or staff to order necessary preventive services or to write behavioral contracts for patients. Printed reminder postcards can be mailed to patients so that they can schedule a reexamination. The Public Health Service's *Clinician's Handbook of Preventive Services* [19] is a particularly useful guide that contains information regarding specific prevention services (e.g., the burden of suffering from the target disorder, recommendations of major authorities, basic information about performing each type of preventive service, scientific references, and patient education resources).

Although paper-based reminder systems do promote preventive care efforts, two controlled studies have found that a computerized reminder system is significantly more effective [17, 18]. Such a reminder system can be designed using demographic data already contained in the usual primary-care computerized billing system. The system can provide health maintenance protocols for specific ages and gender. These protocols should be modified easily to implement new recommendations or patient-specific risk factors. Documentation of patient compliance can be audited easily, and reminder messages can be sent.

Counseling to encourage patients to reduce their cancer risk through smoking cessation or diet improvement is essential to cancer prevention. Successful preventive care hinges on good communication by clinicians about the cooperation and involvement of patients themselves. Recognizing this fact, the Public Health Service, as part of its PPIP program, has designed personal health guides that provide a permanent record of preventive care and valuable basic information about health maintenance. In addition, the American Cancer Society has developed many types of patient education materials. PPIP materials can be ordered from the

Name
D.O.B.
No.

**Adult Preventative Care
Flow Sheet**

ALLERGIES:

Health Counseling

(Circle if appropriate)
1. Alcohol and Drugs
2. Aspirin
3. Dental and Oral Health
4. Hormone Replacement Therapy
5. Domestic Violence
6. Family Planning
7. Folate
8. Injuries (e.g. seat belts, falls)
9. Nutrition
10. Occupational Health
11. Osteoporosis
12. Physical Activity
13. Polypharmacy
14. Self-Exams (skin, breast, testicular)
15. STDs/HIV Infection
16. Tobacco
17. _____
18. _____

| Date |
| Type(s) |
| Date |
| Type(s) |
| Date |
| Type(s) |
| Date |
| Type(s) |
| Date |
| Type(s) |
| Date |
| Type(s) |

Screening and Tests

Suggested Examinations and Tests:*

BLOOD PRESSURE
BREAST EXAM
CHOLESTEROL
COGNITIVE AND FUNCTIONAL IMPAIRMENT

DEPRESSION
DIGITAL RECTAL EXAM
FECAL OCCULT BLOOD
GLAUCOMA
HEARING

HEIGHT/WEIGHT
MAMMOGRAPHY
ORAL CAVITY EXAM
PAP SMEAR/PELVIC EXAM
PLASMA GLUCOSE

PROSTATE EXAM/PSA
SIGMOIDOSCOPY
SKIN EXAM
TESTICULAR EXAM
THYROID FUNCTION/EXAM

TUBERCULIN SKIN TESTING
URINALYSIS
VISION

* Specific preventative protocols should be tailored to the patient's risk factors and based on discussion between the patient and provider

Examinations and Tests   **Schedule**

| Date |
| Result |
| Date |
| Result |
| Date |
| Result |
| Date |
| Result |
| Date |
| Result |
| Date |
| Result |

Immunizations

Immunization/Frequency

Influenza
≥ 65 yrs.
or immunocompromised
Yearly
| Date |
| Manuf. & Lot No. |

Pneumococcal
≥ 65 yrs.
or immunocompromised
One dose
| Date |
| Manuf. & Lot No. |

Varicella
Nonimmune adults
Two doses delivered 4-8 weeks apart if immunized after age 13 years
| Date |
| Manuf. & Lot No. |

Hepatitis B
Adults at increased risk
3- or 4-dose series
| Date |
| Manuf. & Lot No. |

Tetanus and Diphtheria
All adults
Every 10 years
| Date |
| Manuf. & Lot No. |

Rubella
Women of childbearing age and health care workers without evidence of immunity or prior immunization
One dose
| Date |
| Manuf. & Lot No. |

Other Immunizations

| Date |
| Manuf. & Lot No. |
| Date |
| Manuf. & Lot No. |
| Date |
| Manuf. & Lot No. |
| Date |
| Manuf. & Lot No. |
| Date |
| Manuf. & Lot No. |
| Date |
| Manuf. & Lot No. |
| Date |
| Manuf. & Lot No. |

Figure 4.2 Adult preventive care flow sheet for tracking dates and results of preventive care. This form can be individualized for particular age and gender groups and additional screening activities, according to each patient's risk profile. One valuable feature of the record is the inclusion of result codes. (Reprinted from the Public Health Service, "Put Prevention Into Practice" kit. Washington, DC: US Government Printing Office.)

Agency for Healthy Care Policy and Research (AHCPR) at 1-800-358-9295.

PUBLIC POLICY AND PHYSICIAN ADVOCACY

Legislative activities and collaboration among federal, state, and local government, private and not-for-profit public health organizations, and the practicing physician have led to major public health legislation in cancer prevention and control. Three areas of cancer control that will be critically important in the coming decade were summarized in a report by the Institute of Medicine (IOM) [20]: assessment, policy development, and assurance. *Assessment* refers to the concept of community diagnosis, including the tools of public health surveillance and epidemiologic research. Using the results of assessment as a basis, *policy development* is the process by which society makes decisions about health problems through planning, priority and goal setting, policy leadership and advocacy, and provision of public information. *Assurance* is the guarantor function of public health, to ensure that health services and legislative mandates are met according to agreed-on goals [20]. Three recent review articles addressed these areas of cancer control in discussions of the importance of diet and tobacco use [21], the evidence for cancer causation (Table 4.6) [22, 23], and cancer prevention programs, public education campaigns, and government and social policy measures for preventing cancer [23].

The development and assurance of public policy has a central role in cancer prevention. For example, the control of occupational exposure to carcinogens in the United States is an important triumph in primary cancer prevention and demonstrates that systematic regulatory control of the workplace can be an effective cancer prevention measure. Strategies for preventing lung and other tobacco-related cancers are not very different from public health approaches that have worked effectively in the past against scourges such as smallpox and syphilis. The putative cause of these cancers is a class 1 carcinogen-laden product—the cigarette—which contains significant amounts of nicotine, a potent contributor to drug dependence. The vectors of this agent are multi-billion-dollar, multinational tobacco conglomerates, backed by sophisticated marketing and product promotion. To compound the social problem, the tobacco industry is a major employer, all the way from the farm through the manufacturer to the small-business retailer. Thus, the logical intervention method is a consolidated and aggressive government-led campaign [24, 25].

The government-funded social-norm change model is best described by California's tobacco control program [26]. The California experience demonstrates that a comprehensive approach designed to change social norms has an impact much greater than that of a frontal attack designed to market cessation services directly to tobacco users. The goal of this social-norm change approach is indirect influence on current and potential future tobacco users by creating a social milieu and legal climate in which tobacco becomes less desirable, less acceptable, and less accessible than it is currently.

This conditioning influence of society on the individual is as great for behaviors and attitudes related to tobacco as it is for any other human behavior. Two-thirds of cancer deaths in the United States can be linked to tobacco use, diet, obesity, and lack of exercise, all of which can be modified through action at both the individual and societal level. Normative social attitudes (social norms) change over time according to the evolution of events in communities and as a result of intentional human intervention. The California Tobacco Control Program [26] has sought to change the broad social norms that surround tobacco use by pushing tobacco use out of the charmed circle of a normal, desirable practice and characterizing it as an abnormal practice—in short, to denormalize smoking and other tobacco use. Such an effort must engage everyone, both nonsmokers and smokers. Four broad priority areas, or policy themes, were established for use in program planning and funding decisions. These areas, which act in concert to change social norms related to tobacco use, are (1)

Table 4.6 Causes of Cancer in the United States

Risk Factor	Percentage
Tobacco	30
Adult diet and obesity	30
Sedentary lifestyle	5
Occupational factors	5
Family history of cancer	5
Viruses and other biological agents	5
Perinatal factors and growth	5
Reproductive factors	3
Alcohol	3
Socioeconomic status	3
Environmental pollution	2
Ionizing and ultraviolet irradiation	2
Prescription drugs and medical procedures	1
Salt and other food additives or contaminants	1

protecting people from exposure to secondhand tobacco smoke, (2) revealing and countering tobacco industry influence, (3) reducing youth access to tobacco products, and (4) providing cessation services.

The second public policy paradigm for successful government intervention is the effort to prevent mortality by screening mammography. Breast cancer is the most common cancer in women in the United States (approximately 175,000 new invasive cases in 1999) and is second only to lung cancer as a cause of cancer death (nearly 43,000 deaths in 1998). At this time, screening and early detection provide the best opportunity for further mortality reductions. Therefore, the American Cancer Society recommends that women aged 40 years and older undergo annual mammography and clinical breast examinations. However, frequency of occurrence of regular and systematic breast cancer screening relates inversely to income, education, social class, and race: Higher socioeconomic status and being white are associated with more frequent systematic breast screenings. Though the horizontal insurance coverage for breast cancer screening has widened to encompass Medicare, Medicaid, and most privately insured populations, significant near-poor populations historically have not been covered; therefore, some government programs are now targeting these populations. However, reimbursement rates by both the private and public sectors for mammography and clinical breast examination have fallen to levels that either preclude the widespread use of these tests or result in substandard services.

The current managed-care environment has compounded these financial issues by cutting costs and regulating access. Thus, the provision of breast cancer screenings for low-income populations has become a priority of the government at all levels, as the public sector is the major source of health care for such populations. The Breast and Cervical Cancer Control Program of the Centers for Disease Control and Prevention and parallel state-funded efforts bring breast cancer–screening services to low-income women who have no other way to receive such services. Such programs also build the capability to deliver high-quality educational and clinical services to high-risk communities. Allocation of federal funds to states for such national programs should be determined in part by the state's base of the population in need. Also, greater flexibility for states in meeting certain federal program requirements could enable states to use both federal and state resources in complementary ways to provide greater benefit to more women.

Though insurers and other third-party payers have progressively been required to pay for mammography and clinical breast examinations as allowable services and costs, the additional services that result from mammography (follow-up care and treatment costs) are not necessarily covered. Patient tracking and follow-up care are major concerns among the poor and uninsured and especially among such special populations as migrant workers and non-English-speaking people. Thus, funded programs detect breast cancers early in high-risk populations of women who then have no available means for obtaining treatment of these newly detected cancers. The vertical integration issue revolves around ways to meld the function of public health screening programs (such as the Breast and Cervical Cancer Control Program) with the mainstream medical care system. Federal (and state) enabling legislation and adequate appropriations to support treatment costs could provide either for Medicaid entitlement for women in whom breast or cervical cancer is diagnosed or for a program for low-income older women that divides the cost for health care coverage between federal and state governments.

However, even with increased coverage for screening and aftercare, low-income women at highest risk often are unaware of the need for such screening and the services available to them. More important, they must be motivated to take advantage of these programs despite their personal, social, economic, and cultural misgivings. Such an enterprise calls for considerable innovation and sensitivity because, in these women's hierarchy of needs, being screened for breast cancer may rank very low. Even after costs and medical necessity are addressed adequately, issues of cultural biases, transportation, child-care, and time away from work must be tackled. To that end, government programs have set up partnerships involving these indigenous high-risk populations, in order both to establish a public education program and to provide a health care access infrastructure.

Finally, any program must address quality assurance. Numerous concerns involve the entire spectrum, from ensuring that mammography facilities have minimum American College of Radiology–approved standards for equipment, personnel, protocols, and procedures, through to quality control for all the health care providers involved (e.g., physicians, nurses, and radiology technicians). Even something as simple as a clinical breast examination can be fraught with serious errors if the health professionals conducting the examination are not trained to cover systematically the entire breast and are not taught to recognize exactly what they are palpating. Provider education and health professional training are intrinsic parts of these categorical breast cancer screening programs.

Despite all the difficulties inherent in a universal breast cancer–screening program, the strategy of trying to prevent breast cancer deaths appears to be working: Between 1991 and 1995, breast cancer incidence rates essentially plateaued, and breast cancer mortality declined significantly, especially among younger white and African-American women. Undoubtedly, these changes were the result of improved screening, early detection, and treatment.

Physician Advocacy

The practicing physician plays a pivotal role in changing an individual's health risk and modifying behavior through direct contact with patients and their families and by involvement in community-based activities at the state, local, or national level. Physicians were leaders in tobacco coalitions that have instigated increased taxes on tobacco products as a deterrent to smoking by youths and as a fund-raiser for tobacco control programs. Other potential spheres of antitobacco influence exist in school health programs, counseling for pregnant women and their spouses, and the promotion of smoke-free legislation. In addition, physicians can advocate for legislation to mandate mammography standards, healthy-lifestyle school education programs, improved funding for diagnosis and treatment, and an expanded role of managed care in cancer prevention and detection.

American Cancer Society

The American Cancer Society has historically been one of the greatest nationwide change agents in cancer prevention and control. Among the Society's goals for the year 2015 is a 50% cancer mortality reduction and a 25% cancer incidence reduction. Meeting these goals assumes collaboration of the entire cancer prevention and control constituency: individual health care providers and governmental and private cancer organizations. The impact of such a collaboration could dwarf many of our nation's past public health achievements. The American Cancer Society has committed itself to providing the leadership and funding to turn these ambitious goals into a reality.

SUMMARY

To a large extent, cancer is preventable. Most of the burden of prevention lies in an individual's lifestyle. Societal change is important in supporting and motivating personal lifestyle modifications. The largest benefits to be seen in cancer prevention are in the areas of tobacco cessation and dietary change. Control of obesity and a heightened level of physical activity also can contribute to decreased cancer incidence. Environmental causes, although perceived publicly as a major contributor to human ills, have thus far not been shown to be responsible for very many cancers. Nonetheless, the avoidance or removal of known toxic environmental agents is a worthy pursuit. Cancer-causing inherited genes are very uncommon but, even in those persons with highly penetrable, genetically transmitted cancer susceptibility, cancer prevention often is possible (e.g., through removal of the target organ). A goal of genetic research is to discover ways in which to repair the mutated or deleted gene.

The health care professional plays a critical role in cancer prevention and control, whether through successfully counseling patients about lifestyle changes or by encouraging at-risk persons to enter chemoprevention trials. Even when cancer prevention is not possible, prevention of cancer death by promoting cancer screening is an important duty of every health care professional. Finally, primary-care physicians can play an active role by advocating for cancer control policies, by becoming involved in local, state, or national efforts. The successes in tobacco control suggest that we can be successful in bringing about other societal shifts in cancer control awareness (e.g., in promoting a healthy lifestyle). Moreover, for the first time in recent decades, age-adjusted cancer death rates have declined since 1990, raising hopes that a downward trend in rates will persist into the next century.

REFERENCES

1. Chang M-H, Chen C-J, Lai M-S, et al. Universal hepatitis B vaccination in Taiwan and the incidence of hepatocellular carcinoma in children. *N Engl J Med* 336: 1855–1859, 1997.
2. Coulter A, Schofield T. Prevention in general practice: the views of doctors in the Oxford region. *Br J Gen Pract* 41:140–143, 1991.
3. Wechsler H, Levine S, Idelson RK, et al. The physician's role in health promotion revisited—a survey of primary care practitioners. *N Engl J Med* 334:996–998, 1996.

4. US Preventive Services Task Force, US Office of Disease Prevention and Health Promotion. *Guide to Clinical Preventive Services: Report of the U.S. Preventive Services Task Force* (2nd ed). Washington, DC: US Department of Health and Human Services, Office of Public Health and Science, Office of Disease Prevention and Health Promotion, 1996:933.

5. Kottke TE, Solberg LI, Brekke ML, et al. Preventive services rates in 44 midwestern primary care clinics, room for improvement. *Mayo Clin Proc* 72:515–523, 1997.

6. Anderson LM, May DS. Has the use of cervical, breast and colorectal cancer screening increased in the United States? *Am J Public Health* 85:840–842, 1995.

7. McGinnis JM, Lee PR. Healthy People 2000 at mid-decade. *JAMA* 273:1123–1129, 1995.

8. Frame PS, Werth PL. How primary health care providers can integrate cancer prevention into practice. *Cancer* 72:1132–1137, 1993.

9. Frame PS. Health maintenance in clinical practice: strategies and barriers. *Am Fam Physician* 45:1192–1200, 1992.

10. Kottke TE, Brekke ML, Solberg LI. Making "time" for preventive services. *Mayo Clin Proc* 68:785–791, 1993.

11. Solberg LI, Kottke TE, Brekke ML, et al. Using continuous quality improvement to increase preventive services in clinical practice—going beyond guidelines. *Prev Med* 25: 259–267, 1996.

12. Hahn DL, Olson N. The delivery of clinical preventive services: acute care intervention. *J Fam Pract* 48:785–789, 1999.

13. Dietrich AJ, Carney PA, Winchell CW, et al. An office systems approach to cancer prevention in primary care. *Cancer Pract* 5:375–381, 1997.

14. Hulscher ME, Wensing M, Grol RP, et al. Interventions to improve the delivery of preventive services in primary care. *Am J Public Health* 89:737–746, 1999.

15. Solberg LI, Kottke TE, Brekke ML. Will primary care clinics organize themselves to improve the delivery of preventive services? A randomized controlled trial. *Prev Med* 27:623–631, 1998.

16. Leininger LS, Finn L, Dickey L, et al. An office system for organizing preventive ervices: a report by the American Cancer Society Advisory Group on Preventive Health Care Reminder Systems. *Arch Fam Med* 5:108–115, 1996.

17. McPhee SJ, Bird JA, Fordham D, et al. Promoting cancer prevention activities by primary care physicians. Results of a randomized, controlled trial. *JAMA* 266:538–544, 1991.

18. Frame PS, Zimmer JG, Werth PL, et al. Computer-based vs manual health maintenance tracking. A controlled trial. *Arch Fam Med* 3:581–588, 1994.

19. US Office of Disease Prevention and Health Promotion. *The Clinician's Handbook of Preventive Services: Put Prevention into Practice.* Alexandria, VA: International Medical, 1994.

20. Institute of Medicine. *The Future of Public Health.* Washington, DC: National Academy Press, 1998.

21. McGinnis JM, Foege WH. Actual causes of death in the United States. *JAMA* 270:2207–2212, 1993.

22. Colditz G, DeJong W, Hunter D, et al. (eds). *Harvard Report on Cancer Prevention: Cancer Causes and Control,* Vol 7. Cambridge, MA: Harvard University Press, 1996.

23. Colditz G, DeJong W, Emmons K, et al. (eds). *Harvard Report on Cancer Prevention: Cancer Causes and Control,* Vol 8. Cambridge, MA: Harvard University Press, 1997.

24. Bal DG. Designing an effective statewide tobacco control program—California. *Cancer Suppl* 83:2717–2721, 1998.

25. Connolly G, Robbins H. Designing an effective statewide tobacco control program—Massachusetts. *Cancer Suppl* 83:2722–2727, 1998.

26. Lloyd J, Hunter L. *A Model for Change: the California Experience in Tobacco Control.* State of California, Department of Health Services, October 1998.

SUGGESTED READINGS

Epidemiologic Profile: Risk Factors

Block G, Patterson B, Subar A. Fruit, vegetables, and cancer prevention: a review of epidemiological evidence. *Nutr Cancer* 18:1–29, 1992.

Blumberg BS, London WT. Hepatitis B virus and the prevention of primary cancer of the liver. *J Natl Cancer Inst* 74: 267–273, 1985.

de la Chapelle A, Peltomaki P. The genetics of hereditary common cancers. *Curr Opin Genet Dev* 8:298–303, 1998.

Doll R, Peto R. The causes of cancer: quantitative estimates of avoidable risks of cancer in the United States today. *J Natl Cancer Inst* 66:1191–1308, 1981.

Fraumeni JF Jr (ed). *Persons at Risk of Cancer: An Approach to Cancer Etiology and Control.* New York: Academic, 1975.

Frumkin H, Levy BS. Carcinogens. In Levy BS, Wegman DH (eds), *Occupational Health: Recognizing and Preventing Work-Related Disease.* Boston: Little, Brown, 1983:145–750.

Gertig DM, Hunter DJ. Genes and environment in the etiology of colorectal cancer. *Semin Cancer Biol* 8:285–298, 1998.

Knudson AG. Hereditary predisposition to cancer. *Ann NY Acad Sci* 833:58–67, 1997.

Kolodner RD, Tytell JD, Schmeits JL, et al. Germ-line msh6 mutations in colorectal cancer families. *Cancer Res* 59:5068–5074, 1999.

Newman B, Mu H, Butler LM, et al. Frequency of breast cancer attributable to BRCA1 in a population-based series of American women. *JAMA* 279:915–921, 1998.

Perera FP. Molecular epidemiology of environmental carcinogenesis. *Recent Results Cancer Res* 154:39–46, 1998

Potter JD. Colorectal cancer: molecules and populations. *J Natl Cancer Inst* 91:916–932, 1999.

Wong F, Boice JD Jr, Abramson DH, et al. Cancer incidence after retinoblastoma: radiation dose and sarcoma risk. *JAMA* 278:1262–1267, 1997.

Preventive Strategies

APPROACHES TO SMOKING CESSATION

Fiore MC. Methods used to quit smoking in the U.S. *JAMA* 263:2760–2765, 1990.

Fiore MC. The new vital sign: assessing and documenting smoking status. *JAMA* 266:3183–3184, 1991.

Fiore MC, et al. (eds), *Smoking Cessation Guideline*. Rockville, MD: Agency for Health Care Policy and Research, Public Health Service, US Department of Health and Human Services, April 1996. (Several guidelines are available, including *Clinical Practice Guideline* [AHCPR pub. no. 96–0692], *Patient Guide* [AHCPR pub. no. 96–0695], and *Quick Reference for Primary Care Physicians* [AHCPR pub. no. 96–0693].)

Gritz ER, Fiore MC, Henningfield JE. Smoking and cancer. In Murphy GP, Lawrence W Jr, Lenhard RE Jr (eds), *American Cancer Society Textbook of Clinical Oncology* (2nd ed). Atlanta: American Cancer Society, 1995.

Hurt RD. Nicotine patch therapy. *JAMA* 271:595–600, 1994.

Kenford SL. Predicting smoking cessation. *JAMA* 271:589–594, 1994.

Smith SS, Jorenby DE, Fiore MC, Baker JB. Smoking cessation: what's new since the AHCPR guideline? *J Respir Dis* 19:412–426, 1998.

CHEMOPREVENTION

Chelbowski RT, Butler J, Nelson A, et al. Breast cancer chemoprevention: tamoxifen—current issues and future prospective. *Cancer* 72:1032–1037, 1993.

Fisher B, Constantino JP, Wickerham DL, et al. Tamoxifen for prevention of breast cancer: report of the National Surgical Adjuvant Breast and Bowel Project P-l study. *J Natl Cancer Inst* 90:1371–1388, 1998.

Greenwald P. Experience from clinical trials in cancer prevention. *Ann Med* 26:73–80, 1994.

Kelloff GJ, Boone CW, Steels VE, et al. Progress in cancer chemoprevention: perspectives on agent selection and short-term clinical intervention trials. *Cancer Res* 54(suppl):2014–2024, 1994.

Lippman SM, Benner SE, Hong WK. Chemoprevention: strategies for the control of cancer. *Cancer* 72:984–990, 1993.

Lippman SM, Benner SE, Hong WK. Cancer chemoprevention. *J Clin Oncol* 12:851–873, 1994.

Omenn GS, Goodman GE, Thornquist MD, et al. Risk factors for lung cancer and for intervention effects in CARET, the Beta-Carotene and Retinol Efficacy Trial. *J Natl Cancer Inst* 88:1550–1559, 1996.

Powles TJ, Eeles R, Ashley S, et al. Interim analysis of the incidence of breast cancer in the Royal Marsden Hospital tamoxifen randomised chemoprevention trial. *Lancet* 352:98–101, 1998.

Selby JV, Friedman GD, Quesenberry CP Jr, et al. A case-control study of screening sigmoidoscopy and mortality from colorectal cancer. *N Engl J Med* 326:653–657, 1992.

Selby JV, Friedman GD, Quesenberry CP Jr, et al. Effect of fecal occult blood testing on mortality from colorectal cancer. *Ann Intern Med* 118:1–6, 1993.

Sturmer T, Glynn RJ, Lee IM, et al. Aspirin use and colorectal cancer: post-trial follow-up data from the Physicians' Health Study. *Ann Intern Med* 128:713–720, 1998.

Thun MJ, Namboodiri BS, Heath CW. Aspirin use and reduced risk of fatal colon cancer. *N Engl J Med* 325:1593–1596, 1991.

Veronesi U, Maisonneuve P, Costa A, et al. Prevention of breast cancer with tamoxifen: preliminary findings from the Italian randomized trial among hysterectomized women. *Lancet* 352:93–97, 1998.

DIET AND PHYSICAL ACTIVITY

American Cancer Society 1996 Advisory Committee on Diet, Nutrition and Cancer Prevention. Guidelines on diet, nutrition and cancer prevention: reducing the risk of cancer with healthy food choices and physical activity. *Cancer* 46:325, 1996.

Henderson CW. Prescription foods to prevent cancer. *Cancer Weekly Plus* 9:1999.

McGinnis JM, Foege WH. Actual causes of death in the United States. *JAMA* 270:2207–2212, 1993.

National Academy of Sciences Committee on Diet Nutrition and Cancer Diet Nutrition and Cancer. Washington, DC: Assembly of Life Science, National Academy Press, 1982.

US Department of Agriculture. *The Food Guide Pyramid.* [Home and Garden Bull. 252.] Washington, DC: US Department of Agriculture, 1992.

Work Study Group on Diet, Nutrition and Cancer. American Cancer Society guidelines on diet, nutrition and cancer. *Cancer* 41:334–338, 1991.

World Cancer Research Fund and American Institute for Cancer Research. *Food Nutrition and the Prevention of Cancer: A Global Perspective.* Washington, DC: American Institute for Cancer Research, 1997.

IDENTIFYING AND INCLUDING HIGH-RISK PATIENTS

Elder DE, Goldman LI, Goldman SC, et al. Dysplastic nevus syndrome. *Cancer* 46:1787–1794, 1984.

Li FP. Phenotypes, genotypes and interventions for hereditary cancers. *Cancer Epidemiol Biomarkers Prev* 4:579–582, 1995.

Nichols KE, Li FP, Haber DA, Deller L. Childhood cancer predisposition: applications of molecular testing and future implications. *J Pediatr* 132:389–397, 1998.

President's Commission for the Study of Ethical Problems in Medicine and Biomedical and Behavioral Research. *Screening and Counseling for Genetic Conditions: A Report on the Ethical, Social and Legal Implications of Genetic Screening, Counseling and Education Programs.* Washington, DC: US Government Printing Office, 1983.

Wijnen JT, et al. Clinical findings with implications for genetic testing in families with clustering of colorectal cancer. *N Engl J Med* 339:511–518, 1998.

Public Policy and Physician Advocacy

Bal DG, Nixon DW, Foerster SB, Brownson RC. Cancer prevention. In Murphy GP, Lawrence Jr W, Lenhard Jr RE (eds), *American Cancer Society Textbook of Clinical Oncology* (2nd ed). Atlanta: American Cancer Society, 1995.

Bronson RC, Bal DG. The future of cancer control research and translation. *J Public Health Manage Pract* 2(2):70–78, 1996.

Brownson RC, Reif JS, Alavanja MCR, Bal DG. Cancer. In Brownson RC, Remington PL, Davis JR (eds), *Chronic Disease Epidemiology and Control.* Washington, DC: American Public Health Association, 1993:137–167.

Doll R, Peto R. *The Causes of Cancer: Quantitative Estimates of Avoidable Risks of Cancer in the United States Today.* New York: Oxford University Press, 1981.

Giovino GA, Henningfield JE, Tomar SL, et al. Epidemiology of tobacco use and dependence. *Epidemiol Rev* 17:48–65, 1995.

Nestle M, Bal DG, Birt DF, et al. Guidelines on diet, nutrition, and cancer prevention: reducing the risk of cancer with healthy food choices and physical activity. *CA Cancer J Clin* 46:325–341, 1996.

Wingo PA, Ries LAG, Giovino GA, et al. Annual report to the nation on the status of cancer 1973–1996, with a special section on lung cancer and tobacco smoking. *J Natl Cancer Inst* 9:675–690, 1999.

Wingo PA, Ries LAG, Rosenberg HM, et al. Cancer incidence and mortality, 1973–1995: a report card for the US. *Cancer* 82:1197–1207, 1998.

Woolam G, Bal DG, Eyre H, et al. *Report of the Blue Ribbon Advisory Group on Community Cancer Control to the Board of Directors of the American Cancer Society: Society-Wide Recommendations for Community Cancer Control.* Atlanta: American Cancer Society, 1997.

Wynder EL, Graham EA. Tobacco smoking as a possible etiologic factor in bronchiogenic carcinoma. A study of six hundred and eighty-four proved cases. *JAMA* 143: 329–336, 1950.

5

Cancer Detection

■ ■ ■

Robert A. Smith
Curtis J. Mettlin

PRIMARY PREVENTION IS THE PREFERRED strategy for reducing the disease burden of cancer. When the underlying etiology of a particular malignancy accounts for a large proportion of the attributable risk and is avoidable, such as the association between tobacco use and lung cancer, a method for primary prevention is obvious. However, few cancers have such a clear prevention strategy. Although some behaviors have been associated with a protective effect for certain cancers (e.g., regular physical activity, a healthy diet, and avoiding sun exposure and certain occupational exposures), the mechanism for these protective effects as observed in epidemiologic studies is not well understood. Few explicit and indisputable behaviors that ought to be avoided or adopted have been associated with a predictable and certain reduction in disease risk for individuals. Thus, at this time, the control of cancer primarily depends on successful treatment.

In general, cancer prognosis is better and treatment more successful if the disease is detected when still localized. This finding is not true for all cancers but for some prevalent cancers, including cancers of the skin, breast, cervix, endometrium, ovary, testis, colon and rectum, prostate, and lung, a more favorable prognosis associated with early detection has led to secondary prevention strategies. In some instances, these have been successful. Secondary prevention is distinguished from primary prevention in that it is intervention focused on altering the natural history of the disease, thus avoiding disease-related adverse outcomes. Screening for cancer is a secondary prevention strategy that contributes to morbidity and mortality reduction by either identifying and treating precursor lesions known to be predictive of eventual malignancy, thus preventing progression to invasive disease, or by diagnosing invasive disease at an early stage when treatment is more successful, thus preventing death or avoiding morbidity. Screening is "the application of various tests to apparently healthy individuals to sort out those who probably have risk factors or are in the early stages of specified conditions" [1].

DECISION TO SCREEN

The observation that a particular cancer has a more favorable prognosis if diagnosed while still localized is only one element of a more complex decision matrix used to determine whether to offer cancer screening to an asymptomatic population [1–4]. Cancer screening currently is considered for only a few cancers. In general, the following questions should be asked in the determination of whether to screen a particular population for a given type of cancer [5]:

- Is the disease an important health problem, as measured by morbidity, mortality, and other measures of disease burden?
- Does the disease have a detectable preclinical phase?
- Does treatment of disease detected before the onset of clinical symptoms offer benefits compared with treatment after the onset of symptoms?
- Does the screening test meet acceptable levels of performance in terms of accuracy and cost?
- Is the screening process acceptable to individuals at risk and their health care providers?

Such questions are fundamental when deciding to offer screening to a healthy population. Because many healthy individuals must be tested to find the few who may have disease, these considerations not only are the basis for decisions about whether to implement a screening program but form the basis for continuing efforts to improve cost-effectiveness. Each of these criteria is described in greater detail later.

It will also become apparent that there are no threshold criteria for any of the preceding program considerations alone or—more important—in combination [6, 7]. A disease may not be an important cause of mortality but may account for significant morbidity. Likewise, a disease may account for significant mortality, but if disease onset and death typically occur very late in life, screening may have limited impact on life extension. Additionally, a cancer with a lower mortality rate but early average age at onset may account for many more years of premature mortality than would a cancer with higher mortality but late average age at onset. A high false-positive rate may be acceptable in screening for cancers at some organ sites but not at others because of the costs (both human and financial) associated with diag-

nostic testing after receipt of abnormal screening examination results. Finally, it is important to remember that values and population concerns, as well as scientific evidence, play a role in policy decisions about screening [7].

DISEASE BURDEN

Cole and Morrison [2] observed that a disease is suitable for screening if it has serious consequences that are recognized by the target population. On the basis of this initial criterion, fatal diseases or those that cause significant morbidity (or both) are potentially suitable for screening. Accordingly, this criterion includes nearly all cancers [2]. The American Cancer Society (ACS) estimated that in 2000, invasive cancer will be diagnosed in more than 1.2 million individuals [8]. This estimate does not include basal and squamous cell cancers of the skin, nor does it include important in situ melanoma or in situ lesions of the cervix and breast, all of which account for well more than an additional 1 million new cases. The ACS also estimated that in 2000, approximately 552,000 individuals were expected to die from cancer (nearly 25% of all deaths). Cancer is the second leading cause of death among men and women in the United States [8].

The importance of cancer as a public health problem can be expressed also by other measures of disease burden. Among men, the lifetime risk of developing cancer is 44.7%, and the lifetime risk of dying from cancer is 23.61%; among women, the lifetime risk of developing cancer is 38%, and the lifetime risk of dying from cancer is 20.5% [9]. Cancer is also a leading cause of premature mortality, expressed as average (i.e., expected) longevity for a given age at the time of death from cancer. The National Cancer Institute (NCI) estimated that cancer accounted for 8.2 million years of premature mortality in 1995. Although death from heart disease accounted for slightly more person-years of life lost, the average years of life lost from cancer is higher (15.2 years) than that from heart disease (11.7 years) [9].

CHARACTERISTICS OF THE DISEASE

Even though a disease is judged to be an important health problem, it must meet additional disease-specific criteria to justify screening. These criteria include the nature of the disease latency period and the degree to which treatment before the onset of clinically apparent disease truly improves prognosis, compared with that achieved with later treatment.

The detectable preclinical phase (DPCP), also known as the *sojourn time,* is the estimated duration of time during which an occult tumor can be detected with a screening test before symptom onset [10]. For a screening program to have an adequate yield, there should be a sufficient prevalence of detectable occult disease to justify screening large numbers of healthy individuals. Thus, the issue is not the prevalence of disease in the general population but rather the prevalence of detectable disease in the group being screened [2].

Most cancers have a long preclinical phase, which technically begins after the first reproduction of malignant cells. The length of the DPCP is a function of disease and host characteristics and the sensitivity of the screening test.

With the onset of screening, the incidence rate will increase, owing to the additional detection of occult cancers in the prevalent pool of individuals with undiagnosed cancer. That pool includes those who present with symptoms and those with asymptomatic detectable disease. The incidence and mortality rates and the duration of the DPCP influence prevalence of detectable cancers in a population. For any incidence rate, the longer the DPCP, the greater the prevalence of disease at the initial screening. For screening to be successful, the DPCP should be sufficiently long to ensure that periodic screening provides the opportunity to detect most disease in the target population before the onset of symptoms. *Lead time* is the amount of time gained before symptoms develop by detecting cancers through screening; thus, the average lead time always will be shorter than the average DPCP.

Both the DPCP and the lead time vary by cancer site; for any malignancy, the DPCP may vary by age and gender within the population being screened, and individual and histologic variations may be seen in tumor growth rates. For example, analyses of breast cancer trial data have shown that the mean DPCP and mean lead time vary by age and (in postmenopausal women) by histologic features [11]. Tabar et al. [12, 13] have estimated that the mean DPCP is 1.7 years in women aged 40 to 49, 3.3 years in women aged 50 to 59, and 3.8 years in women aged 60 to 69. On the basis of these observations, recent changes in Swedish breast cancer screening policy now include the recommendation to screen women aged 40 to 55 every 18 months and women aged 55 and older every 24 months [14].

Knowledge of the DPCP is important for determining screening intervals, because the DPCP defines the upper limit of the lead time that might be gained [10, 15]. The goal of screening is to advance the lead time, thereby reducing the incidence rate of advanced disease. A screening interval nearly equal to or exceeding the mean DPCP creates increased potential for a higher rate of interval cancers (cancers that arise and present with clinical manifestations between regularly scheduled screenings) and, thus, poorer prognosis in that subset of the incident cases. If prognosis remains relatively unchanged while the disease is in the DPCP, the timing of cancer detection during the preclinical phase is of little importance. Conversely, if a significant proportion of disease detected in the preclinical period is advanced, that finding may necessitate shortening the screening intervals to a period considerably less than the average DPCP. The regular examination of the stage distribution of cancers detected by screening, as well as the interval cancer rate, can provide valuable insights into the efficacy of particular screening intervals, and thus improve the performance of screening programs. Early evidence of the influence of the DPCP on the interval cancer rate was seen in the two-county study, which reported nearly twice the interval cancer rate in women aged 40 to 49 compared with women aged 50 and older when women in both groups were screened at intervals of 24 or more months [16]. To achieve similar screening outcomes, Swedish investigators concluded that premenopausal women should be screened at shorter intervals than postmenopausal women.

Treatment of screening-detected cancers should offer advantages over treatment of disease that presents with symptoms. These advantages may be measured by any one outcome or combination of outcomes: lower mortality, lower morbidity, or improved quality of life (or all). Detection of occult disease should not be equated with better outcomes, as this may not always be the case or the entirety of the benefit may not be sufficient to warrant screening the population [17]. Likewise, if a significant proportion of screening-detected cancers in asymptomatic individuals no longer are localized and have poor prognosis, screening may not be sufficiently beneficial. This is especially the case if changes in the screening interval are not feasible or no alternative early detection technology exists. Then again, if a shorter but still practical screening interval were possible or if a screening test with better performance emerges, the potential to screen for occult disease may be reconsidered.

EFFECTIVENESS OF SCREENING TESTS

A screening test can have four possible results, any of which is based on the true disease status of the individual and the test outcome (Table 5.1). A healthy individ-

Table 5.1 Measures of Screening Performance

Screening Test Results	Disease Status	
	Present	Not Present
Positive	a	b
Negative	c	d

Sensitivity = $a/(a + c)$; specificity = $d/(b + c)$; positive predictive value = $a/(a + b)$.

ual may be labeled correctly as not having a disease (true-negative) or may be labeled incorrectly as possibly having the disease (false-positive). Conversely, an individual with occult disease may be labeled correctly as possibly having the disease (true-positive) or may be labeled incorrectly as not having the disease (false-negative). The measurement of these outcome categories is complicated because screening tests are not in themselves definitive; final resolution of the accuracy of the original interpretation may take weeks, months, or even years or may not occur at all if an individual is lost to follow-up. By convention, screening outcomes are measured as follows:

- True-positive (TP): Cancer or precursor lesion diagnosed within a specified period after an abnormal screening examination result.
- False-positive (FP): No known cancer or precursor lesion diagnosed within a specified period after an abnormal screening examination result
- True-negative (TN): No known cancer or precursor lesion diagnosed within a specified period after a normal screening examination result
- False-negative (FN): Cancer or precursor lesion diagnosed within a specified period after a normal screening examination result; false negatives generally become apparent when symptoms develop during the interval between regularly scheduled examinations (e.g. interval cancers).

Because most members of the screened population are healthy, the majority of screening test results are normal (true-negative). However, an otherwise healthy individual undergoing screening also may receive an indeterminate interpretation, which may be resolved with further testing at the time of screening or within several weeks of the original test or after follow-up testing recommended at an intermediate interval (i.e., 6 months). For purposes of evaluation, individuals with an indeterminate finding may be classified on the basis of the original interpretation (true-positive or false-positive) or of the subsequent interpretation (true-

positive or true-negative), but one strategy should be chosen and used consistently to measure screening program outcomes. Based on patient considerations (i.e., days, weeks, or months living with uncertainty) and program costs, it could be argued that all indeterminate cases not resolved on the day of screening and not determined to be cancer within the specified interval (as described) should be labeled as false-positives. In this situation, the recommendation for interim testing is, in effect, an abnormal finding that has costs both for individuals (anxiety, additional time away from normal activities, etc.) and for the health care system (additional testing and costs).

The summary categories in Table 5.1 are the basic building blocks of screening program evaluation. They measure various parameters of test accuracy and performance, in particular sensitivity, specificity, and positive predictive value (PPV).

Sensitivity

The sensitivity of a screening test is the probability that it will detect cancer among all asymptomatic individuals who actually have the disease. Sensitivity indicates the proportion of all individuals with the disease (true-positives and false-negatives) who were identified correctly by the screening test (true-positives only) within a specified period of time, usually the screening interval. Sensitivity is calculated as follows: TP/(TP + FN). Measuring sensitivity is a challenge because the identification of false-negatives depends on the ability to follow a population over a prolonged period so as to identify cancers diagnosed within the follow-up period after a normal examination result [17]. Furthermore, the potential for misclassification is real because a cancer diagnosed within the follow-up period after a normal examination result is assumed to have been detectable during the initial examination; likewise, a cancer that truly was missed but not diagnosed within the predefined follow-up period will not be labeled as a false-negative. This approach to classification does not require reinterpretation of the previous screening test both for practicality and because of the potential bias of knowing that a patient had cancer at the time of the reference examination. Day and Walter [18] proposed an alternative approach to estimating sensitivity, based on the proportional incidence of interval cancers (i.e., the ratio of the number of observed cancers that are not screening-detected [interval cases] to the expected incidence in the absence of screening). The complement of this fraction is the program sensitivity.

Specificity

The specificity of a screening test is the probability that the test will correctly identify healthy individuals as not having the disease. Specificity is the proportion of all individuals without the disease (true-negatives and false-positives) who were identified correctly by the screening test (true-negatives only) within a specified period, usually the screening interval, as noted. Specificity is calculated as follows: TN/(TN + FP). Measuring specificity depends on the various definitions of a false-positive outcome, each of which has meaning for program evaluation. Specificity will be lower (indicating poorer test performance) if the definition of a false-positive is based on initial test results, which even though initially abnormal or indeterminate, may be resolved to a normal interpretation with some additional testing. Conversely, the measure of specificity may be more favorable if it is based on biopsy results, which ultimately will result in a smaller number of false-positives from which to calculate specificity [19].

Because specificity will vary on the basis of the definition of a false-positive, the criteria for false-positives in specificity measures must be delineated and the criteria must have meaning for program evaluation. Furthermore, there is no inherent reason to choose one measure or another, so long as the underlying measurement factors are specified. In fact, specificity based on initial screening test results and eventual biopsy outcomes are each important measures for evaluating cost-effectiveness. Lowering the false-positive rate may be a higher priority in one screening program as compared with another, owing to differences in patient harms and financial costs associated with a diagnostic workup.

Positive Predictive Value

The PPV of a screening test is the proportion of all positive screening cases that result in a diagnosis of cancer. As a measure of screening program performance, the value of the PPV, like specificity, varies directly with the definition of a false-positive examination. The PPV is calculated as follows: TP/(TP + FP). The PPV is influenced by the sensitivity of the screening test, but the greatest influence on PPV derives from the specificity of the screening test and from the magnitude of the underlying prevalence of disease in the population undergoing screening [2]. Thus, a screening test for a particular cancer may have equivalent sensitivity and specificity among all groups being screened, but the PPV will be lower in the group with lower disease prevalence.

Consider the following hypothetical example: A disease has a prevalence at screening of 500 cases per 100,000 individuals; 400 cases were identified correctly by the screening test, so sensitivity is 80%; 100 cases were missed by screening, so the false-negative rate is 20%. The large majority of individuals who did not have the disease tested normal, but 995 individuals (1%) had positive test results, resulting in a 99% specificity. Based on this example (400/[400 + 995]), PPV = 29%. If sensitivity improves from 80% to 90%, only a 2% improvement occurs in the PPV. Conversely, a decline in specificity of 1% results in a decline in PPV from 29% to 17%. The influence of specificity on PPV becomes apparent in considering that a small change in the false-positive rate influences large numbers of healthy individuals who will have, or avoid, additional testing.

As mentioned, PPV is influenced also by the underlying prevalence of disease, and this influence is entirely on the numerator in the calculation. Even if a screening test is highly accurate, PPV will vary with the prevalence of disease. If sensitivity and specificity remain the same (80% and 99%, respectively) and the prevalence of disease in this example is doubled (i.e., from 500 cases to 1,000 cases), PPV would increase to 44%; if disease prevalence in the population is only 250 cases, PPV would be 18% [20].

Screening Test Performance: Summary Considerations

Summary measures of screening efficacy, such as sensitivity, specificity, and PPV, are relatively uninformative about the contribution of the underlying factors that influence each rate. A general caution is to avoid accepting these estimates uncritically as measures of the maximum achievable test performance.

Sensitivity, specificity, and PPV are the basic indices of screening program performance. Since the majority of individuals who undergo screening examinations do not have cancer or have cancer that is within the DPCP, nearly all normal result interpretation (true-negatives) are accurate. Generally, true-positives are identified soon after an abnormal screening examination finding and are measured by biopsy results. False-negatives or false-positives are based on the assumption that cancer would have been detected, or was not present, at the initial screening examinations on the basis of the presence or absence of histologic confirmation of disease within the specified evaluation period (usually one year).

The sensitivity and specificity of a screening test may be influenced by factors other than simply the ability of the test to detect cancer or to rule out cancer. These factors can be thought of as falling along a continuum. At one end of the continuum are factors that may be outside the influence of screening program modifications or improvements in quality assurance (i.e., these factors are idiosyncratic). In the presence of a wide variation in individual DPCPs, some rate of interval cancers in a screening program is unavoidable, since these cases are not attributable to any source of error during the previous screening examinations. Such cases appear as interval cancers simply because of faster tumor growth rates. Other individual characteristics also may render screening of some individuals a greater challenge: For example, mammography is less useful in women who have such significant breast density that very little mammographic contrast is discernible in the breast parenchyma. Finally, certain disease characteristics challenge the limits of current technology.

At the other end of the continuum are factors that affect test performance through screening program and quality assurance influences. These factors include tailoring screening programs to the estimated DPCP, adhering to test quality-control recommendations, improving the quality of test interpretation and reducing human error, and establishing appropriate interpretive thresholds for a positive test result.

As mentioned, the PPV is a summary measure of screening program efficiency. In evaluating the PPV and comparative rates of PPV, the underlying goal of screening for that particular disease must be considered. A low PPV may indicate lower specificity, lower disease prevalence, or a combination of these two influences. Likewise, a higher PPV may indicate higher specificity or higher disease prevalence (or both) [2]. Obviously, a high PPV is preferred, but a high PPV may not be indicative of good performance. If disease prevalence is high and specificity is very high, a test with relatively poor sensitivity still may have a PPV better than that of a screening test with high sensitivity for a disease of lower prevalence (as in the foregoing example). Alternately, focusing screening on a higher-risk subpopulation may increase PPV by increasing disease prevalence but, again, may be accomplished at the cost of the overall detection rate. PPV is a useful measure of program performance only when it is evaluated in the context of other performance indices, such as the stage distribution of screen-detected cancers and the interval cancer rate. The issue of whether a low PPV is acceptable should be considered by weighing the human and pro-gram costs of a false-positive examination and the recall rate required to reduce significantly the incidence rate of advanced disease.

Cost-Effectiveness

Screening large numbers of healthy people for occult disease can be expensive. In addition to the cost of screening tests are costs associated with diagnostic evaluations and the cost of treatment for screen-detected disease that may never have become clinically apparent. Because of these costs, decisions about screening should be made only after careful consideration of whether the implementation of a screening test meets well-defined criteria related to disease burden, benefit of early detection, test performance, acceptability to the population, and costs. Put another way, does the potential exist for a favorable balance between the benefits of screening and its limitations and costs? In today's managed-care environment, program costs and outcomes receive scrutiny greater than that in any previous period [21].

Two basic models are available for the evaluation of costs and outcomes: cost-benefit analysis (CBA) and cost-effectiveness analysis (CEA). Each model emphasizes measuring costs and benefits, but the two differ in their methods of measuring outcomes. In a CBA, benefits are expressed in monetary terms, whereas benefits in a CEA are expressed as health outcomes [22]. Benefits in a CBA may be based on a human capital model that assigns a monetary "value" to a life. However, assigning a dollar value to health outcomes—a life saved, a reduction in disability, peace of mind, and the like—is both inherently difficult and arbitrary and, as Garber et al. [22] observed, naturally offends sensibilities. An alternative and more accepted approach in CBA is to assign benefit on the basis of an individual's willingness to exchange dollars for a health benefit, an approach that favors those with higher incomes over those with fewer discretionary resources but in any case assumes a rational ability to assess the comparative worth of an "investment" in health against a benefit or odds of a benefit. If costs exceed benefits, the intervention is judged to be non-cost-beneficial and therefore unjustified. CBA is essentially a go/no go equation.

In contrast, cost-effectiveness studies in medicine are focused on the unit or net cost of achieving a particular health-related outcome [23]. In cancer screening, cost-effectiveness can be expressed in terms of the cost to detect one cancer, prevent one death, add a year of life, or add a quality-adjusted year of life. At the most basic level, the most appropriate and intuitive estimate of the cost-effectiveness of cancer screening is an estimate of the marginal cost-per-year of life saved (MCYLS). The marginal costs of screening are the costs incurred by implementing a screening program minus the costs of case detection and management without screening. The marginal effectiveness is the years of life expected and gained in the screened group minus the years of life expected in the group not screened. The MCYLS is the fraction of the marginal costs of screening divided by the marginal effectiveness. In general, if a screening test achieves a benchmark of less than $40,000 per MCYLS, costs are judged to be within acceptable limits of cost-effectiveness [22]. Of course, achieving this benchmark does not preclude additional efforts to improve cost-effectiveness. Likewise, since the benchmark is arbitrary, MCYLS that exceed $40,000 do not necessarily mean that screening is too expensive to be offered to the public, especially if there is a potential to improve cost effectiveness.

CEA offers the potential to measure the value of an intervention against alternatives, which could be the cost of not having the intervention, or alternative interventions focused on the same general outcome (i.e., which of two screening tests is more cost-effective, etc.). A review of the cost-effectiveness literature reveals a broad range of methodologic approaches and the application of different model assumptions and inputs focused on more similar outcomes (e.g., years of life saved). This observation underscores the importance of recent recommendations from the United States Public Health Service Panel on Cost-Effectiveness in Health and Medicine [24]. The overarching purpose for assembling the panel was review of the theoretic foundations of cost-effectiveness analyses and issuance of methodologic recommendations to improve the practice and comparability of cost-effectiveness analyses, especially the latter. The important conclusion from the panel's recommendations is that any summary estimate of the MCYLS must be evaluated by taking into consideration the model inputs and assumptions (e.g., screening costs, expected benefit, timing of benefit, screening intervals, discount rates, and adjustment for health status).

Cost analyses of cancer screening rarely result in a favorable cost-benefit ratio, which is why most cancer screening evaluations are based on cost-effectiveness models. However, as a society, we place a premium on health as a commodity worth the expenditure of surplus value. The most cost-effective screening model merely provides the most benefit for the smallest cost;

it also may be the least beneficial intervention for individuals and thus comparatively less acceptable than more expensive alternatives. In this respect, the statement that a program is or is not cost-effective merely reflects an ad hoc judgment regarding the value of expenditures for a particular benefit. Society may choose a less cost-effective program if it provides greater benefits to individuals undergoing screening.

Acceptability

Participation in screening depends on the acceptance of its value by providers and the public. Low participation in cancer screening among both sectors can be due to low awareness, low perceptions of risk, costs, low access, and aversion to the test or to test results. However, most investigations have shown that each of these barriers can be overcome for the large majority of the population. What is clear is that high levels of participation in a screening program depend on compliance with key roles by both providers and individuals.

Studies have shown consistently that the single most important factor in whether individuals have ever had a screening test or have been screened recently is a recommendation from their health care providers [25–27]. Although public education campaigns may raise awareness and interest in screening, health care providers still play the pivotal role in legitimizing the importance of screening, assisting with informed decisions, performing cancer screening tests, and making referrals for screening outside the primary-care setting [25]. Even more important, the referring provider can serve as a point of reminder for periodic cancer screening.

The single biggest obstacle to regular screening is the lack of provider referral. Because average physician-patient encounters are short and typically occur for acute care, they generally are not conducive to cancer screening or discussions about cancer screening or preventive health counseling [28]. In addition, such other factors as physician-patient ratios, the organization of a practice, lack of preventive health orientation and reminder tools (flow sheets, patient data systems, etc.), neglect, physician specialty, and the like variously have been identified as "structural" barriers to screening [29,30]. Such barriers can lead to a situation in which screening commonly occurs opportunistically rather than regularly.

When screening is organized, however, individuals have a greater likelihood of receiving routine screening. Tools that have been shown to enhance screening include flow sheets, chart reminders, computerized tracking and reminder systems, and group practices [31–34]. In a recent report, Somkin et al. [35] observed that women who received mailed reminders were more likely to have had a recent Papanicolaou (Pap) test and mammogram than were women who had not received reminders. Finally, referring providers are in the key position to help patients to prepare for a screening test, to understand screening results that are abnormal, and to manage follow-up care.

In the United States, considerable resources are dedicated to educating individuals about the importance of early cancer detection. Commonly, these messages derive from the assumption that individuals take action when they perceive a behavior's importance for their health [36]. On the basis of this model, health education related to screening generally communicates the risk of disease, explains the value of screening, and concludes with the recommendation that affected individuals talk with their doctors about testing. Because primary-care providers either conduct the test or provide the referral, this approach targets the "demand side" to achieve cancer screening. Since the majority of individuals are not reminded through a centralized surveillance system to have regular screening, compliance with screening still often depends on patient inquiries [33, 37]. Even with a comprehensive tracking and monitoring system in place, individuals must comply with routine screening invitations and, even more important, with recommendations for follow-up of abnormal test results. The latter, however, should be viewed as a joint responsibility between physicians and patients [19].

METHODOLOGIC ISSUES: EVALUATING EARLY-DETECTION PROGRAMS

The determination of whether a screening intervention is effective may appear to be a simple matter. Theoretically, one only need observe whether persons live longer or have a lesser risk of dying from the disease in question as a result of application of a screening test. Case reports or anecdotal evidence of good outcomes after cancer detection in asymptomatic persons, however, should not be trusted as evidence of screening effectiveness. Screening tests evaluated outside the context of a rigorous research design (described later) are subject to many biases that may, and usually do, invalidate the conclusions being drawn. Included among these complicating factors are lead-time and length biases, subject self-selection, and overdiagnosis.

Lead Time Bias

As described, the interval between the moment in which a condition can be detected by a screening test and the moment in which that condition would have been identified by patient awareness of signs or symptoms is known as the lead time. Unless lead time is accounted for, comparisons of survival rates in screened and unscreened populations will be misleading. Bias always operates toward better survival rates in the screened group, because the length of the lead time advances the point at which survival begins to be measured. Possibly, earlier detection only advances the time of a patient's diagnosis, without moving back the time of death.

Length Bias

As described earlier, the period in the natural history of a cancer during which the tumor may be detected before symptoms appear is the DPCP. The DPCP is the practitioner's "window of opportunity" to advance the point of detection. Different types of cancer offer windows of different length because of variations in tumor growth rates and other biological characteristics. Because of the greater opportunity for detection, more of the cancers with a long preclinical phase will be detected when a population is screened. A tumor with a longer preclinical phase probably also has a longer clinical phase and will be a more indolent and less threatening lesion. This bias toward detection of less threatening cancers is *length bias*. It will complicate the interpretation of outcome differences between cancers detected by screening and those found outside the screening program, because the cancers most likely to escape detection may be the very cancers that have the greatest likelihood of causing death.

Overdiagnosis

The purpose of early detection examinations is to find cancers (and, in some cases, precursor lesions) at an early stage, on the assumption that occult disease eventually will become clinical disease. However, some lesions detected in a screening program may not have the same biological propensity to progress and cause death; in the absence of a screening program, these lesions would remain indolent and would not progress to the point at which symptoms would be apparent. Overdiagnosis is an extreme example of length bias. Because early detection interventions theoretically are more likely than is symptom recognition to yield lesions that might never become clinically significant cancers, survival statistics for screening detected cancers may be biased by the inclusion of a biologically benign subset.

Patient Self-Selection

Persons who elect to undergo early detection tests may differ from those who do not in ways that could affect their survival or recovery. For example, users of early detection services may be more health-conscious, more likely to control such risk factors as smoking or diet, more alert to the signs and symptoms of disease, more adherent to treatment, or generally healthier. Any of these factors could produce a longer survival from cancer independent of early detection, and the better survival observed in screened patients compared with that in the general population could be due more to the selection of patients than to the effect of early detection.

RESEARCH DESIGNS FOR SCREENING EVALUATION

Researchers use several approaches to study cancer screening effectiveness, including descriptive studies, case-control studies, and randomized controlled trials. Each of these strategies has certain strengths and weaknesses. Some methods are more powerful than are others in dealing with the biases described, in particular the randomized clinical trial, but no single approach can provide all the answers needed for the evaluation of screening efficacy. Assessing effectiveness almost always requires combining evidence from multiple sources based on different research methodologies. By this means, the weakness of one method may be compensated by the strengths of another.

Descriptive Studies

Uncontrolled studies based on the experience of physicians, hospitals, and non-population-based registries can yield important information about screening. Often, screening evaluation measures such as sensitivity, specificity, and PPVs are reported first from descriptive studies. The first evidence that screening may be successful is an increase in the number of early cancers, with shifts toward more favorable stage at diagnosis and increased survival rates; later, a reduction in deaths may occur. Descriptive studies, however, do not establish efficacy because of the absence of an appropriate control group and the influence of the previously described potential biases.

Case-Control Studies

Retrospective case-control studies can provide additional evidence of screening effectiveness. The advantage of a case-control approach is that it is a low-cost strategy that may provide evidence more quickly than do prospective studies when the screening procedure already is in clinical use [38]. Although mortality reduction can be an end point measured in these studies, case-control studies are subject to bias and confounding from uncontrolled factors [38]. The case-control design also is not useful for screening tests that have no history of use; therefore, it is unsuited for completely new technologies.

Randomized Clinical Trials

The most rigorous assessment of screening is obtained from randomized clinical trials that primarily measure cancer-specific mortality reduction. In a randomized clinical trial, the distorting effects of self-selection are bypassed through random assignment to either an experimental group invited to receive screening or to another, uninvited group. The mortality end point is not subject to the effects of lead time or length biases.

End results are based on comparisons between invited and uninvited groups rather than on comparisons of the screened and unscreened groups. In effect, the design of a randomized clinical trial of screening evaluates the effect of an invitation to screening rather than screening per se. The distinction is important, because noncompliance with the invitation to screening in the experimental group and contamination in the control group (i.e., participation in screening) has an effect on the magnitude of the observed outcome. Random assignment to a study and control group does not guarantee full compliance with an individual's group assignment, and noncompliance erodes study power and reduces the estimated effect of the intervention. Although randomized clinical trials are most desirable from a methodologic perspective, the sample sizes required, the expense, and their long duration have tended to limit the number of screening trials.

CANCER SCREENING GUIDELINES

The ACS, the United States Preventive Services Task Force (USPSTF), the American Medical Association, the American College of Physicians, and other organizations periodically review the state of the science related to screening for a particular cancer site to issue disease-specific screening guidelines or to endorse guidelines developed by other organizations. Recommendations about cancer screening also result from expert groups, such as those assembled by the National Institutes of Health (NIH) Office of Medical Applications of Research to address clinical practice dilemmas identified as a persistent source of uncertainty among health care providers and patients. The ACS cancer screening guidelines are shown in Table 5.2.

Guidelines can help policy makers, clinicians, and the public to reach decisions about appropriate cancer screening [39]. Although the intent of cancer screening is to reduce mortality, because of the expense of population-based screening and the potential harm to some individuals, in recent years increasing emphasis has been placed on the importance of following an evidence-based process and on articulating the values and evidence-based criteria underlying the final recommendations. Although the issues often seem straightforward, organizations and expert groups can and do reach different conclusions about the value of screening for a particular cancer, about the appropriate target population, about which tests should be used, and about the frequency of testing. These differences can prove to be an obstacle if the lack of consensus causes providers and the public to question the certitude of the recommendation.

Since few objective thresholds are available for making decisions about cancer screening, understanding the rationale for or against a recommendation for cancer screening depends on whether an organization includes a clear description of the process, evidence, and rationale that form the basis for the recommendation. This is especially true for those criteria that pertain to test efficacy, as most guideline differences among organizations are attributable to differences in judgments about whether the evidence regarding the effectiveness of a screening test is sufficiently strong to recommend population-based testing.

The single best source of evidence of the efficacy of a cancer screening test is a randomized clinical trial with a mortality end point. However, there are few of these studies because of the high costs (financial costs and study duration). These costs include the multiple rounds of screening and years of follow-up needed to accumulate sufficient numbers of disease-specific deaths for comparison between the experimental and control groups. Although some organizations may be prepared to draw inferences from evidence from other study designs, other organizations have required data from a randomized trial as the ultimate arbitrator of whether screening can be recommended. Uncertainty is a reasonable basis for an organization's decision not to recommend screening, but favorable as well as unfavorable aspects of the uncertainty should be detailed, as dismissive summary statements about the lack of "scientific" evidence do little to advance understanding of the state of the evidence. An organization may choose to issue a cancer screening recommendation based on available data and inference, as the burden of disease cannot be set aside until the ideal evidence for establishing policy is available. Organizations may be especially inclined to follow this route if no study is underway or even planned. For these reasons, end users will be served better with detailed descriptions of the evidence, how it was reviewed, and how it shaped the final guideline.

Guideline differences between organizations also may be due simply to the timing of the review of new data. The release of clinical practice guidelines, or updates, is based on the accumulation of evidence judged to be sufficient to consider careful review before recommending screening or modifying existing screening guidelines. However, organizations generally are not poised to react at the first sign of new evidence; thus, they may have different guidelines simply owing to the timing of their process of acting on new evidence. However, once new evidence is available, a guideline may become outdated. For this reason, organizations that issue guidelines must review new data often, to ensure that guidance to the public and to the provider community is based on the most current evidence.

Individuals puzzling over differences in guidelines should appreciate that timing, values, and criteria for how evidence is considered are factors that explain differences in current recommendations among organizations. The Agency for Health Care Research Quality (AHCRQ; formerly the Agency for Health Care Policy and Research [AHCPR]) has a listing of cancer screening guidelines (the full text of the organization's guidelines appears on the World Wide Web at http://www.guidelines.gov.).

Table 5.2 American Cancer Society Recommendations for the Early Detection of Cancer in Average-Risk, Asymptomatic People

Cancer Site	Population	Test or Procedure	Frequency
Breast	Women ≥ 20 years old	Breast self-examination Clinical breast examination (CBE)[a] Mammography	Monthly, ≥ 20 years old Every 3 years, 20–39 years old; Annual, ≥ 40 years old Annual, ≥ 40 years old
Colon-rectum	Men and women ≥ 50 years old	FOBT and flexible sigmoidoscopy[b] *or* Double-contrast barium enema[b] *or* Colonoscopy[b]	Annual FOBT and flexible sigmoidoscopy every 5 years beginning at age 50; Double-contrast barium enema every 5–10 years beginning at age 50; Colonoscopy every 10 years beginning at age 50
Prostate	Men ≥ 50 years old	Digital rectal examination and prostate-specific antigen test	Both should be offered annually to men 50 years and older[c]
Cervix	Female ≥ 18 years old	Papanicolaou (Pap) test and pelvic examination	All women who are, or have been, sexually active, or have reached age 18, should have an annual Pap test and pelvic examination. After a woman has had 3 consecutive satisfactory normal examination results, the Pap test may be performed less frequently at the discretion of her physician.
Cancer-related checkup	Men and women ≥ 20 years old	The cancer-related checkup should include examination for cancers of the thyroid, testicles, ovaries, lymph nodes, oral cavity, and skin and health counseling about tobacco, sun, exposure, diet and nutrition, risk factors, sexual practices, and environmental and occupational exposures.	Examinations every 3 years at ages 30–39; annually at ages 40 and older

FOBT = fecal occult blood test.
[a]Beginning at age 40, an annual CBE should be done prior to mammography.
[b]Digital rectal examinations should be done at the time of sigmoidoscopy, barium enema, and colonoscopy.
[c]Health care providers should provide patients with information about the potential risks and benefits of early detection and treatment and assist them with making informed decisions about testing.

DISEASE-SPECIFIC RECOMMENDATIONS: EVIDENCE AND METHODS

Breast Cancer

DISEASE BURDEN

Breast cancer is the most common malignancy diagnosed in American women. It accounts for nearly one in three new diagnoses of cancer [8, 40]. According to ACS estimates, invasive breast cancer will be diagnosed in 182,800 women in 2000, and ductal carcinoma in situ (DCIS) will be diagnosed in an additional 42,600 women [8, 40]. The large number of new cases of DCIS is a relatively new phenomenon, mostly attributable to the increase in the use of mammography. Presently, the estimated incidence of DCIS and invasive disease exceeds the combined estimated incidence of respiratory, colorectal, endometrial, and ovarian cancer. DCIS has been regarded as a nonobligate precursor of invasive breast cancer, representing a continuum of risk based on tumor heterogeneity similar to that observed with invasive disease, with both prognosis and risk of recurrence associated with the histologic characteristics of the lesion [41, 42]. However, results from the National Surgical Adjuvant Breast and Bowel Project B-17 trial [43] observed that recurrence with invasive disease was associated with all grades of DCIS. The exact proportion of detected but untreated DCIS that would progress to invasive breast cancer is not known but has been estimated to be between 25% and 50% [41].

Breast cancer is the second most common cause of cancer mortality among women, accounting for nearly one in five cancer deaths. Among US women, death from breast cancer also is a leading cause of premature mortality. On average, a woman dying of breast cancer has lost 19.2 years of expected life [9].

Breast cancer is rare among men. The ACS estimated that 1,400 new cases of male breast cancer will occur in 2000 and that 400 deaths will result, less than 1% of the annual incidence and mortality among women [40]. Men are not included in screening recommendations for breast cancer because the disease is so rare in men. However, clinicians should be sensitive to clinical signs of symptomatic disease in men because they are identical to those seen in women.

The overall five-year survival rate for breast cancer cases diagnosed in 1990 is 85% [9]. When calculated by extent of disease at diagnosis, five-year survival is much improved if breast cancer is diagnosed while still localized (97%) and is progressively poorer for regional (77%) and distant disease (22%).

SCREENING RECOMMENDATIONS

The first breast cancer screening guidelines were issued by the NCI in 1977 after a consensus conference focused on questions about age-specific benefits from breast cancer screening and concerns about radiation exposure during mammographic examinations [44]. These first guidelines recommended annual mammography for women aged 50 years and older and mammography for women aged 40 to 49 only if they had a personal history of breast cancer or a first-degree relative with breast cancer. The ACS endorsed this core recommendation and added recommendations for routine clinical breast examination (CBE) and breast self-examination (BSE). In subsequent years, new data have led to modifications in breast cancer screening guidelines, with changes in screening intervals, targeted age groups, and

a new emphasis on surveillance for high-risk groups [45, 46]. One noteworthy feature of this period has been the recurring controversy over screening women aged 40 to 49. Although some organizations have endorsed screening this group, others have not [47–50].

The ACS recommends that women begin monthly BSE at age 20 and that women between ages 20 and 39 undergo a clinical breast examination every three years (see Table 5.2). Beginning at age 40, women should have an annual mammogram and CBE. The ACS also stressed that CBE should take place prior to mammography and that a short interval should separate the two examinations. The reason given is that if a mass is present, it can be brought to the attention of the radiologist and a diagnostic evaluation can be considered. If CBE follows mammography and discloses a mass undetected on a mammogram, the patient would have to return for additional directed imaging. CBE before mammography avoids potential waste of resources. The ACS breast cancer screening guidelines impose no upper age limit, as long as women are in good health. Women at significantly higher risk for breast cancer should consult with their health care providers about beginning screening earlier. Recommendations for women at higher risk because of significant family history were recently developed by the Cancer Genetics Studies Consortium [51].

The most recent change in guidelines followed several international consensus conferences that took place during 1996 and 1997. On January 21, 1997, the NIH Office of Medical Applications of Research and the NCI jointly sponsored a Consensus Development Conference on Breast Cancer Screening for women aged 40 to 49 [52]. The NIH conference was organized in response to new breast cancer screening data presented in March 1996 at an international conference in Falun, Sweden sponsored by the Swedish Cancer Society and the Swedish National Board of Health and Welfare [53]. At the conclusion of the NIH conference, the panel's overriding conclusion was "that the data currently available do not warrant a universal recommendation for mammography for all women in their forties. Each woman should decide for herself whether to undergo mammography" [52].

The panel also recommended that a woman's decision about whether to undergo mammography should be based not only on the scientific evidence but on her medical history, her perception of risk and benefit, and her method of dealing with uncertainty. The outcome of the meeting was highly controversial as measured initially by extensive media coverage and subsequently by the inclusion of a dissenting minority report published with the final report [52]. Several months after the NIH meeting, the ACS reviewed the same data and reached a different conclusion (as noted earlier), revising its breast cancer screening guidelines on the basis of the new data from the world's trials, in particular new data about differences in tumor growth rates in premenopausal and postmenopausal women [54]. The American College of Radiology and the American Medical Association also have modified their guidelines and issued the same breast cancer screening recommendation as that of the ACS [55, 56]. The NCI revisited their guidelines after the NIH meeting, and on the advice of the National Cancer Advisory Board, rejected the conclusion of the NIH panel and recommended that women should begin mammography in their forties and should undergo a mammogram every one to two years; after age 50, a woman should have a mammogram every one to two years. The NCI did not take a position on CBE or BSE [57]. In its most recent guidelines statement, the USPSTF conceded insufficient evidence to recommend for or against breast cancer—screening for women younger than age 50 or older than age 70 and recommended mammography every one to two years for women between the ages of 50 and 69. However, the most recent revision of the USPSTF guidelines occurred in 1996 and therefore was issued prior to the availability of more recent data from randomized clinical trials supporting the efficacy of mammography in women aged 40 to 49 [50].

SCREENING AND DIAGNOSTIC METHODS

The single most effective tool for the early detection of breast cancer is mammography. Guidelines for early breast cancer detection emphasize a combination of BSE, CBE, and mammography as a complete program of surveillance. After age 40, the principle roles of BSE and CBE are to identify masses that were not detected on mammography due to test limitations, rapid tumor growth, or human error.

Breast Self-Examination
BSE should begin at age 20 and should be performed monthly. Women may follow various techniques for BSE, but the choice of any technique probably can be made on the basis of personal preference. As with clinical examinations, BSE should be performed systematically and should include both manual palpation and a visual inspection of the breasts. Because some premenopausal women experience breast discomfort near the time of menstruation, they may find that BSE is more comfortable 8–10 days after the beginning of the menses.

Clinical Breast Examination
CBE is the physical palpation of the breast by a trained clinician. Today, its role in early breast cancer detection is defined primarily by a woman's age. Between the ages of 20 and 40, CBE is the clinical complement to BSE, and its performance every three years is recommended. Beginning at age 40, women should undergo CBE annually and ideally near and prior to the time of their annual mammogram. Technique is important and should be systematic. A competent physical examination includes palpation in small segments, from the nipple to the periphery of the breast, including the axilla [58].

Mammography
Screening mammography is a radiographic examination of the breasts to detect abnormalities that may be breast cancer. Modern mammography has evolved from the use of general purpose x-ray equipment to today's dedicated imaging equipment. During the last decade, significant resources have been devoted to lowering radiographic dose and to improving image quality. Average breast dose per view has been reduced from several centiGrays (cGy, or rads) to 1–2 mGy (0.1–0.2 rads) per view [59]. Image quality and interpretive skills also have been improved through early and ongoing efforts by the American College of Radiology's Mammography Accreditation Program, and subsequently through the passage of the Mammography Quality Standards Act of 1992, which requires a facility to meet a broad range of technical and personnel standards to be certified by the US Food and Drug Administration (FDA) as a provider of mammography services [60, 61].

A screening mammogram involves two views of each breast: a craniocaudal view and a mediolateral oblique view. Prior to obtaining the radiograph, a radiologic technologist positions a woman's breast in a compression device. The purpose of compression is to equalize the thickness of the breast, to separate breast tissues that may obscure a lesion, to permit even penetration, to prevent motion blur, to improve contrast (by decreasing radiation scatter), and to reduce radiation dose to the breast. Compression may cause some discomfort but is essential to ensure sensitivity. After the examination, an interpreting physician (nearly always a radiologist) examines the films for abnormalities. Generally, the rate of abnormal findings is higher for first screening examinations, but overall, the average range of initial abnormal screening results is 5–10% [62].

In most instances, abnormalities are resolved through additional diagnostic mammography imaging with special views, or ultrasonography. Under new FDA rules,

Table 5.3   American College of Radiology Breast Imaging and Reporting Data System (BI-RADS) Assessment Categories

Category 0	**Need Additional Imaging Evaluation:**
	Finding for which additional imaging evaluation is needed. This is almost always used in a screening situation and should be used rarely after a full imaging evaluation. Includes the use of spot compression, magnification, special mammographic views, and ultrasound. The radiologist should use judgment in determining how vigorously to pursue previous studies.
Category 1	**Negative:**
	There is nothing on which to comment. The breasts are symmetrical and no masses, architectural disturbances, or suspicious calcifications are present.
Category 2	**Benign Findings:**
	There is also a negative mammogram, but the interpreter may wish to describe a finding. Involuting calcified fibroadenomas, multiple secretory calcifications, fat-containing lesions such as oil cysts, lipomas, galactoceles, and mixed-density hamartomas all have characteristic appearances and may be labeled with confidence. The interpreter might wish to describe intramammary lymph nodes, implants, and the like while still concluding that there is no mammographic evidence of malignancy.
Category 3	**Probably Benign Findings; Short-Interval Follow-up Suggested:**
	A finding placed in this category should have a very high probability of being benign. It is not expected to change over the follow-up period. At the present time, most approaches are intuitive. These will likely undergo future modification as more data accrue as to the validity of an approach, the interval required, and the type of findings that should be followed.
Category 4	**Suspicious Abnormality; Biopsy Should Be Considered:**
	These are lesions that do not have the characteristic morphologies of breast cancer but have a definite probability of being malignant. The radiologist has sufficient concern to urge a biopsy. If possible, the relevant probabilities should be cited so that the patient and her physician can make the decision on the ultimate course of action.
Category 5	**Highly Suggestive of Malignancy; Appropriate Action Should Be Taken:**
	These lesions have a high probability of being cancerous.

Note: Category 0 is regarded as an incomplete assessment; categories 1–5 are final assessments.
Source: Modified with permission from the American College of Radiology, *Illustrated Breast Imaging Reporting and Data System* (3rd ed). Reston, VA: American College of Radiology, 1998.

the results of screening must be reported to the referring physician and directly to patients in lay language [63]. The American College of Radiology has developed the Breast Imaging Reporting and Data system (BI-RADS) in an effort to standardize mammography reporting, to improve communication with referring physicians and other radiologists, and to standardize data for mammography practice audits, required by FDA as an ongoing source of practice internal review for self-improvement (Table 5.3) [64]. Generally, abnormalities that cannot be resolved with additional imaging will be biopsied using fine-needle aspiration, ultrasonography or radiographically directed core needle biopsy, or will be surgically excised.

At present, no other imaging modality is recommended for primary screening for breast cancer. Ultrasonography may be used to resolve palpable abnormalities that are not seen on a mammogram, to differentiate cystic from solid masses, and (in some rare instances) to screen for nonpalpable masses when the breast contains such dense parenchyma that screen-film mammography is not useful [65]. Other imaging modalities that likely will have a role in breast imaging in the future are digital mammography and magnetic resonance imaging [66–70]. Light scanning (diaphanography and transillumination), thermography, and xeromammography are not recommended for breast cancer screening [71].

EVIDENCE OF EFFECTIVENESS

Mammography

No other cancer screening test has been studied as extensively as has mammography. When experimental work with x-rays early in the 20th century by Salomon and others demonstrated the detection of occult breast disease, the potential for diagnosis before the onset of clinical symptoms was established [72, 73]. Since it was well established by this time that disease prognosis was more favorable with early detection, these discoveries ushered in both the technology and the public health impetus to screen for breast cancer.

The first trial of breast cancer screening, the Health Insurance Plan (HIP) of New York study, was initiated in December 1963 [74]. It was the first randomized, controlled trial to evaluate the efficacy of breast cancer screening with CBE and mammography. Approximately 62,000 women aged 40 to 64 were randomly assigned to two groups: The experimental group would be offered annual CBE and two-view mammography (craniocaudal and mediolateral views) for four years, and the control group would receive usual care. Ten years into the study, the study group demonstrated approximately 30% fewer breast cancer deaths than did the control group [75]. The favorable results of the HIP study led the ACS and the NCI to launch the Breast Cancer Detection Demonstration Project (BCDDP) to determine whether mammography screening could be applied successfully in the community [76]. To answer these questions, the BCDDP screened more than 280,000 women at 29 centers between 1973 and 1980. The results were consistent with what had been observed in the HIP study: Specifically, the breast cancer stage distribution was much more favorable among study participants than among incident cases in the NCI's Surveillance, Epidemiology, and End Results program during the same period, and overall long-term survival likewise has been better over the duration of follow-up using this same comparison population [77]. These results, in combination with the findings from the HIP study, were sufficiently persuasive to justify promotion of routine breast cancer screening, a public health initiative that continues to be a high priority. In addition to the HIP and BCDDP studies, seven randomized trials in Sweden, the United Kingdom, and Canada have contributed evidence related to screening for breast cancer with mammography (Table 5.4) [78–82].

During the last two decades, a debate over the value of mammography among women younger than 50 has dominated deliberations about breast cancer screening and has been a source of an ongoing and, at times, highly visible debate in the United States and in Europe [47, 83–89]. Although many leading medical organizations in the United States endorsed breast cancer screening for women aged 40 to 49, some equally prominent organizations did not. For the most part, the dispute over screening policy for women younger than age 50 was based on the lack of clear evidence from the world's trials that mammography screening for women aged 40 to 49 was effective.

Before 1997, two trials—the HIP trial of Greater New York and the Swedish two-county trial—had shown a statistically significant reduction in breast cancer mortality among women aged 50 and older, but no statistically significant reduction in deaths had been observed from an individual trial for women aged 40 to 49 [78, 90]. Although indirect evidence suggested a benefit from both the trials and observational studies, until recently no trial or meta-analysis had shown a statistically

significant reduction in breast cancer deaths among women who were in their forties at the time of random assignment to screening. Some researchers were persuaded by the absence of definitive evidence of a benefit, but others argued that the absence of a statistically significant mortality reduction was an artifact of methodologic shortcomings in trials, in particular low statistical power for subgroup analysis [91]. As seen in Table 5.4, each trial followed a somewhat different protocol that in some instances, based on the accumulation of data over the last several decades, has important implications for the interpretation of study results. These factors include the study methodology, the clinical protocol (screening interval, number of views, etc.), participation rates in the study group (compliance), screening rates in the control group (contamination), and the number of screening rounds before an invitation was extended to the control group [92, 93].

To overcome the limitations of small sample sizes in the group of women aged 40 to 49, investigators began to conduct meta-analyses of trial data, combining age-specific results from the various studies [94–98]. In 1995, Smart et al. [97] published the first meta-analysis showing a statistically significant reduction in deaths for women in the aged 40 to 49 group. The most recent meta-analysis using the most current trial data results, with average follow-up of 12.7 years, results in a relative risk (RR) of 0.82 (18% fewer breast cancer deaths in the study group) when all trials are combined, a RR of 0.74 (26% fewer deaths in the study group) when only population-based trials are combined (i.e., excluding the National Breast Screening Study [NBSS]-1), and an RR of 0.71 (29% fewer deaths in the study group) for all five Swedish randomized, controlled trials [98]. Each point estimate is statistically significant at the 95% confidence level, although the all-trial meta-analysis has the lowest RR of breast cancer mortality owing to the excess rate of breast cancer deaths in the NBSS-1 among the group invited to screening (see Table 5.4). The meta-analysis of Swedish trials is included in this comparison because those trials represent a more homogeneous group and because they include the two second-generation trials (i.e., Gothenburg and Malmö), which applied more advanced screening protocols and observed 44% and 36% fewer breast cancer deaths (statistically significant) in the invited groups as compared with the control groups. The consistency of results in the other meta-analyses and the recent results from Gothenburg and Malmö indicate that the potential benefit of screening in premenopausal and postmenopausal women is more similar than different. More recent analyses of trial data have provided important insights

Table 5.4 Randomized Controlled Trials of Breast Cancer Screening

Study (Duration)	Screening Protocol	Frequency, no. of rounds	Study Population				Follow-up (years)	RR (95% CI)
			Age (years)	Subgroup	Invited	Control		
HIP Study (1963–1969)	2 VMM CBE	Annually, 4	40–64	40–49	14,432	14,701	18	0.77 (0.53–1.11)
				50–64	16,568	16,299	18	0.80 (0.59–1.08)
Edinburgh[a] (1979–1988)	1 or 2 VMM	24 months, 4 rounds	45–64	45–49	11,755	10,641	12.6	0.81 (0.54–1.20)
				50–64	11,245	12,359	10	0.85 (0.62–1.15)
Kopparberg (1977–1985)	1 VMM	24 months, 4 rounds	40–74	40–49	9,650	5,009	15.2	0.67 (0.37–1.22)
				50–74	28,939	13,551	11	0.58 (0.43–0.78)
Ostergotland (1977–1985)	1 VMM	24 months, 4 rounds	40–74	40–49	10,240	10,411	14.2	1.02 (0.59–1.77)
				50–74	28,229	26,830	11	0.73 (0.56–0.97)
Mälmo[b]	1 or 2 VMM	18–24 months, 5 rounds	45–69	45–49	13,528	12,242	12.7	0.64 (0.45–0.89)
				50–69	17,134	17,165	9	0.86 (0.64–1.16)
Stockholm (1981–1985)	1 VMM	28 months, 2 rounds	40–64	40–49	14,185	7,985	11.4	1.01 (0.51–2.02)
				50–64	25,815	12,015	7	0.65 (0.4–1.08)
Gothenburg (1982–1988)	2 VMM	18 months, 5 rounds	39–59	39–49	11,724	14,217	12	0.56 (0.32–0.98)
				50–59	9,276	16,394	5	0.91 (0.62–1.52)
NBSS-1 (1980–1987)	2 VMM CBE	12 months, 45 rounds	40–49	40–49	25,214	25,216	10.5	1.14 (0.83–1.56)
NBSS-2 (1980–1987)	2 VMM CBE	12 months, 45 rounds	50–59	50–59	19,711	19,694	7.0	0.97 (0.62–1.52)

RR = relative risk; CI = confidence interval; HIP = Health Insurance Plan; 1 VMM = one-view mammography of each breast; 2 VMM = two-view mammography of each breast; CBE = clinical breast examination; NBSS = National Breast Screening Study.

[a]The Edinburgh trial included three separate groups of women 45–49 years old at entry: In the first were 5,949 women in the invited group and 5,818 in the control group (with 14 years follow-up); the second was composed of 2,545 in the invited group and 2,482 in the control group (12 years follow-up); and the third included 3,261 in the invited group and 2,341 in the control group (10 years follow-up) [81]. Only the results of the first group had been previously reported.

[b]The Mälmo trial included two groups of women aged 45–49 years old at entry: One group (MMST-I) received first-round screening in 1977–1978 and included 3,954 women in the invited group and 4,030 women in the control group. The second group (MMST-II) received first-round screening from 1978 to 1990 and was composed of 9,574 women in the invited group and 8,212 women in the control group [79]. Only the results of the first group had been previously reported.

about screening in different age groups of women and have helped to explain why early trial results provided less favorable results in premenopausal women [53, 99].

As noted, in the individual trials a mortality benefit begins to appear relatively early (approximately five years) for women who were aged 50 and older at randomization, whereas it occurs much later for women who were aged 40 to 49 at randomization. Second, with accumulating years of follow-up in the aged 40 to 49 group, the RR of mortality steadily improves. Some have argued that the delayed benefit in women aged 40 to 49 was a function of small sample sizes and overall better survival in younger women as compared with older women [100]. Conversely, others have argued that the observed delay in benefit was an artifact of trial design, in which mortality reductions attributed to women in their forties actually were due to diagnoses after age 50 among women randomly assigned in their forties (i.e., a woman assigned at age 49 reaches age 50 in the second year of the trial, etc.) [101]. Recent analysis of the two-county data provides a clearer and more clinically intuitive explanation for the delay in benefit based on the interrelationship among tumor histology, the DPCP, and age [99]. As described, the mean breast cancer DPCP (i.e., potential lead time) is shorter (1.7 years) in women younger than age 50, compared with women older than age 50 (3.3+ years) [102, 103]. Because the majority of the world's trials screened women aged 40 to 49 at an interval of 24 months, faster tumor growth rates in women in their forties meant that they were less likely to benefit from mammography than were women aged 50 and older. The organizers of the Falun meeting concluded that the screening interval of 24 or more months was differentially effective in reducing mortality among women aged 40 to 49 versus women aged 50 and older. Among the groups invited to screening, the 24-month interval was equally effective in women younger and older than age 50 for grade 2, medullary, and invasive lobular tumors, and it was effective in reducing deaths among grade 3 tumors diagnosed in women aged 50 and older. However, the 24-month interval was not effective for grade 3 tumors diagnosed in women aged 40 to 49, and women with diagnosed high-nuclear-grade tumors accounted for a significant proportion of deaths observed early in the trial (i.e., soon after diagnosis).

Other recent data reveal the importance of tailoring the DPCP to screening intervals. New results from the Gothenburg trial, which screened women aged 39 to 49 at 18-month intervals, show that the timing of the benefit, which appears at six to eight years, is similar to that observed for women aged 50 and older [82]. In the Gothenburg trial, which screened women aged 40 to 49 every 18 months and showed a 44% reduction in breast cancer mortality, the proportional interval cancer incidence was 18% in the first 12 months after a negative screen result and increased to more than 50% in the period 12 to 18 months [82].

In the University of California at San Francisco screening program, a similar pattern has been observed. Sensitivity declined at twice the rate in the interval between one and two years for women in their forties, compared with women aged 50 and older, reflecting faster tumor growth rates for women in their forties [104]. According to Sickles [104], interval cancer rates for women aged 40 to 49 who are screened annually are approximately equivalent to interval cancer rates in women aged 50 years and older screened every two years.

If the screening interval is greater than the mean DPCP, the potential for the program to reduce the rate of advanced disease will be reduced, since a higher proportion of cancers will progress undetected to the point at which they become clinically evident and appear as interval cancers. Although adherence to recommended screening intervals is important to the success of any breast cancer screening program, it is an especially important factor for reducing the rate of advanced disease in premenopausal women.

The sensitivity and specificity of mammography fall within acceptable parameters and vary somewhat by age, with sensitivity, specificity, and PPV improving in successive age groups of women. Historically, reports of sensitivity and specificity have been influenced by the debate over the value of screening women younger than age 50 leading to the erroneous conclusion that sensitivity, specificity, and PPV were uniform within premenopausal and postmenopausal women and were measurably poorer in premenopausal versus postmenopausal women [49, 105]. Sensitivity measures available from the trials were influenced also by the screening interval, especially for women younger than age 50. More recent data examining sensitivity, specificity, and PPV by age have shown a continuum of improvement with increasing age and have demonstrated that performance in adjacent decades of life is more similar than different [106, 107].

Physical Examination
Over time, mammography has superseded physical examinations as the most sensitive and important examination for the early detection of breast cancer. Before mammography became available, suspicious abnormalities were detected by physical examinations by clinicians or by the women themselves (including self-detection apart from systematic examination). Indeed, the origins of breast cancer detection through palpation has led to the common characterization of any breast abnormality detected during screening as a "lump," even though a majority of mammographic abnormalities are not palpable.

No randomized trials have tested the efficacy of CBE as a single screening modality. CBE has been included in some randomized trials of mammography, but any estimation of the sensitivity of CBE in these early studies must be interpreted in the historical context of the sensitivity of mammography at that time. In the HIP study, two-thirds of the breast cancers detected were palpable, and nearly half were detected only by palpation [108]. Some trials have examined the combined modality of mammography and CBE and have revealed that a small percentage of palpable masses are not seen on mammography. These factors have led to guidelines that include routine CBE, ideally near to and prior to the occasion of the mammogram, as part of the screening regimen [109, 110]. A patient with a palpable mass detected prior to her screening mammogram is no longer asymptomatic, and a screening mammogram is inappropriate. A negative mammogram finding in the presence of a palpable mass does not rule out breast cancer; the AHCRQ has recommended strongly that problem-solving techniques such as ultrasound and directed biopsy be considered in such instances [71]. In one study of breast cancer litigation, the majority of cases were due to failure to respond appropriately to a palpable mass; in a significant percentage, a negative mammogram result was judged to be definitive [111].

Since mammography use has become more common and constitutes a primary emphasis of health education messages about breast cancer, concerns have been raised about the adequacy of CBE training in medical school and about use and quality of CBE in the primary-care setting [112, 113]. In particular, male physicians were more likely to report that perceived embarrassment among female patients was a factor in determining how often they performed CBE, which is consistent with findings from another study that showed that the patients of male physicians had higher rates of breast cancer screening with mammography only compared with female physicians' patients [113].

BSE has obvious appeal as a screening test because it is simple and convenient, presents no financial cost to participants, is noninvasive, and is intended to lead to earlier awareness of the presence of symptoms. However, recommendations for BSE have been controversial due to a lack of definitive evidence of its efficacy and to concerns about harms, including (1) the possibility of distracting from the importance of mammography, (2) false reassurance, (3) heightened anxiety about breast cancer, (4) anxiety during the examination, and (5) false-positive results [114–118]. Findings about efficacy have been mixed. Some studies have shown improvements in breast cancer survival among women who practiced BSE, whereas others have not [119, 120]. Results of studies of the association between tumor size and BSE also have been mixed; some studies showed average tumor size as smaller among practitioners of BSE, compared with nonpractitioners, whereas other studies showed no advantage [117, 118]. Moreover,

some studies have suggested that although BSE per se may have limited efficacy, highly proficient BSE may be effective in reducing the incidence rate of advanced disease or death from breast cancer [121, 122]. Several randomized trials of BSE have been initiated, but summary findings have not been published [123, 124].

KEY ISSUES

Commonly, age-specific comparisons of the efficacy of breast cancer screening have compared an under-50 age group with an over-50 age group (ages 40–49 compared with age 50 and older). If both disease burden and screening performance were homogeneous among women older than 50, logic would justify these comparisons. Yet, as the data show, this broad-brush approach obscures similarities between women in smaller, proximate age groups. Given the size of these cohorts, comparing and evaluating screening performance by decade of life is more appropriate and interesting. Evaluation of screening performance by decade of life shows only small differences in the performance of mammography in successive age groups [125].

Much of the controversy over BSE is easily set aside if the value and potential of BSE are placed in context. BSE is not a substitute for mammography; thus, health education messages must be clear about the unique advantages of mammography as compared with physical examinations. During the relatively low-incidence period (between ages 20 and 40), routine BSE may result in earlier detection among regular and proficient practitioners than among women not practicing BSE. BSE advocates cite as one its chief advantages the creation of a heightened awareness of breast changes, detectable during BSE or at any other time [126]. After age 40, BSE is a safety net for breast abnormalities that may be missed on mammography or may arise in the interval between examinations. Just as women should be instructed that mammography offers them the greatest advantage for early detection, they should be counseled that the appearance of symptoms after a normal mammogram finding must not be discounted. Finally, to the extent that some women experience anxiety about BSE and during BSE, they should receive proper training in the technique, and clinicians should be prepared to evaluate BSE performance periodically.

Breast cancer screening has been shown to reduce mortality in clinical trials, and increasing rates of screening during the last 15 years have been associated with recent declines in breast cancer death rates in the United States [127]. Greater benefits from mammography are possible if improvements in quality assurance are achieved and if breast cancer screening can evolve from opportunistic screening to organized screening. In addition, health education messages must evolve to inform women fully about the benefits and limitations of screening.

Colorectal Cancer

DISEASE BURDEN

Colorectal cancer is the third most common cancer diagnosed among men and among women and is the third leading cause of cancer mortality within each group. The ACS estimated that in 2000, colorectal cancer will be diagnosed in 130,200 men and women and that 56,300 will die of this disease [8, 40]. Incidence and mortality rates increase with age, are somewhat higher for men than for women, and are higher in blacks than in whites. Incidence and mortality rates have been declining in recent years among whites but have increased among blacks. More favorable disease trends among whites are likely attributable to both declining incidence and more favorable survival.

Among those with diagnosed colorectal cancer, survival is highly dependent on disease stage at diagnosis. Five-year survival is 91% if the disease is diagnosed while still localized (i.e., confined to the wall of the bowel) but is only 66% for regional disease (i.e., disease with lymph node involvement) and is 9% in the presence of distant metastases. However, to date, use of colorectal screening procedures has been low; thus, between 1990 and 1995, only one in three colorectal cancers were diagnosed while still localized.

SCREENING RECOMMENDATIONS

Most organizations recommend that average-risk adults be screened regularly for colorectal cancer, beginning at age 50. As shown in Tables 5.2 and 5.5, the ACS recommends three options: a fecal occult blood test (FOBT) and flexible sigmoidoscopy (FSIG), with FOBT repeated annually and FSIG repeated every five years after the initial screening; double-contrast barium enema (DCBE) every 5–10 years; or colonoscopy every 10 years. Annual digital rectal examination (DRE) no longer is recommended due to low sensitivity, but DRE should be performed prior to FSIG, DCBE, or colonoscopy. A multidisciplinary expert panel convened by the AHCRQ also issued similar guidelines in 1997, including two additional routine screening alternatives: annual FOBT alone (without periodic FSIG) or FSIG every five years (without annual FOBT). These guidelines have been endorsed by the American College of Gastroenterology, the American Gastroenterological Association, the American Society of Colon and Rectal Surgeons, the American Society for Gastrointestinal Endoscopy, the Crohn's and Colitis Foundation of America, the Oncology Nursing Society, and the Society of American Gastrointestinal Endoscopic Surgeons [128]. The ACS also has endorsed these guidelines but does not recommend periodic FSIG without annual FOBT, or FOBT alone unless FSIG is not available in the community, because each examination alone is less sensitive than are the two combined [129]. The USPSTF recommends annual FOBT beginning at age 50, or periodic FSIG, although an interval is not specified [130]. The USPSTF declined to recommend alternatives to FOBT and FSIG, finding insufficient evidence to recommend for or against periodic DCBE or colonoscopy [130].

Table 5.5 shows guidelines for higher-risk individuals. Such individuals include those with a family history or individual history of adenomatous polyps or colorectal cancer, a family history of familial adenomatous polyposis, a family history of hereditary nonpolyposis colorectal cancer (HNPCC), or a personal history of inflammatory bowel disease [129]. In general, colorectal cancer screening guidelines for higher-risk individuals recommend earlier surveillance and more complete examinations.

SCREENING AND DIAGNOSTIC METHODS

Fecal Occult Blood Test

The FOBT detects the presence of blood in stool that may derive from colorectal cancer or from large polyps (> 2 cm). Small polyps do not tend to bleed, and bleeding from cancers or large polyps is intermittent, observations that argue in support of annual testing and the obtaining of serial specimens during the annual test [131]. A positive FOBT result is the basis for a diagnostic workup to identify the source of bleeding by examining the entire colon with either DCBE or colonoscopy.

The most common FOBTs in use today are guaiac-based (Hemoccult II and Hemoccult SENSA), followed by immunochemical tests (HemeSelect and HemoQuant). Guaiac-based tests detect blood in the stool through the pseudoperoxidase activity of heme, or hemoglobin, whereas the immunochemical tests react with human hemoglobin. Hemoccult II and Hemoccult SENSA test results can be obtained in a physician's office, whereas the immunochemical test results are

Table 5.5   American Cancer Society Guidelines for Screening and Surveillance for the Early Detection of Colorectal Polyps and Cancer, by Risk Category

Risk Category and Description	Recommendation	Age (years) to begin	Screening Interval and Recommendations
Average			
Men and women ≥ 50 years old without moderate and high-risk characteristics (as described below)	One of the following: FOBT plus flexible sigmoidoscopy[a] *or* TCE[b]	50 50	FOBT every year and flexible sigmiodoscopy every 5 years[c] Colonoscopy every 10 years or DCBE every 5–10 years
Moderate			
People with single, small (< 1 cm) adenomatous polyps	Colonoscopy	At the time of initial polyp diagnosis	TCE within 3 years after initial polyp removal; if normal, follow recommendations for average-risk individuals
People with large (≥ 1 cm) or multiple adenomatous polyps of any size	Colonoscopy	At the time of initial polyp diagnosis	TCE within 3 years after initial polyp removal; if normal, TCE every 5 years
Personal history of curative-intent resection of colorectal cancer	TCE	Within 1 year after resection	If normal, TCE in 3 years; if second TCE result is normal, TCE in 5 years
Colorectal cancer or adenomatous polyps in first-degree relative younger than age 60, or in at least first-degree relatives of any age	TCE	Age 40 or 10 years before the youngest case in the family, whichever is earlier	Every 5 years
Colorectal cancer in other relatives (not first-degree)	Follow recommendations for average-risk individuals		
High			
Family history of FAP	Early surveillance with endoscopy, counseling to consider genetic testing, and referral for specialty care	Puberty	If genetic test result is positive or polyposis is confirmed, consider colectomy; otherwise, continue endoscopy every 1–2 years
Family history of HNPCC	Colonoscopy and counseling to consider genetic testing	21	If untested, or genetic test result is positive, colonoscopy every 2 years until age 40; after age 40, colonoscopy annually
Inflammatory bowel disease	Colonoscopy with biopsies for dysplasia	8 years after the start of pancolitis; 12–15 years after the start of left-sided colitis	Colonoscopy every 1–2 years

FOBT = fecal occult blood test; TCE = total colon examination; DCBE = double-contrast barium enema; FAP = familial adenomatous polyposis; HNPCC = hereditary nonpolyposis colorectal cancer.

[a]Digital rectal examination should be done at the time of each sigmoidoscopy, colonoscopy, or DCBE.

[b]TCE includes either colonoscopy or DCBE. Flexible sigmoidoscopy should be added to DCBE in those instances when the rectosigmoid colon is not well visualized; DCBE should be added to the examination in those instances when the entire colon cannot be visualized by colonoscopy.

[c]FOBT and flexible sigmoidoscopy should begin at age 50. *Repeat* FOBT annually and flexible sigmoidoscopy every 5 years.

Source: Adapted from T Byers, B Levin, D Rothenberger, et al. American Cancer Society guidelines for screening and surveillance for early detection of colorectal polyps and cancer: update 1997. *CA Cancer J Clin* 47:154–160, 1997.

obtained in a laboratory. Rehydration of specimens improves sensitivity but remains controversial because of the associated increase in false-positive outcomes. The reported sensitivity of a single FOBT varies considerably, from less than 50% to approximately 90%.

Improving the performance of FOBT is highly dependent on following a recommended protocol [132, 133]. Whether a nonrehydrated or rehydrated test is used, the test is best performed at home, following a mildly restricted diet for 72 hours prior to initiating testing. Red meats, poultry, fish, raw vegetables, and medications including vitamin C and iron should not be consumed in the period prior to testing. Nonsteroidal anti-inflammatory drugs and aspirin should be avoided unless an individual is taking low doses of aspirin for vascular disease. Specimens should be collected over a three-day period from successive bowel movements, with two samples placed on each test card. Once three samples have been collected, FOBT cards should be returned according to the provider's instructions. A one-sample FOBT with stool collected on DRE during an office visit is especially not recommended. Although convenient, this particular protocol has very poor sensitivity, and false-positive results may ensue from DRE-related trauma [133].

Sigmoidoscopy

Sigmoidoscopy is a relatively simple procedure that requires minimal preparation. Sigmoidoscopes used in screening may be rigid (25 cm) or flexible (35 or 60 cm), although the sigmoidoscope used most commonly is flexible and approximately 60 cm long. Operator visualization is achieved through either a fiberscope or a videoscope. The flexible scope is preferable because of less patient discomfort, greater visualization of the mucosa, and greater range [128]. Patient preparation involves use of a saline enema one to two hours before the examination, and the test generally is performed without sedation. Prior to beginning FSIG, the examiner should perform a DRE [129]. A skilled examiner can complete the examination in less than 10 minutes. If the test result is positive, patients usually are referred for colonoscopy. Biopsy during sigmoidoscopy is rare for two reasons. First, the presence of polyps in the distal bowel signals an elevated risk for polyps or cancer in the proximal bowel. Second, biopsy with electrocautery poses the risk of explosion of ignited hydrogen or methane in the incompletely prepared bowel. For patient safety and greater test sensitivity, total colon examination (TCE) is generally postponed until a full bowel preparation can be accomplished prior to colonoscopy [128].

Barium Enema

Barium enema is a radiologic examination of the bowel that derives contrast from barium (a single-contrast study) or from the combination of barium and instilled air (a double-contrast study). DCBE is more sensitive than is the single-contrast study for both malignancies and polyps. Bowel preparation for DCBE is more thorough than that required for FSIG. Generally, patients will begin a clear liquid diet 24 hours before the examination, followed by liquid laxatives and enemas. Competent bowel preparation is critical to test sensitivity and specificity because residual stool can mask lesions or can lead to false-positive results. As with FSIG, the patient should have a DRE at the time of the examination. Prior to the examination, a flexible tube is inserted into the rectum to introduce barium to the bowel. Fluoroscopic examination monitors the progress of the barium through the bowel (patients may be required to roll and assume various positions to ensure that bowel cavities will be coated with barium). Once the bowel is coated completely, x-rays may be taken. If a patient has a positive test result, the next step is a colonoscopy.

Colonoscopy

Like DCBE, colonoscopy is a TCE and requires extensive bowel preparation. The modern colonoscope is capable of examining the entire bowel, with the examination terminating at the cecum. Colonoscopes have sufficient flexibility to maneuver through the bends and folds of the colon without significant looping that would not only impair progress but would cause significant discomfort to the patient. The instrument is far more complex than a sigmoidoscope because it must be capable of air insufflation, irrigation, and suction and the passage of biopsy forceps and polypectomy snares [134]. Like sigmoidoscopes, the tip of the instrument is equipped with a small video camera and light to provide high-resolution visualization of the bowel wall. Generally, patients begin a liquid diet one or more days before the examination, followed by a repeated oral ingestion of special fluids to stimulate bowel movements until the bowel is clean. After this cleansing procedure, usually performed at home, patients are advised not to eat or drink anything 8 to 10 hours before the procedure. Commonly, patients receive a mild sedative prior to the procedure; however, for many the discomfort is not so great as to require a sedative. Usually, colonoscopy is performed in a hospital, but it can also be done in an outpatient setting. The examination is more complicated than sigmoidoscopy, with a higher risk of complications [123, 135]. A skilled operator can complete an uncomplicated examination in approximately 30 minutes [134].

EVIDENCE OF EFFECTIVENESS

The goal of screening for colorectal cancer is both the detection of early stage adenocarcinomas and the detection and removal of adenomatous polyps, generally accepted as precursors in the development of colorectal cancer. Reduction in colorectal cancer morbidity and mortality through screening is achieved through a combination of more favorable stage at diagnosis of occult disease and disease prevention resulting from removal of precursor lesions.

Polyps are common in adults older than 50 years. Since most will not develop into adenocarcinoma, histology and size determine their clinical importance as precursor lesions [136]. The most common and clinically important polyps are adenomatous polyps, which represent approximately half to two-thirds of all colorectal polyps and are associated with the greatest risk of colorectal cancer [137]. Other polyps, which include hyperplastic polyps and inflammatory polyps, are not believed to have clinical significance in the development of colorectal cancer.

The evidence of the importance of colorectal polyps in the development of colorectal cancer is largely indirect but nonetheless convincing. First, adenomatous polyps and adenocarcinomas in the colon and rectum have a similar anatomic distribution, and the average age at which polyps begin to appear in adults precedes the age-incidence distribution of colorectal cancer [138]. Average polyp dwell time is believed to be very long. On the basis of a range of estimates from different kinds of observational studies and modeling efforts, the AHCRQ panel estimated that 10 years was a reasonable estimate for the time required for an adenomatous polyp smaller than 1 cm to become an invasive lesion [128]. Second, a strong association exists between polyp size and the grade of dysplasia, with higher-grade dysplasias observed more commonly in large polyps [136]. Third, epidemiologic evidence has shown higher risks of colorectal cancer after 14 years among individuals who had large polyps removed from the rectum or sigmoid colon and subsequently received no follow-up testing [137]. Fourth, individuals with familial adenomatous polyposis have a nearly 100% probability of developing colorectal cancer, and they experience earlier onset and extensive distribution of polyps throughout the colon and rectum [139]. Fifth, epidemiologic evidence has shown a lower incidence of colorectal cancer among individuals who have had large adenomatous

polyps removed than among the general population [140, 141]. As will be seen later, the protection offered by screening and removal of adenomatous polyps extends only to the area of the bowel that has been examined.

Fecal Occult Blood Testing

The observation that cancers detected through FOBT had a more favorable stage and better survival than did cases diagnosed with symptoms has led to prospective trials in Europe and the United States evaluating the efficacy of FOBT in reducing deaths from colorectal cancer. Two such trials are described here. In the Minnesota trial, 46,551 asymptomatic participants aged 50 to 80 were assigned randomly to one of three groups: a group that would receive an annual invitation to screening, a group that would receive an invitation to biennial (every two years) screening, and a control group that would receive usual care [142]. Participants with a positive FOBT result received a TCE with colonoscopy. After 14 years of follow-up, the 13-year cumulative mortality in the group offered annual screening was 5.33 per 1,000, compared with 8.33 per 1,000 in the biennially screened group and 8.83 in the usual care (control) group. Annual screening was associated with a statistically significant 33% reduction in deaths from colorectal cancer compared with usual care. The reduction in deaths associated with biennial screening compared with usual care was not statistically significant at the time of initial follow-up. In a subsequent analysis of Minnesota trial data with 18 years of follow-up, Mandel et al. [143] still observed a more favorable reduction in deaths from annual screening compared with biennial screening; however, with additional years of follow-up, the group that was screened biennially had a statistically significant 21% lower mortality than did the control group, a finding comparable with findings observed in the European trials. In the Nottingham trial, 150,251 individuals were assigned randomly to FOBT every two years or to usual care, with positive tests evaluated with colonoscopy [144]. After an average of eight years of follow-up, a statistically significant 15% reduction in deaths from colorectal cancer was observed in the group who underwent biennial screening.

Estimates of the sensitivity and specificity of the FOBT vary considerably and can be influenced by the type of occult blood test, by whether the specimen is rehydrated (i.e., adding a drop of water to the slide window before processing, to increase test sensitivity), and by variations in interpretation, specimen collection, number of samples collected per test, the screening interval, and other factors [133]. Under the best of circumstances (i.e., in a research setting with repeated testing), nonrehydrated Hemoccult tests have a sensitivity for cancer between 72% and 78% and a specificity of 98%, whereas rehydrated Hemoccult tests have an increased sensitivity of 88% to 92% but a decrease in specificity to 90–92% [128]. Although it improves sensitivity, rehydration of specimens leads to an increase in the false-positive rate. As estimated by the AHCRQ panel, for every cancer detected using a nonrehydrated test, 6 to 10 patients will undergo TCE, whereas for every cancer detected with a rehydrated test, between 17 and 50 patients will undergo TCE [128].

Newer FOBT tests appear to improve specificity while still maintaining higher sensitivity [133]. One unique feature of colorectal cancer screening, however, is that the higher program costs associated with false-positive results can be viewed as an investment against future screening costs among those individuals with false-positive examination results. Because screening intervals are longer for DCBE (5–10 years) and colonoscopy (10 years), an individual with a false-positive result on the FOBT followed by a TCE result judged to be normal may not require rescreening for 5–10 years [128, 129, 133].

Flexible Sigmoidoscopy

The advantage of FSIG over FOBT is that it allows examiners to visualize the distal bowel directly and has higher sensitivity and specificity for both adenocarcinomas and polyps. The disadvantage of FSIG is that the length of the scope permits visualization of only approximately half the bowel.

Several uncompleted randomized trials of FSIG are under way; thus, current evidence for the efficacy of FSIG derives from case-control investigations. Selby et al. [145] examined the screening histories of patients who died from colorectal cancer with controls matched for age and gender. Evaluation of patient records revealed that a history of rigid sigmoidoscopy was associated with 59% fewer deaths from colorectal cancer lesions in the region of the bowel within reach of the sigmoidoscope. Consistent with this interpretation was the finding that sigmoidoscopy offered no protective effect for death due to cancers developed in the proximal colon (i.e., that part of the colon outside the reach of the instrument). Newcomb et al. [146] observed a 79% reduction in colorectal cancer mortality in patients who had a history of one or more sigmoidoscopies compared with patients who never had undergone a sigmoidoscopy. Muller and Sonnenberg [147] showed also that patients with colorectal cancer were less likely to have undergone sigmoidoscopy than were matched controls,

a finding consistent with the hypothesis that endoscopic examinations provide for the opportunity to identify and remove adenomatous polyps and thereby eliminate potential precursor lesions. Kavanagh et al. [148] recently reported similar results from a prospective cohort study of approximately 25,000 men aged 40 to 75. Screening endoscopy was associated with a 48% lower incidence of colorectal cancer overall, a 60% lower incidence of cancer in the distal colon or rectum, and a 44% lower risk of death from colorectal cancer.

Combined FOBT and FSIG

FOBT and FSIG each represent lower-cost alternatives for colorectal cancer screening as compared with DCBE or colonoscopy. Since a majority of invasive lesions and large adenomatous polyps bleed at least intermittently, FOBT aims to detect occult blood in stool. FOBT offers little direct potential to prevent colorectal cancer because it is insensitive to smaller, potential precursor lesions. FSIG is far more sensitive and specific, provides direct visualization of the distal bowel, and therefore leads to the detection of both cancers and polyps, although the length of the instrument is a limiting factor. The combination of FOBT annually and FSIG every five years is superior to either FOBT or FSIG alone insofar as the two examinations together constitute a quasi-TCE. FOBT provides for some surveillance in the proximal colon (outside the reach of FSIG), and FSIG in the distal colon has higher sensitivity and specificity than does FOBT and provides an opportunity to visualize cancer and polyps. The combination of FOBT and sigmoidoscopy was evaluated in a controlled trial that randomly assigned asymptomatic individuals aged 40 and older to a group that would receive annual screening with rigid sigmoidoscopy plus FOBT or rigid sigmoidoscopy alone. After 5–11 years of follow-up, the investigators observed fewer colorectal cancer deaths in the group receiving annual FOBT and sigmoidoscopy, compared with those in the group receiving sigmoidoscopy alone (0.36 versus 0.63 per 1,000; $p = .53$) [149]. A study in Nottingham also has shown favorable early results from combination FOBT and FSIG [150]. After one screening examination, 12.2 adenomas larger than 1 cm and 1.5 cancers were detected per 1,000 individuals in the group receiving combination testing, compared with 3.1 adenomas and 0.5 cancers per 1,000 persons in the group receiving FOBT alone [150].

Barium Enema

Radiographic screening for colorectal cancer can be carried out through contrast studies using barium alone (single-contrast) or barium and air (double-contrast).

The DCBE is used more commonly as a screening test because of its superiority at detecting smaller lesions and polyps. Because the addition of air into the colon can cause some discomfort, the single-contrast study may be used for patients who would be anticipated to tolerate DCBE poorly.

The evidence for the efficacy of DCBE is largely indirect, based on the performance of DCBE in detecting small malignant lesions and polyps and the known benefits of early detection and polypectomy for reducing mortality. In one trial, DCBE with sigmoidoscopy was compared with colonoscopy alone among a group of 383 symptomatic patients [151]. Colonoscopy was more sensitive for the detection of polyps smaller than 9 mm, but the combination of DCBE plus sigmoidoscopy performed equally well for lesions larger than 9 mm, those believed to have greater clinical significance [151]. In a small percentage of cases (5–10%), complete visualization of the bowel is not possible; in such cases, endoscopy must be added to ensure that the patient has a complete examination.

Colonoscopy

Colonoscopy has unique advantages among all screening tests: Visualization of the entire bowel is possible, and clinically significant adenomas can be identified and removed. Evidence for the effectiveness of colonoscopy is indirect; no large trials with mortality end points have been conducted to evaluate the efficacy of screening with colonoscopy. However, as is the case with DCBE, the high sensitivity of the test has been regarded as sufficient for colonoscopy to be included among recommended screening tests. In the large majority of screening procedures ($> 90\%$), the cecum can be visualized; when colonoscopy is incomplete, the examination may be repeated or the total colon may be examined using DCBE [152]. In a case-control study of 32,702 veterans, patients who had undergone colonoscopy were significantly less likely to develop colorectal cancer (odds ratio = 0.61, 95% confidence interval [CI] = 0.48–0.77) compared with individuals who had not had colonoscopy, and those who had undergone colonoscopy with polypectomy demonstrated evidence of an even greater protective effect from colorectal cancer (odds ratio = 0.48, 95% CI = 0.35–0.66) [147]. In the Telemark Polyp Study, 400 asymptomatic men and women aged 50 to 59 and 399 controls were selected randomly from the Telemark, Norway population registries [141]. The experimental group was offered flexible sigmoidoscopy, and participants with detected polyps received colonoscopy with polypectomy and two subsequent rounds of colonoscopy. After 13 years of follow-up, the relative risk of colorectal cancer in the group receiving colonoscopy and polypectomy was 0.2 (95% CI = 0.03–0.95, $p = .02$) [141].

KEY ISSUES

An Office of Technology Assessment study of the cost-effectiveness of colorectal screening (subsequently refined by the AHCRQ panel) concluded that each alternative for colorectal screening fell below the $40,000 MCYLS dollar benchmark [128, 153]. Although each alternative is "cost-effective" and will save lives, alternative screening strategies are not equal in their potential to reduce morbidity and mortality. FSIG alone has the poorest performance as a screening test. Under various assumptions of polyp dwell time, combination screening of annual FOBT and either FSIG or DCBE every 10 years is similarly cost-effective to more frequent schedules. However, if most colorectal cancers develop from adenomas and if the dwell time is 10 years or longer, the conclusion was that screening with colonoscopy had the greatest potential if the unit cost could be reduced to $300 or less [153].

Currently, the efficacy of various screening alternatives has not resulted in equal access to the different tests, as DCBE and colonoscopy are not supported by definitive evidence and require larger outlays of resources by third-party payers. Today, participation in colorectal cancer screening by average-risk adults aged 50 or older is low. The low rates of screening among US adults are regrettable because screening is effective and patients have shown varying interest and acceptability for the different screening tests [27].

Data from the 1992 National Health Interview Study revealed only 33% of adults aged 49 and older reported having an FOBT in the previous three years, and only 33% reported ever having had sigmoidoscopy [27]. A 1998 ACS national survey of adults aged 50 and older indicated that approximately half of adults had never been screened for colorectal cancer; among those persons, only 12% reported that a health care provider had recommended screening [154].

Although the demand for colorectal cancer screening is low, an untested assumption is that the public avoids colorectal screening because of embarrassment and distaste. In fact, the current literature suggests that the public is highly compliant with physician recommendations for colorectal screening and appreciates its advantages for both early detection and prevention [27]. Although individuals may regard the elements and process of colorectal screening as distasteful, little evidence supports the conjecture that low screening rates are due to aversion. Rather, low screening rates are attributable to low awareness of the importance of colorectal cancer screening, low rates of provider recommendations for screening, and limited access. Today's situation is reminiscent of the period more than a decade ago in which public health outreach targeted women with health education messages about the importance of regular mammography. Inasmuch as routine screening has the potential to reduce deaths from colorectal cancer by more than 50%, the challenges to achieve widespread screening are no less than urgent.

Prostate Cancer

DISEASE BURDEN

Because of the prevalence of the disease, its serious threat to life, and the association of early diagnosis with improved survival, prostate cancer is a good candidate for improved control through early detection. It is the most common cancer (excluding skin cancer) of American men and is a significant public health problem. Diagnosis of an estimated 180,400 new cases of prostate cancer was anticipated in the United States in 2000, and an estimated 31,900 men in the United States were expected die of this disease [8, 40]. Prostate cancer accounts for some 11% of all male cancer-related deaths and is exceeded only by lung cancer as a cause of cancer-related death in men. Although the prognosis is good when diagnosis reveals cancer still localized to the prostate, nearly one-third of prostate cancers are diagnosed when the tumor already has spread locally; in 1 in 10 cases, the disease is metastatic at diagnosis. The five-year survival rate for men with advanced prostate cancer is only 31% [9].

SCREENING RECOMMENDATIONS

In 1992, the ACS published a recommendation that men older than 50 be tested annually for prostate-specific antigen (PSA) by DRE [155]. The American Urological Association made a similar recommendation. The ACS recommendation was reviewed in 1997, and the most recent guideline is that both a PSA blood test and DRE should be offered annually, beginning at age 50, to men who have at least a 10-year life expectancy and to younger men who are at high risk (see Table 5.2) [156]. The ACS also recommends that information be given to patients regarding potential risks and benefits

of early detection and treatment so as to aid informed decisions about testing. Men in high-risk groups, such as those with two or more affected first-degree relatives (father and a brother, or two brothers) or black men may consider screening at an age younger than 50 [156].

SCREENING AND DIAGNOSTIC METHODS

Digital Rectal Examination

The simplest screening test for prostate cancer is DRE, in which an examiner's gloved, lubricated finger is inserted into a patient's rectum to feel for any irregular or abnormally firm area on the periphery of the prostate gland. Palpable asymmetry of the gland and, particularly, hard nodular areas are classic criteria that prompt further diagnostic evaluation. Despite the possibility of detecting prostate cancer by DRE in asymptomatic men, studies in which DRE was the only modality used have yielded disappointing results [157, 158]. The majority of palpable cancers are not early cancers, and many clinically important cancers located in regions of the gland are inaccessible to digital palpation. Although it is limited by its poor sensitivity, DRE is recommended as one component of screening because it may detect cancers missed by other tests, it is a low-cost procedure, and it has value in evaluating other prostate abnormalities, such as benign prostate hyperplasia [159].

Prostate-Specific Antigen Blood Test

PSA is a protein produced by cells in the prostate gland [160]. It was used first to monitor disease recurrence or progression in patients after treatment for prostate cancer. Strong evidence of its value in detecting early prostate cancer in men with no symptoms or signs of prostate disease was reported beginning in 1989 [161, 162]. In the ensuing years, large numbers of men in the United States and elsewhere underwent this test and, as is to be expected of an effective test, the annual incidence rate of prostate cancer increased markedly. The principal strengths of the PSA test are its superior sensitivity, reasonable cost, and high patient acceptance. The principal drawback of the test is its imperfect specificity because common conditions, such as benign prostatic hyperplasia and prostatitis, can cause borderline or markedly abnormal test results. These false-positive results can lead to further, expensive diagnostic evaluation and unwarranted patient anxiety. At the other extreme, the high sensitivity of the test can result in overdiagnosis; small, indolent cancers that might require no treatment can be gathered in the same net as the aggressive, potentially life-threatening forms.

Several variations on the basic PSA test have been proposed as means of improving test specificity. The percentage of free PSA ratio relates the amount of unbound PSA circulating in the blood to the amount bound with other blood proteins [163]. A low percentage of free PSA (e.g. 25% or less) is more suggestive of the presence of cancer. Some estimate that use of this test for men with borderline PSA results could eliminate 20% of prostate biopsies [164]. PSA density (PSAD) is determined by dividing the PSA number by the prostate volume (its size as measured by transrectal ultrasonography) [165, 166]. This calculation has the effect of adjusting for PSA elevation associated with benign gland enlargement. A higher PSAD indicates greater likelihood of cancer. Age-specific PSA reference ranges are another way to interpret PSA test results [167]. PSA levels are known to be normally higher in older men than in younger men, even in the absence of cancer. Some of the cancers missed in older men using age-referenced norms, however, may be lethal; therefore, the use of PSA reference ranges has not gained widespread acceptance. A low PSA level that increases with time may be more suggestive of cancer than is a moderately elevated PSA that does not change. PSA velocity is the rate at which the PSA level rises over time and has been proposed as another means by which to improve the specificity of the PSA test [168]. Although these test variations are still being investigated, the evidence to date suggests that they offer only marginal improvements over the basic PSA test.

Transrectal Ultrasonography

Transrectal ultrasonography (TRUS) places a small rectal probe against the prostate gland to image the entire gland. Often, areas of the gland with differing morphology yield different images. However, cancer has no unique and reliably assessed ultrasonographic signature, and TRUS has been shown to have poor specificity when it is the sole screening modality [169]. It does, however, play a very important role in the early detection process. It is a means of measuring gland dimensions accurately and of calculating total gland volume. This information is useful in evaluating borderline elevations in PSA using PSAD. More important, TRUS is the means for guiding needle biopsies of the prostate gland for diagnostic purposes. The biopsies can be directed to suspicious areas palpated by DRE or seen on TRUS imagery. More commonly, TRUS is used to guide systematic biopsies of different sections of the entire gland (e.g., sextant biopsy).

EVIDENCE OF EFFECTIVENESS

Evidence supporting the effectiveness of PSA alone or in combination with DRE and TRUS is available from several sources. Early comparative studies showed that PSA and related testing could increase prostate cancer detection in asymptomatic men. In addition, the stage distribution of screen-detected cancers was demonstrated to be much more favorable than that which occurred in the general, unscreened population. The ACS National Prostate Cancer Detection Project showed that after five years of annual testing by PSA, DRE, and TRUS, 91.7% of detected cancers were localized to the prostate, compared with 66.0% in a contemporaneous national database covering men of the same age [169].

After widespread implementation of PSA testing in the late 1980s and early 1990s, prostate cancer incidence in the United States increased significantly, consistent with the pattern expected after introduction of a more sensitive screening test [170]. At the same time, the mean age at diagnosis of prostate cancer was lowered by two years (70.7 to 68.8 years) [171]. Numerous cancer registries reported the shift toward detection at an earlier disease stage predicted by the early cohort studies. This increase in the number of early stage prostate cancers also had a significant impact on the numbers of patients treated with curative intent. Between 1974 and 1993, the proportion of men with diagnosed prostate cancer treated by radical prostatectomy tripled (9.2% to 29.2%) [172].

Changing the ultimate disease outcome is a critical criterion in evaluating the effectiveness of any screening program, and the impact of PSA and related testing on mortality was not immediately apparent from the early studies. No randomized controlled trials of PSA-based prostate cancer screening had been performed before it became a widespread practice. The observed increase in detection and the stage shift without an eventual impact on mortality would be evidence that prostate cancer screening actually was ineffective. However, currently accruing evidence demonstrates that mortality is decreasing. Between 1990 and 1995, the prostate cancer death rate in the United States for white men younger than 75 years old decreased more than 14% [173]. It is possible that this change is only coincidental to the preceding increase in PSA use, but few other changes in treatment or diagnosis would account for the decrease in death rates.

More specific evidence of mortality reduction is provided by a randomized controlled trial conducted in Quebec [174]. Comparing the death rates in 8,137 screened men and 38,056 unscreened men after seven years of follow-up yielded a 69.2% reduction in the prostate cancer death rate. This study had a compliance rate of only 23.1%, and 6.5% of men assigned to the control group were actually screened. However, even when analyzed on an intent-to-treat basis, a mortality reduction continued to be observed. A large trial of prostate cancer screening in the United States is under way [175]. The results of this study may shed further light on the potential of prostate cancer screening to affect disease outcomes.

KEY ISSUES

Many uncertainties surround the early detection of prostate cancer. Several scientific and medical organizations including the American Society of Internal Medicine, the National Cancer Institute, the Centers for Disease Control and Prevention, the American Association of Family Physicians, and American College of Preventive Medicine do not recommend that providers routinely offer prostate cancer screening to their patients [176]. The American College of Physicians has a guideline similar to the recommendations of the ACS (i.e., that physicians should be prepared to discuss the benefits and known harms of screening, diagnosis, and treatment and then to assist men in making decisions) [177]. The recommendations of the ACS and American College of Physicians acknowledge disease burden in the presence of uncertainty and that individual preferences should be taken into account. From some perspectives, the lack of randomized controlled trial data justifies limiting introduction of screening, but for most, the key issue relates to potential overdiagnosis [178–180].

Unlike many other cancers, prostate cancers generally develop and progress slowly. Given that the disease typically occurs late in life, some cancers detecting by screening are unlikely to be life-threatening. This possibility is confirmed by the fact that autopsy studies have shown that many men have clinically occult prostate cancers at the time of their death from other causes. To have detected and treated these cancers could not have yielded benefit. In addition, observation alone is an accepted treatment option for some early prostate cancers, especially in older men. Observing older patients for signs of progression to more advanced cancer offers one alternative to early detection followed by aggressive treatment. Future research may yield prostate cancer screening tools that have greater specificity in the detection of tumors that clearly warrant immediate intervention.

Lung Cancer

DISEASE BURDEN

Lung cancer is the second most common cancer, and the leading cause of death from cancer, among both men and women in the United States. The ACS estimated that in 2000, 164,100 new cases of lung cancer will be diagnosed, and that there will be 156,900 deaths [8, 40]. Incidence rates are higher in men than in women and are higher in whites than in blacks. Lung cancer is relatively uncommon before age 50, with rates increasing rapidly after that age. Age-specific incidence rates peak in the seventies [9]. Since 1973, incidence rates have declined 2.5% in men but have increased 123% in women, the direct result of increasing rates of cigarette smoking among females beginning in the 1940s. Since 1992, a decline in incidence among both men (-10.1%) and women (-0.7%) has been observed. Although mortality rates have declined in men (-0.3%), they still are increasing in women (2.9%) [9]. These trends reflect the historically different population patterns of cigarette smoking in men and women in the last 50 years.

Overall, lung cancer has a very poor prognosis. The most recent five-year survival statistics show only 14% of patients surviving five years, with nearly 60% of patients succumbing within the year of diagnosis. Five-year survival is measurably better (49%) when the disease is diagnosed while still localized, but only 15% of cases are diagnosed without regional disease or distant metastases [9].

The majority of lung cancers develop in individuals with a history of cigarette smoking. Stopping smoking results in a decline in risk with time, but the lung cancer risk remains elevated in former smokers compared with those who never smoked, even after 10 years. Still, the magnitude of the remaining lower relative risk should be considered in the context of the underlying risk of lung cancer in those who never smoked, which is very small [181].

SCREENING RECOMMENDATIONS

At this time, no organization recommends routine screening for lung cancer among the general adult population or among individuals who are at higher risk owing to tobacco or occupational exposures [50, 180–184]. Historically, attempts have been made to evaluate the potential to screen for lung cancer, but studies to date generally are regarded as negative or at least inconclusive, but in either case not sufficiently strong to warrant a recommendation for screening.

Currently, because of limitations of earlier studies, a large NCI trial evaluating the effectiveness of chest radiography in the early detection of lung cancer is underway [185]. However, because of the magnitude of disease burden and because early stage disease is associated with longer survival, interest remains high in developing a technology that would detect tumors at a more favorable stage and thereby reduce mortality.

SCREENING AND DIAGNOSTIC METHODS

The technologies available for detecting lung cancer at an early, more favorable stage include imaging modalities and cytologic and molecular evaluations of lung sputum. Chest radiographs have some, although limited, potential in screening, especially in comparison with new imaging technologies that achieve higher resolution. Normally, two images are taken, a posteroanterior view and a lateral view. The sensitivity of chest radiographs depends on the size and location of the lesion, quality assurance factors related to image quality, and the interpretation skills of a physician [186]. Failure to detect lesions at a favorable size, or even when larger, can occur because the mediastinum and other aspects of chest structure obscure them; commonly, detection failures occur due to errors in perception on the part of an interpreter [187]. Low-dose computed tomography (CT) (i.e., spiral or helical CT) produces multiple images of the lung conventionally in 5-mm multiplanar slices that can produce a three-dimensional display of the lung. Low-dose CT is more sensitive than are chest radiographs in the detection of small pulmonary nodules, which also poses challenges to establish protocols for triaging cases with malignant potential.

Sputum cytology was believed to have potential to detect early lung cancer but showed little added advantage over chest radiographs in the NCI cooperative trials and was not associated with any reduction in deaths from lung cancer. In the trials, approximately one in four cancers was detected by sputum cytology alone, and the majority of these were squamous cell carcinomas diagnosed at a favorable stage. However, attempts to refine the use of sputum cytology are continuing [188]. One disadvantage of sputum cytology is that other methods must be applied to identify the location of the cancer.

Attempts to identify a group at appreciable risk for lung cancer beyond smoking history have focused on molecular risk assessment in current and former smok-

ers. Evaluation of lung epithelium for evidence of accumulated genetic damage through polymerase chain reaction techniques is another new area of investigation [189].

EVIDENCE OF EFFECTIVENESS

Lung cancer is unique among the cancers discussed in this chapter because a secondary prevention strategy to reduce deaths from lung cancer would be entirely unnecessary if primary prevention (i.e., avoiding beginning smoking) were entirely successful. However, the current public health challenge includes current and former smokers who began smoking before the health hazards were understood widely and those who subsequently began cigarette smoking despite warnings about the health hazards. Too often, marketing messages from the tobacco companies have been more persuasive than health education messages about the dangers of use of tobacco products.

To date, prospective studies of lung cancer screening have not demonstrated persuasively that screening for lung cancer with chest radiography alone or in combination with sputum cytology saves lives. In the early 1970s, the NCI supported three randomized prospective trials in the United States through the Cooperative Early Lung Cancer Detection Program [190]. The first of these trials, the Mayo Lung Project (1971–1983), randomly assigned 9,211 men who had been heavy cigarette smokers to either an experimental group or a control group. Men in the experimental group would receive an invitation to have a chest radiograph and sputum cytology every four months, whereas those in the control group would be advised to have an annual chest radiograph without receiving reminders [191]. Prior to random assignment, all individuals were screened, resulting in diagnosis of 91 cancers (8.3 per 1,000), of which half were resectable. The lung cancer five-year survival rate among prevalent cases was 40% [192]. Over the duration of the study, 206 cancers were detected in the experimental group compared with 160 lung cancers in the control group. Only 18 cases were detected with sputum cytology. Compliance in the study group was 75%, but significant contamination also was seen in the control group, with 53% receiving chest radiographs in the final year of the study and 73% receiving at least one chest radiograph in the final two years. Although five-year lung cancer survival in the experimental group was better (33%) than that in the control group cases (15%), no significant difference was observed in lung cancer mortality.

The second two prospective trials in the NCI study program evaluated the added advantage of sputum cytology to chest radiography for early lung cancer detection. The Memorial Sloan-Kettering Lung Project (1974–1982) randomly assigned 10,040 men who were aged 45 and older and smoked an average of one pack of cigarettes a day to an experimental group that would receive annual chest radiographs and sputum cytology every four months or to a control group that would receive only annual chest radiographs [193]. The investigators concluded that chest radiography was superior to sputum cytology in the detection of early lung cancer. Forty percent of the cancers were detected at stage 1, and two-thirds of these patients did not die of their disease. Overall five-year survival among study cases was 35%, compared with 13% in the general population. However, the intent of the study was to evaluate the added value of cytology, and the investigators conceded no overall reduction in lung cancer deaths between the dual-screen and the radiographs-only groups [193, 194]. The Johns Hopkins Lung Project (1973–1982) had a design similar to that of the Memorial Project, in which 10,384 men who were aged 45 and older and had a significant smoking history were assigned randomly to an experimental or a control group. Men in the experimental group would receive an annual chest radiograph and sputum cytology every four months, whereas controls received only an annual chest radiograph only [195]. No difference in lung cancer mortality was observed between the study and the control groups, and the investigators concluded that sputum cytology added to chest radiography offered no benefit in reducing deaths from lung cancer [196].

The Czech Study on Lung Cancer Screening (1976–1983) randomly assigned 6,364 male current smokers aged 40 to 64 to an experimental group and a control group after a prevalent screen. The experimental group members received an invitation to undergo chest radiography every six months, whereas controls were offered a chest radiograph at the end of three years [197]. Both experimental and control groups received annual screening in the three years after the six-year study period. Survival was better in the experimental group than in controls for cases diagnosed in the first three years of the study, but comparisons for all years taken together showed no mortality benefit among cases diagnosed in the experimental group compared with the control group [198, 199].

Newer technology for the early detection of lung cancer appears to be more promising than are conventional chest radiographs. The Early Lung Cancer Action Project is designed to evaluate screening with low-dose CT [200]. In a report of the baseline experience with 1,000 volunteers who were aged 60 or older, had a smoking history of at least 10 pack-years, and would be acceptable candidates for thoracic surgery, low-dose CT significantly outperformed conventional chest radiography in the detection of small pulmonary nodules. Low-dose CT identified 233 participants with noncalcified nodules and 27 malignancies, of which 26 were resectable and 23 were stage I disease. In contrast, conventional chest radiographs identified 68 noncalcified nodules, of which seven were malignant and four were stage I. Workup of positive CT results was based on the size of the nodule and the change observed on repeat screening. Based on the average tumor size in the Early Lung Cancer Action Project, the investigators projected five-year survival of 80% for cases diagnosed using low-dose CT [200]. Other promising methods for the early detection of lung cancer include fluorescent bronchoscopy and molecular screening for transformation of bronchial epithelial cells.

Although these results of prospective trials have been disappointing in the presence of such significant disease burden, they also were methodologically limited at inception in their ability to demonstrate a benefit from screening. Although none of the studies showed fewer deaths in the experimental group than in the control group, none of the studies compared disease outcome in a group offered screening and a group not invited to screening. Such a study is underway (the multicenter prostate, lung, colorectal, and ovarian trial sponsored by the NCI) [175]. Furthermore, chest radiography alone and in combination with sputum cytology improved the stage at diagnosis and was associated with more favorable survival, which also has been observed in case-finding series. Despite these limitations, a predominant and rather uncritical belief is that lung cancer screening is not effective, whereas, if it is more appropriate to conclude that insufficient data are available to recommend for or against lung cancer screening. An International Conference on Prevention and Early Diagnosis of Lung Cancer, held in Varese, Italy in December 1998 reviewed the historical data and information on new technologies for the early detection of lung cancer. Conference participants endorsed a statement concluding that data were insufficient to recommend for or against screening but that individuals at risk for lung cancer should be informed about the differences in results from trials and case-finding series. Others have concluded also that case finding is a reasonable approach for individuals at high risk [201].

KEY ISSUES

Both in the United States and around the world, the burden of tobacco-related illness is high and is increasing. Despite the limitations of the existing scientific literature to provide a clear basis for public policy on early detection, a persistent dogma holds that screening for lung cancer is ineffective [202]. Survival of patients with lung cancer detected in the earliest stages is five times greater than that of patients whose cancer is diagnosed after symptoms develop. The emergence of new, more sensitive technology marks not only the potential for a new direction in screening, but serves to heighten the urgency for testing since the current lung cancer disease burden is so great. Delays in initiating prospective evaluation mean that studies may encounter difficulties in participant enrollment if the technology becomes available in the clinical setting before trials are initiated.

Cervical Cancer

DISEASE BURDEN

The ACS estimated that in 2000, 12,800 new cases of invasive cervical cancer will be diagnosed among US women and 4,600 deaths from cervical cancer will occur [8, 40]. Since 1973, the incidence of invasive disease has declined by 43.3%, with an estimated average annual percentage change of -2.3% [9]. Incidence rates per 100,000 women are higher among blacks than among whites (11.8 versus 7.4), as are mortality rates (6.1 versus 2.5). Five-year survival is very good for women with diagnosed localized disease (90.4%) but declines considerably for disease diagnosed regionally (50.9%) and for distant metastasis (11.6%).

The comparatively small number of expected incident cases compared with other cancers reflects not only the success of the Pap test, but is a reminder that the purpose of screening for cervical cancer is less for the detection of invasive disease than for the detection of cytologic abnormalities indicating the presence of cervical intraepithelial neoplasia (CIN) [203]. It has been estimated that approximately 10% of the estimated 50 million Pap tests performed annually show abnormal results at some level, and that half of these (2.5 million) disclose at least low-grade cytologic abnormalities [204]. However, no current, reliable population-based study can estimate the expected number or rate of in situ lesions because of variations in nomenclature and their application over time was highly variable within and between geographic areas. Without the ability to ensure the reliability of data with reasonable costs, the NCI and state registries chose to discontinue collection of such data [205]. Variation is also seen in laboratory reports and convenience samples have been used to estimate the distribution of precursor lesions, reflecting differing underlying population characteristics and variations in local patterns of cytologic reporting. However, a recent report using data from the Centers from Disease Control and Prevention's National Breast and Cervical Cancer Early Detection Program summarized findings from participants throughout the United States. Data from 312,858 women screened for cervical cancer showed an overall abnormality rate of 3.8%, a 9:1 ratio of CIN3—carcinoma in situ to invasive disease, and an 18.5:1 ratio of CIN2 or worse to invasive disease [206].

SCREENING RECOMMENDATIONS

A broad, general consensus exists for screening recommendations for cervical cancer [130, 182, 207–209]. The ACS recommends that women should begin annual screening at the age of 18 or after the onset of sexual activity, whichever comes first. After three consecutive negative Pap test results, screening can be performed less frequently at the discretion of a physician (see Table 5.2) [207]. The ACS does not set an upper age limit for screening. The USPSTF recommends that screening begin after the onset of sexual activity and that Pap smears should be repeated every three years. Although the USPSTF conceded there was insufficient evidence to recommend for or against an upper age limit for screening, they concluded that screening could be discontinued after age 65 in women who had consistently normal Pap smear results [130]. Most organizations link the beginning of testing either to the onset of sexual activity or to the age of 18 if a patient's sexual history is believed to be unreliable. Overall, these guidelines reflect the strong evidence that the underlying etiology of cervical cancer is associated with sexually acquired viral infections and that the disease has a long latency period [130, 210–213].

SCREENING AND DIAGNOSTIC METHODS

The Pap test is the cancer-screening test used most widely throughout the world. The procedure is simple but, as with all cancer-screening tests, errors that compromise test accuracy can occur with inattention to quality assurance. Basically, the Pap test involves the collection of exfoliating epithelial cells from the cervical squamocolumnar junction, or transformation zone.

Both the cervix and endocervix should be sampled. Various collection tools are available (spatula, cotton swab, cytobrush, cervix brush, cytopick, etc.) for specimen collection. Boon et al. [214] evaluated various approaches to specimen collection and found that the combination of spatula and cytobrush, or the cytopick, offered the best performance as measured by presence of endocervical cells. They also concluded that the spatula alone or the combination of spatula and cotton swab showed poor performance and was not recommended [214]. The two samples (cervical and endocervical) should be applied to one side of a glass slide and fixed quickly (usually with a spray fixative) to prevent air-drying. Then the slide is examined under a microscope by a cytotechnologist.

In an effort to improve the accuracy and cost-effectiveness of the Pap smear, several new Pap test-based technologies have evolved, with a particular emphasis on sensitivity. Each takes a somewhat different approach to correcting some shortcomings—mainly sampling and detection errors—of the conventional Pap smear. Sampling error is estimated to account for some two-thirds of false-negative test results, and errors in interpretation account for the remaining one-third [215]. ThinPrep® uses thin-layer cytology to reduce false-negative results due to sampling error. Instead of being placed on a glass slide first, the sample is suspended in a fixative solution, after which it is dispersed, filtered, and distributed on a glass slide in a monolayer. Accuracy is increased because fewer artifacts (blood, mucus, etc.) can interfere and because cells are not overlapping. Placing the sample directly into fixative solution also avoids air-drying artifacts from delayed fixation of conventionally prepared smears. The test has been shown to have higher sensitivity, especially in populations with a lower prevalence of cytologic abnormalities [215].

PAPNET applies neural network technology to identify false-negatives among the pool of Pap smears interpreted as normal. A computerized algorithm identifies slides likely to contain abnormal cells. Suspicious areas are targeted, and a cytotechnologist then decides whether the slide should be reviewed. AutoPap also targets interpretation error through computer algorithms that select slides that have exceeded a preset and adjustable threshold for abnormalities. Each of these technologies increases the sensitivity of the Pap smear, but each is also a more expensive screening test. A comparative review of these new technologies concluded that their application was more cost-effective when incorporated into protocols of less frequent screening and that cost-effectiveness was higher in populations of higher dis-

ease prevalence [216]. Added to annual screening, they offer little advantage to life expectancy over the conventional Pap smear.

Other tests have been used both for primary screening and for diagnostic workup of cervical abnormalities. Commonly, colposcopy is used as a diagnostic adjunct to Pap smear screening. The colposcope allows for visualization of the cervix and transformation zone under magnification of ×10 to ×20. Prior to colposcopy, the transformation zone is bathed in a 3–5% acetic acid solution that accentuates abnormalities (mosaicism, punctation, etc.) for biopsy. As a procedure for screening, it may be used in combination with the Pap smear to achieve added sensitivity but generally has been judged to be impractical and not cost-effective [217].

Cervicography is another "visual" approach to screening and basically is merely the photographically captured image of the cervix that clinicians would see through the colposcope [218, 219]. To date, cervicography has not been shown to have sufficient accuracy to be considered as an alternative to the Pap test.

Because of the strong association between infection with particular subtypes of human papillomavirus (HPV) and cervical cancer, HPV testing has been proposed as a strategy for screening, for triaging mildly abnormal Pap smear results, or for risk assignment to distinguish a high-risk group for more aggressive surveillance [220–225]. Current testing for HPV DNA uses the Hybrid Capture method and was approved by the FDA in 1996 for commercial use [226]. However, the potential for such testing rests on the assumption that infection with particular subtypes of HPV (in particular, HPV types 16 and 18) was a necessary, not merely sufficient, etiologic factor in CIN [227]. Although researchers are not certain that HPV infection is strictly necessary for the development of CIN, it is apparently at least an important cofactor in nearly all cervical cancers, as demonstrated by a 93% prevalence of HPV DNA in a review of 1,000 cervical cancer specimens [228].

At this time, routine HPV testing as a basis for identifying a high-risk group would be problematic for several reasons beyond the lack of complete certainty of its status as a necessary precursor to cervical cancer. First, HPV infection may be active, latent, or transient and thus the potential for misclassification at testing is high. Second, and even more problematic for a program of risk assessment with cross-population screening, is the fact that exposure opportunities vary in individuals over time. Apart from the fact that persons may test negative because an infection is latent or the viral load is low, they also may acquire an infection in the period after testing [228]. Third, since HPV infection is com-

Table 5.6   Cervical cytology classification schemes

Classification System (year) [reference]	Diagnostic Terminology							
	Within Normal Limits	Benign Cellular Changes	Epithelial Cell Abnormalities					
The Bethesda System (TBS) (1993) [229]	Normal	Infection Reactive Repair	ASCUS	Squamous Intraepithelial Lesion (SIL)				Invasive carcinoma
				Low Grade (LSIL)		High Grade (HSIL)		
Richart (1973) [223]			Condyloma	Cervical Intraepithelial Neoplasia (CIN)				
				CIN 1	CIN 2	CIN 3		
Reagan–WHO (1979) [232]		Atypia		Mild Dysplasia	Moderate Dysplasia	Severe Dysplasia	In situ Carcinoma	
Papanicolaou (1972) [231]	I	II	III			IV		V

ASCUS = atypical squamous cells of undetermined significance; WHO = World Health Organization.

Source: Adapted from the Agency for Health Care Policy and Research. *Evaluation of Cervical Cytology. Evidence Report/Technology Assessment No. 5,* Rockville, MD: AHCPR, 1999 [215].

mon in adults who have had more than one sexual partner and as most individuals with HPV infection do not develop cervical cancer, public health education would face an enormous challenge to avoid stigma associated with testing positive for a sexually acquired infection. Finally, HPV testing as a primary screening test or adjunct to the Pap smear would have to meet similar, basic performance criteria described for any screening test. Although these caveats do not rule out the potential role of HPV testing, additional epidemiologic and clinical research currently are needed before HPV infection status is likely to play a key role in secondary prevention strategies for cervical cancer.

After years of evolution in cytologic classification systems for Pap smear results, the NCI sponsored a 1988 meeting to develop a new system both to standardize cytologic nomenclature and to address shortcomings in the various systems in use. These shortcomings included uneven cytologic-histologic correlation, low reliability, and confusion in communication between referring physicians, both in the use of different systems and in inconsistent use of nomenclature within a system. This new system, known as the Bethesda System, was intended to provide ". . . a uniform format for cytopathology reports that is intended to communicate clinically relevant information using standardized terminology" [229]. It has been adopted widely since that time. One important contribution of the Bethesda System was its incorporation of specimen adequacy into the nomenclature; another was the incorporation of term-

inology to classify atypical squamous and glandular cells of undetermined significance, with the intent to reduce the false-negative rate resulting from inadequate workup of these abnormalities [207]. A historical comparison of the evolution of different cytologic reporting systems is shown in Table 5.6 [215, 230–233].

EVIDENCE OF EFFECTIVENESS

Cervical cancer is marked by a long period of preclinical disease progressing through a number of well-defined premalignant stages. This progression also is not certain, with evidence indicating that a significant proportion of premalignant lesions will regress [234]. Age-specific incidence data previously available from NCI's Surveillance, Epidemiology, and End Results program and cross-sectional studies from small geographic areas or clinical populations are consistent with the following observations: (1) The prevalence of precursor dysplastic lesions is greater among younger women than among older women; (2) carcinoma in situ of the cervix peaks in the mid thirties; and (3) the incidence of invasive disease peaks in the mid forties, remaining relatively constant among white women and continuing to rise among black women [235]. These reports have shown considerable variation according to classifications of risk, with prevalence rates of atypia, CIN1, and CIN2 being higher than average among women attending sexually transmitted disease clinics [236, 237]. These findings are consistent with epidemiologic studies that have shown strong associations between reproductive behaviors and risk, including early age at first intercourse, number of sexual partners, and history of sexually transmitted disease [238].

It is generally accepted that screening for cancer of the cervix, specifically precancerous lesions, is effective in reducing both the incidence of and mortality from cervical cancer. Although no randomized trial has tested the efficacy of screening for cervical cancer, it has been observed that cytologic screening was an accepted part of medical care among both women and providers prior to the point when the randomized trial with a mortality end point had become the standard by which the efficacy of a screening test is evaluated [1]. Even so, the logic of cytologic screening always has measured up well against criteria applied to the value of a screening test. Screening with the Pap smear is comparatively inexpensive and is accepted widely both by the public and by providers. Cervical cancer is characterized by a long lead time, with potentially cancerous lesions progressing through a succession of identifiable stages prior to becoming invasive. If the disease is detected before it progresses to invasive disease, a variety of treatment options are available, and the disease is almost certainly curable.

Perhaps the most widely cited evidence for the contribution of cytologic screening to the reduction in cervical cancer mortality is the long-term decline since the 1930s in the death rate from cervical cancer in the United States (down nearly 80%), which is coincident with the introduction of the Pap smear, although it has been noted that rates had begun to decline prior to widespread use of the test, perhaps due to an increase in the hysterectomy rate, trends in the underlying epidemiology of disease, and other factors [239]. However, few would oppose the argument that cytologic screening primarily has influenced this downward trend in the death rate.

Scientific evidence for the efficacy of cervical cytology exists in nonexperimental studies, specifically observational and case-control studies. The best examples of observational studies are the evaluations of cervical cancer mortality rates in five Nordic countries before and after the introduction of screening programs [240–244]. A comparison of mortality rates before and after introduction of cytologic screening between two time periods, 1963 to 1967 and 1978 to 1982, revealed mortality reductions between 8% and 73% [240]. Factors underlying this wide range of mortality reductions are consistent also with a screening effect. In Norway, where participation rates were lowest, mortality remained comparatively unchanged, whereas in Iceland,

which organized an aggressive screening program with high rates of participation, the mortality reduction (73%) was greatest among the five countries [240, 242, 244]. Numerous examples of case-control studies also show a benefit from cervical cancer screening, typically examining the screening histories of women with diagnosed invasive disease and those in matched control groups [245, 246].

Although the Pap smear is simple, its accuracy is highly dependent on achieving a high level of quality in specimen collection, slide preparation, and microscopical examination and interpretation. Even under the best of circumstances, the Pap smear has a significant error rate [224]. A technology assessment of cervical cytology by the Duke University Center for Clinical Health Policy Research conducted for the AHCRQ concluded that conventional Pap-smear screening had a specificity of 98% but a sensitivity of only 51% [215]. Sensitivity is higher when the threshold of a positive test result is lower (i.e., a low-grade squamous intraepithelial lesion or atypical cells of undetermined significance versus a high-grade squamous intraepithelial lesion).

KEY ISSUES

Performing a Pap test during a routine gynecologic examination is relatively simple. For a majority of premenopausal women, it is an annual event. The argument about annual versus less frequent Pap testing cannot be separated from the larger question of how frequently otherwise healthy women need a gynecologic checkup. In the average provider's mind, perhaps, is the concern that a three-year interval could easily become a 4–6-year interval or could lead to a loss of contact with the patient altogether. Furthermore, in the United States, liability concerns among practicing physicians cannot be overlooked.

The question of risk further complicates the issue of screening intervals. Many would argue that those at high risk (i.e., women with documented early initiation of sexual intercourse, multiple sexual partners, history of sexually transmitted diseases, etc.) should have annual examinations indefinitely. However, ascertaining risk is both practically and socially difficult, and many women unknowingly are placed at greater risk because of the behaviors of prior and current partners. Even though they may be few in number collectively, they may represent a large number of prior exposures. One could assume that these risk profiles would ensure more frequent testing in this group of women because of the lower likelihood of serial normal Pap test results.

However, when providers have knowledge of these risk factors or are practicing in a high-risk population, concerns about undetected disease and compliance with less frequent testing probably lead them to regard annual testing as the only acceptable practice. In general, though the epidemiologic literature supports less frequent testing for women whose prior tests suggest no presence of disease, the lack of widespread acceptance for less frequent testing indicates that, as yet, neither the systems nor medical culture support this practice.

Endometrial Cancer

DISEASE BURDEN

Cancer of the endometrium is the most common cancer of the female reproductive organs in the United States. The ACS estimates for 2000 predicted that 26,100 new cases of endometrial cancer will be diagnosed in the United States and that 6,500 women will die of this disease [8, 40]. Incidence increased from 1973 to 1978 because of an association with unopposed estrogen replacement therapy, but no associated increase was registered in mortality [247]. In fact, the endometrial cancer mortality rate has declined 27% in the last two decades [9]. Prognosis is associated very much with stage at diagnosis. From 1986 to 1993, the five-year relative survival rates among US white women were 96% for localized disease, 69% for regional disease, and 29% for distant disease. Black women have poorer survival at each stage of disease and are more likely to receive diagnoses of late-stage endometrial cancer [248].

SCREENING RECOMMENDATIONS

Endometrial cancer can progress to an advanced stage before symptoms appear. Although the disease has a preclinical phase at which earlier intervention could be beneficial, no routine screening tests for endometrial cancer have proved effective in altering disease outcome. In the presence of elevated risk for this disease, screening tests may be considered, although as yet no randomized prospective studies are available for screening in higher-risk women. Use of tamoxifen for breast cancer prevention or after breast cancer treatment has been associated with a two- to three-fold increase in risk of endometrial cancer [249]. The American College of Obstetricians and Gynecologists has recommended that screening by annual endometrial sampling in women taking tamoxifen may be performed at the discretion of individual patients and gynecologists [250].

In addition, results from three HNPCC registries have shown a 10-fold increased risk of endometrial cancer in women who carry the HNPCC genetic abnormality, compared with women in the general population who do not carry this abnormality; the cumulative risk for endometrial cancer is 43% by age 70 [251]. Additional investigation is needed to determine the appropriate monitoring for endometrial cancer in HNPCC carriers.

SCREENING AND DIAGNOSTIC METHODS

A Pap test may identify endometrial abnormalities fortuitously, but it is not sensitive enough in detecting endometrial cancer to be used as a screening technique [252]. Sampling of endometrium tissue is indicated for women who present with unexplained uterine bleeding. Intrauterine sampling may be by aspiration, biopsy, or curettage of the endometrium [155]. When tissue specimens are nondiagnostic, transvaginal ultrasonography (TVS) to evaluate postmenopausal bleeding has demonstrated a high sensitivity for detecting endometrial cancer and endometrial disease according to a threshold for abnormal endometrial thickening [253, 254]. A study using a 5-mm threshold to define such thickening revealed abnormal endovaginal ultrasonographic results in 96% of women with cancer and 92% of women with endometrial disease [255].

EVIDENCE OF EFFECTIVENESS

Routine screening of asymptomatic women for endometrial cancer has not been proved to be beneficial. Large-scale, rigorous controlled studies of potential screening techniques have not been performed; thus, recommendations for screening certain groups of women at high risk for endometrial carcinoma are based chiefly on expert opinion.

KEY ISSUES

In the absence of a sensitive screening test for endometrial cancer in asymptomatic individuals, emphasis should be placed on women's recognition of the significance of early signs and symptoms (e.g., abnormal vaginal bleeding, spotting, pelvic pain, and unexplained weight loss). Additional research is needed in evaluating endometrial tissue sampling in women at higher risk. More evidence regarding this issue may be provided from the endometrial cancer studies as part of the NCI Breast Cancer Prevention Trial.

Ovarian Cancer

DISEASE BURDEN

Ovarian cancer is the fifth most common cancer and the fifth leading cause of cancer death among US women. Diagnosis of an estimated 23,100 new cases of ovarian cancer was anticipated in 2000, and thought to result in approximately 14,000 deaths [8, 40]. Ovarian cancer accounts for 4% of all cancers in women, and it has the highest mortality rate of all gynecologic cancers. Approximately 76% of ovarian cancer patients survive one year after diagnosis, and only 50% are alive five years after diagnosis [9]. The prognosis for survival from ovarian cancer, however, is largely dependent on the extent of disease at diagnosis. Women diagnosed with local disease are more than three times more likely to survive five years than are women with distant disease. However, only one-fourth of women present with localized disease at diagnosis [9]. Ovarian cancer would appear to fit the criteria required to qualify a disease for early detection intervention. It is a prevalent disease with a high risk of death, and patients benefit from early treatment.

SCREENING RECOMMENDATIONS

Despite the suitability of the disease as a target for screening interventions, no such interventions have sufficient sensitivity and specificity for use in the general population at risk for ovarian cancer. The ACS recommends annual pelvic examinations beginning at age 18 (or earlier for sexually active persons). During this examination, the ovaries should be palpated for abnormalities of size, shape, or consistency [3]. An NIH Consensus Panel concluded in 1994 that no blood tests or imaging studies can be recommended for ovarian cancer screening of women who are not at significantly elevated risk of the disease [256]. To determine risk, all women should have a comprehensive family history recorded. According to the Panel's conclusion, women with two or more affected first-degree relatives should be offered counseling about their ovarian cancer risk by a gynecologic oncologist (or other specialist qualified to evaluate family history and to discuss hereditary cancer risks), since these women have a 3% chance of being positive for an ovarian cancer hereditary syndrome. Women with a known hereditary ovarian cancer syndrome, including breast-ovarian cancer syndrome, site-specific ovarian cancer syndrome, and HNPCC, should receive annual rectovaginal pelvic examination, CA-125 determinations, and TVS until childbearing is completed or at least until age 35, at which time prophylactic bilateral oophorectomy is recommended to reduce this significant risk [256]. Although women with these hereditary syndromes are estimated to represent only 0.05% of the female population, they have a 40% estimated lifetime risk of ovarian cancer.

SCREENING AND DIAGNOSTIC METHODS

Bimanual Pelvic Examination

The sensitivity and specificity of pelvic examination for the detection of ovarian cancer are defined imprecisely but certainly are poor. Many small but potentially life-threatening tumors cannot be felt by palpation, nor can such examination differentiate benign from malignant conditions. An estimated 10,000 pelvic examinations are required to detect one ovarian cancer, which may also not be an early tumor when detected. Generally, detection by bimanual pelvic examination reveals advanced disease.

Ultrasonography

Abdominal ultrasonography has been used in ovarian cancer screening with poor results, owing to very low specificity. However, TVS is capable of detecting small ovarian masses and may discriminate some benign masses from malignant adnexal masses. Even this more proximal examination, however, still only poorly predicts which masses are cancers and which are due to benign diseases of the ovary. Color Doppler ultrasonography may improve the specificity of TVS further, but current data are insufficient to suggest that this or any other imaging modality is useful as a screening tool in evaluating average-risk, asymptomatic women. Nevertheless, with these limitations in mind, TVS may be appropriate for women with a high risk for ovarian cancer, as noted.

CA-125

The most extensively studied ovarian cancer serum marker is CA-125. It is a tumor-associated antigen, and its main value is its use in surveillance of women who already have had surgery to remove an epithelial ovarian cancer. Levels of CA-125 are increased in many women with ovarian cancer, but noncancerous diseases of the ovaries also can increase the blood levels of CA-125. Additionally, some ovarian cancers may not produce enough CA-125 to elicit a positive test result. Although testing for CA-125 is not accurate enough for use in the general population, as with TVS, it has been recommended for women at high risk for this disease [256].

EVIDENCE OF EFFECTIVENESS

Much of the evidence concerning the effectiveness of ovarian cancer screening has come from cohort studies. The results to date have not been sufficiently promising to compel conduct of a true randomized controlled trial. In one study, 5,479 self-referred, asymptomatic women underwent periodic screening with abdominal ultrasonography; 326 participants had positive test results, and early ovarian cancer was diagnosed in only five patients [257]. TVS was used in a study of 3,220 asymptomatic, postmenopausal women and yielded only two early ovarian cancers [258].

A case-control study of CA-125 using stored sera reported a specificity of 100% for the most commonly used cutoff level, but sensitivity was only 57%. Einhorn et al. [259] studied CA-125 in a single screening of 5,550 women. Among 175 women undergoing further evaluation, six cancers were detected, two of which were advanced at diagnosis. Jacobs et al. [260] studied the feasibility of ovarian cancer screening with CA-125 and transabdominal ultrasonography in 22,000 women. The group invited to screening was offered three annual screenings with both tests. Women with CA-125 of 30 units/ml were recalled for ultrasonography; among 468 women with elevated levels of CA-125, 29 were referred for a gynecologic opinion and, among this group, six received diagnoses of ovarian cancer. During the follow-up period, 10 women in the group invited to screening developed ovarian cancer; overall, 20 cases were diagnosed in the group not invited to screening. Average survival time was greater in the group invited to screening than in the control group (72.9 versus 41.8 months); although mortality was lower and a favorable stage shift was observed for the group invited to screening, no statistically significant difference between the two groups was detected in the mortality rate or stage distribution. The investigators concluded that the investigation supports the feasibility of offering screening (given high compliance) and that a larger randomized trial with adequate sample sizes should be considered.

KEY ISSUES

Ovarian cancer clearly is a disease that might be controlled better by more effective screening interventions. The key issue that prevents affirmative recommendations for ovarian cancer screening is the poor performance of the screening tools evaluated so far. An ongoing NCI multicenter trial is testing the utility of TVS and CA-125 measurement in reducing mortality from ovarian cancer. Results from this and other studies may more clearly delineate high-risk groups that may be suitable targets for systematic screening. Basic research is needed to develop superior tumor marker or imaging tests.

Testicular Cancer

DISEASE BURDEN

The ACS estimates anticipated that 6,900 new cases of testicular cancer will be diagnosed in 2000 and that 300 men in the United States will die of the disease [8, 40]. Testicular cancer accounts for approximately 1% of all cancers in men and is 4.5 times more common among white men than among black men. Although it is uncommon overall, it is the most common malignancy among men aged 15 to 35. The majority of testicular cancers are diagnosed at the localized stage. Recent advances in the treatment of testicular cancer have permitted cure of the disease even when it is diagnosed at an advanced stage. Five-year survival has improved dramatically in the last three decades, from 63% for testicular cancers diagnosed between 1960 and 1963 to 95% for those diagnosed between 1988 and 1995 [9]. As a result, US testicular cancer mortality has declined by 60% in recent years, without much change in the distribution of stage of disease at diagnosis. Among all invasive cancers, only thyroid malignancies have a higher overall five-year survival rate (96%).

SCREENING RECOMMENDATIONS

The ACS recommends examination of the testicles during a cancer-related checkup every three years for men older than 20 and annually after age 40 [182]. The American Academy of Family Physicians recommends palpation of the testicles for men who are aged 13 to 39 and fall into a higher risk group due to a history of cryptorchidism, orchiopexy, or testicular atrophy [183]. The USPSTF conceded insufficient evidence to recommend for or against routine screening of asymptomatic men [130]. None of these organizations recommends routine testicular examination.

SCREENING AND DIAGNOSTIC METHODS

Generally, testicular cancer is detected through physician palpation or self-detection. No available tests can detect testicular cancer at an asymptomatic stage. Suspicious masses may be evaluated further through ultrasonography and biopsy.

EVIDENCE OF EFFECTIVENESS

No randomized trials have tested the efficacy of testicular examination either by physicians or by individuals. Some advantage is seen in detecting testicular cancer at an early stage in that it may reduce the need for toxic treatment or major surgery. For this reason, examination of the testicles for lumps or nodules or any change in the size, shape, or consistency of the testes may be included in routine general physical examinations performed by health professionals. Patient delay after awareness of a testicular abnormality has been associated with poorer survival, and health education to promote seeking medical care promptly may be beneficial [261].

The issue of regular testicular self-examination by asymptomatic men is more controversial. Performance of periodic self-examination is infrequent even by men educated about the technique, and self-palpation of the testes has low specificity and predictive value [262–264]. Because self-examinations or clinical examinations result in additional provider encounters to evaluate suspicious findings (which are not cancer), false alarms do burden the health care system and can be costly. The scientific literature does not provide much insight into the effectiveness of self-examination of the testicles or an examination by a health care provider, but what evidence does exists suggests that palpation and palpation combined with ultrasonography meet conventional benchmarks for accuracy. Data about the likelihood of false-positive results are less plentiful, but if the rate in the targeted group was as low as 1% because of detection of other masses in the scrotum, based on the underlying risk of disease (3 per 100,000), the ratio of false alarms to cancers detected would be 997 to 1.

KEY ISSUES

Testicular cancer is a poor candidate for control by screening and early detection. The disease is highly treatable and usually is curable. Even if a test were developed to detect testicular cancer during a preclinical phase, aside from basic issues of disease burden and cost-effectiveness, the infrequency of deaths from the disease prohibits documenting any decrease in mortality associated with screening. Although routine screening through self-examination or by a physician is not recommended, delays in diagnosis appear to arise primarily from a lack of awareness of the disease. For this reason, the ACS has endorsed awareness campaigns that inform the public of the signs and symptoms of testicular cancer so as to prompt physician evaluation of an abnormality sooner rather than later.

Melanoma and Nonmelanoma Skin Cancer

DISEASE BURDEN

Combined, melanoma and nonmelanoma skin cancers are the most common cancers, accounting for nearly half of all malignancies. Approximately one million cases of nonmelanoma skin cancer and more than 40,000 melanoma cases are diagnosed in this country each year. Melanoma accounts for only some 4% of skin cancer cases but causes the majority of skin cancer deaths. The ACS predicted that in 2000, approximately 1,900 deaths will result from nonmelanoma and 7,700 deaths from melanoma skin cancer [8, 40]. The number of new melanomas diagnosed in the United States is increasing. Since 1973, the rate of new melanomas diagnosed per year has doubled from 6 per 100,000 to 12 per 100,000 [9]. Late diagnosis is associated with poor prognosis, which in the case of melanoma generally is measured by the thickness of the lesion.

SCREENING RECOMMENDATIONS

The ACS recommends skin examination by a trained health professional every three years for those aged 20 to 39 and annually after age 40 as part of a periodic checkup [265]. The American College of Preventive Medicine recommends periodic total cutaneous examinations for targeted populations at high risk for malignant melanoma [176]. High-risk factors include white race, fair complexion, and the presence of pigmented lesions (dysplastic or atypical nevus) with several large nondysplastic nevi, with many small nevi, with moderate freckling, or with familial dysplastic nevus syndrome [266–268]. The American Academy of Dermatology, the Skin Cancer Foundation, and an NIH Consensus Conference on Early Melanoma recommended annual screening for all patients with familial dysplastic nevus syndrome. The NCI, the Canadian Task Force on the Periodic Health Examination, the USPSTF, the American Academy of Family Physicians, and the American College of Obstetrics and Gynecology variously recommend periodic examination of the skin for those at high risk [50, 176].

SCREENING AND DIAGNOSTIC METHODS

Skin cancer screening involves a 2–3-minute visual inspection of a patient's entire body, including the scalp, hands, and feet. It also may involve patient attention to sun exposure, sun protection, and family history. The principal aim is early identification of melanoma because of the greater life-threatening potential of this disease. Identification of nonmelanoma skin cancer and precursor lesions is an additional potential benefit that may be achieved by total skin examination. A total examination is preferable to examining only the sun-exposed areas of the body because skin cancers often occur at anatomic sites that are not directly exposed to sources of risk. One study reported a sensitivity of 93.3%, a specificity of 97.8%, a PPV of 54%, and a negative predictive value of 99.8% when the screening was performed by dermatologists [269].

The ACS and other organizations also have encouraged monthly skin self-examinations. Individuals are encouraged to check their skin by standing in front of a full-length mirror (and to use a hand-mirror for areas not easily seen) to become familiar with patterns of freckles, moles, and other marks on the skin and to be alert for changes. Friends and relatives also can be alert to changes or to appearance of new or abnormal-appearing areas on the skin.

EVIDENCE OF EFFECTIVENESS

Lack of sufficient evidence prohibits establishing whether routine examination of the skin produces a decrease in mortality. No randomized clinical trial has evaluated the effectiveness of periodic screening in reducing melanoma mortality. Given that visual inspection of the skin is an intervention that is available to all with eyesight, conducting a truly randomized trial would appear impossible. Persons in both intervention and control groups would have the capability to identify suspicious lesions and contaminate the randomization to the extent that the outcomes might be uninterpretable. Evidence relevant to skin cancer—screening recommendations is based primarily on results from community-wide screenings, case-control studies, and observational studies. Studies of high-risk populations report that patients routinely screened by dermatologists have a mean tumor thickness of detected malignant melanoma less than that of historical or population-based controls [270]. The American Academy of Dermatology—ACS program of skin cancer screening examined 500,000 people in various risk categories between 1985 and 1991 and diagnosed more

than 35,000 nonmelanoma skin cancers and 3,500 presumed melanomas, most of them in the early stages [271]. The effectiveness of skin cancer screening may be increased if it is targeted to those persons at high-risk (e.g., whites who are older than age 20 and have atypical mole syndrome or congenital melanocytic nevi; persons with specific phenotypic traits; or those with a history of nonmelanoma skin cancer), but no rigorous comparisons of screening in different risk groups has been done.

In addition to the outcomes, benefits presumably associated with early detection are reduced medical costs. A high proportion of patients with thin melanoma lesions may be treated simply by local excision that can be performed on an outpatient basis.

KEY ISSUES

The evidence in support of the effectiveness of visual screening for skin cancer is weak, but screening recommendations may be justified on the grounds that the intervention is so inexpensive and carries such low risk that any benefit will outweigh risks and costs. In addition, melanoma incidence has been rising worldwide, and the severity and prevalence of the disease may be of sufficient public health importance to warrant community-level action [272, 273]. Evaluation of screening effectiveness is complicated by the fact that skin examination does not identify cases at an asymptomatic stage. Possibly, the most rapidly progressing lesions are those most likely to be brought to medical attention by the patient, leaving more indolent tumors to be detected in screening. Thus, a more favorable stage distribution in a screened population may be a manifestation of length bias.

CANCER-RELATED CHECKUPS

In the late 1970s, the ACS initiated an evidence-based assessment of tests for the early detection of cancer in asymptomatic individuals. Based on the results, *Guidelines for the Cancer-Related Checkup: Recommendations and Rationale* was published in 1980 [3]. In the ensuing years, guidelines for routine screening have changed, as new data have become available. Apart from participating in screening that can be recommended as part of a population-based initiative, the ACS has viewed the patient's periodic encounters with clinicians as having potential for health counseling and a cancer-related checkup. Health counseling may include guidance about smoking cessation, diet, physical activity, and the benefits and risks of undergoing various screening tests. Also, these encounters may result in case-finding examinations of the thyroid, testicles, ovaries, lymph nodes, oral region, and skin.

CONCLUSION

In the very near term, the greatest potential to reduce deaths from cancer is early detection of occult disease (i.e., preclinical malignancies and precursor lesions that have been growing for many years). Ultimately, prevention is the preferred solution to the disease burden of cancer. Adopting healthier lifestyles, in particular eliminating tobacco use, is believed to offer a potential greater than that of early detection in the long run, but the fulfillment of that potential is uncertain at this time. However, the potential for the fullest benefit of applied early-detection strategies also remains uncertain, because screening is integrated poorly into routine health care. Screening under opportunistic conditions rather than through a system is inefficient at both individual and population levels; moreover, absence of a system obviates readiness to implement any new early detection technology that could improve disease control. A comprehensive system of early detection potentially leads not only to high levels of participation but ensures that all the elements of a program of early detection and intervention are highly competent, interrelated, and interdependent. A system has the potential not only to increase quality but to reduce the volume of small errors that contribute to incremental erosions of efficiency and to reduce the gross failures that result in avoidable death. Although many practical barriers must be overcome to establish true population-based screening programs, a system of organized screening holds the greatest potential for realizing the benefits of reducing the incidence rate of advanced cancers.

REFERENCES

1. Morrison A. *Screening in Chronic Disease.* New York: Oxford University Press, 1992.
2. Cole P, Morrison AS. Basic issues in cancer screening. In Miller AB (ed), *Screening in Cancer.* Geneva: International Union Against Cancer, 1978.
3. Eddy D. Guidelines for the cancer related checkup: Recommendations and rationale. *CA Cancer J Clin* 30:3–50, 1980.
4. Miller AB. Fundamentals of Screening. Miller AB, ed. *Screening for Cancer.* Orlando, FL: Academic Press, 1985;3–24.
5. Prorok P, Chamberlain J, Day N, et al. UICC Worksop on the evaluation of screening programs for cancer. *Int J Cancer* 34:1–4, 1984.
6. Smith RA. Screening fundamentals. *Monogr Natl Cancer Inst* 22:15–22, 1997.
7. Shapiro S. Screening for secondary prevention of disease. In Armenian HK, Shapiro S (eds), *Epidemiology and Health Services.* New York: Oxford University Press, 1998,183–206.
8. Greenlee RT, Murray T, Bolden S, Wingo PA. Cancer statistics, 2000. *CA Cancer J Clin* 50:7–33, 2000.
9. Ries L, Kosary C, Hankey B, et al. *SEER Cancer Statistics Review, 1973–1996.* Bethesda, MD: National Cancer Institute, 1999.
10. Duffy SW, Chen HH, Tabar L, Day NE. Estimation of mean sojourn time in breast cancer screening using a Markov chain model of both entry to and exit from the preclinical detectable phase. *Stat Med* 14:1531–1543, 1995.
11. Tabar L, Fagerberg G, Chen HH, et al. Tumour development, histology and grade of breast cancers: prognosis and progression. *Int J Cancer* 66:413–419, 1996.
12. Tabar L, Fagerberg G, Chen HH, et al. Efficacy of breast cancer screening by age. New results from the Swedish Two-County Trial. *Cancer* 75:2507–2517, 1995.
13. Tabar L, Duffy SW, Chen HH. Re: Quantitative interpretation of age-specific mortality reductions from the Swedish Breast Cancer-Screening Trials (letter; comment). *J Natl Cancer Inst* 88:52–55, 1996.
14. Sweden National Board of Health and Welfare. *Mammography Screening for Early Detection of Breast Cancer in Sweden.* NBHW: 1998.
15. Duffy SW, Chen HH, Tabar L, et al. Sojourn time, sensitivity and positive predictive value of mammography screening for breast cancer in women aged 40–49. *Int J Epidemiol* 25:1139–1145, 1996.
16. Tabar L, Faberberg G, Day NE, Holmberg L. What is the optimum interval between mammographic screening examinations? An analysis based on the latest results of the Swedish two-county breast cancer screening trial. *Br J Cancer* 55:547–551, 1987.
17. Miller AB. Fundamental issues in screening for cancer. In Schottenfeld D, Fraumeni JF (eds), *Cancer Epidemiology and Prevention* (2nd ed). New York: Oxford University Press, 1996.
18. Day NE, Walter SD. Simplified models of screening for chronic disease: estimation procedures from mass screening programmes. *Biometrics* 40:1–14, 1984.
19. Bassett LW, Hendrick RE, Bassford TL, et al. *Quality Determinants of Mammography.* Clinical Practice Guidelines, No. 13, Publication No. 95–00632. Rockville, MD: AHCPR Agency for Health Care Policy and Research Public Health Service, US Department of Health and Human Services, 1994.
20. Smith R. Principles of successful cancer screening. *Surg Oncol Clin North Am* 8:1–23, 1999.
21. Gold M. Recommendations of the panel on cost-effectiveness in health and medicine. *JAMA* 276:1253–1258, 1996.
22. Garber AM, Weinstein MC, Torrance GW, Kamlet MS. Theoretical foundations of cost-effectiveness analysis. In

Gold MR, Siegel JE, Russell LB, Weinstein MC (eds), *Cost-Effectiveness in Health and Medicine.* New York: Oxford University Press, 1996.

23. Eisenberg JM. Clinical economics. A guide to the economic analysis of clinical practices. *JAMA* 262:2879–2886, 1989.

24. Siegel J, Weinstein M, Russell L. Recommendations for reporting cost-effectiveness analysis. *JAMA* 276:1339–1341, 1996.

25. National Cancer Institute Breast Cancer Screening Consortium. Screening mammography: a missed clinical opportunity? Results of the NCI breast cancer screening consortium and national health interview survey studies. *JAMA* 264:54–58, 1990.

26. Horton JA, Romans MC, Cruess DF. Mammography attitudes and usage study, 1992. *Womens Health Issues* 2:180–186, discussion 187–188, 1992.

27. Vernon SW. Participation in colorectal cancer screening: a review (see comments). *J Natl Cancer Inst* 89:1406–1422, 1997.

28. Kiefe CI, Funkhouser E, Fouad MN, May DS. Chronic disease as a barrier to breast and cervical cancer screening (see comments). *J Gen Intern Med* 13:357–365, 1998.

29. Smith RA, Haynes S. Barriers to screening for breast cancer. *Cancer* 69(suppl 7): 1968–1978, 1992.

30. Rimer BK. Current use and how to increase mammography screening in women. *Surg Oncol Clin North Am* 6:203–211, 1997.

31. McPhee SJ, Bird JA, Fordham D, et al. Promoting cancer prevention activities by primary care physicians. Results of a randomized, controlled trial. *JAMA* 266:538–544, 1991.

32. Dietrich JJ, Woodruff CB, Carney PA. Changing office routines to enhance preventive care. The preventive GAPS approach. *Arch Fam Med* 3:176–183, 1994.

33. Gann P, Melville SK, Luckmann R. Characteristics of primary care office systems as predictors of mammography utilization. *Ann Intern Med* 118:893–898, 1993.

34. Garr DR, Ornstein SM, Jenkins RG, Zemp LD. The effect of routine use of computer-generated preventive reminders in a clinical practice. *Am J Prev Med* 9:55–61, 1993.

35. Somkin CP, Hiatt RA, Hurley LB, et al. The effect of patient and provider reminders on mammography and Papanicolaou smear screening in a large health maintenance organization. *Arch Intern Med* 157:1658–1664, 1997.

36. Fulton JP, Buechner JS, Scott HD, et al. A study guided by the health belief model of predictors of breast cancer screening among women ages 40 and older. *Public Health Rep* 106:410–420, 1991.

37. Horton JA, Cruess DF, Romans MC. Compliance with mammography screening guidelines: 1995 Mammography Attitudes and Usage Study Report. *Womens Health Issues* 6:239–245, 1996.

38. Cronin KA, Weed DL, Connor RJ, Prorok PC. Case-control studies of cancer screening: theory and practice. *J Natl Cancer Inst* 90:498–504, 1998.

39. Gaus CR. Guideline development and use. In Bassett LW, Hendrick RE, Bassford TL, et al. (eds), *Quality Determinants of Mammography. Clinical Practice Guidelines,* No. 13, Publication No. 95–00632, vol 13. Rockville, MD: AHCPR Agency for Health Care Policy and Research Public Health Service, US Department of Health and Human Services, 1994.

40. American Cancer Society. *American Cancer Society Facts and Figures.* Atlanta: American Cancer Society, 1999.

41. Page DL, Jensen RA. Ductal carcinoma in situ of the breast: understanding the misunderstood stepchild (editorial, comment) (see comments). *JAMA* 275:948–949, 1996.

42. Morrow M. Understanding ductal carcinoma in situ: A step in the right direction. *Cancer* 86:375–377, 1999.

43. Fisher ER, Dignam J, Tan-Chiu E, et al. Pathologic findings from the National Surgical Adjuvant Breast Project (NSABP) eight-year update of protocol B-17. *Cancer* 86:429–438, 1999.

44. National Cancer Institute. *Consensus Development Meeting on Breast Cancer Screening.* Bethesda, MD: U.S. Department of Health, Education, and Welfare; Public Health Service, 1977.

45. Dodd GD. American Cancer Society guidelines on screening for breast cancer. An overview. *Cancer* 69(suppl 7):1885–1887, 1992.

46. Smith RA. Breast cancer screening guidelines. *Womens Health Issues* 2:212–217, discussion 217–219, 1992.

47. American Cancer Society. *Mammography: Two Statements of the American Cancer Society.* New York, 1983.

48. Eddy DM, Hasselblad V, McGivney W, Hendee W. The value of mammography screening in women under age 50 years. *JAMA* 259:1512–1519, 1988.

49. Fletcher SW, Black W, Harris R, et al. Report of the International Workshop on Screening for Breast Cancer (see comments). *J Natl Cancer Inst* 85:1644–1656, 1993.

50. U.S. Preventive Services Task Force. *Guide to Clinical Preventive Services.* Baltimore: Williams & Wilkins, 1996.

51. Burke W, Petersen G, Lynch P, et al. Recommendations for follow-up care of individuals with an inherited predisposition to cancer. I. Hereditary nonpolyposis colon cancer. Cancer Genetics Studies Consortium. *JAMA* 277:915–919, 1997.

52. National Institutes of Health Consensus Development Panel. National Institutes of Health Consensus Development Conference Statement: Breast Cancer Screening for Women Ages 40–49, January 21–23, 1997. National Institutes of Health Consensus Development Panel. *J Natl Cancer Inst* 89:1015–1026, 1997.

53. Organizing Committee and Collaborators. Breast cancer screening with mammography in women aged 40–49 Years. Report of the organizing committee and collaborators, Falun meeting, Falun, Sweden (21 and 22 March, 1996). *Int J Cancer* 68:693–699, 1996.

54. Leitch AM, Dodd GD, Costanza M, et al. American Cancer Society guidelines for the early detection of breast cancer: update 1997. *CA Cancer J Clin* 47:150–153, 1997.

55. Feig SA, D'Orsi CJ, Hendrick RE, et al. American College of Radiology guidelines for breast cancer screening. *AJR Am J Roentgenol* 171:29–33, 1998.

56. Short MP, Nielsen NH, Young DC, Kahn M. Council on Scientific Affairs. *Mammography Screening for Asymptomatic Women: Report of the Council on Scientific Affairs.* Chicago: American Medical Association, 1999.

57. National Cancer Institute. *Statement from the National Cancer Institute on the National Cancer Advisory Board Recommendations on Mammography.* Bethesda, MD: NCI, 1997.

58. Donegan WL. Diagnosis. In Donegan WL, Spratt JS (eds), *Cancer of the Breast.* (4th ed). Philadelphia: W. B. Saunders Company, 1995:157–205.

59. Hendrick RE. Quality assurance in mammography. Accreditation, legislation, and compliance with quality assurance standards. *Radiol Clin North Am* 30:243–255, 1992.

60. Hendrick RE. Quality control in mammography: The American College of Radiology's Mammography Screening Accreditation Program. *Curr Opin Radiol* 1:203–211, 1989.

61. Food and Drug Administration. *Quality Mammography Standards; Final Rule,* vol 62, edition 208. Rockville, MD: Department of Health and Human Services, 1997, 55851–55901.

62. May DS, Lee NC, Nadel MR, et al. The National Breast and Cervical Cancer Early Detection Program: report on the first 4 years of mammography provided to medically underserved women (see comments). *AJR Am J Roentgenol* 170:97–104, 1998.

63. Food and Drug Administration (CDRH). *Compliance Guidance: The Mammography Quality Standards Act: Final Regulations.* Bethesda, MD: U.S. Department of Health and Human Services, 1999.

64. American College of Radiology BI-RADS Committee. *Illustrated Breast Imaging Reporting and Data System (BI-RADS).* Reston, VA: American College of Radiology, 1998.

65. Jackson VP, Hendrick RE, Feig SA, Kopans DB. Imaging of the radiographically dense breast. *Radiology* 188:297–301, 1993.

66. Lewin JM, Hendrick RE, D'Orsi CJ, et al. *Clinical evaluation of a full-field digital mammography prototype for cancer detection in a screening setting—work in progress.* Presented at the 84th scientific assembly and annual meeting of the RSNA, 1998.

67. Qian W, Clarke L. Digital mammography: Computer-assisted diagosis method for mass detection with multiorientation and multi-resolution wavelet transforms. *Acad Radiol* 4:724–731, 1997.

68. Feig SA, Yaffe MJ. Clinical prospects for full-field digital mammography. *Semin Breast Dis* 2:64–73, 1999.

69. Vyborny CJ, Giger ML. Computer vision and artificial intelligence in mammography. *AJR Am J Roentgenol* 162:699–708, 1994.

70. Orel SG. High-resolution MR imaging for the detection, diagnosis, and staging of breast cancer. *Radiographics* 18:903–912, 1998.

71. Bassett L, Hendrick R, Bassford T, et al. *Quality Determinants of Mammography.* Clinical Practice Guideline No. 13. Bethesda, MD: Agency for Health Care Policy and Research, Public Health Service, U.S. Department of Health and Human Services, 1994.

72. Bassett LW, Gold RH, Kimme-Smith C. History of the technical development of mammography. In Haus AG, Yaffe MJ (eds), *Syllabus: A Categorical Course in Physics: Technical Aspects of Breast Imaging.* Second editon. Chicago: Radiological Society of North America, 1993:9–20.

73. Donegan WL. Introduction to the history of breast cancer. In Donegan WL, Spratt JS (eds), *Cancer of the Breast* (4th ed). Philadelphia: W. B. Saunders Company, 1995:1–15.

74. Shapiro S. Periodic breast cancer screening in seven foreign countries. *Cancer* 69(suppl 7):1919–1924, 1992.

75. Shapiro S, Venet W, Strax P, et al. Ten- to fourteen-year effect of screening on breast cancer mortality. *J Natl Cancer Inst* 69:349–355, 1982.

76. Baker L. Breast Cancer Detection Demonstration Project: Five year summary report. *CA Cancer J Clin* 32:196–229, 1982.

77. Smart CR, Byrne C, Smith RA, et al. Twenty-year follow-up of the breast cancers diagnosed during the Breast Cancer Detection Demonstration Project (see comments). *CA Cancer J Clin* 47:134–149, 1997.

78. Tabar L, Fagerberg CJ, Gad A, et al. Reduction in mortality from breast cancer after mass screening with mammography. Randomised trial from the Breast Cancer Screening Working Group of the Swedish National Board of Health and Welfare. *Lancet* 1: 829–832, 1985.

79. Andersson I, Aspegren K, Janzon L, et al. Mammographic screening and mortality from breast cancer: the Malmo mammographic screening trial. *BMJ* 297:943–948, 1988.

80. Miller AB, Baines CJ, To T, Wall C. Canadian National Breast Screening Study: 1. Breast cancer detection and death rates among women aged 40 to 49 years (published erratum appears in *Can Med Assoc J* 148:718, 1993) (see comments). *Can Med Assoc J* 147:1459–1476, 1992.

81. Alexander FE, Anderson TJ, Brown HK, et al. The Edinburgh randomised trial of breast cancer screening: results after 10 years of follow-up. *Br J Cancer* 70:542–548, 1994.

82. Bjurstam N, Bjorneld L, Duffy SW, et al. The Gothenburg breast screening trial: first results on mortality, incidence, and mode of detection for women ages 39–49 years at randomization (see comments). *Cancer* 80:2091–2099, 1997.

83. Bailar JC. Mammography before age 50 years? (editorial). *JAMA* 259:1548–1549, 1988.

84. Eddy DM. Screening for breast cancer (see comments). *Ann Intern Med* 111:389–399, 1989.

85. Fletcher S, Black W, Harris R, et al. *Report of the International Workshop on Screening for Breast Cancer.* Bethesda, MD: National Cancer Institute, 1993.

86. Forrest AP, Alexander FE. A question that will not go away: at what age should mammographic screening begin? (editorial, comment). *J Natl Cancer Inst* 87:1195–1197, 1995.

87. Eckhardt S, Badellino F, Murphy GP. UICC meeting on breast-cancer screening in pre-menopausal women in developed countries. Geneva, 29 September-1 October 1993. *Int J Cancer* 56:1–5, 1994.

88. Shapiro S. The call for change in breast cancer screening guidelines (editorial). *Am J Public Health* 84:10–11, 1994.

89. Eddy DM. Breast cancer screening in women younger than 50 years of age: what's next? (editorial). *Ann Intern Med* 127:1035–1036, 1997.

90. Shapiro S, Strax P, Venet L. Periodic breast cancer screening in reducing mortality from breast cancer. *JAMA* 215:1777–1785, 1971.

91. Hurley SF, Kaldor JM. The benefits and risks of mammographic screening for breast cancer. *Epidemiol Rev* 14: 101–130, 1992.

92. Hurley SF, Jolley DJ, Livingston PM, et al. Effectiveness, costs, and cost-effectiveness of recruitment strategies for a mammographic screening program to detect breast cancer. *J Natl Cancer Inst* 84:855–863, 1992.

93. Kopans DB. An overview of the breast cancer screening controversy. *J Natl Cancer Inst Monogr* 22:1–3, 1997.

94. Wald N, Chamberlain J, Hackshaw A. Report of the European Society of Mastology Breast Cancer Screening Evaluation Committee (published erratum appears in *Tumori* 80: 314, 1994). *Tumori* 79:371–379, 1993.

95. Elwood M, Cox B, Richardson A. The effectiveness of breast cancer screening by mammography in younger women: correction (letter). *Online J Curr Clin Trials* 1994; Doc. No. 121: (385 words; 4 paragraphs).

96. Kerlikowske K, Grady D, Ernster V. Benefit of mammography screening in women ages 40–49 years: current evidence from randomized controlled trials (letter) (see comments). *Cancer* 76:1679–1681, 1995.

97. Smart CR, Hendrick RE, Rutledge JH III, Smith RA. Benefit of mammography screening in women ages 40 to 49 years. Current evidence from randomized controlled trials (published erratum appears in *Cancer* 75(11):1995). *Cancer* 75:1619–1626, 1995.

98. Hendrick RE, Smith RA, Rutledge JH III, Smart CR. Benefit of screening mammography in women aged 40–49: a new meta-analysis of randomized controlled trials. *J Natl Cancer Inst Monogr* 22:87–92, 1997.

99. Tabar L, Duffy SW, Vitak B, et al. The natural history of breast carcinoma: what have we learned from screening? *Cancer* 86:449–462, 1999.

100. Kopans DB. Mammography screening and the controversy concerning women aged 40 to 49. *Radiol Clin North Am* 33:1273–1290, 1995.

101. de Koning HJ, Boer R, Warmerdam PG, et al. Quantitative interpretation of age-specific mortality reductions from the Swedish breast cancer-screening trials (see comments). *J Natl Cancer Inst* 87:1217–1223, 1995.

102. Tabar L, Chen HH, Fagerberg G, et al. Recent results from the Swedish Two-County Trial: the effects of age, histologic type, and mode of detection on the efficacy of breast cancer screening. *J Natl Cancer Inst Monogr* 22:43–47, 1997.

103. Duffy SW, Day NE, Tabar L, et al. Markov models of breast tumor progression: some age-specific results. *J Natl Cancer Inst Monogr* 22:93–97, 1997.

104. Sickles EA. Breast cancer screening outcomes in women ages 40–49: clinical experience with service screening using modern mammography. *J Natl Cancer Inst Monogr* 22:99–104, 1997.

105. Kerlikowske K, Grady D, Barclay J, et al. Effect of age, breast density, and family history on the sensitivity of first screening mammography (see comments). *JAMA* 276:33–38, 1996.

106. Linver MN, Paster SB. Mammography outcomes in a practice setting by age: prognostic factors, sensitivity, and positive biopsy rate. *J Natl Cancer Inst Monogr* 22:113–117, 1997.

107. Linver MN, Rosenberg RD. Callback rate after screening mammography. *AJR Am J Roentgenol* 171:262–263, 1998.

108. Shapiro S, Venet W, Strax P, Venet L. *Periodic Screening for Breast Cancer: The Health Insurance Plan Project and its Sequelae.* Baltimore: Johns Hopkins Press, 1988.

109. Feig SA, Shaber GS, Schwartz GF, et al. Thermography, mammography, and clinical examination in breast cancer screening. Review of 16,000 studies. *Radiology* 122:123–127, 1977.

110. Burns PE, Grace MG, Lees AW, May C. False negative mammograms causing delay in breast cancer diagnosis. *J Can Assoc Radiol* 30:74–76, 1979.

111. Guthrie TH Jr. Breast cancer litigation: A retrospective analysis. *Breast J* 1:376–379, 1995.

112. Lee KC, Dunlop D, Dolan NC. Do clinical breast examination skills improve during medical school? *Acad Med* 73:1013–1019, 1998.

113. Desnick L, Taplin S, Taylor V, et al. Clinical breast examination in primary care: perceptions and predictors among three specialties. *J Womens Health* 8:389–397, 1999.

114. O'Malley MS, Fletcher SW. US Preventive Services Task Force. Screening for breast cancer with breast self-examination. A critical review. *JAMA* 257:2196–2203, 1987.

115. Smith RA. Point-counterpoint: Is breast self-examination being emphasized too much? *Oncology Times*, 1994, 42.

116. Cassileth BR. Point-counterpoint: Is breast self-examination being emphasized too much? *Oncology Times*, 1994, 42.

117. Costanza MC, Foster RS Jr. Relationship between breast self-examination and death from breast cancer by age groups. *Cancer Detect Prev* 7:103–108, 1984.

118. Dowle CS, Mitchell A, Elston CW, et al. Preliminary results of the Nottingham breast self-examination education programme. *Br J Surg* 74:217–219, 1987.

119. Foster RS Jr, Lang SP, Costanza MC, et al. Breast self-examination practices and breast-cancer stage. *N Engl J Med* 299:265–270, 1978.

120. Mant D, Vessey MP, Neil A, et al. Breast self examination and breast cancer stage at diagnosis. *Br J Cancer* 55:207–211, 1987.

121. Newcomb PA, Weiss NS, Storer BE, et al. Breast self-examination in relation to the occurrence of advanced breast cancer. *J Natl Cancer Inst* 83:260–265, 1991.

122. Harvey BJ, Miller AB, Baines CJ, Corey PN. Effect of breast self-examination techniques on the risk of death from breast cancer. *Can Med Assoc J* 157:1205–1212, 1997.

123. Semiglazov VF, Moiseenko VM. Breast self-examination for the early detection of breast cancer: a USSR/WHO controlled trial in Leningrad. *Bull World Health Organ* 65:391–396, 1987.

124. Thomas DB, Gao DL, Self SG, et al. Randomized trial of breast self-examination in Shanghai: methodology and preliminary results (see comments). *J Natl Cancer Inst* 89:355–365, 1997.

125. May D, Lee N, Nadel M, et al. The National breast and cervical cancer early detection program: report on the

first 4 years of mammography provided to medically underserved women. *Am J Radiol* 170:97–104, 1998.

126. Foster RS Jr, Worden JK, Costanza MC. Breast self-examination (letter). *JAMA* 258:1332–1333, 1987.

127. Chu KC, Tarone RE, Kessler LG, et al. Recent trends in U.S. breast cancer incidence, survival, and mortality rates (see comments). *J Natl Cancer Inst* 88:1571–1579, 1996.

128. Winawer SJ, Fletcher RH, Miller L, et al. Colorectal cancer screening: clinical guidelines and rationale (see comments) (published errata appear in *Gastroenterology* 112:1060, 1997 and 114:625, 1998). *Gastroenterology* 112:594–642, 1997.

129. Byers T, Levin B, Rothenberger D, et al. American Cancer Society guidelines for screening and surveillance for early detection of colorectal polyps and cancer: update 1997. *CA Cancer J Clin* 47:154–160, 1997.

130. US Preventive Services Task Force. *Guide to Clinical Preventive Services.* Baltimore: Williams & Wilkins, 1996.

131. Young G, St. John J. Selecting an occult blood test for use as a screening tool for large bowel cancer. *Front Gastrointest Res* 18:135–156, 1991.

132. American College of Physicians. Suggested technique for fecal occult blood testing and interpretation in colorectal cancer screening. *Ann Intern Med* 126:808–810, 1997.

133. Ransohoff DF, Lang CA. Screening for colorectal cancer with the fecal occult blood test: a background paper. American College of Physicians (see comments). *Ann Intern Med* 126:811–822, 1997.

134. Waye JD. Colonoscopy (see comments). *CA Cancer J Clin* 42:350–365, 1992.

135. Waye JD, Lewis BS, Yessayan S. Colonoscopy: a prospective report of complications. *J Clin Gastroenterol* 15:347–351, 1992.

136. O'Brien M, Winawer S, Zauber A, et al. The National Polyp Study. Patient and polyp characteristics associated with high-grade dysplasia in colorectal adenomas. *Gastroenterology* 98:371–379, 1990.

137. Atkin WS, Morson BC, Cuzick J. Long-term risk of colorectal cancer after excision of rectosigmoid adenomas (see comments). *N Engl J Med* 326:658–662, 1992.

138. Stryker S, Wolff B, Culp C, et al. Natural history of untreated colonic polyps. *Gastroenterology* 93:1009–1013, 1987.

139. Rustgi A. Hereditary gastrointestinal polyposis and non-polyposis syndromes. *N Engl J Med* 331:1694–1702, 1994.

140. Winawer SJ, Zauber AG, Ho MN, et al. Prevention of colorectal cancer by colonoscopic polypectomy. The National Polyp Study Workgroup (see comments). *N Engl J Med* 329:1977–1981, 1993.

141. Thiis-Evensen E, Hoff GS, Sauar J, et al. Population-based surveillance by colonoscopy: effect on the incidence of colorectal cancer. Telemark Polyp Study I. *Scand J Gastroenterol* 34:414–420, 1999.

142. Mandel JS, Bond JH, Church TR, et al. Reducing mortality from colorectal cancer by screening for fecal occult blood. Minnesota Colon Cancer Control Study (published erratum appears in *N Engl J Med* 329:672, 1996) (see comments). *N Engl J Med* 328:1365–1371, 1993.

143. Mandel JS, Church TR, Ederer F, Bond JH. Colorectal cancer mortality: effectiveness of biennial screening for fecal occult blood (see comments). *J Natl Cancer Inst* 91:434–437, 1999.

144. Hardcastle JD, Chamberlain JO, Robinson MH, et al. Randomised controlled trial of faecal-occult-blood screening for colorectal cancer (see comments). *Lancet* 348:1472–1477, 1996.

145. Selby J, Friedman GD, Quesenberry CP Jr, Weiss NS. A case controled study of screening sigmoidoscopy and mortality from colorectal cancer. *N Engl J Med* 326:653–657, 1992.

146. Newcomb PA, Norfleet RG, Storer BE, et al. Screening sigmoidoscopy and colorectal cancer mortality. *J Natl Cancer Inst* 84:1572–1575, 1992.

147. Muller AD, Sonnenberg A. Prevention of colorectal cancer by flexible endoscopy and polypectomy. A case-control study of 32,702 veterans (see comments). *Ann Intern Med* 123:904–910, 1995.

148. Kavanagh AM, Giovannucci EL, Fuchs CS, Colditz GA. Screening endoscopy and risk of colorectal cancer in United States men. *Cancer Causes Control* 9:455–462, 1998.

149. Winawer SJ, Flehinger BJ, Schottenfeld D, Miller DG. Screening for colorectal cancer with fecal occult blood testing and sigmoidoscopy (see comments). *J Natl Cancer Inst* 85:1311–1318, 1993.

150. Bennett DH, Robinson MR, Preece P, et al. Colorectal cancer screening: the effect of combining flexible sigmoidoscopy with faecal occult blood test. *Gut* 36(suppl 1): T91, 1995.

151. Rex DK, Weddie RA, Lehman GA, et al. Flexible sigmoidoscopy plus air contrast barium enema versus colonscopy for suspected lower gastrointestinal bleeding. *Gastroenterology* 98:855–861, 1990.

152. Rex DK, Lehman GA, Hawes RH, et al. Screening colonoscopy in asymptomatic average-risk persons with negative fecal occult blood tests (see comments). *Gastroenterology* 100:64–67, 1991.

153. Wagner JL, Tunis J, Brown M, et al. Cost-effectiveness of colorectal cancer screening in average-risk adults. In Young G, Levin B (eds), *Prevention and Early Detection of Colorectal Cancer.* London: Saunders, 1996.

154. American Cancer Society. *Adults' Knowledge and Experience with Testing for Colorectal Cancer: a Study of Adults Age 50 and Over.* Atlanta: American Cancer Society, 1998.

155. Mettlin C, Jones G, Averette H, et al. Defining and updating the American Cancer Society guidelines for the cancer-related checkup: prostate and endometrial cancers (see comments). *CA Cancer J Clin* 43:42–46, 1993.

156. von Eschenbach A, Ho R, Murphy GP, et al. American Cancer Society guideline for the early detection of prostate cancer: update 1997. *CA Cancer J Clin* 47:261–264, 1997.

157. Chodak GW, Keller P, Schoenberg HW. Assessment of screening for prostate cancer using the digital rectal examination. *J Urol* 141:1136–1138, 1989.

158. Schroder FH, van der Maas P, Beemsterboer P, et al. Evaluation of the digital rectal examination as a screening test for prostate cancer. Rotterdam section of the Euro-

pean Randomized Study of Screening for Prostate Cancer (see comments). *J Natl Cancer Inst* 90:1817–1823, 1998.

159. Basler JW, Thompson IM. Lest we abandon digital rectal examination as a screening test for prostate cancer (editorial, comment). *J Natl Cancer Inst* 90:1761–1763, 1998.

160. Wang MC, Valenzuela LA, Murphy GP, Chu TM. Purification of a human prostate specific antigen. *Invest Urol* 17:159–163, 1979.

161. Catalona WJ, Smith DS, Ratliff TL, et al. Measurement of prostate-specific antigen in serum as a screening test for prostate cancer (published erratum appears in *N Engl J Med* 325:1324, 1991) (see comments). *N Engl J Med* 324:1156–1161, 1991.

162. Mettlin C, Lee F, Drago J, Murphy GP. The American Cancer Society National Prostate Cancer Detection Project. Findings on the detection of early prostate cancer in 2,425 men. *Cancer* 67:2949–2958, 1991.

163. Stenman UH, Leinonen J, Zhang WM. Standardization of PSA determinations. *Scand J Clin Lab Invest* 221(suppl): 45–51, 1995.

164. Mettlin C, Chesley AE, Murphy GP, et al. Association of free PSA percent, total PSA, age, and gland volume in the detection of prostate cancer. *Prostate* 39:153–158, 1999.

165. Benson MC, Whang IS, Olsson CA, et al. The use of prostate specific antigen density to enhance the predictive value of intermediate levels of serum prostate specific antigen. *J Urol* 147(3 Part 2):817–821, 1992.

166. Benson MC, Whang IS, Pantuck A, et al. Prostate specific antigen density: a means of distinguishing benign prostatic hypertrophy and prostate cancer. *J Urol* 147(3 Part 2):815–816, 1992.

167. Oesterling JE. Prostate-specific antigen. Improving its ability to diagnose early prostate cancer (editorial, comment) (see comments). *JAMA* 267:2236–2238, 1992.

168. Carter HB, Pearson JD, Metter EJ, et al. Longitudinal evaluation of prostate-specific antigen levels in men with and without prostate disease (see comments). *JAMA* 267:2215–2220, 1991.

169. Mettlin CJ, Murphy GP, Babaian RJ, et al. Observations on the early detection of prostate cancer from the American Cancer Society National Prostate Cancer Detection Project. *Cancer* 80:1814–1817, 1997.

170. Stephenson RA, Stanford JL. Population-based prostate cancer trends in the United States: patterns of change in the era of prostate-specific antigen. *World J Urol* 15:331–335, 1997.

171. Mettlin CJ, Murphy GP. Why is the prostate cancer death rate declining in the United States? (editorial) (published erratum appears in *Cancer* 82:1802, 1998). *Cancer* 82:249–251, 1998.

172. Mettlin C. Changes in patterns of prostate cancer care in the United States: results of American College of Surgeons Commission on Cancer studies, 1974–1993. *Prostate* 32:221–226, 1997.

173. Ries L, Kosary C, Hankey B, et al. *SEER Cancer Statistics Review, 1973–1995.* Bethesda, MD: National Cancer Institute, 1998.

174. Labrie F, Candas B, Dupont A, et al. Screening decreases prostate cancer death: first analysis of the 1988 Quebec prospective randomized controlled trial. *Prostate* 38:83–91, 1999.

175. Kramer BS, Gohagan J, Prorok PC, Smart C. A National Cancer Institute sponsored screening trial for prostatic, lung, colorectal, and ovarian cancers. *Cancer* 71(suppl 2):589–593, 1993.

176. Ferrini R, Woolf SH. American College of Preventive Medicine practice policy. Screening for prostate cancer in American men. *Am J Prev Med* 15:81–84, 1998.

177. American College of Physicians. Screening for prostate cancer. *Ann Intern Med* 126:480–484, 1997.

178. Collins MM, Barry MJ. Controversies in prostate cancer screening. Analogies to the early lung cancer screening debate (see comments). *JAMA* 276:1976–1979, 1996.

179. Hall RR. Screening and early detection of prostate cancer will decrease morbidity and mortality from prostate cancer: the argument against. *Eur Urol* 29(suppl 2):24–26, 1996.

180. Albertson PC. Screening for prostate cancer is neither appropriate nor cost-effective. *Urol Clin North Am* 23: 521–530, 1996.

181. Halpern MT, Gillespie BW, Warner KE. Patterns of absolute risk of lung cancer mortality in former smokers (see comments). *J Natl Cancer Inst* 85:457–464, 1993.

182. American Cancer Society. *The American Cancer Society Guideline for the Cancer-Related Checkup: An Update.* Atlanta: American Cancer Society, 1993.

183. American Academy of Family Physicians. *Age Charts for the Periodic Health Examination.* American Academy of Family Physicians, 1994.

184. Eddy D. *Screening for Lung Cancer.* Philadelphia: American College of Physicians, 1991.

185. Gohagan J, Prorok P, Kramer B. The prostate, lung, colorectal and ovarian cancer screening trial of the National Cancer Institute. *Cancer* 75:1869–1873, 1995.

186. Black WC. Lung Cancer. In Kramer BS, Gohagan JK, Prorok PC (eds), *Cancer Screening: Theory and Practice.* New York: Marcel Dekker, Inc., 1999: 327–377.

187. Muhm JR, Miller WE, Fontana RS, et al. Lung cancer detected during a screening program using four-month chest radiographs. *Radiology* 148:609–615, 1983.

188. Petty TL. The identification of lung cancer by sputum cytology. Dominioni L, Strauss G (eds), *International Conference on Prevention and Early Diagnosis of Lung Cancer* 1998:115–116.

189. Hittelman WH: Molecular risk assessment in current and former cigarette smokers. Dominioni L, Strauss G (eds), *International Conference on Prevention and Early Diagnosis of Lung Cancer,* 1998:117–120.

190. Berlin NI: Overview of the NCI cooperative early lung cancer detection program, Dominioni L, Strauss G (eds), *International Conference on Prevention and Early Diagnosis of Lung Cancer,* 1998:11–14.

191. Fontana RS, Sanderson DR, Woolner LB, et al. Screening for lung cancer. A critique of the Mayo Lung Project. *Cancer* 67(suppl 4): 1155–1164, 1991.

192. Fontana RS. The Mayo lung project: a perspective. Dominioni L, Strauss G (eds), *International Conference on Prevention and Early Diagnosis of Lung Cancer,* 1998: 15–20.

193. Melamed MR, Flehinger BJ, Zaman MB, et al. Screening for early lung cancer. Results of the Memorial Sloan-Kettering study in New York. *Chest* 86:44–53, 1984.

194. Melamed MR. Lung cancer screening results in the New York study. Dominioni L, Strauss G (eds), *International Conference on Prevention and Early Diagnosis of Lung Cancer,* 1998:21–28.

195. Frost JK, Ball WC Jr, Levin ML, et al. Early lung cancer detection: results of the initial (prevalence) radiologic and cytologic screening in the Johns Hopkins study. *Am Rev Respir Dis* 130:549–554, 1984.

196. Tockman MS. What did we learn from the Johns Hopkins Lung Project, Dominioni L, Strauss G (eds), *International Conference on Prevention and Early Diagnosis of Lung Cancer,* 1998:29–33.

197. Kubik A, Polak J. Lung cancer detection. Results of a randomized prospective study in Czechoslovakia. *Cancer* 57:2427–2437, 1986.

198. Kubik A, Parkin DM, Khlat M, et al. Lack of benefit from semi-annual screening for cancer of the lung: follow-up report of a randomized controlled trial on a population of high-risk males in Czechoslovakia. *Int J Cancer* 45:26–33, 1990.

199. Kubik A, Haerting J. Survival and mortality in a randomized study of lung cancer detection. *Neoplasma* 37:467–475, 1990.

200. Henschke CI, McCauley DI, Yankelevitz DF, et al. Early Lung Cancer Action Project: overall design and findings from baseline screening (see comments). *Lancet* 354:99–105, 1999.

201. Wolpaw DR. Early detection in lung cancer. Case finding and screening. *Med Clin North Am* 80:63–82, 1996.

202. Smith IE. Screening for lung cancer: time to think positive (comment). *Lancet* 354:86–87, 1999.

203. Koss LG. The Papanicolaou test for cervical cancer detection. A triumph and a tragedy (see comments). *JAMA* 261:737–743, 1989.

204. Kurman R, Henson D, Herbst A, et al. Interim guidelines for management of abnormal cervical cytology. *JAMA* 271:1866–1869, 1994.

205. American Association of Central Cancer Registries. *Working Group on Pre-invasive Cervical Neoplasia and Population-based Cancer Registries: Final Subcommittee Report.* AACCR, 1993.

206. Lawson H, Lee N, Thames S, et al. Cervical cancer screening among low-income women: results of a national screening program, 1991–1995. *Obstet Gynecol* 92:745–752, 1998.

207. Shingleton HM, Patrick RL, Johnston WW, Smith RA. The current status of the Papanicolaou smear. *CA Cancer J Clin* 45:305–320, 1995.

208. American College of Physicians. Screening for cervical cancer. In Eddy D (ed), *Common Screening Tests.* Philadelphia: American College of Physicians, 1991:413–414.

209. Canadian Task Force on the Periodic Health Examination. *Canadian Guide to Clinical Preventive Health Care.* Canadian Communications Group, 1994.

210. Eifel PJ, Berek JS, Thigpen JT. Cancer of the cervix, vagina, and vulva. In Devita VT, Hellman S, Rosenberg SA (eds), *Cancer: Principles and Practice of Oncology,* vol 1, (5th ed). Philadelphia: Lippincott-Raven, 1997.

211. Gefeller O, Windeler J. Risk factors for cervical cancer: comments on attributable risk calculations and the evaluation of screening in case-control studies (letter, comment). *Int J Epidemiol* 20:1140–1143, 1993.

212. Nakagawa S, Yoshikawa H, Onda T, et al. Type of human papillomavirus is related to clinical features of cervical carcinoma. *Cancer* 78:1935–1941, 1996.

213. Thomas DB, Ray RM. Oral contraceptives and invasive adenocarcinomas and adenosquamous carcinomas of the uterine cervix. The World Health Organization Collaborative Study of Neoplasia and Steroid Contraceptives. *Am J Epidemiol* 144:281–289, 1996.

214. Boon ME, de Graaff Guilloud JC, Rietveld WJ. Analysis of five sampling methods for the preparation of cervical smears. *Acta Cytol* 33:843–848, 1989.

215. Agency for Health Care Policy and Research. *Evidence Report on Evaluation of Cervical Cytology,* 1999.

216. Brown AD, Garber AM. Cost-effectiveness of 3 methods to enhance the sensitivity of Papanicolaou testing. *JAMA* 281:347–353, 1999.

217. Giles JA, Hudson E, Crow J, et al. Colposcopic assessment of the accuracy of cervical cytology screening. *BMJ (Clin Res Ed)* 296:1099–1102, 1988.

218. Hall JB, McGee JA Jr, Marroum MC, Dee L. Evaluation of the cerviscope as a screening instrument. *Gynecol Oncol* 20:17–22, 1985.

219. Tawa K, Forsythe A, Cove JK, et al. A comparison of the Papanicolaou smear and the cervigram: sensitivity, specificity, and cost analysis. *Obstet Gynecol* 71:229–235, 1988.

220. Cox JT, Lorincz AT, Schiffman MH, et al. Human papillomavirus testing by hybrid capture appears to be useful in triaging women with a cytologic diagnosis of atypical squamous cells of undetermined significance. *Am J Obstet Gynecol* 172:946–954, 1995.

221. Cuzick J, Szarewski A, Terry G, et al. Human papillomavirus testing in primary cervical screening (see comments). *Lancet* 345:1533–1536, 1995.

222. Kiviat NB, Koutsky LA, Critchlow CW, et al. Prevalence and cytologic manifestations of human papilloma virus (HPV) types 6, 11, 16, 18, 31, 33, 35, 42, 43, 44, 45, 51, 52, and 56 among 500 consecutive women. *Int J Gynecol Pathol* 11:197–203, 1992.

223. Koutsky LA, Holmes KK, Critchlow CW, et al. A cohort study of the risk of cervical intraepithelial neoplasia grade 2 or 3 in relation to papillomavirus infection. *N Engl J Med* 327:1272–1278, 1992.

224. Schneider A, Koutsky LA. Natural history and epidemiological features of genital HPV infection. *IARC Sci Publ* 119:25–52, 1992.

225. van Muyden RC, ter Harmsel BW, Smedts FM, et al. Detection and typing of human papillomavirus in cervical carcinomas in Russian women: a prognostic study. *Cancer* 85:2011–2016, 1999.

226. Jenkins D, Sherlaw-Johnson C, Gallivan S. Assessing the role of HPV testing in cervical cancer screening. *Papilloma Rep* 9:89–101, 1998.

227. Franco EL, Rohan TE, Villa LL. Epidemiologic evidence and human papillomavirus infection as a necessary cause of cervical cancer. *J Natl Cancer Inst* 91:506–511, 1999.

228. Bosch FX, Manos MM, Munoz N, et al. Prevalence of

human papillomavirus in cervical cancer: a worldwide perspective. International biological study on cervical cancer (IBSCC) Study Group (see comments). *J Natl Cancer Inst* 87:796–802, 1995.

229. Broder S. Rapid communication - The Bethesda system for reporting cervical/vaginal cytologic diagnoses - report of the 1991 Bethesda workshop. *JAMA* 267:1892, 1992.

230. National Cancer Institute Workshop. The Bethesda System for reporting cervical/vaginal cytologic diagnoses: revised after the second National Cancer Institute Workshop, April 29–30, 1991. *Acta Cytol* 37:115–124, 1993.

231. Nyirjesy I. Atypical or suspicious cervical smears. An aggressive diagnostic approach. *JAMA* 222:691–693, 1992.

232. Reagan JW, Fu YS. Histologic types and prognosis of cancers of the uterine cervix. *Int J Radiat Oncol Biol Phys* 5:1015–1020, 1979.

233. Richart RM. Cervical intraepithelial neoplasia. *Pathol Annu* 8:301–328, 1973.

234. Miller A, Knight J, Narod S. The natural history of cancer of the cervix and the implications for screening policy. In Miller A, Chamberlain J, Day N, et al. (eds), *Cancer Screening.* Cambridge: Cambridge University Press, 1991.

235. Celentano DD, de Lissovoy G. *Assessment of Cervical Cancer Screening and Follow-up Programs.* Atlanta: Centers for Disease Control, 1990.

236. Briggs RM, Holmes KK, Kiviat N, et al. High prevalence of cervical dysplasia in STD clinic patients warrants routine cytologic screening. *Am J Public Health* 70:121–124, 1980.

237. Tavelli BG, Judson FN, et al. Cost-yield of routine Papanicolaou smear screening in a clinic for sexually transmitted diseases. *Sex Transm Dis* 12:110–113, 1985.

238. Harris RW, Brinton LA, Cowdell RH, et al. Characteristics of women with dysplasia or carcinoma in situ of the cervix uteri. *Br J Cancer* 42:359–369, 1980.

239. Gardner JW, Lyon JL. Efficacy of cervical cytologic screening in the control of cervical cancer. *Prev Med* 6:487–499, 1977.

240. Laara E, Day NE, Hakama M. Trends in mortality from cervical cancer in the Nordic countries: association with organised screening programmes. *Lancet* 1:1247–1249, 1987.

241. Hakama M. Effect of population screening for carcinoma of the uterine cervix in Finland. *Maturitas* 7:3–10, 1985.

242. Johannesson G, Geirsson G, Day N. The effect of mass screening in Iceland, 1965–74, on the incidence and mortality of cervical carcinoma. *Int J Cancer* 21:418–425, 1978.

243. Hakama M, Magnus K, Petterson F. *Effect of Organized Screening on the Risk of Cervical Cancer in the Nordic Countries.* Cambridge: Cambridge University Press, 1991.

244. Magnus K, Langmark F, Andersen A. Mass screening for cervical cancer in Ostfold county of Norway 1959–77. *Int J Cancer* 39:311–316, 1987.

245. Celentano DD, Klassen AC, Weisman CS, Rosenshein NB. Cervical cancer screening practices among older women: results from the Maryland Cervical Cancer Case-Control Study (see comments). *J Clin Epidemiol* 41:531–541, 1988.

246. Olesen F. A case-control study of cervical cytology before diagnosis of cervical cancer in Denmark. *Int J Epidemiol* 17:501–508, 1988.

247. Jick H, Walker AM, Rothman KJ. The epidemic of endometrial cancer: a commentary. *Am J Public Health* 70:264–267, 1980.

248. Barrett RJ II, Harlan LC, Wesley MN, et al. Endometrial cancer: stage at diagnosis and associated factors in black and white patients. *Am J Obstet Gynecol* 173:414–422, discussion 422–423, 1995.

249. Fisher B, Costantino JP, Redmond CK, et al. Endometrial cancer in tamoxifen-treated breast cancer patients: findings from the National Surgical Adjuvant Breast and Bowel Project (NSABP) B-14 (see comments). *J Natl Cancer Inst* 86:527–537, 1994.

250. American College of Obstetricians and Gynecologists (ACOG) committee on Gynecologic Practice. Committee opinion: tamoxifen and endometrial cancer, number 169. *Int J Gynaecol Obstet* 53:197–199, 1996.

251. Aarnio M, Mecklin JP, Aaltonen LA, et al. Life-time risk of different cancers in hereditary non-polyposis colorectal cancer (HNPCC) syndrome. *Int J Cancer* 64:430–433, 1995.

252. Burk JR, Lehman HF, Wolf FS. Inadequacy of papanicolaou smears in the detection of endometrial cancer. *N Engl J Med* 291:191–192, 1974.

253. Osmers R, Volksen M, Schauer A. Vaginosonography for early detection of endometrial carcinoma? (see comments). *Lancet* 335:1569–1571, 1990.

254. Varner RE, Sparks JM, Cameron CD, et al. Transvaginal sonography of the endometrium in postmenopausal women. *Obstet Gynecol* 78:195–199, 1991.

255. Smith-Bindman R, Kerlikowske K, Feldstein VA, et al. Endovaginal ultrasound to exclude endometrial cancer and other endometrial abnormalities (see comments). *JAMA* 280:1510–1517, 1998.

256. National Institutes of Health Consensus Development Conference Statement. *Ovarian Cancer: Screening, Treatment, and Follow-up.* NIH Consensus Statement 1994. Bethesda, MD: National Institutes of Health, 1994.

257. Campbell S, Bhan V, Royston P, et al. Transabdominal ultrasound screening for early ovarian cancer (see comments). *BMJ* 299:1363–1367, 1989.

258. DePriest PD, van Nagell JR Jr, Gallion HH, et al. Ovarian cancer screening in asymptomatic postmenopausal women. *Gynecol Oncol* 51:205–209, 1993.

259. Einhorn N, Sjovall K, Knapp RC, et al. Prospective evaluation of serum CA 125 levels for early detection of ovarian cancer. *Obstet Gynecol* 80:14–18, 1992.

260. Jacobs IJ, Skates SJ, MacDonald N, et al. Screening for ovarian cancer: a pilot randomised controlled trial (see comments). *Lancet* 353:1207–1210, 1999.

261. Moul JW, Paulson DF, Dodge RK, Walther PJ. Delay in diagnosis and survival in testicular cancer: impact of effective therapy and changes during 18 years. *J Urol* 143:520–523, 1990.

262. Sheley JP, Kinchen EW, Morgan DH, Gordon DF. Limited impact of testicular self-examination promotion. *J Community Health* 16:117–124, 1991.

263. Buetow SA. Testicular cancer: to screen or not to screen? (see comments). *J Med Screen* 3:3–6, 1996.

264. Westlake SJ, Frank JW. Testicular self-examination: an argument against routine teaching. *Fam Pract* 4:143–148, 1987.

265. McDonald CJ. American Cancer Society perspective on the American College of Preventive Medicine's policy statements on skin cancer prevention and screening (comment). *CA Cancer J Clin* 48:229–231, 1998.

266. Tucker MA, Halpern A, Holly EA, et al. Clinically recognized dysplastic nevi. A central risk factor for cutaneous melanoma (see comments). *JAMA* 277:1439–1444, 1997.

267. Mihm MC Jr, Barnhill RL, Sober AJ, Hernandez MH. Precursor lesions of melanoma: do they exist? *Semin Surg Oncol* 8:358–365, 1992.

268. U. S. Department of Health and Human Services. *Breast Cancer Deaths Decline Nearly 5 Percent.* Bethesda, MD: National Cancer Advisory Board, 1995.

269. Rampen FH, Casparie-van Velsen JI, van Huystee BE, et al. False-negative findings in skin cancer and melanoma screening. *J Am Acad Dermatol* 33:59–63, 1995.

270. Tiersten AD, Grin CM, Kopf AW, et al. Prospective follow-up for malignant melanoma in patients with atypical-mole (dysplastic-nevus) syndrome. *J Dermatol Surg Oncol* 17:44–48, 1991.

271. McDonald CJ. Status of screening for skin cancer. *Cancer* 72(suppl 3): 1066–1070, 1993.

272. Koh HK, Geller AC, Miller DR, Lew RA. The early detection of and screening for melanoma. International status. *Cancer* 75(suppl 2): 674–683, 1995.

273. Koh HK, Geller AC. Melanoma control in the United States: current status. *Recent Results Cancer Res* 139:215–224, 1995.

6

Pathologic Evaluation of Neoplastic Diseases

■ ■ ■

JOHN D. PFEIFER
MARK R. WICK

MANY PHYSICIANS THINK OF THE PATHOLOGY laboratory only as an unpleasant area of the medical school where they first were exposed to museum specimens of human disease, including neoplasia. Accordingly, too often they forget that abnormalities in these mummified or soggy tissues explained many of the physical findings associated with disorders of living human beings. They are advised to remember the often-quoted statement of Sir William Osler regarding this topic: "To know Pathology is to know Medicine."

In reality, the modern specialties of pathology and laboratory medicine are dynamic facets of medical practice, in which physicians skilled at laboratory analysis actively contribute to the care of patients. Even the autopsy can be included in this statement, because its aim is to serve as a quality assurance measure to be used in a prospective educational manner by clinicians. Other areas of pathology and laboratory medicine regularly involved in the precise definition of disease and in the monitoring of therapeutic results include surgical pathology, cytopathology, neuropathology, dermatopathology, hematopathology, blood banking, clinical chemistry, and microbiology.

The pathologist's understanding of oncologic disorders has progressed far beyond the recognition of abnormal tissues with the microscope, although this activity still retains primary importance in the diagnosis of cancer. Today, laboratory specialists play an integral role in eliminating incorrect differential diagnostic considerations, determining prognostic factors, evaluating treatment outcomes, and supporting the multidisciplinary care of oncology patients. The range of ancillary tests available to assist pathologists in these activities has been expanded markedly by recent technologic advances, but new tests must be used prudently with knowledge of their strengths and weaknesses.

The authors gratefully acknowledge the excellent secretarial assistance of Fran Buhr.

This chapter presents a practical introduction to the diverse analyses that are performed by pathologists and have an impact on the diagnosis and treatment of patients with malignant neoplasms. In addition to discussing gross tissue examination, tissue processing, and conventional microscopical examination with its allied methods, this chapter outlines more specialized procedures used in the pathologic analysis of malignant tumors, including immunohistochemistry, flow cytometry, and molecular probe analysis.

INTERACTIONS BETWEEN CLINICIANS AND PATHOLOGISTS

To use the services of pathologists optimally, clinicians must be familiar with the strengths and limitations of the technical procedures employed in the laboratory. Oncologists and surgeons are not merely "consumers" of pathologic data; rather, they should be interactive participants in the generation of such information. Much of what the pathologist is able to say about a particular case depends on receipt of pertinent clinical facts, prompt and proper submission of specimens, and adequacy of a tissue sample itself. A rapid and confident pathologic diagnosis is ensured only when these factors receive proper attention.

Therefore, wise clinicians consult with the pathology laboratory when scheduling many of the invasive diagnostic procedures that yield pathologic specimens. Then discussion can address the amount of tissue required for diagnosis, the possible need for intraoperative frozen sections, special processing requirements, and the role of adjunctive pathologic analyses for diagnosis or prognosis. For example, if lymphoma is suspected in a patient with lymphadenopathy, the best approach is to perform an excisional lymph node biopsy instead of fine-needle aspiration; conversely, the latter procedure usually yields adequate tissue for diagnosis in most cases of probable metastatic carcinoma. In addition, karyotyping, flow cytometric immunophenotyping, and certain immunohistochemical studies can be performed only on fresh tissue and are precluded if the specimen is placed in fixative solution before dispatch to the pathology laboratory. Likewise, effective communication regarding anatomic orientation of a specimen often is essential for adequate interpretation of the completeness of tumor resection (i.e., involvement of the margins), which in turn influences decisions regarding adjuvant irradiation, chemotherapy, and additional surgical procedures.

DEFINITIONS OF TUMOR TYPES

Current tumor classification systems include terms that are based on biological behavior, cellular function, histologic makeup, embryonic origin, anatomic location, and eponyms (Table 6.1). Although hardly requiring mention, nomenclature is important because it is the means by which pathologists communicate a diagnosis and because specific tumor designations carry specific clinical implications.

Neoplasms (literally, new growths) may be benign or malignant. They consist of the proliferating tumor cells themselves and a supportive stroma containing connective tissue and blood vessels. An abundant stromal collagenous response to a neoplasm (most often malignant) is called *desmoplasia*.

The most important features used to define a tumor as benign or malignant are its empirically known biological behavior and its microscopical appearance. Generally, benign neoplasms are innocuous and slow-growing, whereas malignant lesions often exhibit more rapid proliferation, invade adjacent tissues, and metastasize. Often, malignant neoplasms manifest mitotic activity, abnormal nuclear chromatin, cellular pleomorphism, an abnormal or haphazard-appearing arrangement of cells, and areas of necrosis, whereas benign neoplasms lack these features and often have a bland microscopical appearance. However, exceptions to these generalizations abound. Benign neoplasms can kill an affected patient if located inopportunely (e.g., an ependymoma blocking the aqueduct of Sylvius), and some can metastasize (e.g., benign giant-cell tumor of bone). Malignant neoplasms, on the other hand, may have a bland, mature cellular microscopical appearance, as seen in small lymphocytic lymphoma.

Malignant neoplasms of epithelial origin are called *carcinomas*. If predominantly glandular or ductal, they are termed *adenocarcinomas;* if derived from a stratified squamous epithelium, they are termed *squamous cell carcinomas;* lesions with hybrid features of glandular and squamous carcinomas are known as *adenosquamous carcinomas*. Neoplasms originating in a specific organ may be named accordingly; hence, the terms *hepatocellular* or *adrenocortical carcinomas*. Malignant neoplasms of mesenchymal origin are designated *sarcomas;* a sarcoma differentiating toward fat cells is termed a *liposarcoma;* toward fibrous tissue, a *fibrosarcoma;* toward smooth muscle, a *leiomyosarcoma;* toward blood vessels, an *angiosarcoma;* and so on. Malignant tumors do not necessarily have benign counterparts, and the converse applies as well.

Often, modifiers used in diagnosis reflect prognostic

Table 6.1 Nomenclature Pertaining to Neoplastic Diseases

Origin Cell or Tissue	Benign	Malignant
Tumors of epithelial origin		
Squamous cells	Squamous cell papilloma	Squamous cell carcinoma
Basal cells	—	Basal cell carcinoma
Glandular or ductal epithelium	Adenoma	Adenocarcinoma
	Cystadenoma	Cystadenocarcinoma
Transitional cells	Transitional cell papilloma	Transitional cell carcinoma
Bile duct epithelium	Bile duct adenoma	Cholangiocarcinoma
Liver cells	Hepatocellular adenoma	Hepatocellular carcinoma
Melanocytes	Nevus	Malignant melanoma
Renal epithelium	Renal tubular adenoma	Renal cell carcinoma
Skin adnexal glands		
Sweat glands	Sweat gland adenoma	Sweat gland carcinoma
Sebaceous glands	Sebaceous gland adenoma	Sebaceous gland carcinoma
Tumors of mesenchymal origin		
Hematopoietic-lymphoid tissue	—	Leukemias, lymphomas, Hodgkin's disease, multiple myeloma
Neural and retinal tissue		
Nerve sheath	Neurilemoma, neurofibroma	Malignant peripheral nerve sheath tumor
Nerve cells	Ganglioneuroma	Neuroblastoma
Retinal cells (cones)	—	Retinoblastoma
Connective tissue		
Fibrous tissue	Fibroma; fibromatosis	Fibrosarcoma
Fat	Lipoma	Liposarcoma
Bone	Osteoma	Osteogenic sarcoma
Cartilage	Chondroma	Chondrosarcoma
Muscle		
Smooth muscle	Leiomyoma	Leiomyosarcoma
Striated muscle	Rhabdomyoma	Rhabdomyosarcoma
Endothelium and related tissues		
Blood vessels	Hemangioma	Angiosarcoma, Kaposi's sarcoma
Lymph vessels	Lymphangioma	Lymphangiosarcoma
Synovium	—	Synovial sarcoma
Mesothelium	—	Malignant mesothelioma
Meninges	Meningioma	Malignant meningioma
Other origins		
Uncertain	—	Ewing's sarcoma/peripheral neuroectodermal tumor
Renal anlage	—	Wilms' tumor
Germ cells (testes and ovaries)	Mature cystic teratoma (dermoid cyst) in women	Seminoma (dysgerminoma); embryonal carcinoma; endodermal sinus tumor; mature teratoma in men
Trophoblast	Hydatidiform mole	Choriocarcinoma

Note: This list is not exhaustive but is intended to provide an introduction to tumor nomenclature.
Source: Adapted with permission from MW Lieberman, RM Lebovite, Neoplasia. In I Damjanov, J Linder (eds), *Anderson's Pathology* (10th ed). St Louis: Mosby, 1996:517.

information, as in *poorly differentiated adenocarcinoma.* Neoplasms with biologically ambiguous names always should include a precise modifier (e.g., *malignant schwannoma* versus *benign schwannoma*). Generally, non-specific anatomic names should be avoided (e.g., *bron-chogenic carcinoma of the lung* could refer to *squamous cell carcinoma, adenocarcinoma, small-cell neuroendocrine carcinoma,* or other tumor types).

Usually, neoplasms of the hematopoietic system have no benign analogs. Consequently, the terms *leuke-*

mia and *lymphoma,* together with appropriate modifiers (e.g., *chronic myelogenous leukemia* and *follicular, predominantly small cleaved-cell lymphoma*) always refer to malignant proliferations. Similarly, *melanoma* is used always to describe a malignant melanocytic neoplasm.

Finally, time-honored but idiosyncratic eponyms remain. For example, Warthin's tumor is a benign lesion of the salivary glands; a Brenner tumor is an epithelial neoplasm of the ovary that has both benign and malignant forms.

MACROSCOPIC EXAMINATION OF TISSUE SPECIMENS

As a discipline, pathology had its beginnings in the careful gross examination of diseased tissues at the autopsy table. Even before the microscope had come into general use, several disorders were well recognized at a macroscopic level, including malignant melanoma and various carcinomas. The current rush to introduce molecular techniques to diagnostic medicine tends to minimize the power and importance of simple, deliberate macroscopic examination. However, all subsequent tissue processing and testing is meaningless if the presence of a tumor is overlooked, if representative neoplastic tissue is not sampled for microscopic examination, if tumor extension to a surgical margin is not recognized, and so on. How critical a thorough gross examination is to all subsequent steps in the pathologic evaluation of neoplasia cannot be overstated.

Pathologists grossly examine all resected tumors submitted to the laboratory, keeping several objectives in mind. First, the presence of representative lesional tissue is confirmed, and the areas of the specimen that are best suited to further study are identified. Second, the margins of excision are labeled with indelible ink to retain the orientation of the specimen for subsequent histologic analysis. Third, the specimen is opened and sectioned with a scalpel or sharp knife, at which time the pathologist notes the consistency, color, and extent of the neoplastic growth. Then, on the basis of differential diagnosis of a neoplasm, generated by integration of its macroscopic characteristics and clinical history, appropriate tissue samples are collected; although tissue sections are fixed in formalin for routine processing, flow-cytometric analysis and cytogenetic studies require fresh tissue; some immunohistochemical stains require fresh-frozen tissue; tissue for electron-microscopical study must be fixed in a special preservative, and so on. Not uncommonly, macroscopic features alone are sufficient to suggest a final diagnosis. Figure 6.1 shows a

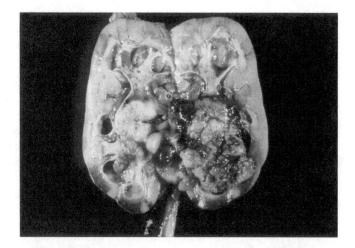

Figure 6.1 Renal pelvic tumor with macroscopic characteristics typical of transitional cell carcinoma, including a papillary configuration.

renal pelvic tumor from an adult patient, the gross attributes of which are characteristic of transitional cell carcinoma. In Figure 6.2, the darkly colored mandibular mass from a child is macroscopically typical of a pigmented neuroectodermal tumor.

The anatomic orientation of excised tissues should be a routine part of the information submitted to the pathology department. This inclusion allows not only for an accurate description of the extent of the tumor but for the precise localization of sites at which tumor is present at the margin of resection. Also imperative is that the pathologist examine the entire resected tumor before it is subdivided for other purposes (e.g., before a portion of a neoplasm is sent to a research laboratory for investigational purposes). When careful inspection of the lesional borders is important, violation of the tissue margins before they can be examined adequately for pathologic information is an obvious disservice to patient care. For example, for some types of follicular thyroid lesions and thymic neoplasms, a tumor is diagnosed as malignant rather than as benign on the basis of whether it penetrates capsular boundaries; obviously, receipt of a partial specimen in the gross pathology laboratory prevents proper examination of such lesions.

MICROSCOPIC (HISTOPATHOLOGIC) EXAMINATION OF TISSUE SPECIMENS

The light microscope continues to serve as the cornerstone of surgical pathology. Assuming that the foregoing tissue-processing requirements have been met, the

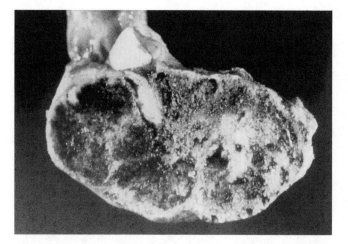

Figure 6.2 Pigmented neuroectodermal tumor of infancy involving the mandible. The appearance is virtually diagnostic in light of the tumor's location and the dense pigmentation evident macroscopically.

use of the simple hematoxylin and eosin (H&E) staining method on paraffin-embedded tissue sections is sufficient to make the diagnosis with most malignant neoplasms. What should be noted, however, is that certain clinical procedures (e.g., vigorous compression of tissue specimens during endoscopic biopsy or extensive use of electrical or thermal cautery during resection) have the potential to interfere with diagnosis because they can damage microscopic anatomy severely.

For the morphologic features of a tissue to be visualized optimally by routine light microscopy, the specimen must undergo proper preparation and processing. First, a minimum period of fixation in formalin (or an alternative mordant) is required; depending on the overall size of the specimen, this interval varies from one to two hours to more than 12 hours. After fixation, pathologists complete the gross examination of the specimen and excise slices of the tissue, which then are subjected to additional automated processing. This additional processing includes further fixation, dehydration of the tissue, and saturation with hot paraffin wax; when these steps are taken together, their completion requires at least several hours. Finally, the processed tissue slices must be embedded in paraffin, sectioned on a microtome, and stained by histotechnologists in the pathology laboratory. Routine processing of tissue, therefore, requires at least an overnight interval (often longer), a fact appreciated by the general public [1].

If special studies are needed for diagnosis (e.g., routine histochemistry, immunohistochemistry, electron microscopy, or flow cytometry), obviously additional time is required. Knowledge of the sequence of events involved in proper processing of tissue should prevent frustration on the part of clinical physicians, who often wonder why their receipt of microscopical interpretation is so long delayed after a specimen has been submitted to the laboratory. Although a quicker method of histologic examination does exist—the frozen section procedure (see later)—it is not appropriate in many situations, is technically difficult, and yields microscopical preparations inferior to those procured with conventional processing; consequently, it is used sparingly for the routine evaluation of neoplasia.

When examining the stained slides, pathologists employ knowledge of histology and cytology to recognize changes related to neoplasia and other diseases. Tissue growth patterns, the degree of cellular differentiation, and details relating to prognosis (e.g., adequacy of excision) are assessed. Ideally, a firm diagnosis of cancer always would be possible by brief examination of routinely processed and stained tissue. However, this expectation is unrealistic, and a difficult case often affords no substitute for painstaking study of the slides, additional specialized stains, and collegial consultation among laboratory physicians.

Several potential reasons explain uncertainty in the interpretation of biopsy or resection specimens. One important reason relates to the natural history of any given pathologic process: Tissue may be obtained at a time when a neoplastic lesion is not developed fully and therefore lacks diagnostic histologic features of malignancy. Such treatments as irradiation or chemotherapy often alter the pathologic characteristics of the tissue, and crush or cautery artifacts may distort tissue histology. In addition, a frequent question is whether the tissue is a representative sample of the entire lesion. Two especially important sources of uncertainty are so-called borderline or minimal deviation malignancies (epithelial, mesenchymal, or melanocytic), which, by their very nature, are characterized by microscopic features differing minimally from those of benign neoplasms or reactive processes [2], and pseudoneoplastic processes, which likewise can arise from many different tissues and differ minimally from malignant processes [3].

In the course of diagnosis, pathologists should discuss pertinent findings with the appropriate clinicians. Ultimately, a written report is issued for the specimen and includes the tumor type and any additional information that can be used by oncologists to assign a stage to the malignancy, to assess prognosis, or to plan further therapy. Discussions with clinicians about the case may be distilled into a summary in the report that includes comments on the expected behavior of the tumor and recommendations for subsequent management.

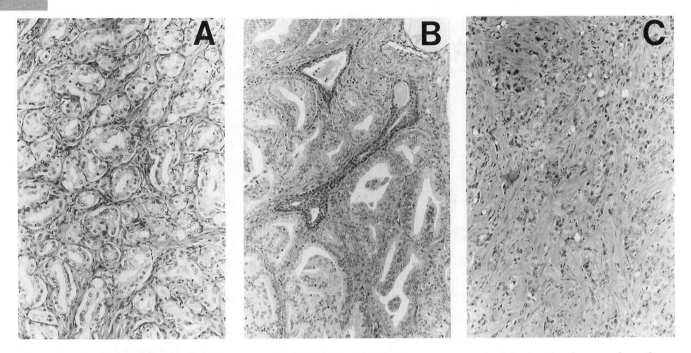

Figure 6.3 Adenocarcinoma of the prostate. (A) Well-differentiated (tumor composed of single, closely spaced, uniform glands). (B) Moderately differentiated (tumor composed of irregular glands showing cribriform epithelium and infiltration of nonneoplastic prostate). (C) Poorly differentiated (tumor showing no glandular differentiation with individually infiltrating cells). (Courtesy of Dr. Peter Humphrey, Department of Pathology, Washington University School of Medicine, St. Louis, MO.)

Grade and Stage

Microscopic examination of routinely processed and stained tissue is used also to determine tumor stage and grade, which together offer important prognostic information and allow for comparison of therapeutic results using various cooperative treatment protocols. Tumor grading is based primarily on the degree of differentiation of the malignant cells (Figs. 6.3, 6.4), nuclear features, and an estimate of the rate of growth as indicated by the mitotic rate. The correlation between histologic appearance and biological behavior is imperfect, and grading criteria vary greatly for different neoplasms. Nonetheless, all grading criteria attempt to describe the extent to which the tumor cells resemble their normal tissue counterparts. Accurate grading is complicated by variations in differentiation from area to area in large tumors, site-related considerations, and the clonal evolution of a tumor that occurs with time.

Tumor stage is based on features of the untreated primary lesion (including size and extent of tissue invasion) and on the presence of lymph node or hematogenous metastasis as determined by microscopic examination [4]. The staging systems of the American Joint Committee on Cancer and the Union Internationale Contre le Cancer (International Union Against Cancer) now provide identical definitions and stage groupings and are based on the TNM classification scheme (for primary *t*umor features, presence and extent of lymph *n*ode involvement, and distant *m*etastasis) [4].

The details of staging and grading procedures for specific tumors are considered elsewhere in this text. However, two examples will illustrate how their importance can vary for the assessment of prognosis for different tumor types. First we consider squamous cell carcinoma of the uterine cervix.

The tumor stage of squamous cell carcinoma of the uterine cervix is an extremely important prognostic variable. The clinical significance of tumor size (i.e., the T substage) is indicated by combined studies showing a 0.3% incidence of pelvic lymph node metastasis in microinvasive squamous cell carcinomas with no more than a 3-mm depth of stromal invasion (tumor stage T1a1) as compared with a 7.4% incidence of lymph node metastasis in squamous cell carcinomas that have a 3.1- to 5.0-mm depth of stromal invasion (tumor stage T1a2). Further, patients with stage T1a1 squamous cell carcinomas have a recurrence rate of only 0.2%, whereas those with stage T1a2 lesions have a recurrence rate of 5.4% [5]. This greater than 10-fold dif-

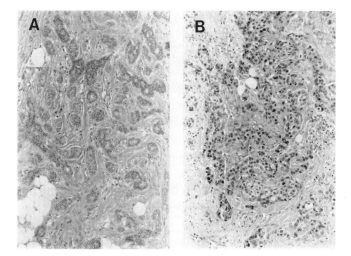

Figure 6.4 Infiltrating ductal carcinoma of the breast. (A) Well-differentiated (tumor forms tubules with clearly visible lumina, and the nuclei are regular, with little variation in size and shape). (B) Poorly differentiated (tumor grows as sheets and cords of cells with no tubule formation, and the nuclei show marked variation in size and shape; several mitoses are present, some atypical).

ference in the presence of lymph node metastasis and the recurrence rate between even two substages demonstrates the strong correlation of stage and clinical outcome for squamous cell carcinomas of the cervix. However, a noteworthy factor is that the histologic grade of cervical squamous cell carcinoma generally has no influence on survival of patients in any staging group [6–8].

In contrast, adenocarcinoma of the prostate is an example of a tumor for which microscopical grading is one of the best predictors of prognosis because it is correlated strongly with biological behavior, including invasiveness and metastatic potential [9]. The grading system [10] is based on the degree of glandular differentiation and pattern of growth, as evaluated by low-power microscopic examination (see Fig. 6.3). Although the histologic grade correlates well with both clinical stage and the mortality rate within each stage, a combination of microscopic grade and clinical stage provides the best prognostic information.

Intraoperative Consultation and Frozen Sections

The term *frozen section* is synonymous with an intraoperative microscopical consultation; frequently, such a consultation also involves gross specimen examination, which helps pathologists to assess which tissue areas or margins are sampled most appropriately, the need for collecting fresh tissue for special studies, and so on. For the actual frozen section itself, the tissue sample first is frozen (the most widely used method involving rapid cooling in a refrigerated bath of organic liquid). Histologic sections then are prepared using a cryostat (refrigerated microtome), are stained with H&E, and then are examined microscopically. The entire procedure, including thorough histologic study, usually can be accomplished in approximately 10 to 15 minutes. Consequently, frozen sections are of great practical value in clinical situations that require an immediate answer to questions affecting proper patient therapy. Proper interpretation requires a complete gross examination of the tissue prior to sectioning and requires a well-trained pathologist with experience. Informative, interactive communication with the surgeon, including salient details of the clinical history, also are essential for optimization of this process.

As with all diagnostic procedures, frozen-section consultation has specific indications. In general, these indications include tissue identification; identification of the presence and nature of a lesion (a determination that can help to define the appropriate pathologic workup so that representative tissue can be placed in appropriate fixatives or media for ancillary testing that may be required); confirmation that excised material is sufficient for diagnosis; definition of the extent of disease; demonstration of metastasis; and assessment of the adequacy of surgical margins [11]. Frozen sections should not be used merely to satisfy the curiosity of surgeons, to compensate for inadequate preoperative evaluation, or as a mechanism to communicate information more quickly to patients or their families.

Although histopathologic interpretation of frozen sections is technically limited and more difficult than diagnosis using formalin-fixed paraffin-embedded tissues, frozen sections are a useful means of intraoperative consultation. However, some diagnoses are well known to be tenuous by frozen section; consequently, the use of frozen sections is totally inadvisable in some settings (e.g., distinguishing benign from malignant breast lesions or distinguishing benign from malignant follicular thyroid tumors) [11–13]. The accuracy of frozen-section diagnosis commonly is reported to be in the range of 94% to 98%, but this figure varies, depending on the tissue type and the reason for consultation [11, 14]. Because frozen-section diagnoses often have a significant influence on a surgical procedure being performed, intraoperative microscopical consultations must be used wisely by both surgeons and pathologists.

Cytopathologic Assessment

Cytopathology is the practice of morphologic examination of individual cells and clusters of cells for the purpose of diagnosis. Suitable specimens are collected in three basic ways: exfoliation from an epithelial surface (e.g., cervical smears obtained with a spatula or brush; bronchial washings or brushings; spontaneously shed urinary tract cells in the urine); aspiration of fluid from body cavities (e.g., cerebrospinal fluid, pleural fluid, peritoneal fluid); and fine-needle aspiration (FNA) of cysts, inflammatory swellings, and neoplasms (e.g., tumors of virtually any organ including the breast, lymph nodes, lung, and thyroid). After collection, the cytologic preparation is spread on a glass slide, is fixed, and is stained. If several slides are available, more than one type of stain often is used. In most instances, a Papanicolaou stain yields the greatest clarity of nuclear detail, but a Romanowsky stain often yields better cytoplasmic detail. Special investigations also may be carried out on cytologic specimens (e.g., routine histochemistry, immunohistochemistry, static cytometry, and even molecular pathology studies), but the need for ancillary testing must be anticipated before sample procurement, because special preparations may be needed for such analyses.

Because exfoliative cytology is noninvasive, often it is used to screen for precursor lesions in asymptomatic populations (e.g., the Papanicolaou test, which has been extremely successful in lowering the mortality associated with cervical cancer over the last 50 years) or to follow up patients at high risk (e.g., to detect recurrence in women who have a history of cervical dysplasia or to detect recurrent urinary tract lesions such as dysplasia or transitional cell carcinoma). However, it must be realized that exfoliative cytology shares the major problem inherent in all screening tests: the need to balance sensitivity and specificity. Though fewer cases of neoplasia will be missed with a lower threshold for a diagnosis of atypia (higher sensitivity), the trade-off is that more patients without neoplastic disease will undergo additional, often costly, follow-up testing (lower specificity).

Although generalizations are difficult, the cytomorphologic evaluation of possible malignancy is predicated on a systematic assessment of each cellular compart-

ment (including specific features of the nucleus and cytoplasm) and of intercellular relationships and the overall background. The most helpful nuclear changes for a diagnosis of malignancy include anisonucleosis (marked variation in nuclear size and shape), irregular chromatin distribution (with clearing or coarse clumping), hyperchromasia, abnormal nucleoli, and abundant or abnormal mitoses (Fig. 6.5). The most helpful cytoplasmic changes indicating malignancy are a significant increase in the volumetric nucleus-to-cytoplasm ratio and tight molding of the cell membrane around the nucleus. Anisocytosis (marked variation in cellular size and shape) and decreased cohesiveness are abnormalities of intercellular relationships indicative of malignancy, although other intercellular relationships (e.g., the formation of sheets or ducts) also provide important clues to the nature of the cells being evaluated. The presence of a so-called tumor diathesis (consisting of inflammatory cells, erythrocytes, and cellular debris) is a background feature that strongly suggests an invasive malignancy. Because reactive cellular changes (due to inflammation, infection, irradiation, or cytotoxic chemotherapy) can be confused easily with malignant proliferations, a complete clinical history is essential for ac-

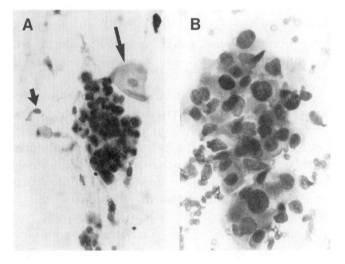

Figure 6.5 (A) Exfoliative cytology specimen (bronchial washings) from a 60-year-old woman with a lung mass. Note the cluster of cells demonstrating pronounced nuclear and cellular pleomorphism, diagnostic of malignancy. Normal superficial squamous cell (*large arrow*) and a normal ciliated columnar cell (*small arrow*) (magnification, 400×) are present. (B) Fine-needle aspiration cytology specimen from a 49-year-old woman with a breast mass. The cluster of cells shows marked nuclear and cellular pleomorphism, diagnostic of malignancy (magnification, 1,300×).

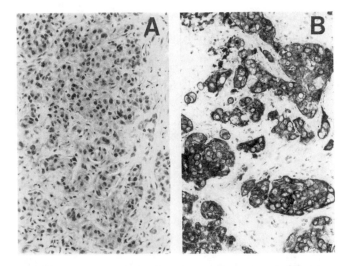

Figure 6.6 Poorly differentiated neoplasm involving paratracheal lymph nodes in a woman with a history of breast carcinoma. (A) Large malignant cells are seen growing in sheets and nests. (B) Immunoreactivity for cytokeratin identifies the tumor as metastatic adenocarcinoma.

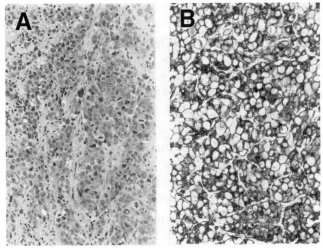

Figure 6.7 Poorly differentiated neoplasm involving paratracheal lymph nodes in a woman with a history of breast carcinoma and transitional cell carcinoma. (A) Large pleomorphic malignant cells are seen growing in sheets and vague nests. (B) Immunoreactivity for leukocyte common antigen identifies the tumor as a lymphoma (confirmed by molecular analysis that demonstrated a clonal T-cell receptor gamma-chain rearrangement).

curate cytologic diagnosis. Often, cytology and biopsy can improve the likelihood of diagnosing malignancy in a single procedure [15, 16].

FNA is a technique used widely to obtain a sample of cells for immediate cytologic evaluation. For many years, FNA has been a safe and reliable method for the diagnosis of cysts, inflammatory swellings, and palpable masses. However, the use of ultrasonography and radiologic imaging modalities for needle guidance recently stimulated application of FNA for the diagnosis of deep-seated lesions of internal organs (e.g., liver, lung, pancreas). In the appropriate clinical settings, it has several advantages over conventional biopsy. For patients, FNA is safe, results in little pain (anesthesia often being unnecessary), and can be performed on an outpatient basis. For pathologists and their clinical colleagues, FNA is performed easily and provides a specimen that often is sufficient for rapid and accurate diagnosis. Although the reliability of FNA clearly depends on the tissue and type of lesion [12, 17], the technique is particularly well suited for the diagnosis of metastasis, recurrence, and disease staging.

Cytology has a high degree of reliability when morphologic interpretations are performed by experienced, well-trained individuals. Although an effort often is made to confirm the diagnosis by conventional biopsy prior to definitive treatment, some exceptions exist. For example, diagnosis of many primary carcinomas, diag-

nosis of metastatic carcinoma in cerebrospinal or pleural fluids, or imaging-guided FNA of lesions of the liver or other organs rarely is followed by an open biopsy prior to definitive treatment. In addition, cytologic evaluation of clinically suspicious masses can identify nonneoplastic lesions without incurring the expense or morbidity of open biopsy.

SPECIAL PATHOLOGIC PROCEDURES

In approximately 10% of all oncology cases, routinely assessed microscopical features are insufficiently conclusive for a firm diagnosis. For example, malignant melanomas and anaplastic carcinomas are maddeningly similar histologically, often mandating the use of immunohistochemical studies or electron microscopy to distinguish the two through elucidation of submicroscopic, cell lineage–related features (Figs. 6.6, 6.7). Similarly, spindle cell sarcomas of soft tissue may resemble one another so markedly that adjuvant analyses are necessary for final diagnosis (Fig. 6.8).

Of course, such evaluations require additional time for implementation and interpretation. These techniques merit further discussion, as they are used widely and provide extremely useful information.

Histochemical Stains

When H&E staining of paraffin-embedded tissue sections is insufficient to make a firm diagnosis of a malignant neoplasm, additional histochemical staining often provides sufficient information for definitive diagnosis. Because many of these specialized histochemical stains can be applied to formalin-fixed paraffin-embedded tissue, often they do not require the extra time and expense of many of the more specialized pathologic diagnostic procedures (e.g., electron microscopy or flow cytometry). However, because some special stains have specific requirements for uncommon tissue fixation and processing, pathologists must anticipate the possible need for special stains on the basis of clinical history and the initial gross examination to ensure that adequate tissue samples are appropriately processed. Table 6.2 lists the more common special histochemical stains. The widespread application of immunohistochemical stains (see later) has limited the usefulness of many histochemical stains and has rendered others obsolete.

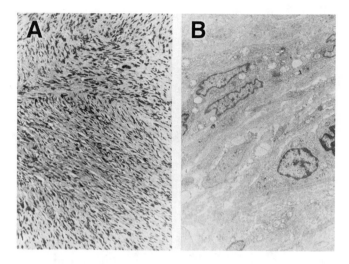

Figure 6.8 Histologically indeterminate malignant spindle-cell neoplasm of soft tissue. (A) The differential diagnosis includes leiomyosarcoma, fibrosarcoma, and malignant peripheral nerve sheath tumor on the basis of light-microscopical attributes. (B) Electron microscopy shows attenuated overlapping cytoplasmic processes, indicating the diagnosis of malignant peripheral nerve sheath tumor.

Electron Microscopy

Electron microscopy is performed after tissue is processed in special fixative, is embedded in epoxy (plastic) resin, is sectioned thinly (producing sections < 0.1 mm thick), and is impregnated with heavy metals. These heavy-metal stains enable differential absorption of a focused electron beam passed through the specimen en route to specialized photographic film. The photographic negative is developed and printed to provide an image of the specimen in which the extracellular space, cell membrane, and intracellular contents can be evaluated (magnified 200,000 times or more). On the basis of the presence of certain cytoplasmic organelles and other features listed in Table 6.3, pathologists may be able to distinguish one malignant cell type from another [18–20]. Ultrastructural features, however, are not used to distinguish benign from malignant tumors. Electron microscopy can be especially helpful when other specialized techniques do not provide a definitive diagnosis [21, 22].

Immunohistochemistry

Current practical immunohistochemistry is based on an indirect, antibody-enzyme method known in common parlance as the *immunoperoxidase procedure*. In this technique, a rehydrated, deparaffinized tissue section, or a frozen tissue section, is overlaid with a specific, well-characterized primary antibody directed at an antigen of diagnostic value. After controlled incubation and subsequent removal of the primary reagent, the tissue section is incubated with a second antibody having generic specificity for the first. Usually, the latter antibody is conjugated with biotin, providing a bridge for the subsequent binding of an avidin-biotin horseradish peroxidase complex that completes the immunochemical assembly (Fig. 6.9). The peroxidase enzyme then can be used to catalyze an oxidation-reduction reaction of a dye that is precipitated at the site of antibody binding. After a counterstaining procedure designed to highlight morphologic details, the presence of the antigen of interest can be visualized at a light-microscopical level within the tissue section (see Figs. 6.6, 6.7).

With few exceptions, the antigenic determinants that are the targets of immunohistochemical stains are not absolutely tissue- or tumor-specific. Therefore, pathologists must employ panels of primary antibodies in the study of a tumor, building an antigenic fingerprint that allows for a final interpretation. A sampling of commonly assessed antigens is listed in Table 6.4. On the basis of relative tissue specificities of these antigens, algorithms can be constructed to enable the resolution of differential diagnostic problems that often arise with

Table 6.2   Selected Specialized Histochemical Stains of Value in the Diagnosis of Neoplasia

Stain	Specificity	Sample Uses and Comments
Alcian blue	Acid mucosubstances	Demonstration of stromal mucin production by mesotheliomas
Periodic acid–Schiff	Glycogen (with appropriate control); neutral mucosubstances	Demonstration of mucus or glycogen production
Oil red-O	Neutral lipids	Demonstration of lipids (useful for distinguishing, for example, between ovarian fibroma and thecoma); cannot be used on paraffin-embedded tissue
Fontana-Masson (argentaffin)	Catecholamines or indolamines	Demonstration of neurosecretory differentiation and of melanin; some modifications require special fixative
Grimelius (argyrophilic)	A subset of neurosecretory granules	Demonstration of neurosecretory differentiation
Trichrome	Nuclei, cytoplasm, and collagen	Nonspecific; often can demonstrate immature skeletal muscle cells (myoblasts) in poorly differentiated mesenchymal tumors
Leder	Requires the presence of enzyme choloacetate esterase	Demonstration of cells of myeloid lineage and mast cells (actually an enzymatic histochemical technique)
Congo red	Amyloid	Demonstration of amyloid deposition in neuroendocrine tumors or associated with plasma cell tumors, immunocyte dyscrasias (e.g., multiple myeloma), chronic inflammatory conditions, chronic renal failure, etc.

Table 6.3   Valuable Selected Electron-Microscopic Features in the Diagnosis of Neoplasms

Finding	Predominant Distribution	Diagnostic Use
Intercellular junctions	Epithelial cells; selected mesenchymal nonlymphoid tumors	Distinction between lymphoma and carcinoma
External pericellular basal lamina	Epithelial cells; selected mesenchymal nonlymphoid tumors	Distinction between lymphoma and carcinoma; identification of some soft-tissue sarcomas
Intracellular or intercellular lumina	Glandular epithelium	Identification of adenocarcinomas
Microvillous core rootlets	Glandular epithelium of alimentary tract	Identification of gastrointestinal origin of metastatic carcinomas
Cytoplasmic tonofibrils	Squamous epithelium	Identification of squamous differentiation in epithelial tumors
Premelanosomes	Melanocytic cells	Identification of melanomas
Neurosecretory granules	Neuroendocrine cells	Identification of neuroendocrine neoplasms
Thick and thin filament complexes	Striated-muscle cells	Identification of rhabdomyosarcomas
Thin filament dense body complexes	Smooth-muscle cells	Identification of leiomyomas and leiomyosarcomas
Birbeck granules	Langerhans cells	Identification of Langerhans cell proliferations (e.g., histiocytosis X)
Cytoplasmic mucin	Secretory glandular epithelium	Distinction between malignant mesothelioma and adenocarcinoma; localization of origin for some adenocarcinomas

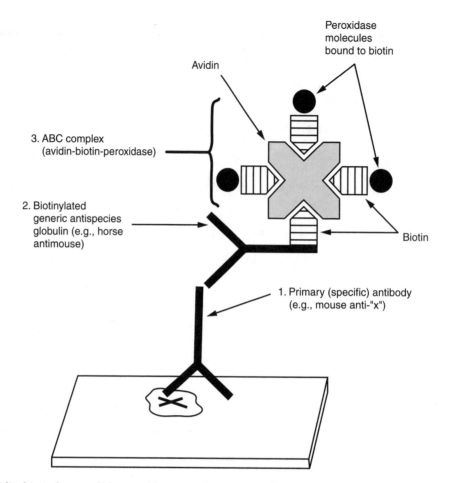

Peroxidase
molecules
bound to biotin

Avidin

3. ABC complex
(avidin-biotin-peroxidase)

2. Biotinylated
generic antispecies
globulin (e.g., horse
antimouse)

Biotin

1. Primary (specific) antibody
(e.g., mouse anti-"x")

Figure 6.9   The avidin-biotin horseradish peroxidase complex (ABC) technique of immunohistochemistry. A primary antibody to an antigen of interest is incubated with tissue sections, followed sequentially by a biotinylated secondary antibody and ABC complex. If the primary antibody binds (i.e., if the antigen is present in the tissue), the ensuing sequence of reagent linkages provides the substrate for chromogen localization and light-microscopic visibility of the reaction products. In this manner, antigens of diagnostic value can be detected in tissue.

histologically similar neoplasms (Figs. 6.10, 6.11). What must be emphasized is that, with the exception of establishing monoclonality of lymphoid proliferations, immunohistochemistry is not used to differentiate benign from malignant lesions.

Immunohistochemistry is used also to demonstrate components of a neoplasm's phenotype that may affect prognosis and treatment but that are not evident on routine light microscopy. As an example, many studies have shown that overexpression of the erb-B2 oncoprotein (encoded by the *HER2/neu* oncogene) is associated with a greater risk of relapse and death in patients with breast cancer [23], even in the subset of patients with low-stage and low-nuclear-grade tumors, a group generally believed to have a rather uniformly good prognosis [24]. Identification of erb-B2 overexpression is used also to select women who have metastatic breast cancer and are likely to benefit from treatment with

trastuzumab (Herceptin), a monoclonal antibody that binds to erb-B2 and inhibits its stimulation of cell proliferation. Immunohistochemical analysis of cell proliferation markers (e.g., Ki-67 or proliferating cell nuclear antigen), hormone receptors (e.g., estrogen receptor and progesterone receptor), oncoproteins (e.g., erb-B2 and BCL2), and tumor suppressor genes products (e.g., *p53*), either alone or in combination, also can provide prognostic information in a variety of other tumor types [25–27].

Flow Cytometry

Flow cytometry allows for the rapid quantitative measurement of cellular characteristics, such as size, surface marker expression, and DNA content. Flow-cytometric analysis of tumors is performed to identify cellular sub-

Table 6.4   Selected Antigenic Moieties of Diagnostic Value in Practical Immunohistochemistry

Antigen	Predominant Distribution	Common Diagnostic Uses
Cytokeratin	Epithelial cells	Distinction of carcinoma from lymphoma or melanoma
Cytokeratin isoforms	Epithelial cells	Determination of primary site of metastatic carcinoma (pattern of expression of various isoforms is related to site of origin)
Epithelial membrane antigen	Epithelial cells	Distinction of carcinoma from melanoma
Leukocyte common antigen	Leukocytes	Distinction of lymphoma from carcinoma or melanoma
Desmin	Myogenous cells	Identification of smooth-muscle or skeletal muscle tumors
Muscle-specific actin	Myogenous cells	Identification of smooth-muscle or skeletal muscle tumors
Prostate-specific antigen	Prostatic epithelium	Identification of metastatic prostatic carcinoma
Calcitonin	Parafollicular thyroid epithelium	Distinction of medullary thyroid carcinoma from other thyroid tumors
Carcinoembryonic antigen	Endodermally derived epithelium	Identification of gastrointestinal and lung adenocarcinomas; distinction of adenocarcinoma from mesothelioma
Placental alkaline phosphatase	Placental tissue and germ-cell tumors	Identification of possible germ-cell and trophoblastic tumors
Alpha-fetoprotein	Neoplastic hepatocytes and selected germ-cell tumors	Identification of hepatocellular carcinoma, endodermal sinus tumor, and other germ-cell tumors
β–Human chorionic gonadotropin	Placental tissue; trophoblastic and germ-cell tumors	Identification of trophoblastic differentiation in germ-cell tumors
CA-125	Müllerian epithelium	Identification of possible female genital tract carcinomas
CA-19–9	Alimentary tract epithelium	Identification of gastrointestinal and pancreatic carcinomas
Gross cystic disease fluid protein–15	Mammary epithelium and apocrine glands	Identification of metastatic breast carcinoma
Estrogen receptor and progesterone receptor	Mammary epithelium	Identification of metastatic breast carcinoma; prediction of clinical response to hormonal therapy in breast carcinoma
HMB-45	Melanocytic cells	Identification of melanoma
Chromogranin-A	Neuroendocrine cells	Identification of neuroendocrine carcinomas
Synaptophysin	Neuroendocrine cells	Identification of neuroendocrine carcinomas and neuroectodermal tumors
CD31	Vascular endothelium	Identification of vascular neoplasms
CD34	Vascular endothelium and some soft-tissue tumors	Identification of vascular neoplasms, solitary fibrous tumors, dermatofibrosarcoma protuberans
erb-B2 (gene product of *HER2/neu*)	Epithelium	Level of expression can provide prognostic information for breast carcinomas

populations within a specific histologic tumor type already stratified by stage and grade. Typically, these subpopulations are not evident on routine histopathologic examination and, to be clinically relevant and therefore useful, their identification must correlate with prognosis or response to treatment.

Briefly, the principle of flow cytometry is as follows. A monodispersed cell sample is stained with appropriate fluorochromes and then is suspended in an aqueous buffer and passed through a flow chamber designed to align the stream of cells so that they are struck individually by a focused laser beam (or beams). The scattered light and fluorescent emissions from each cell are separated according to wavelength by appropriate filters and mirrors and are directed to detectors that convert the emissions into electronic signals that are analyzed and

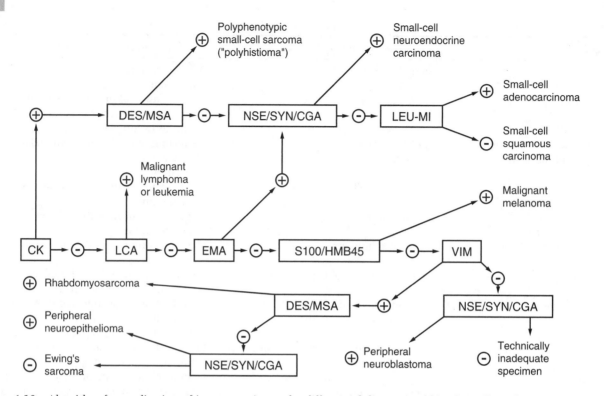

Figure 6.10   Algorithm for application of immunostains to the differential diagnosis of histologically indeterminate small-cell malignancies. *CK* = cytokeratin; *DES* = desmin; *MSA* = muscle-specific actin; *LCA* = leukocyte common antigen; *EMA* = epithelial membrane antigen; *NSE* = neuron-specific enolase; *SYN* = synaptophysin; *CGA* = chromogranin-A; *LEU-M1* = CD15 antigen; *S100* = S-100 protein; *VIM* = vimentin.

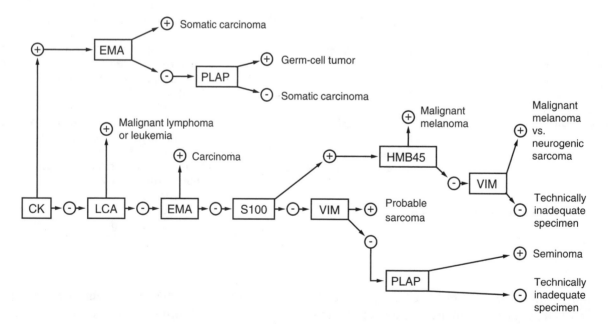

Figure 6.11   Algorithm for application of immunostains to the differential diagnosis of histologically indeterminate large-cell malignancies. *CK* = cytokeratin; *EMA* = epithelial membrane antigen; *LCA* = leukocyte common antigen; *PLAP* = placental alkaline phosphatase; *S100* = S-100 protein; *VIM* = vimentin.

stored by a computer. The data can be displayed as a frequency histogram (number of cells versus intensity of fluorescence) for single-parameter analysis or as a scattergraph for multiparametric analysis. Through the process of gating (the placement of electronic boundaries around specific areas in the frequency distribution), computer analysis can be performed on the data from only the subset of cells within the gated region, a method that can be used to take full advantage of multiparametric analysis [28].

The fluorochromes used to stain cells in flow cytometry include compounds that bind stoichiometrically to DNA, that label both DNA and RNA but fluoresce at different wavelengths for each type of nucleic acid, or that can be attached covalently to antibodies against specific cell antigens. Simultaneous multiparametric analysis is possible using two or more fluorochromes that emit light of different wavelengths.

In vivo single-cell suspensions, such as peripheral blood or bone marrow, can be analyzed easily by flow cytometry. Solid tissues, including lymph nodes and solid tumors, require additional preparation (usually gentle enzymatic, detergent, or mechanical treatment) to achieve a monodispersed sample. Methods have been developed also for analysis of single-cell suspensions derived from archival tissue that has been formalin-fixed and embedded in paraffin [28].

The recently developed technique of slide-based laser-scanning cytometry [29], admittedly still largely experimental, uses appropriate fluorochromes to stain cells in routine tissue sections or cytology preparations. The slides then are viewed using a microscope coupled to a computer, a laser, and hardware necessary to collect and analyze fluorescence emissions. Thus, tissue architecture and cell morphology can be correlated with the marker profile of individual cells within the neoplastic population.

SURFACE MARKER ANALYSIS

The role of cell-surface antigen analysis in diagnosis of neoplasia is illustrated best for lymphoid and other hematopoietic malignancies [30]. Multiparametric evaluation with a panel of monoclonal antibodies against surface antigens (Fig. 6.12, Table 6.5) facilitates classification of different subtypes of lymphoma and leukemia and has become a routine facet of diagnosis. Worth noting is that although flow-cytometric quantitation of intracellular constituents (e.g., the tumor suppressor *p53*) is possible, such procedures remain largely experimental because the correlation with detection by immunohistochemistry is low [31].

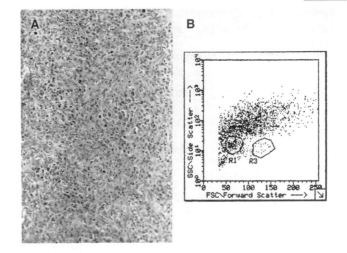

Figure 6.12   Example of the classification of a lymphoma by flow cytometry (see Table 6.5). (A) Section of spleen from a 61-year-old woman showing effacement of the parenchyma by large malignant lymphocytes. (B) Scattergram of the malignant infiltrate obtained by flow cytometry. Note the presence of two gated regions corresponding to small lymphocytes and large lymphocytes (arbitrarily labeled *R1* and *R3*, respectively). The results of multiparametric analysis of the cells within region R3 (see Table 6.5) when combined with the morphology of the tumor are diagnostic of large-cell lymphoma, B-cell type.

DNA MEASUREMENTS

Although many flow-cytometric studies have examined DNA ploidy as a prognostic factor, several variables complicate interpretation. For example, very few, if any, malignant tumors have a chromosomal complement normal in number and structure; therefore, the many diploid-range malignancies actually represent a heterogeneous group of lesions with chromosomal abnormalities below the level of resolution of flow cytometry. In addition, a small population of aneuploid cells may not be detected by flow-cytometric measurements. Some tissues, such as liver, normally contain tetraploid and even octaploid cells, and aneuploid cellular populations can be observed in several benign neoplastic and reactive soft-tissue lesions [32, 33]. Flow-cytometric cell-cycle analysis is directed primarily at calculation of the proportion of S-phase cells (the percentage of cells undergoing DNA synthesis) and is used to identify rapidly dividing neoplasms.

Arriving at summary statements is difficult as regards the correlation of flow-cytometric data on DNA ploidy or S-phase fraction with prognosis, but published reports suggest that consistent relationships do exist for specific forms of tumors. A careful prospective study of

Table 6.5 Example of the Use of Selected Monoclonal Antibodies for the Classification of a Lymphoma by Flow Cytometry

Antibody (Cluster Designation)	Specificity	Percentage of Positive Cells in Gated Regions of Figure 6.12*	
		R1	R3
T-cell markers			
CD3	Pan T cell	58	8
CD4	Helper-inducer T-cell subset	26	7
CD8	Cytotoxic-suppressor T-cell subset	26	7
B-cell markers			
CD19	B cells	14	93
HLA-DR	B cells, activated T cells (major histocompatibility complex class II antigen)	62	100
Anti-IgM	B-cell subset (immunoglobulin heavy-chain isotype M)	2	38
Anti-lambda	B-cell subset (lambda light chain)	13	68

*The staining pattern is diagnostic only for the region of the scattergram containing the large atypical lymphocytes (the gated region labeled *R3*). The cells in the R3 region stain positive for HLA-DR, CD19, and lambda immunoglobulin light chain, consistent with a monoclonal B-cell population. See Figure 6.12.

renal cell carcinoma has documented increased survival in patients with tumors having homogeneously diploid or near-diploid DNA content, as opposed to those with an aneuploid DNA profile [34]. For carcinoma of the breast, combined results generally confirm that the S-phase fraction influences disease-free survival but that aneuploidy is not a significant independent prognostic variable [35]. However, for many neoplasms, the correlation between DNA content or S-phase fraction and prognosis is uncertain. For many neoplasms, differences in standardization of S-phase fraction and ploidy measurements, differences in tissue preservation (i.e., fresh, frozen, or paraffin-embedded), and differences in patient population and outcome end points render comparison of conflicting results extremely difficult.

Diagnostic Molecular Genetics

The development of molecular techniques for evaluating tumors is a direct result of the tremendous advancements over the last two decades in molecular biology and in our understanding of the genetic mechanisms of neoplasia. The sensitivity and wide applicability of the techniques has rendered them useful not only in the diagnosis of malignancy but in the determination of prognosis, in monitoring the effect of therapy, and in genetic screening. The major techniques in current use are presented in the following sections, along with a few examples of their diagnostic utility.

The fundamental principle underlying these molecular tests is that cancer is a clonal process. As the original transformed cell proliferates, the DNA mutations it has accumulated are transmitted to its descendants. The expanding population of progeny cells, therefore, constitutes a clone in which all the cells are genetically identical to the founder cell (except for additional DNA mutations that may accumulate).

IN SITU HYBRIDIZATION AND FLUORESCENCE IN SITU HYBRIDIZATION

In situ hybridization (ISH) is performed to detect RNA or DNA and, therefore, can provide a measure of gene expression. One technical advance that allowed for a wide application of ISH to diagnostic pathology was the development of methods for labeling DNA probes with radioactive or nonradioactive compounds. Traditionally, nucleic acid probes were labeled by incorporation of a radioisotope of phosphorus. However, biotin can be incorporated into a nucleic acid probe by employing biotinylated derivatives of uridine triphosphate or deoxyuridine triphosphate during probe synthesis; the labeled nucleic acid probe exhibits denaturation and renaturation kinetics that are equivalent to those of an unsubstituted template. Through the use of avidin that has been complexed to fluorescent marker molecules, such chromogenic enzymes as horseradish peroxidase or alkaline phosphatase, or electron-opaque plastic spheres, the probe can be detected after ISH. Other methods for nonradioactive labeling of probes include the direct incorporation of fluorochromes or haptens. Because the labeled probes can be hybridized to the endogenous nucleic acid sequences in paraffin-embedded tissue sections and cytologic smears, the reaction product is localized to specific cells or even to subcellular compartments. Thus, the major advantage of ISH is that it permits simultaneous evaluation of morphology and the ISH result.

The technique of fluorescence in situ hybridization (FISH) involves the hybridization of DNA probes to metaphase chromosomes deposited on microscope slides or to chromatin within intact interphase cells [36]. Because the DNA probes are coupled to a fluorochrome, hybridization is detected by routine fluorescence microscopy. The technique can be used on formalin-fixed, paraffin-embedded tissue; therefore, FISH also permits correlation of morphology with the nuclear hybridization pattern of individual cells. The high resolution of FISH renders the technique suitable for detection of a variety of chromosomal abnormalities, including gene deletion, gene amplification, and chromosomal rearrangements.

Both ISH and FISH can be useful aids for diagnosis, for the identification of patient populations at increased risk of developing malignancies, or for the assessment of prognosis [36–38]. Some recent examples of the application of these molecular pathology techniques follow.

ISH has been used widely in the detection of human papillomaviruses (HPVs), of which more than 75 variants have been identified. The majority of cervical neoplasia, dysplasia, and carcinoma can be attributed to HPV infection; specific HPV types (i.e., 16, 18, 31, 33, 35, 45, 51, 52, 56, and 58) are highly correlated with high-grade dysplasia and malignancies of the cervix. Because the viral capsid antigen of all types is identical, immunohistochemical techniques are of little value in typing them. However, ISH has been used successfully to identify specific HPV types in cervical tissue [39, 40], demonstrating the utility of the method for identification of patients who have HPV infection and are at increased risk for progression to uterine cervical carcinoma. In this regard, a predominance of HPV types 6, 11, 16, and 18 also has been documented in carcinomas of the oral cavity, larynx, lung, nasal sinuses, anus, and esophagus [41].

FISH can be used to detect amplification of the *HER2/neu* oncogene, either alone or in combination with immunohistochemical techniques that demonstrate overexpression of the oncoprotein itself. In studies of breast carcinoma patients, FISH demonstration of an increased *HER2/neu* copy number has been correlated with lymph node metastasis. Patients who had tumors with more than five gene copies generally did not survive as long as those with lesions lacking gene amplification, and *HER2/neu* amplification may have greater prognostic value than most currently used predictive factors, including hormone-receptor status and size of primary tumor [23, 42].

SOUTHERN BLOT AND NORTHERN BLOT HYBRIDIZATIONS

For Southern blots, DNA is extracted from cells, digested with a restriction endonuclease, subjected to electrophoresis in an agarose gel to separate the fragments on the basis of size, and transferred to a filter on which it can be hybridized to a radiolabeled DNA probe. Southern blots are used to detect genomic rearrangements, especially those of genetic loci involved in consistent karyotypic abnormalities of certain tumors. Northern blots (which are completely analogous to Southern blots except that RNA is extracted from cells) are employed to detect abnormal gene expression in the absence of gross karyotypic abnormalities or to determine cell lineage on the basis of gene expression. The versatility and high sensitivity of Southern and Northern blots are, in practical terms, offset by the time required to obtain the result (usually five days or longer).

Analysis of Neuroblastomas

Amplification of the *N-myc* oncogene is a seemingly independent prognostic factor associated with advanced stage and rapid progression of neuroblastomas; the estimated 18-month patient survivals are 70%, 30%, and 5% for patients with tumors having 1, 3 to 10, and more than 10 *N-myc* copies, respectively [43]. Traditionally, Southern blot analysis has been the standard method by which amplification of *N-myc* in neuroblastomas is quantified, but recently the detection of *N-myc* amplification by FISH was shown to correlate well with results of Southern blotting [44].

Analysis of Hematopoietic Malignancies

The biological basis for the use of Southern blotting in the diagnosis and classification of lymphomas is the rearrangement of antigen receptor genes (the immunoglobulin heavy- and light-chain genes in B cells versus the T-cell receptor genes in T cells) that occurs in the normal progenitors from which lymphoid neoplasms arise. With the use of appropriate probes, the identification by Southern hybridization of a discrete nongermline band is evidence of the presence of a clonal population, a characteristic of lymphoid populations encountered only rarely in benign infiltrates (Fig. 6.13).

In addition to its use in differentiating monoclonal from polyclonal lymphoproliferative diseases, Southern blotting can detect rearrangements associated with chromosome translocations in chronic myelogenous leukemia (CML), to identify minimal residual disease

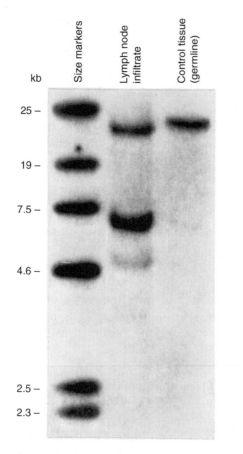

Figure 6.13 Southern blot of DNA extracted from a lymph node that histologically contained an atypical lymphoid infiltrate (DNA digested with the restriction enzyme EcoRI; immunoglobulin heavy-chain J region probe). A discrete set of restriction fragments is detected, indicating that the lymphoid proliferation is monoclonal and suggesting a diagnosis of lymphoma. kb = kilobases.

POLYMERASE CHAIN REACTION

A powerful advance in molecular biology that has revolutionized the use of molecular techniques in the pathologic evaluation of neoplasia has been the development of the polymerase chain reaction (PCR). Because PCR-based methods provide a means to amplify specific target DNA or RNA sequences, PCR has an extreme sensitivity in many diagnostic situations. PCR can be performed on fresh or paraffin-embedded tissue and, provided the target DNA or RNA has not been degraded, the quantity of tissue required often is minute.

To perform PCR, the nucleotide sequence flanking the DNA region of interest must be known, to which complementary oligonucleotide primers are synthesized. These oligonucleotide primers are added in vast excess to the target DNA sample, along with a thermostable DNA polymerase. If the target DNA sequence is present, the primers will hybridize and initiate DNA synthesis by the polymerase. After completion of the first polymerization cycle, the reaction mixture is heated to denature the DNA and is cooled to re-anneal the primers and the target DNA; thus, another cycle of DNA synthesis begins. The 20 to 30 cycles of a typical PCR, therefore, result in exponential amplification of the target DNA. The PCR products are assessed by gel electrophoresis and usually can be visualized directly using special stains; however, Southern blot hybridization can be performed with a conventional radiolabeled probe for the expected PCR product, to increase specificity by verifying the identity of the PCR product or to achieve more sensitive detection of the PCR product. In fact, PCR followed by Southern blotting routinely can detect one neoplastic cell in a background of 10^5 nonneoplastic cells. Because the DNA sequence of the PCR product can be determined easily by standard methods, even point mutations can be detected.

Reverse transcriptase PCR (RT-PCR) is a modification of the standard PCR technique and allows for amplification of target sequences from RNA. Cellular RNA first is transcribed into single-stranded cDNA by the enzyme reverse transcriptase, and the cDNA then is subjected to standard PCR for amplification of the target region. RT-PCR can be used to detect novel transcripts from fusion genes produced by chromosomal translocations, a method that has found wide applicability in the diagnosis of hematolymphoid and solid-tissue malignancies (as discussed later).

Correlation of tissue morphology with the PCR result can be achieved in two ways. Traditionally, areas of tumor (or even individual cells) are simply microdissected

during clinical remission, and to demonstrate the relationship between a recurrent malignancy and the original clonal population. In these settings, Southern blot analysis is very sensitive and can detect a clonal population that represents only 1% to 5% of the analyzed lymphoid cells [45]. The diagnostic utility of immunogenotyping lymphoid proliferations is indicated by the finding that Southern blot analysis (with probes for the immunoglobulin heavy chain, immunoglobulin light chain, and a T-cell receptor locus) resolved diagnostic problems in more than 50% of cases in which morphology and immunophenotyping yielded indeterminate results [46].

from a routinely prepared tissue slide or cytology slide; the nucleic acids then are extracted from the collected cells and are subjected to amplification as usual. Alternatively, using the technique known as *in situ PCR*, amplification is performed directly on the tissue slide itself; the product DNA within the tissue then is detected by ISH, allowing straightforward correlation of morphology and the PCR result [47].

Diagnosis of Leukemia

Detection of chromosome translocations by PCR has proved useful for the diagnosis and subclassification of hematolymphoid malignancies. For example, 95% of CMLs and 15% to 20% of acute lymphocytic leukemias contain the Philadelphia chromosome (Ph[1]), a t(9;22) translocation of the *bcr* gene from chromosome 22q11 to the *abl* oncogene from 9q34. Detection of the *bcr-abl* fusion gene transcript is considered pathognomonic for CML, and the use of RT-PCR exceeds the sensitivity of cytogenetic analysis [48].

Diagnosis of Lymphoma

The diagnosis of lymphomas by PCR is based on the detection of antigen receptor gene rearrangements. Because no practical immunohistochemical or flow-cytometric methods can detect T-cell clonality, PCR methods for the diagnosis of T-cell lymphomas, especially from paraffin-embedded tissue, are especially useful [49, 50]. As compared with Southern blot analysis, PCR is up to 50 times more sensitive, with no loss of specificity [51, 52].

However, the analysis of B-cell clonality by PCR amplification of immunoglobulin rearrangements is less definitive. A low sensitivity and specificity (especially a high false-positive rate) by PCR analysis suggests that, though it may provide adjunct information on clonality, the PCR result must be interpreted in the context of the clinical setting and histologic profile of the B-cell infiltrate [53, 54].

Diagnosis of Solid-Tissue Malignancies

The recent description of strikingly consistent cytogenetic abnormalities in soft-tissue tumors and some pediatric tumors (Table 6.6) has provided additional settings in which PCR-based techniques have been used as adjuncts for the classification and diagnostic workup of neoplasms [55]. For example, in the pediatric setting, tumors composed of small, round blue cells that are extremely similar morphologically (e.g., Ewing's sarcoma/primitive neuroectodermal tumor, alveolar rhabdomyosarcoma, and desmoplastic small round-cell tumor) can

be classified (Fig. 6.14) by detection of specific fusion transcripts by RT-PCR [56, 57].

MEDICAL, LEGAL, AND ETHICAL ISSUES

Worth emphasizing is that special diagnostic procedures, as with all clinical and laboratory tests, must be used only in appropriate circumstances. Most molecular genetic tests are labor-intensive and expensive as compared with routine histopathologic workup and immunohistochemistry. Though many of the special procedures offer extremely high sensitivity, especially the DNA- and RNA-based molecular techniques, none is absolutely specific [58]. Unlike immunohistochemistry, much of molecular genetic testing does not allow for direct correlation with morphology. Consequently, special tests should be ordered only after a specific differential diagnosis has been generated on the basis of integration of the clinical history and the microscopic findings in routinely prepared slides. Specialized tests never should be used as the basis for assigning a diagnosis in vacuo.

In fact, the sensitivity of PCR has raised several important clinical questions that remain unanswered. For example, PCR methods can detect residual leukemic cells in many patients who are in remission on the basis of standard clinical and histologic tests; however, the utility of such testing remains questionable because residual disease detected only by PCR is not considered a reliable predictor for relapse [59]. Again, both immunohistochemistry and PCR can detect in lymph nodes microscopic tumor metastases that are not evident by standard microscopic examination [60–63]; though a definite survival disadvantage is associated with these occult metastases in most studies, questions of specificity remain [64, 65], and serial sectioning followed by immunohistochemical staining or PCR is far too labor-intensive and expensive for routine use. These illustrations show how easily the newest technologies can outpace their application in a knowledgeable and practical way.

The advent of molecular testing also has entangled pathologists in a number of medicolegal debates. For example, faced with increased patient empowerment and patient-driven demand for specialized testing, should physicians alone continue to define the standard of care for specialized testing? In a situation where the diagnosis is certain but based on routinely prepared slides, should a pathologist be held liable if additional confirmatory specialized testing is not performed [66]? Cost-effectiveness analyses have been applied to several

Table 6.6   Selected Tumor-Specific Cytogenetic Abnormalities in Malignancies

Tumor Type	Cytogenetic Changes	Involved Genes
Leukemias		
CML	t(9;22)(q34;q11)	*BCR abl*
B-cell ALL	t(9;22)(q34;q11)	*BCR abl*
	t(1;19)(q23;p13)	*PBK1 E2A*
	t(8;14)(q24;q32)	*myc IGH*
	t(2;8)(p11;q24)	*IGK myc*
	t(8;22)(q24;q11)	*myc IGL*
	t(4;11)(q21;q23)	*AF4 MLL*
T-cell ALL	t(1;14)(p32;q11)	*TAL1 TCRD*
	t(1;14)(p34;q11)	*LCK TCRD*
	t(8;14)(q24;q11)	*myc TCRA*
Non-Hodgkin's lymphomas		
Follicular small cleaved-cell lymphoma	t(14;18)(q32;q21)	*IGH bcl2*
Burkitt's lymphoma	t(8;14)(q24;q32)	*myc IGH*
	t(2;8)(p11;q24)	*IGK myc*
	t(8;22)(q24;q11)	*myc IGL*
Mantle-zone lymphoma	t(11;14)(q13;q32)	*bcl1 IGH*
Solid tumors		
Neuroblastoma	Amplification	*N-myc*
Breast carcinoma	Amplification	*HER2/neu*
Ewing's sarcoma/primitive neuroectodermal tumor	t(11;22)(q24;q12)	*FLI1 EWS*
	t(21;22)(q22;q12)	*ERG EWS*
	t(7;22)(p22;q12)	*ETV1 EWS*
	t(17;22)(q12;q12)	*E1AF EWS*
	t(2;22)(q33;q12)	*FEV EWS*
Alveolar rhabdomyosarcoma	t(2;13)(q35;q14)	*PAX3 FKHR*
	t(1;13)(p36;q14)	*PAX7 FKHR*
Myxoid round-cell liposarcoma	t(12;16)(q13;p11)	*CHOP TLS*
	t(12;22)(q13;q11–12)	*CHOP EWS*
Desmoplastic small round-cell tumor	t(11;22)(p13;q12)	*WT1 EWS*
Synovial sarcoma	t(X;18)(p11.2;q11.2)	*SSX1 SYT*
		SSX2 SYT
Clear-cell sarcoma	t(12;22)(q13;q12)	*ATF1 EWS*
Extraskeletal myxoid chondrosarcoma	t(9;22)(q22;q12)	*CHN EWS*
Dermatofibrosarcoma protuberans: giant-cell fibroblastoma	t(17;22)(q22;q13)	*PDGFB COL1A1*
Other		
Endometrial stromal sarcoma	t(7;17)(p15–21;q12–21)	—

CML = chronic myelogenous leukemia; ALL = acute lymphocytic leukemia.
Note: This table is not an exhaustive compilation of karyotypic changes in human malignancies; rather, it is intended to illustrate a subset of tumor-specific chromosomal abnormalities of use in molecular diagnosis.

aspects of the pathologic evaluation of surgical specimens [13, 67]: Should a purely economic analysis define the standard of care for specialized testing? The latter question is especially relevant considering the changes in health care financing under way in the United States.

Finally, the recent advances in the genetics of cancer, in molecular diagnostics, and in the detection of DNA abnormalities within tissue specimens have raised several ethical issues. Should informed consent for presymptomatic diagnostic testing for cancer genes differ from consent for conventional diagnostic and therapeu-

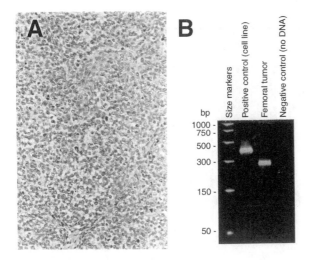

Figure 6.14 Femoral tumor in a 15-year-old girl. (A) Tumor is composed of small, round cells morphologically diagnostic of a Ewing's sarcoma/primitive neuroectodermal tumor. (B) Reverse transcriptase–polymerase chain reaction analysis based on the expected t(11;22) cytogenetic abnormality using oligonucleotide primers for *FLI1* (on chromosome 11) and *EWS* (on chromosome 22); the presence of a band from the femoral tumor confirms the diagnosis. The band size of 277 base pairs indicates a fusion between exon 7 of *EWS* and exon 6 of *FLI1* in the femoral tumor; the band size of 343 base pairs (bp) indicates a fusion between exon 7 of *EWS* and exon 5 of *FLI1* in the positive control cell line.

tic measures [68, 69]? How can patient confidentiality be maintained and discrimination be avoided, given the likely increased pressure from certain sectors (e.g., insurance companies and employers) for access to test results? What is the appropriate venue in which extremely sensitive genetic tests should be offered? Are such specialized tests to remain the responsibility of pathologists and other health care professionals, or should they be offered on a more informal, commercial basis? All physicians, not just pathologists, need to consider their obligation to provide effective, culturally sensitive, nondirective counseling to their patients regarding these issues.

Cytogenetics

As noted, specific chromosomal abnormalities are consistently associated with certain malignant neoplasms and often have diagnostic, therapeutic, and prognostic relevance. Though the application of molecular biology techniques to the detection of chromosomal abnormalities has defined a new level of cytogenetic analysis, rou-

tine karyotypic analysis of a tumor often is the only procedure available to probe chromosome structure [70]. Because standard karyotypic studies require culture of viable tumor cells, the need for this type of genetic analysis must be anticipated in advance. The most common karyotypic abnormalities detected by cytogenetic analysis are translocations, gene amplifications, and deletions.

The classic example of a balanced translocation is the Philadelphia chromosome that (as noted previously) is present in most cases of CML. Because cases of CML lacking the Ph[1] chromosome tend to resist therapy and have a less favorable prognosis, karyotypic analysis can provide clinically relevant information. For hematologic malignancies in general, cytogenetic analysis often plays an integral role in providing information of diagnostic and prognostic value.

The karyotypic manifestations of gene amplification include homogeneously staining regions (HSR) of single chromosomes and double minutes (DM), which are small, paired, extrachromosomal chromatin fragments. As an example, although the predominant genetic abnormalities in neuroblastoma are rearrangements and deletions of the terminal portion of the short arm of chromosome 1, the majority of neuroblastomas also have HSR and DM. Usually, the HSR and DM represent amplification of the *N-myc* oncogene, and a strong correlation exists among the degree of amplification, clinical stage, and prognosis.

Because of a decreased sensitivity as compared with other molecular techniques, karyotypic analysis of chromosomal deletions often plays less of a role in the diagnosis of a neoplasm or medical syndrome [71]. Nonetheless, recurring deletions have been described for many neoplasms, including deletions of the long arm of chromosome 22 in benign meningiomas, of the short arm of chromosome 3 in small-cell carcinomas of the lung, of the long arm of chromosome 13 in retinoblastomas, and of the short arm of chromosome 11 in Wilms' tumors. Whether these karyotypic abnormalities will be discovered to provide independent prognostic information remains a subject of investigation.

Tumor Markers

A tumor marker is a biochemical indicator of the presence of a neoplastic proliferation. In clinical usage, the term *tumor marker* refers to a molecule that can be detected in serum, plasma, or other body fluids. Often, sensitive methods of measurement are required for optimum usefulness—usually radioimmunoassay or en-

Table 6.7 Selected Tumor Markers and Applications in Diagnostic Medicine

Tumor Marker	Commonly Associated Malignant Neoplasms	Nonneoplastic Diseases
Hormones		
Human chorionic gonadotropin (HCG)	Gestational trophoblastic disease, gonadal germ-cell tumors	Pregnancy
Calcitonin	Medullary cancer of thyroid	—
Catecholamines and metabolites	Pheochromocytoma	—
Oncofetal antigens		
Alpha-fetoprotein	Hepatocellular carcinoma, gonadal germ-cell tumors (especially endodermal sinus tumor)	Cirrhosis, toxic liver injury, hepatitis
Carcinoembryonic antigen	Adenocarcinomas of colon, pancreas, stomach, lung, breast, ovary	Pancreatitis, inflammatory bowel disease, hepatitis, cirrhosis, tobacco abuse
Isoenzymes		
Prostatic acid phosphatase	Adenocarcinoma of prostate	Prostatitis; nodular prostatic hyperplasia
Neuron-specific enolase	Small-cell carcinoma of lung; neuroblastoma	—
Specific proteins		
Prostate-specific antigen	Adenocarcinoma of prostate	Nodular prostatic hyperplasia, prostatitis
Monoclonal immunoglobulin	Multiple myeloma	Monoclonal gammopathy of unknown significance
CA-125	Epithelial ovarian neoplasms	Menstruation, pregnancy, peritonitis
CA-19-9	Adenocarcinoma of pancreas or colon	Pancreatitis; ulcerative colitis

zyme-linked immunosorbent assay. No tumor marker is specific; all are present at low levels in the normal physiologic state or in nonneoplastic disease, and virtually any given marker may be seen in conjunction with a variety of neoplasms. Tumor markers can be divided into two broad categories: tumor-derived moieties and tumor-associated (or host-response) markers. Useful tumor markers and associated neoplasms are presented in Table 6.7.

Tumor-derived markers include oncofetal antigens (alpha-fetoprotein and carcinoembryonic antigen); hormones (β–human chorionic gonadotropin, human placental lactogen, antidiuretic hormone, parathyroid hormone, calcitonin, insulin-like growth factor, catecholamine metabolites); tissue-specific proteins (immunoglobulins, prostate-specific antigen [PSA], gross cystic disease fluid protein-15); enzymes (gamma-glutamyl transpeptidase); isoenzymes (prostatic acid phosphatase, placental alkaline phosphatase, neuron-specific enolase); oncogene products; various polyamines; sialic acid; and glycolipids.

Tumor-associated markers include interleukin-2, tumor necrosis factor, immune complexes, acute-phase reactants (C-reactive protein, α_2-macroglobulin), and enzymes (lactate dehydrogenase, creatine kinase BB isoenzyme, glutamate dehydrogenase). Most often, tumor-associated markers are used together with tumor-derived markers.

Only one tumor marker, PSA, has demonstrated specificity and sensitivity adequate for the screening detection of malignancies in the general population. The measurement of serum PSA levels in widespread screening programs has resulted in the diagnosis of earlier-stage prostate adenocarcinoma in younger men, a shift that could influence mortality. The utility of serum PSA measurement is demonstrated by the fact that it has become part of the program for early cancer detection recommended by the American Cancer Society [72].

The primary utility of most tumor markers has been determination of the response to therapy (i.e., the detection of residual disease or relapse). As Figure 6.15

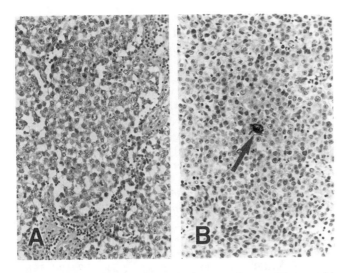

Figure 6.15 Sections of a testicular mass from a 57-year-old man. Preoperative workup demonstrated an increased serum β-human chorionic gonadotropin level. (A) Routine histopathologic examination shows a classic seminoma. Note the uniform malignant cells with abundant clear cytoplasm, arranged in nests divided by fibrous bands; a lymphocytic stromal infiltrate is present. No trophoblastic elements are noted. (B) Immunohistochemical stain for human chorionic gonadotropin demonstrates isolated, strongly reactive mononuclear cells (*arrow*), confirming the presence of trophoblastic elements in the tumor.

demonstrates, the serologic detection of a tumor marker also may suggest additional steps in the pathologic evaluation of a neoplasm. Because of the lack of specificity of the markers individually, the utility of test panels is an area of active investigation. In current practice, however, the use of tumor markers for follow-up after treatment usually is limited to markers known to have been present before treatment.

SUMMARY

This overview has covered a number of conventional and recent techniques available to pathologists for use in the evaluation of neoplastic diseases. Knowledge of the potential uses and abuses of these procedures is important to both clinicians and pathologists to help to ensure that patient care is not hindered through the omission or misapplication of pertinent studies. An understanding of the pathologic evaluation of tumors also emphasizes the need for cooperation between pathologists and oncologists for optimal diagnosis and management of oncology patients.

REFERENCES

1. Altman LK. Baseball: Strawberry's surgery is termed successful. *New York Times,* 148(51,300):sec. 8, October 4, 1998:8.
2. Koss LG. Minimal neoplasia as a challenge for early cancer detection. In Grundmann E, Beck L (eds), *Minimal Neoplasia: Diagnosis and Therapy.* Berlin: Springer, 1988:1–8.
3. Wick MR, Ritter JH. Pseudoneoplastic lesions: an overview. In Wick MR, Humphrey PA, Ritter JH (eds), *Pathology of Pseudoneoplastic Lesions.* Philadelphia: Lippincott-Raven, 1997:1–24.
4. Fleming ID, Cooper JS, Henson DE, et al. (eds), *AJCC Cancer Staging Manual* (5th ed). Philadelphia: Lippincott-Raven, 1997:3–18.
5. Anderson MC. Premalignant and malignant squamous lesions of the cervix. In Fox H, Wells M (eds), *Obstetrical and Gynaecological Pathology* (4th ed). New York: Churchill Livingstone, 1995:273–322.
6. Sevin BU, Lu Y, Bloch DA, et al. Surgically defined prognostic parameters in patients with early cervical carcinoma. A multivariate survival tree analysis. *Cancer* 78: 1438–1446, 1996.
7. Comerci G, Bolger BS, Flannelly G, et al. Prognostic factors in surgically treated stage IB–IIB carcinoma of the cervix with negative lymph nodes. *Int J Gynecol Cancer* 8:23–26, 1998.
8. Finan MA, DeCesare S, Fiorica JV, et al. Radical hysterectomy for stage IB1 vs IB2 carcinoma of the cervix: does the new staging system predict morbidity and survival? *Gynecol Oncol* 62:139–147, 1996.
9. Bostwick DG. Evaluating prostate needle biopsy: therapeutic and prognostic importance. *CA Cancer J Clin* 47: 297–319, 1997.
10. Gleason DF, Mellinger GT. Prediction of prognosis for prostatic adenocarcinoma by combined histological grading and clinical staging. *J Urol* 111:58–64, 1974.
11. Challis D. Frozen section and intra-operative diagnosis. [Broadsheet no. 41.] *Pathology* 29:165–174, 1997.
12. Boyd LA, Earnhardt RC, Dunn JT, et al. Preoperative evaluation and predictive value of fine-needle aspiration and frozen section of thyroid nodules. *J Am Coll Surg* 187:494–502, 1998.
13. Esserman L, Weidner N. Is routine frozen section assessment feasible in the practice environment of the 1990s? *Cancer J Sci Am* 3:266–267, 1997.
14. Wang KG, Chen TC, Wang TY, et al. Accuracy of frozen section diagnosis in gynecology. *Gynecol Oncol* 70:105–110, 1998.
15. Scucchi LF, Di Stefano D, Cosentino L, Vecchione A. Value of cytology as an adjunctive intraoperative diagnostic method. *Acta Cytol* 41:1489–1496, 1997.
16. Zardawi I. Fine needle aspiration cytology vs. core biopsy in a rural setting. *Acta Cytol* 42:883–887, 1998.
17. Arisio R, Cuccorese C, Accinelli G, et al. Role of fine-needle aspiration biopsy in breast lesions: analysis of a series of 4,110 cases. *Diagn Cytopathol* 18:462–467, 1998.
18. Mierau GW, Weeks DA, Hicks MJ. Role of electron microscopy and other special techniques in the diagnosis of

childhood round cell tumors. *Hum Pathol* 29:1347–1355, 1998.

19. Erlandson RA, Woodruff JM. Role of electron microscopy in the evaluation of soft tissue neoplasms, with emphasis on spindle cell and pleomorphic tumors. *Hum Pathol* 29:1372–1381, 1998.

20. Dardick I, Herrera GA. Diagnostic electron microscopy of neoplasms. *Hum Pathol* 29:1335–1338, 1998.

21. Ordoñez NG, Mackay B. Electron microscopy in tumor diagnosis: indications for its use in the immunohistochemical era. *Hum Pathol* 29:1403–1411, 1998.

22. Kandel R, Bedard YC, Gan QH. Value of electron microscopy and immunohistochemistry in the diagnosis of soft tissue tumors. *Ultrastruct Pathol* 22:141–146, 1998.

23. Walker RA, Jones JL, Chappell S, et al. Molecular pathology of breast cancer and its application to clinical management. *Cancer Metastasis Rev* 16:5–27, 1997.

24. Battifora H, Gaffey M, Esteban J, et al. Immunohistochemical assay of neu/c–erbB-2 oncogene product in paraffin-embedded tissues in early breast cancer: retrospective follow-up study of 245 stage I and II cases. *Mod Pathol* 4:466–474, 1991.

25. van Diest PJ, Brugal G, Baak JPA. Proliferation markers in tumours: interpretation and clinical value. *J Clin Pathol* 51:716–724, 1998.

26. Fern M. Prognostic factors in breast cancer: a brief review. *Anticancer Res* 18:2167–2172, 1998.

27. Taylor CR, Cote RJ. Immunohistochemical markers of prognostic value in surgical pathology. *Histol Histopathol* 12:1039–1055, 1997.

28. Koss LG, Czerniak B, Herz F, Wersto RP. Flow cytometric measurements of DNA and other cell components in human tumors: a critical appraisal. *Hum Pathol* 20:528–548, 1989.

29. Kamentsky LA, Burger DE, Gershman RJ, et al. Slide-based laser scanning cytometry. *Acta Cytol* 41:123–143, 1997.

30. Jennings CD, Foon KA. Recent advances in flow cytometry: application to the diagnosis of hematologic malignancy. *Blood* 90:2863–2892, 1997.

31. Benini E, Costa A, Abolafio G, Silvestrini R. *p53* Expression in human carcinomas—could flow cytometry be an alternative to immunohistochemistry? *J Histochem Cytochem* 46:41–47, 1998.

32. Saeter G, Lee CZ, Schwartze E, et al. Changes in ploidy distributions in human liver carcinogenesis. *J Natl Cancer Inst* 80:1480–1485, 1988.

33. RuB S, Comino A, Fruttero A, et al. Flow cytometric DNA analysis of cirrhotic liver cells in patients with hepatocellular carcinoma can provide a new prognostic factor. *Cancer* 78:1195–1202, 1996.

34. Ljungberg B, Stenling R, Roos G. DNA content in renal cell carcinoma with reference to tumor heterogeneity. *Cancer* 56:503–508, 1985.

35. Donegan WL. Tumor-related prognostic factors for breast cancer. *CA Cancer J Clin* 47:28–51, 1997.

36. Werner M, Wilkens L, Aubele M, et al. Interphase cytogenetics in pathology: principles, methods and applications of fluorescence in situ hybridization (FISH). *Histochem Cell Biol* 108:381–390, 1997.

37. McNicol AM, Farquharson MA. In situ hybridization and its diagnostic applications in pathology. *J Pathol* 182:250–261, 1997.

38. Jin L, Lloyd RV. In situ hybridization: methods and applications. *J Clin Lab Anal* 11:2–9, 1997.

39. Southern SA, Graham DA, Herrington CS. Discrimination of human papillomavirus types in low and high grade cervical squamous neoplasia by in situ hybridization. *Diagn Mol Pathol* 7:114–121, 1998.

40. Unger ER, Vernon SD, Lee DR, et al. Detection of human papillomavirus in archival tissues: comparison of in situ hybridization and polymerase chain reaction. *J Histochem Cytochem* 46:535–540, 1998.

41. zur Hausen H. Papillomavirus infections—a major cause of human cancers. *Biochim Biophys Acta* 1288:F55–F78, 1996.

42. Slamon DJ, Clark GM, Wong SG, et al. Human breast cancer: correlation of relapse and survival with amplification of the HER-2/neu oncogene. *Science* 235:177–182, 1987.

43. Seeger RC, Brodeur GM, Sather H, et al. Association of multiple copies of the *N-myc* oncogene with rapid progression of neuroblastomas. *N Engl J Med* 313:1111–1116, 1985.

44. Hachitanda Y, Saito M, Mori T, Hamazaki M. Application of fluorescence in situ hybridization to detect *N-myc* (*MYCN*) gene amplification on paraffin-embedded tissue sections of neuroblastomas. *Med Pediatr Oncol* 29:135–138, 1997.

45. Grody WW, Gatti RA, Naeim F. Diagnostic molecular pathology. *Mod Pathol* 2:553–568, 1989.

46. Kamat D, Laszewski MJ, Kemp JD, et al. The diagnostic utility of immunophenotyping and immunogenotyping in the pathologic evaluation of lymphoid proliferations. *Mod Pathol* 3:105–112, 1990.

47. Long AA. In-situ polymerase chain reaction—foundation of the technology and today's options. *Eur J Histochem* 42:101–109, 1998.

48. Kawasaki ES, Clark SS, Coyne MY, et al. Diagnosis of chronic myeloid and acute lymphocytic leukemias by detection of leukemia-specific mRNA sequences amplified in vitro. *Proc Natl Acad Sci USA* 85:5698–5702, 1988.

49. Greiner TC, Raffeld M, Lutz C, et al. Analysis of T cell receptor–γ gene rearrangements by denaturing gradient gel electrophoresis of GC-clamped polymerase chain reaction products. Correlation with tumor-specific sequences. *Am J Pathol* 146:46–55, 1995.

50. Ashton-Key M, Diss TC, Du MQ, et al. The value of the polymerase chain reaction in the diagnosis of cutaneous T-cell infiltrates. *Am J Surg Pathol* 21:743–747, 1997.

51. Yu RC, Alaibac M. A rapid polymerase chain reaction–based technique for detecting clonal T-cell receptor gene rearrangements in cutaneous T-cell lymphomas of both the αβ and γδ varieties. *Diagn Mol Pathol* 5:121–126, 1996.

52. Benhattar J, Delacretaz F, Martin P, et al. Improved polymerase chain reaction detection of clonal T-cell lymphoid neoplasms. *Diagn Mol Pathol* 4:108–112, 1995.

53. O'Sullivan MJ, Ritter JH, Humphrey PA, Wick MR. Lymphoid lesions of the gastrointestinal tract. A histologic, immunophenotypic, and genotypic analysis of 49 cases. *Am J Clin Pathol* 110:471–477, 1998.

54. Ritter JH, Wick MR, Adesokan PN, et al. Assessment of clonality in cutaneous lymphoid infiltrates by polymerase

chain reaction analysis of immunoglobulin heavy chain gene rearrangement. *Am J Clin Pathol* 108:60–68, 1997.

55. Mentzel T, Fletcher CDM. Recent advances in soft tissue tumor diagnosis. *Am J Clin Pathol* 110:660–670, 1998.

56. Downing JR, Khandekar A, Shurtleff SA, et al. Multiple RT-PCR assay for the differential diagnosis of alveolar rhabdomyosarcoma and Ewing's sarcoma. *Am J Pathol* 146:626–634, 1995.

57. de Alava E, Ladanyi M, Rosai J, et al. Detection of chimeric transcripts in desmoplastic small round cell tumor and related developmental tumors by reverse transcriptase polymerase chain reaction. A specific diagnostic assay. *Am J Pathol* 147:1584–1591, 1995.

58. Thorner P, Squire J, Chilton-MacNeil S, et al. Is the EWS/FLI-1 fusion transcript specific for Ewing's sarcoma and peripheral primitive neuroectodermal tumor? A report of four cases showing this transcript in a wider range of tumor types. *Am J Pathol* 148:1125–1138, 1996.

59. Faderl S, Estrov Z. The clinical significance of detection of residual disease in childhood ALL. *Crit Rev Oncol Hematol* 28:31–35, 1998.

60. Shivers SC, Wang X, Li W, et al. Molecular staging of malignant melanoma. Correlation with clinical outcome. *JAMA* 280:1410–1415, 1998.

61. Liefers GJ, Cleton-Jansen A-M, van de Velde CJH, et al. Micrometastases and survival in stage II colorectal cancer. *N Engl J Med* 339:223–228, 1998.

62. Izbicki JR, Hosch SB, Pichlmeier U, et al. Prognostic value of immunohistochemically identifiable tumor cells in lymph nodes of patients with completely resected esophageal cancer. *N Engl J Med* 337:1188–1194, 1997.

63. Dowlatshai K, Fan M, Snider HC, Habib FA. Lymph node micrometastases from breast carcinoma. Reviewing the dilemma. *Cancer* 80:1188–1197, 1997.

64. Bustin SA, Dorudi S. Molecular assessment of tumour stage and disease recurrence using PCR-based assays. *Mol Med Today* 4:389–396, 1998.

65. Bostick PJ, Chatterjee S, Chi DD, et al. Limitations of specific reverse-transcriptase polymerase chain reaction markers in the detection of metastases in the lymph nodes and blood of breast cancer patients. *J Clin Oncol* 16:2632–2640, 1998.

66. Dehner LP. On trial: a malignant small cell tumor in a child. Four wrongs do not make a right. *Am J Clin Pathol* 109:662–668, 1998.

67. Raab SS. The cost-effectiveness of routine histologic examination. *Am J Clin Pathol* 110:391–396, 1998.

68. National Advisory Council for Human Genome Research. Statement on use of DNA testing for presymptomatic identification of cancer risk. Commentary. *JAMA* 271:785, 1994.

69. Elias S, Annas GJ. Generic consent for genetic screening. *N Engl J Med* 330:1611–1613, 1994.

70. Humphrey GME, Squire R, Lansdown M, et al. Cytogenetics and the surgeon: an invaluable tool in diagnosis, prognosis and counselling of patients with solid tumours. *Br J Surg* 85:725–734, 1998.

71. Malcolm S. Microdeletion and microduplication syndromes. *Prenat Diagn* 16:1213–1219, 1996.

72. von Eschenbach A, Ho R, Murphy G, et al. American Cancer Society guideline for the early detection of prostate cancer: update 1997. *CA Cancer J Clin* 47:261–264, 1997.

7

General Approach to Cancer Patients

■ ■ ■

RAYMOND E. LENHARD, JR.
ROBERT T. OSTEEN

THIS CHAPTER IS AN INTRODUCTION TO THE disease- and organ-specific sections that follow. It focuses on general principles of cancer management and emphasizes the philosophy and reasoning that lie behind many of the recommendations for diagnosis, treatment, rehabilitation, and overall management discussed in depth later in this book.

The most successful approach to cancer control is prevention. Several healthy lifestyle behavioral modifications, such as tobacco avoidance, dietary modification, maintenance of a normal body weight, and physical activity, should be employed as preventive measures that can diminish one's risk of developing cancer. In addition, clinical trials of chemoprevention in breast, head, neck, and other cancers are the first of many trials during the coming years that will take advantage of knowledge of the biology of cancer to target specific high-risk populations.

If cancer prevention fails, detecting cancer as early as possible is important. For many primary sites of cancer, early detection is a reasonable goal and will result in less intense treatment and improved treatment results. In every instance, a well-conceived management plan is critical.

Modern disease diagnosis and treatment and rehabilitation of the patient with cancer or suspected cancer rely heavily on the classic principles of the doctor-patient relationship. For health care personnel, understanding the fears and concerns of patients and their families is as important as having detailed information about specific cancer treatments. The former requires that doctors and other caregivers have the discipline to truly listen to their patients and to lead them through this medically complex, emotionally daunting experience. The scientific information can be obtained from a variety of current data sources, such as the National Cancer Institute's PDQ system; the American Cancer Society's National Cancer Information Center; textbooks; meetings; and consultations with oncologists.

Often, primary-care physicians are in the best position to establish an early diagnosis. In careful history taking, clues that may be detected (often of minor symptoms) can alert physicians to evaluate their patients for possible cancer. In past years, a number of these clues were brought to the attention of the public in the form of the American Cancer Society's seven danger signals. However, many of these commonly known signs and symptoms are evidence of advanced disease, and our efforts to detect cancer in its curative stages must, therefore, emphasize screening of asymptomatic people.

When cancer is suspected, a logical and direct approach must be taken to establish a diagnosis. At the time of diagnosis, the patient must be evaluated completely, so that a comprehensive plan of action can be developed. Cancer patients have a disease that is both medical and emotional. Throughout the course of the illness, the diagnosis creates anxiety in patients, family members, and friends; in the physician, who must tell affected patients the consequences of the diagnosis; and in the physician's office or hospital staff, who see and interact with the patient. Physicians must conduct a calm, directed, logical evaluation of patients and present as optimistic a plan as possible, based on a consideration of all the treatment modalities available.

Both local and distant control of the disease are primary objectives to maintain or improve quality of life and to extend survival, with an emphasis on disease-free survival. An overall strategy for accomplishing these objectives should consider financial costs associated with the diagnosis and treatment of the disease process and other, less tangible costs to patients, their families, and society.

INTERDISCIPLINARY EVALUATION AND PLANNING

A major advance during the last few years has been the development of a greater appreciation of the value of an interdisciplinary approach to patient management. Once a clue of the presence of a cancer is obtained, the specific professional talents that are needed should be identified. Often, such skills cannot be provided by a single individual. The hallmark of modern clinical oncology is the involvement of physicians from several disciplines and of nurses, social workers, nutritionists, and other members of the health care team in the early phases of the management of a cancer patient. Although the plan for evaluation and treatment usually requires the efforts of an interdisciplinary team to ob-

tain optimal results, leadership in this enterprise still necessitates a perceptive and knowledgeable coordinating physician who may be an oncologist, the primary-care physician, an internist, or a general surgeon. In addition, patients with premalignant conditions or a genetic predisposition for cancer may need expert counseling regarding risks, availability of screening, and options for prophylaxis.

In addition to individual consultations, interdisciplinary considerations may be provided by a tumor board conference, wherein an interchange of ideas helps to focus the plan. Though some patients may be treated by a representative of only one discipline, in most situations the ideal treatment program requires a combination of health care providers representing various oncologic specialties.

At each step, the responsible physician should consider the effect that a proposed therapy would have on subsequent interventions. For example, at the time of operation, an appropriate step may be for the surgeon to modify the approach to render subsequent radiotherapy more effective or less harmful to normal organs. Placement of radiopaque clips around the area from which a mass has been resected may provide critical guidance for planning radiotherapy fields. The radiation oncologist may plan the treatment area to spare bone marrow for later chemotherapy. The medical oncologist may need to consider the risks from prolonged low white blood cell or platelet counts in patients who have a partially obstructed intestine and who may require surgery. These treatment-planning decisions are examples of the multidisciplinary approach and the need for periodic review of the plan at specific decision points during treatment.

DIAGNOSIS AND STAGING

Although the primary focus of the initial physical examination is on the presenting symptoms, patients who are being evaluated for the presence of cancer require a complete physical examination and the recording of a complete history so as to elucidate possible sites of metastatic spread of the cancer. Questions asked during compilation of a complete medical history might raise the suspicion of metastasis and could lead to a focus on specific aspects of the physical examination outside the original area of concern. Although blood tests and imaging studies have refined our diagnostic capabilities, a thorough history and physical examination still are critical first steps. Specific attention should be devoted to the chief complaint. It provides a clue to deranged physiology or a malfunctioning organ system and identifies a problem that must be solved, a symptom that must be alleviated. By concentrating on the chief complaint, physicians convey to patients the message that the symptom is important and that it can be relieved either by eliminating the cause or by appropriate symptomatic treatment.

Establishing the Diagnosis

The general philosophy guiding the diagnosis and staging of various cancers is that these efforts should be both efficient and cost-effective. A biopsy of any potential cancer site should be performed early in the process, as it establishes the basis for staging and treatment. A number of biopsies (fine-needle aspiration biopsy, superficial lymph node biopsy, some endoscopic biopsies) can be carried out promptly and with minimal preparation.

Though performing a biopsy immediately after initial history taking and physical examination may be appropriate for superficial masses, most clinical presentations require additional diagnostic tests before a biopsy can be considered. To minimize patient discomfort and limit cost, physicians should avoid tests that have a low likelihood of providing useful information and should avoid any tests that provide information similar to that obtained from other tests already performed or planned. An example of such duplication of diagnostic effort is the use of two slightly different, but expensive, radiologic techniques when the diagnostic information provided from both approaches is similar (e.g., abdominal computed tomography and magnetic resonance imaging; transhepatic cholangiogram and endoscopic retrograde cholangiopancreatogram).

All tests must be relevant to the decision that must be made. Generally, we recommend doing the least expensive tests first. However, a relatively expensive but highly informative test done early in the diagnostic workup may shorten the process and, in the long run, might be the most cost-effective. Before ordering complex or expensive diagnostic examinations, physicians should consider how the result would affect the overall treatment plan. This caution applies to tests performed both to help establish a diagnosis and to aid in the staging process.

Cancer Staging

Establishing a precise stage for each patient with cancer is important. The primary reason for staging is to help to provide optimal treatment selection and planning for individual patients. Assigning a stage is also a way to determine a patient's eligibility for and entry into a clinical research trial. Staging may stratify patient groups or may be used to standardize treatments to assist in more accurate comparisons of results in patients undergoing two or more treatments that are being compared. Though many different staging systems have been employed over the years, the trend has been toward the development of a unified staging nomenclature for all primary sites.

The practice of dividing cancer cases into groups arose from the observation that survival rates were higher for cases in which the tumor was localized than for those in which the disease had extended beyond the organ or site of origin. Often, these groups were termed *early cases* and *late cases,* respectively, suggesting disease progression with time. The late cases were divided into *regional* (those involving the regional nodes) and *distant* (those in which the cancer had spread to distant sites).

Over the last 40 years, the American Joint Committee on Cancer has carried out retrospective studies of outcome on most anatomic sites of cancer and has reviewed staging protocols reported in the literature. The effort has progressed to an international collaboration between the Union Internationale Contre le Cancer and the American Joint Committee on Cancer that resulted in agreement on one system of staging that is used worldwide [1].

Cancer staging accomplishes the following objectives:

- It aids clinicians in the planning of treatment for each patient.
- It assists in the evaluation of treatment modalities.
- It facilitates exchange of information between treatment centers worldwide.
- It evaluates the outcome of treatment (i.e., patient survival).
- It estimates the prognosis or outcome for each patient by stage and treatment.

Modern staging systems use clinical, surgical, pathologic, and biochemical parameters to define extent of disease and to direct treatment. Prognostic variables have been delineated clearly from pathologic findings in surgical specimens removed as part of the treatment process, and this information is valuable when combined with clinical staging to direct treatment planning. Specific definitions of the extent of the local neoplasm, or tumor (T), have been defined for each type of cancer, and definitions have been developed for categorizing regional lymph node spread (N). Distant metastases (M) may be found in many anatomic sites. This system, known as the *TNM staging system*, and its application to each anatomic site are discussed in detail in the site-oriented chapters.

THERAPEUTIC GOALS

Cure

The first decision regarding treatment is whether the cancer can be cured or whether palliation is the only practical goal. The potential for cure is increased if the cancer is localized sufficiently so that it can be eliminated by surgery or irradiation. Cure is also possible in some cancers even when the disease is widespread. Surgery, radiotherapy, chemotherapy, or combinations of these treatments may be used for both palliation and cure.

Disease-Free Interval and Survival Time

The consideration of several time intervals is important as a patient's treatment plan is being formulated. Increased duration of survival is important, but often equally relevant to patients is the time that they are free of disease. Many issues of quality of life revolve around this point. Cost-versus-benefit measures include both length of survival and "performance status," quantified by using one of the several measures that rate activities of daily living (e.g., the Karnofsky scale or the Eastern Cooperative Oncology Group activity and performance standards). Aggressive, highly toxic chemotherapy, radiotherapy, or surgical procedures can be justified if they result in complete regression of the cancer and a prolonged, disease-free survival time after treatment. From this group of patients come those who remain well for the duration of their lives and are cured. However, even in the event of later recurrence of cancer, a long period free of known cancer after primary treatment contributes positively to quality of life.

Overall survival data are a key factor in the selection of treatments. Some treatments remove or diminish the visible cancer but do not change expected survival time. Consideration of both survival and the expected clinical response to therapy is important in the development of a treatment strategy. A thorough understanding of oncology forms the basis for establishing the chances for prolonged, disease-free survival and overall survival time, which must be balanced against cost in terms of physical discomfort, mental distress, family upheaval, and financial loss.

Prevention of Local Recurrence

The optimal extent of surgical resection, appropriate placement of the radiotherapy fields and dosimetry, and skilled use of adjuvant irradiation or chemotherapy after surgery variously contribute to successful control of local disease. Although a cancer may recur at a distant site and can be the cause of death, often control at the original primary site figures prominently in the overall success of a treatment and in a patient's quality of life. Local obstruction (bowel, ureter, airway) and pain arising from locoregional progression of cancer are major medical problems requiring palliation. Initial treatment that is likely to prevent these late complications is well worth the extra effort, even if overall survival time is not extended.

Palliation

In many circumstances, palliation is the only practical goal of treatment. Ideally, initial treatment should be potentially curative or life-extending; however, many patients at the time of diagnosis have advanced disease or a cancer that is poorly responsive to treatment. Such patients benefit greatly from an intelligent and sensitive approach to both their medical and emotional problems. The best control of pain associated with cancer may be achieved by a local surgical procedure or by effecting a limited regression of the cancer with irradiation or chemotherapy. Bypass surgical procedures for various obstructions also may provide significant improvement in a patient's quality of life. The rate of clinical progression of the cancer and the extent of life-threatening metastases or the presence of other medical problems usually dictate the treatment course to be taken.

Patients whose cancers are not curable with currently available therapies do not always need to be treated when the cancer is first discovered. However, if the cancer is progressing and a decision to treat is made, the treatment should be vigorous, with a goal to prevent or relieve symptoms and to decrease the size of the tumor mass. This approach may be best for palliation of symptoms and also may result in prolonged, disease-free survival.

In the palliative mode, the physician's focus changes from treatment directed to the cancer to management of patients' overall medical and psychosocial problems. Symptoms may be caused by the cancer or by entirely unrelated medical problems. For example, patients with an incurable, slowly progressive cancer may suffer significant distress from an unrelated medical problem, such as bladder obstruction due to benign prostate enlargement. Not only might this offer an obstacle to future administration of effective pain medication, but surgical relief of this problem may be the one thing that can be done to relieve the symptom of most significance to such patients. Transurethral resection may be an appropriate procedure in such patients' management and should not be overlooked simply because the patient has incurable cancer.

Also important is avoiding a search for sites of metastasis that do not threaten life or function or for other diseases for which no effective treatment exists. Diagnostic evaluations pursued to prove which of two equally untreatable conditions is present are counterproductive. Patients and families often focus on the outcome of these tests and will be disappointed to find that considerable time and money have been invested in a futile search that may answer an interesting question but will not influence outcome.

TREATMENT STRATEGIES
Locoregional Treatment

Staging is directed toward identifying patients who have localized disease that can be treated with curative intent. If the primary lesion appears to be localized and suitable for curative treatment by either surgical resection or radiotherapy, treatment should begin promptly.

Optimal locoregional control of disease implies treatment of the local disease and any regional extensions that may be present. Whether the approach is surgery or irradiation, usually a margin of normal tissue is included in the treatment plan to ensure total eradication at the local site. For surgical procedures and radiotherapy ports, this approach usually means that a margin of several centimeters of grossly normal tissue is resected or irradiated in continuity. In the case of surgical resection, the pathologist can confirm that the margin of resection is clear of microscopic extension of the neoplasm. This technique is not feasible in assessing the adequacy of radiotherapy treatment ports. If the margins around the primary tumor are designed well, however, both irradiation and surgery have a reasonable chance of controlling local disease.

When regional lymph nodes are involved by cancer, similar therapeutic principles are employed in either lymphatic dissection or radiotherapy to the lymphatic bed. Anatomically, treatment of regional lymphatics is accomplished more easily in some sites (axilla or neck) than in others (intraabdominal). In some instances, surgery followed by irradiation of a wider margin of tissue offers optimal opportunity for local control or cure.

Often, strategies for locoregional treatment combine surgery and radiotherapy to preserve function and cosmetic appearance while eradicating the cancer. The use of surgery to remove the visible tumor and the use of irradiation to eliminate microscopic residual disease has been particularly successful in limb-sparing treatment of soft-tissue sarcomas and in avoiding mastectomy for breast cancer, improving cosmetic and functional outcome while providing survival rates equivalent to more extensive surgical approaches. Such combined therapy requires careful, knowledgeable cooperation between surgeons and radiation oncologists to maximize effectiveness and to minimize complications.

Systemic Treatment

Systemic chemotherapy has curative potential for some neoplastic diseases, including acute leukemia (especially in children), embryonal carcinoma of the testis, uterine choriocarcinoma, large-cell lymphoma, and Hodgkin's disease. In these and other highly responsive cancers, treatment with curative intent should begin as soon as possible after the diagnosis is established. More commonly, systemic chemotherapy and hormonal therapy have proved to be beneficial in a palliative role, in controlling symptoms, and in extending survival and disease-free survival. Adjuvant chemotherapy combined with either surgery or radiotherapy to increase both the disease-free interval and survival also has emerged as an important treatment strategy.

Oncologists know that carefully quantifying the disease is basic to the conduct of good clinical research. This process also significantly affects physicians' ability to make decisions at every step in clinical patient management. Nearly all decisions that relate to the efficacy of treatment are based on knowing the size and anatomic location of the cancer and its metastases and on quantifying the rate of either progression or regression of tumor masses or other biological measures of the activity of the disease. Therefore, the primary cancer and selected representative metastases should be measured, and these data should be recorded in patients' records. Prognosis in an individual patient is based on changes in these tumor measurements.

The choice of any patient's initial treatment plan is based on statistics derived from national studies that predict response and outcome for all patients with this stage of a particular cancer type and with similar pathologic findings, but the evaluation of the correctness of the treatment plan selected for any one patient is based on that individual's response. If the measured tumor masses progress during treatment or stop regressing despite use of the same doses of chemotherapy that previously were successful, five possible strategies may be pursued: One might (1) escalate the doses of these medications, (2) switch to another class of chemotherapy (other drugs alone or in combination), (3) employ radiotherapy, (4) use palliative surgery, (5) or discontinue treatment. Each subsequent treatment plan applied will yield a lower response rate, as predicted by studies of groups of similar patients, but the response of each patient may vary from the norm. Therefore, individualizing treatment based on the rate of regression and dose-response effect will dictate future treatment.

Numerous common cancers (e.g., lung, colon, stomach, kidney, liver) have a low rate of response to chemotherapy. The majority of patients with these diagnoses have a low probability of benefit from treatment and are likely to endure the addition of toxicity from the treatment to any symptoms that they may have from the cancer. Research in the use of biological tests that predict which patients may respond to a specific chemotherapeutic agent or regimen continues to be an important avenue in exploring ways to improve clinical decision making. These studies focus on tumor growth rate, metastatic potential, and intrinsic drug resistance. Until we can define more precisely those groups of patients who can benefit from treatment, patients with cancers that have a predictable low response to treatment with conventional chemotherapy should be enrolled in a research clinical trial.

If the therapeutic intent is not curative and the anatomic position of metastases is not life-threatening or causing local symptoms, time can be allotted for assessing disease progression before treatment begins. Some cancers are indolent and may not progress for long periods. Risk of treatment of these tumors includes not only the toxicities of the therapy but the emergence of chemotherapy-resistant populations of tumor cells. Treatment of a nonprogressive, asymptomatic cancer that cannot be cured cannot be recommended for the majority of patients.

When the cancer no longer is regressing or when toxicity, as assessed by the patient, exceeds the potential for long-term positive effect, treatment should be stopped. From the outset, patients and physicians should agree on this point: Beginning a therapeutic course does not commit patients to lifelong treatment; rather, patients can elect to stop treatment without jeopardizing their relationship with their doctor. Failure of conventional treatment may prompt some patients to embark on expensive travel from cancer center to cancer center or to seek treatment from practitioners who use alternative methods. Failure to achieve either regression of the tumor or meaningful palliation is a reason to discontinue treatment. Nonetheless, practitioners owe it to their patients to provide psychological support and to avoid the patients' perception of discontinuation of treatment as abandonment of either the patient or hope.

CLINICAL RESEARCH

If we are to make significant progress in the diagnosis and treatment of cancer, all patients should be considered as potential candidates for inclusion in a research clinical trial. Much of the progress that has been made in oncology in the last several decades has been based on carefully controlled observations in well-designed clinical trials. Not all patients either qualify for or will choose to be part of a clinical trial, but the option should be offered to all that are eligible.

Conveying to patients the concept of selecting an investigational treatment by the statistical process of randomization is particularly difficult but, in many important studies, it is the cornerstone of good design. Selection bias by either patients or doctors can influence outcome and may lead to inappropriate treatment for countless patients in the future. One reason given for the limited number of patients entered in clinical trials is the inability of both patients and treating physicians to accept the principle of random selection as a method for choosing treatments. Such a concern implies that one of them knows which treatment arm of a randomized trial actually is best. Obviously, if that is the case, carrying out the study is inappropriate, as the result already is known. If, in fact, the answer to the question posed by the study is unknown, a clinical trial is the most appropriate choice for treatment, as a state-of-the-art therapeutic course is being compared with a potentially superior (but possibly inferior) regimen. The philosophic barrier to research posed by lack of understanding of the value of clinical trials should be the subject for education for both patients and physicians.

Information about specific studies that are available

is found easily in the National Cancer Institute's PDQ listing of national clinical trial protocols or by contacting a National Cancer Institute–designated cancer center (1-800-4-CANCER). The inclusion of community-based oncologists in the research activities of cancer centers and cooperative clinical trial groups has facilitated patient access to clinical research. Practicing physicians should develop a relationship with local research facilities that have ties to these national study groups so as to be able to offer their patients this valuable treatment option.

FOLLOW-UP CARE

Follow-up may be defined as a planned checkup on a regular basis after cancer therapy has been completed. The benefits of regular checkups are many, including the following:

- The diagnosis and treatment of long-term complications of cancer treatment
- The opportunity to institute preventive strategies (e.g., diet modification or assistance with tobacco cessation).
- Screening for and early detection of a second cancer (e.g., multicentric precancerous lesions that are common in the head and neck, a second cancer in the opposite breast, a second cancer in the colon).
- The diagnosis and treatment of locally recurrent cancer. In some cases, therapy may be possible for cure and, in others, for palliation. Examples would be the recurrence of a skin cancer the cure of which is most likely, or an in-breast recurrence of cancer after breast-conserving therapy wherein resection for cure is possible.
- Screening for metastases. Although systemic metastases from most solid tumors cannot be cured, some special situations are favorable. Liver metastases from colorectal cancer are potentially resectable and result in long-term disease-free survival. Similarly, pulmonary metastasis from soft-tissue sarcomas sometimes can be resected, and prolonged survival can ensue.
- The detection of a functional or physical disability (or both), offering the opportunity to undertake corrective measures. For example, when stomal care is imperfect, proper instruction by the enterostomal therapist or a visit by another patient with a stoma or to a support group can be helpful.

In this era of managed care and cost containment, the benefits of follow-up are being reassessed and studied. How frequently a patient is seen by nurse or doctor and which tests are performed have a direct bearing on cost. If early testing and frequent visits can be translated into better survival, fewer symptoms, or less severe complications, a close follow-up plan is justified. In many instances, little evidence suggests that early treatment of a recurrence affects any of these outcomes. Nonetheless, extending the time between follow-up visits and limiting the tests performed may diminish the potential for achieving the benefits listed and also may have detrimental psychological effects on patients and a negative impact on the doctor-patient relationship.

A single physician should assume responsibility for follow-up care. In many cases, patients will receive two or more therapeutic modalities, and multiple physicians will want to follow up such patients. In far too many situations, however, patients receive no continuity of care. In some cases, patients live a substantial distance from the specialized cancer center where treatment was performed, and so the primary-care physician must carry out the follow-up function and be the common pathway for information and follow-up strategies.

Recurrences may be locoregional, disseminated, or both. The most important predictors of recurrent cancer are stage at the time of initial therapy and histologic findings. The mode of detection of recurrence may be by physical examination or such tests as roentgenography, computed tomographic scans, bone scans, ultrasonography, biological markers, and the like. A workup for recurrent cancer may detect a second cancer in a paired organ or in a residual organ, such as the colon.

When a new mass is detected in patients who were treated for cure or in patients who have experienced a stable remission but whose clinical status seems to be deteriorating, an important factor is to establish by biopsy that the cancer that was originally treated successfully has actually relapsed. Other, more treatable causes of clinical deterioration should be considered. Infection, tissue necrosis, cancer-related metabolic abnormalities, and diseases unrelated to the cancer variously can cause symptoms of generalized weakness, pain, disorientation, and other signs that can be misinterpreted as cancer progression. For example, hypercalcemia can mimic brain metastases or bowel obstruction. Anemia arising from a benign duodenal ulcer can mimic bone marrow infiltration. Some cancers produce metabolically active polypeptides that mimic organ dysfunction. A second primary cancer, some of which may be curable or more responsive to treatment than the original disease, can be interpreted incorrectly as a metastasis. A disciplined search for these alternatives to the more common diagnosis of recurrent cancer always should be considered.

REHABILITATION

In cancer rehabilitation, the medical care team is concerned with the physical, social, and emotional needs of patients and their families. Modern cancer rehabilitation should be available and offered to all. It often is needed over months or years, starting at the time of cancer diagnosis. A team effort is required, with collaboration among patients, families, and health professionals.

Most patients cope well; others manage poorly or not at all. The inability to cope may reflect a lifelong pattern or can be related acutely to the diagnosis or its prognosis. Psychological and emotional barriers may result in a failure to comply with treatment or to tolerate its side effects and may lead to inappropriate behavior within the family or rejection by fellow employees or by management on return to work. A good support system is critical to getting patients through this crisis.

The success of helping patients and families to cope with cancer has improved dramatically in the last two decades. Quality of life during and after treatment now is a major concern. Complex social problems may surface and can involve such diverse issues as loss of body function; disruption of family and other significant relationships; financial security; employment and insurance; psychological implications related to cancer and its treatment; and problems that relate to coexisting medical conditions. Patterns of cancer care are changing rapidly, with a shift of treatment delivery from the hospital to the outpatient setting and home care and with the expanded use of support groups and hospice.

Not every patient will require the services of a rehabilitation team because personal needs, desires, and resources vary. Nonetheless, physicians should be alert to the potential need for services. Emphasis should be placed on the facts that the need for rehabilitative care does not cease when patients leave the hospital and that coordination for continuing care is essential before a patient's discharge.

A physiatrist may be required to assist in the strengthening of muscles, in the use of artificial limbs, and in retraining for activities of daily living. A pharmacist may be needed to help in pain management and the use of patient-controlled analgesia pumps. Oncology nurses can provide psychosocial support and a variety of educational programs for patients before, during, and after treatment. They also play a major role in at-home care and rehabilitation and assist patients and family members to deal with the many psychosocial issues involved in cancer.

A physical therapist should be involved from the outset in the care of some patients. For example, patients with breast cancer often need some assistance with arm exercises, whether the treatment is primarily surgical or radiotherapeutic. Often, physical therapy can be instituted before primary treatment of the cancer actually is begun.

Social workers are important in a total rehabilitation effort and can help in planning personal and family activities, in identifying and using community resources, and in finding appropriate vocational counselors. Social workers often are called on to provide emotional support and guidance. In addition, a member of the clergy or a lay volunteer also may be helpful in providing assistance and advice in both personal and religious matters. Psychologists and other mental health professionals may be called in for help with the stress and emotional problems that are so common among cancer patients and their families.

Home health care agencies and services are available in most communities. For patients with advanced cancer, hospices provide invaluable services. Such services include pain management and supportive care in an institutional setting and at home.

BEYOND DIAGNOSIS AND TREATMENT
Communication Between Doctor and Patient

For cancer patients, one of the most disturbing aspects of cancer is fear of the unknown. Primary physicians involved in coordinating the diagnostic and evaluation phase cannot afford to delay communications to affected patients until all the facts regarding diagnosis and treatment are known. This precaution may be unsettling, but it is not nearly as frightening as the absence of any information. To feel comfortable with the process, patients must understand both the reasons for the specific diagnostic tests and the treatment options available once a more definitive diagnosis is established. In general, repeated and continued counseling throughout the evaluation and treatment-planning process is reassuring, rather than frightening, to the patient; confidence in the doctor is established; and patients become effective participants in the management team.

Over the years, there has been a healthy and appropriate shift away from the philosophy of hiding the facts of cancer. The diagnosis, treatment implications, and survival potential have practical implications to the patient beyond any that may be perceived immediately by the doctor. What are the patient's plans? Is the patient preparing to assume long-term business debt, to get married, or to become pregnant? The estimated prognosis of survival and the expectation, timing, and severity of symptoms from either the cancer or the treatment are vitally important to patients, though often doctors may find predicting them difficult.

To carry out an effective discussion of treatment, physicians, patients, and affected families must have a clear understanding of the clinical situation, an estimate of what can be accomplished, and some idea of the costs of the proposed actions. The role of physicians is to assess the clinical goals, the limitations of various approaches, and the potential outcomes; to present them to patients clearly; and to make a recommendation for action. Physicians need to allot sufficient time for this process to allow patients and their families to ask questions.

The most difficult issue to discuss with patients is their expectation for survival. Published statistical survival information is based on an analysis of all patients with a specific diagnosis and stage of disease and may not predict the outcome for particular patients. Usually, accurate subsets of data that relate to clinical stage, distribution of metastases, histologic grade of the cancer, and other newer methods of predicting outcome are not available. In addition, few of the published data take into consideration variations in rate of tumor growth or response to treatment.

One needs to assess what factors are important to individual patients and how much risk they are prepared to take to extend life. How can symptom-free survival be maximized, and can the benefit after intense treatment be translated into a prolonged period of quality life after the treatment has been concluded? Patients may question the value of a few additional months of life if this is accompanied by progressive pain from the cancer or by debilitating symptoms resulting from treatment.

Patients will make the ultimate decision regarding treatment options, and physicians must be prepared to accept the possibility that patients' decisions may not be those proposed by the doctor. If physicians see patients' decisions as not in their best interests, physicians should try to persuade without becoming confrontational. Each of us makes decisions that affect our lives, our careers, and important events in our lives differently. A slim chance for success may be embraced by one person and rejected by another. This fact argues for as full a disclosure as possible. Fear of hospitalization, surgery, irradiation, or chemotherapy may cause patients to choose a plan that will result in shorter survival but less toxicity. Doctors do, however, have a responsibility not to follow through with a program if they think that a patient's decision will not result in a good outcome, and it may be necessary to assist such a patient in finding a replacement doctor to direct his or her care. Establishing patients' confidence in the treatment team will be absolutely necessary for the days and weeks of treatment that lie ahead once the treatment program has begun.

Assessment of Impact on the Family

In the early phase of evaluation of patients and, subsequently, as the dynamics of the diagnosis and treatment evolve, doctors, nurses, and other members of the treatment team should be aware of a patient's occupational and family responsibilities. What will happen if the patient is admitted to the hospital, becomes ill with the acute effects of surgery, irradiation, or chemotherapy, or experiences progression of the disease? Who will care for the family, who cooks the meals, and from where does the family income come? Such issues require assessment at the outset. They help to explain why patients may make some choices and not others, and why a specific treatment option may be selected. Many community and personal support resources exist to serve these needs. These services are accessible and promoted by the American Cancer Society through the National Cancer Information Center (800-ACS-2345) and through the National Cancer Institute via its Cancer Information Service telephone response program (1-800-4-CANCER).

Financial Implications

Not the least of the problems facing patients with cancer is the fact that most of the services that the medical care system has to offer are expensive. Although the hospital or other treating facility will collect personal and financial information as part of the process of admission to the facility, doctors must be aware of the current and changing financial status of their patients. What will be the cost of treatment above that covered by insurance? Will the proposed diagnosis and treatment plan change the financial stability of the family and potentially lower their standard of living forever? If physicians understand the facts and the dynamics of the situation, they are in a better position to offer strong patient and family support.

CONCLUSION

We have outlined a philosophy of cancer management from the perspective of physicians who are primarily responsible for the patient. Details of specific strategies of care are developed more fully by the authors of chapters that follow. We emphasize that clinicians' approach to patients who have or are suspected of having cancer should not differ from the organized approach used to analyze other clinical problems. The doctor-patient relationship must be established with an honest but optimistic discussion of treatment alternatives to ensure an environment of confidence and trust.

A multidisciplinary medical team should be involved with planning from the outset; however, a single physician should serve as the patient's primary contact and be available to discuss, explain, and lead. Also critical is that discussions and diagnostic evaluation lead to a coordinated plan. The tumor board format can facilitate this process, and all hospitals should try to establish

themselves as approved by the American College of Surgeons Commission on Cancer Programs. To follow the plan, physicians should gather and record in the chart as much information as possible about the cancer to be able to evaluate treatment progress or progression of the disease and to be prepared to shift course as circumstances dictate.

Primary physicians should be acquainted with the availability of consultants, cancer centers, and national databases, and the opportunities available to patients to participate in clinical research.

Finally, modern oncology emphasizes treatment of the entire patient, always keeping rehabilitation and prompt return to activities of daily living in the forefront of thinking. Although many cancers can be cured, much can be done for all patients with this disease, regardless of outcome.

Reference

1. Fleming ID, Cooper JS, Henson DE, et al. (eds). *AJCC Cancer Staging Manual* (5th ed). Philadelphia: Lippincott-Raven, 1997:83–90.

8

Basis for Current Major Therapies for Cancer

A. Introduction

■ ■ ■

THEODORE E. YAEGER
LUTHER W. BRADY

Over the last 100 years, cancer therapy research has nurtured the development of a recognized number of primary treatment options. The growth of surgery and radiotherapy to treat local and locoregional disease has been followed by increasingly effective systemic chemotherapy. Although these disciplines initially were viewed as independent arms in the war on cancer, their complementary natures now are being appreciated. Surgery, radiotherapy, and chemotherapy form the basic foundation for treating cancer patients, but important new modalities, including immunotherapy, are joining an expanding armamentarium of tools for cancer diagnosis, therapy, and support. This chapter provides a detailed review of the four current major therapies for treating cancer: the development, implementation, and integration of surgery, radiotherapy, chemotherapy, and immunotherapy are presented.

After the advent of anesthesia and prior to 1920, the mainstay of cancer therapy was surgical intervention. The evolution of radiotherapy and radium placement likewise remained under the influence of surgeons. Much as with surgery, irradiation was thought to be used best by the use of ablative doses (i.e., destruction of the tumorous area and normal surrounding tissue, followed by a surgical repair if possible) [1]. Patients presenting with metastatic disease could be treated only with supportive care and the generous use of morphine, when available [2].

From the 1920s to the 1940s, tremendous progress was made in both surgery and radiotherapy. The contributions from pioneers of both fields were being used and improved widely. Dr. William Stewart Halsted's concept of a radical resection quadrupled the cures of breast cancer [3]. The use of fractionated irradiation, as developed mainly by the Curie Institute, led to the birth of clinical radiotherapy and its ability to cure even those patients whose cancers were considered inoperable [4]. In 1934, therapeutic radiology became a specialty certification from the American Board of Radiology [5]. Still, patients with metastases mostly could hope only for comfort, as little advance had been made in the management of metastatic diseases except for early attempts at palliative therapeutic interventions [6].

From the 1940s to the 1960s, radiotherapy made significant advances, owing to improvements in the technology available for treatment. High-energy gamma sources and, ultimately, linear accelerators were introduced into clinical practice. The American Society for Therapeutic Radiology and Oncology began in 1959 with 111 active members and has grown to today's 5,493. Radiobiology and irradiation physics were developing standards that would allow reproducible treatment results in a variety of cancers [7]. High cure rates for advanced Hodgkin's disease were being reported [8–10]. Antisepsis and antibiotics made surgery ever more possible, and classic surgical interventions were being modified with good results. Better anesthesia and modern blood banking allowed more prolonged surgical times, and extended explorations became the rule [11]. Metastatic cancer symptoms were being treated using improved opioids and more effective radiotherapy. However, not much progress had been achieved for patients developing or presenting with metastases [12].

From the early 1960s to the present, great advances have been made in virtually every field of cancer treatment. Chemotherapy became a reliable and effective intervention, surgery now focuses on less radical, organ-sparing procedures whenever possible, and irradiation techniques have developed as an alternative for conservation of normal organs and function in almost every major cancer site. Additionally, bone marrow transplantation to allow ablative chemotherapy has become practical [13–15]. Diagnostic radiology now plays a significant role in the staging processes.

The diagnosis of cancer has become precise without the use of debilitating invasive procedures. Equally important, computed axial tomography followed by magnetic resonance imaging and sophisticated nuclear medicine technology [16] has opened new possibilities for staging options and accurate follow-up. Palliative treatments [17] and supportive care, spearheaded by national hospice groups, provide state-of-the-art terminal care and bereavement support for affected patients and their loved ones.

Most recently, oncologists have enjoyed a new collaboration with specialists from all the major disciplines; these specialists are working cooperatively to treat many cancers. Conservation surgery, in conjunction with irradiation and chemotherapy, allows cancer patients an ever-higher cure rate and greater potential to lead normal lives with intact bodies [18]. Now, even patients with metastatic disease can experience prolonged remissions with the use of combined systemic therapies. Pain control as a specific multimodality discipline has become part of the oncology armamentarium [19]. Administration of biological agents now can support cancer patients' hematologic reserves to allow continued tolerance of high-dose therapy [20]. Three-dimensional computed simulation [21] is helping us to discover new horizons in radiotherapy. Manipulation of the basic biological processes through immunotherapy and gene-based strategies also has opened new vistas of creative treatment.

New concepts and applications are being revealed in rapid succession to expand the frontiers of cancer therapy. Each of the following major sections of this chapter presents the mechanisms used in each major treatment modality—surgery, radiotherapy, chemotherapy, and immunotherapy—and explains the rationale of their past and present applications and potential developments for the near future.

B. Surgical Therapy

■ ■ ■

IRVIN D. FLEMING

BACKGROUND

Prior to the nineteenth century, cancer generally was considered to be a systemic disorder; thus, remedies were systemic. An example of this tendency was that described by Galen of Pargamum (approximately 130–200 AD). Galen proposed that cancer was caused by an excess of "black bile" and recommended such remedies as bleeding, purging, and dietary restrictions [22]. John Abernethy [23], an English surgeon and anatomist (1814), was one of the early investigators to consider

Table 8.1 Changing Role of Surgery in Cancer Treatment

Before 1850	Early heroic attempts to resect cancer
1850–1950	Development of standard surgical techniques for resection
1950–1960	Extended radical surgical procedures
1960–1980	Exploration of combined-modality treatment
1980–2000	Improved organ preservation and survival with combination therapy with surgical resection

that malignant tumors could be a local phenomenon and thus proposed the possibilities of treatment by surgical resection. Through the nineteenth century, isolated reports mentioned surgical resection for cancer. These attempts were considered heroic and rarely were associated with long-term cure (Table 8.1).

With the advent of general anesthesia in 1846 [24] and antisepsis in 1867 [25], pioneer surgeons attempted resection of malignant tumors in a variety of sites. Reports cited successful surgical resection of cancer in such sites as breast [26], stomach [27], colon, and ovary [28]. In 1894, William Stewart Halstead [29] published his classic results demonstrating the advantage of radical resection of breast cancer incorporating radical resection of the breast with regional lymph nodes. The radical resection was associated with superior local control and improved three-year survival when compared with previous surgical attempts with local excision of breast tumors. The procedure demonstrated that improved survival could be achieved by the more radical surgery [29].

Improved surgical technical ability, along with better anesthesia, safe blood transfusions, and other supportive measures, ushered in an era of routine resection of cancer in most common sites. In the 1950s, more radical resections were attempted to improve survival. Eventually, these attempts led to a point at which increasingly radical surgical procedures did not produce increasing cure rates but began to be associated with increasing morbidity and a negative impact on quality of life. The problem was simply that more radical surgery could not control metastatic disease effectively in other anatomic sites. Other options were explored, such as combining surgical resection with other forms of cancer therapy. With the development of effective radiotherapy came attempts to increase local control by applying preoperative or postoperative radiotherapy. The focus was use of combination therapy to increase organ sparing and the preservation of anatomic function in such neoplasms as

breast cancer, extremity sarcoma, laryngeal cancer, and rectal cancer, all without decreasing survival. In some areas, these efforts were successful; in others, the combined therapy had minimal impact on local control or overall cure.

The discovery and use of antitumor chemotherapeutic agents for advanced cancer led to the logical development of strategies to use chemotherapy in combination with surgical resection or irradiation (or both) to reduce the incidence of local recurrence and distant metastasis, thereby improving survival. Such combinations of adjuvant therapy have been developed and now are being used effectively in a number of cancer sites, including head and neck, breast, colorectal region, ovaries, and lung (small-cell cancers). Currently, many examples demonstrate success derived from using combined therapy by reducing morbidity with increased local control and survival. One such example is breast conservation surgery. Women presenting with small breast carcinomas (stages I and II) can be treated effectively with complete local resection, axillary lymph node dissection, and breast irradiation with results that equal that of a radical mastectomy [30]. Also, when appropriate, the risk of subsequent metastasis can be reduced by adjuvant systemic chemotherapy. This procedure achieves cure rates equal to those of mastectomy using breast preservation surgery in combination with irradiation and chemotherapy [31].

Other examples include anal sphincter preservation for anal carcinoma. The major morbidity of anal carcinoma was resection of the anal sphincter, with resulting permanent colostomy. Historically, this procedure produced a cure rate of 20–30%. Use of combined chemotherapy and irradiation has increased the survival rate for anal carcinoma patients to 75%, with preservation of anal continence in the majority of patients [32].

Historically, major sarcomas of bone and soft tissues were treated by radical surgical resection that usually required a major limb amputation. Through use of a combination of complete en bloc resection of the tumor, radiotherapy, and chemotherapy, the amputation rate has been reduced to less than 15% without decrease in local control or survival [33].

Combination therapy now has been proved to increase survival in a number of pediatric malignancies, including Wilms' tumor, neuroblastoma, rhabdomyosarcoma, and osteogenic sarcomas [34]. Currently, many ongoing clinical research protocols seek to determine the most effective combinations of surgical resection, radiotherapy, and chemotherapy along with other treatment modalities for the cure of childhood malignancies and at the same time seek to reduce the long-term side effects of therapy.

DIAGNOSIS

Historically, the management of a malignant tumor began with surgical resection, and other treatment (e.g., radiotherapy or chemotherapy) was added after the surgery. However, with many effective new forms of combination therapies, the diagnosis and stage may be established first, followed by other treatment and subsequent surgical resection. The goal of initial biopsy and evaluation is to obtain sufficient tissue and information to diagnose and stage a cancer and then to begin therapy. Biopsy can be accomplished by fine-needle aspiration, large-core needle biopsy, or open surgical biopsy. In certain situations, the histologic diagnosis is established by resection of the tumor itself (e.g., gastrointestinal neoplasms). However, with more effective preresection diagnostic capabilities, such as endoscopy and fine-needle biopsy, definitive resection often is undertaken with a well-established pathologic diagnosis. If a suspected neoplasm is to be treated by any modality other than surgical resection (i.e., radiotherapy or chemotherapy), an essential factor is to establish an accurate histologic diagnosis and stage prior to beginning treatment. Also, sufficient biopsy material must be obtained prior to treatment to allow for assessment of tumor biological markers, special immunohistochemical staining, and genetic studies of the tumor, as these factors may influence treatment and prognosis.

CLINICAL AND PATHOLOGIC STAGING

After a diagnosis of cancer has been made, effective treatment cannot be planned without knowledge of the extent of tumor spread. Essential elements in evaluating the extent of the cancer stage are (1) size and extent of the primary tumor (T); (2) extent of regional spread in lymph nodes (N); and (3) evidence of distant metastatic spread (M). Using this TNM classification, the American Joint Committee on Cancer, in cooperation with the Union Internationale Contre le Cancer, established staging criteria for common cancer sites [35]. This effort was undertaken to ensure that a single system of staging is used worldwide. This common staging system allows physicians to plan treatment and to compare end results of therapy throughout the world.

Often, modern cancer treatment calls for combina-

tion therapy, especially for high-risk tumors that may not respond completely to a single treatment modality. Treatment protocols, including surgery, radiotherapy, and chemotherapy, usually are directed by the type of cancer (histologic classification) and stage of the tumor to be treated. In summary, accurate staging is essential to planning effective therapy, conducting clinical trials, and evaluating end results.

Cancer staging embodies two categories. The clinical stage is determined by clinical evaluation of the tumor supplemented by information from appropriate diagnostic studies. The pathologic stage is determined by study of the removed tumor, other removed tissue, or biopsies. (A classic example would be the number of positive axillary lymph nodes removed with a modified radical mastectomy for breast cancer.) Every physician and treatment facility undertaking the management of patients with malignant neoplasms should evaluate the end results of treatment on the basis of the stage of disease at diagnosis. This evaluation is accomplished by accurate staging and use of a database (tumor registry) with patient follow-up. Evaluation of the end results of cancer treatment can be meaningful only with long-term follow-up.

SURGICAL RESECTION

Currently, in 90% of patients in whom solid malignant tumors are cured, the cure is achieved by surgical resection alone or in combination with other modalities (Table 8.2). The role of a surgeon is to remove the malignant tumor completely with an appropriate margin of normal tissue. The extent of the required surgical margins varies with the type and location of the tumor. Visceral organs involved with cancer (e.g., esophagus, stomach, pancreas, colon) require sufficient margins of resection to ensure complete tumor resection while minimizing changes in the physiologic status of a patient. On evidence of high risk of regional lymphatic spread, the regional lymph nodes usually are resected along with the primary tumor (e.g., axillary node dissection for breast carcinoma, mesenteric resection for bowel cancer). The removal of clinically involved lymph nodes is termed *therapeutic lymph node dissection*.

However, in the event of a known risk of lymph node spread without clinical evidence of tumor involvement, the term *prophylactic lymph node dissection* is used. On some occasions, lymph node dissections are performed in discontinuity with the primary tumor resection, as in the case of malignant melanoma of the trunk or extremity with lymph node involvement. In recent

Table 8.2 Common Cancer Sites Requiring Surgical
Resection as an Essential Component of Curative Therapy

Site	*Survival*	
	Local (%)	All Stages (%)
Breast	96	85
Colon and Rectum	90	61
Melanoma (skin)	95	88
Kidney	88	60
Ovary	95	50
Endometrium (uterus)	95	84
Liver	15	5
Pancreas	18	4
Lung	49	14

Source: Data from *Cancer Facts and Figures 2000.* Atlanta: American
Cancer Society, 2000:14.

years, considerable interest and research have been
devoted to determining whether removing a sentinel
node, identified to be the node most likely to be affected
first by tumor spread, has merit as an indicator of lymph
node spread. The sentinel node is identified by lymphoscintigraphy with radionuclide or vital dye.

Lymph node mapping is used to identify the pattern
of spread from the primary tumor site. Then the sentinel node is removed and studied for evidence of metastasis. This approach is being evaluated in a variety of
tumor sites, such as melanoma and breast cancer. The
information from such sentinel node excisions is being
used to determine the impact of tumor involvement of
the sentinel node on prognosis and the ways that the
findings should influence the type of surgery and other
treatment [36].

At one time, researchers believed that as more extensive surgical resection was feasible, improved cure
rates would follow. However, this anticipated result has
not always proved to be true. The chief cause of failure
in the surgical treatment of many cancers is distant
spread of disease. In recent years, the trend has been
toward complete but less radical surgical resection of
the tumor in combination with radiotherapy, systemic
chemotherapy, or both.

Classic examples of this approach are seen in breast
conservation surgery that combines surgery with radiotherapy and in the treatment of sarcoma of soft tissue
or bone that attempts to avoid amputation by using
combination therapy [33]. Despite great strides made
with combination therapy, few carcinomas and sarcomas are cured today without some form of surgical removal of a primary tumor (see Table 8.2).

Palliative Surgical Procedures

On many occasions, patients may present at the time of
initial diagnosis with a primary carcinoma that is surgically nonresectable or that already has metastasized.
Such advanced tumors may be associated with increasing symptoms, such as intestinal obstruction, pain, or
bleeding. Frequently, these symptoms require surgery
for effective palliation even though the cancer cannot
be cured. Management of a cancer obstruction or a
bleeding lesion by intestinal bypass or resection has
been shown to enhance affected patients' quality of life
and to improve the clinical situation to allow other
measures of cancer treatment to be used. Considerable
clinical judgment is needed to determine how aggressive the palliative surgical management approach
should be [37].

Resection of Visceral Metastasis

In some clinical settings, resection of isolated visceral
metastasis of certain tumors is associated with long-
term disease-free control and possibly a cure. Surgical
resection of visceral metastasis requires consideration of
the following important factors: (1) type of primary tumor, (2) interval between primary diagnosis and metastasis, (3) number and location of the metastases, (4)
technical feasibility of a clear margin of resection, (5)
performance status of affected patients, and (6) ability
to treat such patients further with additional antitumor
therapies. Tumors presenting with isolated pulmonary
metastasis that might be considered for surgical resection include Wilms' tumor, osteogenic sarcoma, soft-
tissue sarcomas and, occasionally, colorectal carcinoma
[38]. Likewise, some tumors presenting with isolated
liver metastasis that might be controlled by resection include colorectal cancer and carcinoid tumors [39].

Surgical Support for Patients Receiving
Other Therapies

Aggressive systemic chemotherapy or modern radiotherapy requires considerable support to manage such
complications as poor nutrition, neutropenia, sepsis,
and opportunistic infections. Many current chemotherapeutic agents cause severe toxicity and local tissue
slough if extravasated from intravenous (IV) injection.
The need for frequent blood sampling and IV drug administration requires a reliable venous access. Likewise,
if patients are to complete their therapy successfully,

long-term nutritional support via the parenteral or enteric route can be accomplished by a long-standing venous line inserted in a central vein (e.g., the superior vena cava) and brought through the skin by way of a subcutaneous tunnel to avoid infection. The alternative is a central venous catheter attached to a subcutaneous injectable port, which can be accessed by needle either for administration of chemotherapy or for obtaining venous blood samples. With proper placement and care, the lines and ports can be used for months or years if necessary.

Both chemotherapy and head and neck radiotherapy are associated with oral stomatitis, ulceration, and severe nutritional problems. Occasionally, supplemental alimentation via the gastrointestinal tract or total parenteral nutrition is required in patients receiving antineoplastic therapy. Another clinical management problem requiring surgical support is removal of pleural fluid or ascites for symptomatic relief or for diagnosis.

POSTTREATMENT EVALUATION OF TUMOR STATUS

Occasionally in the clinical setting, a tumor site must be reevaluated subsequent to treatment to plan further therapy or to determine whether to discontinue therapy. Re-exploration with appropriate biopsy or other techniques may be necessary. Results of diagnostic imaging, such as computed tomography, may have to be clarified further before subsequent therapy can be selected. Also, some cases of local recurrent or residual tumors can be managed successfully by surgical resection with the hope of long-term control or cure.

LONG-TERM COMPLICATIONS OF CANCER TREATMENT

Now that an increasing number of cancer patients are being cured, delayed complications of tumors or of tumor treatment are being recognized. Occasionally, irradiation of the abdomen is associated with such bowel complications as intestinal strictures, malabsorption, and fistula formation. These complications may occur up to 10 years after treatment [40]. Second primary malignant tumors are seen with increasing frequency in patients treated with both irradiation and chemotherapy. Young women who are long-term survivors of Hodgkin's disease are reported to experience a remarkable increase in the incidence of breast cancer [41]. Thyroid deficiency and thyroid neoplasm have pre-

sented in 10–30% of patients irradiated in the head and neck [42]. These problems challenge involved surgeons and those who see cancer patients in long-term follow-up to be alert to the increased risk of cancer recurrence, new primary tumors, and delayed treatment complications.

REHABILITATION AND SUPPORT

At present, some 50–60% of all patients in whom cancer is diagnosed either are cured or achieve long-term control of their disease. "Cured" cancer patients have unique problems requiring both physician and community support. Many rehabilitation concerns have been addressed by such organizations as the American Cancer Society. The Society has sponsored numerous programs, including the Reach to Recovery Program for patients treated for breast cancer, the Ostomy Support Programs for colostomy and enterostomy patients, the Lost Cord Program for laryngectomy patients, and self-help programs for cancer survivors and their families. Physicians caring for cancer patients should be aware of such programs and should encourage patient participation. Surgeons and others in the treatment team also should play an active role in the development and maintenance of community rehabilitation programs.

Because approximately 35% of cancer patients will present at some time with nonresectable, recurrent, or metastatic cancer, treating physicians must be knowledgeable about palliation and symptom relief for advanced cancer. Pain, nausea, anorexia, insomnia, problems of infection, and bleeding are some symptoms associated with advanced cancer. Also, depression, anxiety, exhaustion, and frustration are frequently encountered by both cancer patients and their families. Often, these problems tax the ability of attending physicians, but physicians' ability to address such issues effectively in a caring and compassionate manner is the true art of medicine.

PARTICIPATION IN CLINICAL TRIALS

New methods of cancer treatment are the outgrowth of basic and clinical research. All new methods of cancer treatment must be tested through controlled clinical trials. Although certain active studies of cancer treatment are open for accrual for virtually all major cancer sites, fewer than 4% of adult cancer patients presently are entered in clinical trials [43]. In many of these clinical cancer research studies, the surgical resection of tumor in combination with other forms of therapy is the basis for all new approaches to cancer treatment.

Surgeons have three clearly defined roles in the area of clinical trials: first, participation in the development of good clinical research trials that incorporate surgical resection with other modes of therapy; second, monitoring the quality of surgical resection in these studies, as poor surgical resection may be more of a factor in a poor outcome than is the type of adjuvant therapy; and third—and most important—referring appropriate patients into clinical trials. Today, many cancer clinical trials are performed in a community hospital setting. Some researchers have pointed out that approximately half of clinical research protocols of cooperative group studies now are being conducted in community hospital oncology programs [44].

HOSPITAL CANCER PROGRAMS

More than 1,500 hospitals in the United States have in place a cancer program that is surveyed and approved by the Commission on Cancer of the American College of Surgeons. These voluntary programs on the part of the hospital are designed to upgrade the care of cancer patients. Hospitals with American Cancer Society–approved cancer programs treat more than 75% of cancer patients in this country. The elements of an effective, approved hospital cancer program include an active cancer committee and a database (tumor registry) that accesses all cancer patients, provides for cancer staging, and maintains long-term follow-up. In addition, these cancer programs have sponsored ongoing cancer educational components, tumor conferences for presentations and discussion of cancer cases, and in-depth patient treatment evaluation of selected cancer sites. Another aspect of hospital cancer programs is the promotion of community cancer control activities through public and professional education and community cancer-screening activities. Surgeons interested in good cancer care should support the development of such programs and should participate actively in community cancer prevention and early detection activities.

SURGICAL ONCOLOGISTS

The vast majority of surgical procedures in cancer patients are performed by well-trained general surgeons experienced in treating cancer, working with other on-cologists specialized in the treatment of the more common cancer sites. The subspecialty of surgical oncology embraces surgeons who, on completion of general surgical training, have obtained additional training and experience in a university surgical oncology training program or a major cancer center and have made a career commitment to the surgical treatment of cancer. Surgical oncologists have developed expertise in the management of less common cancers at unusual sites. Usually, they are experienced in resection of head and neck cancer, pelvic tumors, and unusual bone and soft-tissue tumors. The training of surgical oncologists includes an in-depth knowledge of other nonsurgical cancer treatment modalities and is designed to encourage the most effective combination of treatment. Surgical oncologists are a resource for community surgeons in dealing with unusual or complicated neoplasms. Usually, such specialists are active in professional cancer education programs and in the development of cancer treatment protocols and other cancer control activities.

CONCLUSION

The role of surgeons in modern cancer management has continued to evolve from heroic and radical operations to remove extensive tumors to an integrated approach combining a variety of cancer treatment modalities: surgery, radiotherapy, and chemotherapy. Of course, the best opportunity for cure is sought while reducing associated morbidity and mortality. The real key to reducing mortality from cancer lies in prevention and early detection. Involved surgeons should be active participants in these and other cancer control efforts to reduce morbidity and mortality from cancer.

C. Radiotherapy

■ ■ ■

GLENN B. MIESZKALSKI
LUTHER W. BRADY
THEODORE E. YAEGER
REINER CLASS

X-rays were first described in 1895 by Roentgen [45], and the Curies reported their discovery of radium approximately three years later [46]. The biological effects of this ionizing radiation soon were realized, and they

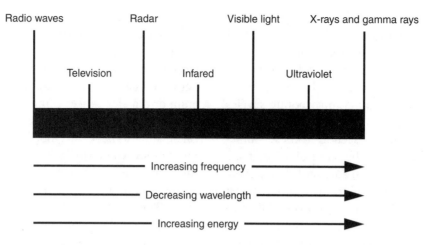

Figure 8.1 The electromagnetic spectrum comprises visible light, radio waves, radiant heat (infrared), x-rays, and gamma rays. X-rays and gamma rays have shorter wavelengths and, thus, higher energies. This higher energy enables them to break chemical bonds and produce biological damage.

were used promptly to treat a variety of malignant and nonmalignant conditions. During the next decades, technologic advances accumulated rapidly. By 1922, 200-kV x-rays were available for treating patients.

Clinical evidence regarding the effects of ionizing radiation on both normal tissue and malignant tumors also accumulated rapidly. At the 1922 International Congress of Oncology in Paris, Coutard [47] presented evidence that advanced laryngeal cancer could be cured by protracted, fractionated radiotherapy without disastrous, treatment-induced sequelae. This event marked the beginning of clinical radiotherapy as a medical discipline.

By 1934, Coutard [48] had developed a protracted, fractionated scheme that remains the foundation of radiotherapy today. The scheme was based largely on clinical observations, since basic radiobiologic knowledge was lacking. The science of radiobiology advanced slowly during the first half of the twentieth century. It was not until the mid-1950s that in vivo and in vitro assays for mammalian cells, both neoplastic and normal, were developed. This advance permitted the quantitation of irradiation effect by counting surviving cells [49–51]. During the next three decades, radiobiologic science experienced a period of exponential growth. Experiments using cultured mammalian cells led to a wealth of knowledge of the means by which irradiation produces biological injury and the factors that might modify this response. These observations substantiated the basis of modern irradiation biology.

PHYSICAL BASIS OF RADIOTHERAPY

Ionizing radiation used in radiotherapy includes both electromagnetic "waves" and particulate radiation. Comprehension of the biological effects of such radiation is necessary for a basic understanding of what this radiation is, how it is produced, and how it reacts with tissue. Electromagnetic waves are part of a broad spectrum that includes radio waves, microwaves, visible light, x-rays, and gamma rays (Fig. 8.1). In radiotherapy, x-rays and gamma rays are used. These two types of radiation possess the same general properties, differing only in their source and energy. X-rays are produced when energetic, charged particles (usually electrons) impinge on a target and react with either atomic nuclei or orbital electrons. Gamma rays are produced during the decay of an unstable nucleus in a radioactive element. In quantum physics, x-rays and gamma rays may be represented conveniently as particles called *photons*. The energy of a photon (E) is determined using the relationship $E = h\nu$, where h is the constant of proportionality known as *Planck's constant* and ν is the frequency of the wave. Substituting for the frequency, this equation becomes $E = hc/\lambda$, where c is the speed of light and λ is the wavelength.

Particulate radiation includes electrons, protons, neutrons, alpha particles, negative pi-mesons, and heavy ions. Due to cost and size constraints, heavy-particle radiation research is conducted at a limited number of institutions. Currently, only electrons are commonly used in radiotherapy.

Radiation may be directly or indirectly ionizing; charged particles are *directly ionizing:* If they have sufficient energy, they may directly disrupt the atomic or molecular structure of the material through which they pass and produce chemical and biological changes. Electromagnetic radiation and neutrons are *indirectly ionizing:* When they are absorbed in tissue, they give up their energy to produce fast-moving charged particles that then inflict the damage. In the case of electromagnetic radiation, fast-recoil electrons are produced. Neutrons give up their energy to yield fast-recoil protons, alpha particles, and heavier nuclear fragments.

In tissue, gamma rays and x-rays may interact in several ways, including coherent scattering, photoelectric effect, Compton effect, pair production, and photodisintegration. The dominant reaction will vary with the energy of the radiation in use. At the energies commonly used in radiotherapy, the dominant reaction is the Compton effect, in which a photon interacts with a loosely bound orbital electron (Fig. 8.2). Part of the energy of the incident photon is transferred to the electron as kinetic energy. This Compton electron then may interact with other electrons in the surrounding tissue. The remaining energy is carried away by another photon, which is less energetic than the original photon. The probability of Compton interactions essentially is independent of the atomic number of the target tissue, depending rather on the electron density of the target tissue. Thus, the amount of radiation absorbed is roughly the same whether the target is bone or soft tissue. In contrast, diagnostic x-rays are of lower energy and react predominantly by the photoelectric effect. The photoelectric effect is highly dependent on atomic number; therefore, bone and soft tissue appear fairly different on a diagnostic x-ray film.

Protons, neutrons, and other heavy particles interact with the nucleus of an atom rather than with the orbital electrons. Heavy particles dislodge various lower-energy showers of densely ionizing protons, neutrons, and others and deposit a large amount of energy over a short distance. This is the concept of linear energy transfer (LET), which depends on the type of radiation used. Photons and electrons have a low rate of energy transfer (low LET). Heavy particles tend to deposit their energy in a track over a relatively short distance, a process classified as high-LET radiation.

In general, radiation is administered in one of two ways. When the distance between the radiation source and the target is short, the term *brachytherapy* is used. Brachytherapy allows for a rapid falloff in dose away from the target volume, as predicted by the inverse square law $I \propto 1/d^2$, where I is the intensity and d is the distance from the source. When the radiation source is at a distance from the target (generally 80–100 cm), the term *teletherapy* is used. Teletherapy allows for a more uniform dose across the target volume.

BIOLOGICAL BASIS OF RADIOTHERAPY

Radiobiology is the study of the action of ionizing radiation on organisms. The first recorded experiment in this field was conducted in 1901, when Becquerel inadvertently left a container with 200 mg of radium in his pocket for six hours. Subsequently, he described the skin erythema that appeared two weeks later and the ulceration that developed, which required several weeks to heal. During the early part of this century, radiobiologic experiments were conducted with simple biological systems. These included measurement of lethal doses in animals, destruction of germination capabilities of seeds, retardation of growth in plants and their roots, and observation of the degree of skin erythema and mucositis [52]. In the 1950s, in vivo and in vitro techniques to culture mammalian cells led to a period of intense investigation.

Despite advances in knowledge, some doubt remains as to how radiation causes cell death. The energy from radiation is deposited throughout the cell without interference from intracellular structures. Generally, DNA is believed to be the critical target for lethal injury [53].

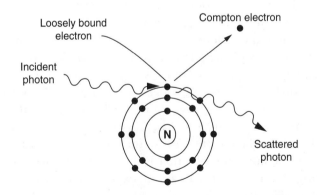

Figure 8.2 The Compton effect is the dominant reaction at the photon energies commonly used in radiotherapy. In this reaction, a loosely bound orbital electron interacts with the incident photon. Part of the photon's energy is transferred to the electron as kinetic energy. This "recoil" electron may then interact with other electrons in the surrounding tissue. The remaining energy is carried away by the scattered photon. *N* = nucleus.

In addition, damage to cell membranes and microtubules may be supplementary mechanisms of cell death [54].

Radiation may injure the DNA molecule directly or indirectly. When any form of radiation is absorbed in a cell, possibly it will interact directly with a critical intracellular structure and cause biological damage. This direct action is the dominant process in high-LET radiation, such as that involving neutrons and alpha particles. With x-rays or gamma rays, the dominant process is an indirect action. Approximately one-third of the damage may be due to the direct interaction of a recoil electron with a target molecule. The remaining two-thirds of the damage will be due to indirect action. In this case, the recoil electron reacts with water (the makeup of approximately 70% of most cells) to produce hydroxyl radicals, which then may interact with a target molecule. Various substances alter the lifetime and, thus, the effectiveness of hydroxyl radicals. Electron-affinic molecules (e.g., nitroimidazoles) prolong the life of the radicals and increase the radiation effect (radiosensitization). Such free radical scavengers as sulfhydryl molecules shorten the life of the radicals and decrease the radiation effect (radioprotection).

The actual damage to the DNA may take several forms: possible change or loss of a base, rupture of hydrogen bonds between DNA strands, dimerization, cross-link formation, and single-strand breaks or double-strand breaks. On the chromosomal level, postradiation abnormalities usually are due to chromosome breaks and errors in rejoining postreplication chromosomes. This result may lead to chromatid aberrations, such as dicentrics, rings, anaphase bridges, and acentric fragments [55–59]. These changes would require two separate damaging events; therefore, they depend on the square of the dose. The improper segregation of DNA with chromosomal damage during mitosis is the most likely cause of radiation-induced mitotic death.

The events involved in biological injury from radiation display a wide disparity in time course. The physical process of radiation absorption is completed in roughly 10^{-15} seconds. Hydroxyl radicals will remain for approximately 10^{-5} seconds, during which they may inflict damage. The time course between this physical damage and the appearance of biological damage varies. If a nonessential area of the cell is damaged, no measurable biological effect may exist. If the damage is lethal, it may be expressed hours to days later, when the cell attempts to divide. If the damage is oncogenic, its expression may be delayed 40 or more years. Finally, if the damage is a mutation, particularly a recessive muta-

tion, it may not be expressed for many generations.

Radiation dose is quantified using the amount of energy absorbed per unit mass. The standard unit for reporting dose is the gray (Gy), defined as one joule per kilogram. Older publications may refer to dose in terms of the rad, which is equal to 0.01 Gy or 1 centigray (cGy). Very little energy actually is absorbed from a given dose of radiation. For example, the energy absorbed from a whole-body dose of 4 Gy would be 67 calories (roughly the same amount of energy as would be absorbed from drinking a sip of warm coffee). Yet a whole-body dose of 4 Gy will result in bone marrow suppression and death within approximately a month. The potential for damage from ionizing radiation is due to the way in which the energy is deposited: Energy from x-rays is deposited in discrete packets, each large enough to break a chemical bond and thus cause biological damage.

SURVIVAL CURVES

A cell survival curve expresses the relationship between radiation dose and the proportion of cells that survive. Generally, *cell death* is defined as the loss of reproductive integrity in proliferating cells. In differentiated cells that no longer divide, it may be considered to be a loss of a specific function. Cell survival curves are obtained by exposing a population of cells to incremental doses of radiation and counting the number of surviving cells. The resulting data are plotted using a logarithmic scale for surviving fraction on the ordinate and a linear scale for dose in the abscissa. The overall shape of such curves is nearly the same for all mammalian cells, with some variation in the slope for different cell lines and for different types of radiation. With low-LET radiation, the curve usually begins with a shoulder in the low-dose region before beginning a logarithmic decline. The presence of the shoulder suggests that cells may accumulate some injury without dying. This "sublethal" damage then could be repaired. In contrast, high-LET radiation yields a survival curve that is a straight line from the origin. Survival is essentially an exponential function of dose (Fig. 8.3).

Survival curves may be described using one of two models. First, the curves may be said to have an initial slope D_1 owing to single-event killing and a final slope D_0 owing to multiple-event killing (Fig. 8.4A). The quantities D_1 and D_0 represent the doses that will decrease survival to 37% of the original. On average, this dose will deliver one inactivating event per cell. The

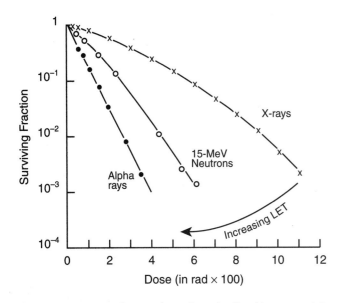

Figure 8.3 Survival curve for cultured cells of human origin exposed to 4-MeV α-particles, 15-MeV neutrons, and 250-kVp x-rays. The slope of the fractional survival curves becomes steeper with increasing linear energy transfer (*LET*) of the radiation, whereas the size of the shoulder diminishes. (Reprinted with permission from E Hall, *Radiobiology for the Radiologist* [4th ed]. Philadelphia: Lippincott, 1994:159.)

shoulder of the curve may be represented by the extrapolation number (n) or the quasi-threshold dose (D_q). The extrapolation number is obtained by extrapolating the straight portion of the curve back through the *y* axis. In general, curves with a large extrapolation number will have broad shoulders, and curves with a small extrapolation number will have narrow shoulders. The quasi-threshold dose is obtained by extrapolating backward from a line extending from the straight portion of the curve to the *y* axis at a survival fraction of unity. A threshold dose is one below which no effect is produced. However, since no radiation dose can be given without producing an effect, the quasi-threshold dose is used instead.

An alternative method of describing survival curves is the linear quadratic model (see Fig. 8.4B). This model assumes two components to cell killing: one proportional to dose and the other proportional to the dose squared. The survival curve is described by the equation $S = e^{-\alpha D} - \beta^{D2}$, where *S* is the fraction of cells surviving a dose *D* and α and β are constants. The linear (α) and quadratic (β) portions of cell killing are equal when the dose is equal to the ratio of α to β. This ratio gives an indication of a cell's ability to repair itself. In general, cells from clinically radiosensitive tumors have higher

α-to-β ratios than do cells from radioresistant tumors. In addition, tumors with lower α-to-β ratios have a higher dependence on dose per fraction and dose rate than do radiosensitive tumors.

Although the general shape of the survival curve is the same for all mammalian cells, considerable variation is seen in the inherent radiosensitivity of different cell lines and tumors. These variations are expressed mainly in the width of the initial shoulder and in the slope of the curve. Differences may occur also in survival for the same cell lines irradiated under different conditions. In addition, survival is influenced by reoxygenation of hypoxic cells, repair of sublethal damage, repopulation by new cells, and reassortment in the cell cycle. Collectively, these factors often are termed the *four Rs of radiation biology.*

Oxygen Effect and Reoxygenation

The effect of oxygen on cells subjected to irradiation has been well documented [60–62]. The ratio of the doses needed to produce the same biological effect whether oxygen is present or absent is the *oxygen enhancement ratio* (OER). In general, the presence of oxygen enhances the effect of ionizing radiation (Fig. 8.5). The degree of enhancement varies with the type of radiation. For sparsely ionizing radiation, such as x-rays and gamma rays, the OER ranges from 2.5 to 3.0. For densely ionizing radiation, such as alpha particles, the OER approaches 1.0 (no oxygen effect). For radiation of intermediate ionizing density, such as neutrons, the OER is approximately 1.6 [63]. Although the OER generally has been accepted to be independent of dose, evidence suggests that the OER for x-rays and gamma rays may be closer to 2.0 at doses of less than 200 cGy [64]. Evidence also indicates that dose rate may affect the OER for x-rays and gamma rays [65, 66].

The exact nature of the oxygen effect is not known, but oxygen generally is believed to aid in the production of cell damage via radiation-induced free radicals. This theory is consistent with the observation that the oxygen effect is much greater with radiation that acts via free radicals than with densely ionizing high-LET radiation. The mechanism is believed to involve combining the electron-affinic oxygen with an unpaired electron in the outer shell of a free radical, yielding a peroxide that is a nonrestorable form of the target material [67]. Since the lifetime of a free radical is short, oxygen must be present in the nucleus at the time of exposure or within milliseconds of radiation exposure. If

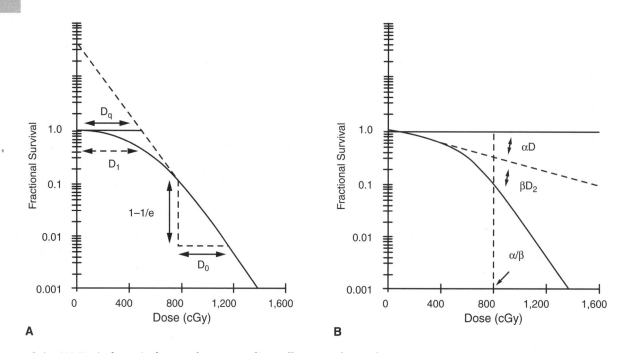

Figure 8.4 (A) Typical survival curve for mammalian cells exposed to radiation (x-rays or gamma rays) of low linear energy transfer (low-LET). The curve is described by the initial slope D_1, the final slope D_0, and some expression of the width of the shoulder (either n, the extrapolation number, or D_q, the quasi-threshold dose). (B) Typical survival curve for mammalian cells exposed to low-LET radiation, expressed in terms of the linear-quadratic model. In this model, two components contribute to cell killing: One is proportional to dose (αD), and the other is proportional to the square of the dose (βD_2). The ratio at which these two components are equal is the ratio of α/β.

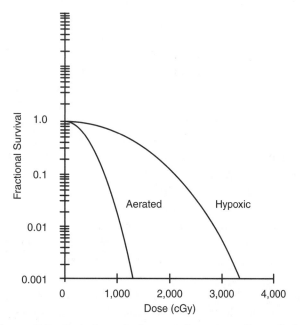

Figure 8.5 Typical survival curves for mammalian cells irradiated during aerobic and hypoxic conditions. Note the smaller shoulder and steeper slope of the cells irradiated under aerobic conditions.

bacterial cells are irradiated under anoxic conditions and oxygen is added immediately after the radiation exposure, some sensitization will occur up to approximately 2 milliseconds after irradiation [68]. However, if bacterial cells are exposed to oxygen 5–10 milliseconds after irradiation, no biological injury will occur above that produced under anoxic conditions [68, 69].

Oxygen must be present also in sufficient quantities to have a radiosensitizing effect. Below a partial pressure of 20 mm of Hg, cells will have significant protection from radiation damage. Most normal tissues have oxygen concentrations in the range of 40 mm of Hg and, therefore, are not protected from radiation damage. Tumors, on the other hand, often have areas of poor blood supply and oxygen-deficient cells. A decreasing gradient of oxygen occurs with increasing distance from a vascular capillary. Beyond 150–200 mm from a capillary, the oxygen tension is essentially zero [70]. Tumor cells farther than approximately 160 mm from a capillary become necrotic and die [70]. Between the regions of well-oxygenated viable cells and hypoxic necrotic cells, a reasonable expectation would be an area in which the oxygen tension was high enough to allow cells to remain clonogenic but low enough to be protected from radiation and thus provide a nidus for regrowth of a tumor.

Further evidence for the role of hypoxia in limiting the curability of human tumors is found in reports of improved results with irradiation after the correction of anemia [71] or the use of hyperbaric oxygen [72]. Despite this evidence, not all researchers agree that hypoxia is a common cause of treatment failure in radiotherapy [73]. This outcome may be due to reoxygenation; tumor cells that are hypoxic one day may be well oxygenated on subsequent days [74, 75].

Repair

Individual cells exposed to a dose of radiation may respond in several ways. If no damage occurs at any critical site within the cell, the cell will be unaffected. If sufficient damage does occur at a critical site, the cell will die during one of its subsequent divisions (lethal damage). Finally, cells may experience sublethal damage that may be repaired if the cell is given sufficient time, energy, and nutrients. This repair of sublethal damage allows cells to tolerate higher total doses of radiation when it is administered in multiple small fractions. The shoulder of the survival curve reflects the repair of sublethal damage [76]. The capacity for repair varies in different normal tissue and tumors. Slowly responding tissues, such as the spinal cord, tend to repair damage slowly (over 6–8 hours), but the repair is essentially complete. In contrast, rapidly responding tissues (e.g., skin, mucosa, and bone marrow) often experience incomplete repair. This outcome may be due to continued stress on the cell to divide, which results in fixation, rather than repair, of the injury [77]. An important implication is that slowly responding tissues are spared more by using multiple small fractions of radiation than are acutely responding tissues. Clinically, one may capitalize on this reaction by administering multiple small fractions of radiation daily, with a separation of 68 hours between fractions to permit repair of normal tissue [78, 79].

Reassortment

Individual cells will vary in their radiosensitivity throughout the cell cycle. After plotting survival curves for Chinese hamster cells irradiated at various stages of the cell cycle, Sinclair [80] found cells to be most sensitive during mitosis (M) and least sensitive during the late phase of nucleic acid synthesis (S). In addition, if the first gap phase (G_1) was of an appreciable length, a resistant period would occur in early G_1, followed by a sensitive phase in late G_1. Finally, the second gap phase (G_2) was found to be a sensitive phase, with a sensitivity that may approach that of the M phase.

The reasons for changes in radiosensitivity during the cell cycle are not understood well. Radiosensitivity does not appear to be related to oxygen, as studies by Legrys and Hall [81] and Hall et al. [82] have shown no difference in the OER for various stages of the cell cycle. One possible explanation is involvement of sulfhydryl compounds, which are free radical scavengers and, therefore, are natural radioprotectors. Intracellular levels of sulfhydryl compounds tend to be highest during S phase and lowest near mitosis [83].

Repopulation

Both tumors and normal tissue may undergo cell division during a course of fractionated radiotherapy. Normal tissue may respond to damage by recruiting inactive stem cells and shortening the duration of the cell cycle [84]. Commonly, this reaction is seen in irradiation of the skin and oral mucosa, during which new, growing tissue can be seen within the treatment field. Repopulation is beneficial because it reduces overall injury to the normal tissue.

In a given tumor, treatment with a cytotoxic agent (e.g., radiation) may cause cells to divide faster than before treatment. This effect is known as *accelerated repopulation*. One of the earliest demonstrations of tumor regeneration during irradiation was by Hermens and Barendsen in 1969 [85]. They reported a rapid exponential increase in clonogen number in rat rhabdomyosarcoma after a delay of approximately one volume-doubling time. Evidence also points to the possibility of accelerated repopulation in human tumor cells. Withers et al. [86] reviewed the literature on radiotherapy in head and neck tumors and estimated the dose needed to achieve local control in 50% of cases as a function of treatment time. These investigators determined that clonogen repopulation in head and neck cancer accelerates approximately 28 days after the start of fractionated radiotherapy. To compensate for this accelerated growth, they suggested that an increase of approximately 60 cGy per day would be required.

These data demonstrate that for head and neck cancer (and most likely for other tumors), radiotherapy should be completed as soon after the initiation of treatment as is feasible. Also, delaying the start of treatment may be better than imposing a delay during treatment.

Finally, with a prolonged course of fractionated irradiation, the later dose fractions will be less effective because the surviving clonogens will be undergoing accelerated repopulation.

DOSE, TIME, AND FRACTIONATION

The standard multifraction treatment regimens in common use today were based largely on French experiments in the 1920s and 1930s [87]. At that time, sterilizing a ram with a single dose of radiation to the testes was found to be impossible without producing extensive damage to the skin of the scrotum. However, if the radiation was spread out over a series of daily doses, sterilization was possible without unacceptable skin reactions. By 1934, Coutard [48] had developed a protracted fractionated scheme that still is used commonly today. Only now, more than 60 years later, can we explain the efficacy of fractionated irradiation based on well-designed radiobiologic experiments.

Dose-time considerations constitute a complex function that expresses the interdependence of the total dose, time, and number of treatments in the production of a biological effect in a given tissue volume. This is based on the four *R*s of radiobiology: Fractionating a dose spares normal tissue by allowing for repair of sublethal damage and repopulation of cells between fractions. Also, tumor damage increases, owing to reoxygenation of hypoxic cells and reassortment of cells into more sensitive phases of the cycle.

Several fractionation schemes are used today. In each, the benefits of sparing acute reactions and allowing reoxygenation of tumors must be weighed against allowing surviving tumor cells to proliferate during treatment. *Standard fractionation* for radiotherapy consists of five equal fractions weekly. This schedule evolved without solid biological basis and was based to a large degree on empiricism and convenience. *Hyperfractionation* involves giving a larger number of smaller-than-conventional doses (approximately 100–120 cGy twice a day). The goal of hyperfractionation is to provide a higher total dose and, it is hoped, a higher probability of tumor control without increasing the risk of late complications. *Accelerated fractionation* consists of multiple daily fractions of 150–200 cGy per fraction. This schedule decreases the overall treatment time; however, because the total dose per day is high, some reduction in overall dose is necessary. *Hypofractionation* involves a smaller number of larger fractions. Again, the large daily dose necessitates a reduction in overall dose

to avoid serious complications. *Split-course irradiation* consists of larger daily fractions (usually > 250 cGy/day) with a planned break in the middle of the course to permit acute reactions to subside. Generally, split-course regimens are not advisable unless the overall treatment time is decreased.

CLINICAL CONSIDERATIONS

Many factors enter into treatment planning in radiotherapy. The aim of therapy should be defined prior to the onset of treatment. In curative irradiation, patients are projected to have a probability of surviving after administration of adequate treatment. In contrast, palliative treatment offers no hope for cure or extended survival. In curative cases, a certain probability of significant side effects, though undesirable, may be acceptable. The goal of palliative irradiation, however, is to improve affected patients' quality of life by relieving some symptom or by preventing some tumor-related complication that could impair such patients' self-sufficiency. Thus, no major iatrogenic complications should be seen.

In a curative setting, an extremely important factor for radiation oncologists is to deliver the highest possible dose to the tumor volume to ensure maximum potential for tumor control while minimizing the incidence of severe sequelae in normal surrounding tissue. Determination of the optimal dose necessitates examination of the dose-response curves for normal tissue and tumors (Fig. 8.6). The farther these two curves diverge, the more favorable is the therapeutic ratio (TR), which can be defined as the percentage of tumor control with therapy A versus therapy B divided by the percentage of major complications with therapy A versus therapy B. Higher TRs are found with more efficient radiation technologies.

Improvements in radiotherapy require increased TRs. In other words, the increase in biological effectiveness must be greater in the tumor than in normal tissue. This outcome would result in a divergence of the probability curves for tumor control and complications and an increase in the TR. Radiosensitizers increase the TR by rendering tumor cells more susceptible to the effects of radiation, thereby shifting the tumor control curve to the left. Radioprotectors increase the TR by rendering normal tissue less susceptible to the effects of radiation, thereby shifting the curve for complications to the right. Since the curves for tumor control and complications are sigmoidal, small changes in the midrange of tumor

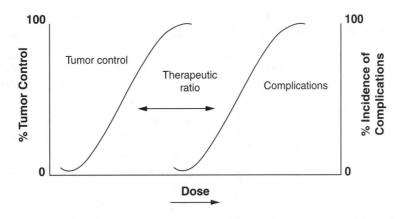

Figure 8.6   Curves for tumor control and normal tissue complications are plotted together. The therapeutic ratio is directly related to the distance between the two curves. Factors that increase the separation between the curves will increase the therapeutic ratio: For example, radiosensitizers shift the tumor control curve to the left, and radioprotectors shift the tissue complications curve to the right.

control probability (where the curve is steepest) can provide significant changes in outcome.

This observation presents two additional implications. First, if a treatment change produces a modest difference in the percentage of tumor control or complications, that change should not be interpreted as a substantial change in the biological effectiveness of the dose. Second, a small change in a biologically effective dose possibly can translate into a large therapeutic gain or loss.

At approximate incidences of effect of less than 10% or greater than 90%, the curves are relatively flat, and any additional dose is relatively inefficient. For example, if the tumor control probability already stood at 90%, no therapeutic gain would accrue from dose increases if the incidence of severe complications already equaled no less than 5%, because the probability of complications would increase much faster than would the chance of cure. In view of the proximity of the dose-response curves for normal tissue and most human tumors, patients cannot be treated with curative intent without the production of complications. In general, radiation oncologists attempt to limit serious complications to no more than 5%. The total dose that will produce a 5% chance of a serious complication at five years after treatment is termed the $TD_{5/5}$ (Table 8.3) [88].

Tumor control is related directly to total dose. For every increment of irradiation dose, a certain fraction of cells will be killed. Thus, the total number of surviving cells will be proportional to the initial number present and the fraction killed with each dose. What becomes apparent is that various levels of radiation yield a differ-

ent probability of tumor control, depending on the number of clonogenic cells present. For subclinical disease, which would represent less than 10^6 cells/mm^3, 4,500–5,000 cGy is believed to be adequate to control the disease in more than 90% of patients. This finding is based on studies of squamous cell carcinoma of the upper respiratory tract [89] and of adenocarcinoma of the breast [90]. For microscopically detected disease, which represents more than 10^6 cells/mm^3, doses of 6,000–6,500 cGy are required for epithelial tumors. For clinically palpable tumors, doses in the range of 6,000 cGy for T1 tumors up to 7,500–8,000 cGy for T4 tumors are required. Again, these doses reflect squamous cell carcinoma and adenocarcinoma, respectively [91–94].

The so-called shrinking-field technique makes use of this concept of different doses for different volumes of tumor. In this technique, portals that are progressively reduced in size are used to give progressively higher doses of radiation to the central portion of a tumor, where more clonogenic cells are present. In comparison, the periphery of a tumor, where a lower number of cells is present, receives a lesser dose. This technique minimizes the amount of normal tissue receiving high-dose irradiation.

TUMOR RESPONSE

Radiocurability refers to the eradication of tumor at the primary or regional site and reflects a direct effect of the irradiation, which may not parallel affected patients' ultimate outcome. *Radiosensitivity* expresses tumor re-

Table 8.3 Doses for Whole-Organ Irradiation That Result in a 5% Incidence (TD$_{5/5}$) and a 50% Incidence (TD$_{50/5}$) of Severe Complications at Five Years

Organ	Fractionated Dose (cGy)
Testes	100–200
Ovary	600–1,000
Eye (lens)	600–1,200
Lung	2,000–3,000
Kidney	2,000–3,000
Skin	3,000–4,000
Thyroid	3,000–4,000
Liver	3,500–4,000
Heart	4,000–5,000
Bone marrow	4,000–5,000
Gastrointestinal	5,000–6,000
Spinal cord	5,000–6,000
Brain	6,000–7,000
Peripheral nerve	6,500–7,700
Mucosa	6,500–7,700
Bone and cartilage	> 7,000
Muscle	> 7,000

Source: Modified from P Rubin, L Constantine, D Nelson, Late effects of cancer treatment: radiation and drug toxicity. In C Perez, LW Brady (eds), *Principles and Practice of Radiation Oncology.* Philadelphia: Lippincott, 1992.

sponse to irradiation. No significant correlation exists between radiosensitivity and radiocurability. Thus, a tumor may be fairly radiosensitive yet incurable. Conversely, a radioresistant tumor may well be curable.

Tumor response to irradiation is not necessarily a good measure of radiosensitivity. Most tumors contain a proportion of rapidly proliferating tumor cells and inflammatory cells that show an early response to irradiation. The response of a tumor to irradiation will depend on the programmed lifetime of terminally differentiated cells within the tumor, the proliferation kinetics of the malignant clonogens, and the removal rate of dead cells. In general, local control for rapidly regressing tumors will be slightly higher than that for slowly regressing tumors. Despite this observation, reduction in total dose on the basis of tumor response is not warranted [95].

The interpretation of slow tumor regression is somewhat more complex. Slow regression can be due to slow tumor proliferation and cell loss kinetics. It also may indicate a mass of residual stroma without viable tumor cells, as is commonly seen in Hodgkin's disease, pituitary adenomas, and choroidal melanomas. Finally, slow regression may be due to persistent tumor. The issue is clouded further by the fact that a small proportion of most tumor types will regress slowly even though the majority regress quickly. In view of the heterogeneity of tumor response, obtaining early postirradiation biopsies of a slowly regressing tumor often is unnecessary and sometimes is misleading [95] because of the impossibility of distinguishing sterilized but still living tumor cells from those that have retained their reproductive integrity. Since early postirradiation biopsies are associated with considerable risk of tissue necrosis, the advisable approach usually is to avoid performing such biopsies if a tumor continues to regress; often, they are not indicated sooner than three months after therapy.

Radiation oncologists are much like surgeons in that they attempt to cure disease in affected patients by local eradication of a tumor. This concept represents local control, implying that the tumor never will return to the treated area; on providing local control, a higher probability of cure would be expected [96]. Oncologists tend to evaluate therapies in terms of response rates. A *complete response* is defined as the absence of clinically detectable tumor, whereas a *partial response* is defined as a greater than 50% reduction in tumor mass. Radiation oncologists tend to place less emphasis on response rates than do their peers on other oncologic specialties, as a complete response does not necessarily translate into a cure and a partial response most likely will translate into a complete failure.

SUMMARY

Many advances in radiation oncology have occurred since the discovery of x-rays in 1895. Initially, radiation oncology was based largely on empiricism and clinical observations. Modern radiobiology provides a rationale for both normal-tissue and tumor response to irradiation. These responses are based largely on the four *R*s of radiobiology: reoxygenation of hypoxic cells, repair of sublethal damage, repopulation of cells between fractions, and reassortment of cells to more sensitive phases of the cell cycle.

Since cell killing is a random process, no single dose of radiation will guarantee a cure. Radiation oncologists attempt to provide the highest probability of tumor control while minimizing the risk of serious complications. Thus, radiation oncologists are searching constantly for ways to increase the TR and to improve patient care. Today, advances in all aspects of oncology have led to a realistic possibility of cure of more than 50% of newly diagnosed cases of cancer [97, 98]. Researchers hope that future advances will continue to improve radiation oncology and cancer care for all.

D. Systemic Therapy

■ ■ ■

M. ROBERT COOPER
MICHAEL R. COOPER

Medical oncology is a discipline that specializes in the use of systemic forms of treatment for the management of patients with malignancies. This focus of medical oncology on systemic therapy distinguishes it from surgical and radiation oncology, which are best suited for treating malignancies while they still are localized. The systemic treatment of malignancies began in the early 1940s when nitrogen mustard was first used to obtain a brief remission in a patient with lymphoma [99]. This historic event demonstrated the potential of cytotoxic agents in the treatment of malignancies and ushered in the modern era of chemotherapy. In 1948, Farber et al. [100] demonstrated the activity of antifolate compounds in the treatment of leukemia. This finding was followed in 1949 by the synthesis of methotrexate (MTX), which proved to be the first drug capable of curing an advanced human malignancy (gestational choriocarcinoma) [101]. Improvements in therapy arose from the continued introduction of new cytotoxic drugs, and from the demonstration that combinations of cytotoxic drugs are often superior to single-agent therapy. The superiority of combination chemotherapy to single-agent therapy was first demonstrated in the treatment of Hodgkin's disease [102]. Combination chemotherapy has subsequently proven successful in the treatment of childhood acute lymphocytic leukemia (ALL), testicular carcinoma, and intermediate and high-grade lymphomas.

Further improvement in the systemic therapy of cancer has evolved from the hypothesis that giving cytotoxic or hormonal agents (or both) in the adjuvant setting (i.e., after definitive local therapy) and in the absence of overt metastatic disease can cure a subset of patients whose disease would otherwise recur. This idea was tested first in the management of women with resectable breast cancer who at the time of mastectomy were found to have axillary nodal metastases. The presence of axillary nodal metastases is a strong predictor of the later development of recurrent, metastatic breast cancer. Randomized clinical trials have demonstrated a modest but clear increase in both disease-free and overall survival resulting from adjuvant chemotherapy and adjuvant hormonal therapy, and these benefits have been extended to women with even less advanced breast cancers [103]. More recently, adjuvant treatment with fluorouracil-based chemotherapy has been shown to improve the survival of patients with resectable colorectal cancer [104].

Cytotoxic and hormonal agents are the current mainstay of systemic cancer treatment. Efforts continue in the search for new cytotoxic drugs, with the taxanes and topoisomerase I inhibitors being examples of recent successes in this field. Likewise, more selective hormonal agents also are being developed, primarily with the intent of reducing their effects on normal tissues. However, medical oncology is just now beginning to profit from an explosion of new knowledge in molecular and structural biology, specifically from the identification of the genes and gene products that are responsible for the malignant phenotype. The expectation is that the novel agents of the future will more selectively target these molecular aberrations, and yield treatment that is both more effective and less toxic. A brief overview of some of these new therapies will be given at the end of this section, but most attention will be given to the cytotoxic and hormonal agents that are of immediate clinical relevance.

CELL-CYCLE KINETICS

Cancer is a disease characterized by abnormal regulation of cellular growth and proliferation. The kinetics of tumor growth are important in understanding how chemotherapy may thwart the growth of malignant neoplasms; in some instances, tumor growth kinetics may also help to explain why such treatment so often fails. Although from a clinical perspective a tumor's growth is described most relevantly as that of an entire tissue, the concepts of tissue growth are built on observations regarding the growth of individual cells. The kinetics of cellular growth are therefore examined first.

The familiar model of cellular proliferation, equally applicable to normal and malignant cells, is the result of studies combining tritiated thymidine (^{3}H-TdR) labeling of cells with autoradiography [105]. Thymidine, the nucleoside precursor of the DNA nucleotide deoxythymidine monophosphate, is essential for the synthesis of DNA; a cell replicating its genome in preparation for mitosis incorporates thymidine into its nucleus. In a typical experiment, ^{3}H-TdR is injected into an animal or a patient, and fresh tissue then is obtained by biopsy at serial intervals. The tissue so exposed to the isotope is overlaid with a photographic emulsion; the low-energy beta particles emitted by the tritium have a very short range, so only the silver grains lying directly above labeled nuclei are activated.

Additional techniques now are available to determine the DNA content of cells and the cell-cycle characteristics of neoplastic populations. Laser-based flow cytometry is a more rapid and simpler technique for measuring the DNA content of cells and provides information for ploidy analysis and cell-cycle kinetic studies. The use of ^{3}H-TdR requires radioactive materials and fresh tissue and is a tedious process. Flow cytometry is a highly automated procedure that can measure the DNA content of both fresh and frozen tissues in paraffin-embedded specimens. This technique now is widely available for clinical purposes and provides useful prognostic information for patients with breast cancer [106]. Current studies indicate that a high proportion of tumor cells actively duplicating their DNA (i.e., a high S-phase fraction) is associated with an increased risk of recurrence and with mortality for patients with both node-negative and node-positive invasive breast cancer.

Bromodeoxyuridine (BrdU) labeling of DNA also can provide an assessment of the DNA synthesis of neoplastic tissues. The amount of BrdU incorporated into DNA can be quantitated by either flow cytometry or microscopic techniques. The use of BrdU labeling techniques is hampered somewhat by the need for fresh tissue and for dual fluorescent staining techniques. Both flow cytometry and BrdU labeling can measure DNA content, but the former is simpler and yields more reproducible results.

The first critical observation to be made from such investigations was that DNA synthesis is not a continuous process from one mitosis to the next but rather occurs during a discrete period of the intermitotic time, know as the *S phase* [107]. The intermitotic time has been subdivided further into a total of five phases (Fig. 8.7). G_1, the time or "gap" between mitosis and S phase, is the portion of the cell cycle dedicated to fulfilling the specialized functions of a given cell type. During G_1, the cell's energy is directed toward the synthesis of RNA and protein designed to execute these functions. G_1 is also the phase of the cell cycle in which the cell prepares for and eventually commits to replication of its DNA. G_2, the gap between the end of S phase and mitosis, represents the usually brief time required to organize the nucleus for the events of mitosis. The onset of mitosis is marked by chromosomal condensation and is followed by chromosomal segregation and cell division, yielding two daughter cells. The fifth phase of the cell cycle, G_0, often is depicted as lying outside the loop connecting one mitosis with the next. This designation is used because cells in G_0, in contrast to cells in G_1, do not

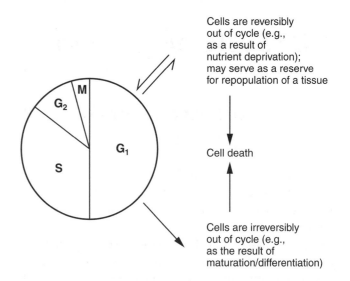

Figure 8.7 Diagrammatic representation of the cell growth cycle, emphasizing the relationships between proliferating and nonproliferating cell populations. M = mitosis; S = DNA synthesis phase; G_1 = the time or "gap" between mitosis and S phase; G_2 = the gap between the end of S phase and mitosis.

respond to the signals that normally prompt the initiation of DNA synthesis. However, cells in G_0 are by no means dead: they continue to synthesize RNA and protein and so may carry out some of the normal functions of a particular cell type. In addition, G_0 cells often act as a reserve population that, given the appropriate cues (e.g., increased availability of nutrients), can reenter the pool of proliferating cells and thus repopulate a tissue.

Measurement of the duration of the various phases of the cell cycle is conceptually simple. Because thymidine is either incorporated into DNA or is metabolized rapidly and excreted, only cells that are in S phase at the time of ^{3}H-TdR administration will demonstrate the development of grains over their nuclei on an autoradiograph. A cohort of cells labeled in S phase can be followed by first obtaining serial biopsy specimens of tissue for autoradiography after ^{3}H-TdR injection and then recording the percentage of mitoses that are labeled in each specimen [108]. When the percentage of labeled mitoses (PLM) is plotted against the time after ^{3}H-TdR injection, a curve such as the one in Figure 8.8 is obtained. Cells at the very end of S phase during ^{3}H-TdR labeling will be the first to produce labeled mitoses; the elapsed time between exposure to ^{3}H-TdR and the appearance of these first labeled mitotic cells is the length of G_2. Cells poised at the beginning of S phase during labeling are the last to appear in mitosis, so the width of the wave reflects the duration of S phase (T_s). If tissue samples subsequently are examined, waves of

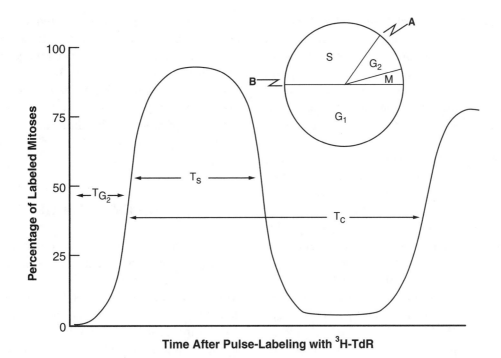

Figure 8.8 Determination of cell cycle times using the percentage-of-labeled-mitosis method. Only cells in S phase become labeled at the time of ^{3}H-thymidine (^{3}H-TdR) administration. Those cells at the very end of S phase (*point A*) are the first to appear in mitosis, and those just beginning to enter S phase (*point B*) are the last to do so. The time lag between ^{3}H-TdR pulsing and the appearance of the first labeled mitosis represents the time required for cells to pass through G_2 (T_{G2}). The width of the waves of labeled mitosis gives the duration of S phase (T_s), and the time separating one wave from the next yields the total cell-cycle time (T_c). M = mitosis; S = DNA synthesis phase; G_1 = the time or "gap" between mitosis and S phase; G_2 = the gap between the end of S phase and mitosis.

labeled mitoses appear while the daughter cells of those originally labeled pass through mitosis. The time separating the beginning of one wave from the beginning of the next yields the total cell-cycle time (T_c). When the cell-cycle kinetics of mammalian cells are examined in vivo using the PLM method, the durations of S, G_2, and M phases are found to be remarkably similar (approximately 7 hours, 3 hours, and 1 hour, respectively). Moreover, in most instances, no significant difference is seen in the duration of these phases between normal and malignant tissues. The longest and most variable phase is G_1, ranging from two to three hours to several days. Surprisingly, the intermitotic time (T_c) for most normal human cells is one to two days, whereas that of most malignant cells is approximately two to three days [109].

Obviously, cell-cycle kinetics alone are inadequate for describing the growth of tumors. First, despite rather similar values for T_c, different malignancies have distinctly different growth rates. For example, T_c has been estimated at roughly 2.5 days for acute myelogenous leukemia (AML) and approximately 2.0 days for squa-

mous cell carcinoma of the skin [109]; yet, untreated AML results in death within weeks of diagnosis, whereas squamous cell carcinoma takes a more indolent course, usually measured in years. Second, if tumor growth were determined solely by the cell-cycle time, tumors would double in volume every two to three days. Although Burkitt's lymphoma approximates this rate of growth, clearly it is an exception rather than the rule. To resolve these apparent incongruities, tumor growth must be described in the context of an entire tissue.

TISSUE GROWTH KINETICS

When tumors are examined as entire tissues, what quickly becomes obvious is that not all the cells are proliferating (i.e., not all are "in cycle"). In fact, only a minority are proliferating, with the bulk in phase G_0, differentiated to the point at which they no longer have the potential to replicate, or simply dead. The fraction of tumor cells that is in cycle can be calculated by ^{3}H-

TdR autoradiography. First, the labeling index (LI) is determined—the proportion of cells synthesizing DNA at the time of exposure to the isotope (the proportion of cells developing labeled nuclei). Then, if T_s and T_c are known for the cells of that tissue, as might be estimated by the PLM method, the fraction of proliferating cells in the tumor, called the *growth fraction* (GF), is determined as follows: $GF = LI \times T_c/T_s \times \lambda$. By itself, the LI does not give the fraction of proliferating cells, as not all cells will be in S phase at the time of ^{3}H-TdR exposure; hence, the term T_c/T_s to make the correction. The constant λ (always close to 1) is necessary to make adjustment for the fact that the distribution of cells in different phases of the cell cycle is not strictly equal (each cell undergoing mitosis yields two daughter cells, so the relative number of cells in each phase of the cell cycle decreases from G_1 to mitosis). When the LI has been determined for a variety of solid tumors, it generally has been low, ranging from 1% to 8% [109]. These results should be compared with the LI of the epithelium of the normal gastrointestinal tract, which is roughly 16%.

In addition to having a low GF, most tumors suffer from a high rate of cell loss, further limiting their rate of growth [110]. The percentage of newly produced daughter cells that die is high, in part a result of the inherent genetic instability of malignant cells. Moreover, tumors tend to outstrip their vascular supply and so develop large areas of ischemic necrosis. Given this general tendency for low growth fractions and high rates of cell loss, obviously most tumors are not what, on the surface, they appear to be: seething masses of rapidly dividing cells. Yet the nature of tumor growth is progressive, so clearly the rate of cell loss ultimately lags behind that of cell production. This imbalance between cell production and cell loss—the fact that tumors are not checked appropriately by the homeostatic mechanisms that maintain a predetermined number of cells in normal tissue—lies at the heart of tumor progression.

The importance of this imbalance between cell production and cell loss is well demonstrated by comparing AML with chronic myelogenous leukemia (CML) [109]. AML is rapidly progressive, killing patients within a matter of weeks to months if untreated. On the other hand, CML usually follows an indolent course over several years. Surprisingly, the LI for the myeloblasts in AML is approximately 5–11%, whereas that for myeloblasts of CML generally is up to 43%. The difference is that the myeloblasts of CML in all but its terminal stages are able to differentiate to more mature progeny (e.g., neutrophils) with brief life spans. The myeloblasts of AML rarely produce more mature successors and, given their longer life span as compared with mature cells, they accumulate rapidly. Even in the terminal phase of CML (blast crisis), when the percentage and number of myeloblasts increase rapidly, the LI does not change. The problem at this point in the illness is that the myeloblasts no longer are able to differentiate and mature further; consequently, the clinical course of the disease becomes similar to that of AML.

GOMPERTZIAN GROWTH

The concepts presented thus far describe tumor growth at only one point during the tumor's life span. Yet the growth of a tumor changes drastically with time, a fact with important implications for cancer treatment in general and for cancer chemotherapy in particular. An English insurance actuary named Gompertz developed a mathematical model to describe the relationship between an individual's age and expected time of death. The asymmetric sigmoidal curve produced by this model comes close to describing accurately the growth of a tumor over its entire life span (Fig. 8.9). The gompertzian equation used to calculate the time required for a tumor to reach 10^9 cells estimates that most human malignancies originate less than two years prior to their clinical detection [111]. The exact mechanisms influencing the shape of the gompertzian curve are not well understood, but the slowing of growth in larger tumors undoubtedly is due in part to (1) hypoxia, as tumors outstrip their fragile vascular supply; (2) decreased availability of nutrients and hormones; (3) accumulation of toxic metabolites, and (4) inhibitory cell-to-cell communication.

During the early phases of a tumor's life span, both the rate at which cells are produced and the rate at which cells are lost from the tumor are proportional to the number of cells in the tumor at a given time. Because cell number and tumor volume (V) are proportional, $d_v/d_t = (K_P - K_L) \times V$, where *dv/dt* equals the rate of change in tumor volume per unit time, K_P equals the rate constant for cell production, and K_L equals the rate constant for cell loss. This relationship, on rearrangement and integration, gives the following more useful relationship: $V = V_0 \exp[(K_P - K_L)(t_2 - t_1)]$, where V_0 represents the volume of the tumor at time zero and V represents the volume of the tumor after the time interval $t_2 - t_1$ has elapsed. In short, for a significant portion of its life, a tumor grows exponentially. This simple exponential relationship allows a simple calculation of the doubling time of the tumor (T_D): $Ln\ 2/(K_P - K_L) = T_D$.

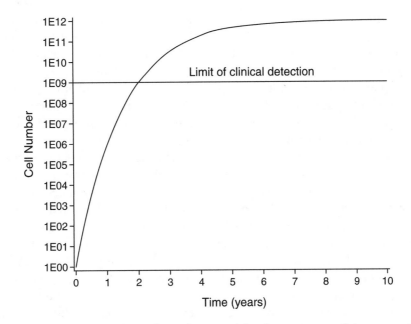

Figure 8.9 The gompertzian growth curve. During the early stage of development, growth is exponential. As a tumor enlarges, its growth slows. By the time a tumor becomes large enough to cause symptoms and is clinically detectable, most of its growth has already occurred, and the exponential phase is complete.

Measuring the time required for a tumor to double in size should allow an estimate of the time required for the tumor to achieve a given size from its beginning as a single cell. When such calculations are made using clinical measurements of T_D, one concludes that tumors start 10–20 years prior to their clinical detection.

Such calculations are fundamentally flawed. With occasional exceptions, by the time a tumor becomes clinically detectable, it has achieved a mass of approximately 1 g, or 10^9 cells. To have reached this size, the tumor already has undergone some 30 doublings, and its growth is no longer exponential. The additional 10 doublings required to produce 10^{12} cells, or a 1 kg lesion—a tumor burden at which most patients succumb—occur much more slowly than do the previous 30 doublings and represent a fraction of the tumor's growth.

Most chemotherapeutic agents in clinical use exert their antitumor effects (and the bulk of their toxicities) by interfering directly with the synthesis or function of DNA. Not surprisingly, these drugs generally are more toxic to proliferating cells than to those incapable of replication or in phase G_0, and so are more effective against tumors with high GFs [112]. By the time tumors are clinically detectable, they lie "high on the gompertzian curve," where their GFs are low. However, if the number of cells in a tumor can be reduced, as might occur by surgical debulking or radiotherapy, the tumor

will have been brought to a lower point on the gompertzian curve. Cells previously in phase G_0 reenter the cell cycle, the GF of the tumor increases, and the growth rate of the tumor may be similar to the rate of a tumor that had just attained the same size from a single cell. If effective chemotherapy against the tumor is available, it would now likely be even more effective. This concept of moving tumors down on the gompertzian curve prior to the delivery of chemotherapy is part of the rationale behind adjuvant chemotherapy [113]. Thus, chemotherapy may be given to patients who have no overt evidence of residual disease after local treatment (e.g., surgery or radiotherapy for a primary breast cancer) but for whom experience with similar patients indicates a high chance of relapse from the presence of undetectable micrometastatic disease.

STEM CELL MODEL OF TUMOR GROWTH

A further impediment to effective chemotherapy is the conclusion that proliferating cells—those that should be most vulnerable to the toxic effects of chemotherapy—are not necessarily the cells that must be eliminated to eradicate a tumor. Instead, the critical cell population responsible for the persistence and growth of a tumor often is largely in phase G_0. The reasons for this apparent paradox are found in the stem cell model of tissue growth.

The stem cell model of tissue growth has been elaborated most extensively for cells of the bone marrow, which are depicted as components of a complex hierarchy. At the top of the hierarchy are relatively undifferentiated cells with an unlimited capacity for self-replication and for replenishing the marrow with all its elements. Yet these cells are virtually unable to perform the ultimate functions of the marrow (i.e., oxygen transport, hemostasis, and defense against infection). At the bottom of the hierarchy are mature, highly specialized cells (e.g., neutrophils, erythrocytes, and platelets) that can execute these tasks but are unable to divide and renew themselves. Although proliferative rates for the immediate descendants of stem cells tend to be high (the LI for myeloblasts and myelocytes is 40% and 20%, respectively; the LI for early erythroid precursors ranges between 30% and 75%), the stem cells themselves, unless provoked by an appropriate stimulus (e.g., blood loss or infection), tend to proliferate slowly [109].

The sluggish proliferation of marrow stem cells has been inferred by the extent to which their numbers are reduced by the administration of very high doses of ^{3}H-TdR, a technique dubbed *thymidine suicide*. As in ^{3}H-TdR autoradiography, only cells synthesizing DNA (those in S phase) will accumulate the isotope in their nuclei. However, in the thymidine suicide experiments, the doses of ^{3}H-TdR are high enough to be lethal to these cells.

The original stem cell assays of bone marrow were performed in mice [113]. If a mouse is given a sufficiently large dose of radiation, it will fail to recover hematopoietic function; both the mature cells and the stem cells of the marrow will be damaged irrevocably. If, however, this lethally irradiated mouse is transfused with marrow from a nonirradiated syngeneic mouse, its marrow will repopulate, and hematopoiesis will resume. In addition to repopulating the bone marrow, the transfused marrow will establish colonies of hematopoiesis in the spleen, each colony derived from a single stem cell. These spleen cell colonies contain granulocytes, erythrocytes, platelets, and their less mature precursors, so the founding stem cell is termed *pluripotent* (i.e., capable of giving rise to cells of all three lineages). When normal bone marrow is exposed to high doses of ^{3}H-TdR and then is transfused into a lethally irradiated, syngeneic mouse, the number of spleen colonies formed is reduced only slightly compared with the number obtained with transfusion of marrow not exposed to the isotope. The conclusion is that the marrow's stem cells are not proliferating rapidly (i.e., most

are in G_0). Yet, if the donor marrow is stimulated to proliferate, as might occur if the donor were rendered anemic by phlebotomy, exposure of that marrow to ^{3}H-TdR before transplantation results in a more pronounced reduction in the number of spleen colonies formed [114]. Thus, the induction of anemia caused the stem cells to move out of phase G_0 and back into the cell cycle, so that the deficit in erythrocytes might be corrected.

The stem cell model of tissue growth has been extended to describe the growth of nonhematopoietic tissues, including tumors. Several lines of evidence argue for the propriety of applying this model to malignant tissues. First, nearly all tumors arise from a single pluripotential, albeit aberrant founding (stem) cell. The monoclonal origin of human tumors was suggested strongly by the unique paraprotein of multiple myeloma and by cytogenetic studies in leukemia (the best example of which is the 9;22 translocation in CML); it was established most firmly by the finding of a single glucose-6-phosphate dehydrogenase (G-6-PD) isoenzyme in tumor cells of women heterozygous at the G-6-PD locus. Second, like bone marrow, tumors contain cells of varying degrees of differentiation. The more differentiated cells have low rates of proliferation and, when transplanted, are incapable of establishing new tumors. The less differentiated cells have higher proliferative rates (just as the LI is higher for myeloblasts than for myelocytes) and are more efficient at founding new tumors. Indeed, the more anaplastic tumors tend to have higher GFs and follow a more fulminant course if left without effective treatment. The third point in favor of the stem cell model is the response of some human tumors to radiotherapy. Radiotherapy can cure tumors that arise spontaneously in humans at doses that would be incapable of curing experimental tumors of the same size in mice. The increased sensitivity of the spontaneous human tumors appears to reflect a smaller population of stem cells.

Stem cells in tumors have been measured directly through (1) mouse spleen colony assays (e.g., injection of lymphoma cells into a mouse with the ensuing appearance of lymphoma colonies in the spleen), (2) the enumeration of metastatic lung colonies after IV injection of tumor cells into mice, and (3) tumor colony formation in vitro. The last method has been applied to human tumors, with somewhat mixed results [115]. The impetus for developing an in vitro assay of human tumor stem cells was the hope that it would enable more rational drug therapy. Notation of the effect of varying concentrations of chemotherapeutic agents on stem cell colony formation might allow prediction of the drugs that would be most likely to have activity in vivo. However, although such assays are good at predicting which drugs will not be effective, they fail to predict accurately which drugs will succeed (this topic is discussed more extensively later in this section). Nonetheless, the stem cell assay has provided insight into tumor growth. It has demonstrated that only 1 in 1,000 to 1 in 10,000 cells in a tumor is capable of forming colonies of cancer cells in vitro. Although this poor cloning efficiency could be due in part to technical problems related to growing cells in tissue culture, it more likely reflects the fact that most cells in a tumor have a very limited (if any) potential for self-renewal.

Controversy exists over the proliferative status of stem cells in human tumors, some studies indicating that they spend less time in phase G_0 than do their bone marrow counterparts [116, 117]. Nonetheless, it is clear that the proliferating cells of a tumor—perhaps the cells that respond most dramatically to chemotherapy and yield clinical, albeit transient, regression of disease—are not necessarily the cells that must be eradicated to effect a cure. Thus, when cure is the objective, the tumor's response to a drug is best assessed by measuring the survival not of all tumor cells but rather only of clonogenic or stem cells.

RELATIONSHIPS BETWEEN TUMOR CELL SURVIVAL AND DRUG DOSE

For many of the commonly used chemotherapeutic agents, the relationship between tumor cell survival and drug dose is exponential. The number of cells surviving a given dose of drug is proportional to both the drug dose and the number of cells at risk for exposure to the drug: $dN \propto NdD$, where N = number of cells in the tumor and D = drug dose, or $dN = -KndD$, where the proportionality constant –K is introduced with a negative sign because the number of cells decreases with increasing drug dose. Rearranging and integrating the foregoing equation yields the following more useful formula: $N = N_0exp-K(D - D_0)$, where the subscript 0 indicates the initial dose and cell number.

A simple exponential relationship such as this implies that the death of a tumor cell is the consequence of a simple interaction between the drug molecule and its target in the cell. Of more immediate clinical relevance, exponential cell killing implies that multiple courses of therapy will be needed to eradicate the tumor, because each dose of drug produces the same *proportion* of cells killed, not the same number of cells killed. It also implies that small changes in the drug dose may translate into large changes in cell survival. Imag-

ine that at the beginning of treatment, a tumor contains 10^{10} cells. If each course of treatment results in the death of 99.9% of these cells and if one log of cell growth occurs between courses of treatment, five courses of treatment are required to eliminate the last cell (Fig. 8.10).

Note that this reasoning assumes an ideal situation in which all cells are equally sensitive to the drug, cells resistant to the drug are absent at the onset of therapy, and no cells develop drug resistance during therapy. These assumptions are not entirely valid, of course, during the treatment of spontaneous human tumors; indeed, nonkinetic forms of drug resistance are the major impediment to the successful treatment of human tumors. Nonetheless, the example makes the point that repeated courses of treatment are necessary. It also demonstrates that complete clinical remission, typically achieved when the number of tumor cells falls below 10^9, does not equal a cure; treatment must be continued despite the absence of an overt tumor. This thinking un-

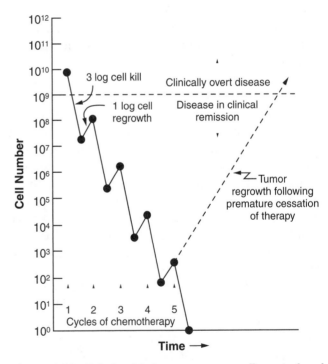

Figure 8.10 Relationship between tumor cell survival and administration of chemotherapy. The exponential relationship between drug dose and tumor cell survival dictates that a constant proportion, not number, of tumor cells is killed with each treatment cycle. In this example, each cycle of drug administration results in 99.9% (3 log) of cell kill, and 1 log of cell regrowth occurs between cycles. The broken line indicates what would occur if the last cycle of therapy were omitted: despite complete clinical remission of disease, the tumor ultimately would recur.

derlies the standard practice of delivering two additional cycles of chemotherapy to patients with Hodgkin's disease or other potentially curable lymphomas after the achievement of a complete clinical remission. Continued treatment with potentially toxic drugs when no tumor is clinically evident is difficult for both patients and oncologists. Only rarely do oncologists have the benefit of being able to follow sensitive and specific tumor markers (as are often available for the management of men with non-seminomatous testicular cancers) to monitor the effect of treatment beyond the point of complete remission.

The disproportionate increase in cell survival that results from a decrease in drug dose is shown readily with a simple example. Assume that a tumor before any treatment contains 10^{11} cells. Also assume that the proportionality constant -K is -5 for the alkylating agent cyclophosphamide when used in the treatment of this particular tumor. If a dose of 1.5 g cyclophosphamide is delivered, the tumor will be left with 5.5×10^7 cells: N $= N_0 \exp{-K}(D - D_0)$; $N_0 = 10^{11}$ when $D_0 = 0$ and N $= 10^{11}\exp{-5}(1.5 - 0) = 5.5 \times 10^7$ cells. If the oncologist chooses to administer 0.75 g of cyclophosphamide instead of 1.5 g, $N = 10^{11}\exp{-5}(0.75 - 0) = 2.4 \times 10^9$ cells and the result is that a 50% decrease in dose has translated into a 98% increase in cell survival.

Often, a reduction in the drug dose is unavoidable because of undue toxicity to normal tissues (e.g., myelosuppression, mucositis). Nonetheless, attempting to administer drugs in full dosages (which implies both the amount and frequency with which a drug is given) is an important goal in treating patients. Retrospective analyses of the dose intensity of chemotherapy and the outcome of treatment (e.g., response rates, response duration, and survival) have suggested such a correlation for 5-fluorouracil (5-FU) in colon cancer, doxorubicin in breast cancer, and cisplatin in ovarian cancer [118, 119]. Similar analyses of the treatment of Hodgkin's disease have indicated a benefit in maintaining the dose intensity of cytotoxic therapy [120, 121]. However, the retrospective nature of these analyses leaves them open to a number of criticisms. For example, the inability to deliver chemotherapy at a high dose-intensity could be related to patient- or tumor-related factors that were themselves predictive of a poor outcome. More recently, the Cancer and Leukemia Group B conducted a prospective study of the importance of dose intensity in the treatment of women with stage II, node-positive breast cancer, using the cytoxan, doxorubicin, and 5-FU (CAF) regimen [122]. The women in this study were allocated randomly to three dose levels of CAF, and a significant dose-response effect, measured in terms of disease-free and overall survival, was observed, but only in those women whose primary breast tumors expressed high levels of the c-erb-B2 (HER2/neu) oncogene. A possible explanation for this correlation between a benefit from dose-intense chemotherapy and increased c-erb-B2 expression is that c-erb-B2 expression is a marker for relative resistance to one or more of the drugs in the CAF regimen, and that higher doses were needed to overcome this resistance. Indeed, high expression of c-erb-B2 is associated with increased intracellular concentrations of topoisomerase II, the major target of doxorubicin. Although this study lends support to the idea of dose intensity, it also points out that not all patients will benefit from more aggressive treatment: the patients with c-erb-B2-negative breast cancers did not fare better with the more dose-intensive CAF regimens.

Plots of cell survival as a function of drug dose have rarely been constructed for human tumors under treatment in vivo. Such curves have been constructed, however, for animal tumors using the spleen colony assay or a metastatic lung nodule assay, and for both animal and human tumor cell lines cultured in vitro. It is important to note that these experimental systems measure the survival only of clonogenic tumor cells as a function of drug dose; as emphasized earlier, clonogenic cells are of interest since it is their elimination that is ultimately required for a cure.

In the spleen colony assay tumor cells (e.g., from a murine lymphoma) are injected into a lethally irradiated syngeneic mouse following exposure of the tumor to varying doses of the drug in question [123]. The number of tumor cell colonies that subsequently appear in the spleen reflects the number of clonogenic cells surviving drug exposure. Some tumors will form metastatic lung nodules following IV injection, and stem cell survival can be assayed in this manner as well. The first conclusion to be drawn from such studies and the analogous in vitro cell culture assays is that the slope of the cell survival vs. drug dose curve is much steeper for rapidly proliferating cells (Fig. 8.11A) (i.e., tumors whose clonogenic cells are more often "in cycle" [not in G_0] are more sensitive to a given drug dose) [124]. Only a handful of drugs—cisplatin, the nitrosoureas, nitrogen mustard, and bleomycin show little increased toxicity for proliferating cells [125].

The second conclusion to be drawn from these experiments is that some chemotherapeutic agents exhibit a plateau in cell killing as the dose is further increased (Fig. 8.11B). Drugs behaving in this manner have their exclusive or major effect during a single phase of the cell cycle, characteristically during the S phase. To in-

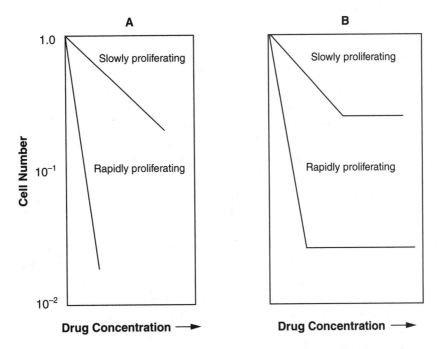

Figure 8.11   Relationship between the proliferative rate of tumor cells and sensitivity to chemotherapy. (A) Cell populations are exposed briefly to varying concentrations of drug, with subsequent determination of clonogenic cell survival. Rapidly proliferating cells (i.e., cell populations with few cells in G_0) are more sensitive to a given drug dose than are slowly proliferating cells. The drugs used in these experiments have no significant specificity for any phase of the cell cycle. (B) These experiments were performed as in part A but with drugs that are specific for one phase of the cell cycle (e.g., S phase). Again, rapidly proliferating cells are more sensitive to a given drug than are slowly proliferating cells. However, now a plateau occurs in survival with increasing drug dose for both types of cell populations. Further decline in cell survival can be achieved only by prolonging the duration of exposure to the drug, allowing more cells to enter the susceptible phase of the cell cycle.

crease cell kill beyond the plateau level, the duration of exposure must be prolonged to allow more tumor cells to enter the susceptible phase of the cell cycle. The antimetabolites, drugs structurally similar to normal precursors of DNA and RNA synthesis, and that disrupt cell function by competing with these precursors in critical metabolic pathways, are the most notable drugs of this type and include cytosine arabinoside, thioguanine, mercaptopurine, methotrexate, 5-FU, and hydroxyurea. Recognition of the plateau in the cell survival versus dose curve for the antimetabolites has greatly influenced the manner in which antimetabolites are administered to patients, with most treatment strategies attempting to achieve prolonged exposure of the tumor to the drug.

PHARMACOKINETIC DETERMINANTS OF RESPONSE TO CHEMOTHERAPY

Although the pharmacokinetics of individual chemotherapeutic agents are important in suggesting doses and schedules of drug administration that may be most effective in the clinic, such agents usually are not subjected to therapeutic drug monitoring as is often the case for a number of other drugs commonly used in clinical practice (e.g., aminoglycosides, digoxin, theophylline, anticonvulsants, and some antiarrhythmic agents). For example, because of its cell-cycle phase specificity (toxicity to only those cells in S phase) and because of its brief elimination half-life, cytosine arabinoside is given by continuous IV infusion over a period of seven days when used in the treatment of AML; however, measuring plasma concentrations of cytosine arabinoside during its administration is uncommon. Likewise, measurement of platinum concentrations is uncommon, but the well-described renal clearance of carboplatin has resulted in the use of various formulas to estimate the concentration-versus-time exposure to carboplatin as a function of the estimated glomerular filtration rate. Perhaps the only routine application of therapeutic drug monitoring in oncology occurs with the use of high-dose MTX, which has very limited applications.

For all the other chemotherapeutic agents used in current clinical practice, measurement of serum drug concentrations is merely a research tool. Rather than measuring drug concentrations, oncologists typically titrate drug doses to achieve a given degree of myelosuppression. This approach is highly appropriate for drugs (e.g., alkylating agents) with antitumor and myelosuppressive effects that are directly proportionate to dose and to the total area under the concentration-versus-time curve (AUC) rather than to instantaneous plasma drug concentrations. However, many agents currently being developed as potential anticancer drugs are not myelosuppressive. Many are directed toward interference with aberrantly expressed signal transduction molecules and likely will interact with their targets in a reversible manner. Therefore, the antitumor activity and toxicity of such compounds will likely depend not so much on total cumulative exposure (total AUC) as on tissue concentrations and the exposure time to such concentrations. Thus, therapeutic drug monitoring may in the future play a greater role in the judicious use of systemic cancer therapies.

GENETIC MODELS OF DRUG RESISTANCE

To this point, the models used to describe the results of cytotoxic chemotherapy have been useful in predicting outcome in some selected settings, but the shortcomings of these models are obvious in light of what occurs in the majority of patients with solid tumors. Given that most chemotherapeutic agents are more toxic to rapidly proliferating tumors, and given that a tumor's proliferative rate should increase as its size decreases, a tumor that responded favorably to an initial course of chemotherapy would be expected to become increasingly sensitive to treatment during subsequent courses of therapy. However, this scenario rarely, if ever, transpires. More typically, tumors regress and may become clinically undetectable during the initial courses of chemotherapy, but later resurge with vigor despite continuation of the same therapy. Tumor growth kinetics clearly fail to explain this sequence of events.

Most often, mechanisms other than a tumor's growth fraction or a cell's location in the cell cycle explain why malignancies are resistant to chemotherapy. First, tumor cells may reside in so-called sanctuary sites inaccessible to most drugs. Often, the central nervous system (CNS) and testes are impervious to drugs that distribute freely to other tissues; cancers in these sites frequently relapse, notwithstanding successful treat-

ment elsewhere. A major advance in the treatment of childhood ALL came with the recognition that the meninges often were a site of recurrent disease and that prophylactic treatment of the CNS, either with radiation or intrathecal MTX, could increase the chances for cure in those children who had achieved a complete remission of the disease with systemic therapy. Second, drug resistance also may seem greater than it is, such as when a drug is absorbed incompletely, is metabolized rapidly and excreted, or fails to be converted to its active form. In many treatment protocols, these forms of "pseudoresistance" are circumvented (at least partially) by escalation of drug doses until mild to moderate normal tissue toxicity occurs. However, by far the most important forms of drug resistance—the most typical explanations for treatment failure—lie in the genetic and biochemical makeup of malignant cells.

The genetic basis of drug resistance in malignant cells has been well established from several lines of evidence. Even before gene transfer experiments were performed, researchers applied to tumor cells cultured in vitro the same procedures used to prove that bacterial resistance to antibiotics arises as the result of spontaneous mutation and subsequent selection. The rate of development of drug resistance calculated from such experiments is consistent with known rates of spontaneous mutation: roughly one of every 10^6 to 10^7 cells. Therefore, a tumor that has just reached a size sufficient for it to be detected clinically (e.g., 10^9 cells) is likely to contain 10^2 to 10^3 drug-resistant cells. If the rate of spontaneous mutation is constant, the larger the tumor, the greater the number of drug-resistant cells it will harbor. What is not so intuitively obvious is that the relationship between tumor size and the probability of finding drug-resistant cells in it is exponential, such that $P_0 = 1/\exp^{\alpha\,(N-1)}$, where P_0 equals the probability of finding no drug-resistant cells within a tumor containing N cells and having a spontaneous rate of mutation α [126, 127]. This relationship predicts that the curability of a tumor—here equated with the probability that no drug-resistant cells are found—does not decline gradually as the tumor grows larger but instead falls precipitously as the tumor approaches a critical size determined by its rate of spontaneous mutation. A tumor containing 10^6 cells and having a spontaneous mutation rate of 10^{-7} stands only a 10% chance of containing drug-resistant cells. However, if the tumor is allowed to grow 1.5 logs (to 5×10^7 cells), this chance increases to more than 99%. The clinical message behind this model of tumor growth, the *Goldie-Coldman model*, is that curing smaller tumors is easier, and that the best moment for effective treatment is as soon after detection as possible. Delay in treatment, by allowing a modest increase in the tumor burden, can result in a large increase in the probability of encountering drug-resistant cells, thereby possibly forfeiting affected patients' chances for cure or, at least, for meaningful disease regression. Although the reasoning is different from that provided by kinetic concepts, the message is the same.

An extension of the Goldie-Coldman model argues that affected patients should benefit from the use of multiple, non-cross-resistant drugs. The use of multiple chemotherapeutic agents in combination has been responsible for much of the success achieved in the treatment of childhood ALL, Hodgkin's disease, some non-Hodgkin's lymphomas, and testicular carcinoma; single-agent chemotherapy clearly is inferior for the treatment of these malignancies. The superiority of multiple drugs over single agents is not so clear in treating some of the more common solid tumors of adults, such as colon cancer. The failure of multiple agents in the treatment of these tumors is not so much a failure of the Goldie-Coldman model as it is a reflection of these tumors' inherently high levels of resistance to all currently available chemotherapeutic agents. Also, practical limits dictate how far the theoretic advantages of combination chemotherapy can be taken. Two or even three drugs may be active against a given tumor, but if all produce similar normal tissue toxicities, combining them in the clinic will be difficult. Either the combination will result in excessive morbidity and mortality or the drug doses will be reduced to levels at which none is particularly effective.

The problem of tumor drug resistance is amplified further by the inherent genetic instability of malignant neoplasms. The genetic instability of tumors is manifested grossly by the multiple chromosomal defects—breaks, deletions, translocations, inversions, and extrachromosomal double minutes—that tend to increase in number and complexity over their life spans. Chemotherapeutic agents may add to this genetic instability by acting as mutagens themselves. Thus, new subclones of malignant cells appear routinely. Those with an increased capacity for self-renewal and proliferation gradually replace the slower growing, better differentiated cells in the tumor, and drug-resistant clones replace sensitive clones in the face of systemic treatment. Classic examples of disease evolution include Richter's syndrome, wherein the patient with chronic lymphocytic leukemia develops an aggressive diffuse large-cell lymphoma; and the progression of CML, initially an indolent myeloproliferative disorder with a single chromosomal abnormality (the 9;22 translocation), to a more fulminant disease (blast crisis) still accompanied by the 9;22 translocation but heralded by the accumulation of additional chromosomal abnormalities.

BIOCHEMICAL MECHANISMS OF DRUG RESISTANCE

Although an important strategy for overcoming drug resistance is to treat affected patients with several agents that have nonoverlapping toxicities and different mechanisms of action, the phenomenon of multidrug resistance may thwart this strategy. In this scenario, successive generations of cells exposed to sublethal concentrations of a cytotoxic chemotherapeutic agent become resistant not only to that drug but to other chemotherapeutic agents with different mechanisms of action and different chemical structures [128]. This phenomenon is described best for several natural products used as chemotherapeutic agents (e.g., the anthracyclines, vinca alkaloids, epipodophyllotoxins, taxanes, and dactinomycin). The only common feature of these diverse agents is that all possess planar aromatic rings and a ternary nitrogen atom. The cause of this phenomenon is the increased expression of a protein in the plasma membrane of the tumor cell, known as the *P170 glycoprotein*, the effect of which is to decrease intracellular accumulation of these compounds by increasing their efflux from the cell [129]. P170 glycoprotein is expressed widely in normal tissues and probably represents a generalized defense mechanism for decreasing the exposure of cells to environmental toxins. A number of agents have been identified that can interfere with the ability of the P170 glycoprotein to pump chemotherapeutic agents from the cell: cyclosporin A and various nonimmunosuppressive analogs; calcium channel blockers; hormonal agents (tamoxifen, progestins); amiodarone; quinidine; and aprotic polar solvents. Researchers have attempted to use these agents in the clinic to enhance the sensitivity of tumor cells to cytotoxic compounds, but thus far their clinical utility has not been proved. More recently, a second protein, known as the *multidrug resistance protein,* was identified [130]. Although genetically distinct from the P170 glycoprotein, it also appears to mediate the efflux of natural-product chemotherapeutic agents.

Drug efflux proteins are not the only mechanisms whereby tumor cells can become resistant to chemotherapeutic agents. For example, glutathione, a naturally occurring intracellular thiol, can assist in the detoxification of oxygen-free radicals, and elevated concentrations of glutathione have been shown to reduce the sensitivity of tumor cells to a number of chemotherapeutic agents, including bleomycin, doxorubicin, melphalan, and cisplatin [131]. One strategy being examined to circumvent this form of drug resistance is to impair the synthesis of glutathione with DL-buthionine sulfoximine, an inhibitor of the enzyme γ-glutamylcysteine synthetase, which catalyzes the rate-limiting step in glutathione synthesis [132]. In addition to generating high intracellular concentrations of glutathione, cells can develop resistance to alkylating agents by developing an enhanced ability to repair DNA damage. High levels of the DNA repair enzyme O^6-alkyl-guanine alkyl transferase predict resistance to nitrosoureas, dacarbazine, and temozolomide, which damage DNA by alkylating the O^6 position of guanine [133]. A strategy that is being evaluated in the clinic and that has proved successful in preclinical models is to blunt the ability of O^6-alkyl-guanine alkyl transferase to effect DNA repair by treating patients, prior to administering an alkylating agent, with O^6-benzylguanine, which has obvious structural similarity to the site of alkylation in the DNA molecule.

Resistance to chemotherapeutic agents can result from a mutation in the target of the drug or resistance may arise from amplification of the targeted enzyme, as occurs when the dihydrofolate reductase (DHFR) is overexpressed in cells resistant to MTX. Clearly, the biochemical mechanisms of drug resistance are legion. What is not clear is that attempts to circumvent any *one* mechanism of resistance will prove successful in increasing the therapeutic index of a cytotoxic agent.

Although pessimism in the field of cancer drug resistance has been generated by the diversity of mechanisms that tumor cells possess for reducing the toxicity of chemotherapeutic agents, excitement has been heightened by the recent recognition that cells share a common mechanism for orchestrating their death, even though the inciting events may be diverse. In the past, cell death has been viewed as a simple result of the inability of cells to maintain their structural and functional integrity, such that dying cells were cells that literally "fell apart," victims of entropy. In fact, however, in many circumstances cell death requires the active participation of the cells in initiating and executing a program of events that ultimately causes their demise, a process now termed *apoptosis* [134].

Apoptosis requires both energy and protein synthesis and is a necessary part of the normal development of multicellular organisms and of the maintenance of normal tissues and organs. Though the details of the apoptotic cascade still are being delineated, already several components of its control with clinical relevance have been identified. For example, overexpression of *bcl-2* inhibits apoptosis and explains the cellular accumulation responsible for the slow progression of low-grade B-cell lymphomas and chronic lymphocytic leukemia [135]. Additionally, activation of the apoptotic cascade in response to both chemotherapy and irradiation has been shown to be a *p53*-requiring process [136]. Because many tumor cells possess mutated *p53*, they not only have dysregulated control of the cell cycle but are resistant to drug- and radiation-induced apoptosis. Efforts are underway to attack this form of drug resistance by identifying compounds that can activate the apoptotic pathway or by reintroducing the missing control element (e.g., by inserting the wild-type *p53* gene into tumor cells using a viral vector).

CLINICAL DEVELOPMENT OF COMBINATION CHEMOTHERAPEUTIC REGIMENS

Given the wide array of antineoplastic agents available for use in the treatment of malignancies and given their diverse mechanisms of action, those who are not accustomed to using these drugs experience difficulty in understanding the apparent "alphabet soup" of chemotherapeutic regimens in current use. Although some regimens have a pharmacologic rationale behind them, most regimens have been developed empirically from clinical experience.

Despite the empiricism of combination chemotherapy regimens, certain principles help to guide their development. Typically, the initial approach begins with compounds that have proven activity as single agents in the disease being targeted. Alternatively, two drugs may be used in combination, because one of the drugs is known to modulate the activity of the other. An example of the latter situation is the use of leucovorin in combination with 5-FU: the effect of leucovorin is to enhance the ability of 5-FU to inhibit its target enzyme, thymidylate synthase.

Another critical factor is knowledge of the normal tissue toxicities of the agents being combined, so that overlapping toxicities are avoided. Nonetheless, many regimens combine drugs that individually cause myelosuppression. Such myelosuppressive combinations are possible because myelosuppression is reversible, because good therapy is available for support of affected patients during the period of myelosuppression, and because the relationship between dose and myelosuppression is roughly linear.

Yet another important factor is a sense of the kinetics of drug-induced toxicities. For example, combining doxorubicin and cytoxan is fairly straightforward, because both drugs produce a pattern of myelosuppression that allows them to be delivered every 21 days. However, if an attempt were made to combine doxorubicin with melphalan, the doxorubicin probably could not be delivered every 21 days because of the more delayed onset of and recovery from melphalan-induced myelosuppression.

If possible, an attractive technique is using multiple drugs that do not exhibit cross-resistance; even more attractive is the combination of drugs that exhibit synergistic antitumor effects. Conversely, an additional precaution is that agents can interact in an antagonistic manner. For example, when paclitaxel is given prior to cisplatin, additive or synergistic antitumor effects are obtained, but administration of cisplatin before paclitaxel produces less than an additive antitumor effect. Alternatively, one chemotherapeutic agent may influence another's pharmacokinetics in such a way as to enhance toxicity. For example, combining MTX and cisplatin certainly is possible but, because cisplatin is nephrotoxic and MTX is cleared by the kidneys, obvious potential pitfalls are inherent in attempting to do so.

PREDICTION OF INDIVIDUAL PATIENT TUMOR SENSITIVITY TO CHEMOTHERAPEUTIC AGENTS

An intellectually attractive alternative to the empirically gained knowledge behind selection of drugs for treating various neoplasms is to assess the sensitivity of individual patients' tumors to an array of agents in vivo before actually treating such patients. In vitro chemosensitivity testing of patient-derived tumor specimens has been and still is performed but has proved to be of limited clinical value. Often, propagating human tumor specimens in vitro is difficult. If the tumor can be grown in vitro, the cells that grow often represent only 1% or fewer of all of the cells in the original specimen. Are these cells representative of the tumor as a whole? Are they, in fact, the clonogenic cells (i.e., the stem cells that are ultimately responsible for the tumor's continued proliferation)? The artificiality of the in vitro system obviously poses additional limitations on its ability to predict in vivo responses. Is the concentration versus time exposure achieved in vitro similar to that which can be achieved in a patient? Is the degree to which the chemotherapeutic agent can gain access to the tumor lim-

ited (i.e., by virtue of poor tumor vascularity) or is the agent less active in the hypoxic, acidic tumor environment? Is the chemotherapeutic agent itself active, or does it function as a prodrug requiring in vivo activation?

Of course, additional problems are associated with obtaining tumor specimens in many patients whose disease is not readily accessible to biopsy. Another problem is the two to three weeks required to obtain an answer from the in vitro chemosensitivity testing. The human tumor clonogenic assay has demonstrated a 96% true-negative rate and a 62% true-positive rate; in other words, it is good at predicting which agents will prove ineffective in the clinic, but it is not particularly useful in predicting which agents will work [137].

An alternative strategy to the human tumor clonogenic assay is to approach the problem of chemosensitivity and resistance from a mechanistic perspective. If the drug's biochemical target in the cell is known, perhaps the activity of the drug can be predicted from knowledge regarding the presence or absence of the target in the cell. The best example of this approach is the prediction of response to antiestrogen therapy in treating breast cancer, based on the presence or absence of estrogen (and progesterone) receptor proteins in the tumor specimen.

NEW DRUG DEVELOPMENT AND CLINICAL TRIALS

As mentioned, there is an ongoing search to discover new cytotoxic and noncytotoxic therapies for the treatment of malignancies. Noncytotoxic therapies include biological response modifiers, which typically are macromolecules exerting an effect on the immune system of affected patients. Such therapies currently include the interferons and interleukins, colony-stimulating factors (e.g., G-CSF and granulocyte macrophage-CSF), monoclonal antibodies, and tumor vaccines. Another class of potentially noncytotoxic agents just starting to enter the clinic are molecules that may interfere with aberrant signal transduction or gene expression. Great interest also surrounds the genetic manipulation of tumors, although there are formidable obstacles to the practical application of this theoretically attractive approach to cancer treatment.

The National Cancer Institute of the United States long has provided leadership in the development of new anticancer therapies, and it continues to do so. However, private industry is becoming increasingly engaged in the development of new molecules and strategies for cancer treatment; given the costs involved in bringing new treatments to the clinic, this activity should be encouraged. Nonetheless, resources are limited for all involved; thus, government, academic, and industrial leaders must work together to ensure that the best ideas for new therapies are brought forward and that their clinical development is performed expeditiously, ethically, and with the best scientific underpinnings possible. Typically, a new anticancer treatment must proceed through three general phases of development before it can be made available for widespread use.

Phase I

The traditional phase I trial of a new cytotoxic drug has as its objective the definition of the maximally tolerated dose of the drug and of the dose that will be recommended for subsequent evaluation of its efficacy (the focus of the phase II trial). Separate groups of patients are treated with increasing doses of the experimental agent until dose-limiting toxicity (DLT) occurs. During this trial, an attempt is made to describe the pharmacokinetics of the drug, the determinants of its toxicity and, if possible, the effect on the drug's presumed biological target.

Phase I trials of cytotoxic agents focus on the determination of the maximum tolerated dose because dose intensity is considered to be important for cytotoxic drugs. However, in the course of evaluating other types of anticancer agents, increasing the dose to the point of toxicity may not be rational. A more generally useful idea is that of an optimum biological dose. In the case of a cytotoxic chemotherapeutic agent, the optimum biological dose and the maximum tolerated dose may be very similar. Conversely, if the agent is a receptor antagonist, as is the case for many hormonal therapies (e.g., tamoxifen), the dose administered would be increased only to the point at which the receptor was blocked completely. Increasing the dose further would not be expected to increase the drug's efficacy, but might produce increased toxicity.

Phase II

Once an acceptable dose and schedule for a new treatment have been determined from its phase I evaluation, the next step is to evaluate the potential effectiveness of the new treatment. In the typical phase I study, patients with a variety of tumor types are included; they need only have acceptable hematologic, hepatic, and renal function and a reasonable performance status. Because of the heterogeneity of the patient population studied in phase I and because many patients in the phase I evaluation are treated at suboptimal doses, making conclusions about the treatment's antitumor activity is difficult. Certainly the observation of tumor regression in the course of the treatment's phase I evaluation is encouraging, and it may suggest appropriate tumor types for subsequent investigation. However, it is the phase II study that formally attempts to gauge a therapy's antitumor activity by delivering it via an optimal dose and schedule to a group of patients with a single type and stage (extent) of tumor.

Selection of the tumor type to be studied in the phase II clinical trial may be influenced by a number of factors, including the activity of the therapy in preclinical tumor models, responses observed during the therapy's phase I evaluation, and similarity of the new compound to compounds with known activity in specific tumor types. Marketing considerations also may influence strongly the choice of the population to be targeted. The patients to be evaluated in a phase II clinical trial should have measurable tumor, a satisfactory performance status and, ideally, no or minimal prior treatment. Although for most cytotoxic agents such patients will be required to have evidence of good hematologic function, the requirements regarding other major organ function may not be as stringent as they were in a phase I trial. For example, if the phase I evaluation of a new drug determines that it is eliminated exclusively by the hepatobiliary system, the phase II trial may permit enrollment of patients with moderately impaired renal function.

A dilemma for phase II trials is that for many of the common adult solid tumors (e.g., lung cancer, colorectal cancer, breast cancer) certain standard chemotherapeutic regimens have known—albeit variably limited—activity and impact on overall survival. If a novel therapy is given only to patients in whom standard therapy has failed, the likelihood that the novel therapy will be able to exhibit antitumor activity is diminished. In many instances, this dilemma is unavoidable. However, in some situations, an ethical approach may be to treat patients first with the novel therapy prior to giving standard treatment, particularly when the disease is not immediately life-threatening and the impact of standard treatment on survival is slight. In a patient with newly diagnosed Hodgkin's disease, supporting this approach would be difficult, but it has been used successfully, with no impact on overall survival, in treating patients with advanced breast and lung carcinomas.

Phase III

Phase III clinical trials are often called *pivotal studies* because they help to establish the ultimate place of a new treatment in the standard therapy of a given disease. Typically, phase III trials are randomized studies comparing a new treatment against established therapy. Fundamental to the proper execution of phase III trials is the idea that patients should be randomly assigned prospectively to receive either the experimental or the standard treatment to eliminate bias. Methods may be used to ensure that the allocation of patients to either standard or experimental therapy is balanced in terms of prognostically important pretreatment characteristics. Phase III studies may be performed in the adjuvant setting, wherein an agent or group of agents is used in an attempt to reduce the rate of disease recurrence after definitive surgery or radiotherapy (or both). Such adjuvant studies may require that patients be assigned randomly to an untreated or placebo arm.

CHEMOTHERAPEUTIC AGENTS

It is beyond the scope of this section to describe each standard chemotherapeutic agent in detail and to give specific guidelines for its proper clinical use. This critical information is readily available from several sources [138, 139]. Rather, the current discussion will introduce the major classes of cytotoxic drugs, emphasizing their mechanisms of action, pharmacology, and unique toxicities. Selected agents will be described in some detail either because they are commonly used or because their pharmacology is particularly interesting.

Alkylating Agents

An alkylating agent, mechlorethamine, was the first nonhormonal cytotoxic drug found to be useful in the treatment of malignant disease. Although structurally diverse, all alkylators have, or generate via intermediates, reactive functional groups that are electron-deficient and that form covalent bonds with electron-rich (nucleophilic) groups in nucleic acids, proteins, and an array of smaller molecules. Despite the wide range of groups with which alkylating agents can form covalent bonds (amino, imidazole, carboxyl, sulfhydryl, and phosphate), the bases in DNA are by far the most important, particularly the electron-rich N-7 position of guanine. DNA alkylation produces a variety of defects (depurination, double-stranded and single-stranded breaks, interstrand and intrastrand cross-links) that sometimes permanently disrupt DNA replication and transcription. If it cannot be repaired efficiently, this fundamental alteration in the information coded in the DNA molecule may be expressed in cellular death, mutagenesis, or carcinogenesis. The primacy of DNA base alkylation in mediating these effects is underscored by the heightened susceptibility to alkylating agents of cells known to be deficient in DNA repair enzymes. Conversely, an increased ability to repair such damage represents one form of resistance to these drugs.

In contrast to the antimetabolites, which interfere with the pathways leading to the synthesis of new DNA (and RNA), alkylating agents react with preformed nucleic acids. Thus, they tend to be active throughout all phases of the cell cycle. Although most alkylating agents are more toxic to proliferating than to nonproliferating cells, the distinction is not as pronounced as it is for the antimetabolites; in fact, for a subset of the alkylating agents, the nitrosoureas, the distinction hardly exists at all [123]. This ability to kill nonproliferating cells renders attractive the use of alkylators against tumors with low growth fractions (e.g., multiple myeloma). Moreover, alkylating agents have an almost infinite number of potential sites in DNA for disruption and, lacking the cell-cycle specificity or cell cycle-phase specificity of antimetabolites, they typically do not exhibit a plateau in cell kill with increasing dose. These features render them theoretically attractive for testing the notion of drug intensity—the idea that the logarithmic relationship between drug dose and cell survival can be exploited to clinical advantage—as in high-dose chemotherapy followed by bone marrow rescue.

However, the same properties that render alkylating agents effective anticancer drugs produce a set of unique long-term toxicities. Their ability to kill the slowly cycling stem cells of tumors also translates into toxicity for the stem cells of the bone marrow. In contrast to the predictable and short-lived myelosuppression of drugs that merely destroy the more mature cells of the marrow (e.g., myeloblasts, myelocytes, metamyelocytes, and neutrophils), alkylators often are responsible for producing delayed, prolonged, and even permanent marrow failure. Stem cell toxicity also is manifested by the frequent development of amenorrhea in women and of oligospermia or azoospermia in men, often causing irreversible infertility. Finally, the most feared stem cell toxicity of alkylating agents is their mutagenic (and ultimately carcinogenic) effect on bone marrow stem cells, culminating in a form of AML that is relatively refractory to treatment. The risk of developing AML is directly proportional to the total drug dose administered to affected patients and to the length of follow-up; for one group of patients having ovarian carcinoma and followed up for 10 years after completing alkylator therapy, the risk of AML was as high as 5–10% [140].

The oldest group of alkylating agents, the nitrogen mustards, includes mechlorethamine (the prototype), melphalan, chlorambucil, cyclophosphamide, and ifosfamide. Mechlorethamine is a highly reactive and unstable molecule, liable to cause irritation at the site of injection; its clinical use has become rather limited to the four-drug regimen (mechlorethamine, vincristine [Oncovin®], procarbazine, and prednisone [MOPP]) used to treat Hodgkin's disease and, occasionally, other lymphomas. The other nitrogen mustards are derivatives of mechlorethamine; all contain ring structures that render them more stable and, with the exception of ifosfamide, all are available as oral preparations. Chlorambucil has a very narrow spectrum of activity, being restricted to the treatment of slowly growing lymphoid neoplasms, such as chronic lymphocytic leukemia, Waldenström's macroglobulinemia, and indolent non-Hodgkin's lymphomas. Although in the past melphalan has played a role in the treatment of breast and ovarian carcinomas, now it is used primarily for managing multiple myeloma. Melphalan is notorious for its erratic gastrointestinal absorption: 20–50% of an oral dose can be recovered in the feces. Intravenous administration of melphalan can circumvent this problem, but the usual clinical practice is to titrate the oral dose of the melphalan to point where mild hematologic toxicity occurs.

Cyclophosphamide, the most versatile alkylating agent, is unique among the nitrogen mustards on several accounts. First, cyclophosphamide is itself inactive, requiring hepatic metabolism to 4-hydroxycyclophosphamide before yielding active alkylating metabolites. 4-Hydroxycyclophosphamide (in equilibrium with its acyclic isomer, aldophosphamide) is transported into cells where it spontaneously decomposes into phosphoramide mustard and acrolein. The former species is thought to be primarily responsible for the antitumor alkylating effects of cyclophosphamide, while the latter species is excreted into the urine and is responsible for the urothelial toxicity of the drug. Second, the metabolites of cyclophosphamide have a more selective toxicity for proliferating cells than do other alkylators: prolonged myelosuppression does not occur; cumulative toxicity to the marrow is unusual; and leukemogenesis appears to be less of a problem than with other alkylat-

ing agents [141]. These advantages, coupled with the drug's activity against a very broad spectrum of tumors, have caused it to be the alkylating agent administered most commonly.

The peculiar toxicity of cyclophosphamide and its newer analog, ifosfamide, is an acute sterile hemorrhagic cystitis. As mentioned, the metabolite acrolein is thought to be the culprit. Hemorrhagic cystitis largely can be prevented by simply maintaining a high urine output, thereby reducing the exposure of the urothelium to this toxic metabolite. However, with high-dose administration of either drug, consideration should be given to the co-administration of either N-acetylcysteine (Mucomyst) or sodium 2-mercaptoethanesulfonate (mesna), thiol compounds that neutralize acrolein.

The pharmacokinetics of cyclophosphamide have not been described fully because of the difficulty in detecting some of its metabolites in plasma. Nonetheless, both the parent compound and its metabolites clearly are excreted by the kidneys. Renal failure results in prolonged blood levels but usually not in increased toxicity, probably because renal clearance of the parent drug is normally low and can be maintained even in patients with marginal renal function. Because cyclophosphamide requires activation by hepatic microsomal enzymes, liver dysfunction would be anticipated to prompt a change in dose. Systematic data regarding the influence of renal and hepatic dysfunction on the choice of dose is lacking, however. Common sense would suggest attenuated doses of cyclophosphamide in patients with severe renal failure.

There are four other chemical classes of alkylating agents: (1) the nitrosoureas (carmustine, lomustine, semustine, streptozotocin); (2) the alkyl sulfonates (busulfan); (3) the triazines (dacarbazine, or DTIC); and (4) the ethylenimines (thiotepa, hexamethylmelamine). The nitrosoureas are distinguished by their lipid solubility—suggesting a potential role in the treatment of intracranial tumors—and by their lack of cross-resistance with other alkylating agents. Their clinical usefulness has been limited, however, by a tendency to cause myelosuppression that is more delayed, prolonged, and cumulative than that of other alkylators. Busulfan, the only alkyl sulfonate in clinical use, deserves mention for its long-standing role in CML, a role based on a high degree of selectivity for the myeloid cells of the bone marrow. In some cases, busulfan can produce a period of drug-free, albeit always impermanent, clinical remission in CML.

Platinum Compounds

CISPLATIN

The discovery of cisplatin was fortuitous. During experiments on the effect of electrical currents on bacterial growth, growth inhibition was observed in a zone immediately adjacent to platinum electrodes. Of numerous platinum compounds in solution, the active substance was demonstrated to be cisplatin. Subsequent work demonstrated its activity against a variety of tumors.

Cisplatin (*cis*-diaminodichloroplatinum II) is an inorganic planar coordination complex, the platinum atom coordinated to two amine groups on one side and two chlorine atoms on the other. Cytotoxicity arises from mechanisms similar to those of classic alkylating agents. The chlorine atoms of the complex function as leaving groups, displaced by nucleophiles, such as the bases in DNA. In actuality, the chlorine atoms first must be displaced by water molecules, producing a charged platinum complex, prior to nucleophilic addition. The substitution of water for chlorine proceeds slowly in the presence of a high chloride concentration, as is present in plasma; theoretically then, formation of the active, charged complex should occur intracellularly, where the chloride concentration is low. As with classic alkylating agents, the preferred site for binding of cisplatin to DNA is the N-7 position of guanine. Being bifunctional (having two leaving groups), cisplatin can form interstrand DNA cross-links, the number of which correlates with the drug's cytotoxicity. The *trans*-isomer of cisplatin, which is inactive, produces DNA-protein cross-links but cannot form DNA interstrand cross-links at clinically relevant concentrations. Interstrand cross-links form slowly and are opposed by the enzymatic mechanisms of excision and repair; resistance to the drug may arise from these processes. Cisplatin is most active in phase G_1 but behaves predominantly in a phase-nonspecific manner.

Cisplatin is given intravenously, although it can also be given intraperitoneally for treatment of ovarian carcinoma. By IV injection, approximately 90% of the drug becomes rapidly bound to proteins and is cleared from the plasma slowly. That proportion of the dose that remains as free drug—the active form of cisplatin—is cleared rapidly; 90% of this free drug is cleared from the plasma during the first two hours after injection. Cisplatin is cleared almost exclusively by the kidneys, primarily the result of glomerular filtration. The rate of cisplatin clearance can be accelerated by maneuvers aimed at increasing urinary output (e.g., saline or mannitol diuresis), explaining in part the protective effect of diuresis against the drug's toxicities.

The major dose-limiting toxicity of cisplatin is renal damage; it is a direct tubular toxin, preferentially affecting the proximal straight tubule and the distal and collecting tubules. In addition to experiencing a decline in glomerular filtration rate, many patients waste magnesium and other electrolytes as a result of tubular dysfunction. Usually, acute nephrotoxicity attributable to cisplatin therapy is reversible; with repeated dosing, however, cumulative damage of a more permanent nature does occur. Ensuring rapid clearance of the free drug by saline or mannitol diuresis is one way of minimizing nephrotoxicity. However, an even greater degree of protection is needed in administering very high doses of cisplatin. A simple means of providing additional protection is to administer the drug in 3% (hypertonic) saline; not only is a diuresis established but the generation of a high urinary chloride concentration slows the formation of toxic, charged, water-substituted complex in the lumen of the renal tubule. Other toxicities of cisplatin include ototoxicity (tinnitus, high-frequency hearing loss), peripheral neuropathy (usually in the form of a stocking-glove-distribution sensory loss with paresthesias), and relatively severe nausea and vomiting. In contrast to the classic alkylating agents, cisplatin is only mildly myelotoxic, rendering it an attractive drug for many combination regimens.

Cisplatin is the most active single agent against both seminomatous and nonseminomatous testicular cancers; when combined with VP16 and bleomycin, it is usually curative. It has clear activity in its gynecologic counterparts, the germ-cell tumors of the ovary. Cisplatin also forms the cornerstone for regimens used in the treatment of advanced ovarian carcinoma, typically being combined with a taxane or an alkylating agent, such as cyclophosphamide. Cisplatin is also an important component of regimens used to treat both small- and non-small-cell lung cancers, transitional cell carcinoma of bladder, head and neck cancer, and tumors of the upper gastrointestinal tract.

CARBOPLATIN

Carboplatin (diaminocyclobutane-dicarboxylatoplatinum [II]), as implied by its name, is a platinum-containing compound closely related to cisplatin. It differs from cisplatin in that its dose-limiting toxicity, like that of a typical alkylating agent, is myelosuppression. In conventional doses, it causes much less nausea and vomiting and renal toxicity, neurotoxicity, and ototoxicity than does cisplatin. Like cisplatin, carboplatin is eliminated largely by glomerular filtration, and it is now common to adjust carboplatin dosing according to the individual patient's estimated creatinine clearance. The formula used most commonly is one that was proposed initially by Calvert et al. [142] and then was modified by Jodrell et al. [143]: AUC (carboplatin) = dose/(creatinine clearance + 25), where AUC ("area under the curve") is the total concentration-versus-time exposure resulting from a single dose of the drug (mg-min/ml), dose is expressed in total milligrams (*not* mg/m²), and creatinine clearance is measured in milliliters per minute. Though some high-dose regimens requiring peripheral blood stem cell or marrow support may target the delivery of AUCs as high as 18 mg-min/ml, in conventional regimens doses are administered with the intention of producing AUCs in the range of 5–7 mg-min/ml.

Although carboplatin and cisplatin are related closely, they are not always interchangeable. Not only do they have different toxicities, but their spectrums of antitumor activity differ as well. For example, compared with cisplatin, carboplatin yields inferior results in the treatment of nonseminomatous testicular carcinoma. In contrast, preliminary results from the Southwest Oncology Group [144] suggest that it may be equivalent in the treatment of advanced ovarian carcinoma.

Antimetabolites

Interest in antimetabolite development followed the discovery that folic acid antagonists were effective in the treatment of childhood ALL. Elucidation of the biochemical pathways leading to DNA and RNA synthesis permitted the proliferation of a large number of drugs fashioned to be structurally similar to critical intermediates (metabolites) in these pathways. Antimetabolites function either by competing with normal metabolites for the catalytic or regulatory site of a key enzyme or by substituting for a metabolite that normally is incorporated into an important molecule (e.g., DNA or RNA). Because most antimetabolites interfere with nucleic acid synthesis (rather than with preformed nucleic acids, as do the alkylating agents), they have little, if any, effect on cells in phase G_0 and usually exhibit maximum activity during S phase. The enzymes inhibited by antimetabolites are fewer than the sites potentially available to alkylating agents (i.e., the almost innumerable bases of DNA), and complete inhibition of these enzymes may occur at clinically achievable drug levels.

Such relatively complete target inhibition, coupled with specificity for cells in a single phase of the cell cycle, explains the plateau in cell survival with increasing drug dose. Also in contrast to the alkylating agents, antimetabolites are not associated with delayed or prolonged myelosuppression, and they appear to present a minimal risk of leukemogenesis or carcinogenesis.

FOLIC ACID ANALOGS

A number of folic acid analogs have been produced that inhibit the enzyme DHFR. However, only MTX is used commonly as an anticancer drug. DHFR is responsible for the generation of reduced folates, molecules occupying key positions in nucleic acid synthesis. Reduced folates are required for the transfer of methyl groups during the biosynthesis of purines. Moreover, inhibition of DHFR blocks the production of N_5,N_{10}-methylene tetrahydrofolate, a reduced folate coenzyme that participates with thymidylate synthetase in the conversion of 2-deoxyuridylate to thymidylate (dTMP). DNA synthesis ceases as a result of this lack of dTMP and purines.

Plasma MTX is approximately 50% bound to plasma proteins and is eliminated primarily by the kidneys without extensive metabolism. Disappearance of MTX from the plasma is essentially biphasic: The initial distribution phase has a half-life of 20 minutes to 3 hours, while the final phase has a half-life of 8–10 hours. The terminal phase is prolonged in the face of renal dysfunction. A third elimination phase, which occurs very slowly, also has been described and is attributed to enterohepatic recirculation of the drug. The renal excretion of MTX can be inhibited by coadministration of weak organic acids (e.g., aspirin or penicillin). Aspirin therapy can compound toxicity further by displacing MTX from its binding site on albumin, increasing the concentration of free drug.

The cytotoxicity of MTX depends critically on the duration of exposure of a tissue to the drug above a certain threshold value rather than on the peak level of drug in the tissue [145]. Irrespective of the duration of exposure to MTX, toxicity for many tissues does not occur until the level of drug exceeds 10^{-8} M. Conversely, exceedingly high levels of MTX may be tolerated well by normal tissues provided exposure is limited to 24–36 hours. The availability of a reduced folate "antidote" in the form of 5-formyltetrahydrofolate (leucovorin or citrovorum factor) allows the duration of MTX-induced dTMP and purine depletion to be controlled precisely; the ability to measure serum MTX levels allows one to determine how much leucovorin to administer and when leucovorin rescue may be safely discontinued.

An appreciation of these details of MTX pharmacology has permitted MTX to be delivered in doses 10–100 times greater than given conventionally. The major impetus to administration of such high doses is the theoretic possibility of thereby overcoming some forms of MTX resistance: defects in active transport of the drug might be overcome by passive diffusion; increased amounts of DHFR from gene amplification might be inhibited more completely; intracellular levels of the drug might remain high despite decreased polyglutamation; and even enzymes with reduced affinity for MTX might be inhibited. Moreover, high-dose MTX followed by leucovorin rescue can achieve tumoricidal drug levels in the CNS and, if performed properly, is not associated with myelosuppression. This latter advantage would also permit more frequent drug administration.

These theoretical advantages explain the inclusion of high-dose MTX with leucovorin rescue in experimental protocols for such diseases as ALL, lymphomas, and tumors of the head and neck. Yet the only disease for which high-dose MTX with leucovorin rescue has become standard is osteogenic sarcoma. Indeed, responses to high-dose MTX are observed rarely in patients whose tumors are refractory to conventional doses. The supposition is that the resistance of in vivo human tumors to MTX has less to do with the mechanisms of resistance cited heretofore and perhaps more to do with the limited potential of a drug that depends so heavily on DNA synthesis for its toxicity in the treatment of tumors with low growth fractions. The exquisite sensitivity of rapidly proliferating gestational trophoblastic neoplasia to conventional doses of MTX lends additional credence to this argument. Enthusiasm for high-dose regimens is tempered also by (1) the propensity of MTX in high doses to precipitate in the renal tubules (avoided by maintaining a high urine output and by alkalinizing the urine, all of which typically require hospitalization); (2) the tendency of MTX in high doses to accumulate significantly within third-space fluid compartments (e.g., pleural and peritoneal effusions) and thereafter to diffuse out of them slowly, producing prolonged exposure to the drug; (3) the need to measure plasma MTX levels; and (4) the cost of such treatment.

With standard doses of MTX, given without leucovorin rescue, myelosuppression is frequent but generally mild to moderate. The time to the nadir is slightly shorter than that with alkylating agents and is followed by rapid recovery. Usually, nausea and vomiting are absent or mild, but mucositis can be disabling, involving the entire oral and gastrointestinal mucosa and posing the risk for secondary superinfection and, rarely, perforation. Diarrhea is also seen occasionally. Infrequently,

patients may have transient elevation of liver function test results, but hepatic damage is uncommon except in patients receiving a long-term, low oral dosage, in whom fibrosis and cirrhosis have been reported. Pulmonary complications, allergic reactions, and significant alopecia are uncommon.

MTX enjoys a wide spectrum of antitumor activity but rarely is used as a single agent. However, as cited earlier, it is often curative as a single agent in the treatment of gestational trophoblastic neoplasia. MTX is included in many combination regimens for ALL, lymphomas, carcinoma of the breast, and tumors of the head and neck. It is particularly useful as an intrathecal agent in treating leptomeningeal tumor infiltrates.

PYRIMIDINE ANALOGS

The pyrimidine analogs include 5-FU, 5-fluorodeoxyuridine (5-FUdR), cytosine arabinoside (Ara-C), and gemcitabine.

5-Fluorouracil

5-FU resembles both uracil and thymidine. Phosphorylation of 5-FU to 5-fluorouridine triphosphate (5-FUdTP) allows the analog to be incorporated into RNA; nuclear processing of messenger and ribosomal RNA is disrupted, and the fraudulent pyrimidine may cause errors in base pairing during RNA transcription. 5-FU also is converted to 5-fluorouridine monophosphate (5-FUdMP), a compound that irreversibly inhibits thymidylate synthetase; DNA synthesis is brought to a halt because of thymidine depletion. These two mechanisms of cytotoxicity allow 5-FU to be active throughout the cell cycle, not just in S phase. A single IV bolus of 5-FU has a plasma half-life of only 10–30 minutes, and no drug can be detected in plasma after three hours; however, intracellular levels may persist for hours. Because of the short plasma half-life of the drug and because its effects on DNA synthesis are expressed only in cells undergoing S phase, it sometimes is administered by continuous IV infusion. In one study, a prolonged continuous infusion schedule of 5-FU, when compared with standard bolus therapy, did yield a higher response proportion in metastatic colorectal carcinoma (30% versus 7%, respectively), but this higher response proportion did not translate into improved survival [146].

5-FU has been given orally, but its low oral bioavailability precludes the routine use of this method. Research continues to identify strategies for increasing the drug's bioavailability, either by the administration of prodrugs (e.g., ftorafur) or by the coadministration of compounds that inhibit the catabolism of 5-FU (e.g., uracil). Solutions and creams containing fluorouracil also are available and have been used for patients with premalignant keratoses and malignant lesions of the skin. In addition, 5-FU and its closely related analog, 5-FUdR, have been used for intraarterial therapy, most notably in patients with hepatic metastases from colorectal carcinoma.

5-FU is not significantly emetogenic but can be fairly toxic to the gastrointestinal epithelium. Stomatitis and diarrhea can result in life-threatening intravascular volume depletion and gram-negative septicemia. Generally, leukopenia and thrombocytopenia are mild, with nadirs occurring in these counts some 7–14 days after drug administration. Recovery from myelosuppression is usually rapid. Significant alopecia is rare. The drug is associated occasionally with hyperpigmentation of the nail beds and superficial veins. Cerebellar ataxia is an unusual but significant complication of 5-FU seen after very large doses or infusions; it typically subsides spontaneously after discontinuation of therapy. Another unusual complication of the drug is its ability to precipitate cardiac ischemia, particularly in patients with known coronary artery disease.

The type of toxicity observed with 5-FU therapy depends on the regimen used for its administration. For example, giving the drug daily for five consecutive days once every three to four weeks primarily produces myelosuppression. In contrast, the dose-limiting complication of 5-FU given as a once a week injection more commonly is diarrhea. Low-dose, continuous-infusion 5-FU regimens also are more likely to produce stomatitis and diarrhea and are associated with the development of painful erythema of the palms and soles (so-called hand-foot syndrome).

5-FU as a single agent exhibits only modest activity in solid tumors. Recently, the effectiveness of 5-FU appears to have been enhanced modestly by the concomitant administration of leucovorin. When 5-fluorouridine monophosphate binds to thymidylate synthetase, it forms part of a ternary complex that includes N_5,N_{10}-methylenetetrahydrofolate, the normal coenzyme for thymidylate synthetase. Although this ternary complex is covalent, it dissociates with a half-life of two to three hours in the absence of excess N_5,N_{10}-methylenetetrahydrofolate. High levels of N_5,N_{10}-methylenetetrahydrofolate, derived from leucovorin, produce optimal conditions for the formation of this complex and deter its subsequent degradation. Clinical trials have shown that the combination of 5-FU and leucovorin has activity greater than that of 5-FU alone in the treatment of advanced colon cancer. However, although the response proportion in colon cancer is higher when leucovorin is added to 5-FU, little evidence suggests a survival advantage [146].

Cytosine arabinoside

Cytosine arabinoside (Ara-C) differs from deoxycytidine only in its sugar moiety, with arabinose replacing deoxyribose. Ara-C penetrates cells via a carrier-mediated process shared with deoxycytidine. Once inside the cell Ara-C, like deoxycytidine, can follow one of two major paths: deamination to the non-toxic compound, Ara-U, or sequential phosphorylation to Ara-CTP, the active form of the drug. The toxicity of Ara-CTP arises from its ability to competitively inhibit the binding of the normal substrate, dCTP, to DNA polymerase; DNA synthesis is thereby arrested. Ara-CTP also may be incorporated into DNA and cause defective ligation or incomplete synthesis of DNA fragments. Both effects are consistent with the selective toxicity of this drug for cells in S phase.

Following IV injection, Ara-C is rapidly inactivated to Ara-U by cytidine deaminase, an enzyme widely distributed throughout the body. After a single bolus injection Ara-C has a plasma elimination half-life of only 7–20 minutes. Single bolus injections of Ara-C tend to be non-toxic to normal marrow and are ineffective in treating leukemia as well. However, if the drug is administered in two divided doses separated by 12 hours, a significant number of patients with leukemia respond. The greater effectiveness of the q 12-hour regimen lies in the fact that the S phase of AML blasts lasts approximately 18–20 hours. If a leukemia cell is in the cell cycle but not in S phase at the time of a bolus injection of Ara-C, it escapes toxicity, since the half-life of Ara-C is so brief. And if the next bolus of Ara-C is not administered until 24 hours later, the same cell may have already passed through S phase and so evade the drug's effects altogether. Yet when Ara-C is given on a q 12-hour schedule, no cycling cell can pas through a complete S phase without being exposed to the drug. If all leukemia cells were in cycle (i.e., if none were in G_0), then from a purely kinetic perspective it would be possible to kill all cells by delivering Ara-C as a bolus every 12 hours or as a continuous infusion over the time required to complete one cell cycle. But many leukemia cells are indeed in G_0, so Ara-C must be administered for a longer period (5–7 days) to allow as many of these cells as possible to enter the proliferating pool and pass through S phase.

Most drug combinations in current use have evolved empirically, and the sequence in which the drugs are administered usually reflects little more than an attempt to avoid overlapping toxicities. The sequential use of Ara-C and asparaginase to induce remission in patients with refractory or relapsed AML represents an important exception that shows how the sequence of drug administration can be critical.

Asparaginase is an enzyme derived from bacterial sources. When given intravenously it hydrolyzes serum asparagine and deprives leukemia cells of an amino acid they themselves cannot synthesize; normal cells are spared because they generally have the ability to synthesize their own asparagine. When studied in a murine model of leukemia, pharmacologic antagonism occurred when both drugs were administered concurrently or when the asparaginase treatment preceded delivery of Ara-C [147]. The explanation for this antagonism is that asparaginase depletion shuts down protein synthesis, which inhibits the progression of tumor cells from G_1 into S phase. Since Ara-C is active only in cells in S phase, asparaginase pretreatment is actually protective. However, if asparaginase is given after Ara-C, synergistic killing of leukemia cells is observed, associated with increased formation of Ara-CTP and Ara-C-containing DNA. For unclear reasons, asparaginase treatment also lowers the cellular pool of the normal metabolite, dCTP, and thus reduces the amount of the normal substrate against which Ara-C must compete. These laboratory observations led to the design of a clinical trial comparing high-dose Ara-C alone to high-dose Ara-C followed by asparaginase treatment in patients with refractory or relapsed AML. The preclinical pharmacologic considerations bore fruit: the use of sequential high-dose Ara-C and asparaginase resulted in a complete remission rate of 42%, while high-dose Ara-C alone achieved a complete remission rate of only 12% [148].

Purine Analogs

There are two guanine analogs in clinical use: 6-mercaptopurine (6-MP) and 6-thioguanine (6-TG). These two drugs are very similar to one another, and resistance to one drug usually predicts resistance to the other. Both parent compounds are inactive until they undergo metabolic conversion to their respective monophosphate ribonucleotides, a result of the enzyme hypoxanthine-guanine phosphoribosyl transferase (HGPRTase), whose normal function is to salvage purines for nucleic acid synthesis by adding ribose phosphate to them. The monophosphate nucleotides are capable of inhibiting de novo purine synthesis (i.e., the formation of adenylic and guanylic acids from inosinic acid). Further phosphorylation gives rise to the respective triphosphate nucleotides. In the case of 6-TG, conversion to the deoxyribonucleotide allows significant amounts of the drug to be incorporated into DNA, the extent of which correlates with the production of strand breaks and cellular cytotoxicity.

In experimental tumors it has been possible to show that resistance to these two purine analogs can ensue from a deficiency in the activating enzyme, HGPRTase. However, leukemia cells are not typically deficient in this enzyme, and other mechanisms of resistance must be important (e.g., rapid dephosphorylation of the active nucleotides by a membrane-bound alkaline phosphatase).

6-MP and 6-TG are used almost exclusively to treat leukemias; they have no signficant activity against solid tumors. Because of their use in the treatment of leukemia, it is important to understand the differences in their catabolism. 6-MP is oxidized to 6-thiouric acid by xanthine oxidase. The concomitant administration of allopurinol, an inhibitor of xanthine oxidase used to prevent hyperuricemia and acute uric acid nephropathy during rapid leukemia cell lysis, may increase the toxicity of 6-MP by impairing its degradation. The dose of 6-MP is therefore reduced by 75% if allopurinol is to be coadministered. The catabolism of 6-TG follows a different pathway and no dose reduction is required in the presence of allopurinol.

Adenosine Analogs

Several adenosine analogs exist, but their clinical use is restricted to specific lymphoid malignancies. Pentostatin (2-deoxycoformycin) is an adenosine analog produced by a species of *Streptomyces*. It is a powerful inhibitor of adenosine deaminase (ADA), an enzyme that deaminates adenosine to inosine and deoxyadenosine to deoxyinosine. Accumulation of adenosine and deoxyadenosine is toxic to cells, particularly to those of the lymphoid system, as suggested by the severe lymphopenia of children with congenital ADA deficiency. Pentostatin is used primarily in the treatment of hairy cell leukemia. Fludarabine is an adenosine analog that is relatively resistant to deamination by adenosine deaminase. It is used in the treatment of chronic lymphocytic leukemia and low-grade lymphomas.

Topoisomerase I Inhibitors

The currently available topoisomerase I inhibitors topotecan and irinotecan belong to a class of compounds known as the *camptothecins*. The parent compound of this group of drugs, camptothecin, was derived from a Chinese tree, *Camptotheca acuminata*. Camptothecin and all of its analogs are lactones that normally exist in a pH-dependent equilibrium with their corresponding hydroxycarboxylic acids. The lactone forms of these compounds are the more biologically active species.

Camptothecin itself is poorly soluble in water, and initial clinical trials of camptothecin conducted in the early 1970s used the salt of the corresponding hydroxycarboxylic acid. When camptothecin was delivered in this manner, it caused unpredictable hematologic and urothelial toxicities; thus, attempts at further development were abandoned. Most likely, the variability in hematologic toxicity arose from variable conversion of the hydroxycarboxylic acid back to the lactone, because the pH of the solution was not controlled. The hemorrhagic cystitis that occurred may have been due to renal excretion of large amounts of relatively inactive hydroxycarboxylic acid that were converted back to the active lactone in the acidic environment of the urine. Addition of hydrophilic substituents to the parent camptothecin structure has permitted the creation of more water-soluble compounds that can be administered in their lactone forms and that have more predictable clinical effects.

The mechanism of action of the topoisomerase I inhibitors is unique. In fact, the use of the term *inhibitor* is somewhat misleading. Topoisomerase I is a constitutively expressed enzyme found in all mammalian cells and involved in DNA replication and recombination and in RNA transcription. For these processes to occur, the normally supercoiled, double-stranded DNA molecule must be relaxed or unraveled at the appropriate locus. Topoisomerase I binds preferentially to supercoiled, double-stranded DNA and cleaves the phosphodiester bond of the DNA backbone, resulting in a single-strand nick. This action allows relief of torsional strain in the DNA molecule by permitting the intact strand to pass through the single-strand nick or by facilitating rotation around the intact strand's phosphodiester bond. Once the torsional strain has been relieved and the relevant DNA process has been completed, the topoisomerase I enzyme catalyzes the reverse reaction (i.e., the repair or religation of the single-stranded DNA nick). Typically, this sequence of DNA nicking, relief of torsional strain, and religation is rapid, and detecting the topoisomerase I enzyme in association with DNA is difficult. The camptothecins perturb this sequence of events by inhibiting the process of religation.

Stated differently, the camptothecins stabilize the normally transient complex of topoisomerase I with single-stranded nicks in the DNA molecule. Although single-stranded DNA breaks are not themselves lethal, when a replication fork encounters a persistent single-stranded nick, the result may be a double-stranded DNA break. These double-stranded breaks are more often lethal for the cell. This explanation for the toxicity of camptothecins, known as the *fork collision model*, predicts that the toxicity of topoisomerase I inhibitors should be expressed primarily in cells undergoing DNA replication (i.e., those in S phase). Both preclinical and clinical information support the cell cycle-phase specificity of the biological effects of topoisomerase I inhibitors.

CPT-11 (IRINOTECAN)

CPT-11 is the first camptothecin derivative to have been successfully developed in the clinic. Although it has a broad spectrum of antitumor activity (colorectal cancer, small and non-small cell lung cancer, cervical cancer, ovarian cancer), its use in the United States has been primarily limited to the treatment of patients with metastatic colorectal cancer, first in the treatment of 5-FU-refractory disease, and more recently as first-line therapy for metastatic colorectal cancer in combination with 5-FU.

CPT-11 is a prodrug that requires enzymatic cleavage of a side chain moiety by a ubiquitous carboxylesterase converting enzyme to yield the biologically active metabolite, SN-38. Both CPT-11 and SN-38 undergo non-enzymatic hydrolysis of their lactone rings to form the less biologically active open-ring carboxylate species. The pharmacokinetics of CPT-11 are complex. Approximately 22% of the drug is eliminated unchanged into the urine. The SN-38 lactone has an elimination half-life of approximately seven hours, and is excreted into the bile either as SN-38 or as the non-toxic SN-38 glucuronide. The amount of non-glucuronidated SN-38 that is excreted into the bile and from thence into the gastrointestinal tract is thought to be primarily responsible for the severe, late-onset diarrhea that can accompany treatment with CPT-11. While it is difficult to predict the likelihood that an individual patient will experience late-onset diarrhea as the result of CPT-11 therapy, therapy with high-dose loperamide has been effective in ameliorating this problem.

Two regimens have been commonly used for CPT-11 therapy. In Japan and the United States CPT-11 was developed using a weekly schedule of drug administration (e.g., 100–125 mg/m²/week for four of six weeks, and in Europe CPT-11 has more commonly been given as a single 350 mg/m² infusion once every three or four weeks). In addition to the unpredictable late-onset diarrhea, therapy with CPT-11 is associated with myelosuppression (primarily neutropenia), nausea and vomiting (which can often be protracted), fatigue, elevated liver function tests (reversible), and rarely with pulmonary toxicity.

A randomized trial of irinotecan plus supportive care versus supportive care alone was performed after 5-FU failure in patients with metastatic colorectal cancer [149]. Patients with proven metastatic colorectal cancer that had progressed within six months of treatment with 5-FU were assigned randomly to receive either 300–350 mg/m² of irinotecan every three weeks with supportive care or to receive supportive care alone. The overall survival was significantly better for those patients who received irinotecan, with a 36.2% one-year survival compared with 13.8% in those in the supportive care only group. A quality-of-life analysis supported the use of irinotecan when compared with supportive care only.

Another study compared irinotecan, 350 mg/m² infused every three weeks, with 5-FU by continuous infusion in patients who had failed to respond to first-line 5-FU or whose disease had progressed after treatment with first-line 5-FU therapy [150]. Survival at one year was increased from 32% in those in the 5-FU group to 45% in those in the irinotecan group. Median survival was 10.8 months for the irinotecan group and 8.5 months for the 5-FU group. Quality-of-life assessment was similar in both groups. Irinotecan is now used with 5-FU in the first-line therapy of metastatic colorectal cancer.

TOPOTECAN

Topotecan is relatively water soluble compared with the parent camptothecin molecule. After IV infusion, topotecan is cleaved rapidly and nonenzymatically to the corresponding hydroxycarboxylic acid, such that exposure to lactone represents only 18–33% of total drug exposure. The pharmacokinetics of topotecan are linear. The lactone has an elimination half-life of approximately 1.7–3.4 hours, and total drug is eliminated with a half-life of 2.9–4.3 hours. Topotecan carboxylate is cleared primarily by the kidneys, and current recommendations are to reduce the dose of the drug given to patients with impaired renal function. In patients with a creatinine clearance of 40 ml/min or greater, no reduction in dose is suggested; in those with a creatinine clearance of 20 ml/min or less, the recommendation is that topotecan not be given at all. For those patients with creatinine clearances between 21 and 39 ml/min, it is suggested that the topotecan dose be reduced by 50%.

No information is available to indicate that the dose of topotecan should be reduced if the hepatic function is impaired. Topotecan binds insignificantly to plasma proteins (< 20%), a fact that may account in part for its relatively high penetrance into the CNS. Cerebrospinal fluid concentrations of topotecan lactone are approximately one-third of simultaneous plasma concentrations.

When given in its current US Food and Drug Administration (FDA)–approved dose and schedule of 1.5 mg/m²/day infused daily over a 30-minute period for five consecutive days and repeated every three weeks, the primary dose-limiting toxicity of topotecan is neutropenia, although thrombocytopenia is more common than with CPT-11. In general, clinical trials of topotecan have used relatively aggressive definitions of dose-limiting toxicity; thus, at this dose and schedule, severe neutropenia (absolute neutrophil count < 500/mm³) is common. The neutrophil nadir occurs around day 10, and recovery is complete by day 21, allowing cycles of therapy to be given on an every three-week basis. Nonhematologic toxicities with this dose and schedule of topotecan administration are infrequent and typically mild. They include nausea and vomiting, alopecia, mucositis, elevated hepatic transaminases, skin rash, and fever.

Topotecan is approved by the US FDA for the treatment of patients with advanced ovarian cancer that has recurred in spite of previous platinum-based chemotherapy [151], and in the second-line treatment of small-cell lung cancer.

Antitumor Antibiotics

The antitumor antibiotics—the anthracyclines, anthracenediones, dactinomycin, bleomycin, and mitomycin C—are a structurally diverse group of compounds derived from microbial fermentation. Their cytotoxicity precludes their use as antibacterial agents, but they have proved to be valuable in treating a broad spectrum of tumors.

ANTHRACYCLINES

Doxorubicin, the anthracycline administered most commonly, consists of a planar, four-ring anthraquinone attached to an amino sugar, daunosamine. The related compound, daunorubicin, differs from doxorubicin only by the substitution of a methoxy for a methyl group in the anthraquinone ring; daunorubicin is used almost exclusively in the treatment of acute leukemia.

The structure-function relationships of doxorubicin and other anthracyclines have been examined widely because they are among the most effective antitumor agents available, yet they produce dose-limiting cardiotoxicity. The clinical benefit of separating the two effects would be substantial. The mechanisms underlying anthracycline cytotoxicity are complex. First, the anthraquinone ring can intercalate base pairs of DNA, the stability of this complex being enhanced by the attraction of the amino group of daunosamine for the phosphate groups of the DNA backbone. DNA intercalation results in disruption of DNA replication and RNA transcription; what is uncertain is just how important intercalation is to anthracycline cytotoxicity. Normally, DNA is organized and folded into chromatin and perhaps is protected from this type of drug interaction. Second, anthracyclines can produce single-stranded and double-stranded DNA scission and thereby impair DNA repair. The process of DNA scission may be facilitated by base pair intercalation or by an interaction with topoisomerase II. A third mechanism for generating both DNA breaks and other forms of damage is the creation of free radicals. The quinone ring of the anthracyclines can assume a semiquinone form with an unpaired electron; this species reacts with molecular oxygen (O_2) to generate superoxide (O_2^-), which disrupts a wide variety of cellular structures, including DNA. However, doxorubicin retains toxicity under hypoxic conditions when superoxide radicals cannot be formed. Finally, anthracyclines tend to bind to almost everything with which they come into contact, and possibly kill cells through disruption of the cell membrane. In fact, in one experimental system in which doxorubicin was attached to small beads, cell death occurred despite the inability of the drug to enter cells, lending credence both to the notion of direct membrane disruption and to the importance of free radical formation [152]. Nonetheless, a large body of literature supports the idea that anthracycline toxicity in many systems depends on the drug's ability to enter cells; witness their susceptibility to the phenomenon of multidrug resistance, characterized by increased efflux of anthracyclines and other natural products across the cell membrane. As might be anticipated, given their wide-ranging effects, the anthracyclines exhibit activity throughout the cell cycle, although effects are most pronounced for cells in S or G_2 phase.

Doxorubicin is administered intravenously and is distributed widely in the body. It binds extensively to plasma proteins and other tissues. Plasma clearance is triphasic: the half-lives of the three phases are 8–25 minutes, 1.5–10.0 hours, and 24–48 hours. The second phase is attributed to hepatic metabolism of the drug to yield an active metabolite (doxorubicinol) and a number of metabolites (aglycones) that have no antitumor effect but may contribute to cardiac and other toxicities. The final phase reflects release of drug from tissue binding sites. Because doxorubicin and its metabolites are excreted through the bile, dosage reduction is mandatory for patients with biliary obstruction.

The major toxicity of doxorubicin is myelosuppression, with granulocytes being affected more severely than are platelets. Usually, the nadir count occurs one to two weeks after the drug has been administered, with a typically rapid return to normal pretreatment levels. Total alopecia is almost always observed. Nausea, vomiting, and stomatitis are moderate. The drug must be administered with great caution because leakage into tissues can cause severe necrosis, which on occasion has led to limb loss. In a small percentage of patients, a reddish hue and flare may be noted in the vein used for drug administration, a rapidly resolving side effect not indicative of a drug leakage. Hyperpigmentation has also been noted. An insignificant but frequently alarming side effect is the passage of red urine, owing to renal excretion of the parent drug. Usually, this reaction occurs within hours of drug administration and is of no clinical consequence. "Recall" reactions, consisting of erythema and occasional skin ulceration at sites that have received prior radiation, can occur months after therapy has been completed.

As mentioned, the unique toxicity of doxorubicin is damage to heart muscle, a problem that increases in incidence with an increasing cumulative dose of the drug. As the total dose of doxorubicin approaches 550 mg/m², the incidence rate of chronic congestive heart failure becomes 1–4%; above this cumulative dose, the incidence rises more dramatically. Thus, most protocols dictate that the lifetime cumulative doxorubicin dose does not exceed 450 mg/m². Patients who receive significant doses of doxorubicin should be monitored for cardiotoxicity. The gold standard for assessing doxorubicin-induced cardiac toxicity is the endomyocardial biopsy. Although this procedure reflects drug-related myocardial damage in a manner that is linear with dose, it is neither practical nor widely available. Most commonly, the left ventricular ejection fraction is determined by radionuclide cineangiography at serial total doses of the drug, with cessation of doxorubicin therapy if the left ventricular ejection fraction drops significantly below the baseline value. Also important is an awareness of the increased risk of anthracycline-induced cardiotoxicity in the presence of other cardiac insults (e.g., prior mediastinal irradiation, systemic hypertension, and the coadministration of mitomycin C or high doses of cyclophosphamide). Elderly patients often have clinically occult myocardial disease, and a common reaction in older patients is the development of left ventricular dysfunction at lower cumulative doses of doxorubicin.

Several doxorubicin analogs have been studied extensively in phase II trials, including epirubicin, esorubicin (deoxydoxorubicin), and menogaril. To date, these analogs have not proved superior to the parent compound, and all are potentially cardiotoxic. As mentioned, the ability of anthracyclines to generate free radicals has been implicated in the production of cardiotoxicity. Clinical trials of the free radical scavengers vitamin E and N-acetylcysteine, which lessen the cardiotoxicity of doxorubicin in some animal systems, were unsuccessful. However, several clinical trials involving women with metastatic breast cancer receiving long-term therapy with doxorubicin indicate that the ethylenediaminetetraacetic acid analog dexrazoxane can reduce the cardiotoxicity of doxorubicin in humans without clearly reducing its antitumor activity. Dexrazoxane inhibits free radical formation by chelating iron. Anthracyclines can bind ferric iron that, when reduced to ferrous iron, can react with O_2^-, H_2O_2, and OH^-. The cardiotoxicity of doxorubicin also can be reduced by altering the schedule of administration. For example, administering doxorubicin by a slow continuous IV infusion (e.g., as a 96-hour infusion) or as a set of low-dose weekly infusions is less cardiotoxic than is administering the same dose as a single bolus infusion once every three to four weeks. This finding suggests that doxorubicin-induced cardiotoxicity is not simply a function of total drug exposure (AUC) but is related also to higher acute drug concentrations. A strategic alternative to moderating the cardiotoxicity of doxorubicin is to incorporate it into a liposome. Liposomal formulation alters the tissue distribution of doxorubicin in such a way that very little drug accumulates in cardiac tissues.

ANTHRACENEDIONES

Mitoxantrone, an anthracene derivative, binds to nucleic acids by intercalation, resulting in DNA strand excision. Its spectrum of action is similar to that of doxorubicin. The major toxicity is myelosuppression, with nadir counts occurring approximately two weeks after treatment. Nausea, vomiting, and mucositis are seen but generally are much milder than with doxorubicin. Alopecia is almost non-existent. Cardiotoxicity can occur but generally only after large cumulative dosages; at an equally myelosuppressive dosage, mitoxantrone appears less cardiotoxic than doxorubicin. Nonetheless, appropriate periodic cardiac monitoring should be performed in mitoxantrone-treated patients whose cumulative dose exceeds 100 mg/m^2.

ACTINOMYCIN D

This is a cell cycle-specific agent with optimum activity in the G_1 and S phases, which interferes with both DNA and RNA synthesis. The drug is given intravenously and, after equilibrating in body tissue, is cleared slowly from the plasma and is excreted in the bile and urine. Dose modifications should be considered for patients with severe hepatic or renal disease. The major toxicity is myelosuppression, which generally occurs one to two weeks after treatment, with the nadir at three weeks. Thrombocytopenia may be profound and may precede leukopenia. The drug must be administered with caution, as skin infiltration causes severe necrosis. Nausea and vomiting are moderate to severe. Large doses may result in substantial mucositis involving the entire alimentary tract. Skin changes are frequent, with acne-like rashes observed most commonly. As seen with the anthracyclines, an unusual property of actinomycin D is its ability to cause erythema and occasional skin ulceration in sites that have received prior radiotherapy (irradiation recall). This effect may occur as late as several months after treatment. Alopecia is moderate.

BLEOMYCIN

Bleomycin is a mixture of several different peptide subtypes, is cell cycle-specific, and exhibits major activity in the G_2 and M phases. The drug can be administered by the IV or intramuscular route, and it is used occasionally as an intracavitary agent in patients with malignant effusions. Bleomycin is metabolized rapidly in all tissues except for the skin and lung, the two organs most likely to be involved in toxic reactions. Up to 20–40% of the drug is excreted in the urine over a 24-hour period, and dose modifications are recommended in patients with severe compromise of renal function.

Common toxicities include febrile reactions, which usually occur several hours after administration. Concurrent use of corticosteroids may prevent this toxicity. Anaphylactic reactions have been reported but are rare. Nevertheless, appropriate precautions should be taken in patients receiving bleomycin; epinephrine, hydrocortisone, and diphenhydramine should be available at the bedside. Skin reactions are common and occasionally are dose-limiting. Frequently, erythema and inflammation are seen in the hands and over pressure points, such as the elbows. Hyperpigmentation also is common, although it rarely results in protocol modification. Severe stomatitis may occur.

The major complication of bleomycin therapy is pulmonary fibrosis, which is more common in patients older than 70 years, in those with prior chest or mediastinal irradiation, or in those who have received more than 500 mg of the drug. However, a small percentage of patients may develop lethal damage even after very small doses. Early detection rests on the clinical finding of fine basilar rales on chest auscultation, which frequently precede chest radiographic evidence of disease. Commonly, pulmonary function tests show a decreased vital capacity, with the diffusion capacity being the first and most sensitive indicator of alveolar damage. Patients who require surgery and have received bleomycin previously must have their inspired oxygen content closely monitored, as high PO_2 levels may enhance subclinical pulmonary damage, increasing the probability of serious or fatal pulmonary toxicity.

MITOMYCIN C

Mitomycin C probably functions as an alkylating agent, resulting in cross-linking of DNA strands. It tends to be active throughout all phases of the cell cycle but appears to be most active in the G_1 and S phases. It must be administered intravenously and is metabolized mainly in the liver, although a small percentage is excreted in the urine. The major toxicity is myelosuppression, which is cumulative. Generally, nadirs are seen at three to four weeks and, once toxicity is observed, recovery may be very slow, possibly as long as four to six weeks. Usually, nausea, vomiting, and stomatitis are not major problems. As with doxorubicin and dactinomycin, severe skin damage may result from drug leakage, and meticulous attention to its administration is necessary. On rare occasions, affected patients may develop severe alopecia, liver function abnormalities, or pulmonary toxicities. Nephrotoxicity is uncommon but has been reported. The current use of mitomycin C in several adjuvant programs, mainly for gastrointestinal carcinoma, has been associated with reports of an adult hemolytic-uremic syndrome consisting of microangiopathic hemolytic anemia and progressive glomerular damage. This syndrome, although uncommon, usually has been progressive and has resulted in death in most cases reported. Caution must be recommended in using mito-

mycin C in patients with a favorable long-term prognosis until the pathophysiology of this unusual but more frequently reported syndrome is defined.

PLANT ALKALOIDS
Vincristine and Vinblastine

Extracts of the periwinkle plant, long believed in folklore to have medicinal value, were found to cause myelosuppression in rats and led to the isolation of two active alkaloid anticancer compounds, vincristine and vinblastine. These two compounds are complex, multiringed molecules of nearly identical structure. Vinblastine differs from vincristine only by the substitution of a formyl group for a methyl group at one point in a side chain of the parent molecule; nonetheless, this seemingly minor structural variation results in a very different pattern of toxicity and antitumor activity.

Vincristine and vinblastine share a common mechanism of cytotoxicity in that they both bind to tubulin, a dimeric protein. Normally, tubulin polymerizes to form the microtubular apparatus along which chromosomes migrate during mitosis, and it serves as a conduit for neurotransmitter transport along axons. Binding of the vinca alkaloids to tubulin prevents the protein's polymerization. The results are cytotoxicity, manifested by an arrest of cells in metaphase with subsequent lysis, and neurotoxicity, characterized by depressed deep-tendon reflexes and paresthesias if mild, and by motor weakness, cranial nerve palsies, and paralytic ileus if severe.

The dose-limiting toxicity of vincristine is neurotoxicity; myelosuppression is infrequently observed with conventional doses. Vinblastine, on the other hand, is decidedly myelotoxic and produces less neurotoxicity. Vincristine is an important component of regimens used to induce remission in childhood ALL, and it is used in a variety of combination chemotherapeutic regimens for other malignancies, especially for lymphomas. Vinblastine has made a major contribution to combination chemotherapy for testicular carcinoma.

Both vincristine and vinblastine are given by IV injection and display similar pharmacokinetics. Both are bound extensively to proteins, producing rapid biphasic clearance from the plasma as they are distributed into body tissues. The terminal phase of plasma clearance is long (20–30 hours) and reflects elimination of the drugs and metabolites via the biliary tract. A common practice is to reduce the dose of vincristine and vinblastine in the presence of obstructive liver disease.

Etoposide

Etoposide (VP-16) is a semisynthetic derivative of podophyllotoxin, a cytotoxic drug isolated from the root of the May apple plant and used for years in the topical treatment of condylomata acuminata. Like podophyllotoxin and the vinca alkaloids, VP-16 causes metaphase arrest. Unlike these other alkaloids, VP-16 does not inhibit microtubule assembly, apparently the result of a sugar moiety that is absent in the other compounds. However, VP-16 can induce strand breaks in DNA, an effect that is mediated by its interaction with topoisomerase II.

VP-16 is most often administered intravenously, its absorption after oral administration being fairly variable. However, larger doses by the oral route can achieve equal systemic effects, and an oral gelatin capsule is available. The pharmacokinetics of VP-16 have not been well sorted out but, under normal circumstances, some 40–60% of a dose appears to be excreted in the urine as unchanged drug and metabolites. Nonetheless, normal clearance of VP-16 has been described in a patient with end-stage renal disease. Similarly, hepatic dysfunction does not seem to alter clearance. The only peculiar toxicity of VP-16 is a tendency to produce transient hypotension if administered by rapid IV injection; this problem is avoided by infusing the drug over a period of 30 minutes or longer.

VP-16 currently enjoys a wide range of clinical use. It is a key component of curative combination chemotherapy for testicular carcinoma. The drug is also included in several combination regimens directed against aggressive forms of non-Hodgkin's lymphoma. Finally, VP-16 probably is the most active single agent used in treating small-cell lung cancer.

Taxanes

The taxanes are a relatively new class of cytotoxic agents, the clinical development of paclitaxel having been initiated in the mid-1980s. The discovery of paclitaxel, however, was made years earlier as part of the National Cancer Institute's program to screen thousands of plant extracts for antitumor activity. In 1963, a crude extract of the bark of the Pacific yew, *Taxus brevifolia,* was found to possess antitumor activity; in 1971, paclitaxel was identified as the active component of that extract. Initially, the supply of paclitaxel was limited because of the need to isolate it from the bark of this slowly growing evergreen tree, a relatively ancient and rare species. Isolation of the precursor of paclitaxel— 10-deacetyl baccatin III—from other parts of the tree (e.g., the needles) and from other *Taxus* species, such as the European yew, has made the semisynthetic production of paclitaxel and docetaxel in adequate quantities feasible.

Paclitaxel and docetaxel are similar in their primary mechanisms of action. Both bind to microtubules and inhibit the depolymerization of those microtubules into tubulin dimers. This effect is precisely opposite to that of the vinca alkaloids, which prevent microtubule assembly. Alteration of the normal tubulin dimer-microtubule equilibrium disrupts a number of processes within the cell, most notably the process of mitosis. Relatively low concentrations of paclitaxel (e.g., 50 nmol/liter) are effective in enhancing tubulin polymerization, and most preclinical studies suggest that the drug's biological effects correlate best with the duration of exposure above a concentration threshold rather than with peak concentration or total exposure (AUC). Docetaxel differs from paclitaxel in that it binds to tubulin with higher affinity. This property may render some of its biological effects less schedule-dependent than those of paclitaxel.

PACLITAXEL

In the early stages of its clinical development, paclitaxel administration was characterized by a high frequency of hypersensitivity reactions. To decrease the frequency and severity of hypersensitivity reactions, the infusion duration was prolonged to 24 hours, and patients were premedicated routinely with corticosteroids and with both H_1- and H_2-receptor antagonists. However, clinical trials have demonstrated that when paclitaxel is given as a three-hour infusion and is preceded by the same premedication regimen, the incidence of hypersensitivity reactions is similar to that incurred with the 24-hour infusion. In addition, the antitumor activity of the three-hour infusion appears to be similar to that of the 24-hour infusion. Nonetheless, because of the preclinical data suggesting that the duration of exposure above a concentration threshold is important in maximizing the antitumor activity of paclitaxel, investigators are exploring paclitaxel regimens that infuse the drug over 96 hours or even longer periods.

The pharmacokinetics of paclitaxel are somewhat complex. When the drug is given as a relatively prolonged infusion (i.e., over a six-hour period or longer), the plasma concentration-versus-time decay curve is biphasic, with half-lives of 0.34 and 5.8 hours for distribution and elimination phases, respectively. However, when paclitaxel is given as a three-hour (or shorter) infusion, its pharmacokinetic effects are found to be dose-dependent. Paclitaxel is eliminated primarily by hepatic metabolism involving cytochrome P450 mixed-function oxidases and biliary excretion. Renal clearance accounts for only 5–10% of total body clearance. The steady-state volume of distribution for paclitaxel is greater than is the volume of total body water, which implies extensive distribution or protein binding (or both). Paclitaxel is highly (95%) bound to plasma proteins, but this binding appears to be reversible and of low affinity.

Several important drug interactions are related to paclitaxel. Because the primary route of clearance involves metabolism by P450 mixed-function oxidases, other drugs metabolized by this system can alter paclitaxel clearance and thus exposure. Both phenytoin and phenobarbital accelerate the metabolism of paclitaxel in human microsomal studies, and clinical data suggest that this action occurs in vivo. Conversely, a number of drugs have been implicated in the reduction of paclitaxel clearance, including diazepam, erythromycin, ketoconazole, and fluconazole. H_2-receptor antagonists as cimetidine and famotidine, which are administered as part of the premedication regimen, do not have an appreciable effect on paclitaxel clearance.

Paclitaxel has been combined successfully with other cytotoxic chemotherapeutic agents, most notably with platinum compounds and with anthracyclines. However, the sequence in which these drugs is given is important. In the case of the paclitaxel-cisplatin combination, administering the cisplatin first induced more neutropenia than did the reverse sequence of drug administration [153]. Therefore, most regimens delivering either cisplatin or carboplatin in combination with paclitaxel deliver the paclitaxel first. The reasons for this sequence dependence of the regimen's hematologic toxicity are not entirely clear. Cisplatin (but not carboplatin) can modulate the activities of P450 mixed-function oxidases so that altered paclitaxel clearance may be part of the explanation [154]. With the combination of doxorubicin and paclitaxel, doxorubicin's clearance is reduced by approximately one-third when paclitaxel is given first, and the result is increased mucositis [155, 156]. In the case of the combination of cyclophosphamide and paclitaxel, administering the cyclophosphamide first results in greater hematologic toxicity.

When paclitaxel is administered as a single agent in conjunction with premedication with dexamethasone and both H_1- and H_2-receptor antagonists, the incidence of major hypersensitivity reactions is between 1% and 2.0%. The principal toxicity of paclitaxel is neutropenia, with an onset at some 8–10 days after drug infusion and with an ensuing rapid recovery completed by days 15–21. This reaction allows cycles of therapy to be delivered on an every three-week basis. In the absence of hematopoietic growth factor support, doses up to 175–200 mg/m^2 can be delivered on this schedule. Though the use of G-CSF does permit delivery of higher doses, a persuasive case for dose intensification of paclitaxel administration has not yet been made.

Paclitaxel has relatively modest nonhematologic toxicities. Perhaps the most common toxicity is asymptomatic bradycardia during infusion of this drug. More serious bradyarrhythmias have been observed, including Mobitz I and Mobitz II second-degree heart blocks and third-degree heart block, but the reported incidence of these is only on the order of 0.1% [157]. Though paclitaxel clearly can cause bradyarrhythmias, what is not clear is whether it is associated with atrial or ventricular tachyarrhythmias. One clinical trial [158] involving the administration of paclitaxel and doxorubicin in combination demonstrated a higher-than-expected frequency of congestive heart failure, suggesting that paclitaxel may enhance anthracycline-induced cardiac dysfunction. Though this result is not conclusive, prudence in this context dictates evaluation of left ventricular function at lower cumulative anthracycline doses than is standard practice when administering anthracyclines alone or in combination with other agents.

Paclitaxel can cause mucositis, and this toxicity is particularly common with prolonged infusion regimens (e.g., > 96 hours). As would be expected with an agent affecting microtubule function, paclitaxel can cause neurologic toxicity. This effect is expressed most commonly as a predominantly sensory peripheral neuropathy, and it can be dose-limiting when paclitaxel is given by brief (1–3-hour) infusion. Alopecia occurs almost universally in patients receiving conventional doses of paclitaxel; in contrast to many other cytotoxic agents, it involves all body hair sites, so that patients lose eyebrows, eyelashes, and pubic and axillary hair. This drug has only a minor tendency to cause nausea or vomiting.

DOCETAXEL

Docetaxel is a semisynthetic derivative of 10-deacetyl baccatin III, also the precursor of paclitaxel. This material is extracted from the needles of the European yew, *Taxus baccata*, which is both readily available and renewable. The similarities between paclitaxel and docetaxel are many.

The most common schedule used for docetaxel administration is a one-hour infusion repeated every three weeks. Although cardiac conduction disturbances have not been linked to docetaxel infusion, acute hypersensitivity reactions have been. For this reason, as with paclitaxel, patients are treated with dexamethasone before and after docetaxel infusion, although histamine-receptor antagonists are not required. Corticosteroid therapy not only reduces the incidence and severity of acute hypersensitivity reactions but tends to reduce the cumulative fluid retention observed with repeated courses of docetaxel therapy.

Like paclitaxel, docetaxel is highly protein-bound and is cleared primarily through hepatic metabolism and biliary excretion. Although not examined as extensively as with paclitaxel, hepatobiliary dysfunction and P450-active drugs would be expected to alter the clearance of docetaxel. Like paclitaxel, the pharmacokinetics of docetaxel are characterized by a large steady-state volume of distribution and a high clearance rate, but with doses as high as 115 mg/m^2, no deviation from first-order elimination has been observed.

The primary and dose-limiting toxicity of docetaxel is myelosuppression and, as with paclitaxel, primarily the neutrophils are affected. The neutrophil nadir occurs by approximately day 9 after docetaxel administration, and recovery is complete by days 15–21. Myelosuppression appears to be less schedule-dependent than with paclitaxel, a result likely arising not from differences in the pharmacokinetics of this drug but rather from their differing affinities for microtubular binding.

Cumulative fluid retention resulting from repeated courses of docetaxel administration appears to result from the drug's ability to increase capillary permeability. This problem is not ordinarily observed with cumulative doses of less than 400 mg/m^2 but quickly increases in incidence and severity above this level. Cumulative fluid retention is reduced by using lower single doses of docetaxel and by corticosteroid premedication and postmedication.

Dermatologic toxicity may be more frequent with docetaxel than with paclitaxel. Between 50% and 75% of patients treated with docetaxel develop some form of dermatologic toxicity, most commonly an erythematous, maculopapular rash involving the hands and forearms. Nail changes occur and include brown discoloration, ridging, onycholysis, soreness, and brittleness of the fingernails. Docetaxel therapy has been associated also with palmar-plantar erythrodysesthesia. Corticosteroid premedication appears to reduce the incidence and severity of these dermatologic toxicities.

The peripheral neuropathy associated with docetaxel therapy appears to be similar to that seen with the use of paclitaxel. However, drug-induced malaise is more common with docetaxel and, on rare occasions, has required dosage reduction or cessation of treatment.

SELECTED PROTECTIVE AGENTS USED IN COMBINATION WITH CYTOTOXIC CHEMOTHERAPY

A number of agents have been recently added to the chemotherapeutic armamentarium are not cytotoxic themselves but instead have the potential to increase the therapeutic index of certain cytotoxic agents by protecting normal—rather than neoplastic—tissues from the damaging effects of specific cytotoxic drugs. Three such agents are G-CSF, amifostine, and dexrazoxane.

Granulocyte Colony-Stimulating Factor

G-CSF belongs to a large family of molecules known as the *hematopoietic colony-stimulating factors*. These factors are acidic glycoproteins that bind to corresponding cell-surface receptors present on hematopoietic progenitors. The effects that follow binding of these factors to their receptors are varied and include stimulation of hematopoietic progenitor proliferation, differentiation, and functional enhancement of the more differentiated progeny of these cells. G-CSF exerts its primary influence on progenitor cells that already are committed to granulocytic differentiation. The most obvious effect of G-CSF is its increase of the number of mature granulocytes in the bone marrow and peripheral blood. However, besides increasing the granulocytic mass, G-CSF causes an earlier release of granulocytes into the circulation, it enhances the ability of granulocytes to mediate antibody-dependent cytotoxicity, and it augments the bactericidal capacity of granulocytes by increasing their production of superoxide anions.

The most common use of G-CSF is to attenuate the duration of severe granulocytopenia associated with the administration of cytotoxic chemotherapy. Typically, the cytotoxic drugs are delivered first, then G-CSF is administered subcutaneously as a once-daily injection beginning some 24–48 hours thereafter. The duration of therapy with G-CSF varies with the chemotherapeutic regimen being used; however, the daily injections generally are continued through the period of most severe granulocytopenia and then are stopped once myeloid recovery is complete. When used in this fashion after substantially myelosuppressive chemotherapy, G-CSF does not prevent severe granulocytopenia but rather shortens its duration.

Randomized studies of dose-intensive chemotherapy administered with and without prophylactic G-CSF support have demonstrated the ability of G-CSF to help maintain the dose intensity of several combination chemotherapeutic regimens and to reduce the incidence of febrile granulocytopenia and hospitalization [159]. It is important, however, to understand the rationale behind G-CSF therapy and to avoid indiscriminate use in all patients receiving myelosuppressive chemotherapy. G-CSF support makes most sense when it is used to preserve the dose intensity of a treatment that has curative or significantly palliative potential. Otherwise, it may be equally efficacious and less expensive simply to reduce the doses of the chemotherapeutic agents being given. Also, the appropriate approach in many situations may be to avoid giving prophylactic G-CSF therapy with the first cycle of treatment and instead to use this first cycle to gauge a patient's need for such support. The practice of initiating therapy with G-CSF after the development of severe chemotherapy-induced granulocytopenia is of very limited utility; investigators have experienced difficulty in demonstrating that use of G-CSF in this setting has an appreciable impact on clinically significant outcomes.

For prophylaxis against chemotherapy-induced granulocytopenia, G-CSF is administered most commonly in a dose of 5 μg/kg/day by subcutaneous injection. It can be given intravenously but appears to be less effective when delivered in this manner, a fact that is probably a reflection of its rapid elimination from plasma. Administering G-CSF by the subcutaneous route produces lower plasma concentrations but longer exposure. G-CSF is well-tolerated in most patients. The most frequent adverse effect is bone pain, which occurs most often near the time of maximal hematopoiesis (i.e., when peripheral blood granulocyte counts are rebounding). The simultaneous administration of myelosuppressive chemotherapy and G-CSF actually may aggravate the ensuing granulocytopenia, particularly in the instance of cytotoxic agents having relatively greater activity against proliferating cells.

G-CSF has little, if any, effect on the marrow progenitor cells that give rise to erythrocytes, monocytes, and platelets. Erythropoietin, which has been so successful in increasing the red blood cell mass in patients with renal failure, can reduce transfusion requirements in selected patients receiving chemotherapy.

Amifostine

Amifostine is a compound that has been in existence for many years, having been developed by the US Army as a protector against radiation injury. A well-developed preclinical body of literature documents the ability of amifostine to protect normal tissues—but not neoplastic tissues—from the DNA damage resulting from radiation, alkylating agents, and organoplatinum compounds.

Amifostine is a prodrug that is dephosphorylated in vivo by plasma membrane alkaline phosphatase to the free thiol, called WR-1065. This free thiol then is postulated to bind to the active species of alkylating agents or platinum compounds, to donate hydrogen to DNA radicals, and to scavenge oxygen-free radicals. WR-1065 accumulates in normal tissues to a degree greater than in neoplastic tissues for at least two reasons. First, higher concentrations of alkaline phosphatase are found in the capillaries and cell membranes of normal cells compared with neoplastic cells. Second, both the lower vascularity and lower pH of neoplastic tissues work to lower the inherent activity of the alkaline phosphatase enzyme. As a consequence, the concentration of the free thiol can be as much as 100-fold greater in normal organs (e.g., bone marrow, kidney, and heart) than in tumor tissue.

Although a great deal of preclinical work has been performed to demonstrate the ability of amifostine to increase the therapeutic index of alkylating agents, perhaps more important are the clinical trials that confirm this effect. A controlled trial demonstrated that amifostine pretreatment decreased both the degree and duration of the neutropenia associated with cyclophosphamide therapy [160]. Additionally, in a phase I trial of carboplatin combined with amifostine, the maximally tolerated dose of carboplatin was increased above that which had been observed with carboplatin alone [161]. Interestingly, in this latter study, more than one dose of amifostine was delivered because of the long elimination half-life of carboplatin (approximately 90 minutes). The pivotal phase III trial that permitted US licensure of amifostine was a randomized trial of cyclophosphamide plus cisplatin without or without amifostine, in patients with advanced ovarian carcinoma. Though tumor response rates were equivalent in the two arms, patients receiving the amifostine had less myelosuppression, nephrotoxicity, and neurotoxicity [162].

One of the problems with the clinical use of amifostine is that it has a relatively brief half-life. More than 90% of the parent compound is cleared from the plasma in six minutes. However, the pharmacologically relevant species, the free thiol, is present for at least 90 minutes after infusion. Typically, amifostine is delivered as a 15-minute infusion, beginning 30 minutes prior to the administration of chemotherapy. In the case of cytotoxic agents with long half-lives (e.g., carboplatin, as cited), delivering an additional dose of amifostine may be necessary after the chemotherapeutic agent has been given to achieve optimal protection.

Generally, amifostine is well tolerated, but it does have significant short-term side effects. Its administration is associated with nausea, vomiting, hypotension, sneezing, a warm or flushed feeling, mild somnolence, a metallic taste during the infusion, and occasional allergic reactions. The emesis associated with amifostine clearly is dose-related and can be severe. However, vigorous prophylactic antiemetic therapy (e.g., serotonin antagonist plus glucocorticoid plus lorazepam) is fairly successful in preventing this problem.

The most clinically significant side effect of amifostine is transient hypotension. However, systolic blood pressure decreases of more than 20 mm of Hg lasting longer than five minutes, or symptomatic decreases in blood pressure, occur in fewer than 5% of patients. The median time to the onset of hypotension is 14 minutes; by the time this problem occurs, most of the amifostine has been given. The mechanism whereby amifostine causes hypotension is not known, and prolonging the duration of the infusion actually may exacerbate its tendency to lower blood pressure. Patients are hydrated routinely prior to amifostine treatment. If they can do so safely, patients who routinely take antihypertensive medications are instructed to discontinue their use for 24 hours prior to amifostine treatment; then they resume antihypertensive therapy immediately after amifostine treatment is completed. Transient hypocalcemia has been reported rarely and is related both to inhibition of parathyroid hormone secretion and direct inhibition of bone resorption.

Dexrazoxane

A great deal of effort has been expended in developing less cardiotoxic analogs of doxorubicin, but none has gained widespread acceptance as being both equally efficacious and less cardiotoxic. Preclinical data suggest that the mechanisms underlying the antitumor effects of doxorubicin may be different from those responsible for its cardiotoxicity. It is now generally accepted that doxorubicin (and other anthracyclines) disrupt mitochondrial function in cardiac myocytes by the generation of free radicals. Cardiac myocytes are especially sensitive to free radical-mediated damage, in part because they have levels of superoxide dismutase and catalase lower than those of other tissues. The production of free radicals by anthracyclines requires the presence of iron. Dexrazoxane is a cyclic analog of ethylenediaminetetraacetic acid that, once inside the cell, undergoes hydrolytic ring opening. The open-ring form of the drug is able to chelate iron, reducing the amount available for the formation of oxygen radical-forming iron-doxorubicin complexes. The selective protection of myocytes afforded by dexrazoxane may arise not only from the relative lack of superoxide dismutase and catalase in the myocytes, but from differential metabolism of dexrazoxane in normal and malignant cells [163].

Currently, dexrazoxane is approved for use only in women who have metastatic breast cancer, have received a lifetime cumulative doxorubicin dose greater than 300 mg/m², and would benefit from continuation of therapy with doxorubicin [164]. Typically, dexrazoxane is not used from the outset of therapy with doxorubicin because of lingering concerns that its coadministration may slightly compromise the antitumor activity of doxorubicin. Dexrazoxane dosage is based on the dose of doxorubicin to be administered. The recommended dosage ratio is 10:1 (500 mg/m² of dexrazoxane; 50 mg/m² of doxorubicin). Dexrazoxane is given as a slow IV push or as a rapid IV infusion 30 minutes before doxorubicin is administered. Dexrazoxane is well tolerated but can itself produce mild suppression of the white blood cell and platelet counts.

HORMONES AND HORMONE ANTAGONISTS

Just as hormones influence the growth of many normal tissues, many malignant cells retain a degree of hormonal sensitivity characteristic of their tissue of origin [165]. This tendency is particularly true of carcinomas of the breast, prostate, and endometrium. To date, the only clinically useful hormonal manipulations have involved, directly or indirectly, the steroid hormones. Steroid hormones mediate their effects by binding to specific intracellular receptors and, as steroid hormone-receptor complexes, interact with DNA to stimulate or repress transcription of specific sequences of messenger RNA, ultimately modulating cellular function and growth. Manipulation of this sequence of events has produced important treatment modalities.

A direct correlation between response and receptor activity is observed in most hormone-responsive malignancies, with estrogen and progesterone receptors being the most common receptor proteins analyzed [166]. Techniques are available also for measuring androgen and glucocorticoid receptors, but measurement of these receptors is not part of clinical practice in the selection of hormonal agents. Patients whose tumors contain both estrogen and progesterone receptors are most likely to respond to hormonal therapy. Those patients whose breast cancer contains both estrogen and progesterone receptors or who have very large quantities of receptors are more likely to respond than are those whose tumors contain estrogen receptors only [167]. Estrogen and progesterone receptors should be measured in all patients with breast cancer and in selected patients with endometrial carcinoma. For some patients with ovarian cancer, determining receptor status may be helpful in selecting treatment. Immunohistochemistry can be used for accurate determination of receptor status from archival tumor tissue in paraffin-embedded blocks.

Tamoxifen

Tamoxifen, perhaps the most important and the most extensively used of the hormonal agents, competes with estradiol for binding to a high-affinity estradiol receptor. The binding of tamoxifen to the estrogen receptor does not result in an estrogenic response in most tissues and renders cells refractory to further estrogen stimulation. A growing body of evidence indicates that the long-term adjuvant administration of tamoxifen (i.e., after local treatment) in postmenopausal women with stage II carcinoma of the breast improves their survival [168].

Tamoxifen is given orally and is mainly excreted via the liver. It has an initial $t_{1/2}$ of 7–14 hours followed by a long secondary $t_{1/2}$ that lasts from days to weeks. Low levels of tamoxifen may be detectable for four to six weeks after discontinuation of the drug, and estrogen receptor measurements in patients taking this drug may be difficult to interpret unless several months have elapsed since discontinuation.

Unlike the estrogens, androgens, and glucocorticoids, which may result in substantial toxicity, tamoxifen is generally well tolerated and is associated with only minimal side effects [169]. A small percentage of patients experience gastrointestinal disturbances, but this rarely leads to discontinuation. Some patients, especially those who are perimenopausal, experience hot flushes, which usually resolve even when the drug is continued. Breast cancer patients with bone and soft-tissue metastases may experience a 'flare' reaction consisting of an increase in bone pain, inflammation of locally recurrent lesions, and occasional hypercalcemia. These 'flare' reactions occasionally occur soon after treatment has started, and they tend to subside in one to two weeks. Patients who have 'flare' reactions frequently experience an excellent response to treatment. It may be difficult to separate tumor progression from the 'flare' reaction, and careful observation is mandatory to prevent discontinuation of a potentially beneficial treatment modality. An increased incidence of thrombophlebitis is associated with tamoxifen use. In the adjuvant setting, about 1% of patients who are given tamoxifen for five years or longer develop thromboembolic complications.

The major toxicity associated with tamoxifen is endometrial carcinoma, which is noted in about 1% of women who take the drug for periods of five years or longer [170]. Ocular changes, including cataracts, are uncommon. Retinopathy has been reported, but is rare. The available data show that liver cancer and other malignancies are no more common in tamoxifen-treated patients than in controls.

Other new antiestrogens are now commercially available, including toremifene (Fareston) for treament of metastatic breast cancer, and raloxifene for treatment of osteoporosis. These agents are likely to have similar effectiveness to tamoxifen in breast cancer management, but they may have fewer stimulatory effects on the endometrium. 'Pure antiestrogens' (e.g., ICI 182,780, Faslodex), which have no estrogen-agonist activity, are now being used in clinical trials for breast cancer.

Gonadotropin-Releasing Factors (LHRH Agonists)

Depletion of steroid hormone in a tumor may be effected indirectly. Prostate carcinoma depends heavily, at least in its early stages, on androgenic stimulation; indeed, the disease does not develop in castrated males. Androgen depletion can be achieved directly with orchiectomy and by administering diethylstibestrol (DES). Although DES may have some slight direct effect on prostate carcinoma, its major effect is to suppress the pituitary's release of luteinizing hormone (LH), which normally stimulates testicular androgen secretion. Neither orchiectomy nor DES is an ideal form of hormonal manipulation: the former approach is emotionally unacceptable for some men, and DES is associated with excessive cardiovascular toxicity. Since the 1970s, a group of synthetic gonadotropin-releasing hormone (GnRH) agonists has been developed that offers an important alternative form of hormonal treatment. At first glance, logic would argue against using an agent that should elicit increased secretion of LH. The GnRH agonists initially may cause a surge of LH secretion and thus a flare in the disease; however, they eventually desensitize the pituitary to the effects of GnRH by decreasing the number of GnRH receptors. The end result is the same as that observed in therapy with DES-decreased secretion of LH, but without the associated cardiovascular morbidity and mortality. The most commonly used LHRH agonists are goserelin (Zolodex®) and leuprolide (Lupron®). Administration is achieved by subcutaneous or intramuscular injection using depot preparations that need to be given every one to three months. Generally, toxicity is mild and includes hot flushes, depression, and loss of libido.

Progestins

Progestins are synthetic compounds structurally related to the naturally occurring human steroid progesterone. Commonly used progestin derivatives include medroxyprogesterone acetate (Provera®), oral; Depo-Provera®, intramuscular; megestrol acetate (Megace®), oral; and hydroxyprogesterone caproate (Delalutin®), intramuscular. Progestins can be given by both the oral and intramuscular routes and are metabolized rapidly by the liver but may display prolonged biological activity. Pharmacologic plasma levels may persist four to six weeks after administration of hydroxyprogesterone acetate and for one to three days after oral megestrol acetate.

Occasionally, progestins cause serious side effects. Patients may experience fluid retention, increased appetite, and a gain in body weight. Higher doses of progestins, notably megestrol acetate, are effective in the management of patients with cancer cachexia [171, 172]. Progestins occasionally cause impaired hepatic function, with enzyme changes characteristic of cholestasis. On withdrawal, all the agents may cause vaginal bleeding, and they should be used with caution in patients with previous phlebitis. Uncommonly, patients with breast cancer and bone metastases may develop hypercalcemia after progestin use.

At present, no form of hormonal therapy can cure established tumors in affected patients. Hormonal therapy causes tumor regression in approximately 30% of patients with endometrial cancer, in 30–40% of patients with breast cancer, and in 80% of those with prostate cancer. Although tumors regress and on occasion shrink below the limits of clinical detection, and although some tumors may respond to a series of different hormonal treatments, ultimately they become refractory to further hormonal manipulation. Evidence now points to the fact that, from the outset, even hormone-responsive tumors contain populations of both hormone-dependent and hormone-independent cells. Moreover, the natural history of most tumors is to become increasingly anaplastic (poorly differentiated) and, thus, less likely to depend on hormonal stimulation for growth.

STRATEGIES FOR IMPROVING THE OUTCOME OF SYSTEMIC CANCER THERAPY
Adjuvant Chemotherapy

When an agent or group of agents produces a high number of responses in overtly metastatic tumors, efforts are made to incorporate them into the treatment of earlier stages of disease, particularly in the adjuvant setting. For several reasons, residual micrometastatic tumor after definitive local therapy (e.g., with surgery or irradiation or both) should be more susceptible to systemic therapy than is clinically detectable tumor. The micrometastatic disease should have a better vascular supply, enabling better drug penetration; it should have a higher proliferative rate; and a smaller number of drug-resistant cells should be present. The rationale for adjuvant treatment of cancer with systemic chemotherapy (and hormonal therapy) was validated first in the treatment of early stage breast cancer and has been shown to increase the cure rate in resectable colorectal carcinoma. Recognizing the impossibility of predicting recurrence definitively in the individual patient in the adjuvant setting is important. The strategy is rather to select populations of patients known to be at high risk for disease recurrence and to treat large numbers of such patients with the intention of producing increases in disease-free and overall survival.

There is also interest in the use of chemotherapeutic agents prior to surgery or radiotherapy (neoadjuvant therapy) in patients with advanced but locally confined malignancy (e.g., carcinoma of the head and neck, breast, bone [osteogenic sarcoma], and cervix). Chemotherapy given prior to radiation or surgery has several advantages. First, the tumor vasculature has not been disturbed by surgery, radiotherapy, or other local procedures. Second, affected patients generally have a good performance status and are not recovering from the side effects of other treatment. Third, involved physicians may assess treatment results directly, rather than having to infer them from subsequent rates of relapse. Last, by shrinking locally advanced tumors, neoadjuvant chemotherapy may render them more amenable to treatment with surgery or radiation. In treating osteosarcoma, such an approach has generated impressive preliminary results and has demonstrated prolonged survival in patients who have little or no evidence of malignancy after histologic examination of their resected primary lesion [173, 174]. Such therapy has shown great promise also in breast cancer, head and neck cancer, and esophageal cancer, and trials underway are investigating its use in treating squamous cell cancers of the vulva and cervix. The precise role of neoadjuvant therapy has yet to be determined, but conceptually this strategy has great promise.

Dosage Intensification

The most extreme example of the dose-intensity concept is found in the use of myeloablative doses of chemotherapy followed by rescue with either peripheral blood progenitor (stem) cells or bone marrow. Much of the logic in this strategy lies in the fact that alkylating agents exhibit extramyeloid toxicities at doses two to seven times higher than those required for myeloablation and that, for alkylating agents, the dose-response curve does not achieve a plateau as quickly as it does for other classes of cytotoxic compounds. Similar observations apply to radiation, and so alkylating agents and radiation often are combined in this technique.

A successful approach to circumventing the prolonged myelosuppression or permanent marrow ablation that results from high-dose chemotherapy is the technique of marrow transplantation. Transplanted marrow may be allogeneic (from an antigenically distinct individual), syngeneic (from an identical twin), or autologous (from patients themselves). Allogeneic and syngeneic marrow transplantation after high-dose chemotherapy (with or without total body radiation) currently is used in the successful treatment of several hematologic malignancies, including CML, AML, and ALL. The success of this approach must be attributed not only to the high-dose chemoradiation but to an antileukemic effect arising from the transplanted allogeneic marrow.

Transplantation of allogeneic marrow produces the undesirable phenomenon of graft-versus-host disease, but a useful consequence of this problem is a graft-versus-leukemia effect. High-dose chemotherapy has been applied successfully also in the treatment of recurrent Hodgkin's disease and of intermediate and high-grade non-Hodgkin's lymphoma. In such cases, autologous marrow has been used more commonly, and the treatment's positive effects on disease control are more clearly attributable to the dose-intense chemotherapy. Although hematopoietic reconstitution after high-dose chemotherapy was provided originally by the infusion of harvested bone marrow cells, such support now is more commonly given using peripheral blood progenitor cells. Progenitor cells or stem cells normally circulate in small numbers in the peripheral blood, but when the marrow reconstitutes itself after moderate-dose chemotherapy, the number of circulating progenitor cells increases. This phenomenon can be amplified further by the simultaneous administration of hematopoietic colony-stimulating factors (e.g., G-CSF). Circulating progenitor cells are harvested by leukopheresis during this period of myeloid recovery and are reinfused after the administration of high-dose chemotherapy.

In contrast to the successes achieved with some of the hematologic malignancies, the utility of high-dose chemotherapy in managing the more common adult solid tumors is not as well established. As described, the availability of hematopoietic growth factors, particularly G-CSF, has allowed for better preservation of the prescribed dose intensity of many standard chemotherapeutic regimens. However, what is not clear is whether the relatively modest increase in dose intensity afforded by the use of prophylactic G-CSF makes a difference in control of the underlying disease.

Directed Drug Delivery

A major limitation of current cytotoxic drugs is their relative lack of selectivity for malignant cells. The mechanism of action of these agents—disruption of nucleic acid synthesis and function—fails to discriminate between normal and malignant cells. Given the dearth of truly tumor-specific agents, several approaches have been taken to more precisely target cytotoxic agents to tumor cells. The simplest form of directed drug delivery is the instillation of chemotherapeutic agents directly into a body cavity (e.g., the pleural or peritoneal spaces). Usually, tumors are not limited to one cavity, though ovarian carcinoma is an important exception. The spread of ovarian carcinoma beyond the ovary's capsule tends to remain confined to the peritoneal surface until the most advanced stages of its natural history. Intraperitoneal administration of cisplatin can induce a substantial number of responses when the disease has become refractory to systemic cisplatin. For patients who are free of disease or who have minimal residual disease at the time of second-look laparotomy, intraperitoneal therapy theoretically would be an attractive option, but its efficacy in this setting still is unproved. In the advanced-disease setting, a slight survival advantage was observed [175] for intraperitoneal cisplatin plus IV cyclophosphamide versus the delivery of both of these drugs intravenously. However, whether the cost, labor, and complexity of the intraperitoneal route of drug delivery warrant declaring this approach as the new standard of care remains uncertain.

Attempts have been made also to alter drug distribution and uptake favorably by (1) attaching drugs to large molecules, (2) encasing drugs within lipid vesicles, and (3) binding drugs to monoclonal antibodies directed against tumor-associated antigens. Often, tumor cells have a high capacity for endocytosis, leading to preferential uptake of, say, a drug-DNA conjugate; once inside the cell, the drug is released from the DNA by enzymatic cleavage of the bonds joining them. This approach is limited by the instability of drug-DNA complexes, by the difficulty that such large complexes have in penetrating solid tumors, and by the endocytotic capacity of the tumor. Delivering drugs in liposomes causes a preferential distribution of drug to the reticulo-endothelial system: the lungs, liver, and spleen. However, cloaking drugs in liposomes can change the relative availability of a drug to different tissues. For example, in one study, doxorubicin packaged in liposomes and given to mice resulted in decreased drug uptake by the heart and cardiotoxicity, with retention of antitumor activity [176].

Substantial obstacles stand in the way of attaching drugs to monoclonal antibodies directed against tumor-associated antigens. First, tumor-associated antigens often are not tumor-specific; not only is less drug delivered to the tumor, but the drug ultimately may concentrate in tissues that share the antigen, producing unexpected toxicities. Second, the density of tumor-associated antigens on cancer cells often is low; most tumors cannot be shown to bear unique antigenic determinants at all. Finally, the drug-monoclonal antibody complex itself often is immunogenic; if successive doses of the complex are administered, eventually they may be cleared rapidly by the reticuloendothelial system. In spite of these obstacles, there have been some recent successes in this field. IDEC-C2B8, known as Rituximab, is a monoclonal antibody recently approved for use in the treatment of patients with recurrent, low-grade non-Hodgkin's lymphoma. This antibody was created to bind the CD20 antigen, which is commonly expressed on the surface of B-lymphocytes, both malignant and benign. Binding of the antibody the CD20 antigen supports complement-mediated lysis, antibody-dependent cellular cytotoxicity, and may precipitate apoptosis in the targeted cell. The immunogenicity of the antibody has been reduced by constructing it as a chimeric protein: the antigen-binding variable regions are composed of mouse sequences, but the constant regions use human sequences. Rituximab has demonstrated the ability to produce clinically meaningful responses in patients with relapsed, low-grade, non-Hodgkin's lymphomas, and attempts are now being made to extend its use to intermediate grade lymphomas, in combination with chemotherapy. In general, Rituximab is well-tolerated. Apart from acute infusion-related events such as fever and chills, the only major effect is a depletion of normal circulating B-lymphocytes, which has not been clearly associated with an increased incidence of infection.

NOVEL APPROACHES TO SYSTEMIC CANCER TREATMENT

Most of this chapter has been dedicated to a review of cytotoxic chemotherapeutic and hormonal agents, as these drugs represent the bulk of what is currently available for systemic cancer treatment. Despite the importance of these agents, they evolved from an understanding of cancer biology as it existed 20 years ago. Since the mid-1970s, our understanding of the pathogenesis of cancer has grown considerably, specifically through the discovery of the genes underlying the malignant phenotype.

The genes lying at the heart of malignant behavior fall into three classes. The first class of genes to be recognized, known simply as *oncogenes*, is derived from normal genes, called *protooncogenes*, which orchestrate cellular growth and differentiation during the early stages of an individual's life. Mutations in these protooncogenes, rarely expressed in mature individuals, allow for their deranged expression as oncogenes, provoking unbridled and aberrant growth. The second class of genes encompasses what are known as *tumor suppressor genes*, the normal function of which is to restrict cellular proliferation. Mutation in a tumor suppressor gene also may result in uncontrolled growth. Finally, a third set of genes governs the replication and repair of DNA. Dysfunction of these genes and their products likewise can contribute to malignant phenotypes. The protein products of some of these genes have been identified, and researchers hope that they may provide more specific targets for cancer therapy. Novel therapies based on a better understanding of the molecular pathogenesis of cancer are now arriving in the clinic, and several early successes will be described below.

Differentiation Therapy

Since the progressive growth of tumors is a manifestation of their failure to mature and differentiate, investigators have long searched for agents that would not necessarily kill tumor cells but rather force them to "grow up". Unfortunately there have been few clinical successes in this field. Perhaps the most notable example of differentiation therapy is the success of all-trans retinoic acid in the treatment of acute promyelocytic leukemia (APL). This compound exerts its antileukemic effect by causing the malignant promyelocytes of this disease to differentiate into mature neutrophils, which subsequently undergo a normal, apoptotic death. In APL, a retinoid receptor gene located on chromosome 17 is involved in a reciprocal translocation with a transcriptional activator gene, PML, which is located on chromosome 15. The result is a fusion retinoid receptor with reduced affinity for its normal ligand. Binding of all-trans retinoic acid to the fusion retinoid receptor can cause the malignant promyelocyte to once again differentiate into more mature myelocytic cells and thereby produce a temporary remission in the disease.

Monoclonal Antibodies

Although small-molecule inhibitors of oncogene protein function would appear to have many potential advantages, one of the first successes in targeting an oncogene product has come from a monoclonal antibody, the humanized anti-HER2 monoclonal antibody trastuzumab, commonly know as Herceptin. This antibody's target is a transmembrane growth factor receptor known as c-erb-B2 or HER2. The normal function and ligands of this receptor are unknown, but it is overexpressed in 25–30% of breast cancers, suggesting that it is important in driving the growth of these cells. HER2 belongs to a family of transmembrane receptors that includes the epidermal growth factor receptor (EGFR) and the platelet-derived growth factor (PDGF) receptor. When these receptors are bound by their normal ligands, they undergo dimerization. Dimerization of the receptors activates their tyrosine kinase activity (located on the cytosolic side of these proteins), the net result of which is the phosphorylation of other proteins in

a cascade of events that signals the cell to grow and divide.

The hypothesis that HER2 overexpression is important in driving the growth of breast cancer cells was supported by laboratory experiments in which antibodies directed against HER2 blocked such growth. Occasionally, the Herceptin monoclonal antibody that has been developed in the clinic has (by itself) caused objective tumor regression in patients with metastatic breast cancer (complete remission plus partial remission rate = 15%; median duration of response = 8.4 months) [177]. However, this antibody would appear to have its greatest therapeutic value when administered in combination with cytotoxic drugs. In a recently reported phase III study [178], 469 women who had HER2-positive metastatic breast cancer and had not received chemotherapy previously for treatment of metastatic disease were chosen randomly to receive one of two standard chemotherapeutic regimens: either doxorubicin (Adriamycin), 60 mg/m², plus cyclophosphamide, 600 mg/m² (the AC regimen), or paclitaxel, 175 mg/m², given once every three weeks. Half of the patients in each chemotherapy arm were assigned randomly to receive concomitant therapy with Herceptin (4 mg/kg loading dose, followed by weekly maintenance doses of 2 mg/kg). Combining the results of both chemotherapy arms, those women who received Herceptin along with their chemotherapy benefited in several respects: the response rate was higher (49% versus 32%), the duration of responses was superior (9.3 versus 5.9 months), and the median time to disease progression was longer (7.6 versus 4.6 months). Interestingly, the combination of Herceptin with paclitaxel appeared to provide greater benefit than did its addition to the AC regimen. This finding was true both in terms of enhancement of the response rate and in terms of toxicity. An important note is that treatment of women with the AC regimen and Herceptin resulted in an 18% incidence of grade III or grade IV myocardial dysfunction, whereas women treated with AC alone experienced only a 3% incidence of this problem.

Overexpression of EGFR, with the consequence of enhanced cellular proliferation, is a common event in many tumors of epithelial origin (e.g., squamous cell carcinoma of the head and neck). Shutting down the proliferative signal that arises from overexpression of EGFR can be accomplished in at least two ways, both of which are being investigated in the clinic. One approach is to deliver molecules that compete for binding to EGFR with epidermal growth factor and transforming growth factor-α, the normal ligands of this receptor. In an approach similar to that taken with Herceptin, a humanized (chimeric) monoclonal antibody, C225, has been developed to target EGFR. C225 binds to the extracellular domain of EGFR and has a higher affinity for the receptor than the normal ligands. Unlike the normal ligands, when C225 binds to the receptor it fails to stimulate its tyrosine kinase activity. Though it has demonstrated only modest single-agent activity, preliminary data suggest that it may improve the therapeutic index of both radiotherapy and cisplatin-based chemotherapy in patients with advanced head and neck cancer.

Small-Molecule Inhibitors of Tyrosine Kinases

The other way to attack overexpression of EGFR is to develop small molecules that inhibit the tyrosine kinase activity of the receptor. Because all tyrosine kinases have a site that binds adenosine triphosphate (ATP), conventional wisdom maintained for many years the impossibility of developing receptor-specific tyrosine kinase inhibitors directed against that portion of the molecule. However, the small-molecule tyrosine kinase inhibitors being explored in the clinic do in fact target the ATP-binding pocket of these proteins. Apparently, sufficient structural variability exists between the ATP-binding pockets of the different kinases to permit selectivity.

Interestingly, the toxicity associated with inhibition of EGFR activity is similar, whether it is accomplished by blocking the binding of normal ligands to the receptor or by inhibiting the receptor's tyrosine kinase activity. Though researchers always have been concerned that anti-EGFR compounds would result in hepatotoxicity because of the high degree of EGFR expression found in the liver, in practice the organ that is most affected is the skin. In the case of the C225 anti-EGFR monoclonal antibody, affected patients experience an eruption characterized by erythematous papules surmounted by pustules, distributed mainly over the central portions of the face and upper trunk [179]. The resemblance to acne is striking. In most cases, this toxicity is not dose-limiting and, in fact, the rash may improve over time even as the antibody continues to be administered. A similar rash has been observed with small-molecule, EGFR-specific tyrosine kinase inhibitors.

In addition to EGFR-specific tyrosine kinase inhibitors, clinical studies are underway that explore small molecules designed to inhibit the tyrosine kinase activity of other aberrantly expressed signal transduction molecules. A novel tyrosine kinase inhibitor, known as STI 571, has yielded strikingly positive results in the

treatment of patients with CML [180]. The 9:22 chromosomal translocation so characteristic of this disease is known to create an abnormal gene, *bcr-abl*, whose protein product has enhanced tyrosine kinase activity. The enhanced tyrosine kinase activity of the *bcr-abl* fusion protein results in the excessive proliferation of myeloid cells that is characteristic of this disease. STI 571 is a potent and selective inhibitor of the tyrosine kinase activity of both the normal *abl* protein and of the *bcr-abl* fusion protein, and was shown to kill *bcr-abl* expressing cells both in vivo and in vitro. This compound has high oral bioavailability and an elimination half-life of 13–18 hours, which makes it ideal as a long-term therapy. Results of a phase I study of STI 571 in 61 patients with chronic phase CML have now been reported. The doses of STI 71 examined in this trial ranged between 25 and 600 mg/day, and there was a clear dose-response effect, with hematologic responses being observed in all of the 51 patients treated with doses of 140 mg/day or higher. Complete hematologic responses (normalization of the peripheral white blood cell and platelet counts) began to occur at 200 mg/day, and occurred in all patients (31 of 31) receiving 300 mg/day or more. In addition to producing hematologic responses, STI 571 has produced cytogenetic responses (disappearance of the 9:22 chromosomal translocation) in patients receiving doses ≥ 300 mg/day, particularly in those who have received at least five months of treatment. The tolerance of STI 571 therapy has been excellent. While the overall impact of this therapy on patient survival has not yet been determined, all of the current evidence suggests that STI 571 will in fact be a major advance in the treatment of this disease.

Farnesyl:Protein Transferase Inhibitors

Although many signal transduction events begin in cell membranes, the pathways through which these signals are propagated through the cytosol to the nucleus are numerous and complex. The intricacies of signal transduction pathways create many additional opportunities for genetic mistakes that may lead to a malignant phenotype and hence create additional targets for cancer therapy. Perhaps the signal transduction target being evaluated most intensively at the moment is the product of the *ras* oncogene [181]. Between 25% and 30% of all cancers express one of the three *ras* oncogenes in existence.

The normal ras protein is attached to the inner aspect of the plasma membrane through a 15-carbon isoprenoid (lipid) moiety called *farnesyl*. The farnesyl group is added to the ras precursor protein through a series of posttranslational modifications. The modifications occur at one end of the ras precursor protein called the *CAAX box.* Although three steps are involved, the first modification, catalyzed by an enzyme known as farnesyl:protein transferase, is the rate-limiting step. When the ras protein is attached to the inner aspect of the plasma membrane and undergoes phosphorylation by a tyrosine kinase (such as EGFR), it in turn activates other kinases that lie in a chain of events that provoke cell growth. Mutant ras proteins behave like relay switches that are stuck in the "on" position, the result being enhanced cellular proliferation. The approach taken by the pharmaceutical industry has been to develop inhibitors of the farnesyl:protein transferase enzyme, so that although abnormal ras precursor proteins continue to be made by the cancer cell, they cannot localize appropriately to the inner aspect of the plasma membrane and, thus, cannot function.

Despite the elegant rationale that lies behind the development of farnesyl transferase inhibitors, their antitumor activity may be only partly due to inhibition of ras function [182]. For example, cells that express the K-ras oncoprotein should be unaffected, in theory, by treatment with farnesyl:protein transferase inhibitors because this ras protein can have an alternative isoprenoid moiety (geranyl-geranyl) added to it by a different enzyme. However, in fact, treatment of such cells with farnesyl:protein transferase inhibitors does decrease their proliferation. Moreover, farnesyl:protein transferase inhibitors can block the growth of tumor cell lines that have no *ras* mutation at all. In the case of such tumor cells, possibly inhibition of normal *ras* function is effective because the normal ras protein lies downstream of an abnormal mitogenic signal. For example, if the tumor cell is overexpressing EGFR, which sends its signal through *ras,* shutting down *ras* may be as effective as shutting down the tyrosine kinase activity of the receptor. Also, the farnesyl:protein transferase enzyme clearly modifies a large number of proteins in addition to ras. The relevance of these proteins to the antitumor activity of farnesyl:protein transferase inhibitors is being investigated.

The clinical development of farnesyl:protein transferase inhibitors has just begun, with results from an as-yet incomplete phase I trial being reported in the spring of 1999 [183]. R115777 is a benzodiazepine peptidomimetic farnesyl:protein transferase inhibitor that essentially is devoid of any geranyl-geranyl:protein transferase activity [184]. This compound inhibits farnesylation of K-ras, the concentration required to achieve 50% inhibition (IC_{50}) being 7.9 nmol/liter,

but can produce only 40% inhibition of geranyl-geranyl:protein transferase at a concentration of 50 μmol/liter. In tissue culture, R115777 inhibits the growth of human tumor cell lines that bear K-ras mutations, with 50% inhibitory concentrations (IC_{50}s) in the range of 16–22 nmol/liter. In a phase I clinical trial, this compound has been administered by mouth twice a day for 10 days, followed by nine days of rest. A dose of 125 mg orally twice per day has been well tolerated and produces serum concentrations well in excess of those required in vitro for inhibition of the enzyme and inhibition of growth.

As with the Herceptin and C225 humanized monoclonal antibodies, undoubtedly farnesyl:protein transferase inhibitors will be combined with cytotoxic chemotherapeutic agents. Such combinations already have been explored in the laboratory, with the finding that at least one farnesyl:protein transferase inhibitor had additive growth-inhibitory effects with doxorubicin, cisplatin, vinblastine, and 5-FU. Moreover, *synergistic* growth inhibition was observed when this farnesyl:protein transferase inhibitor was combined with paclitaxel or another group of compounds, called epothilones, which stabilize microtubules [185]. The farnesyl:protein transferase inhibitor increased the sensitivity of tumor cells to the metaphase block created by these cytotoxic agents, implying that a farnesylated protein may regulate the mitotic checkpoint. This outcome serves as another example of the manner in which a farnesyl:-protein transferase inhibitor might prove useful in the treatment of tumors that lack a *ras* mutation.

Cyclin-Dependent Kinase Inhibitors

Although correction of the defects created by the loss of tumor suppressor genes would seem to be effected most logically through reintroduction of those genes, tremendous practical obstacles confront gene therapy. An alternative to replacing genes directly is to consider the downstream targets of a gene's normal function and then to develop small molecules to influence those targets.

Of these downstream targets, a group that is now receiving much attention are the cyclin-dependent kinases (CDKs). These regulate the progression of cells through the different phases of the cell cycle. One important pathway regulated by CDKs is that of the retinoblastoma (Rb) protein, which normally blocks the progression of cells from G_1 to S phase. The CDK4/6 protein phosphorylates the Rb protein, the result of which is inactivation of the protein's ability to block G_1 to S progression. The CDKs are themselves regulated by cyclin proteins, with which they complex noncovalently in a 1:1 molar ratio. It is this holoenzyme complex that is catalytically active. Further complexity is added by the regulation of the holoenzyme's activity by endogenous CDK inhibitors. The vast majority of human cancers have abnormalities in some component of the Rb pathway. Abnormalities giving rise to increased cellular proliferation may come from overexpression of positive cofactors (cyclins/CDKs), from a decrease in negative factors (endogenous CDK inhibitors), or from Rb gene mutations.

This complex pathway could theoretically be targeted by a number of strategies, but most research is focused on the development of molecules that inhibit the activity of the catalytic CDK subunit by interacting with the ATP-binding site. Although highly selective CDK inhibitors have not yet entered the clinic, there has been some clinical experience with two compounds that have CDK-inhibitory activity: flavopiridol and 7-hydroxystaurosporine (UCN-01).

Flavopiridol is a semisynthetic flavone that inhibits CDKs and also protein kinase C (PKC). In tumor cells with dysregulated growth, flavopiridol induces growth arrest in the G_1 phase of the cell cycle and does so by inhibiting CDK2 and CDK4 [186, 187]. In a recently completed phase I trial of flavopiridol, the drug was administered to patients with advanced solid tumors as a 72-hour continuous IV infusion [188]. The dose-limiting toxicity of this therapy was secretory diarrhea, although the dose could be escalated further with the addition of loperamide and cholestyramine. The concentrations of flavopiridol achieved with a 72-hour infusion were similar to those required for in vitro inhibition of tumor growth and of CDK activity. Minor responses were observed in two patients with renal cell carcinoma and in one patient with a non-Hodgkin's lymphoma. Also being explored is the use of flavopiridol in combination with paclitaxel, based on the observation that flavopiridol enhances paclitaxel-induced apoptosis in a sequence-dependent fashion [189].

Although UCN-01 is an inhibitor of PKC, it also can inhibit the activity of CDKs [190]. Cyclin B1Cdc2, the cyclin-CDK complex that appears to be the most sensitive to the effects of UCN-01, regulates progression of cells through G_2. One mechanism for tumor cells to be resistant to the effects of DNA-damaging agents is to arrest their growth in phase G_2, which provides more time for DNA repair to occur before entry into mitosis: If DNA repair can occur before the cell proceeds to mitosis, the tumor cell is less likely to undergo apoptosis.

Prolonged arrest of cells in phase G_2 is characteristic of tumors that express mutated *p53*, and UCN-01 potently abrogates this arrest. It would be logical, then, to combine UCN-01 with a DNA-damaging agent such as cisplatin, with the hope of improving the therapeutic index of cisplatin. One problem with UCN-01 not predicted from its preclinical evaluation is that in humans it binds with high affinity to α-1-acid glycoprotein [191]. This binding probably accounts for its extremely long elimination half-life (four weeks) [192] and raises concern about its ability to access its intended target.

Angiogenesis

The growth of a malignant neoplasm depends on many factors. Tumor cells contain multiple genetic lesions that both reflect and give rise to genomic instability. Further, the tumor contains stromal cells, including blood vessels, which are not neoplastic but are necessary for the tumor to proliferate beyond microscopic size. The process by which a tumor increases its supporting vascular supply is called *angiogenesis*, and this process is essential to the development of macroscopic tumors. The process of angiogenesis is governed by a variety of growth factors and cytokines known to normally respond to tissue injury and inflammation. PDGF is known to be released from platelets when they form a vascular plug. Vascular endothelial cell growth factor (VEGF) is a potent stimulator of endothelial cell growth and originally was identified by its effect on vessel permeability. Secretion of such angiogenic factors by tumor cells is one mechanism for locally increasing the concentration of these factors at the site of a tumor. The anti-angiogenic agents currently in clinical trials consist of small-molecules with relatively selective toxicity for endothelial cells and of agents directed at newly defined growth-regulatory molecules in endothelial cells, including matrix metalloproteinase inhibitors.

ANGIOGENESIS INHIBITORS IN CLINICAL TRIALS

TNP-470, a derivative of the fungal product fumagillin, causes selective inhibition of endothelial cell function, with arrest of endothelial cells in phase G_1 of the cell cycle [193]. It appears to interact with a novel target, methionine aminopeptidase [194]; the unique relation of this target to endothelial cell physiology is being clarified. When TNP-470 was administered as a one-hour infusion three times a week or as a four-hour infusion weekly, the dose-limiting toxicity was neurocerebellar. An initial phase II evaluation of this agent's activity in renal cell carcinoma (one-hour infusion three times weekly) revealed one partial remission and five patients with stable disease for more than 16 weeks among 20 patients enrolled [195]. Other phase II evaluations are planned, as are extended infusion schedules and combination studies with cytotoxic agents.

Thalidomide is another molecule with selective toxicity for endothelial cells. Its use as an antiangiogenic agent was suggested when researchers realized that the characteristic phocomelia, the teratogenic consequence of its use in pregnancy, may have resulted from toxicity to vessels in the fetal limb buds. Evidence of a therapeutic biological effect directed against endothelial cells was demonstrated first in AIDS-associated Kaposi's sarcoma: of 44 patients in a series of phase Ib and phase II studies, 15 (34%) were considered to have had a partial remission [196, 197]. Major toxicities have included drowsiness, constipation, and a peripheral neuropathy, with rash, myositis, headache, and depression reported less frequently. Ongoing phase II studies of thalidomide's efficacy have suggested that it may have activity in prostate cancer and in recurrent high-grade glioma.

Researchers hope that more selective effects on endothelial cells will come from agents that are targeted to the unique aspects of endothelial cell biology. Antibody-based therapies directed against angiogenesis include Vitaxin, a monoclonal antibody to the human endothelial cell receptor $\alpha_v\beta_3$ integrin. RhuMab VEGF [198] is a humanized monoclonal antibody that binds to VEGF, which theoretically should remove VEGF from availability to the endothelial cell as a growth promoter. Speaking to the ability of this molecule to interact with its target, bleeding has been an occasional toxicity of therapy with this antibody. Alternatively, one could develop an antibody that binds to the receptor for VEGF but fails to activate it, and which prevents the receptor from binding to its normal ligand; an antibody of this type will soon enter clinical trials. Other investigators are attempting to target the VEGF receptor with a more traditional strategy, developing small molecule inhibitors of the receptor's ATP-binding site. One such small molecule is SU5416 [199].

PRACTICAL APPLICATION OF CANCER CHEMOTHERAPY

Although oncologists eagerly await fulfillment of the promises of novel, more selective, and more efficacious systemic cancer treatments, much can be accomplished by the judicious use of the agents currently available.

Most oncologists spend less of their time prescribing chemotherapy and more of their time establishing patients' diagnosis, evaluating the extent of the disease, and assessing the entirety of such patients' comorbid illnesses to formulate an appropriate plan of care. That plan of care may range from aggressive therapy, carrying with it high morbidity and some risk of treatment-related death, to no specific anticancer treatment.

Curable Cancer

Patients with Hodgkin's disease, ALL, AML, non-Hodgkin's lymphoma, testicular and ovarian germ-cell tumors, choriocarcinoma, and childhood sarcomas, and small percentages of those with ovarian and small-cell lung cancer have malignancies that are potentially curable with current chemotherapeutic programs. For such patients, using the most effective agents in the highest dosage and at the most frequent intervals is essential. As the goal of treatment is cure, the acceptance of greater short-term toxicity is justifiable because of the possibility of long-term benefit. The availability of intensive support given by highly trained personnel is mandatory for achieving the best results. In most of these illnesses, responses are rapid and dramatic, and usually only three to six months of therapy is necessary to achieve maximal benefit. Partial response in such patients will be of only marginal value; ultimately, disease in all partial responders will progress, and they will die of malignancy.

Palliative Treatment

The majority of adults with cancer have primary lesions of the aerodigestive tract that are not amenable to cure. Metastatic breast cancer also fits into this category of incurable cancers. Clinical trials are essential for such patients, especially phase II trials, which identify new agents or multimodality regimens. "Standard" treatment for such illnesses may be associated with substantial response rates, as in most patients with breast cancer and ovarian cancer, or little to no response, as in those with renal cell carcinoma or melanoma. For all patients receiving palliative therapy, the therapeutic index of the treatment program, especially as regards toxicity, is of prime importance. Palliation includes treatment of both psychological and physical symptoms. Some physically asymptomatic patients require treatment to allay anxiety and to reinforce their perception "that all is being done." Others without any physical or emotional distress will have nothing to palliate. The decision for treatment in such patients rests on physicians' clear understanding of affected patients' knowledge and desires, and it mandates close physician-patient rapport. When feasible, such patients always should be offered the opportunity to participate in clinical trials.

E. Immunotherapy

■ ■ ■

RONALD B. HERBERMAN

The field of tumor immunology encompasses the wide variety of interactions between the immune system and tumors, emphasizing the immune system's role in resisting the development or progressive growth of cancer and how it can be manipulated to increase such resistance. Tumor immunology also has important applications to the immunodiagnosis of cancer and understanding of altered immunocompetence in tumor-bearing individuals. The main principles of tumor immunology have emerged from extensive studies performed mainly during the last 30 years.

IMMUNE SYSTEM RECOGNITION OF TUMOR CELLS

A wide variety of tumor cells express molecular structures that differ from normal cells of the same individual and can be recognized by one or more components of the immune system. Most of the immunologic discrimination of tumor cells from normal cells has been attributed to recognition by the host of tumor antigens; additionally, however, tumor cells have been found to have other, nonantigenic differences that may be recognizable by the natural immune system.

Tumor Antigens

Most tumor cells have molecular configurations that can be recognized specifically by immune T cells or by antibodies and thus are termed *tumor antigens*. The most important tumor antigens, in terms of immunodiagnosis or host resistance, have been termed *tumor-associated antigens* (TAAs). They are expressed selectively on tumor cells and are not detectable on normal cells of the same individual. For many years, tumor immunologists sought tumor antigens that would be uniquely present on tumor cells and qualitatively different from antigens on any normal cells, hence called *tumor-specific antigens*. However, most antigens on tumor cells that initially were thought to be tumor-specific have been found, by more extensive evaluation of a wider range of normal tissues and the use of highly sensitive immunoassays, to be expressed in some circumstances, at least in low amounts, in some normal cells. Thus, the operational term *TAA* seems more valid. An important subset of TAA is *tumor-associated transplantation antigens* (TATAs), which can induce immunologically specific resistance to tumor growth in autologous hosts. The immunologic reactions that allow a host to recognize TATAs and thereby to mediate elimination of the tumor cells appear to resemble closely those that mediate rejection of tissue allografts with weak histocompatibility antigenic differences from the host. Tumor cells also contain many normal cellular antigens characteristic of the tissue or organ from which the neoplastic cells are derived or the stage of differentiation of the tumor cells.

Controversy surrounds the issue of whether all or most tumors express TATAs. Although the majority of tumors induced in experimental animals by oncogenic viruses or chemical carcinogens have been shown to have TATAs, some studies of tumors arising spontaneously in aged mice or rats have indicated that most of these spontaneous tumors lacked detectable TATAs. Thus, for most human tumors, which have no known etiology and would be considered spontaneous, it has been suggested that they also lack TATAs [200]. However, as discussed in some detail, such arguments are subject to considerable limitations [201]. Although evidence about the proportion of human tumors that express TATAs still is insufficient, considerable suggestive or circumstantial evidence speaks for the presence of TATAs on many human tumors. During the last several years, a series of TAAs on malignant melanomas has been defined and shown to be mainly normal antigens associated with melanocytes and normal cells [202]. Several of these TAAs appear to function as TATAs and form the basis for therapeutic cancer vaccines.

For a TAA to function as a TATA, it must be recognized by the host's immune system and must elicit immunologic reactivity that results in destruction, or at least growth inhibition, of the tumor. During the last several years, our understanding of how TAAs and other antigens are recognized and elicit specific immune reactivity has increased rapidly. Small peptide portions of antigens (most of which are 9–15 amino acids in length) have been shown to associate physically with class II or class I major histocompatibility complex (MHC) molecules, and such combined structures interact with helper or cytotoxic T cells, respectively [203].

In addition to TAAs that evoke cellular immune response in the host, other categories of TAAs exist, some of which also have considerable practical importance. Any TAA recognized by antibodies in the serum of tumor-bearing hosts or in the sera of animals immunized against the antigen can be used to discriminate between tumor cells and normal cells; this capability may be valuable for immunodiagnosis. TAAs common to a variety of tumors, at least of the same organ or histologic type, are most likely to be useful for diagnostic purposes. Studies in animal model systems have shown that tumors induced by chemical carcinogens and some spontaneous tumors have TATAs that are individually distinct and are not present in other tumors induced by the same agent, even when those tumors arise in the same host. Such antigens would not be helpful diagnostically, because antibodies against one tumor would not be expected to react with any other tumors. Common TAAs have been identified on many tumors, and even those that are not recognized by the immune response of tumor-bearing individuals may be detected readily by antibodies elicited in a different species.

Nonantigenic Differences Between Tumor and Normal Cells

Because detecting individually distinct TAAs on human tumors would be technically difficult, not surprisingly, most of the described human TAAs have been found to be distributed widely, at least on tumors of the same histologic type and with shared class I MHC determinants [203]. TAAs are the targets for recognition by the components of the classic immune system: immune T cells or antibodies (or both). Also, various components of the natural immune system (e.g., natural killer cells or macrophages) can recognize and react selectively with tumor cells. Although the basis for such recognition is not well understood, it may be due to the expression on tumor cells of a variety of cell-surface molecules in larger quantity or in altered form relative to normal cells. These tumor-associated differences do not seem to be restricted to tumor cells, as virus-infected normal cells or other cells also may be recognized by natural effector cells.

Basis for Differences

The molecular basis for antigenic or other differences between tumor and normal cells still is not understood completely. Several different mechanisms appear to be involved.

CLONALLY DISTRIBUTED MOLECULES

Some types of molecules may be highly polymorphic and clonally distributed on normal cells of the population. Because most tumors appear to arise from a single abnormal cell, they may express structurally normal molecules that are characteristic for that clone. The best-known example of this type of TAA is the cell-surface immunoglobulin on malignant B cells. The immunoglobulin genes of both normal and malignant B cells undergo recombinations that generate clonal diversity, particularly in the region of the antigen-combining sites. Such idiotypic structures provide individually specific antigens on each malignant clone, and monoclonal antibodies to such idiotypic determinants on human B-cell lymphoma have been the focus for some attempts at immunotherapy. More recently, vaccine trials have been performed to immunize lymphoma patients actively against their idiotypic proteins [204].

VIRUS-ASSOCIATED ANTIGENS

Tumors induced by an oncogenic virus, even when they differ in morphologic appearance or arise in different organs, share the same TAAs, some of which may function by new genetic information introduced by the virus into the tumor cell. In other cases, the oncogenic virus may induce or alter the expression of oncogenes present within the host genome. In the last several years, the products of mutated or overexpressed oncogenes, such as *p53* and *HER2/neu*, have provided the basis for some promising therapeutic vaccines [205].

TAAS OF CARCINOGEN-INDUCED TUMORS

As noted, tumors induced by chemical carcinogens, ultraviolet irradiation, or other physical agents usually express TATAs that individually are tumor-specific. The basis for such induction is not clear, but these agents share the ability to cause mutations in DNA, and their TAAs may be due to genetic alterations in normal cellular genes. Recently, detailed molecular studies have been performed on a series of TATAs associated with a murine carcinogen-induced tumor, and each has been attributed to a point mutation in unrelated genes [206].

DIFFERENTIATION ANTIGENS

Researchers have known for some time that antigens present on normal fetal cells may be expressed also on a variety of tumor cells, regardless of etiology. Antigens that display this characteristic have been termed *oncofetal* or *carcinoembryonic antigens*. On the basis of more recent and extensive experience, particularly from the extensive analysis of the specificity of antigens detected by various monoclonal antibodies, apparently a more general categorization of such antigens might be that of *differentiation antigens*. Often, tumor cells are arrested at a particular point in the pathway of differentiation for the normal cell type from which they arose. They express antigens characteristic for that stage of differentiation. Antigens of stem cells or of cells at early stages of differentiation may be rare in adults but frequent in fetuses and therefore may appear to be oncofetal in their distribution. Such differentiation antigens may help to classify certain tumors, particularly those derived from hematopoietic cells. In these cells, researchers have achieved considerable elucidation of the antigens associated with the stages of development in the various hematopoietic lineages.

TISSUE ANTIGENS

Large amounts of normal tissue or organ-associated antigens may be expressed in tumor cells derived from that tissue. Especially when the normal cells are relatively infrequent, the tissue antigen may appear to be tumor-associated and may be found to be tissue-associated only on careful examination of the relevant normal cells. As mentioned, several of the recently described human melanoma antigens are shared with normal melanocytes.

IMMUNE SYSTEM'S ROLE IN RESISTING CANCER

Many investigators have proposed that the immune system has a general role in preventing or limiting tumor growth. The central concept, known as the *immunosurveillance hypothesis*, postulates that the immune system is a key factor in resistance against the development of detectable tumors. The first known suggestion along these lines came from Paul Ehrlich in 1909 [207]; the modern formulation of the hypothesis originated from MacFarlane Burnet and Lewis Thomas. When information about thymus-dependent immunity became known—and particularly when T cells were found to play a central role in homograft rejection—Burnet modified the immunosurveillance hypothesis to stress the key role of this effector mechanism in antitumor resistance.

The immunosurveillance hypothesis since has generated many experimental studies and much discussion and controversy. One of the reasons for the controversy is that the concept leads to a series of predictions; most available evidence relates to tests of one or more of these predictions:

- Tumor cells have transplantation-type antigens.
- Resistance against tumors is T-cell-dependent and analogous to the homograft reaction.
- A close evolutionary link exists between malignancy and the development of an immune system with capability for rejection of tumors.
- Immunodepression is associated with, and must precede, development of detectable tumors.
- A requisite action of carcinogens or tumor promoters (or both) might be immunosuppression.

The main support for the immunosurveillance hypothesis has come from evidence related to the foregoing prediction regarding immunodepression, because naturally occurring or induced immunodepression has been associated with a higher incidence in some types of tumors. In experimental animal systems, this theory has been demonstrated most clearly with tumors induced by oncogenic viruses. Neonatal thymectomy and other forms of immunosuppression have been shown to lead to increased susceptibility to polyoma virus-induced tumors in mice and to Marek's disease in chickens.

Considerable clinical evidence shows that immunodeficiency diseases are associated with a much higher incidence of lymphoma and leukemia. Allograft recipients receiving immunosuppressive agents—either prednisone and azathioprine or, more recently, cyclosporin A or other immunosuppressive drugs—have been found also to have an increased incidence (approximately 100-fold) of lymphoproliferative disease or other tumors [208]. Patients who had cancer, arthritis, or other diseases and received chemotherapeutic (mainly alkylating) agents have been found subsequently to develop with relatively high frequency resultant primary malignancies, mainly leukemias and lymphomas. The recent observations of a remarkably high incidence of Kaposi's sarcoma or B-cell lymphoma in young adults with the acquired immunodeficiency syndrome are yet another indication of the association of malignancy with immunodepression.

Although such data support immunosurveillance, the original hypothesis was characterized by several major problems or limitations. The majority of human tumors associated with immunodepression have been leukemias and lymphoproliferative diseases, rather than a complete array of the common types of malignancy. The lymphoproliferative diseases occurring in immunosuppressed patients after organ transplantation have been shown to be associated closely with infection by Epstein-Barr virus [209], derived in at least some cases from the donor organs.

Also, the association between immunodepression and tumors has not been consistent. Neonatally thymectomized mice have been found to have a decreased incidence of mammary tumors, and nude and euthymic mice have similar incidences of spontaneous and carcinogen-induced tumors. Further, most spontaneous tumors of experimental animals lack detectable tumor-associated transplantation antigens [200]. Additionally, apparently an evolutionary dissociation exists between the development of tumors and the appearance of a sophisticated immune system and T cells.

These hypotheses have led to the suggestion that immunosurveillance may be operative only against tumors induced by oncogenic viruses, which have strong transplantation antigens and for which immune T cells have been shown to be important in resistance [210]. The major exceptions to the central role of immune T cells in resistance to tumor growth have even led Prehn and Lappe [211] to formulate a counter-theory of immunostimulation, suggesting that the immune system may have mainly enhancing effects on tumor induction and growth.

A more likely explanation for many of the discordant results is the involvement of a variety of effector mechanisms in host resistance. In the last several years, it has become apparent that natural immunity, as well as specifically induced immune responses, may contribute to host defenses. When T-cell-mediated immunity is viewed as only one of a series of possible host defense mechanisms, the foregoing summarized evidence need not be viewed in such a negative light. Target-cell structures other than tumor-associated transplantation antigens might be involved in recognition by other types of effector cells and, in T-cell-deficient individuals, natural immunity might still be functional and capable of resisting tumor growth. This is the basis for an updated immunosurveillance hypothesis: transformed cells express surface antigens or other structures that one or more components of the immune system can recognize; one or more components of the natural or induced immunologic effector mechanisms (or both) can eliminate the transformed cells or impede the progression and spread of tumors.

This broader hypothesis leads to a somewhat different set of predictions:

- Tumor cells have surface structures that are recognized by one or more effectors.
- Tumor cells will be susceptible to lysis or growth inhibition by one or more effector mechanisms.
- One or more of the relevant effector cells should be able to enter the site of tumor growth.
- Augmentation of relevant effector mechanisms will decrease the incidence of tumors or metastases.
- Depression of relevant effector mechanisms, either by carcinogen or by immunosuppressive treatment, will increase the incidence of tumors or metastases.
- Restoration of depressed effector activity will decrease the incidence of tumors or metastases.

In addition to the immune system's postulated role in surveillance against the development of tumors, considerable evidence points to involvement of both the classic and the natural immune responses in host resistance against the progression and metastatic spread of tumors once they arise. In fact, the evidence for an important role of some components of the immune system (e.g., natural killer cells) is much more compelling in regard to antimetastatic effects than for immunosurveillance. The immune system is complex, and several different components may be important effectors of host resistance against tumors.

Role of T Cells

Substantial evidence suggests that thymus-dependent immune responses are important in resistance to tumors induced by oncogenic viruses. However, the absence of the thymus has not been associated with increased susceptibility to other types of tumors, suggesting a limited role for T-cell immunity in immunosurveillance. Further, the inability to detect tumor-associated transplantation antigens on most spontaneous rodent tumors argues against a major involvement of specific immune responses. Recent evidence indicates, however, the importance of distinguishing between immunogenicity and antigenicity. *Immunogenicity* refers to the ability of a TAA to induce an immune response and appears to depend on the degree of expression of the antigen on the tumor cells and on the expression of MHC antigens and immunologic responsiveness. Ultraviolet light-induced tumors in mice have been found to express strong TATAs but usually are nonimmunogenic in ultraviolet light-irradiated animals because of a specific form of immunosuppression. Some other tumors in mice appear to be nonimmunogenic because they lack expression of MHC antigens.

The reactivity of specifically immune cytotoxic T lymphocytes (CTLs) against TAAs or other cell-surface antigens usually are restricted by the MHC, with cytotoxicity detectable only against target cells that share class I MHC determinants with the CTLs. Recently, considerable progress was made in elucidating the basis for the close association between immunogenicity and MHC expression. Many TAAs or other exogenous antigens must be presented to T cells by antigen-presenting cells in physical association with class II MHC molecules. During the last few years, dendritic cells have been targeted as particularly effective antigen-presenting cells [212]. Before presentation, the antigenic molecules are endocytosed and degraded into short peptides, and a physical complex between such peptides and class II molecules is transported to the cell surface. The T-cell receptors on helper (CD4-positive) T cells specifically can bind to and recognize these MHC-peptide complexes. TAAs also may be degraded into short peptides (8–10 amino acids in length) by proteosomes within the tumor cells themselves, which then form a complex with class I MHC molecules [203]. Such peptide-class I complexes can specifically bind to T-cell receptors on CD8-positive CTLs.

Although most TAAs can be recognized by T cells only when physically associated with MHC molecules, a notable exception has been characterized in detail [213]. CTLs have been detected in the regional lymph nodes of some patients with pancreatic cancer; these lymphocytes can recognize and lyse specifically not only autologous tumor cells but MHC-unrelated pancreatic and breast tumor cells. This lack of MHC restriction has been shown to be due to recognition of repeating peptide subunits on mucin molecules that are preferentially expressed on the tumor cells [213].

During the last few years, increasing evidence indicates that despite their progressive growth and metastasis, many tumors contain specifically immune T cells, termed *tumor-infiltrating lymphocytes*. In studies of human tumors, cultures of these lymphocytes from some malignant melanomas or, less frequently, from other tumor types have been shown to contain CTLs with specific antitumor reactivity. These findings not only provide indications for the immunogenicity of some human tumors but, as discussed later, provide a basis for specific adoptive therapy with such immune cells.

Antitumor CTLs derived from melanoma patients have been used also to identify and characterize the recognized TAA [202]. The CTLs have been shown to recognize a particular peptide in the context of a particular class I molecule (e.g., 2 or A1) [202].

Role of Macrophages

Macrophages have been suggested as important factors in antitumor defenses and might be primarily responsible for immunosurveillance against tumors. This possibility is supported by several lines of evidence. Macrophages can accumulate in considerable numbers in a variety of transplantable tumors and in many primary tumors. They have a natural ability to lyse or inhibit the in vitro growth of a wide variety of transformed cells, an ability that can be activated rapidly. Also, several treatments that can depress the function of macrophages (e.g., silica, carrageenan) have been associated with an increased incidence of tumors and metastases.

Additionally, adoptive transfer of in vitro- or in vivo-activated macrophages was shown to inhibit the metastatic spread of some tumor cell lines. Some carcinogens (e.g., methylcholanthrene, acetylaminofluorene) have been shown to depress reticuloendothelial function. Further, stimulation of macrophage function by various immunomodulators has been associated with decreased tumor growth or a decreased incidence of tumors.

However, some major limitations apply to such evidence. Remarkably little evidence substantiates that macrophages have cytotoxic activity against primary, freshly harvested tumor cells, as opposed to established tumor cell lines. Silica and carrageenan—and virtually all the other depressive treatments that have been used—may not be entirely selective in their effects. In fact, they may increase some functions, particularly suppressor activity, by macrophages or other cells.

Furthermore, the carcinogens shown to depress reticuloendothelial function may also have affected a variety of effector mechanisms, and other carcinogens have demonstrated no detectable effects on macrophage or reticuloendothelial function. In experiments with some transplantable tumors in mice, adoptive transfer of macrophages facilitated the development of metastases rather than conferring resistance to metastasis.

As with specific T-cell-mediated immunity, recent therapeutic studies have produced some evidence suggesting an important antitumor defense role for macrophages. An immunostimulatory agent based on the minimal immunomodulatory unit in mycobacteria and shown to be a fairly selective activator of macrophages has demonstrated substantial therapeutic efficacy against metastatic tumors in mice and dogs and appears to exercise activity against lung metastases of patients with osteosarcoma [214].

Role of Natural Killer Cells

Natural killer (NK) cells are a recently defined subpopulation of natural effector cells. They have the morphologic appearance of large, granular lymphocytes and a characteristic cell-surface phenotype that distinguishes them from T cells or macrophages. For example, most human NK cells are CD3-negative and CD56- and CD16-positive, whereas most T cells are CD3-positive and CD56- and CD16-negative. Against cancer cells, these cells exert spontaneous cytotoxic reactivity that is not dependent on or restricted by the MHC. In fact, recent studies have indicated that target cells deficient in MHC expression may be particularly susceptible to lysis by NK cells. In addition to their spontaneous antitumor reactivity, NK cells secrete a variety of cytokines, and their cytotoxic reactivity is augmented substantially by exposure to cytokines, especially interferons or interleukin-2 (IL-2), or by various biological response modifiers. Most lymphokine-activated killer (LAK) cell activity that is generated on culture of blood or spleen cells with IL-2 is attributable to IL-2-activated NK cells. LAK cells display very potent cytotoxic activity against most tumor cells, including freshly isolated tumor cells from the autologous or allogeneic solid tumors or leukemias.

Substantial evidence indicates the importance of NK cells in in vivo resistance against established tumor cell lines [215]. In addition, some evidence conforms to the predictions of the immunosurveillance hypothesis. For example, NK cells are able to accumulate at sites of inflammation and in both small primary and transplanted tumors NK cells have a natural ability to lyse a variety of primary autochthonous tumors, and this ability can be readily activated. Additionally, NK cells are able to eliminate metastatic tumor cells and thereby resist tumor spread.

Finally, an increased tumor incidence (primarily lymphomas) has been found in beige mice with depressed NK activity, in patients with Chédiak-Higashi syndrome, and in immunosuppressed transplant recipients [208]. Some carcinogens (urethane, gamma- or x-irradiation, and dimethylbenzanthracene) have been shown to cause early, profound depression of NK activity.

The most convincing data relate to the important function of NK cells in host resistance against metastases [215]. The observation that NK cells appear to be mainly responsible for the rapid elimination of intravenously inoculated tumor cells provided the initial indication that this effector mechanism might exert very effective control of hematogenous spread of tumors. Experimental support for this possibility first came from the finding that cells from the lung metastases of a transplantable tumor in mice were more resistant to NK activity than were locally growing tumor cells. Further support has come from observations that suppression or augmentation of NK activity in mice was associated with parallel alterations in resistance to artificial metastases produced by IV inoculation of tumor cells.

The patterns of results obtained in these studies suggested that NK cells may influence metastatic spread of tumors primarily by acting during the phase of hematogenous dissemination, presumably by their ability to eliminate the tumor cells rapidly from the circulation of capillary beds. The association between depressed NK activity and increased metastases was confirmed further by study results that revealed that selective restoration of NK activity in rats by adoptive transfer of highly purified, large, granular lymphocytes was accompanied by increased resistance to pulmonary metastases. Immunotherapy studies with transplantable sarcomas in mice by adoptive transfer of LAK cells have indicated appreciable antimetastatic effects even when therapy was initiated after pulmonary metastases had occurred. Highly purified IL-2-activated NK cells were shown to have more potent antimetastatic therapeutic activity than did unspecified LAK cells, and this effect has been associated with the selective accumulation of transferred effector cells at the tumor sites [216].

Role of Antibodies

In many tumor-bearing and immunized individuals, specific antitumor antibodies can be demonstrated. Antibodies specific for TAAs have been shown to kill tumor target cells in two ways, and some evidence suggests that both mechanisms operate in vivo. The first mechanism involves the fixing of complement-dependent IgG and IgM antibodies to antigenic sites on target cells and consequent activation of the complement cascade. Terminal C8 and C9 components bring about lysis by the classic pathway. The second cytocidal pathway is independent of complement and is known as *antibody-dependent cellular cytotoxicity.* Once antitumor IgG antibody fixes to the target cell membrane, various effector cells with receptors for the Fc portion of IgG, particularly NK cells and macrophages, then can bind to the antibody-coated tumor cells and cause their lysis.

Antitumor antibodies may be detrimental to the host. In experimental situations, antibodies administered before transplantation of tumor or infection by oncogenic virus led to tumor enhancement (afferent limb suppression of response) and thus have been termed *enhancing antibodies.* Other studies suggest that enhancing antibodies attach to the surface of tumor cells, thereby blocking or masking attachment sites for cytotoxic lymphocytes and cytolytic antibodies (efferent enhancement). In some clinical studies, the presence of detectable antibodies or antigen-antibody complexes in the circulation has been associated with the presence of tumor or poor prognosis. However, in other clinical studies, high antitumor antibody titers were seen after complete surgical removal of the tumor, and declining titers were associated with recurrence or metastatic spread.

CANCER AND IMMUNE SYSTEM FUNCTION

The presence of cancer can induce antitumor immune responses involving T cells or antibody-producing B cells (or both). In addition, in many situations, more general alterations in their immune system functioning are found in tumor-bearing individuals. Usually, the direction of modulation of immune function in cancer is negative, with depression of a variety of immunologic activities. This has in part been attributable to the release of immunosuppressive factors by the tumor cells and to the stimulation of suppressor macrophages or T cells.

The various detected deficits in immunocompetence in some tumor-bearing individuals have involved most components of the immune system. These have included decreased cellular immune reactivity, as reflected in vivo by delayed cutaneous hypersensitivity tests and in vitro by lymphoproliferative responses to mitogens or alloantigens, decreased macrophage responsiveness, and decreased NK activity.

The literature about depressed immunocompetence in tumor bearers is particularly extensive at the clinical level. The impairments observed have been most consistent in patients with advanced metastatic disease, but some studies have detected abnormalities even early in the course of disease or in patients with no detectable tumor. In tests for delayed cutaneous hypersensitivity to dinitrochlorobenzene, which involve sensitization by a large dose of antigen and challenge two weeks later with a low dose, the failure of some cancer patients to be sensitized has been a useful prognostic indicator of unresectable disease or early recurrence after surgery. Decreasing the dose used for sensitization would reveal some defects in patients with early Hodgkin's disease, which had previously been detected only in patients with advanced disease.

In vitro assays of cell-mediated immunity have been used also to seek decreased reactivity in cancer patients. As with the skin tests, the proportion of patients who had localized disease and evidence of immunodepression has varied considerably. Assays designed to detect subtle alterations in lymphoproliferative responses to mitogens and antigens and standardization of the procedures for testing and data analysis have yielded substantial evidence for depression in some patients with localized or early disease [217]. In one study of lung cancer patients after surgical removal of their tumors, patients with depressed lymphoproliferative responses in vitro to the mitogen concanavalin A or in mixed lymphocyte cultures experienced a significantly reduced disease-free survival. More recent studies have suggested that poor functional activity of T cells in cancer patients may be due to tumor-induced apoptotic damage and death of the lymphocytes [218].

Depressed NK activity levels also have been observed in some cancer patients. In some studies, this finding has been associated with a poor prognosis and a higher risk for developing distant metastases [219].

In addition to functional assays, enumeration of relative proportions and absolute numbers of T and B cells may be useful in immunodiagnosis. In particular, some findings suggest that many cancer patients, including some with localized disease, have decreased percentages of T-cell subpopulations, as assessed by high-affinity rosette formation with sheep erythrocytes or by flow cytometry with antibodies to CD4-positive T cells.

PRACTICAL APPLICATION OF THE PRINCIPLES OF TUMOR IMMUNOLOGY TO IMMUNOTHERAPY FOR CANCER

Tumor immunology investigations have contributed substantially to our overall understanding of the biology of cancer-host interaction. In addition, the information and insights gleaned from such investigations can be applied in a variety of ways to the detection, diagnosis, classification, prognostic assessment, and treatment of cancer.

Increasing evidence of the immune system's participation in resisting the progression and spread of cancer has raised expectations that manipulation of the immune system might also be a valuable treatment. Such optimism has been fostered by the findings that various cytokines and other biological response modifiers can appreciably stimulate or augment immunologic reactivity against cancer. Some species of genetically engineered interferon have been shown to exert appreciable antitumor effects against experimental tumors and against some clinical malignancies. Interferon-α already has been licensed by the US Food and Drug Administration as an effective treatment of hairy-cell leukemia, Kaposi's sarcoma, and poor-prognosis melanoma [220]. IL-2, particularly in combination with LAK cells (as discussed), has been shown to have strong antimetastatic effects against some experimental tumors in mice and rats. In some cases, IL-2 has induced cures. Analogous therapy in some patients with advanced cancer, particularly with malignant melanoma or renal cell carcinoma, has induced partial or complete regression of detectable metastatic lesions [221]. In detailed studies in an experimental tumor model, optimal results apparently may be achieved by combining cytoreduction therapy (surgery and chemotherapy) with adoptive immunotherapy (IL-2 and LAK cells).

Adoptive therapy specifically involving immune T cells and IL-2 may be even more potent than LAK cells and IL-2, with curative effects induced in some experimental tumor models [222]. Recently, very promising therapeutic results were obtained by specific in vitro sensitization with irradiated lymphoid tumor cells from mice with growing tumors. Clinically, tumor-infiltrating lymphocytes from patients with malignant melanoma have been expanded in culture with IL-2 and appear to have specific cytotoxic reactivity against the autologous tumor cells [223]. These IL-2-expanded cells, when transferred to the patients, have induced some complete tumor regressions. Considerably more efforts in the overall area of adoptive cellular immunotherapy seem warranted, with a focus on defining and purifying the effector cells responsible for the therapeutic effects, determining the conditions for optimally generating them and stimulating their antitumor reactivity, and maximizing their accumulation in all sites of tumor growth.

In addition to the studies of adoptive transfer specifically of immune T cells, the evaluation of strategies for immunotherapy, based on induction in vivo of spe-cific antitumor responses, recently has experienced an upsurge involving "cancer vaccines." Treatment of patients with intact, inactivated tumor cells or with tumor cell extracts has provided some encouraging—although still fairly preliminary—results, mainly in patients with malignant melanoma [224] but also in patients with some other tumor types. In recent studies with several animal tumor models, insertion into tumor cells of genes for cytokines (e.g., interleukin-12, interleukin-4, colony-stimulating factor) has resulted in an impressive increase in immunogenicity and antitumor effects. Clinical trials with such genetically altered tumor cells are in progress and also appear promising.

Infusion of monoclonal antibodies against TAAs has been another major approach for the treatment of metastatic cancer. The main strategy has been to combine the antibodies with toxic moieties, whether radionuclides, toxins, or drugs. The goal is to have the antibodies selectively carry the toxic agents to the tumor site or sites. Although this form of immunotherapy is reasonable and eventually should prove very useful, many technical problems have limited its therapeutic benefits.

In addition to the immunoconjugate approach, some antibodies by themselves appear to have promising therapeutic effects, which might be attributable to such mechanisms as complement-dependent lysis of tumor cells, interactions with effector cells for antibody-dependent cytotoxicity, or such immunoregulatory effects as the induction of antiidiotypic responses or triggering of signal transduction pathways in tumor cells. An example of the therapeutic effects of a monoclonal antibody alone is partial regression of tumor in several patients with advanced disease who were enrolled in a study of antibodies to the GD3 ganglioside in human malignant melanoma. More recently, impressive clinical results were seen with anti-CD20 antibodies in patients with lymphoma and with anti-HER2/neu antibodies in patients with breast cancer.

Other efforts have been directed toward stimulating hosts' immune systems using a wide variety of immunomodulators. These may be either defined chemical substances or, more frequently, such bacterial products as bacillus Calmette-Guérin. Although the latter agents usually are very heterogeneous and ill-defined, they can induce strong stimulation of various components of the immune system, including antitumor effector mechanisms. Bacillus Calmette-Guérin, a low-virulence variant of Mycobacterium tuberculosis, has been found to be very effective in treating superficial recurrent carcinoma of the bladder. A synthetic macrophage activator also has demonstrated therapeutic effects against some experimental tumors and is now being evaluated clinically [214].

CONCLUSION

Although immunotherapy for cancer has been somewhat successful to date, this field is in the earliest stages of development. Most of the promising strategies must be investigated in considerably greater detail, and the optimal doses and conditions for treatment must be defined. This task will require a methodical approach, with close interaction among the researchers conducting in vivo studies and detailed in vitro evaluation of the effects on the immune system.

REFERENCES

1. Janeway H. *Radium Therapy in Cancer at the Memorial Hospital, NY.* New York: Paul B. Hoeber, 1917.

2. Ewing J. Early experiences in radiation therapy. Janeway Memorial Lecture, 1933. *Am J Roentgenol Rad Ther* 31:153–183, 1934.

3. Halsted WS. The results of radical operation for the cure of carcinoma of the breast. *Ann Surg* 46:1–19, 1907.

4. Regaud C, Ferroux R. Influence du "facteur temps" sur la sterilisation des linees cellulaires normales et neoplastiques par la radiotherapie. *Radiophysiol Radiother* 1:343–357, 1927.

5. Forssell G. Role of radiology in medicine. *Radiology* 30:12–18, 1938.

6. Holfelder H. Comparison of medical, surgical and radiological conceptions in relation to treatment of disease. *Br J Radiol* 5:39–58, 1932.

7. del Regato J. Historical changes in time-dose relationship in therapeutic radiology. In Vaeth JM (ed), *Frontiers of Radiation Therapy Oncology,* vol III. Basel: Karger, 1968:1–5.

8. Easson EC, Russell MH. The cure of Hodgkin's disease. *Br Med J* 1:1704–1707, 1963.

9. Peters MV, Middlemiss KCH. A study of Hodgkin's disease treated by irradiation. *Am J Roentgenol* 79:114–121, 1958.

10. Kaplan HS. The radical radiotherapy of regionally localized Hodgkin's disease. *Radiology* 78:557–561, 1962.

11. Martin H. Radical surgery in the cancer of the head and neck. *Surg Clin North Am* 33:329–350, 1958.

12. Steiner P. Evaluation of cancer problems. *Cancer Res* 12:455–464, 1952.

13. Kruskall M. Autologous blood transfusion. In Hoffman R, Banz EJ Jr, Shattil SJ, et al. (eds), *Hematology: Basic Principles and Practice.* New York: Churchill Livingstone, 1995:2063–2067.

14. Anderson KC, Dzik WH. Transfusion medicine in hemopoietic stem cell and solid organ transplantation. In Hoffman R, Banz EJ Jr, Shattil SJ, et al. (eds), *Hematology: Basic Principles and Practice.* New York: Churchill Livingstone, 1995:2074–2087.

15. McSweeney P, Storb R. Bone marrow transplantation for malignant disease. In Rick RR, Fleisher TA, Schwartz BD, (eds), *Clinical Immunology: Principles and Practice.* St Louis: Mosby-Year Book, 1995:1831–1851.

16. Manyak MJ. Clinical applications of radioimmunoscintigraphy with prostate-specific antibodies for prostate cancer. *Cancer Control* 5:493–499, 1998.

17. Brady LW, Heilmann H-P, Kagan AR, Steckel RJ (eds). Practical approaches to cancer invasion and metastases. In *Medical Radiology.* Berlin: Springer, 1994.

18. National Comprehensive Cancer Network. Special proceedings issue. *Oncology* 7:1998.

19. Patt RB, Manfreddi P. Cancer pain emergencies. In Paris WCV (ed), *Cancer Pain Management: Principles and Practice.* Boston: Butterworth-Heinemann, 1997.

20. Bernstein SH, Nadernanee A, Vose J, et al. A multicenter study of platelet recovery and utilization in patients after myeloablative therapy and hematopoietic stem-cell transplants: cytokine growth factors in hematology and oncology. *Blood* 91:3509–3517, 1998.

21. Mackie TR. Radiation therapy treatment optimization. *Semin Radiat Oncol* 9:1–3, 1999.

22. Galen. *On the Natural Faculties.* Great Books of the Western World. Chicago: University of Chicago, Encyclopedia Britannica, 1982:196–197.

23. Abernethy J. *Surgical Observations on the Constitutional Origin and Treatment of Local Diseases.* London: Longman, Hurst, Rees, Orm, and Brown, 1814:180–200.

24. Bigelow HJ. Insensitivity during surgical operations produced by intuition. *Boston Med Surg* 33:309–317, 379–382, 1846.

25. Lister J. On the antiseptic principles in the practice of surgery. *Lancet* 2:353–356, 1867.

26. Moore CH. On the influence of inadequate operations on the theory of cancer. *Med Chir Trans* 50:245–280, 1867.

27. Billroth T. *The Medical Sciences in German Universities.* New York: Macmillan, 1924:244.

28. McDowell E. Three cases of extirpation of diseases ovaria. *Reperatory Analyst Rev* 7:242–244, 1817.

29. Halstead WS. The results of operations for the cure of cancer of the breast performed at Johns Hopkins Hospital from June 1, 1889 to January 1894. *Ann Surg* 20:497–555, 1894.

30. Fisher B, Montague E, Redmond C, et al. Comparison of radical mastectomy with alternative treatments for primary breast cancer. *Cancer* 29(suppl):2827–2838, 1977.

31. Singletary SE. Surgical management of locally advanced breast cancer. *Semin Radiat Oncol* 4:254–263, 1994.

32. Nigro ND. An evaluation of combined therapy for squamous cell cancer of the anal canal. *Dis Colon Rectum* 27:763–781, 1984.

33. Brennan MF, Casper ES, Harrison LB. Soft tissue sarcoma. In DeVita VT Jr, Hellman S, Rosenberg SA (eds), *Cancer: Principals and Practice of Oncology* (5th ed). Philadelphia: Lippincott, 1996:1738.

34. Hays DM, Young DC. Solid tumors in pediatric patients.

In McKennon J, Murphy GP (eds), *Fundamentals of Surgical Oncology.* New York: Macmillan, 1986:806–824.

35. Fleming I, Cooper SJ, Henson DE, et al. (eds). *AJCC Cancer Staging Manual* (5th ed). Philadelphia: Lippincott-Raven, 1997.

36. Morton DL, Wen DR, Wong JH, et al. Technical details of intraoperative lymphatic mapping for early stage melanoma. *Arch Surg* 127:392–399, 1992.

37. Bacon HE, Martin PV. The rationale of palliative resection for primary cancer of the colon and rectum complicated by liver and lung metastasis. *Dis Colon Rectum* 7:211–218, 1964.

38. Wanebo HJ, Chu QD, Vezerdis MD, Soderberg C. Patient selection for hepatic resection of colorectal metastasis. *Arch Surg* 131:322–329, 1996.

39. McCormack P. Surgical resection of pulmonary metastasis. *Semin Surg Oncol* 6:297–302, 1990.

40. Marks G, Mohuidden M. The surgical management of radiation injured intestine. *Surg Clin North Am* 63:81–96, 1983.

41. Kaste SC, Hudson MM, Jones DJ, et al. Breast masses in women treated for childhood cancer: incidence and screening guidelines. *Cancer* 82:784–792, 1998.

42. Schneider AB, Shore-Freedman E, Ryo JY, et al. Radiation induced tumors of the head and neck following childhood radiation. *Medicine (Baltimore)* 64:1–15, 1985.

43. Eyre H. President's roundtable on clinical trials: plenary session. ASCO, Atlanta, GA, 1999.

44. Calabresi P, Antman KH, Mayer DK, et al. Cancer at a crossroad—report of the National Cancer Advisory Board on the National Cancer Program. *Cancer* 76:138–156, 1995.

45. Roentgen WC. On a new kind of rays (preliminary communication). [Translation of a paper read before the Physikalische-medicinischen Gesellschaft of Wurzburg on December 28, 1895.] *Br J Radiol* 4:32, 1931.

46. Curie P, Curie M, Bemont G. Sur une nouvelle substance fortement radioactive contenue dans la pechblende (note presented by M Becquerel). *Compt Rend Acad Sci (Paris)* 127:1215–1217, 1898.

47. Coutard H. Roentgen therapy of epitheliomas of the tonsillar regional hypopharynx and larynx from 1920 to 1926. *Am J Roentgenol* 28:313–331, 1932.

48. Coutard H. Principles of x-ray therapy of malignant diseases. *Lancet* 2:1–8, 1934.

49. Puck TT, Marcus PI. Action of x-rays on mammalian cells. *J Exp Med* 103:653–656, 1956.

50. McCulloch EA, Till JE. Proliferation of hematopoietic colony-forming cells transplanted into irradiated mice. *Radiat Res* 22:383–397, 1964.

51. Withers HR. The dose-survival relationship for irradiation of epithelial cells of mouse skin. *Br J Radiol* 40:187–194, 1967.

52. Read J. Mode of action of x-ray doses given with different oxygen concentrations. *Br J Radiol* 25:336–338, 1952.

53. Elkind MM, Whitmore GF. *The Radiobiology of Cultured Mammalian Cells.* New York: Gordon and Breach, 1967.

54. Alper T. *Cellular Radiobiology.* London: Cambridge University Press, 1979.

55. Bender M. Induced aberrations in human chromosomes. *Am J Pathol* 43:260, 1963.

56. Evans HJ. Chromosomes aberrations induced by ionizing radiation. *Int Rev Cytol* 13:221–321, 1962.

57. Gerard CR. Effects of radiation on chromosomes. In Pizzarello D (ed), *Radiation Biology.* Boca Raton, FL: CRC Press, 1982:83–110.

58. Ishihara T, Sasaki MS (eds). *Radiation-Induced Chromosome Damage in Man.* New York: Alan R. Liss, 1983.

59. Hall EJ. Radiation-induced chromosome aberrations. In *Radiobiology for the Radiologist.* Philadelphia: Lippincott, 1988.

60. Deschner EE, Gray LH. Influence of oxygen tension on x-ray induced chromosomal damage in Ehrlich ascites tumor cells irradiated in vitro and in vivo. *Radiat Res* 11:115–146, 1959.

61. Elkind MM, Alescio T, Swain RW, et al. Recovery of hypoxic mammalian cells from sublethal x-ray damage. *Nature* 202:1190–1193, 1964.

62. Gray LH, Conger AD, Ebert M, et al. The concentration of oxygen dissolved in tissues at the time of irradiation as a factor in radiotherapy. *Br J Radiol* 26:638–648, 1953.

63. Hall EJ. The oxygen effect and reoxygenation. In *Radiobiology for the Radiologist.* Philadelphia: Lippincott, 1988:137–158.

64. Palcic B, Skarsgard LD. Reduced oxygen enhancement ratio at low doses of ionizing radiation. *Radiat Res* 100:328–339, 1984.

65. Hall EJ, Bedford JS, Oliver R. Extreme hypoxia: its effect on the survival of mammalian cells irradiated at high and low dose-rates. *Br J Radiol* 39:302–307, 1966.

66. Hall EJ. Radiation dose-rate: a factor of importance in radiobiology and radiotherapy. *Br J Radiol* 45:81–97, 1972.

67. Ewing D, Powers EL. Oxygen-dependent sensitization of irradiated cells. In Meyn RE, Withers HR (eds), *Radiation Biology in Cancer Research.* New York: Raven Press, 1980:143–168.

68. Michael BD, Adams GE, Hewitt HB, et al. A post effect of oxygen in irradiated bacteria: a submillisecond fast mixing study. *Radiat Res* 54:239–251, 1973.

69. Howard-Flanders P, Moore D. The time interval after pulsed irradiation within which injury to bacteria can be modified by dissolved oxygen: I. A search for an effect of oxygen 0.02 second after pulsed irradiation. *Radiat Res* 9:422–437, 1958.

70. Thomlinson RH, Gray LH. The histologic structure of some human lung cancers and the possible implications for radiotherapy. *Br J Cancer* 9:539–549, 1955.

71. Bush RS, Jenkin RDT, Allt WEC, et al. Definitive evidence for hypoxic cells influencing cure in cancer therapy. *Br J Cancer* 37:302–306, 1978.

72. Cater DB, Silver IA. Quantitative measurement of oxygen tension in normal tissues and in the tumours of patients before and after radiotherapy. *Acta Radiol* 53:233, 1960.

73. Withers HR, Suit HD. Is oxygen important in the radiocurability of human tumors? In Friedman M (ed), *The Biological and Clinical Basis of Radiosensitivity.* Springfield, IL: Thomas, 1974.

74. Thomlinson RH. Reoxygenation as a function of tumor size and histopathological type. In *Time and Dose Relationship in Radiation Biology as Applied to Radiotherapy.* [Brook-

haven National Laboratory Rep. 50203(C-57).] Brookhaven, NY: Brookhaven National Laboratory, 1970:242–254.

75. Kallman RF. The phenomenon of reoxygenation and its implications for fractionated radiotherapy. *Radiology* 105:135–142, 1972.

76. Elkind MM, Sutton H. X-ray damage and recovery in mammalian cells in culture. *Nature* 184:1293, 1959.

77. Hendrickson FR, Withers HR. Principles of radiation oncology. In Holleb AI, Fink DJ, Murphy GR (eds), *American Cancer Society Textbook of Clinical Oncology*. Atlanta: American Cancer Society, 1991:39.

78. Suit HD, Howes AE, Hunter N. Dependence of response of a C3H mammary carcinoma to fractionated irradiation on fraction number and intertreatment interval. *Radiat Res* 72:440–454, 1977.

79. Thames HD, Peters LJ, Withers HR, et al. Accelerated fractionation vs hyperfractionation: rationales for several treatments per day. *Int J Radiat Oncol Biol Phys* 9:127–138, 1983.

80. Sinclair WK. Dependence of radiosensitivity upon cell age. In *Time and Dose Relationships in Radiation Biology as Applied to Radiotherapy*. [Brookhaven National Laboratory Rep. 50203 (C-57).] Brookhaven, NY: Brookhaven National Laboratory, 1969:97.

81. Legrys GA, Hall EJ. The oxygen effect and x-ray sensitivity in synchronously dividing cultures of Chinese hamster cells. *Radiat Res* 37:161–172, 1969.

82. Hall EJ, Brown JM, Cavanagh J. Radiosensitivity and the oxygen effect measured at different phases of the mitotic cycle using synchronously dividing cells of the root meristem of *Vicia faba*. *Radiat Res* 35:622–634, 1968.

83. Sinclair WK. Cysteamine: differential x-ray protective effect on Chinese hamster cells during the cell cycle. *Science* 159:442–444, 1968.

84. Ang KK, Landuyt W, Rijnders A, et al. Differences in repopulation kinetics in mouse skin during split-course multiple fractions per day or daily fractionated irradiations. *Int J Radiat Oncol Biol Phys* 10:95–99, 1985.

85. Hermens AF, Barendsen GW. Changes of cell proliferation characteristics in a rat rhabdomyosarcoma before and after x-irradiation. *Eur J Cancer* 5:173–189, 1969.

86. Withers HR, Taylor JM, Maciejewski B. The hazard of accelerated tumor clonogen repopulation during radiotherapy. *Acta Radiol* 27:131–146, 1988.

87. Hall EJ. Time, dose and fractionation in radiotherapy. In *Radiobiology for the Radiologist*. Philadelphia: Lippincott, 1988:240.

88. Rubin P, Constantine L, Nelson D. Late effects of cancer treatment: radiation and drug toxicity. In Perez C, Brady LW (eds), *Principles and Practice of Radiation Oncology*. Philadelphia: Lippincott, 1992.

89. Mendenhall WM, Million RR, Cassisi NJ. Elective neck irradiation in squamous cell carcinoma of the head and neck. *Head Neck Surg* 3:15–20, 1980.

90. Fletcher GH. The scientific basis of the present and future practice of clinical radiotherapy. *Int J Radiat Oncol Biol Phys* 9:1073–1082, 1983.

91. Fletcher GH (ed). *Textbook of Radiotherapy* (3rd ed). Philadelphia: Lea & Febiger, 1980.

92. Fletcher GH, Shukovsky LJ. The interplay of radiocur-

ability and tolerance in the irradiation of human cancers. *J Radiol Electrol* 56:383–400, 1975.

93. Meoz-Mendez RT, Fletcher GH, Guillamondequi OM, et al. Analysis of the results of irradiation in the treatment of squamous cell carcinomas of the pharyngeal walls. *Int J Radiat Oncol Biol Phys* 4:579–585, 1978.

94. Shukovsky LJ, Baeza MR, Fletcher GH. Results of irradiation in squamous cell carcinomas of the glossopalatine sulcus. *Radiology* 120:405–408, 1976.

95. Suit H, Lindberg R, Fletcher GH. Prognostic significance of extent of tumor regression at completion of radiation therapy. *Radiology* 84:1100–1107, 1965.

96. Suit HD. Potential for improving survival rates for the cancer patient by increasing the efficacy of treatment of the primary lesion. *Cancer* 50:1227–1234, 1982.

97. DeVita VT Jr. Principles of chemotherapy. In DeVita VT Jr, Hellman S, Rosenberg SA (eds), *Cancer: Principles and Practice of Oncology* (2nd ed). Philadelphia: Lippincott, 1985:257–285.

98. Rubin P. The emergence of radiation oncology as a distinct medical specialty. *Int J Radiat Oncol Biol Phys* 11:1247–1270, 1985.

99. Gilman A, Philips FS. The biological actions and therapeutic applications of the B-chloroethyl amines and sulfides. *Science* 103:409–436, 1946.

100. Farber S, Diamond LK, Mercer RD, et al. Temporary remissions in acute leukemia in children produced by folic acid antagonist, 4-aminopteroyl-glutamic acid (Aminopterin). *N Engl J Med* 238:787–793, 1948.

101. Hertz R, Lewis J Jr, Lipsett MB. Five years' experience with the chemotherapy of metastatic choriocarcinoma and related trophoblastic tumors in women. *Am J Obstet Gynecol* 82:631–640, 1961.

102. DeVita VT Jr, Serpick AA, Combination chemotherapy in the treatment of Hodgkin's disease. *Ann Intern Med* 73:881–895, 1970.

103. Early Breast Cancer Trialists' Collaborative Group. Systemic treatment of early breast cancer by hormonal, cytotoxic, or immune therapy: 133 randomised trials involving 31,000 recurrences and 24,000 deaths among 75,000 women. *Lancet* 339:1–15, 71–85, 1992.

104. Moertel CG, Fleming TR, Macdonald JS, et al. Levamisole and fluorouracil for adjuvant therapy of resected colon cancer. *N Engl J Med* 322:352–358, 1990.

105 Cleaver JE. *Thymidine Metabolism and Cell Kinetics*. Amsterdam: North Holland, 1967.

106. Hedley DW, Clark GM, Cornelisse CJ, et al. Consensus review of the clinical utility of DNA cytometry in carcinoma of the breast. *Cytometry* 14:482–485, 1992.

107. Howard A, Pele SR. Nuclear incorporation of P32 as demonstrated by autoradiographs. *Exp Cell Res* 2:178–187, 1951.

108. Quastler H, Sherman FG. Cell population kinetics in the intestinal epithelium of the mouse. *Exp Cell Res* 17:420–438, 1959.

109. Tannock I. Cell kinetics and chemotherapy: a critical review. *Cancer Treat Rep* 62:1117–1133, 1978.

110. Steel GG. Cell loss as a factor in the growth rate of human tumors. *Eur J Cancer* 3:381–387, 1967.

111. Norton L. A gompertzian model of human breast cancer growth. *Cancer Res* 48:7067–7071, 1988.

112. Shackney SE, McCormack GW, Cuchural GJ Jr. Growth rate patterns of solid tumors and their relation to responsiveness to therapy: an analytical review. *Ann Intern Med* 89:107–121, 1978.

113. Till JE, McCulloch EA. Hematopoietic stem cell differentiation. *Biochem Biophys Acta* 605:431–459, 1980.

114. Becker AJ, McCulloch EA, Siminovitch L, Till JE. The effect of differing demands for blood cell production on DNA synthesis by hematopoietic colony-forming cells of mice. *Blood* 26:296–308, 1965.

115. Hamburger AW, Salmon SE. Primary bioassay of human tumor stem cells. *Science* 197:461–463, 1977.

116. Selby P, Buick RN, Tannock I. A critical appraisal of the human tumor stem-cell assay. *N Engl J Med* 308:129–134, 1983.

117. Shimizu T, Motoji T, Oshimi K, Mizoguchi H. Proliferative state and radiosensitivity of human myeloma stem cells. *Br J Cancer* 45:679–683, 1982.

118. Hryniuk WM, Levine MN, Levin L. Analysis of dose intensity for chemotherapy in early (stage II) and advanced breast cancer. *NCI Monogr* 1:87–94, 1986.

119. Levin L, Hryniuk WM. Dose intensity analysis of chemotherapy regimens in ovarian carcinoma. *J Clin Oncol* 5:756–767, 1987.

120. van Rijswijk RE, Haanen C, Dekker AW, et al. Dose intensity of MOPP chemotherapy and survival in Hodgkin's disease. *J Clin Oncol* 7:1776–1782, 1989.

121. Bezwoda WR, Dansey R, Bezwoda MA. Treatment of Hodgkin's disease with MOPP chemotherapy: effect of dose and schedule modification on treatment outcome. *Oncology* 47:29–36, 1990.

122. Muss HB, Thor AD, Berry DA, et al. c-*erbB-2* expression and response to adjuvant therapy in women with node-positive early breast cancer. *N Engl J Med* 330:1260–1266, 1994.

123. Bruce WR, Meeker BE, Powers WE, Valeriote FA. Comparison of the dose- and time-survival curves for normal hematopoietic and lymphoma colony-forming cells exposed to vinblastine, vincristine, arabinosylcytosine, and amethopterin. *J Natl Cancer Inst* 42:1015–1023, 1969.

124. van Putten LM, Lelieveld, P, Kram-Idsenga LKJ. Cell cycle specificity and therapeutic effectiveness of cytostatic agents. *Cancer Chemother Rep* 56:691–700, 1972.

125. Twentyman PR, Bleehen NM. Changes in sensitivity to cytotoxic agents occurring during the life history of monolayer cultures of a mouse tumor cell line. *Br J Cancer* 31:417–423, 1975.

126. Goldie JH, Coldman AJ. A mathematic model for relating the drug sensitivity of tumors to their spontaneous mutation rate. *Cancer Treat Rep* 63:727–733, 1979.

127. Goldie JH, Coldman AJ. The genetic origin of drug resistance in neoplasms: implications for systemic therapy. *Cancer Res* 44:3643–3653, 1984.

128. Biedler JL, Riehm H. Cellular resistance to actinomycin D in Chinese hamster cells in vitro: cross-resistance, radioautographic, and cytogenetic studies. *Cancer Res* 30:1174–1184, 1970.

129. Juliano RL, Ling V. A surface glycoprotein modulating drug permeability in Chinese hamster ovary cell mutants. *Biochem Biophys Acta* 455:152–162, 1976.

130. Kruh GD, Chan A, Myers K, et al. Expression of complementary DNA library transfer establishes mrp as a multidrug resistance protein. *Cancer Res* 54:1649–1652, 1994.

131. Hamilton TC, Winker MA, Lovie KG, et al. Augmentation of adriamycin, melphalan, and cisplatin cytotoxicity in drug-resistant and -sensitive human ovarian carcinoma cell lines by buthionine sulfoximine mediated glutathione depletion. *Biochem Pharmacol* 34:2583–2586, 1985.

132. Somfai-Relle S, Suzukake K, Vistica BP, et al. Reduction in cellular glutathione by buthionine sulfoximine and sensitization of murine tumor cells resistant to L-phenylalanine mustard. *Biochem Pharmacol* 33:485–490, 1984.

133. Scudiero DA, Meyer SA, Clatterbuck BE, et al. Sensitivity of human cell strains having different abilities to repair O6-methylguanine in DNA to inactivation by alkylating agents including chloroethyl nitrosoureas. *Cancer Res* 44:2467–2474, 1984.

134. Green DR, Bissonnette RP, Cotter TG. Apoptosis and cancer. *PPO Updates* 8:1, 1994.

135. Korsmeyer SJ. Bcl-2 initiates a new category of oncogenes: regulators of cell death. *Blood* 80:879–886, 1992.

136. Lowe SW, Ruley HE, Jacks T, et al. *p53*-Dependent apoptosis modulates the cytotoxicity of anticancer agents. *Cell* 74:957–967, 1993.

137. Salmon SE, Alberts DS, Duriel GM, et al. Clinical correlations of drug sensitivity in the human tumor stem cell assay. *Recent Results Cancer Res* 74:300–305, 1980.

138. Dorr RT, Von Hoff DD. *Cancer Chemotherapy Handbook*. Norwalk, CT: Appleton & Lange, 1994.

139. Chabner BA, Longo DL. *Cancer Chemotherapy and Biotherapy: Principles and Practice*. Philadelphia, PA: Lippincott-Raven, 1996.

140. Greene MH, Boice JD Jr, Greer BE, et al. Acute non-lymphocytic leukemia after therapy with alkylating agents for ovarian cancer. *N Engl J Med* 307:1416–1421, 1982.

141. Greene MH, Harris EL, Gershenson DM. Melphalan may be a more potent leukemogen than cylophosphamide. *Ann Intern Med* 105:360–367, 1986.

142. Calvert H, Judson I, van der Vijgh WJ. Platinum complexes in cancer medicine: pharmacokinetics and pharmacodynamics in relation to toxicity and therapeutic activity. *Cancer Surv* 17:189–217, 1993.

143. Jodrell DI, Egorin MJ, Canetta RM, et al. Relationships between carboplatin exposure and tumor response and toxicity in patients with ovarian cancer. *J Clin Oncol* 10:520–528, 1992.

144. Ozols RF, Bundy BN, Fowler J, Clarke-Pearson D, Mannel R, Hartenbach EM, Baergen R: Randomized phase III study of cisplatin (CIS)/paclitaxel (PAC) versus carboplatin (CARBO)/PAC in optimal stage III epithelial ovarian cancer (OC): a Gynecologic Oncology Group Trial (GOG 158). *Proc Annu Meet Am Soc Clin Oncol* 18:A1373, 1999.

145. Bleyer WA. The clinical pharmacology of methotrexate. *Cancer* 41:36–41, 1978.

146. Grem JL, Hoth DF, Hamilton JM, et al. Overview of current status and future direction of clinical trials with 5-

fluorouracil in combination with folinic acid. *Cancer Treat Rep* 71:1249–1264, 1987.

147. Schwartz SA, Morgenstern B, Capizzi RL. Schedule-dependent synergy and antagonism between high-dose 1-β-D-arabinofuranosylcytosine and asparaginase in the L5178Y murine leukemia. *Cancer Res* 42:2191–2197, 1982.

148. Capizzi RL, Davis R, Powell B, et al. Synergy between high-dose cytarabine and asparaginase in the treatment of adults with refractory and relapsed acute myelogenous leukemia: a Cancer and Leukemia Group B study. *J Clin Oncol* 6:499–508, 1988.

149. Cunningham D, Pyrönen S, James RD, et al. Randomized trial of irinotecan plus supportive care versus supportive care alone after fluorouracil failure for patients with metastatic colorectal cancer. *Lancet* 352:1413–1418, 1998.

150. Rougier P, van Cursem E, Bajetta E, et al. Randomized trial of irinotecan versus fluorouracil by continuous infusion after fluorouracil failure in patients with metastatic colorectal cancer. *Lancet* 352:1407–1412, 1998.

151. ten Bokkel Huinink W, Gore M, Carmichael J, et al. Topotecan versus paclitaxel for the treatment of recurrent epithelial ovarian cancer. *J Clin Oncol* 15:2183–2193, 1997.

152. Tritton TR, Yee G. The anticancer drug adriamycin can be actively cytotoxic without entering cells. *Science* 217:248–250, 1982.

153. Rowinsky EK, Gilbert M, McGuire WP, et al. Sequences of Taxol and cisplatin: a phase I and pharmacologic study. *J Clin Oncol* 9:1692–1703, 1991.

154. LeBlanc GA, Sundseth SS, Weber GF, et al. Platinum anticancer drugs modulate P-450 mRNA levels and differentially alter hepatic drug and steroid hormone metabolism in male and female rats. *Cancer Res* 52:540–547, 1992.

155. Sledge GW, Robert N, Goldstein LJ, et al. Phase I trial of Adriamycin and Taxol in metastatic breast cancer (Abstract). *Eur J Cancer* 29A (suppl 6):S81, 1983.

156. Holmes FA, Newman RA, Madden V, et al. Schedule dependent pharmacokinetics (PK) in a phase I trial of Taxol (T) and doxorubicin (D) as initial chemotherapy for metastatic breast cancer (Abstract). In: *Proceedings of the 8th NCI-EORTC Symposium on New Drugs in Cancer Therapy,* Amsterdam, March 15–18, 1994: Dordrecht, Netherlands, Kluwer, 1994:197.

157. Arbuck SG, Strauss H, Rowinsky EK, et al. A reassessment of the cardiac toxicity asssociated with taxol. *Monogr Natl Cancer Inst* 15:117–130, 1993.

158. Gianni L, Straneo G, Capri F, et al. Optimal dose and sequence finding study of paclitaxel (P) by 3 h infusion with bolus doxorubicin (D) in untreated metastatic breast cancer patients (Pts) (Abstract). *Proc Am Soc Clin Oncol* 13:74, 1994.

159. Maher DW, Lieschke GJ, Green M et al. Filgrastim in patients with chemotherapy-induced febrile neutropenia. *Ann Intern Med* 121:492–501, 1994.

160. Glover D, Glick J, et al. WR-2721 protects against the hematologic toxicity of cyclophosphamide: a controlled phase II trial. *J Clin Oncol* 4:584–588, 1986.

161. Budd GT, Ganapathi R, Bauer L, et al. Phase I study of WR-2721 and carboplatin. *Eur J Cancer* 29A:1122–1127, 1993.

162. Kemp G, Rose P, Lurain J et al. Amifostine pretreatment for protection against cyclophosphamide and cisplatin-induced toxicities: results of a randomized controlled trial in patients with advanced ovarian cancer. *J Clin Oncol* 14:2101–2112, 1996.

163. Green MD, Alderton P. Sobol M, et al. ICRF-187 (ADR-529) cardioprotection against anthracycline-induced cardiotoxicity: clinical and preclinical studies. In: Muggi FM (ed), *New Drugs, Concepts, and Results in Cancer Chemotherapy.* Boston: Kluwer Academic, 1992:101–117.

164. Speyer JL, Green MD, Zeleluch-Jacquotte A, et al. ICRF-187 permits longer treatment with doxorubicin in women with breast cancer. *J Clin Oncol* 10:117–127, 1992.

165. O'Malley BW, Schrader WT. The receptors of steroid hormones. *Sci Am* 32:234–243, 1976.

166. Friedman MA, Hoffman PG, Jones HW. The clinical value of hormone receptor assays in malignant disease. *Cancer Treat Rev* 5:185–194, 1978.

167. Barakat RR, Park RC, Grigsby PW, et al. Epithelial tumors. In: Hoskins WJ, Perez CA, Young RC (eds), *Principles and Practice of Gynecologic Oncology.* Philadelphia: Lippincott-Raven, 1997:881–883.

168. Report from the Breast Cancer Trials Committee, Scottish Cancer Trials Office (MRC), Edinburgh. Adjuvant tamoxifen in the management of operable breast cancer: the Scottish trial. Report from the Breast Cancer Trials Committee. *Lancet* 2:171–175, 1987.

169. Robinson E, Kimmick GG, Muss HB. Tamoxifen in postmenopausal women: a safety perspective. *Drugs Aging* 8:329–337, 1996.

170. Barakat RR. The effect of tamoxifen on the endometrium. *Oncology* 9:129–142, 1995.

171. Tchekmedyian NS, Tait N, Moody M, et al. Appetite stimulation with megestrol acetate in cachectic cancer patients. *Semin Surg Oncol* 13:37–43, 1987.

172. Cruz JM, Muss HB, Brockschmidt JK, Evans GW. Weight changes in women with metastatic breast cancer treated with megestrol acetate: a comparison of standard versus high-dose therapy. *Semin Oncol* 17:63–67, 1990.

173. Rosen G, Marcove RC, Caparros B, et al. Primary osteogenic sarcoma: the rationale for preoperative chemotherapy and delayed surgery. *Cancer* 43:2163–2177, 1979.

174. Winkler K, Beron G, Delling G, et al. Neoadjuvant chemotherapy of osteosarcoma: results of randomized cooperative trial (COSS-82) with salvage chemotherapy based on histological tumor response. *J Clin Oncol* 6:329–337, 1988.

175. Alberts DS, Liu PY, Hannigan EV, et al. Intraperitoneal cisplatin plus intravenous cyclophosphamide versus intravenous cisplatin plus intravenous cyclophosphamide for stage III ovarian cancer. *N Engl J Med* 335:1950–1955, 1996.

176. Rahman A, Kessler A, More N, et al. Liposomal protection of adriamycin-induced cardiotoxicity in mice. *Cancer Res* 40:1532–1537, 1980.

177. Cobleigh MA, Voel D, Tripathy NJ, et al. Efficacy and safety of Herceptin (humanized anti-*HER2* antibody) as a single agent in 222 women with *HER2* overexpression who relapsed following chemotherapy for metasatic breast cancer (Abstract 376). *Proc Am Soc Clin Oncol* 17:97a, 1998.

178. Slamon D, Leyland-Jones B, Shak S, et al. Addition of Herceptin (humanized anti-*HER2* antibody) to first line chemotherapy for *HER2* overexpressing metastatic breast cancer (*HER2*+/MBC) markedly increases anticancer activity: a randomized, multinational controlled phase III trial (Abstract 377). *Proc Am Soc Clin Oncol* 17:98a, 1998.

179. Ezekiel MP, Robert F, et al. Phase I study of antiepidermal growth factor receptor (EGFR) antibody C225 in combination with irradiation in patients with advanced squamous cell carcinoma of the head and neck (SCCHN) (Abstract 1522). *Proc Am Soc Clin Oncol* 17:3955a, 1998.

180. Drucker BJ, Talpaz M, Resta D, et al. Clinical efficacy of an abl specific tyrosine kinase inhibitor as targeted therapy for chronic myelogenous leukemia. (Abstract 1639). *Blood* 94 (suppl 10, part 1 of 2): 1999.

181. Gibbs JB, Oliff A. The potential of farnesyl transferase inhibitors as cancer chemotherapeutics. *Annu Rev Pharmacol Toxicol* 37:143–166, 1997.

182. Sepp-Lorenzino L, Ma Z, Rands E, et al. A peptidomimetic inhibitor of farnesyl:protein transferase blocks the anchorage-dependent and -independent growth of human tumor cell lines. *Cancer Res* 55:5302–5309, 1995.

183. Zujewski J, Horak ID, Woestenborghs R, et al. Phase I trial of farnesyl-transferase inhibitor, R115777, in advanced cancer (Abstract 1848). *Proc Am Assoc Cancer Res* 39:270, 1998.

184. End D, Skrzat S, Devine A, et al. R115777, a novel imidazole farnesyl protein transferase inhibitor (FTI): biochemical and cellular effects in H-*ras* and K-*ras* dominant systems (Abstract 1847). *Proc Am Assoc Cancer Res* 39:770, 1998.

185. Moasser MM, Sepp-Lorenzino L, Kohl NE, et al. Farnesyl transferase inhibitors cause enhanced mitotic sensitivity to Taxol and epothilones. *Proc Natl Acad Sci USA* 95:1369–1374, 1998.

186. Parker BW, Kaur G, Nieves-Neira W, et al. Early induction of apoptosis in hematopoietic cell lines after exposure to flavopiridol. *Blood* 15:458–465, 1998.

187. Carlson BA, Dubay MM, Sausville EA, et al. Flavopiridol induces G1 arrest with inhibition of cyclin-dependent kinase (CDK) 2 and CDK4 in human breast carcinoma cells. *Cancer Res* 56:2973–2978, 1996.

188. Senderowicz AM, Headlee D, Stinson S, et al. A phase I trial of flavopiridol (FLA), a novel cyclin-dependent kinase inhibitor, in patients with refractory neoplasms. *J Clin Oncol* 16:2986–2999, 1998.

189. Schwartz GK, Werner P, Maslak L, et al. Flavopiridol enhances the biological effects of paclitaxel: a phase I trial in patients with advanced solid tumors (Abstract 725). *Proc Am Soc Clin Oncol* 17:188a, 1998.

190. Wang Q, Fan S, Eastman A, et al. UCN-01: a potent abrogator of G_2 check-point function in cancer cells with disrupted *p53*. *J Natl Cancer Inst* 88:956–965, 1996.

191. Fuse E, Tanii H, Kurata N, et al. *Alteration of pharmacokinetics of a novel anticancer drug, UCN-01, in rats by human α-1-acid glycoprotein* (Abstract 427). Paper presented at the Tenth NCI-ECORTC Symposium on New Drugs in Cancer Therapy, 1998.

192. Senderowizc AM, Headlee D, Lush R, et al. *Phase I trial infusional UCN-01, a novel protein kinase inhibitor, in patients with refractory neoplasms* (Abstract 426). Paper presented at the Tenth NCI-ECORTC Symposium on New Drugs in Cancer Therapy, 1998.

193. Abe J, Zhou W, Takuwa N, et al. A fumagillin angiogenesis inhibitor, AGM-1470, inhibits activation of cyclin-dependent kinases and phosphorylation of the retinoblastoma gene product but not protein tyrosyl phosphorylation or protooncogene expression in vasculka endothelial cells. *Cancer Res* 54:3407–3412, 1994.

194. Sin N, Meng L, Wang MQW, et al. The anti-angiogenic agent fumagillin covalently binds and inhibits the methionine aminopeptidase MetAP-2. *Proc Natl Acad Sci USA* 94:6099–6103, 1997.

195. Stadler WM, Shapiro CL, Sosmann J, et al. A multi-institutional study of the angiogenesis inhibitor TNP-470 in metastatic renal cell carcinoma (Abstract). *Proc Am Soc Clin Oncol* 17:1192, 1998.

196. Bower M, Howard M, Gracie F, et al. A phase II study of thalidomide for Kaposi's sarcomas: activity and correlation with KSVH DNA load (Abstract 76). *J AIDS Hum Retrovirol* 14:A35, 1995.

197. Politi P, Reboredo M, Losso C, et al. Phase I trial of thalidomide in AIDS-related Kaposi sarcoma (Abstract). *Proc Am Soc Clin Oncol* 17:161, 1998.

198. Gordon MS, Talpaz M, Margolin E, et al. Phase I trial of recombinant humanized anti-vascular endothelial growth factor in patients with metastatic cancer. *Proc Am Soc Clin Oncol* 17:809, 1998.

199. Rosen LS, Kabbinavar F, Rosen P, et al. Phase I trial of SU5416, a novel angiogenesis inhibitor in patients with advanced malignancies. *Proc Am Soc Clin Oncol* 17:843, 1998.

200. Hewitt HB. Animal tumor models and their relevance to human tumor immunology. *J Biol Response Model* 1:107–119, 1982.

201. Herberman RB. Counterpoint: animal tumor models and their relevance to human tumor immunology. *J Biol Response Mod* 2:39–46, 1983.

202. Kawakami Y, Robbins PF, Wang RF, et al. The use of melanosomal proteins in the immunotherapy of melanoma. *J Immunother* 21:237–246, 1998.

203. Castelli C, Rivoltini L, Mazzocchi A, Parmiani G. T-cell recognition of melanoma antigens and its therapeutic applications. *Int J Clin Lab Res* 27:103–110, 1997.

204. Kobrin CB, Kwak LW. Development of vaccine strategies for the treatment of B-cell malignancies. *Cancer Invest* 15:577–587, 1997.

205. Mayordomo JI, Loftus DJ, Sakamoto HJ, et al. Therapy of murine tumors with *p53* wild type and mutant sequence peptide-based vaccines. *J Exp Med* 183:1357–1365, 1996.

206. Boon T. Toward a genetic analysis of tumor rejection antigens. *Adv Cancer Res* 58:177–210, 1992.

207. Ehrlich P. Über den jetzigen Stand der Karzinomforschung. In Himmelweit F (ed), *The Collected Papers of Paul Ehrlich*, vol. II. London: Pergamon Press, 1957:550–562.

208. Penn I, Starzl TR. A summary of the status of de novo cancer in transplant recipients. *Transplant Proc* 4:719–732, 1972.

209. Ho M, Jaffe R, Miller G, et al. The frequency of Epstein-Barr virus infection and associated lymphoproliferative syndrome after transplantation and its manifestations in children. *Transplantation* 45:719–727, 1988.

210. Klein G, Klein E. Rejectability of virus-induced tumors and nonrejectability of spontaneous tumors: a lesson in contrasts. *Transplant Proc* 9:1095–1104, 1977.

211. Prehn RT, Lappe MA. An immunostimulation theory of tumor development. *Transplant Rev* 7:26–54, 1971.

212. Avigan D. Dendritic cells: development, function and potential use for cancer immunotherapy. *Blood* 13:51–64, 1999.

213. Jerome KR, Barnd DL, Boyer CM, et al. Cytotoxic T-lymphocytes derived from patients with breast adenocarcinoma recognize an epitope present on the protein core of a mucin molecular preferentially expressed by malignant cells. *Cancer Res* 51:2908–2916, 1991.

214. Kleinerman ES, Raymond AK, Bucana CD, et al. Unique histological changes in lung metastases of osteosarcoma patients following therapy with liposomal muramyl tripeptide (CGPP 198835A lipid). *Cancer Immunol Immunother* 34:211–220, 1992.

215. Gorelik E, Herberman RB. Role of natural killer (NK) cells in the control of tumor growth and metastatic spread. In Herberman RB (ed), *Cancer Immunology: Innovative Approaches to Therapy*. Boston: Martinus Nijhoff, 1986:151–176.

216. Basse P, Herberman RB, Nannmark V, et al. Accumulation of adoptively transferred adherent lymphokine-activated killer cells in murine metastases. *J Exp Med* 174:479–488, 1991.

217. Dean JH. Application of the microculture lymphocyte proliferation assay to clinical studies. In Herberman RB, McIntire KR (eds), *Immunodiagnosis of Cancer*. New York: Marcel Dekker, 1979:738–769.

218. Reichert TE, Rabinowich H, Johnson JT, Whiteside TL. Mechanisms responsible for signaling and functional defects. *J Immunother* 21:295–306, 1998.

219. Schantz SP, Brown BW, Lira E, Taylor DL. Evidence for the role of natural immunity in the control of metastatic spread of head and neck cancer. *Cancer Immunol Immunother* 25:141–145, 1987.

220. Agarwala SS, Kirkwood JM. Adjuvant interferon treatment for melanoma. *Hematol Oncol Clin North Am* 12:823–833, 1998.

221. Rosenberg, SA. Perspectives on the use of interleukin-2 in cancer treatment (keynote address). *Cancer J Sci Am* 1:s2–s6, 1997.

222. Graeenberg PDD, Klaarnet JP, Kern DE, Cheever MA. Therapy of disseminated tumors by adoptive transfer of specifically immune T cells. *Prog Exp Tumor Res* 32:104–127, 1988.

223. Rosenberg SA, Packard BS, Aebersold PM, et al. Use of tumor-infiltrating lymphocytes and interleukin-2 in the immunotherapy of patients with metastatic melanoma. *N Engl J Med* 319:1676–1680, 1988.

224. Maeurer MJ, Storkus WJ, Kirkwood JM, Lotze MT. New treatment options for patients with melanoma: review of melanoma-derived T-cell epitope-based peptide vaccines. *Melanoma Res* 6:11–24, 1996.

9

Complications of Cancer and Cancer Treatment

■ ■ ■

Paul E. Rosenthal

As MORE PATIENTS ARE CURED OF CANCER, A focus on the cumulative effects of the therapies used to achieve that result becomes increasingly important. For most types of cancer, the "ideal" treatment (i.e., one that guarantees survival without short-term toxicity or long-term complications) does not exist. *All* current cancer therapies exact a definable "cost" against which their benefits (tumor regression, freedom from recurrence, palliation of symptoms) must be balanced.

This chapter presents a practical approach to the common problems that arise with cancer therapy, including complications related to radiotherapy and chemotherapy. In addition, the late complications that can affect cured cancer patients are discussed, as are the therapeutic use of blood components and hematopoietic growth factors.

COMPLICATIONS OF RADIOTHERAPY

For the most part, the side effects of radiotherapy are limited to irradiated tissues. These effects can be acute or chronic, depend on the fraction size and total dose, and can be minimized by blocking normal tissue from the beam and using multiple intersecting portals. As does chemotherapy, radiotherapy most severely affects rapidly reproducing tissue (e.g., gastrointestinal mucosa, mucous membranes, and bone marrow stem cells). Tissues that have a slower turnover rate (e.g., connective tissue and muscle) or that do not repopulate to a significant degree are less likely to manifest acute irradiation toxicity. Side effects from irradiation may be increased in patients who also are receiving chemotherapy, either concurrently or sequentially [1].

All tissues in the body can accommodate a maximum tolerable dose of radiation above which damage is permanent. The imperative is to stay below this threshold to avoid irreversible complications while simultaneously offering the best chance for tumor control.

Table 9.1 Major Acute and Chronic (Dose-Dependent) Side Effects of Radiotherapy

Site	Acute Effects	Chronic Effects
Skin	Redness, itchiness, dryness, moist skin breakdown	Telangiectasia, fibrosis
Hair	Temporary alopecia	Permanent epilation
Gastrointestinal tract	Nausea, vomiting, anorexia, diarrhea	Malabsorption, structures, necrosis
Genitourinary tract	Cystitis, frequency	Radiation-induced nephritis
Oral cavity	Taste alterations, mucositis	Permanent xerostomia, permanent taste alteration, dental caries
Reproductive tract	Temporary sterility, dyspareunia	Permanent sterility, vaginal fibrosis
Respiratory tract	Pneumonitis	Pulmonary fibrosis
Blood	Pancytopenia, anemia	Chronic pancytopenia
Cardiovascular system	—	Pericarditis, fibrosis
Eyes	Irritation, tearing	Cataracts

Patients treated with curative intent may accept a higher rate of complications, whereas those treated for palliation should be given doses consistent with a lower incidence of side effects (Table 9.1). Both acute and chronic effects may vary for each organ system. Acute effects seem to be related to parenchymal cell damage of the organ. Long-term changes are due to alterations in the intrinsic small vessels of the end organs. Research in the field of radioprotection eventually may permit the delivery of higher doses of radiation with a lower risk for such deleterious effects [2].

Fatigue

Although fatigue is a common complaint among patients undergoing radiotherapy and chemotherapy [3], little is known about radiation-induced fatigue and how to manage it. Patients should be informed that fatigue is a common experience, because they may equate treatment-related fatigue with disease progression.

When persons in good health become fatigued, rest will help to restore the previous level of functioning. However, in patients with cancer, this restorative capability is impaired. As rest will not always reduce or abolish the fatigue, such patients' energy should be conserved by resting, pacing their activities, and delegating tasks to others. Rest periods can be set up around those times when fatigue is most severe. Patients can arrange to undergo radiotherapy or other high-priority activities at times when their energy level is at its peak. Family members and friends can be enlisted to carry out such daily activities as shopping, preparing meals, performing household chores, and providing child care. Patients who work full-time or even part-time should consider decreasing the amount of time worked; however, this decision may be difficult, because patients often desire to be as active as possible and family finances may be strained [4].

Usually, fatigue disappears within a few weeks after therapy has been discontinued. If fatigue persists, other possible causes should be investigated (e.g., anemia, thyroid dysfunction, hepatic or adrenal metastases, other sites of disease progression, or depression). Treatment of the reversible causes can lead to significant changes in energy levels and an overall sense of well-being, as has been shown with the use of erythropoietin (to treat anemia) or antidepressant medication [5, 6].

Skin Reactions

Radiotherapy increases the mitotic production of basal cells in the skin, upsetting the balance between cell reproduction and cell destruction. This imbalance leads to acute skin reactions that include dryness, peeling, redness, pruritus, breakdown or desquamation due to moisture, and increased pigmentation. Sites at greatest risk for breakdown include bony prominences and moist skin folds in the axilla, under the breast, and in the groin and perineum. Acute radiation-induced skin reactions are temporary and resolve within a few days. Late effects, such as telangiectasia, fibrosis, and even tissue necrosis, may result from changes in capillary permeability and connective tissue damage, although such reactions are infrequent. To alleviate the problem of dry, itchy skin or scalp, an oatmeal-based colloidal soap (e.g., Aveeno®) can be worked into a lather on the affected area for several minutes before it is rinsed off. If itching is severe, topical hydrocortisone lotion, aloe,

Table 9.2   Skin Care During Radiotherapy

General guidelines

Wash the skin with warm water and pat dry. *Caution:* Patients who do not have permanent skin markings should not wash them off.

Use a mild soap that does not contain perfume or deodorant.

Avoid using creams or lotions that contain perfume or deodorant.

Use water-based creams or lotions to prevent dryness and irritation. Pure vitamin E oil, aloe from a plant, or cocoa butter also are beneficial.

Do not expose irradiated skin to the sun while receiving therapy and for one year after treatment.

Do not wear tight-fitting clothing that can rub or press against the skin.

Do not use heating pads or hot water bottles on an irradiated area.

Radiotherapy to the pelvis

Do not use cornstarch in the groin or buttock folds.

Do not use enemas, suppositories, or rectal thermometers during the course of therapy (possible exception: steroid suppositories to manage proctitis).

Moist skin breakdown

Gently cleanse or irrigate the skin with normal saline, Hydrogel, or dermal wound cleanser.

Dress the site with a nonadherent, hydrophilic dressing (e.g., an Adaptic dressing, Duoderm, Aquaphor, or Sorbsan).

Do not use Telfa on an area of moist skin breakdown, as dressings of this type tend to macerate the skin.

For moist skin breakdown in the gluteal fold, use perineal soaks and protective emollients (e.g., Carrington, Hydrogel, Aquaphor, or Silvadene).

vitamin E cream, or a systemic medication (e.g., diphenhydramine) may be indicated. General and specific skin care interventions are listed in Table 9.2 [7].

Alopecia

Hair follicles go through an active period of growth (anagen phase) followed by a resting period (telogen phase). After the telogen phase, hair is shed, and new growth appears in the hair follicle. Irradiation of the scalp causes a change in this cycle. As hair follicle cells in the anagen phase convert prematurely to the telogen phase, the hair begins to drop out at a faster rate. Thinning or complete hair loss will occur at radiation doses above 3,000 cGy, and growth will resume approximately two to six months after therapy is completed. After high-dose irradiation to the scalp (> 5,000 cGy), hair loss often is permanent.

Hair loss due to radiotherapy is distressing, whether it occurs on visible areas, such as the scalp, or hidden areas, such as the pubis. Female patients should select a wig prior to the onset of hair loss, so as best to match the color and style to their own hair. Wearing the wig before they actually need it may ease their psychological adjustment. A turban or scarf may be worn instead of a wig. Men also may obtain psychological benefit from use of a hairpiece [8]. (See the section "Alopecia,"

under "Acute Toxicity of Chemotherapy, Mucocutaneous Toxicity.")

Oral Cavity Changes

Because the cells in tissues of the oral cavity and upper aerodigestive tract divide rapidly, acute toxicity is common in these areas. Frequently, doses of radiation above 3,000 cGy cause mucositis; with doses above 4,500 cGy, permanent, long-term xerostomia may develop secondary to effects on the salivary glands. Such symptoms as changes in taste and hoarseness, dysphagia, and odynophagia often limit food intake and thus have generalized systemic effects on nutrition, although resultant problems may diminish over time.

Before radiotherapy of head and neck cancer is begun, a dentist experienced in oncologic treatment should be consulted about preventive measures, and carious teeth probably should be extracted. Once therapy has commenced, scrupulous oral hygiene is important to minimize dryness and the long-term complication of dental caries. To retard decay, frequent tooth brushing with a soft brush, flossing, and daily fluoride treatments are recommended. Gargling with baking soda or peroxide solutions or commercially available, nonalcoholic mouthwashes may alleviate dryness and pain. The use of artificial saliva between meals also is helpful. Patients should avoid hot spicy foods, alcohol, and cigarettes. Such topical anesthetics as viscous lidocaine (Xylocaine®) or dyclonine can be applied before meals to prevent pain during mastication; owing to this effect, these agents help to maintain food intake and adequate body weight. Oral candidiasis, although an infrequent complication of radiotherapy, should be treated with oral antifungal agents [9].

Effects on Head and Neck Region

A significant number of patients can become hypothyroid when the neck is irradiated in the treatment of lymphomas, tumors of the oropharynx, or lung cancer. Estimates range from 3% to 50% of patients so affected. Serum levels of thyroid hormone and thyroid-stimulating hormone should be monitored, and appropriate therapy should be initiated. Acute otitis externa can be managed with steroid-antibiotic drops. Pruritus of the canals and chronic excessive accumulation of cerumen may be relieved by daily instillation of mineral oil. Chronic hearing loss [9] occurs only after high doses of radiation and is manifest as high-frequency loss. Ocular problems, including acute conjunctivitis, may be treated with topical medications. Such long-term problems as the dry-eye syndrome or cataract formation can be minimized by proper shielding of the eyes.

Upper Gastrointestinal Tract Effects

The esophagus and stomach, which also are lined by rapidly dividing mucosal cells, can tolerate up to 3,000 to 4,000 cGy before symptoms of esophagitis or gastritis occur. Dysphagia and heartburn can be treated with antacids, a bland diet, and (if necessary) such topical anesthetics as viscous Xylocaine® or a "stomatitis cocktail" of sucralfate (Carafate®), antacids, and Xylocaine® plus dextromethorphan (Benylin®). Candidal infection of the esophagus, which may present with a similar constellation of symptoms, can be ruled out by means of barium swallow or diagnostic endoscopy. If present, the infection can be treated effectively with oral antifungal medications. Such chronic effects as esophageal stricture may occur after a dose of 4,500 to 5,000 cGy or with combined-modality therapy. Surgical dilatation offers an effective means of palliation.

Often, the dose to these organs is limited by the level of tolerance of surrounding normal structures, such as the small bowel. Nausea and vomiting may occur if the stomach is in the direct path of the beam. Such pheno-

thiazine antiemetics as thiethylperazine (Torecan®) and prochlorperazine (Compazine®) or, if necessary, ondansetron (Zofran®) are best administered prior to radiation treatment. Ingestion of nonirritating foods with adequate protein and calorie contents and sufficient fluid intake should be encouraged whenever the nausea has subsided [7].

Lower Gastrointestinal Tract Effects

Diarrhea is the major effect of radiotherapy involving the lower gastrointestinal tract. It occurs as a result of malabsorption of fat, carbohydrate, and protein in the small intestine. With increasing doses of radiation, morphologic changes in the small bowel are seen, and the rate of cell loss from the intestinal villi exceeds the reproductive capacity of the crypt cells. Villi become shortened, and the total epithelial surface is reduced. With fat malabsorption, bile salt reabsorption in the terminal ileum is decreased, and an excess of bile salts thus reaches the colon, inhibiting water reabsorption and stimulating peristalsis. Carbohydrate malabsorption contributes to diarrhea by passing unabsorbed sugars into the small bowel, exerting an osmotic effect that leads to dilatation and stimulates peristalsis. When unabsorbed sugars reach the colon, bacterial fermentation occurs, and water and electrolyte reabsorption thus are impaired.

Radiation-induced diarrhea may be managed by a variety of medications, including antispasmodic and anticholinergic agents to decrease bowel spasms. Diphenoxylate (Lomotil®) and loperamide (Imodium®) may be used for moderate diarrhea, whereas such opium derivatives as paregoric and tincture of opium may be used in more severe cases. Dietary changes should include a diet low in roughage, fat, and lactose. In addition, eating small amounts of food at regularly scheduled intervals may be more acceptable to patients than is eating three large meals a day. Occasionally, psyllium (Metamucil®) or other bulk-additive stool softeners may help to normalize bowel movements. If excess flatus or cramping is a problem, simethicone or activated charcoal products can alleviate gastrointestinal distress significantly. Other side effects of radiation to the small intestines include anorexia, nausea, and vomiting. Edema and capillary congestion are characteristic of the acute disease phase [9].

In the chronic phase, injury to the small bowel may result in mucosal ulceration and stricture. Small-bowel obstruction can occur as a result of progressive fibrosis, adhesion formation, and edema, but these effects are rare if the total dose administered is 4,500 cGy or less. Chronic injury to the large intestine is less common, as this organ can tolerate higher total doses of radiation than can the small bowel. The most common long-term complications, however, include increased frequency of bowel movements and radiation proctitis, which can result in rectal bleeding. Often, the latter responds to hemorrhoidal medications or steroid-based creams and suppositories [1].

Genitourinary Tract Effects

The bladder can tolerate higher total doses of radiation than can the small bowel. Generally, patients do not experience side effects until they have received 4,500 to 5,000 cGy of radiation to the bladder. These effects may include frequency, urgency, and burning on urination. Because such symptoms may mask an infection, the latter must be ruled out before proper treatment can be instituted. Pharmacologic measures include such anticholinergics as oxybutynin chloride (Ditropan®) and such antispasmodics as phenazapyridine (Pyridium®) or flavoxate hydrochloride (Urispas®). Ibuprofen may help to relieve acute dysuria. Chronic changes may develop after a dose of 6,500 to 7,000 cGy and usually are due to fibrosis, with diminished bladder capacity and the need for more frequent urination.

The kidneys are among the most radiosensitive organs. Therefore, dosages must be limited to 2,000 to 2,400 cGy to prevent chronic renal failure. When medical reasons necessitate irradiating one kidney above its threshold level of tolerance, tests should be performed to ensure normal function of the remaining kidney [7].

Effects on the Lungs

Lung tissue tolerates radiation exposure poorly. Chronic injury is related to the volume of tissue exposed and to the total dose. The mucus-secreting cells and cilia are damaged acutely, with pulmonary fibrosis being a late complication.

During treatments, thick, tenacious pulmonary secretions may cause a cough, for which decongestants may be useful. As treatment progresses, regression of an obstructing tumor may lead to mobilization of inspissated material and the need for expectorants. More commonly, however, the cough is dry and nonproductive and usually is worse at night. A vaporizer by an affected patient's bedside will provide moisture to the dry airways, and efforts to increase oral hydration are

helpful. The condition may necessitate prescription of cough suppressants containing codeine or oxycodone. Obviously, smoking is to be avoided. Usually, the cough is transient and subsides within weeks after the cessation of radiotherapy.

Radiation pneumonitis can occur if a large portion of one lung is treated with more than 4,000 cGy of radiation or if both lungs receive more than 2,000 cGy. Typically, pneumonitis is manifested as a dry cough, low-grade fever, and dyspnea on exertion 6 to 12 weeks after therapy is completed. The diagnosis is one of exclusion and is based on history, physical examination, and radiographic findings (ground-glass appearance of the lungs). Pulmonary infection must be sought carefully. In most cases, the condition is self-limited and requires no specific therapy. For more severe cases, systemic steroid therapy with prednisone, 40 to 80 mg/day, usually is helpful but should be protracted and tapered slowly. Generally, patients recover without sequelae. An important note is that patients who have been receiving chronic steroid therapy prior to irradiation are at markedly increased risk for radiation pneumonitis, and abrupt steroid withdrawal in such cases may precipitate severe symptoms [1].

After high-dose radiation to the lungs, pulmonary fibrosis may occur, accompanied by radiographic changes and symptoms of dyspnea and cyanosis. Although supplemental oxygen will alleviate symptoms, the pathologic process is irreversible. Treatment with steroids has not been helpful [10].

Cardiovascular Effects

Cardiac toxicity due to irradiation is rare as compared to pulmonary toxicity. Because cardiac muscle cells do not divide, they do not manifest acute changes readily. Usually, injury involves the pericardium, myocardium, or blood vessels; effects on the endocardium are rare, owing to its lack of vasculature. As with other organs showing intermediate and late radiation effects, changes probably are due to alterations in the intrinsic blood vessels and connective tissue of the organ. Below a total dose of 4,500 cGy, radiation-induced damage is uncommon. This dose must be modified, however, if cardiotoxic chemotherapeutic agents have been employed or if a large portion of the heart is to be treated [7].

Doses above 4,500 cGy could cause permanent injury to the cardiac musculature, resulting in cardiomyopathy and symptoms of congestive failure. As with pericarditis of other etiologies, acute radiation pericarditis usually presents with pleuritic chest pain, fever, tachycardia, and electrocardiographic and radiographic changes. Tamponade occurs infrequently. In general, pericarditis is self-limited and responds to conservative therapy and to nonsteroidal antiinflammatory drugs. Chronic pericarditis is uncommon. Acute myocardial infarction, though rare, seems to be associated with the use of irradiation and cardiotoxic chemotherapy [11].

Musculoskeletal Effects

Like cardiac muscle, striated muscle tolerates relatively high doses of radiation. Acute effects seldom are seen and more often are related to damage to the overlying skin. Late tissue changes may manifest themselves as loss of muscle bulk and fibrosis in the irradiated field. Edema of the extremities can be minimized by sparing lymphatics from the radiation portal. If edema occurs, elevation of the limb and the early application of compression stockings will be beneficial. Vigorous massage and physical therapy of the affected area may help to alleviate chronic fibrosis and edema.

In growing bones and limbs, however, irradiation can cause profound and irreversible changes. Growth will be reduced in bones exposed to doses of 2,000 cGy or more, resulting in length discrepancies that require orthopedic surgical correction. Whenever possible, the epiphyseal plate in long bones of growing children should be blocked to minimize this reaction. Conversely, the entire vertebral body generally is included to prevent scoliosis, or irradiation is avoided altogether to minimize these problems.

In adults, the tolerance of bones to x-irradiation is high, with few complications. Occasionally, aseptic necrosis is noted with high doses.

Hematopoietic System Effects

Bone marrow cells are acutely sensitive to the effects of radiation, and risk for myelosuppression is related directly to the amount of marrow in the treatment field. Generally, bone marrow depletion within the portal is transient under total doses of 4,000 cGy, and blood counts are affected substantially only when a large proportion of the skeleton is located within the radiation field, unless the patient is receiving concurrent chemotherapy. In such cases, blood counts must be monitored carefully, and a decision must be made either to interrupt irradiation until counts return to normal or to use growth factors.

Effects on Reproductive Function

The induction of sterility by radiation to the pelvis is dose- and age-dependent in both women and men. In young women, pelvic irradiation of 1,200 to 2,000 cGy (and even lower doses in women in their forties) will result in premature menopause. Repositioning of the ovaries to reduce exposure has been attempted (e.g., in women with Hodgkin's disease), but the efficacy of this approach is unproved, with best results after laparoscopic oophoropexy [12]. Cessation of menses can occur, along with hot flashes, changes in secondary sexual characteristics, and accelerated osteoporosis. Dyspareunia can be due to the onset of menopause but also may be the direct result of the drying effects of radiation on mucous membranes. Vaginal scarring and lack of normal lubrication can interfere with both sexual function and subsequent pelvic examinations.

In women who are sexually active, the regular use of a vaginal dilator both during therapy (when possible) and after therapy has been completed will help to minimize the formation of synechiae. Resumption of sexual intercourse soon after the tissues have healed should be encouraged, and the use of water-soluble lubricants is extremely beneficial. Topical hormonal preparations are contraindicated only in women with hormonally sensitive tumors. Barring any medical contraindication, replacement endocrine therapy also is a possibility [9].

In men, radiation-induced sterility is a function of age and total dose to the testes. Chromosomal aberrations and sterility can be seen after exposure to as little as 100 to 200 cGy. Because the Sertoli and Leydig cells of the testis are more resistant to the effects of radiation, impotence as a result of decreased testosterone production is not as frequent a problem as is sterility, although this effect too is age- and dose-dependent. When fertility is a concern and affected patients' sperm count is adequate, sperm banking should be an important part of pretreatment counseling unless a tumor is growing so rapidly that the time required for this procedure would compromise such patients' well-being. During the treatments themselves, specially designed gonadal shields can be used to minimize the dose to the testes from external scatter radiation. Patients should be told to avoid conception during therapy and for several months thereafter, as chromosomal abnormalities could be transmitted.

Of men who are sexually active prior to pelvic irradiation, approximately half to two-thirds will retain potency after external-beam irradiation. The effects of radiation on small blood vessels may accelerate the onset of impotence in some men. Treatments for impotence (e.g., prosthetic penile implants, vacuum devices, or injections of prostaglandin E–papaverine into the corpus cavernosum) have proved successful in many patients experiencing this reaction. The newer potency drugs, such as Viagra®, have not been studied in this setting but may prove useful.

Nervous System Effects

The risk for cerebral edema, the most common acute effect of brain irradiation, is dose-dependent and usually temporary. Symptomatic relief of radiation-induced brain edema can be achieved with high-dose systemic steroids. Patients who, prior to radiation oncology referral, are already receiving steroid therapy as a way of minimizing tumor-induced swelling should continue these drugs during the early stages of radiotherapy. If such patients remain stable, with no symptoms of increased intracranial pressure, gradual tapering of the steroids is possible during the course of x-irradiation. Antiepileptic medications are not necessary if the risk for seizures is low.

The mature nervous system can tolerate fairly high doses of radiation (brain, 5,000–6,000 cGy; spinal cord, 4,000–4,500 cGy) with little risk for significant long-term toxicity; however, the developing brains of pediatric patients are far more vulnerable, and long-term learning disabilities can result from exposure to relatively modest doses. Endocrine function can be altered years after cranial irradiation, owing to effects on the pituitary-hypothalamic axis. Blood chemistries should be monitored regularly in adults, and children should be followed up closely to detect any delays in growth or development.

After extremely high doses of radiation, as with stereotactic brain irradiation, necrosis of brain tissue can occur in rare circumstances and is treated best with surgical excision if affected patients can tolerate the procedure. Notably, certain chemotherapeutic agents may lower the threshold for radiation-induced central nervous system (CNS) toxicity [7].

Depending on the length and segment irradiated, the spinal cord can tolerate approximately 4,500 cGy of radiation with no acute or permanent untoward effects. Lhermitte's syndrome, however, is an early, transient myelopathy that may be seen during treatment to the cervicothoracic spinal cord. In general, the disorder appears two to four months after the completion of therapy and is manifest as paresthesias of the arms and legs on flexion of the neck. This self-limited process can be present for months but does not cause permanent injury to the spinal cord. No treatment is necessary.

Permanent, irreversible spinal cord injury—myelitis—is related to total dose and fraction size. The symptoms of this devastating problem resemble those in the Brown-Séquard syndrome (hemisection of the cord), and they may not appear until up to two years after treatment. No effective treatment exists for the disorder.

Peripheral nerves can tolerate high doses of radiation. Peripheral neuropathy also is dose-dependent and comes on gradually but, occasionally, affected patients' condition may improve spontaneously [7].

ACUTE TOXICITY OF CHEMOTHERAPY

Chemotherapy has two major limitations: development of drug resistance and toxic side effects. As most chemotherapeutic agents and regimens have a narrow therapeutic ratio, mild to moderate degrees of toxicity are seen in most patients who receive such treatment. The dose and dose rate of chemotherapy are critical to a meaningful antitumor response. If these agents are given in reduced doses or on a haphazard or incomplete schedule, they will cause toxicity without meaningful benefit.

General Principles

Most chemotherapeutic agents are directed against the DNA synthetic mechanism. Not surprisingly, therefore, the majority of acute side effects of chemotherapy are expressed in areas of the body where cell turnover is rapid: the gastrointestinal mucosa, the Sertoli cells of the testis, the hair follicle, and the replicating blood elements in the bone marrow (Table 9.3). A second category of toxicities includes a number of poorly understood effects on parenchymal tissues of organs (e.g., lung, liver, heart). Drug doses and schedules of administration must be based on the specific mechanism of action and clinical pharmacology of each drug and on the time required for normal tissues to recover from their associated acute toxicities. Often, toxicities due to chemotherapy are exacerbated by concomitant medical problems or by the administration of interacting drugs or other therapies (Table 9.4). For example, the myelosuppression produced by a wide variety of chemotherapeutic agents is much more severe in patients who previously have undergone radiation to fields that include

Table 9.3   Emetogenic Potential of Single Chemotherapeutic Agents

Level	Frequency of Emesis (%)	Agent
5	> 90	Carmustine, > 250 mg/m²
		Cisplatin, ≥ 50 mg/m²
		Cyclophosphamide, > 1,500 mg/m²
		Dacarbazine
		Mechlorethamine
		Streptozocin
4	60–90	Carboplatin
		Carmustine, ≥ 250 mg/m²
		Cisplatin, < 50 mg/m²
		Cyclophosphamide, > 750–1,500 mg/m²
		Cytarabine, > 1 g/m²
		Doxorubicin, > 60 mg/m²
		Methotrexate, > 1,000 mg/m²
		Procarbazine (oral)
3	30–60	Cyclophosphamide, ≥ 750 mg/m²
		Cyclophosphamide (oral)
		Doxorubicin, 20–60 mg/m²
		Epirubicin, ≥ 90 mg/m²
		Hexamethylmelamine (oral)
		Idarubicin
		Ifosfamide
		Methotrexate, 250–1,000 mg/m²
		Mitoxantrone, < 15 mg/m²
2	10–30	Docetaxel
		Etoposide
		5-Fluorouracil, < 1,000 mg/m²
		Gemcitabine
		Methotrexate, > 50–250 mg/m²
		Mitomycin
		Paclitaxel
1	< 10	Bleomycin
		Busulfan
		Chlorambucil (oral)
		2-Chlorodeoxyadenosine
		Fludarabine
		Hydroxyurea
		Methotrexate, ≥ 50 mg/m²
		L-Phenylalanine mustard (oral)
		Thioguanine (oral)
		Vinblastine
		Vincristine
		Vinorelbine

Source: Reprinted with permission from PJ Hesketh, MC Kris, SM Grunberg, Chemotherapy emetogenicity. *J Clin Oncol* 15:103–109, 1995.

large volumes of bone marrow. Similarly, in patients in whom radiotherapy has involved the mediastinum and myocardium, cardiomyopathy may develop at lower doses of doxorubicin [13]. In addition, the presence of medical conditions that interfere with the metabolism or excretion of chemotherapeutic agents may increase

their toxicity greatly. Because several chemotherapeutic drugs are metabolized by the biliary system, patients with liver or biliary dysfunction are much more likely to experience severe toxic effects. Likewise, drugs excreted by the kidneys will be more toxic in patients with renal dysfunction.

Drug interactions also are a factor. Salicylates displace methotrexate from its binding sites on albumin and thus can increase this drug's toxicity. Also, because the antileukemic drug 6-mercaptopurine ordinarily is metabolized by the enzyme xanthine oxidase, concurrent administration of the potent xanthine oxidase inhibitor allopurinol can alter this drug's metabolism and increase its toxicity greatly.

Chemotherapeutic agents may interact synergistically with therapeutic x-rays and ultraviolet light. For instance, a "recall reaction" characterized by skin erythema and inflammation may be seen in patients given doxorubicin or dactinomycin shortly after a course of radiotherapy; usually, this inflammation is limited to the area of the body that had been irradiated previously. Several chemotherapeutic agents, notably 5-fluorouracil (5-FU) and methotrexate, may act as photosensitizers, making the patient much more susceptible to inflammation and damage induced by sunlight [13].

Finally, idiosyncratic or allergic reactions may occur with a variety of chemotherapeutic agents. Anaphylaxis has been known to occur in response to the administration of bleomycin, L-asparaginase, and paclitaxel, among others.

Nausea and Vomiting

The act of vomiting is coordinated by receptors in both the gastrointestinal tract and the CNS. These receptors communicate via vagus nerve afferents that connect to the "vomiting center" in the medulla. The chemoreceptor trigger zone in the area postrema of the brain is another important effector of emesis and responds to various chemical stimuli in the blood [14]. Thus, noxious agents may cause vomiting by stimulating receptors in the gastrointestinal tract or in the CNS. Various neurochemicals, such as dopamine, acetylcholine, and serotonin, have been identified as CNS effectors of vomiting. The identification of specific receptor antagonists has allowed more effective drugs to be developed to treat chemotherapy-induced nausea and vomiting [15].

Knowledge of the mechanism of chemotherapy-induced vomiting, of the different patterns of emesis encountered in clinical practice, and of the pharmacology of the various antiemetic drugs should allow tailor-

Table 9.4   Drugs and Treatments That Increase Chemotherapy Toxicity

Chemotherapeutic Agent	Interacting Drug or Treatment	Clinical Result	Mechanism and Comments
Doxorubicin	Irradiation	Skin and soft-tissue inflammation	Radiation recall
Methotrexate	Salicylates	Mucositis	Displacement of methotrexate from albumin-binding sites
Mercaptopurine	Allopurinol	Myelosuppression	Inhibition of xanthine oxidase
Doxorubicin	Paclitaxel	Cardiomyopathy	Concentration of doxorubicin

ing of the antiemetic regimen to individual patients. The most commonly used chemotherapeutic agents in order of their emetogenic potential are listed in Table 9.3.

The emetic patterns most commonly seen in patients receiving chemotherapy are acute emesis, anticipatory emesis, and delayed emesis. Of course, an important factor is to differentiate these patterns from the nausea and vomiting due to increased intracranial pressure, sepsis, gastritis, or bowel obstruction.

In addition to the medications noted later, creation of an environment devoid of noxious stimuli will help to control nausea and vomiting. Maintaining a bland diet, keeping the treatment area calm and quiet, and encouraging the use of relaxation techniques can potentiate the effectiveness of the antiemetic regimen.

ACUTE EMESIS

The severity of acute emesis depends on many factors, the most important of which are affected patients' previous response to chemotherapy and the emetic potential of the drugs employed in the regimen. Table 9.3 lists chemotherapeutic agents according to their potential for causing nausea and vomiting. The dose and route of administration also can alter the emetic pattern.

The newest class of antiemetics, the serotonin antagonists, have proved to be effective either when used as single agents or when combined with steroids. They block the action of serotonin in both the central and the peripheral pathways involved in nausea and vomiting. Ondansetron, the first agent in this class to be used clinically, can be given orally or intravenously. Various regimens are available, including single, high-dose intravenous administration, lower intravenous doses given every 8 hours, or oral doses given three times a day for several days. Granisetron and anastrazole, newer oral agents with a longer half-life, can be given once every 24 hours [16].

Antihistamines, phenothiazines, steroids, tranquiliz-

ers, and antianxiety agents have been used successfully, either alone or in combination, to treat the nausea and vomiting associated with chemotherapy. (Precise dosages and routes of administration may be found in standard pharmacology texts.) However, these drugs are most effective when given prior to chemotherapy; this approach probably allows them to block the emesis receptors and thereby to prevent stimulation by the chemotherapeutic drugs. Their antianxiety properties are helpful also in decreasing anticipatory nausea.

The dopamine-receptor antagonist metoclopramide is effective for cisplatin-induced nausea and vomiting. Usually, it is administered intravenously in high doses (2–3 mg/kg every 2–3 hours). Side effects include extrapyramidal reactions, restlessness, and diarrhea. Haloperidol and droperidol can be given either intravenously or orally (haloperidol). Their side effects are similar to those of metoclopramide and also include sedation.

The phenothiazines (prochlorperazine, chlorpromazine) have a mechanism of action similar to the foregoing agents and may be given intravenously, orally, or as a rectal suppository. Generally, they are less effective for severe emesis but are more convenient to use in an outpatient setting. Side effects are similar to those already listed and also include orthostatic hypotension.

Corticosteroids work by an unknown mechanism and are effective when given either orally or intravenously. Most commonly, dexamethasone is used in doses ranging from 4 to 20 mg. It is most effective when combined with a serotonin antagonist. Most of the major side effects are avoided by employing short courses of steroids.

Lorazepam, a benzodiazepine, is effective when combined with other antiemetic drugs. The usual dose of 1.0 to 1.5 mg/m^2 intravenously is associated with significant sedation.

Cannabinoids have been shown to be as effective as the phenothiazines in randomized trials. Tetrahydrocannabinol (dronabinol) and the synthetic cannabinoid nabilone are administered orally and can cause sedation, dry mouth, and ataxia. Many patients with no prior exposure to cannabinoids report dysphoria, which is why these agents should not be considered as first-line therapy.

Though many of the antiemetics are fairly active when used as single agents, more complete control of nausea and vomiting may be achieved when drugs with different pharmacologic actions are used in combination. Selecting drugs with overlapping toxicities will minimize patient discomfort. Thus, the use of a dopamine-receptor antagonist, such as metoclopramide, combined with a steroid and a benzodiazepine can produce superior emetic control with few side effects.

ANTICIPATORY EMESIS

Anticipatory nausea and vomiting is a conditioned response usually found in patients with poor emetic control after initial chemotherapy. Such patients may begin to experience symptoms on entering the chemotherapy unit or on smelling the alcohol used to prepare the intravenous site. Maximizing the antiemetic regimen during the first course of chemotherapy can prevent this complication. Once established, anticipatory emesis may be treated by desensitization, hypnosis, or relaxation techniques.

DELAYED EMESIS

Although usually not as severe as the acute syndrome, delayed emesis contributes to morbidity by interfering with nutrition and hydration. Most often, it is encountered in patients receiving high-dose chemotherapy and is thought to be caused by residual drug or metabolites. Symptoms are noted 48 hours after chemotherapy administration but may occur up to five days later. Effective treatment includes oral dexamethasone plus oral metoclopramide or a phenothiazine [17].

Hepatotoxicity

Several chemotherapeutic agents are toxic to the liver in varying degrees. Mild effects may be manifest as a transient elevation in hepatic enzymes, whereas severe damage might result in permanent cirrhosis. The nitrosourea compounds (i.e., carmustine [BCNU], lomustine [CCNU], and streptozocin) can cause mild elevations in serum transaminases, alkaline phosphatase, and bilirubin, reflecting liver function abnormalities; however, these levels generally return to normal once the offending agent is withdrawn from the chemotherapeutic regimen.

The antimetabolite methotrexate, a dihydrofolate reductase inhibitor, also is associated with liver dysfunction, often causing elevations in aspartate aminotransferase and lactate dehydrogenase. Patients treated with oral methotrexate are twice as likely to become afflicted with hepatic fibrosis or cirrhosis as are those treated with an intermittent intravenous regimen. Although hepatic fibrosis tends to resolve once treatment is discontinued, the same is not true for cirrhosis, which is a much more serious complication.

Azathioprine and 6-mercaptopurine, antimetabolites that also are used frequently to treat patients with renal transplants or cancer, not only raise the levels of liver enzymes but lead to the development of intrahepatic cholestasis and parenchymal cell necrosis. Liver enzyme levels can be elevated also by the administration of cytosine arabinoside.

The antibiotic mithramycin, used previously to treat testicular carcinoma and hypercalcemia in patients with tumors refractory to therapy, is considered the most hepatotoxic of the chemotherapeutic agents and is, therefore, seldom used. Among its many effects on the liver are significant elevations in aspartate aminotransferase and lactate dehydrogenase, milder elevations in alkaline phosphatase, acute hepatic necrosis, and decreased synthesis of the coagulation factors II, V, VIII, and X. The hepatotoxic effects of L-asparaginase, a drug used frequently in children with acute lymphoblastic leukemia, include fatty changes, decreased serum proteins and coagulation factors, and elevations in liver enzymes. This drug also may cause acute pancreatitis. Administration of floxuridine by hepatic artery infusion has been associated with significant hepatotoxicity [18].

Myelosuppression

Bone marrow suppression is the most important toxic effect of the majority of chemotherapeutic agents and typically is the dose-limiting factor. Death occurring after chemotherapy usually results either from infection related to drug-induced leukopenia or from bleeding related to thrombocytopenia. The onset of myelosuppression varies from drug to drug, although certain general guidelines have been established. For example, the cell cycle–specific chemotherapeutic agents affect the rapidly proliferating pool of blood precursors in the marrow (from myeloblasts to promyelocytes); destruction of this cohort of myeloid precursors leads to a predictable decrease in the peripheral white blood cell count at approximately 10 to 14 days after the drug is administered, after which the white count rapidly returns to normal. Other chemotherapeutic agents affect stem cells, leading to myelosuppression (which occurs later) and to a delay in the recovery of normal blood counts. In most cases, myelosuppression secondary to chemotherapy is relatively short-lived (3–5 days) and is self-limited. The incidence of severe infection rises dramatically when the absolute neutrophil count drops below 1,000 cells/mm³. (The absolute neutrophil count is equal to the total white count multiplied by the percentage of neutrophils.)

Infection in Neutropenic Patients

Infection is a frequent problem associated with chemotherapy-induced leukopenia; probably the most common cause of chemotherapy-related death is sepsis in neutropenic patients. The usual clinical manifestations of infection (e.g., erythema, pain, pulmonary infiltrates, or pyuria) are absent in patients with neutropenia: These patients' lack of polymorphonuclear neutrophils that normally would be recruited to sites of infection incites the inflammatory response.

The hallmark of infection in neutropenic patients is fever. When affected patients' body temperature rises (particularly 7–21 days after chemotherapy, when the leukocyte nadir typically occurs), total white blood cell and neutrophil counts should be assessed immediately. If the absolute neutrophil count is 500 to 1,000/mm³, indicating neutropenia, broad-spectrum antibiotics should be given emergently. Frequently, delay in administering antibiotics in the severely leukopenic patient with infection leads to septic shock, which may be irreversible.

Rarely, infection may develop without fever. In such patients, the sudden onset of weakness, hypotension, or confusion may suggest the diagnosis. Patients receiving chemotherapy may be asked to take their temperature at least twice a day and to report any increase to their physicians without delay.

The evaluation of febrile neutropenic patients should consist of prompt but careful recording of a medical history and a physical examination. The latter should be extended specifically to include the oropharynx, axillae, perineum, and perirectal area and should include venipuncture and intravenous sites. After a chest roentgenogram and appropriate cultures (including blood and urine cultures) have been obtained, broad-spectrum antibiotics should be administered immediately, usually in the emergency department.

Initial infections in the neutropenic patient are typically bacterial and involve such gram-positive organisms as *Staphylococcus aureus* and such gram-negative organisms as *Pseudomonas aeruginosa*, *Escherichia coli*, *Klebsiella*, and *Serratia* species. Often, the source of the infecting organism is previous colonization. Because of variations in the endemic microbial flora, the relative incidence of particular pathogens may vary from hospital to hospital and from year to year. Common sites of infection include the skin, oropharynx, lungs, gastrointestinal and genitourinary tracts, and bloodstream. Particular sites may be at higher risk for infection, owing to the specific malignancy or anticancer therapy (e.g., an obstructive bronchial lesion, radiation-induced esophagitis) [19].

Antibiotic treatment should be based on individual patients' clinical history, the microbial flora, and patterns of antibiotic resistance within the medical institution. Drugs should be selected so as to provide broad coverage against both gram-positive and gram-negative organisms. Specific coverage can be provided when a particular problem is identified, such as potential bowel sepsis requiring anaerobic coverage. Most patients respond to empiric antibiotic therapy. Those with documented infections or unequivocal signs of bacterial infection will require a minimum of 10 to 14 days of antibiotic treatment. Patients who are without documented infections but who reacted with defervescence to antibiotics should continue to be treated until the neutropenia is reversed [19].

For febrile neutropenic patients, the routine use of such recombinant colony-stimulating factors as granulocyte colony-stimulating factor (G-CSF) or granulocyte-macrophage colony-stimulating factor (GM-CSF) in conjunction with antibiotics has not been proved to confer any benefit. Current guidelines suggest using growth factors only in patients who are at high risk for complications from sepsis [20].

Although bacterial infections usually are controlled by prompt administration of antibiotics, treating fungal and viral infections in neutropenic patients is much more difficult. Fungal pathogens may include *Candida*, *Aspergillus*, and *Mucor* species, among others. Patients who are neutropenic and remain persistently febrile despite adequate antibiotic treatment may benefit from a trial of empiric therapy with the antifungal drug amphotericin.

Mucocutaneous Toxicity

ALOPECIA

Hair loss due to chemotherapy is caused by damage to the rapidly dividing cells within the germinal portion of hair bulbs. This complication may affect the scalp hair, eyebrows, and axillary and pubic hair. It is much more common with certain agents (e.g., doxorubicin, actinomycin D, paclitaxel) but is not universal. Such other agents as methotrexate, 5-FU, and cisplatin may cause mild thinning to partial hair loss but rarely produce generalized alopecia. Because hair loss with chemotherapy usually is reversible after treatment has been completed, physicians should make it a point to inform patients about the temporary nature of this side effect. However, normal hair grows as a rate of only perhaps 2 mm a week, so the reversal of alopecia, even after chemotherapy has been discontinued, usually is a slow process. On occasion, for unexplained reasons, some patients show little or no alopecia when it had been expected; in addition, scalp hair occasionally may regrow despite continued chemotherapy.

Patients should be warned before the hair loss becomes significant so they can acquire a suitable hairpiece or wig. Hairpieces can be made to match affected patients' natural hair color and texture. Often, the cost of a wig prescribed by a physician is reimbursed by third-party payers. In addition, patients should be told that their hair may be slightly different in texture and color on regrowth. Although wigs have made social interactions more accessible, personal and especially sexual relations may be affected profoundly. Patients facing this form of chemotherapeutic toxicity require the support of their physicians, families, and friends.

Such preventive measures as the scalp tourniquet, either alone or combined with scalp cooling, have been successful in patients assigned to relatively low-dose chemotherapeutic regimens. However, when higher doses or drugs with longer half-lives are used, these techniques seem only to delay the onset of alopecia or perhaps to lessen its severity slightly. Scalp tourniquets should not be used in patients with such widely disseminated diseases as leukemia or small-cell lung cancer, as they could create a sanctuary for the malignant cells [8].

DRUG EXTRAVASATION

A disastrous and avoidable cutaneous complication of chemotherapy is the local infiltration of a vesicant drug that can cause severe tissue inflammation and necrosis if it escapes from a vein. The major drugs associated with such reactions include doxorubicin, daunorubicin, dactinomycin, mitomycin C, BCNU, dacarbazine (DTIC), nitrogen mustard, vincristine, vinblastine, and vinorelbine. Managing the skin ulceration and inflammation that result from drug extravasation can be extremely difficult. The necrotic process may persist over several months, and excision with skin grafting may be necessary. Therefore, every effort should be made to prevent this complication in the first place. Prevention can be accomplished by injecting the chemotherapeutic agent through the side arm of a freely running intravenous infusion and observing the infusion continuously. On even the suspicion of minimal tissue infiltration, the infusion should be discontinued. An attempt to aspirate the extravasated material should be made through the original intravenous access. Specific antidotes have been defined for some of the drugs, and the appropriate agent should be injected promptly into the site. The routine use of steroids in this setting is not recommended. Central venous catheters and subcutaneous infusion ports markedly reduce the risk for extravasation [21].

CHRONIC SKIN CHANGES

Hyperkeratosis and hyperpigmentation are common during treatment with bleomycin. Bleomycin is a polypeptide antitumor antibiotic used in the treatment of lymphoma, squamous cell carcinoma, testicular cancer, and several other malignancies. It concentrates in squamous tissues and seems to have a unique predilection for the skin, especially affecting the dorsum of the hands and feet and areas of local trauma. Toxicity is related to both total dose level and duration of administration and may be highly symptomatic, disfiguring, and incapacitating. However, the changes slowly reverse when an offending drug is discontinued. Hyperpigmentation of the skin also has been described in association with a number of other chemotherapeutic agents, including 5-FU.

A syndrome of painful palms and soles (*hand-foot syndrome* or *palmar-plantar dysesthesia*) has been described after administration of 5-FU, Ara-C, or capecitabine. The symptoms may be severe and associated with desquamation of the digits. It is reversible on cessation of an offending drug [22].

MUCOSITIS

Ulceration of the mucous membranes can be one of the most painful toxicities induced by antitumor chemotherapy. In patients with concomitant leukopenia and immunosuppression, mucosal ulceration can lead to sepsis and even death. Typically, chemotherapy-induced mucositis is seen with such antimetabolites as 5-FU and methotrexate and with such antibiotics as doxorubicin, dactinomycin, and bleomycin. This form of toxicity occurs earlier than does myelosuppression, commonly four to six days after the start of treatment. Attempts at symptomatic control include attention to good oral hygiene and use of a mixture of an antibiotic (tetracycline) and antifungal agent (nystatin [Myco-statin®]) in a mouthwash. Local anesthetics applied topically can provide brief, partial relief. Severe oropharyngeal mucositis in a patient whose nutritional status is marginal can result in malnutrition or serious nutritional deficiencies, because the condition interferes with oral intake. Typically, mucositis is self-limiting and reversible but still may cause severe symptoms [23].

Pulmonary Toxicity

Although a variety of chemotherapeutic agents have been associated with complications affecting the lung, pulmonary toxicity is seen most commonly with the use of bleomycin and the nitrosoureas. The final result of such injury appears to be pulmonary fibrosis. Early preclinical studies of bleomycin indicated that the drug is concentrated preferentially in squamous tissues, particularly the lung and skin. Electron microscopic studies in humans have shown a decrease in type I pneumocytes and changes in type II pneumocytes after administration of this agent.

Often, pulmonary toxicity due to bleomycin is heralded by a dry, hacking cough followed by dyspnea on exertion. Symptoms may develop during the course of drug therapy or one to three months after treatment ends. The earliest findings on physical examination are fine, crackling, bibasilar rales, although rhonchi and occasionally a pleural friction rub also may be audible. The earliest radiographic manifestations are fine, reticular, bibasilar infiltrates that may progress to alveolar and interstitial infiltrates, progressive involvement of the lower lobe, and lung consolidation. On blood gas analysis, oxygen and bicarbonate concentrations usually are low. Serial pulmonary function tests should be performed in all patients receiving bleomycin. In particular, serial determinations of carbon monoxide–diffusing capacity (D_{co}) may be valuable in monitoring the subclinical pulmonary effects of bleomycin.

Bleomycin-induced lung toxicity is dose-related, increasing significantly at doses in excess of 500 units. In doses of less than 400 to 500 units, the incidence of definite toxicity is constant but low. Risk factors include advanced age, preexisting lung disease, and previous radiotherapy. Concurrent treatment with cyclophosphamide may increase affected patients' susceptibility to such toxicity. Interestingly, when bleomycin is delivered by continuous infusion, the risk for toxicity may be decreased.

A number of other chemotherapeutic agents have been cited as pulmonary toxins, including cyclophosphamide, procarbazine, melphalan, mitomycin C, and BCNU. Methotrexate pulmonary toxicity appears to be related to hypersensitivity to the drug [24].

Cardiotoxicity

Doxorubicin and its related congener, daunorubicin, are the only chemotherapeutic agents frequently associated with cardiac damage. Acute effects on the heart, manifested by electrocardiographic (ECG) abnormalities, may be seen in up to 41% of patients receiving the drug. These ECG changes—primarily nonspecific ST-T wave changes, sinus tachycardia, premature ventricular and atrial contractions, and low-voltage QRS complexes—appear to be more common if such patients previously have had an abnormal ECG, but they do not seem to be predictive of the development of doxorubicin-induced cardiomyopathy. When this type of toxicity occurs, it is associated with mortality as high as 61%. The total dose of doxorubicin administered is the most significant risk factor for the development of drug-induced cardiomyopathy; others include the schedule of drug administration, age, preexisting cardiac disease, prior mediastinal or left chest radiotherapy, and concurrent therapy with cytotoxic drugs. Paclitaxel added to daunorubicin may result in a higher risk of cardiomyopathy even at lower cumulative doses of daunorubicin [25].

Tachycardia may be the first sign of doxorubicin toxicity. Usually, affected patients present with symptoms of congestive heart failure, shortness of breath, or a nonproductive cough. Pathologic findings are nonspecific and can be seen with other cardiomyopathies. The most promising noninvasive method for predicting doxorubicin-induced cardiomyopathy is radionuclide cineangiography. Percutaneous biopsy of the myocardium to assess damage also has been attempted at several centers. Electron microscopy of cardiac biopsy material will reveal vacuolization of myocytes along with dilated mitochondria. Overall, despite a wide variety of tests, no morphologic evidence has been accepted completely as being predictive of doxorubicin-induced heart failure.

Table 9.5   Neurotoxicity of Chemotherapeutic Agents

Drug	Mechanism	Frequency	Clinical Manifestations
Vinca alkaloids			
Vincristine	Axonal damage	Common and dose-limiting	Decreased deep tendon reflexes, paresthesias (numbness and tingling of fingertips)
Vinblastine, etoposide (VP16)	—	Rare	Abdominal pain, constipation, ileus
L-Asparaginase	Drug-induced metabolic disorders	Common	Lethargy, somnolence, confusion
5-Fluorouracil	Cerebellar dysfunction (possible fluorocitrate)	Rare (1–3%)	Ataxia, dysmetria, nystagmus
Procarbazine	Monoamine oxidase inhibition	Uncommon	Sedation, confusion, peripheral neuropathy
Cisplatin	Segmental demyelination	Common	Paresthesias, "stocking-glove" peripheral neuropathy, high-frequency hearing loss
Paclitaxel	Disruption of microtubules	Common	Paresthesias, neuropathy

Cardiomyopathy can be prevented in the majority of affected patients by limiting the dose of doxorubicin. Better methods are needed for identifying patients who have subclinical myocardial damage and therefore are at risk for doxorubicin toxicity. Attempts are being made to develop less cardiomyopathic dose schedules, and the use of alternative anthracyclines is being assessed [26]. Such cardioprotective drugs as dexrazoxane may be useful in preventing toxicity but have not been recommended routinely [27].

Genitourinary Toxicity

Chemotherapeutic agents that cause major renal toxicity include cisplatin, methotrexate, and streptozocin (which damage the tubules). Toxicity depends on the dose of an agent used and the schedule of administration. Cisplatin toxicity may be potentiated by preexisting renal disease or by the concurrent use of other nephrotoxic agents, such as the aminoglycoside antibiotics; it may be avoided by aggressive hydration with normal saline or mannitol [18]. High-dose methotrexate has been associated also with acute renal failure, although this complication can be avoided successfully through the use of hydration and alkalinization schemes. Streptozocin, useful in the treatment of islet-cell tumors, is associated with a syndrome of acute tubular necrosis and renal tubular acidosis related to the dose and rate of drug administration.

Cyclophosphamide and ifosfamide have been associated with hemorrhagic cystitis caused by excretion of the drugs' toxic metabolites in the urine, which may be avoided with adequate hydration prior to administration of these drugs. Symptoms of cystitis include urgency, frequency, dysuria, and a mild microscopic hematuria. Usually, the cystitis is self-limiting, resolving within two to six weeks after cessation of the drug. Severe hemorrhagic cystitis may be a medical emergency, and control may require cystoscopy with clot removal, fulguration of discrete bleeding sites, and instillation of such sclerosing agents as formalin. Liberal use of fluids is recommended both on the day prior to treatment and for 24 hours thereafter, and affected patients should be encouraged to void frequently, particularly at bedtime. The use of mesna, a synthetic sulfhydryl, has reduced significantly the incidence of this complication after the administration of high-dose cyclophosphamide or ifosfamide [28].

Neurotoxicity

Chemotherapeutic agents have been associated also with neurologic toxicities of various sorts (Table 9.5). Best described is the toxicity related to the vinca alkaloids, particularly vincristine. Vincristine is unique among the antineoplastic agents in that its neurotoxicity commonly is dose-limiting. Early manifestations of the neurologic effects of this drug are distal paresthesias and the loss of deep tendon reflexes. Cranial nerve palsy, autonomic neuropathy, and the syndrome of inappropriate antidiuretic hormone secretion are seen with high cumulative doses of vincristine. Typically, toxicity is symmetric, dose-related, and reversible. The peak dose levels obtained after administration appear to correlate better with toxicity than does the overall cumulative dose.

Other drugs reported to cause neurotoxicity are listed in Table 9.5. Cisplatin and carboplatin produce a symmetric sensory neuropathy, particularly at high cumulative doses. Other evidence of neurologic toxicity from cisplatin includes tinnitus and hearing loss, especially in the high-frequency range. 5-FU has been reported to induce cerebellar ataxia, particularly with long-term treatment schedules involving intermittent high doses, and L-asparaginase has been associated with the syndrome of lethargy, confusion, and disorientation [18]. The use of high-dose or intrathecal methotrexate, especially in combination with cranial irradiation, reportedly causes a progressive encephalopathy. Paclitaxel induces a symmetric polyneuropathy that is dose-dependent and is enhanced by combination with cisplatin [29].

LATE COMPLICATIONS OF CHEMOTHERAPY

Recent improvements in cancer treatment have increased the number of long-term, disease-free survivors. As a result, attention has focused on the late toxic effects of chemotherapeutic drugs on the health and quality of life of these survivors. Two major problems that have emerged are gonadal injury from chemotherapy and the development of second malignancies.

Effects on Gonadal Function

Gonadal dysfunction is a common late complication of chemotherapy. The degree of injury is determined by affected patients' age and gender and the total dose of the agent received. Age is important in that the gonads are extremely vulnerable to chemotherapy-related damage during puberty. Men and women differ in their sensitivity to these drugs: Usually, men develop infertility but retain normal Leydig cell function, whereas women may suffer impaired fertility and early ovarian failure. Different classes of drugs vary in their potential for inducing gonadal toxicity. The alkylating agents (nitrogen mustard, cyclophosphamide, melphalan, and many others) produce the most severe effects.

PATIENT AGE AT TIME OF TREATMENT

The gonads of prepubertal children are relatively insensitive to chemotherapeutic drugs because levels of circulating gonadotropins are low prior to puberty. Doses of chemotherapeutic drugs that produce gonadal damage in adolescents and adults have limited effects in the prepubertal child. However, this reduced vulnerability is relative, and high cumulative doses of drugs, especially if associated with irradiation of the gonadal area, may damage the ovaries permanently.

GONADAL DYSFUNCTION IN MEN

Gonadal dysfunction in men consists of infertility and low sperm counts. Because cytotoxic drugs are more damaging to the germinal epithelium (required for sperm production) than to the Leydig cells (responsible for male hormone production), hormonal function and libido remain intact. Qualitative sperm abnormalities (reduced motility, morphologic changes) also may be seen. As many as 90% of postpubertal males treated with combination chemotherapy (mechlorethamine, vincristine [Oncovin®], procarbazine, and prednisone, or MOPP) for Hodgkin's disease may develop irreversible sterility; this incidence may be somewhat lower with drugs used to treat acute leukemia. Prior to the start of chemotherapy, affected male patients at high risk for irreversible sterility should be given the option of sperm banking for later artificial insemination (see Chapter 37).

GONADAL DYSFUNCTION IN WOMEN

Alkylating agents are known to cause ovarian damage similar to that caused by radiotherapy. Frequently, abnormal ovarian function during chemotherapy treatment is manifested as irregular menstrual cycles or amenorrhea. Depending on the total dose of the drug received, young women usually recover normal ovarian function and fertility. However, in women who are within several years of natural menopause, ovarian failure may be irreversible. Gonadal damage may be limited by the use of oral contraceptives during chemotherapy treatment. Biopsy of the ovary after long-term treatment with an alkylating agent frequently reveals the absence of ova and no evidence of follicular maturation. Reversibility of this gonadal failure is related to the total dose and duration of the drug received (see Chapter 37).

Effects on Pregnancy Outcome and Progeny

Despite the frequent adverse effects of chemotherapeutic agents on gonadal function and the documented mutagenicity and teratogenicity of these drugs in animal models, apparently most affected women give birth to normal infants after being treated with chemotherapy and resuming menstruation. Moreover, the incidence of chromosomal or congenital abnormalities does not appear to be greater among the offspring of patients who have received chemotherapy. These facts are helpful in counseling patients about the potential risks to their offspring from anticancer drugs related to their treatment [30] (see Chapter 37).

Second Malignancies and Disorders

The development of acute leukemia as a result of chemotherapy administered for hematologic malignancies, solid tumors, and nonneoplastic disease has become a significant problem. Time from the start of chemotherapy to the onset of leukemia is relatively short, approximately 3¼ to 4¼ years. Often, pancytopenia and increased myeloblasts in the bone marrow precede overt acute leukemia [31].

The usual course of chemotherapy-induced acute leukemia is rapid progression to death within one to two months. Only infrequently does antileukemic therapy produce a complete remission. In Hodgkin's disease, treatment schemes that combine both radiotherapy and chemotherapy seem to act synergistically to increase the risk for leukemia [32]. However, recent studies of the relationship between chemotherapy and irradiation have cast some doubt on the hypothesis that irradiation enhances the leukemogenic effect of chemotherapy [33]. Cases of acute nonlymphocytic leukemia have been known to occur after treatment for such solid tumors as cancer of the breast, ovary, and lung (both small and non-small-cell types) and other tumor types. Of great concern has been the description of acute leukemia after chemotherapy with etoposide and alkylating agents in pediatric patients with various solid tumors [31].

In contrast to acute leukemia, few solid tumors have been described in patients treated with chemotherapy alone. The best-documented solid tumor has been bladder cancer of the type seen after chronic bladder fibrosis induced by cyclophosphamide. However, researchers have discovered that the risk for developing solid tumors is higher than was initially predicted and may continue to rise for more than 15 years after treatment. Those at highest risk are patients who have received both chemotherapy and irradiation. Women who received therapy before age 16 appear to be at greatest risk for developing breast cancer later in life. Other types of tumors seen in this group include cancers of the thyroid, colorectal area, and brain. The evidence should alert clinicians to screen survivors of cancer for the presence of second malignancies. A promising note is that children of survivors do not seem to display an increased risk for cancer [34].

The etiology of chemotherapeutic agent–induced second cancers is not well understood. On the basis of evidence, the mutagenicity of these drugs seems to be a major contributor. Most patients who have developed second malignancies related to chemotherapy have been treated with alkylating agents, which damage the genetic material by cross-linking DNA during the resting phase of the cell cycle. This effect is similar to that of irradiation, and the acute leukemia seen in affected patients is similar to that seen after radiation exposure. Frequently, chromosomal abnormalities are detected in bone marrow cells prior to the development of leukemia, suggesting that direct damage to DNA by the cytotoxic drugs is responsible for the onset of malignancy.

Children who undergo cranial irradiation with or without intrathecal chemotherapy for leukemia and lymphomas have been shown to be at risk for treatment-associated learning disabilities. By means of pretreatment evaluations and periodic reassessments, educators can intervene before disabilities become both functionally and emotionally debilitating. Younger children who receive multimodality therapy during vulnerable periods of brain development have the greatest difficulties with regard to both cognitive and academic functions [35].

BLOOD COMPONENT SUPPORT

Cancer patients may require transfusion of appropriate blood components for many reasons. Some of the more common problems include bone marrow suppression secondary to treatment, acute hemorrhage from mucosal sites or the gastrointestinal tract, poor nutrition, and sepsis.

Red Blood Cells

Packed red blood cells are used preferentially unless life-threatening hemorrhage and hypovolemia are present. One unit of packed red blood cells contains approximately 180 ml of red blood cells and should produce a three-point increase in hematocrit after transfusion.

Minor transfusion reactions include fever, chills, urticaria, and respiratory distress. These effects are caused by sensitivity to donor white blood cells and can be differentiated from major transfusion reactions by the absence of hemolysis. Treatment addresses the symptoms and includes stopping or slowing the transfusion and administering oral acetaminophen, 300 to 600 mg, plus oral or intravenous diphenhydramine, 25 to 50 mg. For persistent symptoms, intravenous hydrocortisone, 50 to 100 mg, may be required. Patients who demonstrate minor reactions should be premedicated for future transfusions. Donor white blood cells may be removed through the use of nylon filters; through removal of the buffy coat after the unit of cells has been centrifuged; or through the use of washed, deglycerolized, frozen red blood cells.

Major transfusion reactions are characterized by lumbar pain, fever, and tachycardia and require immediate cessation of the transfusion while a workup for hemolysis, disseminated intravascular coagulation, or mismatch is begun [36].

Clotting Factors

The use of clotting factors is limited to clinical situations exhibiting a documented coagulopathy. These conditions include disseminated intravascular coagulation, liver failure, or massive hemorrhage.

Platelets

Not all patients with low platelet counts will manifest bleeding complications, so the need for platelet transfusions will depend on the individual clinical setting. In general, patients with platelet counts below 20,000 are at risk for spontaneous bleeding and should be monitored carefully. An initial transfusion of 5 to 10 units of random donor platelets should result in a rise of 10,000 platelets per unit transfused when a count is performed 30 to 60 minutes after transfusion. If the increments in the platelet count are lower after the transfusion, allosensitization may be responsible. Patients with a chronic need for platelet transfusions will benefit from the use of platelets from a single donor who is either ABO-compatible or HLA-matched.

Transfusion reactions to platelets are similar to minor red blood cell reactions and are treated in the same way (see the preceding section). Techniques to remove donor white cells or the use of single-donor platelets will reduce the frequency of these reactions.

White Blood Cells

The use of white blood cell transfusions for neutropenic patients is not considered standard therapy at this time.

Hematopoietic Growth Factors

The recently available cloned human hematopoietic growth factors offer a new dimension in the management of cytopenias associated with cancer and its treatment. Currently, erythropoietin (EPO), G-CSF, GM-CSF, thrombopoietin, and the interleukins are being tested in clinical trials to determine optimal dosage and administration for the treatment of chemotherapy-induced pancytopenia and the bone marrow suppression associated with cancer.

Initially, EPO was used to treat the anemia associated with chronic renal failure. Now it is approved for patients who experience anemia as a result of either chemotherapy or the effects of the underlying malignancy. Care must be taken to rule out other causes of anemia, such as gastrointestinal blood loss, iron deficiency, or vitamin B_{12} deficiency, before EPO therapy is initiated. During the course of treatment, ferritin levels should be monitored closely to prevent rapid depletion of iron stores. Appropriate use of EPO can help cancer patients to achieve a better quality of life and can obviate potentially toxic transfusions [5].

Clinical trials have indicated that both G-CSF and GM-CSF can protect from prolonged neutrophil nadirs those patients undergoing chemotherapy, thereby allowing full drug doses to be delivered on schedule and with less toxicity from bacterial sepsis. Current guidelines suggest that their use be restricted to patients who have demonstrated risk factors for febrile neutropenia. These factors include an episode of febrile neutropenia during a prior cycle of chemotherapy, preexisting neutropenia, or previous bone marrow irradiation [20]. However, neither of these agents affects platelet recovery, and apparently combining the aforementioned colony-stimulating factors with other growth factors will be necessary to provide total hematopoietic protection.

The recent identification and cloning of the platelet-specific growth factor thrombopoietin has allowed its use in clinical trials in which it was shown to elevate platelet counts in patients undergoing chemotherapy [37]. Interleukin-11 has been shown to have a similar effect on platelet counts [38].

Obviously, more experience is needed with these

agents before affected patients will be able to tolerate maximum doses of chemotherapy without the need for blood-product support or prolonged hospital stays to treat side effects. Additionally, the question of their effect on overall survival and their attendant cost have yet to be answered satisfactorily [27].

REFERENCES

1. Chao KSC, Perez C, Brady L. *Radiation Oncology: Management Decisions.* Philadelphia: Lippincott-Raven, 1999: 23–28.

2. Fajando L. Morphology of radiation effects on normal tissues. In Perez C, Brady L (eds), *Principles and Practice of Radiation Oncology.* Philadelphia: Lippincott-Raven, 1998: 143–154.

3. Loge J, Abrahamson A, Ekoberg O, Raasa S. Hodgkin's disease survivors more fatigued than the general population. *J Clin Oncol* 17:253–261, 1999.

4. Cella D, Passik S, Jacobsen P, Breitbort W. Progress toward guidelines for the management of fatigue. *Oncology* 12: 369–372, 1998.

5. Demetri GD, Kris M, Wade J, et al. Quality of life benefit in chemotherapy patients treated with epoietin alpha. *J Clin Oncol* 16:3412–3425, 1998.

6. Miaskowski C, Portenoy R. Update on the assessment and management of cancer related fatigue. *Support Oncol* 1:1–10, 1998.

7. Rubin P, Constine L, Williams J. Late effects of cancer treatment. In Perez C, Brady L (eds), *Principles and Practice of Radiation Oncology.* Philadelphia: Lippincott-Raven, 1998:155–212.

8. Seipp C. Alopecia. In DeVita V, Hollman S, Rosenberg S (eds), *Cancer: Principles and Practice of Oncology* (5th ed). Philadelphia: Lippincott-Raven, 1997:2757–2758.

9. Strohl R. The nursing role in radiation oncology: symptom management of acute and chronic reactions. *Oncol Nurs Forum* 15:429–438, 1987.

10. Rosiello RA, Merrill WW. Radiation-induced lung injury. *Clin Chest Med* 11:65–71, 1990.

11. Shapiro C, Hardenbergh P, Gelman R, et al. Cardiac effects of adjuvant doxorubicin and radiation therapy in breast cancer patients. *J Clin Oncol* 16:3493–3501, 1998.

12. Williams RS, Littell RD, Mendenhall NP. Laparoscopic oophoropexy and ovarian function in the treatment of Hodgkin disease. *Cancer* 85:2138–2142, 1999.

13. Dobelbower R. Principles and practical aspects of radiation therapy. In Skeel R, Lachant N (eds), *Handbook of Cancer Chemotherapy* (4th ed). Boston: Little Brown, 1995:52–70.

14. Grunberg S, Hesketh P. Control of chemotherapy induced emesis. *N Engl J Med* 339:1790–1796, 1993.

15. Hesketh P, Gralla RT, Webb W, et al. Randomized phase II study of the neurokinin I receptor antagonist CJ-11, 974 in the control of cisplatin-induced emesis. *J Clin Oncol* 17:338–343, 1999.

16. Gralla R, Navari R, Hesketh P, et al. Single dose oral granisetron has equivalent antiemetic efficacy to intravenous ondansetron for highly emetogenic cisplatin-based chemotherapy. *J Clin Oncol* 16:1568–1573, 1998.

17. NCCN Antiemesis Practice Guidelines. *Oncology* 11:57–89, 1998.

18. Weiss R. Miscellaneous toxicities. In DeVita V, Hollman S, Rosenberg S (eds), *Cancer: Principles and Practice of Oncology* (5th ed). Philadelphia: Lippincott-Raven, 1997:2796–2806.

19. Macarthur R. Infections: etiology, treatment and prevention. In Skeel R, Lachant N (eds), *Handbook of Cancer Chemotherapy* (4th ed). Boston: Little Brown, 1995:519–531.

20. Update of recommendations for the use of hematopoietic colony-stimulating factors: evidence-based clinical practice guidelines. *J Clin Oncol* 14:1557–1560, 1996.

21. Rudolph R, Larson DL. Etiology and treatment of chemotherapeutic agent extravasation injuries: a review. *J Clin Oncol* 15:1116–1126, 1987.

22. Lokich JJ, Ahlgren JD, Gullo JJ, et al. A prospective randomized comparison of continuous infusion fluorouracil with a conventional bolus schedule in metastatic colorectal carcinoma. *J Clin Oncol* 17:425–432, 1989.

23. Tipton J, Skeel R. Management of acute side effects of cancer chemotherapy. In Skeel R, Lachant N (eds), *Handbook of Cancer Chemotherapy* (4th ed). Boston: Little Brown, 1995:573–589.

24. Stover D, Kaner R. Pulmonary toxicity. In DeVita V, Hollman S, Rosenberg S (eds), *Cancer: Principles and Practice of Oncology* (5th ed). Philadelphia: Lippincott-Raven, 1997: 2729–2739.

25. Percy E. Paclitaxel and cardiotoxicity. *J Clin Oncol* 16: 3481–3482, 1998.

26. Ryberg M, Nielsen D, Skovsgaard R, et al. Epirubicin cardiotoxicity: an analysis of 469 patients with metastatic breast cancer. *J Clin Oncol* 16:3501–3508, 1998.

27. Phillips K-A, Tannock I. Design and interpretation of clinical trials that evaluate agents that may offer protection from the toxic effects of cancer chemotherapy. *J Clin Oncol* 16:3179–3190, 1998.

28. Schuchter L. Current role of protective agents in cancer treatment. *Oncology* 11:505–516, 1997.

29. Rowiasky E, Donebower R. Paclitaxel. *N Engl J Med* 332:1004–1014, 1995.

30. Meistrich M, Vassilopoulou-Sellin R, Lipschultz L. Gonadal dysfunction. In DeVita V, Hollman S, Rosenberg S (eds), *Cancer: Principles and Practice of Oncology* (5th ed). Philadelphia: Lippincott-Raven, 1997:2758–2772.

31. Kushner B, Heller G, Cheung N, et al. High risk of leukemia after short-term dose intensive chemotherapy in young patients with solid tumors. *J Clin Oncol* 16:3016–3020, 1998.

32. Hudson M, Poguette C, Greenwald C, et al. Increased mortality after successful treatment for Hodgkin's disease. *J Clin Oncol* 16:3572–3600, 1998.

33. van Leeuwen F. Second cancers. In DeVita V, Hollman S, Rosenberg S (eds), *Cancer: Principles and Practice of Oncology* (5th ed). Philadelphia: Lippincott-Raven, 1997:2773–2795.

34. Samkila R, Olsen JH, Anderson H. Risk of cancer among offspring of childhood cancer survivors. *N Engl J Med* 338:1339–1344, 1998.

35. Mavey I, Kramer J, Ablin A. Late effects of central nervous system prophylactic leukemia therapy on cognitive functioning. *Oncol Nurs Forum* 13:45–51, 1986.

36. Smith M. Disorder of hemostasis and transfusion therapy. In Skeel R, Lachant N (eds), *Handbook of Cancer Chemotherapy* (4th ed). Boston: Little Brown, 1995:553–572.

37. Prow D, Vadhan-Raj S. Thrombopoietin: biology and potential clinical applications. *Oncology* 12:1579–1608, 1998.

38. Gordon M, McCaskill-Stevens W, Battiato L, et al. A phase I trial of recombinant interleukin-11 in women with breast cancer receiving chemotherapy. *Blood* 87:3615–3624, 1996.

10

Breast Cancer

■ ■ ■

Robert T. Osteen

Breast cancer is the most common malignant tumor among women of the Western world. Approximately 182,800 new cases will be diagnosed in American women in 2000 [1]. The incidence of the disease increased between 1940 and 1987 [2]. Between 1982 and 1986, the rate increased by 4% per year, but since 1987, the incidence rate has been relatively stable. Breast cancer mortality has been stable since 1950, although mortality has increased among women older than 55 years and has decreased among women younger than 55 [3]. To a certain extent, the stable mortality and increasing incidence may reflect an increase in the rate at which carcinoma in situ and small, occult, invasive cancers are being discovered as a result of more widespread use of mammography, or it may indicate a more fundamental change in incidence. Finally, improvements in treatment may have contributed to an increase in the percentage of breast cancers that have been cured over the last 30 years.

These raw statistics mask the broader emotional and financial impact of the disease. For every woman with a diagnosis of breast cancer, another 5 or 10 will have a biopsy that shows benign disease. For every woman who undergoes biopsy, perhaps 10 or more see their physician because of a breast symptom and concern about cancer or have a cancer question raised by an abnormal mammogram.

RISK AND EPIDEMIOLOGIC FACTORS

Among American women, the lifetime risk (birth to some age between 85 and 110 years) for breast cancer is approximately 13%, but the risk of dying from the disease is 3.3%. The risks for a woman developing or dying of breast cancer are affected by the underlying risks for the entire population and the individual risk factors for the patient.

The estimate of an individual's risk is complicated.

The first factor may be an attenuation of risk with time. In other words, the increased risk associated with a particular risk factor may not be constant throughout a woman's life, and the risk of developing breast cancer may be much higher during the first decade after identification of the risk factor than in subsequent decades. For example, a woman with biopsy-proved, atypical ductal hyperplasia has a relative risk of 9.8 during the first decade after the biopsy but a relative risk of 3.6 in the subsequent two decades.

A second factor may be that much of the basic or underlying risk for breast cancer is expressed in old age, and this may be of less concern to a woman than is her immediate cancer risk. For purposes of counseling, 10- and 20-year intervals may be more meaningful than is lifetime risk. For example, the risk that a 35-year-old woman will develop a breast cancer by the age of 55 is 2.5%, and the risk that she will die of cancer during that interval is 0.56% (Table 10.1) [4].

A patient's individual risk factors may multiply that basic risk of the general population. For example, the cumulative risk for a 35-year-old woman with atypical ductal hyperplasia to develop breast cancer by age 45 is calculated by multiplying the baseline risk (from Table 10.1) of 0.88 by the 9.8 relative risk imposed by the

atypical ductal hyperplasia. In this example, the risk of developing breast cancer in the next decade is 8.6, but the risk of dying of breast cancer is 1.3. Patients' perception of their risk may substantially affect their behavior and quality of life [5]. Many patients overestimate their risk, particularly for the pertinent intervals.

Risk factors demonstrated by multiple studies to be important are listed in Table 10.2. Although any family history of breast cancer on either the maternal or paternal side probably increases a patient's risk, the increase is small except in women with a first-degree relative (mother or sister) who had breast cancer. The risk is increased further if the first-degree relative had either premenopausal or bilateral breast cancer. Expressed as cumulative probabilities, the likelihood that a 30-year-old woman will develop breast cancer by age 70 is 8% if either her mother or sister had breast cancer, 18% if two first-degree relatives had breast cancer, and 28% if two first-degree relatives had bilateral breast cancer [6, 7].

Genetic breast cancers occur at a younger age, are more likely to be bilateral, and appear in multiple family members over three or more generations. Perhaps 10% of all breast cancers occur in high-risk families, and several familial breast cancer syndromes exist. They include the breast cancer–ovarian cancer syndrome, the Li-Fraumeni syndrome, and Cowden's disease. Investigation into the genetics of the breast cancer–ovarian

Table 10.1 Cumulative Probability of Eventually Developing and Dying of Breast Cancer, Based on 1985 Estimates of Overall Risk

Age Interval (yr)	Risk of Developing Any Breast Cancer (%)	Risk of Developing Invasive Breast Cancer (%)	Risk of Dying of Breast Cancer (%)
Birth–110	10.2	9.8	3.6
20–30	0.04	0.04	0.00
20–40	0.49	0.42	0.09
20–110	10.34	9.94	3.05
35–45	0.88	0.83	0.14
35–55	2.53	2.37	0.56
35–110	10.27	9.82	3.56
50–60	1.95	1.86	0.33
50–70	4.67	4.48	1.04
50–110	8.96	8.66	2.75
65–75	3.17	3.08	0.43
65–85	5.48	5.29	1.01
65–110	6.53	6.29	1.53

Source: Data from the Surveillance, Epidemiology, and End Results (SEER) Program, white females. In H Seidman, MH Mushinski, SK Gelb, et al., Probabilities of eventually developing or dying of cancer: United States, 1985. *CA Cancer J Clin* 35:36–56, 1985.

Table 10.2 Risk Factors for Developing Breast Cancer

Age
Hereditary factors
  Familial
  Genetic
Prior history of breast cancer
  In situ
  Invasive
Benign breast disease (atypical hyperplasia)
Endogenous endocrine factors
  Age at menarche
  Age at menopause
  Age at first pregnancy
Exogenous endocrine factors
  Postmenopausal estrogen replacement
  Oral contraceptives
Environmental factors
  Region of birth
  Diet
  Alcohol

Source: Reprinted with permission from IC Henderson, Breast cancer. In GP Murphy, W Lawrence Jr, RE Lenhard Jr (eds), *American Cancer Society Textbook of Clinical Oncology* (2nd ed). Atlanta: American Cancer Society, 1995.

cancer syndrome led to the identification and cloning of BRCA1 and BRCA2, two genes that show mutations in some 50% of familial breast cancers. Germline mutations in these cancers are associated with a 50% to 85% lifetime risk of breast cancer, ovarian cancer, or both. BRCA2 mutations also are associated with a substantial increase in the lifetime risk of male breast cancer. Currently, testing for mutations in these two genes is possible, and genetic counseling and testing programs exist in many health care facilities [8, 9].

After women have had breast cancer, the risk of a primary cancer developing in the opposite breast is 0.3% to 0.6% per year. The incidence of subsequent contralateral breast cancer is highest among young women with a long life expectancy and a good prognosis after treatment of breast cancer.

An association has been found between the risk of breast cancer and women's ages during their first full-term pregnancy: That is, the older women are during their first pregnancy, the greater their risk for breast cancer. Although the risk is low among women with multiple pregnancies as compared with women with no or few pregnancies, the age at first pregnancy appears to be the more important factor. Breast feeding has little or no effect on the incidence of breast cancer, independent of the relationship of this disease to parity. Early menarche or late menopause is a minor risk factor for breast cancer [10].

Certain benign, proliferative changes in biopsy specimens are associated with an increased risk for breast cancer [11]. In women with atypical hyperplasia (either ductal or lobular) and a positive family history, the lifetime risk of breast cancer is approximately 20% to 30% [12]. The risk for women with atypical ductal hyperplasia is highest in the first decade after diagnosis and appears to decrease in subsequent decades [13]. Similarly, lobular carcinoma in situ (lobular neoplasia) carries a 20% to 30% lifetime risk for the two breasts. Usually, close follow-up over many years is recommended for patients with these risk indicators.

The preliminary results of a randomized trial comparing tamoxifen to a placebo in patients considered at high risk for breast cancer (patients older than age 60 or ages 35–59 with predicted five-year risk of at least 1.66% or a history of lobular carcinoma in situ) suggested that the risk of breast cancer in these high-risk women can be decreased by some 50% with the administration of tamoxifen [14]. Similar reductions in the incidence of breast cancer were reported from several randomized trials with raloxifene (a selected estrogen receptor modulator) in the management of osteoporosis [15]. Confirmatory trials are ongoing. In addition,

increasing interest has been shown in the systematic evaluation of bilateral prophylactic mastectomies for patients at very high risk for developing breast cancer (e.g., those who have familial breast cancer syndromes). A recent retrospective report suggested up to a 90% reduction in the incidence of breast cancer in high-risk subjects who underwent prophylactic mastectomies [16].

Risk may be related also to the total calorie intake, low physical activity, and weight gain. As women from Oriental countries having a relatively low-fat diet have increased their fat intake or have immigrated to Western countries, their risk of breast cancer has increased. This increased incidence is seen in the immigrants themselves and is even greater in later generations. Although circumstantial evidence links dietary fat consumption and risk for breast cancer, studies have failed to show that dietary changes among mature women will lower their risk of the disease [17, 18]. Moderate alcohol intake (24 g or approximately one ounce of absolute alcohol per day, or approximately two drinks) has been reported to increase the relative risk of developing breast cancer [19].

Several lines of evidence suggest that estrogen plays a role in the genesis of breast cancer. Women whose ovaries have been removed before age 35 have a low risk of subsequent breast cancer. Results of studies correlating the use of oral contraceptives with breast cancer have been conflicting [20]. When the entire population at risk is considered, most studies indicate that oral contraceptives do not increase the risk of breast cancer. If any group is at an increased risk, it probably is young nulliparous women who took birth control pills with a high estrogen content for longer than four years.

The relationship between estrogen replacement therapy (ERT) and the risk for breast cancer remains controversial. Epidemiologic studies, including meta-analyses, still report inconsistent results regarding the use of ERT and increase in breast cancer risk [21]. However, current evidence strongly suggests that taking estrogens for a few years to decrease menopausal symptoms does not increase this risk [22, 23]. In contrast, risk appears to be increased in those women on long-term ERT (10–20 years). Probably the most useful stance is to acknowledge some degree of increased risk for breast cancer but to weigh this against the risk of not receiving long-term ERT. The advantages of ERT are decreased vertebral fractures, decreased coronary artery disease, and decreased hip fractures. The use of progestins with ERT decreases the risk of endometrial cancer but may increase the risk of breast cancer [24]. A conservative but prudent course of action might be to avoid the routine, prolonged use of ERT in those women who are found to be at increased risk for breast cancer.

NATURAL HISTORY AND BIOLOGICAL MAKEUP

Two of the most striking features of breast cancer biology are variable behavior in different patients and a relatively slow growth rate as compared with that of some other tumor types. With the use of conventional forms of treatment, the median survival of patients with metastatic breast cancer is greater than two years [25]. Some patients with metastatic breast cancer live from 10 to 20 years.

The average doubling time for breast cancers is estimated at 100 days. Depending on the size and consistency of the breast, the minimum tumor size that can be palpated is approximately 1 cm. A "sphere" of this size contains 1 to 10 billion cells, the result of 30 to 32 doublings of a single cell. Assuming that a preclinical breast mass grows logarithmically with a doubling time of 100 days, 10 years would be required for the mass to reach a point at which it could be diagnosed by palpation.

Although the point at which metastases occur is unknown, as are the factors that control metastases, the occurrence of metastases seems unlikely during the first 20 doublings. Some cancers may metastasize soon after that point, and the risk of metastasis probably increases steadily the longer the breast cancer grows before detection. Most patients with a diagnosis of breast cancer likely have had the disease for 5 to 10 years prior to diagnosis, and a substantial percentage will have well-established metastases for several years even if metastases cannot be detected by physical examination, roentgenograms, bone scans, computed tomography (CT) scan, or magnetic resonance imaging (MRI).

DETECTION AND EVALUATION

Monthly self-examinations, annual breast examinations by a health professional, and regular mammography are the mainstays of early detection. Of these examinations, mammography plays a central role as it offers the opportunity to find small, highly curable cancers and premalignant conditions.

The ability of mammography to detect cancers before they are apparent on physical examination is indisputable [26]. In recent years, the usefulness of mammography has been enhanced by technical advances that allow increased visualization of the breast parenchyma with less exposure to irradiation, improvements in film quality and processing, refined techniques for imaging, compression, focal size reduction, magnification, and the ancillary use of ultrasonography, better guidelines for the diagnosis of cancer, and greater availability of well-trained mammographers. With these newer techniques, the percentage of cancers detected at a size of less than 2 cm or in a noninvasive stage has increased dramatically [27]. Breast self-examination, which is appealing as a low-cost self-help technique, does not detect small breast cancers and is not a substitute for mammography.

Women should be encouraged to perform regular self-examinations and should be instructed in both proper technique and breast anatomy. Ultrasonography can be used to determine whether lesions seen on mammograms are cysts, but this modality is not a substitute for mammography and should not be employed as an independent screening test. Thermography, which is based on the increased blood flow and increased temperature of some tumors, is not a sensitive test and is not a substitute for mammography. Breast cancer can be detected by CT, but this modality is not superior to mammography, is much more costly, and involves a much greater radiation exposure. MRI avoids radiation exposure but is not more accurate than mammography and is more expensive, and indications for its use are not well established.

Approximately 15% of cancers are not apparent on mammograms; this finding is true of both small and large lesions. Therefore, negative mammograms never should dissuade physicians from performing a biopsy if a suspicious mass has been found on physical examination. The probability of a cancer being undetectable by physical examination or mammogram has been reported to be 3.7% [28].

However, the ability to detect breast cancers at a small size does not ensure that mortality from the disease will be reduced. Mammographic screening simply might detect lethal cancers at an earlier point (lead-time bias), cancers that are growing more slowly and are less likely to be lethal (length-time bias), or tumors that are of questionable malignancy (overdiagnosis bias). Furthermore, patients who participate in screening may be a healthier group than are patients who do not (self-selection bias).

Routine screening mammography appears to reduce breast cancer mortality by approximately 30% [29, 30]. No strategy has been shown to have a larger impact on breast cancer mortality. Because these estimates of benefit were derived from randomized clinical trials, lead-time bias and length-time bias do not confound the results.

Although they provide an overall estimate of the effect of screening, randomized trials leave several important issues unresolved, one of which is the effect of screening within different age groups [26]. Consistently beneficial effects of screening were found in women ages 50 to 69 [28, 29]. A recent meta-analysis of eight randomized trials in women aged 40 to 49 also indicated a benefit for staging in this younger age group [31].

Because breast cancer is substantially less common among younger women, the cost of screening will be proportionally greater relative to any benefit as compared to the cost of screening older patients. There is relatively little information about the value of mammography in women ages 70 or older or about when to stop annual mammograms. The ideal frequency for mammograms in younger women may be higher than that for older women [32], but that hypothesis has not been addressed in properly controlled trials. In the United States, one-year screening intervals generally have been recommended for patients older than 50 years. In other countries, two- and three-year frequencies have been used. A baseline mammogram obtained several years before the start of annual or biannual mammograms at age 40 no longer is recommended. Women who have a strong family history of premenopausal breast cancer should start annual screening earlier than age 40, probably in their midthirties.

The aforementioned screening trials have helped to determine the resources and expenses necessary for an effective screening program. The cost of screening is increased by a considerable number of negative biopsies. The probability that a suspicious but nonpalpable finding on mammography is cancerous is 20% to 30%; thus, screening will result in a large number of negative biopsies. The emotional stress of having a mammographic abnormality with even a very small risk of cancer compels some women to demand immediate biopsy rather than mammographic surveillance.

The high cost and frequency of malpractice suits resulting from perceived delays in the diagnosis of breast cancers places additional pressure on surgeons and diagnostic radiologists to perform biopsies for mammographic abnormalities associated with a low risk for cancer. The cost-benefit ratios for individual women (as viewed by such women and their health care providers) and for the entire population (when viewed as a public

Table 10.3 American Cancer Society Recommendations for Breast Cancer Screening

Age (yr)	Examination	Frequency
20–39	Breast self-examination	Monthly
	Clinical examination	Every 3 yr
≥ 40	Breast self-examination	Monthly
	Clinical examination	Yearly
	Mammography	Yearly

health policy or insurance issue) are different. For individual women, the cost includes lost time from work, discomfort of the procedure, and a small radiation exposure weighed against the advantages of early detection. Recommendations by the American Cancer Society for screening are shown in Table 10.3 and include a recommendation for annual mammography beginning at age 40 [33].

Signs and Symptoms

By far, the most common physical sign of cancer of the breast is a mass that almost always is painless. Any discrete mass should be investigated. Spontaneous, unilateral serous nipple discharge in a nonlactating breast may indicate chronic cystic mastopathy or an intraductal papilloma or, less commonly, cancer. Although a careful search for an occult primary cancer is obligatory if the nipple discharge is bloody, most patients with a bloody discharge have benign disease. Crusting, scaling, erosion, or changes that clinically appear to be persistent dermatitis of the nipple or areola must be subjected to biopsy to rule out Paget's disease. Nipple retraction of recent onset may indicate an underlying carcinoma. Signs of more advanced cancer include dimpling of the skin, changes in the contour of the breast, fixation of a mass to the pectoral fascia or chest wall, edema and erythema of the skin, and axillary adenopathy. If women have any symptoms that suggest metastatic disease, diagnostic workup for those symptoms should be performed.

Physical Examination

Affected patients are examined both supine and seated. While seated, such women are asked to press their hands against the hips to contract the pectoral muscles and then to raise their arms over the head. These maneuvers help to reveal nipple retraction, asymmetry, and areas of skin dimpling. The cervical, supraclavicular, axillary, and infraclavicular lymph nodes are palpated. The examiner palpates the breast by pressing the breast tissue gently against the chest wall or, if the breast is pendulous, against the examiner's hand. While the patient is supine, the ipsilateral arm is raised overhead to flatten the breast parenchyma against the chest wall. The nipple is examined for excoriation and secretions. After the examination is completed, the physician may take the opportunity to review breast self-examination with the patient.

Evaluation of a Palpable Breast Mass

A lesion suspected to be a cyst on physical examination is evaluated best by needle aspiration. If a cyst contains bloody fluid, does not disappear after aspiration of the contents, or recurs after one or more aspirations, biopsy is in order. Fine-needle aspiration of solid masses with cytologic examination of retrieved cells and tissue is an expeditious method of identifying cancer. For suitably large masses, core needle biopsy in the office setting can be an effective way to prove malignancy. A negative pathology report for a sample obtained by using a needle biopsy technique does not prove that the lesion is benign, and an open biopsy should be performed in suspicious cases.

As an outpatient procedure, biopsy of the breast under local anesthesia has virtually no disadvantages. This approach also gives patients with biopsy-proved breast cancer the time to consider therapeutic options. The margins of all excisional biopsies should be defined. Portions of the tissue should be submitted for biochemical or genetic studies such as hormone receptor and *HER2/neu* assays only after a histologic diagnosis of cancer has been made. Especially for small specimens, it is preferable to use immunohistochemical receptor and *HER2/neu* assays that can be performed on sections of the routinely processed tissue. Because of the 4% incidence of occult synchronous cancer in the breast not undergoing biopsy and a 1.5% incidence of occult cancer elsewhere within the breast undergoing biopsy, bilateral mammography is indicated prior to most biopsies (except in women younger than age 30). As stated, a negative result on mammography does not change the requirements for biopsy of a palpable mass. In young women whose dense breast tissue renders examination of the breast difficult, ultrasonography can help with the decision between an irregularity in the surface of the breast tissue and a discrete mass that requires biopsy.

Evaluation of Nonpalpable Mammographic Abnormalities

Screening mammography can detect many small, nonpalpable lesions. Often, mammographic masses and microcalcifications can be subjected to biopsy by a stereotactic core biopsy technique that eliminates the need for an open incision. Discordance between the pathologic results of core biopsy and the mammographic findings must be resolved by open biopsy. Insertion of a fine wire under mammographic control allows precise location densities or clusters of microcalcifications for surgical excision. Although more complicated than biopsy of a palpable mass, wire localization facilitates resection of small lesions with minimal removal of breast tissue and minimal cosmetic deformity. This technique detects more than 90% of target lesions, and a mammogram of the resected specimen will verify that the abnormality has been removed.

The indications for biopsy of nonpalpable mammographic abnormalities are evolving. Although some controversy surrounds the guidelines for determining which lesions should be followed up by serial mammography and which should be subjected to biopsy immediately, the objective should be to minimize the number of biopsies performed on benign lesions while detecting cancers as early as possible.

Screening for Metastatic Disease

Prior to treatment of the primary breast tumor or regional lymph nodes, the possibility of systemic disease should be excluded. Cancer of the breast may spread to any organ of the body, the most common sites being lungs, pleura, bones, and liver. The yield from bone scans in early-stage disease is low, and the false-positive rate is high [34]. For patients with clinical stage III or stage IV disease or with stage II cancer with evidence of lymph node metastases, a bone scan should be obtained; it may reveal metastases weeks to months before lytic lesions can be seen on plain radiographs.

Routine laboratory studies should include chest radiographs and liver function tests. If the liver is not enlarged and liver function is within normal limits, the probability of detecting hepatic metastases by CT or liver scan is low; thus, such scans should not be obtained. Other studies should be selected on the basis of symptoms or findings on physical examination. When patients have clinical stage III or stage IV cancer, an elevated alkaline phosphatase level, or positive results on bone scan, their serum calcium and phosphorus levels

Table 10.4   TNM Staging for Breast Cancer

Classification	Definition
Primary tumor (T)	
TX	Primary tumor cannot be assessed
T0	No evidence of primary tumor
Tis	Carcinoma in situ: intraductal carcinoma, lobular carcinoma in situ, or Paget's disease of the nipple with no tumor
T1	Tumor ≤ 2 cm in greatest dimension
T1mic	Microinvasion ≤ 0.1 cm in greatest dimension
T1a	Tumor > 0.1 but < 0.5 cm in greatest dimension
T1b	Tumor > 0.5 but < 1.0 cm in greatest dimension
T1c	Tumor > 1 cm but < 2 cm in greatest dimension
T2	Tumor > 2 cm but < 5 cm in greatest dimension
T3	Tumor > 5 cm in greatest dimension
T4	Tumor of any size with direct extension to (a) chest wall or (b) skin, only as described below
T4a	Extension to chest wall
T4b	Edema (including peau d'orange) or ulceration of the skin of the breast or satellite skin nodules confined to the same breast
T4c	Both T4a and T4b
T4d	Inflammatory carcinoma
Regional lymph nodes (N)	
NX	Regional lymph nodes cannot be assessed (e.g., previously removed)
N0	No regional lymph node metastasis
N1	Metastasis to movable ipsilateral axillary lymph node(s)
N2	Metastasis to ipsilateral axillary lymph node(s) fixed to one another or to other structures
N3	Metastasis to ipsilateral internal mammary lymph node(s)
Pathologic classification (pN)	
pNX	Regional lymph nodes cannot be assessed (e.g., previously removed, or not removed for pathologic study)
pN0	No regional lymph node metastasis
pN1	Metastasis to movable ipsilateral axillary lymph node(s)
pN1a	Only micrometastasis (none > 0.2 cm)
pN1b	Metastasis to lymph node(s), any > 0.2 cm
pN1bi	Metastasis in 1 to 3 lymph nodes, any > 0.2 cm and all < 2 cm in greatest dimension
pN1bii	Metastasis to 4 or more lymph nodes, any > 0.2 cm and all < 2 cm in greatest dimension
pN1biii	Extension of tumor beyond the capsule of a lymph node metastasis < 2 cm in greatest dimension
pN1biv	Metastasis to a lymph node ≥ 2 cm in greatest dimension
pN2	Metastasis to ipsilateral axillary lymph nodes that are fixed to one another or to other structures
pN3	Metastasis to ipsilateral internal mammary lymph node(s)
Distant metastases (M)	
MX	Distant metastasis cannot be assessed
M0	No distant metastasis
M1	Distant metastasis (including metastasis to ipsilateral supraclavicular lymph node[s])

Note: Paget's disease associated with a tumor is classified according to the size of the tumor.
Source: Used with permission of the American Joint Committee on Cancer (AJCC), Chicago, Illinois. Adapted from ID Fleming, JS Cooper, DE Henson, et al. (eds), *AJCC Cancer Staging Manual* (5th ed). Philadelphia: Lippincott-Raven, 1997:171–180.

should be measured, and a more comprehensive metastatic survey should be initiated.

STAGING

Staging is performed to determine the prognosis, to direct therapies that might be applied on the basis of prognostic categories, and for uniformity of reporting results. The staging system of the American Joint Committee on Cancer Staging and End Results Reporting uses the TNM (*t*umor, *n*ode, *m*etastasis) classification, in which the primary tumor is evaluated on the basis of size and involvement of the skin or underlying structures (Tables 10.4, 10.5). Both physical examination and mammography are used for these determinations. Regional lymph nodes (axillary, supraclavicular, and infraclavicular) are classified according to the likelihood

Table 10.5   AJCC Stage Grouping for Breast Cancer

Stage	T	N	M
Stage 0	Tis	N0	M0
Stage I	T1[a]	N0	M0
Stage IIA	T0	N1	M0
	T1[a]	N1[b]	M0
	T2	N0	M0
Stage IIB	T2	N1	M0
	T3	N0	M0
Stage IIIA	T0	N2	M0
	T1[a]	N2	M0
	T2	N2	M0
	T3	N1	M0
	T3	N2	M0
Stage IIIB	T4	Any N	M0
	Any T	N3	M0
Stage IV	Any T	Any N	M1

[a]T1 includes T1mic.
[b]The prognosis of patients with N1a is similar to that of patients with pN0.
Note: Chest wall includes ribs, intercostal muscles, and serratus anterior muscle but not pectoral muscle.
Source: Used with permission of the American Joint Committee on Cancer (AJCC), Chicago, Illinois. Reprinted from ID Fleming, JS Cooper, DE Henson, et al. (eds), *AJCC Cancer Staging Manual* (5th ed). Philadelphia: Lippincott-Raven, 1997:171–180.

that they contain metastases. Clinical staging is supplemented by the results of the pathologic examination of the resected primary tumor and lymph nodes to arrive at the pathologic stage. Pathologic staging of lymph nodes is recommended for most patients, because it is more reliable than is the clinical assessment of lymph nodes, for which the error rate can be 30% to 40%.

In patients with breast cancer, lymph node status is the most precise prognostic information that can be obtained and is helpful in deciding what adjuvant systemic therapy would be appropriate (see later discussion). Complete axillary node dissection is not needed to distinguish "node-positive" from "node-negative" patients. In patients who have positive nodes, one large study has concluded that at least 10 axillary lymph nodes should be evaluated to separate those in a low-risk group (i.e., fewer than four positive nodes) from those in a high-risk group (i.e., four or more positive nodes) [35]. The incidence of arm edema or other complications is related to the extent of the axillary surgery. When the dissection is limited to nodal tissue lateral to the pectoralis minor muscle, the risk of such complications is low. Sentinel node biopsy (see later discussion) is an attempt to establish the status of the axillary lymph nodes while limiting the risk of arm edema.

PROGNOSIS

Nodal Involvement and Tumor Size

Despite the widespread search for better prognostic factors, no single factor is as predictive as the number of involved lymph nodes or tumor size. The 10-year survival rate in patients without histologically involved lymph nodes is approximately 65% to 70%. Each involved node worsens a patient's prognosis. Patients with larger tumor sizes are more likely to have histologically involved nodes but, within any nodal category, tumor size is an independent prognostic factor.

Patients with noninvasive carcinoma of the breast—regardless of type or size—have an excellent prognosis (> 97% of patients alive and free of disease 10 or more years after diagnosis). Of patients with node-negative invasive cancer, 70% to 80% are alive and free of disease 10 years after completing primary therapy; 64% to 79% remain disease-free after 20 years of follow-up. In most studies of disease at stages I to IIIA, axillary lymph node involvement, as determined by histopathology, is the single most important prognostic factor. More than 50% of node-positive patients treated with modern combined-modality therapy die within 10 years. The 10-year disease-free survival rate ranges between 40% and 65% for those with one to three positive nodes and between 20% and 42% for those with 10 or more positive nodes.

Patients with stage IIIB disease (peau d'orange, inflammatory breast cancer, skin nodules, ulceration, or fixation to the chest wall) have a poor prognosis, with less than 30% remaining disease-free 10 or more years after diagnosis. Generally, prognosis for patients with grossly detectable distant metastatic disease is fairly poor (median survival, 2–3 years). Fewer than 20% of such patients remain alive five or more years after the appearance of distant metastases. However, 2% to 3% of these patients remain in an unmaintained complete remission (i.e., remission in the absence of chemotherapy) more than 10 years after the development of distant spread.

Other Prognostic Factors

Levels of estrogen receptor (ER) and progesterone receptor proteins should be determined for all primary tumor tissue obtained. These levels not only help to predict response to hormonal manipulation in metastatic disease but may have prognostic implications for the primary tumor. Hormone receptor assays can be performed by immunohistochemical techniques on frozen or fixed tissue. ER protein levels increase with age and are markedly higher among postmenopausal women.

Previous staging systems were based on the assumption that stage was related to the length of time that the cancer had been growing prior to diagnosis. For this reason, lower stage numbers were termed *early*. However, the great variability in survival among patients in each stage suggests that intrinsic biological factors are at least as important as the duration of the tumor's growth. For example, the tumor's histologic differentiation (i.e., the degree to which it forms glands and the extent to which any individual cells have cytoplasmic and nuclear characteristics similar to those of normal breast cells) reflects the tumor's invasive and metastatic potential. Undifferentiated tumors are more likely to recur than are well-differentiated tumors, even when they are small and node-negative. Commonly, the Scarf-Bloom-Richardson system or a modification is used [36]. The major drawback of histologic grading is its lack of reproducibility from one pathologist to another.

Measures of increased DNA synthetic activity tend to be associated with a worse prognosis. These measures include the thymidine-labeling index; S-phase fraction as determined by flow cytometry; and increased Ki-67 as measured by immunocytochemistry. However, no generally accepted values define a "good prognostic" or a "bad prognostic" tumor, and the clinical utility of these assays remains uncertain.

In one or more studies, a large number of factors have been reported to have prognostic value [37]. These factors include cathepsin D; *p53; HER2/neu* (erb-B2); epidermal growth factor receptor; transforming growth factor–alpha; heat-shock proteins; proliferating cell nuclear antigen; pS2; haptoglobin-related protein; urokinase plasminogen activator; nm23; tissue ferritin concentrations; laminin receptor expression; cyclic adenosine monophosphate–binding protein; and the monoclonal antibody NCRC11. Of these factors, HER2/neu perhaps has been the most investigated and reproducible prognostic factor. Patients with tumors overexpressing HER2/neu have a higher risk of recurrence and death. Additionally, growing evidence suggests that HER2/neu-overexpressing tumors are relatively resistant to the chemotherapy regimen of cyclophosphamide, methotrexate, and 5-fluorouracil (CMF) and are more sensitive to anthracyclines, especially dose-intensive anthracycline-containing regimens. The availability of a therapeutic monoclonal antibody against HER2/neu increases the impetus to measure that factor [38, 39].

Thus far, none of the factors described in this section except the ERs and the progesterone receptors (and possibly HER2/neu) have been shown reproducibly to predict patients' response to therapy. Therefore, the primary use of these prognostic factors is to define a group of patients whose prognosis is so good after local treatment, without adjuvant systemic therapy, that any degree of toxicity from systemic therapy is unacceptable. Many oncologists would select a prognosis of a 10-year recurrence-free survival of more than 90% as the cutoff point above which systemic therapy is not indicated. None of these factors (singly or in combination) can be used to substitute for measurement of tumor size and the number of histologically involved lymph nodes in making a prognosis.

PATHOLOGIC FEATURES

The majority of invasive breast cancers are infiltrating ductal carcinomas. Infiltrating lobular carcinomas account for approximately 10% of breast cancers and have a prognosis similar to that of the infiltrating ductal type. Tubular, medullary, papillary, and colloid or mucinous carcinomas are uncommon but all have a prognosis better than that of infiltrating ductal or infiltrating lobular carcinomas. The phyllodes tumor (cystosarcoma phyllodes) is a rare, generally benign tumor composed of both epithelial and stromal elements. Phyllodes tumors may be bulky, rarely metastasize, do not spread to lymph nodes, and usually are treated by wide excision or simple mastectomy.

Breast biopsy specimens must be evaluated carefully, particularly now that breast-conserving surgery is selected increasingly as an alternative to mastectomy. Specimens should be processed so that their margins can be identified when visualized under the microscope. Coating specimens with India ink is a technique commonly used for identifying margins. Pathologists should record the dimensions of excised specimens, the size of the tumor, and its gross and microscopical relationships to the specific margins. Such other factors as the amount of associated ductal carcinoma in situ, lymphatic invasion, tumor grade, and histologic type (ductal, lobular, tubular, mucinous, medullary, inflammatory, etc.) may be important in assessing prognosis and selecting treatment.

The two types of carcinoma in situ—lobular and ductal—differ in a number of ways. In both types, malignant-appearing cells are seen under the microscope, but the cells are not invading outside of the lobular or ductal lumen.

Lobular Carcinoma In Situ

Lobular carcinoma in situ (LCIS) never forms a palpable mass, rarely is the cause of an abnormality on a mammogram, and usually is found accidentally on biopsy of some other lesion. LCIS occurs diffusely throughout both breasts and is associated with approximately a 10% to 15% risk of invasive cancer in each breast [40]. The risk of invasive cancer for the breast contralateral to that undergoing biopsy is the same as for the breast with biopsy-proved LCIS. LCIS is viewed as a risk factor for subsequent breast cancer and is related more closely to atypical hyperplasia than to ductal carcinoma in situ (DCIS). Patients with LCIS are given one of two options: observation with careful follow-up or bilateral mastectomies. Most women select observation.

Ductal Carcinoma In Situ

DCIS differs from LCIS in that it may form a mass, although most often today it is diagnosed by biopsy for microcalcifications seen on mammography. Usually, DCIS is unilateral and frequently is found in only one quadrant of one breast. The risk for subsequent cancer is primarily in the quadrant that has undergone biopsy if the DCIS is not eradicated adequately. The natural history of DCIS is not well understood, and it remains unclear how often such lesions progress to invasive cancers. On the basis of nuclear differentiation and the presence or absence of necrosis, several different systems have been devised to divide DCIS into three groups: high-, intermediate-, and low-grade. These systems recognize that different DCIS lesions behave with different potential for microinvasion and for development of microvessel density and have different proliferative rates. Ultimately, a comprehensive system that includes both molecular markers of biological behavior and histologic features likely will provide a meaningful basis for diagnosis and treatment. At the present time, no single system is recognized universally, but the risk for recurrence is considerably lower with low-grade lesions than with high-grade lesions, regardless of whether postoperative irradiation is used.

In the majority of cases, the diagnosis of DCIS can be established readily. Problems arise, however, in differentiating DCIS from lesions at both ends of the spectrum. On the benign end, distinguishing DCIS from atypical ductal hyperplasia can be difficult; on the opposite end, distinguishing some cases of DCIS from DCIS with focal stromal invasion can be difficult. In some instances, DCIS can resemble LCIS.

Mastectomy, long considered the standard treatment for DCIS, is associated with local tumor control and survival rates approaching 100% but is likely to represent overtreatment for many patients. DCIS appears to be a disease of one ductal system. Frequently, it is multifocal within a small area close to the index lesion and rarely is multicentric or present in different parts of the breast distinct and at a distant from the index focus. Holland et al. [41] showed that, in most cases, the disease was confined to one quadrant. These observations provided a rationale for breast-conserving treatment. Eight-year results from a randomized National Surgical Adjuvant Breast and Bowel Project trial (NSABBP-17) showed that local recurrences had been reduced by 55% and that invasive cancers have been reduced by 71% for patients receiving radiotherapy and wide excision as compared with wide excision alone [42].

A reasonable assumption is that low-grade DCIS identified by small areas of microcalcifications and excised with widely negative margins should be treated adequately without radiotherapy. However, selection criteria still are evolving. High-quality mammograms and careful margin assessment are essential to achieve low recurrence rates, regardless of whether the treatment includes radiotherapy. Axillary node dissection is not a standard of care at this time. For patients with extensive high-grade DCIS in which the risk of microinvasion or frank invasion is high, lower axillary dissection may be recommended. Typically, axillary dissection is not recommended for patients with limited DCIS treated with a breast-conserving approach because of the extremely low probability of nodal metastases.

A large randomized trial (NSABBP-24) demonstrated that the addition of tamoxifen to lumpectomy or lumpectomy and radiotherapy further reduced the risk of invasive and noninvasive local recurrences and of the incidence of contralateral breast cancers [43].

THERAPY FOR INVASIVE BREAST CANCER
Conservative Surgery

The major treatment options for patients with early breast cancer are total mastectomy or conservative resection of the tumor followed by radiotherapy. Multiple randomized trials have demonstrated that the 10- to 20-year survival of patients treated with lumpectomy and irradiation is equivalent to that achieved with mastectomy [44]. For example, more than 1,800 women were randomized in an NSABBP trial (NSABBP-06) [45] of treatment with total mastectomy, lumpectomy, or lumpectomy plus radiotherapy. All three groups had node dissection as well. At the end of eight years, significant differences were noted in local failure rates and, to a lesser extent, in distant failure rates, but no difference was seen in overall survival. Because of these results, either a modified radical mastectomy or partial mastectomy and radiotherapy currently is considered optimal local treatment for patients with stage I or stage II breast cancer.

The term *conservative surgery* encompasses several procedures with the shared objective of removing the tumor while preserving enough normal breast tissue for a satisfactory cosmetic result. Such procedures include lumpectomy, partial mastectomy, excisional biopsy, quadrantectomy, and wide local excision, which differ slightly from one another in terms of the amount of tissue removed. The only advantage of conservative surgery and radiotherapy over mastectomy is cosmetic, and the cosmetic results depend, in large part, on the amount of breast tissue that remains postoperatively. Attempts to excise multicentric tumors or tumors that cover large areas of the breast are likely to cause such a large cosmetic defect that complete excision may approach the defect of a mastectomy; therefore, they are treated by mastectomy. Often, tumors characterized by multiple suspicious clusters of microcalcifications scattered throughout the breast are treated preferentially by mastectomy. The extent of local excision should be determined only after careful evaluation and consultation among pathologists, irradiation oncologists, radiologists and mammographers, and surgeons. To confirm adequate removal of a tumor, pathologists must evaluate resected specimens carefully.

Although conservative surgery without radiotherapy has the cosmetic advantages of limited resection of the breast while avoiding the inconvenience and side effects of radiotherapy, this approach may have a local failure rate of more than 30%. The extent to which this high local failure rate might jeopardize survival is unknown but obviously is a matter of concern. As in the case of DCIS, satisfactory, widely accepted selection criteria for avoiding radiotherapy are not available.

Complications after well-executed surgery or radiotherapy are uncommon and, for the most part, involve limitations of shoulder motion, arm edema, or stiffness and pain in the irradiated breast or chest wall affected by surgery. Fatigue and other side effects of radiotherapy may persist for months after treatment, particularly in the elderly.

Stage III breast cancer is advanced locally without apparent distant metastases. The clinical course of patients with stage III cancer indicates that most already have occult metastatic disease and suggests the need for early or initial treatment with systemic chemotherapy. Usually, preoperative or "neoadjuvant" chemotherapy diminishes the local and regional tumor burden, rendering the cancer more amenable to treatment with mastectomy or local excision and radiotherapy. Because patients with stage III cancer generally have a poor prognosis, some institutions favor breast-conserving surgery using chemotherapy and radiotherapy for this group.

The deformity created by mastectomy can be ameliorated by reconstruction with a saline-filled implant or by moving tissue from the back or abdomen (myocutaneous flap). Because of concern about their possible association with the development of connective tissue disorders, silicone-filled implants currently are available to only select women through clinical studies being conducted by the US Food and Drug Administration. Although a large, population-based cohort study failed to show an association between connective tissue disorders and silicone breast implants [46], manufacture of this medically useful product is limited because of the potential expense related to product liability.

The saline-filled implant creates on the chest wall a mound that provides a relatively natural appearance and increases the choice of clothing that can be worn. The myocutaneous flap (a composite of skin, fat, and muscle with its own blood supply) provides a better facsimile of a breast but requires a longer, more complicated operation than does insertion of an implant. Either type of reconstruction can be carried out simultaneously with the mastectomy or at a later date.

Regardless of the treatment of a diseased breast—total mastectomy or partial mastectomy and radiotherapy—sampling of axillary nodes is important to provide tissue for pathologic staging. Dissection of axillary lymph nodes probably contributes little to survival, although it limits the risk of tumor recurrence in the axilla. As discussed, the analysis of axillary lymph nodes is an important prognostic determinant. Many patients who have axillary node dissections experience numbness under the arm and in the skin of the posterior upper arm in the distribution of the intercostal brachial nerve. A small number of patients (5% or fewer) have some degree of swelling of the arm from lymphedema. To minimize further the unpleasant side effects of axillary dissection, a recently devised procedure (sentinel node biopsy) limits nodal sampling to the primary node or nodes draining the tumor [47]. In this procedure, blue dye or a radioisotope (or both) injected into the tumor bed are traced into the axilla to the "sentinel" node, which is identified by its blue color or radioactivity. False-negative rates of nearly 5% to 10% have been reported [48]. Indications for the procedure and patient selection criteria are not well established.

The use of postmastectomy radiotherapy (PMRT) has been controversial. Although PMRT clearly is beneficial for locoregional disease control, recent randomized trials from Denmark and British Columbia indicate a survival benefit also for patients who received PMRT [49, 50]. A consensus summary statement from the American Society of Therapeutic Radiology and Oncology (ASTRO) has recommended the use of radiotherapy for patients with four or more positive nodes. For patients with one to three positive nodes, ASTRO recommended consideration of radiotherapy and a large randomized clinical trial.

Adjuvant Therapy

Patients die of breast cancer because of distant metastases implanted months to years before a primary lesion is diagnosed and treated with surgery or radiotherapy. Mortality can be decreased only if breast cancer is diagnosed before metastases have formed or if metastatic deposits throughout the body can be reached using a systemic therapy. Adjuvant systemic therapy with either chemotherapy or tamoxifen can delay recurrence in many patients and can prolong survival in some. Although the possibility exists for some patients to be cured by systemic therapy, this specific group of patients who can be reliably predicted to benefit from this modality of treatment has not yet been identified.

The relative benefit of such therapies is substantially different in premenopausal women with breast cancer (younger than age 50) and those with postmenopausal breast cancer, but the magnitude of benefit depends on patients' initial age and prognosis. Overall, in women younger than age 50, adjuvant chemotherapy appears to reduce 10-year mortality by nearly 27% of their initial risk. For example, women with a 50% risk of dying without adjuvant chemotherapy experience an approximate 13.5% reduction in mortality (50% × 0.27 = 13.5%). A woman with a 10% risk of death at 10 years can expect her risk to drop to less than 8% (10% × 0.27 = 2.7%; 10% - 2.7% = 7.3%). Obviously, short-term risks (nausea, vomiting, alopecia, anemia) are the

same for all patients, assuming use of the same chemotherapeutic regimen. Thus, recommendations for therapy must include discussions of prognosis, relative benefit, and risk of toxicity.

The relative benefits of adjuvant chemotherapy are smaller in older women. However, this difference in the effect of adjuvant chemotherapy between older and younger women is quantitative, not qualitative. Women at ages 50 to 59 years will have a 14% reduction in mortality, whereas those aged 60 to 69 will have an 8% reduction; both still are statistically significant improvements in outcome. Life will be prolonged for more than four years for younger women and by one to three years for those older than age 50. With regard to chemotherapy, combinations of drugs are more effective than are single agents. Relatively short courses of therapy (4–6 months) appear to be as effective as courses lasting 12 to 24 months.

These results were derived from clinical trials that used combined CMF or variations thereof. More recent regimens have included anthracyclines, either doxorubicin or epirubicin. The most recent meta-analysis of randomized trials indicated that anthracycline-containing regimens yielded a further 11% proportional reduction in mortality as compared to CMF-type regimens [51]. Preliminary results of the first large randomized clinical trial that added paclitaxel sequentially to the doxorubicin-cyclophosphamide combination suggested that this addition resulted in another 22% proportional reduction in mortality as compared to results of doxorubicin-cyclophosphamide alone [52].

Doses of standard chemotherapy should not be reduced. For patients who become neutropenic and have documented infections or febrile episodes requiring antibiotics, the use of granulocyte colony-stimulating factor (G-CSF) decreases the time required for white blood cell recovery and the risk of infection. However, G-CSF should be reserved for these situations; it should not be used routinely in all patients receiving chemotherapy.

Results from pilot trials suggested that very high-dose chemotherapy requiring hematopoietic stem cell support (autologous bone marrow transplantation or peripheral blood progenitor cell reinfusion) might be more advantageous than standard-dose therapy. However, this approach is associated with very high morbidity and with mortality as high as 5%. Randomized trials assessing the relative efficacy of high-dose chemotherapy programs, as compared to standard-dose chemotherapy, have failed to demonstrate a clear superiority for high-dose chemotherapy for treatment of advanced disease or for adjuvant therapy [53–57]. The largest trial of high-dose adjuvant therapy showed an increase in relapse-free and overall survival in the high-dose group but showed a commensurate increase in treatment-related mortality, resulting in equivalent survival [56]. Until compelling data are generated to justify the increased morbidity, mortality, and expense, these treatments should be offered only in the context of hypothesis-testing trials.

Adjuvant tamoxifen will decrease the annual rate of death by perhaps 15%, on the basis of the combined strengths of all randomized clinical trials with tamoxifen. This effect is independent of dose, age, or initial risk but is a function of hormone receptor status and duration of tamoxifen therapy. The reduction in odds of death for women who received five years of adjuvant tamoxifen is 22%, more than twice the reduction observed after only one year. Tamoxifen administered for longer than five years is not more effective than five years of therapy [58]. The benefit from adjuvant tamoxifen is 3- to 10-fold greater for patients with hormone receptor–positive breast cancer as compared with those with hormone receptor–poor tumors. The increase in duration of life for patients treated with five years of tamoxifen is approximately two to three years. The relative benefits of five years of adjuvant tamoxifen in women with ER–positive tumors are similar to those of adjuvant chemotherapy in younger women. The addition of tamoxifen to chemotherapy produces supplemental benefits in women with ER–positive tumors. Similarly, the addition of chemotherapy to tamoxifen results in supplemental benefits as compared to tamoxifen alone. Therefore, recommendations about adjuvant systemic therapy must be based on prognosis, relative benefit, and risk of toxicity.

Approximately 20% to 40% of patients treated with tamoxifen will experience postmenopausal symptoms, including hot flashes, vaginal dryness, sexual dysfunction, and emotional changes. Importantly, reports have demonstrated that treatment with tamoxifen increases the risk for endometrial cancer by two to threefold. The absolute risk of endometrial cancer is low in women who do not receive tamoxifen and, therefore, so is the absolute risk in those receiving tamoxifen. Nonetheless, women should be counseled to report any vaginal bleeding or pelvic symptoms immediately, and they should be evaluated annually with pelvic examinations and Papanicolaou smears.

Short-term toxic effects of chemotherapy include myelosuppression, thrombocytopenia, alopecia, nausea, vomiting, and general fatigue. Alkylating agent–containing regimens also produce permanent amenorrhea in a high proportion of premenopausal women,

especially those older than 40 years. The effects of premature menopause include earlier loss of bone density and the earlier onset of coronary artery disease. The full potential of these agents (especially the alkylating agents) to induce subsequent tumors is still unknown. L-Phenylalanine mustard (melphalan) is associated with an 11-fold increase in the incidence of acute leukemia, whereas cyclophosphamide appears to be less carcinogenic. With the introduction of dose-intensive, doxorubicin-containing regimens into adjuvant trials, a new type of acute leukemia recently was described [59]. These leukemias appear early (within the first 2–3 years after therapy), are mostly of the M-4, M-5 type in the French-American-British classification, and are similar to other leukemias associated with the use of topoisomerase II inhibitors.

In summary, the benefits of adjuvant systemic therapy are substantial. However, to improve on the results of existing treatments, patients are encouraged to participate in ongoing trials designed to test novel drugs and hypotheses, such as dose-intensive therapies. All premenopausal women with node-positive breast cancer should receive some form of adjuvant chemotherapy. Currently, the accepted standard regimens consist of four cycles of doxorubicin (Adriamycin) and cyclophosphamide (AC), or six cycles of 5-fluorouracil, Adriamycin, and cyclophosphamide (FAC), or six months of adjuvant CMF. Postmenopausal women with node-positive breast cancer should also be advised to receive combination chemotherapy with similar regimens in the absence of substantial comorbid conditions that would preclude their administration. Many oncologists would add four cycles of single-agent paclitaxel to the adjuvant therapy of patients with high-risk breast cancer.

All patients with hormone receptor–positive breast cancer, regardless of menopausal or nodal status, should receive adjuvant tamoxifen for five years. Patients with node-negative, hormone receptor–negative breast cancer at a risk high enough to warrant adjuvant systemic therapy should receive combination chemotherapy. The decision to use adjuvant chemotherapy for node-negative, hormone receptor–positive patients should be individualized on the basis of the cancer team's judgment and the wishes of the patient, who should be well informed about the potential risks and benefits.

FOLLOW-UP

The major purposes of routine follow-up evaluation of breast cancer patients are to detect a second primary cancer as early as possible, to detect recurrences in a conservatively treated diseased breast, and to evaluate symptoms for possible metastatic disease. These goals can be achieved by mammography, careful breast examination on each follow-up visit, and breast self-examination. Among the important features of the follow-up examination are a recorded history and a physical examination to detect local and regional recurrent disease or common sites of metastases (e.g., the lung, liver, lymph nodes, bone, and skin). Routine bone, liver, or CT scans are not recommended, because no evidence substantiates that treatment of asymptomatic patients with metastatic disease will provide any survival advantage as compared with treatment begun after symptoms appear [60, 61]. Although the interval for follow-up examinations depends on the prognosis, most patients are seen every three to six months for the first few years and are seen annually thereafter. The follow-up evaluation also should include annual screening for colon, ovarian, and cervical cancers and careful attention to any signs or symptoms of endometrial cancer for women who are receiving or have taken tamoxifen.

TREATMENT OF RECURRENT AND METASTATIC DISEASE

Usually, recurrence within a breast treated with local excision and primary radiotherapy is a local phenomenon and is not necessarily indicative of metastatic disease. Such recurrences are curable by mastectomy or, occasionally, by wide reexcision. Five-year survival rates after surgical treatment of a local recurrence within the breast range from 50% to 75%. Local recurrence after mastectomy, however, is a sign of systemic metastases; overt distant metastases occur in more than 90% of patients within five years of a local recurrence.

Metastatic cancer of the breast is sensitive to a variety of palliative therapies. Biopsy may be required to document the recurrence (especially in the case of a solitary metastasis) and to measure hormone receptor protein levels. Also, an accurate restaging of the extent of metastases to various organ sites is essential, because the treatment strategy and prognosis depend on the extent and location of disease in addition to patients' menopausal status and the disease-free interval.

Endocrine and cytotoxic agents, local and systemic radiotherapy, bisphosphonates, and anti–growth factor therapy, used individually or in combination, variously have been effective in metastatic breast cancer in reducing the size of the tumor and in minimizing symptoms. For patients with a low risk of rapid progression or cata-

strophic complications, a trial of hormonal therapy should be used first. Antiestrogens and selective aromatase inhibitors should be first- and second-choice therapy for postmenopausal patients, with progestins, high-dose estrogens, or androgens reserved for later interventions. Premenopausal women should be treated first with antiestrogens and surgical or medical ovarian suppression (or ablation). Progestins, aromatase inhibitors, and androgens are used for third- and fourth-line therapies. Hormone ablation by adrenalectomy or hypophysectomy is no longer used to treat breast cancer. New agents, such as luteinizing hormone–releasing hormone analogs eventually may replace oophorectomy as well. Often, hormone therapy can provide high-quality palliation for many months without causing incapacitating side effects. Survival may be prolonged by some hormonal interventions, especially the aromatase inhibitors.

Because of the variable response to treatment and prolonged time to response, hormone therapy should not be used in patients with rapidly progressing lymphangitic spread in the lungs or with extensive liver metastases. Approximately 60% of women with tumors positive for ER protein will respond to hormone therapy either with marked reductions in tumor volume (partial or complete response) or with protracted periods of stability. The median survival of patients who respond to primary hormonal approaches is almost four years after treatment. Tamoxifen produces a response in perhaps one-third of all patients with metastatic disease and two-thirds of those with ER protein activity. This drug is effective in both premenopausal and postmenopausal women.

Chemotherapy is indicated as the initial intervention for patients with hormone receptor–negative tumors, for patients with extensive visceral disease, and as the next intervention for patients with hormone receptor–positive tumors that do not respond to sequential hormone therapy. Combination chemotherapy yields a higher response rate and a more extended response than does therapy using a single agent. The overall response rate for chemotherapy is 50% to 60%, but only in 15% to 20% of patients does all evidence of the disease disappear (complete remission). Usually, the response lasts approximately 12 months. The drugs used most commonly are Adriamycin, cyclophosphamide, methotrexate, and 5-fluorouracil in various combinations designated as *CAF* or *CMF.* Recently, paclitaxel (Taxol) and docetaxel (Taxotere) have been approved for first-line and second-line treatment of metastatic breast cancer. Though Adriamycin used to be considered the most effective single agent, the results of a recent randomized trial suggest that docetaxel results in response rates higher than those of Adriamycin, although without prolonged survival.

Various taxane-containing combinations have been developed, although important questions remain concerning the ideal dosages and scheduling. Recently, a docetaxel-doxorubicin combination was reported to produce a response rate significantly higher than that of the standard doxorubicin-cyclophosphamide combination in first-line therapy for metastatic breast cancer. Additional studies of paclitaxel and docetaxel in combination with other drugs are under way in metastatic and early breast cancer.

A novel vinblastine analog, vinorelbine (Navelbine) has substantial activity in metastatic breast cancer. Though this analog has a reproducible 40% to 55% response rate in first-line therapy for metastatic breast cancer, the US Food and Drug Administration has not approved it for this indication. However, owing to its substantial antitumor activity and its excellent tolerability, it is in widespread use both as a single agent and in combination chemotherapy. Another new drug is capecitabine, an oral fluoropyrimidine that results in a slow release of 5-fluorouracil. It is active and well tolerated by the oral route.

Some investigators have reported that combinations of hormone and antineoplastic chemotherapy produce a higher response rate and longer-lasting remission than do either of these therapies alone [62]; however, a survival benefit has not been demonstrated. The use of such combinations precludes successful treatment for long periods with relatively nontoxic hormone therapy alone. For this reason, the separate use of endocrine and antineoplastic drugs is recommended. Continuing therapeutic trials are essential to evaluate new drugs and potential drug combinations that may increase the rate and duration of responses, particularly complete responses.

One important question in the treatment of metastatic breast cancers is whether using more of a drug (increased dose intensity) will yield response rates higher and survival longer than those of standard-dose drug combinations. Recent data from uncontrolled phase I and phase II clinical trials suggest a positive relationship between dose intensity and response [63]. Overall response rates of 80% and complete remission rates of 50% to 65% are seen commonly among patients who have received little or no previous chemotherapy. However, comparison of the results of standard-dose chemotherapy is not possible because of the extensive selection process required for the former and the upstaging that results from extensive testing

[63]. The only randomized trial reported thus far showed an improved response rate, duration, and survival with high-dose therapy as compared with low-dose therapy [64]. However, this study has been criticized because of its size and design, the drug regimens used, and the very poor outcome of the control group.

Marked progress has occurred in improving the benefit-toxicity ratio of high-dose chemotherapy in metastatic breast cancer. Mortality has dropped to 1% to 3% under the guidance of expert hands, and the cost of these interventions also has decreased dramatically. Still unclear, however, is whether any survival extension has occurred and whether the benefits warrant exposing patients with metastatic breast cancer to the toxic effects of such intensive and expensive drug programs.

For several years, overexpression of the *HER2/neu* oncogene has been known to be associated with poor prognosis in both primary and metastatic breast cancers. Moreover, both preclinical and clinical studies suggested that *HER2/neu* oncogene overexpression predicted poor response or resistance to several cytotoxic and, possibly, hormonal agents. For these reasons, several investigators targeted the *HER2/neu* oncogene for novel therapeutic interventions [38, 65]. One of these, trastuzumab (Herceptin), a monoclonal antibody acting against the extracellular domain of the *HER2/neu* oncoprotein, recently was approved by the US Food and Drug Administration for the treatment of metastatic breast cancer overexpressing *HER2/neu* [65]. In patients who have received extensive prior treatment, trastuzumab as a single agent produced objective responses in 13% to 16% of patients, with an additional 25% achieving stable disease. Combined with cytotoxic therapy, this agent improves response rates, time to progression, and survival of patients in this poor prognostic category. This agent is an important new addition to the management of breast cancer. It can be used alone or in combination with paclitaxel or cisplatin in patients with *HER2/neu*-overexpressing breast cancer.

Bone metastases are the most common site of distant spread for breast cancer. They also represent the most common source of morbidity and catastrophic complications (hypercalcemia, pathologic fractures, and spinal cord compression). Bone metastases develop as a result of osteoclast activity caused by a disruption of osteoclast-osteoblast equilibrium. Tumor cells produce and secrete humoral mediators to activate osteoclasts.

Over the last several years, clinical trials have demonstrated that the addition of intravenous bisphosphonates to systemic anticancer treatment (whether hormonal or cytotoxic) reduces the frequency and severity of bone-related complications and prolongs complication-free survival [66]. Therefore, bisphosphonate therapy should be added to the treatment of patients with overt bone metastases. Although preliminary reports suggest that "adjuvant" bisphosphonate therapy might prevent bone metastases, confirmation of these results is needed.

REHABILITATION

The first step toward rehabilitation should be taken at the time of diagnosis, when education about primary treatment options, the disease itself, and follow-up care can cause patients to feel more knowledgeable about and comfortable with the treatment plan. Physicians should try to anticipate patients' cosmetic and emotional concerns after treatment. Providing written or visual reference materials is helpful and will allow affected patients to assimilate information at their convenience.

Though the most important psychological support comes from the patients' immediate families, patients should be told also about the Reach to Recovery Program sponsored by the American Cancer Society and about other rehabilitative programs involving nurses, social workers, therapy groups, and psychiatrists. Physicians should also help patients and their partners to deal with the problems of sexual identity and body image. Episodes of depression are common after a diagnosis of breast cancer. Although such depressions usually do not require medication or psychiatric consultation, both forms of assistance should be available, and the early intervention of social workers or mental health workers should be encouraged. After surgery or irradiation of the breast or axilla, early initiation of an exercise program will help patients to regain the full range of arm and shoulder motion within a few weeks of treatment. Failure to accomplish this, particularly in elderly patients, may result in the permanent loss of shoulder mobility and in long-term discomfort.

Patients should be told of their options regarding breast replacement (i.e., prosthetic external breast forms or surgical reconstruction of the breast after mastectomy). In addition, plastic surgery can recreate subtle breast features such as protuberant nipples and pigmented areolar skin. Breast reconstruction does not increase the risk of local recurrence.

Because metastatic breast cancer can be considered a chronic disease, emotional support should become an integral part of the overall treatment plan rather than being delayed until a crisis occurs. Support by physicians, nurses, and other health professionals over the course of the illness is essential in helping patients to cope with the changes resulting from breast cancer.

REFERENCES

1. Greenlee RT, Murray T, Bolden S, Wingo PA. Cancer statistics, 2000. *CA Cancer J Clin* 50:7–33, 2000.
2. Chu KC, Tarone RE, Kessler LG, et al. Recent trends in U.S. breast cancer incidence, survival, and mortality rates. *J Natl Cancer Inst* 88:1571–1579, 1996.
3. Harris JR, Lippman ME, Veronesi U, Willett W. Breast cancer. *N Engl J Med* 327:319–328, 473–480, 1992.
4. Seidman H, Mushinski MH, Gelb SK, et al. Probabilities of eventually developing or dying of cancer: United States, 1985. *CA Cancer J Clin* 35:36–56, 1985.
5. Kash KM, Holland JC, Halper MS, Miller DG. Physiological distress and surveillance behaviors of women with a family history of breast cancer. *J Natl Cancer Inst* 84:24–30, 1992.
6. Colditz GA, Willett WC, Hunter DJ, et al. Family history, age, and risk of breast cancer. Prospective data: the Nurses' Health Study. *JAMA* 270:338–342, 1993.
7. Ottman R, King MC, Pike MC, Henderson BE. Practical guide for estimating risk for familial breast cancer. *Lancet* 2:556–558, 1983.
8. Blackwood MA, Weber BL. *BRCA1* and *BRCA2:* from molecular genetics to clinical medicine (review). *J Clin Oncol* 16:1969–1977, 1998.
9. Casey G. The *BRCA1* and *BRCA2* breast cancer genes (review). *Curr Opin Oncol* 9:88–93, 1997.
10. Henderson BE. Endogenous and exogenous endocrine factors. In Henderson IC (ed), *Endogenous and Exogenous Endocrine Factors.* Philadelphia: Saunders, 1989:577–598.
11. Page DL, Dupont WD. Anatomic indicators (histologic and cytologic) of increased breast cancer risk (review). *Breast Cancer Res Treat* 28:157–166, 1993.
12. Dupont WD, Page DL. Risk factors for breast cancer in women with proliferative breast disease. *N Engl J Med* 312:146–151, 1985.
13. Dupont WD, Page DL. Relative risk of breast cancer varies with time since diagnosis of atypical hyperplasia. *Hum Pathol* 20:723–725, 1989.
14. Fisher B, Constantino JP, Wickerman DL, et al. Tamoxifen for prevention of breast cancer: report of the National Surgical Adjuvant Breast and Bowel Project P-1 Study. *J Natl Cancer Inst* 90:1371–1388, 1998.
15. Cummings SR, Eckert S, Krueger KA, et al. The effect of raloxifene on risk of breast cancer in postmenopausal women: results from the MORE randomized trial. *JAMA* 281:2189–2197, 1999.
16. Hartman LC, Schaid DJ, Woods JE, et al. Efficacy of bilateral prophylactic mastectomy in women with a family history of breast cancer. *N Engl J Med* 340:70–84, 1999.
17. Howe GR, Hirohata T, Hislop TG, et al. Dietary risk factors and risk of breast cancer: combined analysis of 12 case-control studies. *J Natl Cancer Inst* 82:561–569, 1990.
18. Willet WC, Stampfer MJ, Colditz GA, et al. Dietary fat and the risk of breast cancer. *N Engl J Med* 316:22–28, 1987.

19. Bowlin SJ, Leske MC, Varma A, et al. Breast cancer risk and alcohol consumption: results of a large case-control study. *Int J Epidemiol* 26:915–923, 1997.

20. Romieu I, Berlin JA, Colditz G. Oral contraceptives and breast cancer: review and meta-analysis. *Cancer* 66:2253–2263, 1990.

21. Steinberg KK, Thacher SB, Smith SJ, et al. A meta-analysis of the effect of estrogen replacement therapy on the risk of breast cancer. *JAMA* 265:1985–1990, 1991.

22. Colditz GA, Hankinson SE, Hunter DJ, et al. The use of estrogens and progestins and the risk of breast cancer in postmenopausal women. *N Engl J Med* 332:1589–1593, 1995.

23. Collaborative Group on Hormonal Factors in Breast Cancer. Breast cancer and hormone replacement therapy: collaborative reanalysis of data from 51 epidemiological studies of 52,705 women with breast cancer and 108,411 women without breast cancer. *Lancet* 350:1047–1059, 1997.

24. Schairer C, Lubin J, Troisi R, et al. Menopausal estrogen and estrogen-progestin replacement therapy and breast cancer risk. *JAMA* 283:485–491, 2000.

25. Clark GM, Sledge GW Jr, Osborne CK, McGuire WL. Survival from first recurrence: relative importance of prognostic factors in 1,015 breast cancer patients. *J Clin Oncol* 5:55–61, 1987.

26. Kerlikowske K, Grady D, Rubin SM, et al. Efficacy of screening mammography. A meta-analysis. *JAMA* 273: 149–154, 1995.

27. Osteen RT. Breast cancer. In Steele GD, Osteen RT, Winchester DP, et al. (eds), *National Cancer Data Base: Annual Review of Patient Care.* Atlanta: American Cancer Society and the Commission on Cancer, 1994:56–71.

28. Layfield LJ, Glasgow BJ, Cramer H. Fine needle aspiration in the management of breast masses. In Rosen PP, Fechner RE (eds), *Pathology Annual,* part 2 (vol 24). Norwalk, CT: Appleton & Lange, 1989:23–62.

29. Day NE. Screening for breast cancer. *Br Med Bull* 47:400–415, 1991.

30. Tabar L, Duffy SW, Vitak B, et al. The natural history of breast carcinoma: What have we learned from screening? *Cancer* 86:449–462, 1999.

31. Hendrick RE, Smith RA, Rutledge III JH, Smart CR. Benefit of screening mammography in women aged 40–49: a new meta-analysis of randomized controlled trials *J Natl Cancer Inst Monogr* 22:87–92, 1997.

32. Duffy SW, Day NE, Tabar L, et al. Markov models of breast tumor progression: some age-specific results. *J Naatl Cancer Inst Monogr* 22:93–97, 1997.

33. Leitch AM, Dodd GD, Costanza M, et al. American Cancer Society guidelines for the early detection of breast cancer: update 1997. *CA Cancer J Clin* 47:150–153, 1997.

34. Osteen RT, Cady B, Chmiel JS, et al. 1991 National survey of carcinoma of the breast by the commission on cancer. *Surg Gynecol Obstet* 178:213–219, 1994.

35. Fisher B, Wolmark N, Bauer M, et al. The accuracy of clinical nodal staging and of limited axillary dissection as a determinant of histological nodal status in carcinoma of the breast. *Surg Gynecol Obstet* 152:765–772, 1981.

36. Elston CW, Ellis IO. Pathologic factors in breast cancer: I. The value of histological grade in breast cancer: experience from a large study with long-term follow up. *Histopathology* 19:403–410, 1991.

37. Dickson RB, Lippman ME. Growth factors in breast cancer (review). *Endocrinol Rev* 16:559–589, 1995.

38. Slamon D, Layland-Jones B, Shak S, et al. Addition of Herceptin (humanized anti-HER2 antibody) to first line chemotherapy for HER2 overexpressing metastatic breast cancer markedly increases anticancer activity: a randomized, multinational controlled phase III trial (abstract 377). *Proc Am Soc Clin Oncol* 17:98a, 1998.

39. Muss HB, Thor AD, Berry DA, et al. c-erbB-2 Expression and response to adjuvant therapy in women with node-positive early breast cancer. *N Engl J Med* 330:1260–1266, 1994.

40. Haagemsen CD, Lane N, Lattes R, Bodian C. Lobular neoplasia (so-called lobular carcinoma in situ) of the breast. *Cancer* 42:737–769, 1978.

41. Holland R, Hendricks JHCL, Verbeek ALM, et al. Extent, distribution and mammographic/histologic correlations of breast ductal carcinoma in situ. *Lancet* 335:519–522, 1990.

42. Fisher B, Costantino J, Redmond C, et al. Lumpectomy compared with lumpectomy and radiation therapy for the treatment of intraductal breast cancer. *N Engl J Med* 328:1581–1586, 1993.

43. Fisher B, Dignam J, Wolmark N, et al. Tamoxifen in treatment of intraductal breast cancer: National Surgical Adjuvant Breast and Bowel Project B-24 randomized controlled trial. *Lancet* 353:1991–2000, 1999.

44. Morris AD, Morris RD, Wilson JF, et al. Breast-conserving therapy vs mastectomy in early-stage breast cancer: a meta-analysis of 10-year survival. *Cancer J Sci Am* 3:6–12, 1997.

45. Fisher D, Redmond C, Poisson R, et al. Eight-year results of a randomized clinical trial comparing total mastectomy and lumpectomy with or without irradiation in the treatment of breast cancer. *N Engl J Med* 320:822–828, 1989.

46. Sanchez-Guerrero J, Colditz GA, Karlson EW, et al. Silicone breast implants and the risk of connective-tissue diseases and symptoms. *N Engl J Med* 332:1666–1670, 1995.

47. Giuliano AE, Jones RC, Brennan M, Statman R. Sentinel lymphadenopathy in breast cancer. *J Clin Oncol* 15:2345–2350, 1997.

48. Krag D, Weaver D, Ashikaga T, et al. The sentinel node in breast cancer. A multicenter validation study. *N Engl J Med* 339:941–946, 1998.

49. Overgaard M, Hansen PS, Overgaard J, et al. Postoperative radiotherapy in high-risk premenopausal women with breast cancer who receive adjuvant chemotherapy. *N Engl J Med* 337:949–955, 1997.

50. Ragaz J, Jackson SM, Le N, et al. Adjuvant radiotherapy and chemotherapy in node positive premenopausal women with breast cancer. *N Engl J Med* 337:56–62, 1997.

51. Early Breast Cancer Trialists' Collaborative Group. Polychemotherapy for early breast cancer: an overview of the randomized trials. *Lancet* 352:930–942, 1998.

52. Henderson IC, Berry D, Demitri G, et al. Improved disease free (DSF) and overall survival (OS) from addition of sequential paclitaxel (T) but not from the escalation of doxorubicin (a) dose level in the adjuvant chemotherapy of patients (PTS) with node-positive primary breast cancer (BC) (abstract). *Proc Am Soc Clin Oncol* 17:101a, 1998.

53. Bezwoda WR. Randomized, controlled trial of high dose chemotherapy versus standard dose chemotherapy for high risk surgically treated, primary breast cancer (abstract). *Proc Am Soc Clin Oncol* 18:2a, 1999.

54. Rodenhuis S, Richel DJ, van der Wall E, et al. Randomized trial of high-dose chemotherapy and haemopoietic progenitor-cell support in operable breast cancer with extensive axillary lymph-node involvement. *Lancet* 352: 515–521, 1998.

55. Hortobagyi GN, Buzdar AU, Charmplin R, et al. Lack of efficacy of adjuvant high-dose (HD) tandem combination chemotherapy (CT) for high-risk primary breast cancer (HRPBC)—a randomized trial (abstract). *Proc Am Soc Clin Oncol* 17:123a, 1998.

56. Peters W, Rosner G, Vredenburgh J, et al. A prospective randomized comparison of two doses of combination alkylating agents as consolidation after CAF in high-risk primary breast cancer involving ten or more axillary lymph nodes: preliminary results of CALGB 9082/SWOG 9114/NCIC MA-13 (abstract). *Proc Annu Meet Am Soc Clin Oncol* 18:1a, 1999.

57. The Scandinavian Breast Cancer Study Group 9401. Results from a randomized adjuvant breast cancer study with high dose chemotherapy with CTCb supported by autologous bone marrow stem cells versus dose escalated tailored FEC therapy (abstract). *Proc Annu Meet Am Soc Clin Oncol* 18:2a, 1999.

58. Fisher B, Dignam J, Bryant J, et al. Five versus more than five years of tamoxifen therapy for breast cancer patients with negative lymph nodes and estrogen receptor–positive tumors. *J Natl Cancer Inst* 88:1529–1542, 1996.

59. Diamandidou E, Buzdar AU, Smith TL, et al. Treatment-related leukemia in breast cancer patients treated with fluorouracil-doxorubicin-cyclophosphamide combination adjuvant chemotherapy: the University of Texas MD Anderson Cancer Center experience. *J Clin Oncol* 14:2722–2730, 1996.

60. Rosselli Del Turco M, Palli D, Cariddi A, et al. Intensive diagnostic follow-up after treatment of primary breast cancer. A randomized trial. National Research Council Project on Breast Cancer follow-up. *JAMA* 271:1593–1597, 1994.

61. The GIVIO investigators. Impact of follow-up testing on survival and health-related quality of life in breast cancer patients. *JAMA* 271:1587–1592, 1994.

62. Sledge GW Jr, Hu P, Falkson G, et al. Comparison of chemotherapy with chemohormonal therapy as first-line therapy for metastatic, hormone-sensitive breast cancer: an Eastern Cooperative Oncology Group Study. *J Clin Oncol* 18:262–266, 2000.

63. Antman KH, Rowlings PA, Vaughan WP, et al. High-dose chemotherapy with autologous hematopoietic stem-cell support for breast cancer in North America. *J Clin Oncol* 15: 1870–1879, 1997.

64. Bezwoda WR, Seymour L, Dansey RD. High-dose chemotherapy with hematopoietic rescue as primary treatment for metastatic breast cancer: a randomized trial. *J Clin Oncol* 13:2483–2489, 1995.

65. Baselga J, Tripathy D, Mendelsohn J, et al. Phase II study of weekly intravenous recombinant humanized anti-p185HER2 monoclonal antibody in patients with *HER2/neu*-overexpressing metastatic breast cancer. *J Clin Oncol* 14:737–744, 1996.

66. Hortobagyi GN, Theriault RL, Lipton A, et al. Long-term prevention of skeletal complications of metastatic breast cancer with pamidronate. Protocol 19 Aredia Breast Cancer Study Group. *J Clin Oncol* 16:2038–2044, 1998.

11

Lung Cancer

■ ■ ■

Charles R. Thomas, Jr
Todd E. Williams
Everardo Cobos
Andrew T. Turrisi III

L UNG CANCER IS A MAJOR PUBLIC HEALTH DI-
lemma, accounting for more than 150,000 deaths
in the United States annually. Despite the well-
documented link between tobacco product use and
respiratory diseases, including cancer, the outcome of
such efforts to curb their use have been mixed. Likely,
all socioeconomic groups are aware of the hazards inherent in the use of tobacco products, yet lung cancer
accounts for one-third of all cancer deaths, solidifying
this site as the primary cause of preventable cancer
mortality.

ETIOLOGIC FEATURES AND RISK FACTORS

Cigarette smoking constitutes the greatest risk factor in
the development of lung cancer (Fig. 11.1) [1]. Lung
cancer in nonsmokers is extremely uncommon; the lifetime risk of lung cancer in nonsmokers is estimated to
be less than 1% [2]. This risk increases to as high as
30% in heavy smokers. Approximately 90% of lung
cancers in men and 80% in women are attributed to
cigarette smoking [2]. Other important occupational
and environmental risk factors include asbestos, radon,
and dietary factors. Less common carcinogens include
arsenic, chromium, nickel, ionizing irradiation, vinyl
chloride, chloromethyl ether, and polycyclic aromatic
hydrocarbons. Such lung diseases as pulmonary fibrosis
and chronic obstructive pulmonary disease also are associated with increased lung cancer risk. Recent attention has been focused on the association of molecular
genetic factors and evidence for a familial predisposition
to lung cancer [3].

Asbestos exposure, a known risk factor for mesothe-

The authors thank Ms. Linda Garbett for her help in the preparation of the manuscript.

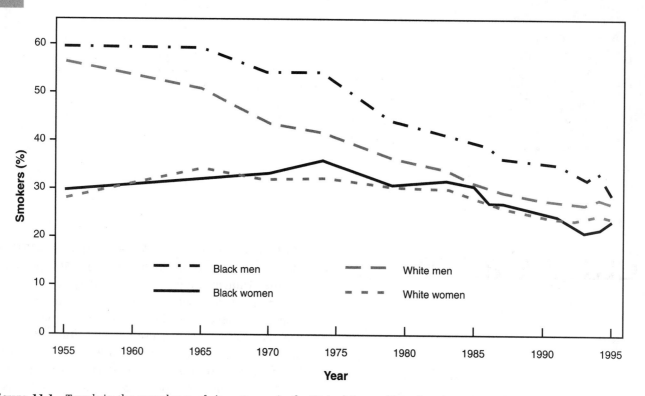

Figure 11.1 Trends in the prevalence of cigarette use in the United States. Note that, in 1992, a change in smoker definition increased estimates by 0.9%.

lioma, significantly increases the risk of lung cancer if individuals smoke tobacco products. The risk of lung cancer in smokers who are exposed to asbestos is increased 60- to 90-fold.

Radon, the decay product of uranium and radium, is a known carcinogen [4]. Conflicting data assess the risk for lung cancer resulting from indoor radon exposure [5, 6], and the determination of risk may, in part, depend on the radon-monitoring technology that is used [7].

Epidemiologic studies demonstrate a reduction in lung cancer risk in individuals who consume large amounts of fruits and vegetables, a benefit theoretically related to higher levels of beta-carotene, vitamin A, and other antioxidants, although adjustment for such other risk factors as tobacco exposure clouds these observations. Results of recent randomized trials evaluating oral supplementation with beta-carotene and retinyl palmitate have not demonstrated a reduction in cancer risk; rather, an adverse effect on lung cancer risk has been observed. Newer ongoing chemopreventive efforts are using agents selectively directed at early molecular targets.

Several published studies suggest that lung cancer can aggregate in some families. This predilection may be due to a genetic predisposition, but the trait (lung cancer) may be expressed only in the presence of its

major predisposing factor, tobacco. Recent research has suggested that the alpha$_1$-antitrypsin deficiency allele may be associated with an increased risk of developing certain lung cancers [8]. Research to isolate other candidate genes for lung cancer predisposition is actively being undertaken [3].

MOLECULAR BIOLOGICAL CONSIDERATIONS

Mutations in selective dominant and recessive genes can lead to a malignant phenotype [9]. Dysregulation, inappropriate expression, or loss of genes can lead to malignancy. Germline alteration of one allele in familial cancer and deletions within the gene in sporadic cancers, such as lung cancer, can be considered relative trademarks of tumor suppressor genes. A common genetic abnormality in lung cancer is the loss of 3p, noted in both small-cell lung cancer (SCLC) and non-small-cell lung cancer (NSCLC). Several of the regions on this chromosome are altered to varying degrees in precancerous lung lesions. Recently, a band (3p14.2) on this chromosome site was found to harbor the fragile histidine triad tumor suppressor gene [10, 11].

In addition to the loss of chromosome 3p, loss of heterozygosity also occurs on chromosomes 5, 9, 13, and 17 and on other sites. Mutations and allelic loss of *p53* and *RB1* tumor suppresser genes also are common, more so with SCLC. Of *p53* mutations that occur in lung cancer, only one-fifth result in altered *p53* protein expression, indicating that our understanding of this critical tumor repressor gene is incomplete [12]. With respect to prognosis, *ras* gene mutations and overexpression of HER-2/*neu* are markers for a worse outcome, especially with respect to adenocarcinoma [13]. Alterations in the expression of the retinoic acid receptor may, in part, contribute to the carcinogenesis of lung cancer [14, 15]. Some of these molecular defects may serve as strategic targets in the design of novel cytostatic agents [16].

PATHOLOGIC CLASSIFICATION

Over the last several decades, multiple revisions and expansions have been made in the various pathologic subtypes of lung cancer (Table 11.1). The current international standard for pathologic classification of lung cancer was devised almost two decades ago with the classification scheme developed by the World Health Organization (WHO) [17]. A practical but unofficial classification used by clinicians separates lung cancer into two distinct subgroups: SCLC and NSCLC.

Small-Cell Lung Cancer

SCLC represents approximately 20% to 30% of all cases of lung cancer. This subtype is associated very strongly with smoking. It tends to arise centrally, presenting in the main-stem or lobular bronchi. SCLC probably arises from the basal neuroendocrine Kulchitsky cells. An aggressive subtype of lung cancer, it metastasizes early to hilar, mediastinal, and distant sites. Without specific treatment, the prognosis of SCLC is dismal. This type of carcinoma is associated with several paraneoplastic syndromes, including the syndrome of inappropriate secretion of antidiuretic hormone, ectopic adrenocorticotropic hormone (ACTH) production with Cushing's syndrome, and Eaton-Lambert syndrome. The current WHO classification of lung cancers recognizes three subtypes of SCLC:

- *Oat-cell carcinomas:* lymphocyte-like cells growing in sheets or nests in sparse connective tissue stroma
- *Small-cell carcinoma, intermediate type:* with polygo-

Table 11.1 World Health Organization Lung Cancer Classification

I. Epithelial tumors
  A. Benign
    1. Papillomas
    2. Adenomas
  B. Dysplasia, carcinoma in situ
  C. Malignant
    1. Squamous cell carcinoma
      a. Spindle-cell variant
    2. Small-cell carcinoma
      a. Oat-cell carcinoma
      b. Intermediate-cell type
      c. Combined oat-cell carcinoma
    3. Adenocarcinoma
      a. Acinar
      b. Papillary
      c. Bronchioloalveolar
      d. Solid carcinoma with mucin formation
    4. Large-cell carcinoma
      a. Giant-cell carcinoma
      b. Clear-cell carcinoma
    5. Adenosquamous carcinoma
    6. Carcinoid tumor
    7. Bronchial gland carcinoma
      a. Mucoepidermoid carcinoma
      b. Adenoid cystic carcinoma
    8. Others
II. Soft-tissue tumors
III. Mesothelial tumors
  A. Benign
  B. Malignant
IV. Miscellaneous tumors
  A. Benign
  B. Malignant
V. Secondary tumors
VI. Unclassified tumors
VII. Tumor-like lesions

nal and fusiform cells larger than typical oat-cell carcinoma and with more abundant cytoplasm
- *Combined oat-cell carcinoma:* oat-cell carcinoma with squamous cell carcinoma or adenocarcinoma (or both).

Little evidence suggests that these subtypes have prognostic relevance. Photomicrographs of SCLC are shown in Figure 11.2 [18].

Non-Small-Cell Lung Cancer

LARGE-CELL CANCER

Large-cell carcinomas represent approximately 10% to 15% of all lung cancers. They are less differentiated

A

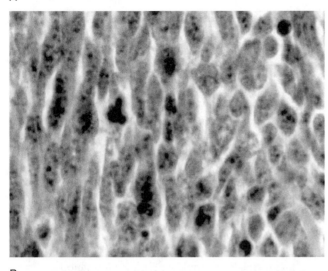

B

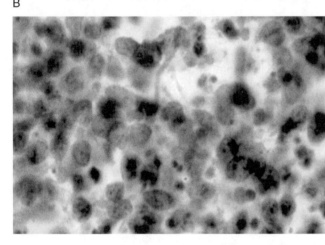

Figure 11.2 (A) Typical histology of small-cell lung cancer. The cells grow in sheets, with no specific architecture. They are small and display scant cytoplasm. Mitoses are numerous, and necrosis is present. The nuclei can be ovoid or elongated and resemble oat cells. (B) Cytologic appearance of similar cells, with indistinct nucleoli. Reprinted with permission of Dr. Pat Connelly (Valley Pathologists, Inc., Dayton, OH).

tumors as compared with squamous cell carcinoma or adenocarcinomas and fail to express either glandular or squamous differentiation on light microscopy. They tend to occur at the periphery of the lung, invading subsegmental bronchi or larger airways. Frequently, they have associated necrosis but typically are not cavitating. Histologically, large-cell carcinomas exhibit epithelial cells with large nuclei, prominent nucleoli, and well-defined cell boundaries. The WHO recognizes two variants of large-cell carcinoma classification: giant-cell and clear-cell types. This subclassification probably has little clinical relevance.

SQUAMOUS CELL CARCINOMA

Previously, squamous cell carcinoma was the most common subtype of lung cancer. A steady decline has been seen in its prevalence over the last 30 years, from representing approximately 50% of all lung cancers in the 1970s to the current 30% to 40% of cases. The reason for the decline is not entirely clear. More than 90% of these cancers arise in the subsegmental or large bronchi. Frequently, they are endobronchial, located centrally, and spread toward the main stem bronchus. Necrosis and cavitation can occur, especially in large tumors.

Microscopical examination shows squamous cell carcinomas composed of sheets of epithelial cells that range from well-differentiated to poorly differentiated. They exhibit evidence of stratification, intercellular bridges, and keratinization with pearl formation (Fig. 11.3) [18]. Most frequently, hypercalcemia is associated with this histologic characteristic, and they tend to be slow-growing and to progress from the in situ stage to a clinically apparent tumor over a period of 3 to 4 years.

ADENOCARCINOMA

Currently, adenocarcinoma is the most common histologic subtype of lung cancer in North America, representing approximately 40% to 50% of all lung cancers. In contrast to squamous cell and small-cell cancers, adenocarcinomas arise predominantly in the periphery of the lung. They can arise in scars or areas of fibrosis and can occur in nonsmokers. Adenocarcinomas can exhibit glandular formation, development of papillary structure, production of mucin, and acinar formation (Fig. 11.4) [18]. The WHO classification divides adenocarcinomas into four subtypes: acinar, papillary, bronchioloalveolar, and solid with mucin production. Immunohistochemical features include expression of carcinoembryonic antigen and epithelial membrane antigen.

In general, adenocarcinomas have a worse stage-for-stage prognosis as compared with squamous cell carcinomas. Adenocarcinomas are the type of lung cancer most commonly seen in women. Digital clubbing and hypertrophic pulmonary osteoarthropathy, though noted in fewer than one-third of cases, are not uncommonly associated paraneoplastic syndromes [19].

Bronchioloalveolar carcinoma behaves as a distinct clinicopathologic entity [20]. It arises from cells growing along the alveolar septa. It exhibits a lepidic type of growth pattern, with preservation of the alveolar architecture [21]. This type of lung cancer can present as a single peripheral nodule, as a multifocal disease, or as a rapidly diffuse pneumonic form that can involve both

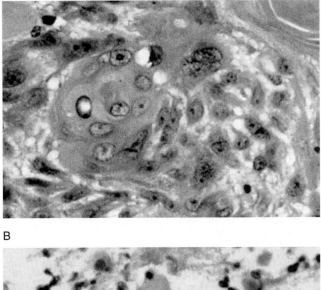

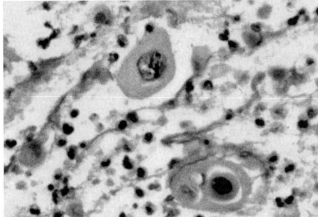

Figure 11.3 (A) Squamous cell carcinoma. The cells have dense cytoplasm and form whorls, with a dense center called *keratin pearls*. Intercellular bridges and spindle formation can be seen. (B) Cytologic representation of squamous cell carcinoma. The cells have dense cytoplasm and prominent borders. Nuclear chromatin is coarse, and nucleoli are variable. The cytoplasm is dense, secondary to cell keratinization. Reprinted with permission of Dr. Pat Connelly (Valley Pathologists, Inc., Dayton, OH).

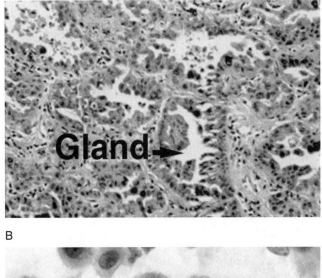

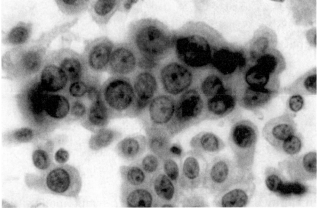

Figure 11.4 (A) Pulmonary adenocarcinoma, glandular formation. The tumor is growing along the alveoli, without distortion of the normal architecture. This latter feature is consistent with bronchioloalveolar carcinoma. (B) Cytologic appearance of an adenocarcinoma. The tumor cells are bigger than normal cells and tend to cluster together. Marked chromatin of the cells and prominent nucleoli are noted. Reprinted with permission of Dr. Pat Connelly (Valley Pathologists, Inc., Dayton, OH).

lungs. Bronchioloalveolar carcinoma also may be more common in women and patients who have smoked less or who never smoked [22].

CARCINOID TUMOR

Carcinoid tumors are uncommon. They are considered part of the spectrum of neuroendocrine tumors, as is the case with SCLC. The lesions must be distinguished via immunohistochemical and/or electron micrograph analysis because light microscopy alone seldom establishes a firm diagnosis. Patients may or may not present with features of carcinoid syndrome (see Chapter 31).

The treatment is not well-defined because the disorder's natural history—primary lung carcinoid tumor—lies between that of SCLC and NSCLC.

CLINICAL PRESENTATION
Symptoms and Signs

The clinical presentation of lung cancer is extremely variable and depends on local manifestations of the tumor, the presence of distant metastases, or associated paraneoplastic syndromes [23–25]. The overwhelming

Table 11.2 Stage-Dependent Presenting Clinical Features of Lung Cancer

Symptoms elicited from medical history
Constitutional (anorexia, fatigue, weight loss)
Gastrointestinal (dysphagia)
Respiratory (cough, hemoptysis, dyspnea)
Musculoskeletal (focal skeletal pain, chest pain)
Neurologic (headaches, syncope, seizures, extremity weakness, recent change in mental status)

Signs noted on physical examination
Bone tenderness
Clubbing
Focal neurologic deficits (papilledema)
Abdominal visceromegaly
Hoarseness
Pleural effusion
Supraclavicular lymphadenopathy
Soft-tissue mass
Superior vena cava syndrome

Routine laboratory test results
Anemia of chronic disease
Elevated alkaline phosphatase, GGT, SGOT, calcium
Space-occupying lesions on head, chest, or abdominal CT scans
Increased radionuclide uptake on bone scintigraphy

GGT = gamma glutamyl transferase; SGOT = serum glutamic oxalo-acetic transaminase; CT = computed tomography.

Table 11.3 Paraneoplastic Syndromes Associated with Lung Cancer

Systemic and constitutional syndromes
Anorexia, cachexia, weight loss
Fever
Nonbacterial thrombotic endocarditis
Orthostatic hypotension
Systemic lupus erythematosus

Dermatologic syndromes
Acanthosis nigricans
Acquired hypertrichosis lanuginosa
Acquired ichthyosis
Acquired palmoplantar keratoderma
Bazex's syndrome (acrokeratosis)
Dermatitis herpetiformis
Dermatomyositis
Erythema annulare centrifugum
Erythema gyratum repens
Exfoliative dermatis (erythroderma)
Extramammary Paget's disease
Florid cutaneous papillomatosis
Pemphigus vulgaris
Pityriasis rotunda
Pruritus
Sign of Leser-Trelat
Sweet's syndrome
Tripe palms
Vasculitis

Endocrine syndromes
Acromegaly
Antidiuretic hormone excess
Carcinoid syndrome
Cushing's syndrome
Ectopic gonadotropin
Galactorrhea
Gynecomastia
Hyperamylasemia
Hypercalcemia
Hypercalcitonemia
Hyperglycemia
Hypertension
Hyperthyroidism
Hypoglycemia
Hyponatremia
Hypophosphatemia
Hypouricemia
Lactic acidosis

Hematologic syndromes
Anemia of chronic disease
Disseminated intravascular coagulation
Dysproteinemia
Eosinophilia
Hypercoagulable state
Leukocytosis
Polycythemia
Red-cell aplasia
Thrombocytopenic purpura

majority of lung cancer patients are symptomatic at the time of diagnosis and most frequently present such signs and symptoms as cough, weight loss, and dyspnea (Table 11.2) [23, 26]. Other findings include chest pain, hemoptysis, bone pain, clubbing, hypertrophic osteoarthropathy, wheezing, dysphagia, or hoarseness. Currently, lung cancer is the most common cause of superior vena cava syndrome. Horner's syndrome (ipsilateral ptosis, miosis, and facial anhidrosis) along with shoulder pain and radicular pain along the ulnar nerve distribution are presenting signs and symptoms of superior sulcus tumors. Other areas of intrathoracic involvement include the pleura and cardiac structures.

Metastatic lung cancer results from hematogenous, lymphangitic, or interalveolar spread. Affected patients' initial clinical presentation may be due to the site of distant metastatic involvement (see Table 11.2) [26]. Common sites of metastatic involvement include the liver, brain, bone, lymph nodes, and adrenal glands. A significant number of paraneoplastic syndromes have been described in association with lung cancer (Table 11.3). These syndromes can manifest as systemic, cutaneous, endocrine, hematologic, neurologic, and renal abnormalities. Some of the more common associated paraneoplastic syndromes are anorexia, cachexia, and

Table 11.3 Paraneoplastic Syndromes Associated with Lung Cancer (*continued*)

Neuromuscular syndromes
  Cerebral encephalopathy
  Lambert-Eaton myasthenic syndrome
  Myasthenia gravis
  Necrotizing myelopathy
  Polymyopathy
  Peripheral neuropathy
  Subacute cerebellar degeneration
  Vision compromise
  Visceral neuropathy

Renal syndromes
  Glomerulopathies
  Tubulointerstitial nephritis

Skeletal
  Clubbing
  Hypertrophic pulmonary osteoarthropathy

Vascular syndromes
  Marantic endocarditis
  Thrombophlebitis (superficial or deep)

weight loss, clubbing, Cushing's syndrome, hypercalcemia, hyponatremia, anemia, peripheral neuropathy, and Eaton-Lambert myasthenic-syndrome.

Diagnostic Workup

The diagnostic workup should include a complete blood count and an electrolyte profile of serum calcium, blood urea nitrogen, creatinine, lactate dehydrogenase (LDH), serum glutamic oxaloacetic transaminase, serum glutamate pyruvate transaminase, total bilirubin, and prothrombin time. For SCLC patients, bilateral bone marrow aspiration and unilateral bone marrow biopsy are recommended unless such patients have obvious extensive-stage disease or have limited-stage disease with a normal LDH value.

Chest radiography remains a reasonable starting point in the workup of lung cancer (Fig. 11.5A) [27]. Thousands of potentially curable lung cancers have been detected via the use of routine chest roentgenography. Screening studies in high-risk populations have shown mixed results in improvement in population outcomes, but patients with smaller lesions consistently survive longer than do those with larger lesions [28, 29].

Computed tomography (CT) scanning has been used in the preoperative staging of patients with lung carcinoma (see Fig. 11.5B, C) [27]. CT scanning also may help to clarify the relationship of the lung mass to its adjacent structures: lymph nodes, esophagus, spinal cord, heart and great vessels, trachea, and chest wall [30]. Intravenous contrast material clarifies the presence of compression or invasion of vascular structures (i.e., pulmonary trunk, aortic arch, or superior vena cava). The sensitivity of the CT scan in predicting the positivity of mediastinal nodes is approximately 60% to 70%. Nodes measuring from 1 to 1.5 cm should be confirmed cytologically or histologically, because approximately one-fifth will prove positive at mediastinoscopy, including nodes in up to 10% and 18% of patients with cT1N0 and cT2N0 disease, respectively [31]. Some large nodes may be found to be benign on pathologic examination. Grossly normal-sized nodes can harbor cancer, and enlarged nodes may be benign. No reliable size or attenuation indicators are pathognomonic for tumor involvement. However, if curative surgery is a possibility, further staging of the mediastinum is paramount. Most chest CT scans also image the upper abdomen adequately enough to visualize obvious liver metastasis and the adrenal glands. Finally, recommending chest CT as a screening tool is premature, despite a preliminary recent report [32].

Magnetic resonance imaging (MRI) can evaluate fairly well the aortopulmonary window vessels and brachial plexus on coronal scan images. However, mediastinal nodes are not well characterized with present-day techniques. Either a CT or an MRI scan of the head should be performed in patients with evidence of distant metastases to other sites or with neurologic symptoms and signs (or both) [23].

Positron emission tomography (PET) scanning is an imaging modality that measures metabolic activity rather than anatomic size to determine disease involvement. It uses short-half-life, radioactive fluorine isotope that binds to glucose. More metabolically active sites consume the glucose, and detectors record its uptake. Because cancers proliferate rapidly and are metabolically active, PET images them as regions with more intense uptake than that of background or nonmalignant masses [33]. The sensitivity of fluorodeoxyglucose PET is greater than 90% for detection of cancer in CT-indeterminate primary lesions [34]. Up to one-tenth of affected patients either may have PET-demonstrated metastases that were not noted with conventional imaging or are shown via PET not to have metastatic disease when conventional imaging had erroneously suggested otherwise [35]. Sensitivity and specificity results for N2 and N3 mediastinal disease are 71% and 97%, respectively [36]. PET technology is becoming a useful tool in detection of lung cancer, although its role, including cost-effectiveness, in the staging paradigm still is evolving [27, 37–39]. For now, its use should comple-

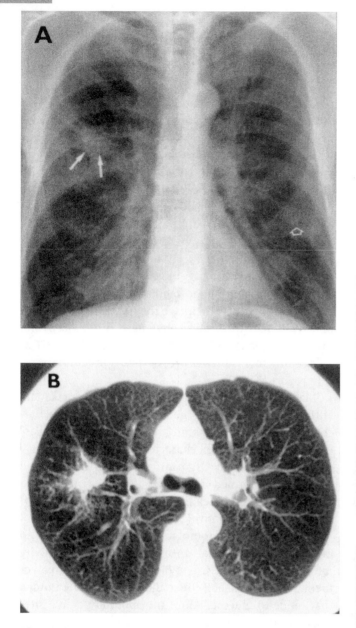

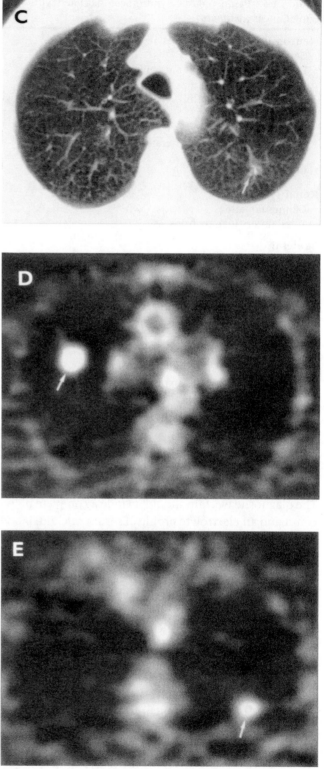

Figure 11.5 (A) Posteroanterior chest radiograph, showing a poorly defined focal opacity in the right upper lobe (*arrows*). The lungs are hyperinflated and emphysematous. The small nodular opacity overlying the middle aspect of the left lung is the nipple shadow (*open arrow*). (B, C) Axial chest computed tomographic cuts confirm a spiculated right upper-lobe mass. A small, irregular focal opacity in the left upper lobe (*arrow*) also is evident. (D, E) Axial positron emission tomographic images show marked fluorodeoxyglucose uptake in both lung lesions (*arrow*).

A

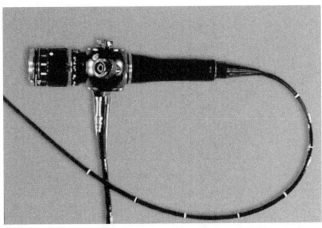

B

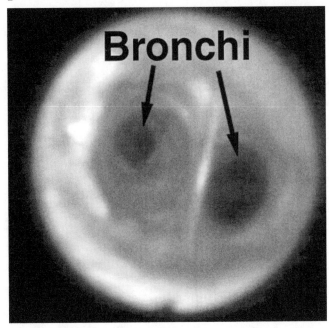

C

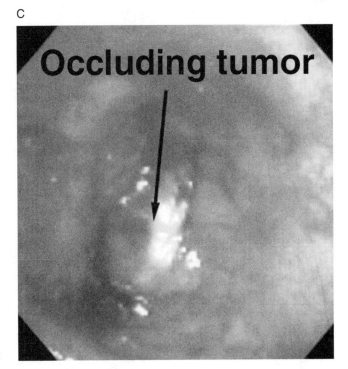

Figure 11.6   (A) Fiberoptic bronchoscope. (B) Bifurcation of the bronchi. (C) An indentation of the lumen, secondary to occlusion by the tumor.

ment, not necessarily replace, CT scanning (see Fig. 11.5D, E) [27].

Bronchoscopy identifies the endobronchial anatomy and distortions by extrinsic compression and commonly yields a pathologic diagnosis (Fig. 11.6A, B) [40]. Combination brushings and biopsy of suspicious lesions are very productive in documenting cancer (see Fig. 11.6C). Transbronchial needle aspiration is useful in sampling subcarinal (level 7) and paratracheal (levels 2R, 4R, and 4L) mediastinal lymph nodes and Pancoast syndrome lesions. The potential for laser and cryosurgical procedures, stent placement, and endobronchial radiotherapy has expanded the role of bronchoscopy.

Transthoracic needle aspiration with CT guidance is commonly used to establish a tissue diagnosis in lesions that are too peripheral for transbronchial needle aspiration. Needle aspiration is also helpful when suspicious hepatic or adrenal lesions (or both) must be submitted to biopsy.

Patients with periesophageal involvement should undergo endoscopy with ultrasonography to determine the presence of esophageal invasion. Endoesophageal ultrasonography varies in usefulness, depending largely on the experience and technical abilities of the operators. Endoscopic ultrasonography has been verified with surgical pathology and has been compared with CT staging of esophageal cancers in several studies [41]. Its staging accuracy in determining depth of invasion is

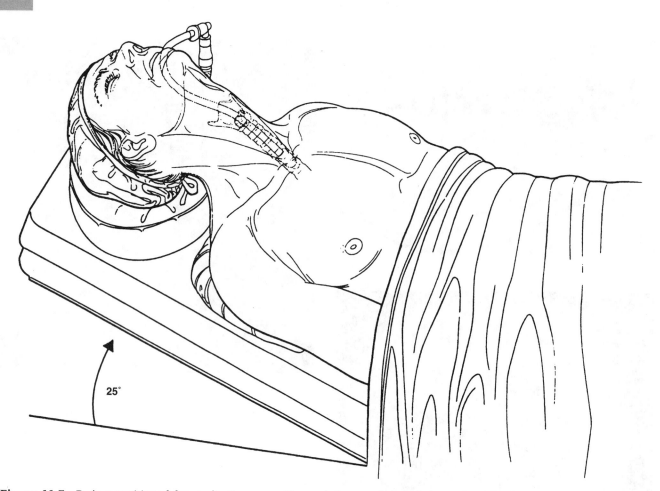

Figure 11.7 Patient positioned for mediastinoscopy. The neck is extended, and the endotracheal tube is draped laterally to avoid the path of the mediastinoscope.

near 90%, which is more accurate than CT, especially for early tumors. Recently, endoscopic ultrasonic identification of mediastinal nodes was claimed to be more accurate than a high-quality CT scan in staging lung cancer [42].

Mediastinoscopy allows assessment of most of the mediastinal nodes (including the pretracheal, paratracheal, subcarinal, and tracheobronchial nodal stations) and determination of whether adjacent mediastinal structures are involved in the tumor. The sensitivity of this test approaches 90%, with a specificity of almost 100%. What should be noted is that mediastinoscopic assessment and mediastinotomy only sample nodes and cannot be considered equivalent to a frank nodal dissection. Because malignant and benign nodes cannot be distinguished reliably by morphologic and pure size criteria on CT scanning, a tissue diagnosis is warranted to determine optimal treatment properly, especially for patients with locally advanced disease (stage III). Contraindications for mediastinoscopy may include a large cervical goiter, significant calcification or aneurysm of the aortic arch or innominate artery, prior radiotherapy, tracheostomy or, possibly, prior mediastinoscopy [43].

Mediastinoscopies are performed via a 3- to 4-cm transverse skin incision centered between the anterior borders of the sternocleidomastoid muscles and just above the sternoclavicular junctions (Figs. 11.7, 11.8) [43]. After careful blunt dissection via the surgeon's finger, the mediastinoscope is advanced into the thorax and facilitates careful identification of nodes that are labeled and sampled promptly (Figs. 11.9–11.11) [43]. Regarding its utility as a prognostic factor, some data are in conflict over whether patients who have positive mediastinal nodes and then are shown to have a pathologically complete response to chemoradiation may do better than those who harbor persistent disease at the time of surgical resection [44, 45]. An anterior or parasternal mediastinotomy permits obtaining a tissue diagnosis of the subaortic and anterior mediastinal nodes (Fig. 11.12) [43].

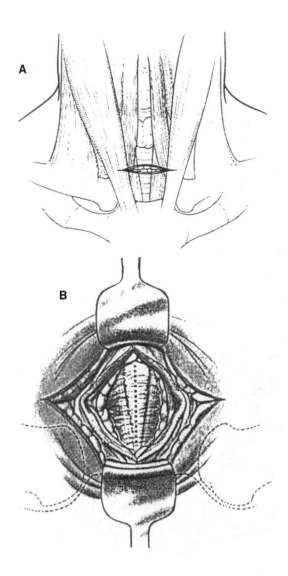

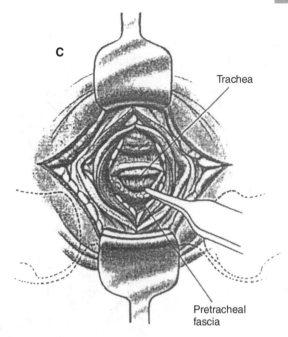

Figure 11.8 Cervical dissection. (A) Skin incision. (B) Vertical midline incision between the sternothyroid muscles after separation of the sternohyoids. (C) Incision and elevation of the pretracheal fascia.

Bone radionuclide and brain CT or MRI scans are not recommended routinely in asymptomatic patients with NSCLC, owing to inconsistent sensitivity and specificity. Cytologic examination of a pleural effusion visible on both chest radiography and CT scanning is recommended for nonsurgical candidates. Often, pleural effusions seen only on chest radiography are too small to accommodate the performance of a thoracentesis.

STAGING SYSTEM

The overriding influence of performance status as a determinant of survival cannot be overemphasized. Generally, weight loss has been considered an important poor prognostic indicator, using a cut-off of 5% to 10% [46]. Female patients have better survival rates than do male patients [47]. Other factors (e.g., LDH, alkaline phosphatase, and serum sodium levels, white blood cell count, loss of blood group antigens, and the ability to stop smoking) have been associated with outcome [48, 49]. Patients with favorable factors are more likely to undergo attempts at curative surgical resection, whereas those with less favorable factors are sent for irradiation. Thus, retrospective comparisons cannot answer questions about which local modality provides superior outcome.

For NSCLC, the TNM (*t*umor, *n*ode, *m*etastasis) staging system described by Mountain [50] in 1986 has been adopted internationally and recently was modified to a minor degree [51]. The American Joint Committee on Cancer also has adopted this classification (Tables 11.4, 11.5), which was derived from evaluation of outcomes from patients treated with surgery.

Size of lesions plays a minor role in the staging system of lung cancer. The 3.0-cm determinant separates T1 lesions from T2 lesions, but criteria of invasion of adjacent lobes, atelectasis, or other nodules in the lobe

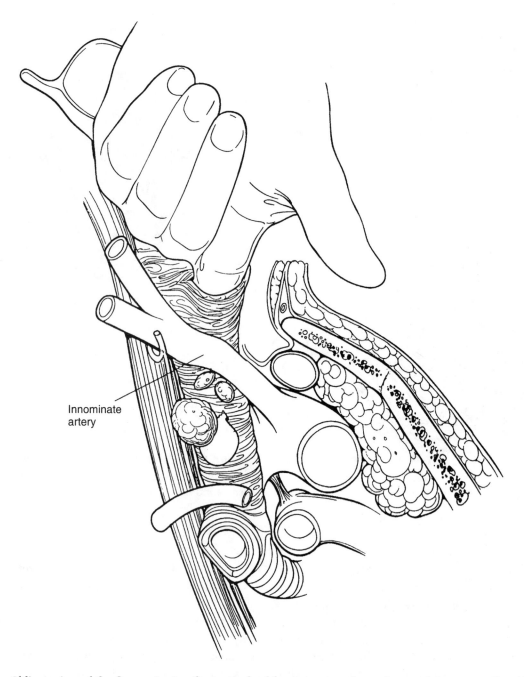

Innominate
artery

Figure 11.9   Oblique view of the finger piercing the pretracheal fascia to enter the node-containing space. Considerable blunt dissection of enlarged lymph nodes can be accomplished with this maneuver.

or lung can influence the T stage. The designation T3 conveys invasiveness into a resectable structure or proximity to the carina, with chest wall involvement, resulting in a prognosis more favorable than that of central lesions that may involve the mediastinal pleura or main stem bronchus [52]. T4 tumors produce cytologically positive pleural effusions or invade adjacent struc-

tures, such as a vertebral body and mediastinal and vascular structures.

The N stage divides nodes into those within the ipsilateral pleural reflection (N1), those within the ipsilateral mediastinum (N2), or those involving the contralateral mediastinum or supraclavicular region (N3; Fig. 11.13) [23, 53]. N3 nodal status is a contraindication for

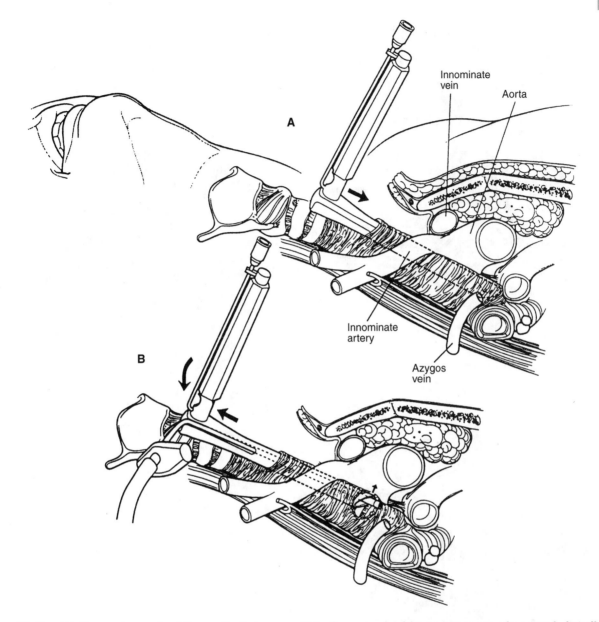

Figure 11.10 (A) The passive angle of the mediastinoscopy within the pretracheal fascia, not previously opened, digitally aims the bevel directly at the trachea. (B) The scope is angled anteriorly to tense fascia so that fascia can be penetrated with a sucker. The innominate artery is subjected to compression during this maneuver.

surgery, because patients at this stage are at higher risk for systemic disease. Nodes outside these regions are considered distant metastases.

The value of surgical staging is for prognosis, because significant discordance occurs between clinical and pathologic stages of NSCLC (Fig. 11.14) [43]. The specific location, number of nodes involved at each level, and presence or absence of nodal capsular extension by tumor cells may influence prognoses [54]. Multiple positive nodes and multiple positive nodal stations are poor prognostic indicators [55].

The staging system used most widely for small-cell carcinoma has been the two-stage system suggested by the Veterans Administration Lung Cancer Group. Limited-stage disease is defined as that which can be encompassed in a tolerable irradiation field. This definition includes tumors confined to one hemithorax and its regional lymph nodes, including the ipsilateral mediastinal, ipsilateral supraclavicular, and contralateral hilar lymph nodes. Extensive stage is any extent of disease beyond that classification.

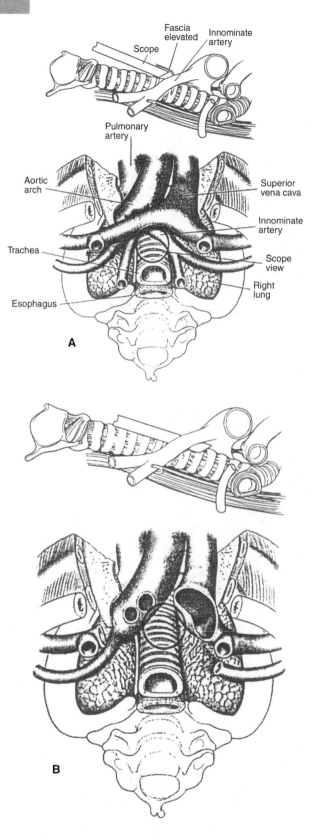

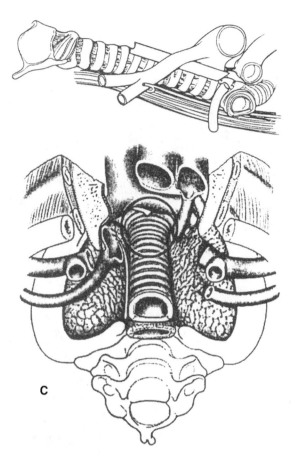

Figure 11.11 Craniocaudal (surgeon's orientation) and corresponding lateral views of superior mediastinal and adjacent structures at three levels: (A) proximal tunnel, (B) midtrachea, and (C) distal trachea and carina. Circles outline potential views through the mediastinoscope at each level, depending on the anteroposterior and lateral angulation of the instrument. (Reprinted with permission from RB Ponn, JA Federico, Mediastinoscopy and staging. In LR Kaiser, IL Kron, TL Spray [eds], *Mastery of Cardiothoracic Surgery*. Philadelphia: Lippincott-Raven, 1998:11–27.)

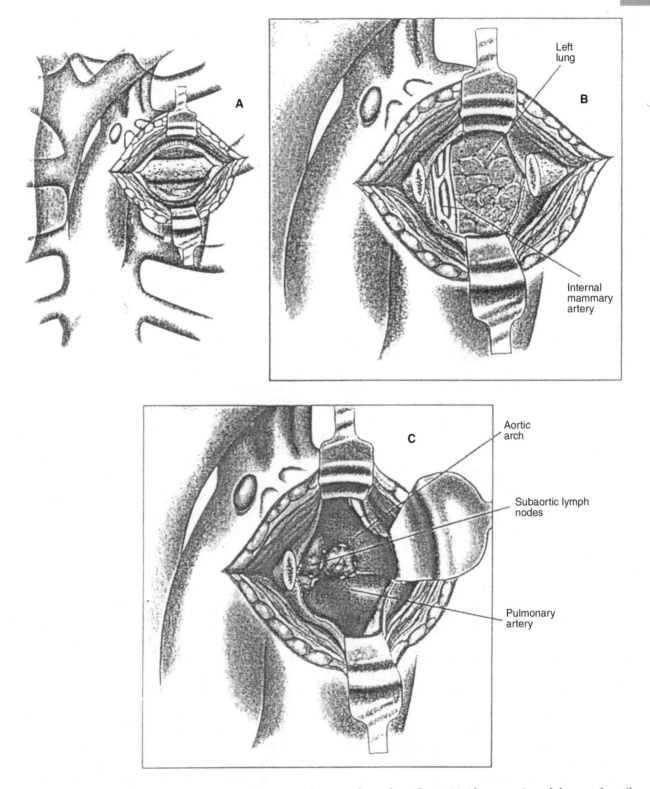

Figure 11.12 Anterior mediastinotomy. (A) Incision over the second costal cartilage. (B) After resection of the costal cartilage. (C) View of enlarged subaortic lymph nodes. (Reprinted with permission from RB Ponn, JA Federico, Mediastinoscopy and staging. In LR Kaiser, IL Kron, TL Spray [eds], *Mastery of Cardiothoracic Surgery*. Philadelphia: Lippincott-Raven, 1998:11–27.)

Table 11.4 TNM Staging for Lung Cancer

Classification	Definition
Primary tumor (T)	
TX	Primary tumor cannot be assessed or tumor proved by the presence of malignant cells in sputum or bronchial washings but not visualized by imaging or bronchoscopy
T0	No evidence of primary tumor
Tis	Carcinoma in situ
T1	Tumor ≤ 3 cm in greatest dimension, surrounded by lung or visceral pleura, without bronchoscopic evidence of invasion more proximal than the lobar bronchus (i.e., not in the main bronchus)
T2	Tumor with any of the following features of size or extent: > 3 cm in greatest dimension; involves main bronchus (≥ 2 cm distal to carina); invades the visceral pleura; associated with atelectasis or obstructive pneumonitis that extends to the hilar region but does not involve the entire lung
T3	Tumor of any size that directly invades any of the following: chest wall (including superior sulcus tumors), diaphragm, mediastinal pleura, parietal pericardium; or tumor in the main bronchus < 2 cm distal to the carina but without involvement of the carina; associated atelectasis or obstructive pneumonitis of the entire lung
T4	Tumor of any size that invades any of the following: mediastinum, heart, great vessels, trachea, esophagus, vertebral body, carina; or separate tumor nodules in the same lobe; or tumor with a malignant pleural effusion
Regional lymph nodes (N)	
NX	Regional lymph nodes cannot be assessed
N0	No regional lymph node metastasis
N1	Metastasis to ipsilateral peribronchial and/or ipsilateral hilar lymph nodes, and intrapulmonary nodes, including involvement by direct extension of the primary tumor
N2	Metastasis to ipsilateral mediastinal and/or subcarinal lymph node(s)
N3	Metastasis to contralateral mediastinal, contralateral hilar, ipsilateral or contralateral scalene, or supraclavicular lymph node(s)
Distant metastasis (M)	
MX	Distant metastasis cannot be assessed
M0	No distant metastasis
M1	Distant metastasis present, including separate tumor nodules in a different lobe (ipsilateral or contralateral)

Source: Used with permission of the American Joint Committee on Cancer (AJCC), Chicago, Illinois. Reprinted from ID Fleming, JS Cooper, DE Henson, et al. (eds), *AJCC Cancer Staging Manual* (5th ed). Philadelphia: Lippincott-Raven, 1997:127–133.

TREATMENT FOR SCLC

Limited-Stage SCLC

Therapy for SCLC is based on chemotherapy and radiotherapy. Two meta-analyses have shown a local control and survival benefit (approximately 5%) with the addition of thoracic radiotherapy (TRT) to chemotherapy [56, 57]. Though selected "stage I" limited-stage patients with isolated coin lesions may undergo surgical resection, the incidence of local relapse is significant [58, 59]. Consequently, adjuvant combination chemotherapy is indicated [60]. Chest irradiation and prophylactic cranial irradiation (PCI) probably should be included in this setting, though few randomized trial data address this clinical scenario. For most patients who have limited-stage disease and are not amenable to initial surgical resection, concomitant radiotherapy and cisplatin-etoposide (PE) combination chemotherapy is a recognized standard [58, 61]. The dose of TRT is 45 to 50 Gy administered in either single daily fractions or twice daily with a 4- to 6-hour interval between 150-cGy fractions [62]. Mature analysis of the US Intergroup Trial comparing a standard TRT fractionation schedule with a hyperfractionated (twice-daily) approach now suggests that survival may be prolonged in selected subsets of individuals receiving the latter schedule [62]. The timing of the combined therapy still is in question, but several prospective, randomized trials suggest that early concurrent therapy is superior [63].

A small subset of select stage I, limited-stage patients—those with isolated coin lesions and no nodes—may benefit from surgical resection [22, 58, 59, 64]. Adjuvant combination chemotherapy is indicated for surgically treated patients [60]. Surgical assessment of the mediastinum before resection is prudent, regardless of CT results. Though useful in a small subset of these patients, surgery remains uncommon in SCLC.

Table 11.5 AJCC Stage Grouping for Lung Cancer

Occult carcinoma	TX	N0	M0
Stage 0	Tis	N0	M0
Stage IA	T1	N0	M0
Stage IB	T2	N0	M0
Stage IIA	T1	N1	M0
Stage IIB	T2	N1	M0
	T3	N0	M0
Stage IIIA	T1	N2	M0
	T2	N2	M0
	T3	N1	M0
	T3	N2	M0
Stage IIIB	Any T	N3	M0
	T4	Any N	M0
Stage IV	Any T	Any N	M1

AJCC = American Joint Committee on Cancer.
Source: Used with permission of the American Joint Committee on Cancer (AJCC), Chicago, Illinois. Reprinted from ID Fleming, JS Cooper, DE Henson, et al. (eds), *AJCC Cancer Staging Manual* (5th ed). Philadelphia: Lippincott-Raven, 1997:127–133.

TRT is considered part of standard therapy for limited-stage SCLC. As with NSCLC, questions that remain unanswered include the relationship between dose, volume, and timing of therapies with survival and local control end points. Timing of modalities embraces two factors: degree of overlap of the modalities (concomitant [both administered at the same time] versus sequential [when no overlap occurs]), and early or late incorporation of the TRT among the cycles of chemotherapy. The alternating strategies provide an amalgam: 1 week of modality A followed by 1 or 2 weeks or more of modality B.

GROWTH FACTOR SUPPORT IN SCLC

Although stem-cell growth factors have been used successfully in extensive-disease SCLC [65], the morbidity requiring this support may vary with the agents used. Cyclophosphamide, etoposide, and vincristine were the combination used to demonstrate that granulocyte colony-stimulating factor decreased morbidity and length of hospital stay. However, the PE regimens produce less hematologic morbidity and at least equal antitumor effect but do not require stem-cell support. The growth factor filgastrim (granulocyte-macrophage colony-stimulating factor) was tested in limited-disease SCLC for its ability to prevent or decrease the duration of neutropenia. Although granulocyte toxicity was reduced modestly, the frequency of grade 4 platelet toxicity unexpectedly increased (25%) [66]. The value of growth factors in this setting is not established.

PROPHYLACTIC CRANIAL IRRADIATION

In most patients who have small-cell carcinoma and achieve a complete clinical response to therapy, the brain is a common site of relapse. Just over half of the affected patients develop clinical brain metastases by 3 years. Such patients benefit from PCI and are at low risk of showing manifestations of brain toxicity (<10% frequency at 3 years). If treatment is delayed until failure, approximately one-half will experience objective responses to palliative whole-brain radiotherapy [67]. Recent European trials have demonstrated that PCI given to patients after achieving a complete response to induction therapy may decrease the relative risk of brain metastasis up to threefold and can result in a 15% reduction in deaths without appreciably increasing late neuropsychiatric sequelae [68–70]. A meta-analysis of seven trials detected a 16% reduction in mortality and a 5.4% increase in 3-year survival in patients who responded completely to induction therapy and went on to receive PCI, as compared to those who did not receive PCI [71]. Late neuropsychiatric changes can be observed in some long-term survivors [72, 73]. A significant portion of such patients may have similar defects prior to receiving PCI [69, 74]. Concomitant brain irradiation and chemotherapy may increase neurotoxicity. Time-dose issues of PCI will be addressed in future clinical trials.

Extensive-Stage SCLC

In patients with extensive-stage disease, (1) PE ± I, (2) cyclophosphamide, doxorubicin, and vincristine (CAV), (3) or alternating PE/CAV is recommended for those with a Zubrod performance status of 2 or less. Recently, topotecan gained US Food and Drug Administration approval [75]. New cytotoxic or cytostatic agents may be appropriate in the context of an investigational clinical trial, especially for those patients with unfavorable prognostic factors. Alternating PE with CAV may yield a survival advantage in selected patients, though randomized studies have yielded conflicting results. For selected patients (i.e., those with brain metastases that may require irradiation as part of their initial treatment), PE or carboplatin plus etoposide may be preferred, owing to the lesser interactive toxicity with concomitantly administered irradiation. Both vinorelbine and the taxanes are active agents in this disease. The addition of TRT may be useful in patients manifesting a complete response in all sites after chemotherapy [76].

Though the general goal of chemotherapy in most

A

B

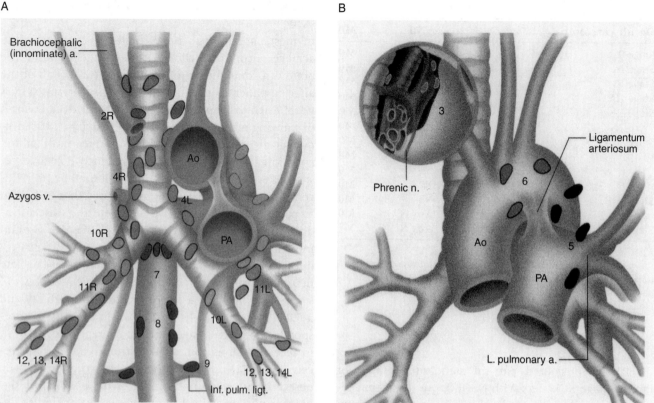

Figure 11.13 (A) Mediastinal lymph nodes and adjacent structures. (B) Aortopulmonary window lymph node region and adjacent structures. *Ao* = aorta; *PA* = pulmonary artery; *Inf. pulm. ligt.* = inferior pulmonary ligament. (C) Lymph node map for TNM staging of lung cancer. **N3 Nodes:** Scalene (or contralateral intrathoracic); **N2 Nodes:** 2R Right upper paratracheal, between the intersection of the innominate artery with the trachea and the lung apex; 2L = Left upper paratracheal, between the top of the aortic arch and the lung apex; 4R = Right lower paratracheal, between the azygos vein and the intersection of the innominate artery with the trachea; 4L = Left lower paratracheal, between the carina and top of the aortic arch, medial to the ligamentum arteriosum; 5 = Aortopulmonary (subaortic and para-aortic), lateral to the aorta, ligamentum arteriosum, or left pulmonary artery and proximal to the first branch of the left pulmonary artery and proximal to the first branch of the left pulmonary artery; 6 = Anterior mediastinal, anterior to the ligamentum arteriosum; 7 = Subcarinal, caudal to the carina and proximal to lower lobe origins; 8 = Paraesophageal, dorsal to trachea, caudal to subcarnial nodes, right or left of midline of esophagus; 9 = Pulmonary ligament, within the pulmonary ligament; 10L = Left tracheobrochial*, between the left upper lobe origin and the carina, medial to the ligamentum arteriosum. **N1 Nodes:** 10R = Right tracheobronchial*, between the right upper lobe origin and the top of the azygos vein; 11 = Interlobar; 12 = Lobar; 13 = Segmental; 14 = Subsegmental. *Classification of the tracheobroncial nodes as N2 or N1 in an area of dispute. Level 10 nodes may be intrapleural on the right but are extrapleural on the left. Hence, the separate categories above. In practical terms for clinical staging, however, we believe that positive nodes accessed by mediastinoscopy, whatever numerical designation one chooses, portend a poor prognosis for primary resection and should prompt consideration of nonoperative or neoadjuvant approaches. (Parts A and B reprinted with permission from American Thoracic Society/European Respiratory Society, Pretreatment evaluation of non-small-cell lung cancer. *Am J Respir Crit Care Med* 156:320–332, 1997. © American Lung Association. Part C reprinted with permission from RB Ponn, JA Federico, Mediastinoscopy and staging. In LR Kaiser, IL Kron, TL Spray [eds], *Mastery of Cardiothoracic Surgery*. Philadelphia: Lippincott-Raven, 1998:11–27.)

C

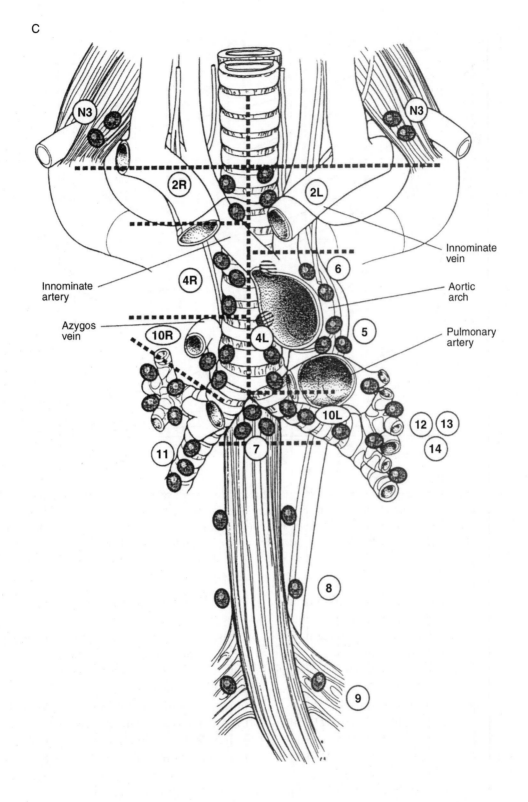

Innominate
vein

Innominate
artery

Aortic
arch

Azygos
vein

Pulmonary
artery

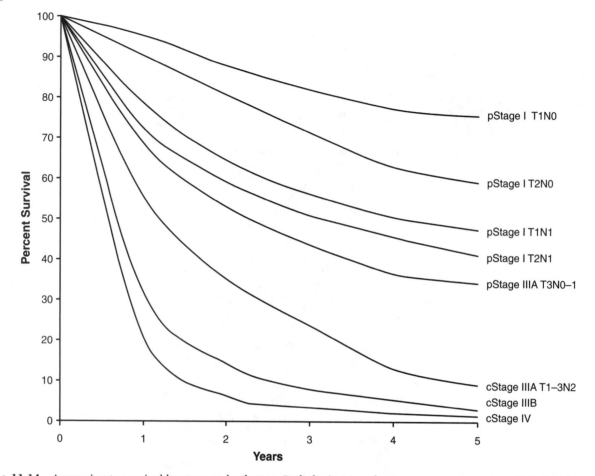

Figure 11.14 Approximate survival by stage and substage. Pathologic (*p*) early stages are contrasted to clinical (*c*) later stages to emphasize the importance of accurate staging. Stage IIIB survival also varies by N3 versus T4, and stage IV survival by intrapulmonary versus intrathoracic metastases. (Reprinted with permission from RB Ponn, JA Federico, Mediastinoscopy and staging. In LR Kaiser, IL Kron, TL Spray [eds], *Mastery of Cardiothoracic Surgery*. Philadelphia: Lippincott-Raven, 1998:11–27.)

patients with extensive-stage disease is effective palliation, some prognostic factors may predict for prolonged objective response and survival. These favorable prognosticators include "regional" metastatic disease, Zubrod performance status of less than 2, normal serum albumin or LDH levels (or both), female gender, presence of "classic" nonneuroendocrine histologic features, age younger than 60 years, and absence of clinical brain metastases [48, 77]. Newer research has suggested that blocking of β_1-integrin-mediated receptors within the stroma of the tumor's extracellular matrix may be the strategy to overcome the drug resistance that develops in most patients [78]. Whether benefit may be derived from "dose-intensive" outpatient chemotherapy and TRT to patients with regional extensive disease (i.e., involving the cervical, ipsilateral axillary, and contralateral supraclavicular nodes; chest wall or pleura-based masses; pericardial or pleural effusions) is under investigation [77].

Elderly Patient Issues in SCLC

Increasing age does not independently predict response to or toxicity and survival from systemic therapy. Single-agent oral etoposide yields response rates in two-thirds of patients, results that may be inferior to those seen with combination chemotherapy. In older patients with a good performance status, combination chemotherapy yields an overall response rate of approximately 70%, with neutropenic sepsis occurring in fewer than 5%. Elderly patients should be treated depending on their general physiologic age. Those with a good performance status and normal renal and hematologic parameters may receive standard chemoradiation for limited-stage disease and combination chemotherapy for extensive-stage disease. For elderly patients who are symptomatic but have other obvious medical co-morbidities, single-agent oral etoposide may be a reasonable option.

TREATMENT FOR NSCLC
Role of Surgery

Surgical resection for early NSCLC remains the treatment of choice. When possible, resection (lobectomy) of the lobe that contains the tumor is the least morbid and most effective procedure and is recommended for most stage I and stage II lesions. The 5-year survival for stage I patients is near 70% [79, 80]. Mortality should be less than 5%. Pneumonectomy is recommended for large, central lesions involving the main stem bronchus or invading the main pulmonary artery. Though accurate staging often may predict whether this operation is necessary, it is common for the intraoperative findings to dictate which definitive operation is required [81]. Morbidity can range from 25% to 50%, with mortality being less than 10% in appropriately selected patients who are operated on by a dedicated thoracic surgical oncologist [82].

A sleeve segmentectomy is a reasonable option to pneumonectomy for lesions extending from the lobar orifice to the main stem bronchus (Fig. 11.15) [83, 84]. Sleeve pneumonectomy is an extended resection that includes the caudal portion of the trachea, carina, tracheobronchial angle, and involved lung parenchyma [83]. The airway is reconstructed by anastomosis of the contralateral main stem bronchus to the caudal trachea. Mortality may approach 15% to 20%.

Lung conservation procedures, such as wedge resection (a nonanatomic removal of involved peripheral lung tissue) or segmentectomy (an anatomic resection that includes the bronchus, pulmonary artery, pulmonary vein, and involved lung parenchyma), are compromises that can be used in some patients with suboptimal pulmonary reserve, but these procedures increase the likelihood of local failure [85].

The role of video-assisted thoracoscopic surgery is being studied both as an invasive diagnostic technique and as a procedure to resect lesions [86]. This procedure avoids thoracotomy, although it remains unclear whether overall operative time, surgical morbidity, and length of hospital stay are as favorable as stated in preliminary reports. Video-assisted thoracoscopic surgery is too new to endorse as an ordinary procedure; its exact role will evolve [87].

Contraindications to surgical resection include extrathoracic metastatic disease, positive contralateral mediastinal or supraclavicular lymph nodes (N3 disease), malignant pleural effusion, compromise of the vocal cords due to recurrent laryngeal nerve impairment, superior vena cava obstruction due to tumor, or suboptimal cardiopulmonary function. Age alone is not a contraindication to potentially curative surgery in early-stage NSCLC. The issue as to whether a patient's race may be a factor in receiving surgery for early-stage NSCLC has been raised [88].

Definitive Radiotherapy

Once the standard treatment for all medically or surgically inoperable (locally advanced or stage III) patients, the role of radiotherapy as a single modality is more limited with the emergence of more effective systemic therapy. The Radiation Therapy Oncology Group study 73–01 compared two methods of 40 to 50 Gy in 5 weeks and 60 Gy in 6 weeks [89, 90]. The 60-Gy dose demonstrated improved short-term results over the lower doses and had been considered a standard. However, a recent failure analysis, which included aggressive post-therapy restaging, documented a 92% local failure rate at 5 years after the use of 60 Gy [91]. Moreover, the use of large-volume TRT ports that cover regional lymphatics in both hila, both sides of the trachea, and (commonly) both supraclavicular nodes limits the effective dose and increases toxicity.

By using three-dimensional treatment-planning technology, the target volume can be delineated more accurately (Color Plate 11.1) [92]. Consequently, the proportion of normal tissue can be decreased within radiotherapy portals.

Patients with multilevel nodes, extracapsular nodes, and clinical involvement at the supraclavicular and central hilar locations are likely to develop distant disease. For medically inoperable stage I NSCLC, definitive radiotherapy has yielded 5-year survival rates of approxi-

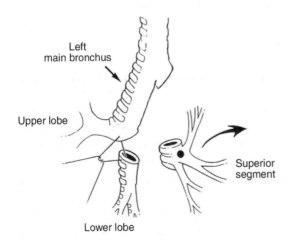

Figure 11.15 Sleeve segmentectomy of superior segment of the left lower lobe.

mately 20% to 40%, still an improvement as compared to past results [93].

Adjuvant (Postoperative) Radiotherapy

TRT is used as an adjunct to potentially curative resection to increase locoregional control. The relative indications for treatment include positive surgical margins, positive regional lymph nodes (N1 and N2), extracapsular lymph node invasion, or lesions that were T3 or T4 (invasion of an adjacent or unresectable structure). A recent meta-analysis reported a significant adverse effect of TRT after resection for patients with disease at stages I, II, N0, and N1 [94]. The statistical limitations inherent in meta-analyses call these results into question [95]. Patients with pathologically negative nodes or a primary tumor confined to the lung parenchyma do not benefit from TRT.

Adjuvant Systemic Therapy for Early-Stage NSCLC

The role of adjuvant systemic chemotherapy for resected stage I and stage II NSCLC remains elusive. A number of randomized trials have been carried out over the last several years, comparing surgery alone with surgery plus adjuvant chemotherapy. At present, adjuvant chemotherapy is recommended best in the context of a clinical trial. With the recent introduction of several drugs with encouraging activity in metastatic NSCLC (e.g., carboplatin, paclitaxel, docetaxel, vinorelbine tartrate, gemcitabine, and irinotecan), clinical trials have been incorporating these agents in an adjuvant setting. Though generating renewed optimism, adjuvant chemotherapy in resectable early-stage NSCLC remains investigational.

Stage III (Locally Advanced) or Regional Disease

Stage III or locally advanced lung cancer accounts for roughly 45,000 cases of the estimated 150,000 cases of lung cancer per year in the United States. Stage III cancer is subdivided into two subtypes: stage IIIA (T1–T2, N2 or T3, N1–N2) and stage IIIB (T4 or N3; see Table 11.5). Stage IIIA disease is associated with a median survival of 12 months and a 5-year survival of 15% to 30%. Though locally advanced, it is potentially a resectable disease. Stage IIIB implies unresectable disease and

is associated with a median survival of 8 months and a 5-year survival of less than 5%. At present, definitive management of stage III disease for patients with acceptable performance status usually involves multi-modality therapy. What constitutes the standard multimodality approach remains controversial and is in a state of flux. Current dilemmas revolve around the role of surgery, the use of induction chemotherapy or chemoradiotherapy, issues regarding sequential or concurrent treatment, and determination of the ideal combination chemotherapeutic regimen. What has become clear is that the extent of N1 and N2 nodal station involvement or chest wall involvement (or both) has a significant bearing on overall prognosis [55, 96–101].

Role of Combined-Modality Approaches

Neoadjuvant combination chemotherapy followed by definitive local therapy in the form of TRT represents an established standard for stage III NSCLC [102, 103]. In good-performance-status patients who experienced less than 5% weight loss and had clinical stage III NSCLC, two cycles of neoadjuvant cisplatin and vinblastine followed by 60 Gy TRT were superior to irradiation alone. A larger trial [104] validated this approach by reporting a 5-year survival of 17% in the treatment arm involving sequential chemotherapy followed by 60 Gy TRT, as compared to a 10% 5-year survival in the cohort treated with 60 Gy alone.

The role of surgical resection in stage III patients is undergoing clarification. Trials have compared the role of surgery alone or chemotherapy (either combined mitomycin, ifosfamide, and cisplatin, or combined cyclophosphamide, etoposide, and cisplatin) before definitive surgery [105, 106]. Both trials' results suggest that surgery alone is not better than what would be expected from TRT alone to 60 Gy. These results support the use of neoadjuvant platinum-based chemotherapy followed by curative surgical resection as one therapeutic option in patients with good performance status.

Concomitant chemoradiotherapy has been used preoperatively. Most phase II studies have not required surgical staging [107]. A North American cooperative group pilot study of surgical stage IIIA and stage IIIB NSCLC patients administered concomitant chemoradiotherapy (45 Gy plus concurrent etoposide-cisplatin) followed by surgery 4 to 6 weeks later. An almost equivalent outcome was observed for both IIIA and IIIB patients [45]. Patients who fail to obtain a complete nodal response to neoadjuvant therapy have a lower survival rate than that of patients who respond completely. These results call into question the value of surgery in this patient population. An ongoing randomized prospective trial of the PE + 45 Gy followed by surgery versus PE + 61 Gy without surgery is attempting to answer this question. Newer cytotoxic agents are being tested with TRT.

Stage IV Metastatic Disease

Patients with disseminated stage IV NSCLC have a dismal prognosis and a median survival of 17 to 20 weeks. The approach is palliative, and treatment options include use of systemic chemotherapy (single-agent versus combination), supportive care, and selective radiotherapy. Controversy continues regarding the role of chemotherapy versus best supportive care. Recent trials and meta-analyses comparing cisplatin-based regimens with best supportive care demonstrate that combination chemotherapy is associated with a modest but significant improvement in survival and that chemotherapy improves quality of life [108]. Therefore, most physicians offer combination chemotherapy to good-performance-status patients. Current chemotherapy regimens include such drugs as carboplatin-taxol, cisplatin-gemcitabine, cisplatin-Navelbine (vinorelbine tartrate), and others [75, 108, 109]. No combination regimen appears convincingly superior to another and, if possible, affected patients should be enrolled in clinical trials. Trials combining some of the aforementioned cytotoxic agents with novel cytostatic compounds directed to specific molecular defects are under way in patients with advanced disease. For patients with compromised performance status and significant weight loss, supportive care probably is a better alternative.

Selective irradiation can be administered also in stage IV patients for symptomatic local sites. Endobronchial laser therapy with either a carbon dioxide or a neodymium–yttrium aluminum garnet (Nd:YAG) laser is indicated if a tumor is obstructing the airway and is unresponsive to standard therapy, if some functional lung tissue remains distal to the obstruction, and if the distal bronchial lumen is identifiable via direct visualization or a probe.

Photodynamic therapy may be used also to palliate large, bulky, obstructing lesions and some early tumors. A hematoporphyrin derivative is administered, localizes to the tumor, and becomes activated with visible light. This modality is not recommended for lesions extending through the bronchial wall or to address mediastinal nodes.

Endobronchial brachytherapy with a ^{192}Ir high-dose-rate remote afterloaded irradiation source temporarily can palliate a mass that is nearly obstructing bronchial lumina. Usually, this form of radiotherapy is recommended for patients with recurrent endobronchial lesions that have received prior external-beam radiotherapy.

Patients presenting with a solitary brain metastasis after a previously resected stage I lesion or individuals presenting with a solitary brain lesion should undergo surgical extirpation followed by external-beam whole-brain radiotherapy. For patients with single or multiple (fewer than five) brain metastases and controlled or absent extracranial disease, stereotactic radiosurgery is a recommended treatment option. Either linear accelerator–based or gamma-knife radiosurgery techniques can be used with equivalent results. Patients with brain lesions and an uncontrolled primary site or a poor performance status (or both) should be started on corticosteroids and should receive palliative whole-brain external-beam radiotherapy [110].

Finally, those patients who develop spinal cord compromise secondary to metastatic disease often can be palliated effectively with short-course external-beam radiotherapy [111]. Those who already have lost bowel or bladder function (or both) or who present with flaccid paralysis are unlikely to regain significant organ function, though many with intact neurologic function may realize a short-term benefit in terms of quality of life.

SUMMARY

Primary lung cancer will continue to be a major public health challenge at the beginning of the twenty-first century. Primary and secondary prevention efforts must continue. Accurate staging and appropriate treatment options can be validated clinically with well-designed clinical trials. Novel breakthroughs involving molecular targeting of malignant cells will help with further definition of optimal diagnostic and treatment paradigms for these common neoplasms.

REFERENCES

1. National Cancer Institute/National Institutes of Health. Stat bite: trends in prevalence of cigarette smoking among U.S. adults. *J Natl Cancer Inst* 91:405, 1999.
2. Schottenfeld D. Epidemiology of lung cancer. In Pass HI, Mitchell JB, Johnson DH, Turrisi AT (eds), *Lung Cancer: Principles and Practice*. Philadelphia: Lippincott-Raven, 1996:305–321.
3. Minna JD. Molecular biology overview. In Pass HI,

Mitchell JB, Johnson DH, Turrisi AT (eds), *Lung Cancer: Principles and Practice.* Philadelphia: Lippincott-Raven, 1996:143–148.

4. Darby SC, Whitley E, Howe GR, et al. Radon and cancers other than lung cancer in underground miners: a collaborative analysis of 11 cases. *J Natl Cancer Inst* 87:378–384, 1995.

5. Lubin JH, Boice JD Jr. Lung cancer risk from residential radon: meta-analysis of eight epidemiologic studies. *J Natl Cancer Inst* 89:49–57, 1997.

6. Auvinen A, Makelainen I, Hakama M, et al. Indoor radon exposure and risk of lung cancer: a nested case-control study in Finland. *J Natl Cancer Inst* 88:966–972, 1996.

7. Alavanja MC, Lubin JH, Mahaffey JA, et al. Residential radon exposure and risk of lung cancer in Missouri. *Am J Public Health* 89:1042–1048, 1999.

8. Yang P, Wentzlaff KA, Katzmann JA, et al. Alpha$_1$-antitrypsin deficiency allele carriers among lung cancer patients. *Cancer Epidemiol Biomarkers Prev* 8:461–465, 1999.

9. Shackney SE, Smith CA, Pollice A, et al. Genetic evolutionary staging of early non–small cell lung cancer: the p53 → HER-2/neu → RAS sequence. *J Thorac Cardiovasc Surg* 118:259–269, 1999.

10. Sozzi G, Sard L, Gregorio L, et al. Association between cigarette smoking and FHIT gene alterations in lung cancer. *Cancer Res* 57:2121–2123, 1997.

11. Tseng JE, Kemp BL, Khuri FR, et al. Loss of FHIT is frequent in stage I non–small cell lung cancer and in the lungs of chronic smokers. *Cancer Res* 59:4798–4803, 1999.

12. Carbone DP. The biology of lung cancer. *Semin Oncol* 24:388–401, 1997.

13. Harpole DH Jr, Marks JR, Richards WG, et al. Localized adenocarcinoma of the lung: oncogene expression of *erbB-2* and *p53* in 150 patients. *Clin Cancer Res* 1:659–664, 1995.

14. Lotan R. Aberrant expression of retinoid receptors and lung carcinogenesis. *J Natl Cancer Inst* 91:989–991, 1999.

15. Picard E, Seguin C, Monhoven N, et al. Expression of retinoid receptor genes and proteins in non-small-cell lung cancer. *J Natl Cancer Inst* 91:1059–1066, 1999.

16. Bunn Jr PA. Imune therapy for lung cancer: Are we getting closer? *Am J Respir Cell Mol Biol* 21:10–12, 1999.

17. World Health Organization. *Histological Typing of Lung Tumors* (2nd ed). Geneva: World Health Organization, 1981.

18. Connelly P. Pathologia Paidion. <http://www.erinet.com/fnadoc/images/pathol~1/lungca~1>

19. Sridhar KS, Lobo CF, Altman RD. Digital clubbing and lung cancer. *Chest* 114:1535–1537, 1998.

20. Okubo K, Mark EJ, Flieder D, et al. Bronchioloalveolar carcinoma: clinical, radiologic, and pathologic factors and survival. *J Thorac Cardiovasc Surg* 118:702–709, 1999.

21. Travis WD, Linder J, Mackey B. Classification, histology, cytology, and electron microscopy. In Pass HI, Mitchell JB, Johnson DH, Turrisi AT (eds), *Lung Cancer: Principles and Practice.* Philadelphia: Lippincott-Raven, 1996:361–395.

22. Fujimori K, Yokoyama A, Kurita Y, et al. A pilot phase 2 study of surgical treatment after induction chemotherapy for resectable stage I to IIIA small cell lung cancer. *Chest* 111:1089–1093, 1997.

23. American Thoracic Society/European Respiratory Society. Pretreatment evaluation of non-small-cell lung cancer. *Am J Respir Crit Care Med* 156:320–332, 1997.

24. Midthun DE, Jett JR. Clinical presentation of lung cancer. In Pass HI, Mitchell JB, Johnson DH, Turrisi AT (eds), *Lung Cancer: Principles and Practice.* Philadelphia: Lippincott-Raven, 1996:421–435.

25. Thomas CR Jr, Rest EB, Brown CR Jr. Rheumatologic manifestations of malignancy. *Med Pediatr Oncol* 18:146–158, 1990.

26. Silvestri GA, Littenberg B, Colice GL. The clinical evaluation for detecting metastatic lung cancer: a meta-analysis. *Am J Respir Crit Care Med* 152:225–230, 1995.

27. Patz EF Jr, Erasmus JJ. Positron emission tomography imaging in lung cancer. *Clin Lung Cancer* 1:42–48, 1999.

28. Salomaa E-R, Liippo K, Taylor P, et al. Prognosis of patients with lung cancer found in a single chest radiograph screening. *Chest* 114:1514–1518, 1999.

29. Strauss GM. The AtBCs of lung cancer screening. *Chest* 114:1502–1505, 1999.

30. Quint LE, Francis IR, Wahl RL, et al. Imaging of lung cancer. In Pass HI, Mitchell JB, Johnson DH, Turrisi AT (eds), *Lung Cancer: Principles and Practice.* Philadelphia: Lippincott-Raven, 1996:437–470.

31. De Leyn P, Vansteenkiste J, Cuypers P, et al. Role of cervical mediastinoscopy in staging of non-small cell lung cancer without enlarged mediastinal lymph nodes on CT scan. *Eur J Cardiothorac Surg* 12:706–712, 1997.

32. Henschke CI, McCauley DI, Yankelevitz DF, et al. Early Lung Cancer Action Project: overall design and findings from baseline screening. *Lancet* 354:99–105, 1999.

33. Chiti A, Schreiner FA, Crippa F, et al. Nuclear medicine procedures in lung cancer. *Eur J Nucl Med* 26:533–555, 1999.

34. Al-Sugair A, Coleman RE. Applications of PET in lung cancer. *Semin Nucl Med* 28:303–319, 1998.

35. Marom EM, McAdams HP, Erasmus JJ, et al. Staging non–small cell lung cancer with whole-body PET. *Radiology* 212:803–809, 1999.

36. Saunders CAB, Dussek JE, O'Dohertly MJ, et al. Evaluation of fluorine-18-fluorodeoxyglucose whole-body positron emission tomography imaging in the staging of lung cancer. *Ann Thorac Surg* 67:790–797, 1999.

37. Vansteenkist JF, Stroobants SG, Dupont PJ, et al. Prognostic importance of the standardized uptake value on 18F-fluoro-2-deoxy-glucose positron emission tomography scan in non-small-cell lung cancer: an analysis of 125 cases. *J Clin Oncol* 17:3201–3206, 1999.

38. Vansteenkiste JF, Stroobants SG, De Leyn PR, et al. Mediastinal lymph node staging with FDG-PET scan in patients with potentially operable non–small cell lung cancer: a prospective analysis of 50 cases. *Chest* 112:1480–1486, 1997.

39. Scott WJ, Shepherd J, Gambhir SS, et al. Cost-effectiveness of FDG-PET for staging non-small cell lung cancer: a decision analysis. *Ann Thorac Surg* 66:1876–1885, 1998.

40. Connelly P. Pathologia Paidion. <http://www.erinet. com/fnadoc/images/pathol~1/lungca~1/bron1a.jpg>

41. Tio TK. Diagnosis and staging of esophageal carcinoma by endoscopic ultrasound. In Meyers MA (ed), *Neoplasms of the Digestive Tract: Imaging, Staging, and Management.* Philadelphia: Lippincott-Raven, 1998:61–70.

42. Gress FG, Savides TJ, Sandler, et al. Endoscopic ultrasonography, fine-needle aspiration biopsy guided by endoscopic ultrasonography, and computed tomography in the preoperative staging of non-small cell lung cancer: a comparison study. *Ann Intern Med* 127:604–612, 1997.

43. Ponn RB, Federico JA. Mediastinoscopy and staging. In Kaiser LR, Kron IL, Spray TL (eds), *Mastery of Cardiothoracic Surgery.* Philadelphia: Lippincott-Raven Publishers, 1998:11–27.

44. De Lyn P, Vansteenkiste J, Deneffe G, et al. Result of induction chemotherapy followed by surgery in patients with stage IIIA N2 NSCLC: importance of pre-treatment mediastinoscopy. *Eur J Cardiothorac Surg* 15:608–614, 1999.

45. Albain KS, Rusch VW, Crowley JJ, et al. Concurrent cisplatin/etoposide plus chest radiotherapy followed by surgery for stages IIIA (N2) and IIIB non-small cell lung cancer: mature results of Southwest Oncology Group phase II study 8805. *J Clin Oncol* 13:1880–1892, 1995.

46. Ihde DC. Non-small cell lung cancer: I. Biology, diagnosis, and staging. *Curr Probl Cancer* 15:61–104, 1991.

47. O'Connell J, Kris M, Gralla R, et al. Frequency and prognostic importance of pretreatment clinical characteristics in patients with advanced non-small cell lung cancer treated with combination chemotherapy. *J Clin Oncol* 4:1604–1614, 1986.

48. Albain KS, Crowley JJ, LeBlanc M, et al. Determinants of improved outcome in small cell lung cancer: an analysis of the 2,580-patient Southwest Oncology Group data base. *J Clin Oncol* 8:1563–1574, 1990.

49. Moore DF Jr, Lee JS. Staging and prognostic factors: non-small cell lung cancer. In Pass HI, Mitchell JB, Johnson DH, Turrisi AT (eds), *Lung Cancer: Principles and Practice.* Philadelphia: Lippincott-Raven, 1996:481–494.

50. Mountain CF. A new international staging system for lung cancer. *Chest* 89(suppl 4):225S–233S, 1986.

51. Mountain CF. Revisions in the international system for staging lung cancer. *Chest* 111:1710–1717, 1997.

52. Detterbeck FC, Socinski MA. IIB or not IIB: the current question in staging non-small cell lung cancer. *Chest* 112:229–234, 1997.

53. Bristol-Myer Co. Bristol-Myer's NSCLC staging sketch [promotional handout for physicians].

54. Vansteenkiste JF, De Leyn PR, Deneffe GJ, et al. Survival and prognostic factors in resected N2 non-small cell lung cancer: a study of 140 cases. *Ann Thorac Surg* 63:1441–1450, 1997.

55. Suzuki K, Nagai K, Yoshida J, et al. The prognosis of surgically resected N2 non-small cell lung cancer: the importance of clinical N status. *J Thorac Cardiovasc Surg* 118:145–153, 1999.

56. Pignon JP, Arriagada R, Ihde DC, et al. A meta-analysis of thoracic radiotherapy early for small-cell lung cancer. *N Engl J Med* 327:1618–1624, 1992.

57. Warde P, Payne D. Does thoracic irradiation improve survival and local control in limited-stage small-cell carcinoma of the lung? A meta-analysis. *J Clin Oncol* 10:890–895, 1992.

58. Ihde D, Souhami B, Comis R, et al. Small cell lung cancer. *Lung Cancer* 17(suppl 1):S19–S21, 1997.

59. Deslauriers J. Surgery for small cell lung cancer. *Lung Cancer* 17(suppl 1):S91–S98, 1997.

60. Angeletti CA, Macchiarini P, Mussi A, et al. Influence of T and stages on long-term survival in resectable small cell lung cancer. *Eur J Surg Oncol* 15:337–340, 1989.

61. McCracken JD, Janaki LM, Crowley JJ, et al. Concurrent chemotherapy/radiotherapy for limited small-cell lung carcinoma: a Southwest Oncology Group study. *J Clin Oncol* 8:892–898, 1990.

62. Turrisi AT III, Kim K, Blum R, et al. Twice-daily compared with once-daily thoracic radiotherapy in limited small-cell lung cancer treated concurrently with cisplatin and etoposide. *N Engl J Med* 340:265–271, 1999.

63. Murray N, Coy P, Hodson I, et al. Importance of timing for thoracic irradiation in the combined modality treatment of limited-stage small-cell lung cancer. The National Cancer Institute of Canada Clinical Trials Group. *J Clin Oncol* 11:336–344, 1993.

64. Eberhardt W, Stamatis G, Stuschke M, et al. Aggressive trimodality treatment including chemoradiation induction and surgery (S) in LD-small-cell lung cancer (LD-SCLC) (Stages I-IIIB)-Long-term results [abstr. no. 1735]. *Proc Am Soc Clin Oncol* 17:450a, 1998.

65. Crawford J, Ozer H, Stoller R, et al. Reduction by granulocyte colony-stimulating factor of fever and neutropenia induced by chemotherapy in patients with small cell lung cancer. *N Engl J Med* 325:164–170, 1991.

66. Bunn PA Jr, Crowley J, Kelly K, et al. Chemoradiotherapy with or without granulocyte-macrophage colony-stimulating factor in the treatment of limited-stage small-cell lung cancer: a prospective phase III randomized study of the Southwest Oncology Group. *J Clin Oncol* 13:1632–1641, 1995.

67. Postmus PE, Haaxma-Reiche H, Gregor A, et al. Brain-only metastases of small cell lung cancer: efficacy of whole brain radiotherapy. An EORTC phase II study. *Radiother Oncol* 46:29–32, 1998.

68. Arriagada R, Le Chevalier T, Borie F, et al. Prophylactic cranial irradiation for patients with small-cell lung cancer in complete remission. *J Natl Cancer Inst* 87:183–190, 1995.

69. Gregor A, Cull A, Stephens RJ, et al. Effects of prophylactic cranial irradiation (PCI) in small cell lung cancer (SCLC); results of UKCCR/EORTC randomized trial. *Proc Am Soc Clin Oncol* 15:A1139, 1996.

70. Arriagada R, Pignon JP, Laplanche A, et al. Prophylactic cranial irradiation for small-cell lung cancer (letter). *Lancet* 349:138, 1997.

71. Auperin A, Arriagada R, Pignon J-P, et al. Prophylactic cranial irradiation for patients with small-cell lung cancer in complete remission. *N Engl J Med* 341:476–484, 1999.

72. Fleck JF, Einhorn LH, Lauer RC, et al. Is prophylactic cranial irradiation indicated in small-cell lung cancer? *J Clin Oncol* 8:209–214, 1990.

73. Lishner M, Feld R, Payne DG, et al. Late neurological complications after prophylactic cranial irradiation in patients with small-cell lung cancer: the Toronto experience. *J Clin Oncol* 8:215–221 1990.

74. Komaki R, Meyers CA, Shin DM, et al. Evaluation of cognitive function in patients with limited small cell lung cancer prior to and shortly following prophylactic cranial irradiation. *Int J Radiat Oncol Biol Phys* 33:179–182, 1995.

75. Pastmus PE, Smit EF. Chemotherapy for brain metastases of lung cancer: a review. *Ann Oncol* 10:753–759, 1999.

76. Jeremic B, Shibamoto Y, Nikolic N, et al. Role of radiation therapy in the combined-modality treatment of patients with extensive disease small-cell lung cancer: a randomized study. *J Clin Oncol* 17:2092–2099, 1999.

77. Murray N. Treatment of small cell lung cancer: the state of the art. *Lung Cancer* 17(suppl 1):S75–S89, 1997.

78. Sethi T, Rintoul RC, Moore SM, et al. Extracellular matrix proteins protect small cell lung cancer cells against apoptosis: a mechanism for small cell lung cancer growth and drug resistance in vivo. *Nature Med* 5:662–668, 1999.

79. Suzuki K, Nagai K, Yoshida J, et al. Prognostic factors in clinical stage I non–small cell lung cancer. *Ann Thorac Surg* 67:927–932, 1999.

80. Harpole DH Jr, Herndon JE II, Yound WG Jr, et al. Stage I non–small cell lung cancer. A multivariate analysis of treatment methods and patterns of recurrence. *Cancer* 76:787–796, 1995.

81. James TW, Faber LP. Indications for pneumonectomy. Pneumonectomy for malignant disease. *Chest Surg Clin North Am* 9:291–309, 1999.

82. Ferguson MK. Preoperative assessment of pulmonary risk. *Chest* 115:58S–63S, 1999.

83. Faber LP. Sleeve resections for lung cancer. *Semin Thorac Cardiovasc Surg* 5:238–248, 1993.

84. Okada M, Tsubota N, Yoshimura M, et al. Extended sleeve lobectomy for lung cancer: the avoidance of pneumonectomy. *J Thorac Cardiovasc Surg* 118:710–714, 1999.

85. Ginsberg RJ, Rubinstein LV. Randomized trial of lobectomy versus limited resection for T1N0 non-small cell lung cancer. Lung Cancer Study Group. *Ann Thorac Surg* 60:615–622, 1995.

86. Landreneau RJ, Mack MJ, Hazelrigg SR. The potential role of video-assisted thoracic surgery in the patient with lung cancer. In Pass HI, Mitchell JB, Johnson DH, Turrisi AT (eds), *Lung Cancer: Principles and Practice*. Philadelphia: Lippincott-Raven, 1996:633–640.

87. Sonett JR. VATS and thoracic oncology: anathema or opportunity. *Ann Thorac Surg* 68:795–796, 1999.

88. Back PB, Cramer LD, Warren JL, et al. Racial differences in the treatment of early-stage lung cancer. *N Engl J Med* 341:1198–1205, 1999.

89. Perez CA, Bauer M, Edelstein S, et al. Impact of tumor control on survival in carcinoma of the lung treated with irradiation. *Int J Radiat Oncol Biol Phys* 12:539–547, 1986.

90. Perez CA, Stanley K, Grundy G, et al. Impact of irradiation technique and tumor control extent in tumor control and survival of patients with unresectable non–oat cell carcinoma of the lung. *Cancer* 50:1091–1099, 1982.

91. Arriagada R, Le Chevalier T, Rekacewicz C, et al. Cisplatin-based chemotherapy (CT) in patients with lo-cally advanced non-small cell lung cancer (NSCLC): late analysis of a French randomized trial. *Proc Am Soc Clin Oncol* 16:A1601, 1997.

92. Leibel SA, Phillips TL (eds), *Textbook of Radiation Oncology*. Philadelphia, Saunders, 1998.

93. Morita K, Fuwa N, Suzuki Y, et al. Radical radiotherapy for medically inoperable non–small cell lung cancer in clinical stage I: a retrospective analysis of 149 patients. *Radiother Oncol* 42:31–36, 1997.

94. PORT Meta-Analysis Trialists Group. Postoperative radiotherapy in non-small-cell lung cancer: systematic review and meta-analysis of individual patient data from nine randomised controlled trials. *Lancet* 352:257–263, 1998.

95. Machtay M, Kaiser LR, Glatstein E. Is meta-analysis really metaphysics? *Chest* 116:539–542, 1999.

96. Yoshino I, Nakanishi R, Osaki T, et al. Unfavorable prognosis of patients with stage II non–small cell lung cancer associated with macroscopic nodal metastases. *Chest* 116:144–149, 1999.

97. Van Velzen E, de la Riviere AB, Elbers HJJ, et al. Type of lymph node involvement and survival in pathologic N1 stage III non–small cell lung carcinoma. *Ann Thorac Surg* 67:903–907, 1999.

98. Riquet M, Manac'h D, Le Pimpec-Barthes F, et al. Prognostic significance of surgical-pathologic N1 disease in non-small cell carcinoma of the lung. *Ann Thorac Surg* 67:1572–1576, 1999.

99. Downey RJ, Martini N, Rusch VW, et al. Extent of chest wall invasion and survival in patients with lung cancer. *Ann Thorac Surg* 68:188–193, 1999.

100. Hagan MP, Choi NC, Mathisen DJ, et al. Superior sulcus lung tumors: impact of local control on survival. *J Thorac Cardiovasc Surg* 117:1086–1094, 1999.

101. York JE, Walsh GL, Lang FF, et al. Combined chest wall resection with vertebrectomy and spinal reconstruction for the treatment of Pancoast tumors. *J Neurosurg (Spine)* 91:74–80, 1999.

102. Dillman RO, Herndon J, Seagren SL, et al. Improved survival in stage III non–small cell lung cancer: seven year follow-up of Cancer and Leukemia Group B (CALGB) 8433 trial. *J Natl Cancer Inst* 88:1175–1177, 1996.

103. Dillman RO, Seagren SL, Propert KJ, et al. A randomized trial of induction chemotherapy plus high-dose radiation versus radiation alone in stage III non–small cell lung cancer. *N Engl J Med* 323:940–945, 1990.

104. Sause WT, Scott C, Taylor S, et al. Radiation Therapy Oncology Group 88–08 and Eastern Cooperative Oncology Group (ECOG) 4588: preliminary results of a phase III trial in regionally advanced, unresectable non–small cell lung cancer. *J Natl Cancer Inst* 87:198–205, 1995.

105. Rosell R, Gomez-Codina J, Camps C, et al. A randomized trial comparing preoperative chemotherapy plus surgery with surgery alone in patients with non-small cell lung cancer. *N Engl J Med* 330:153–158, 1994.

106. Roth JA, Fossella F, Komaki R, et al. A randomized trial comparing perioperative chemotherapy and surgery with surgery alone in resectable stage IIIA non–small cell lung cancer. *J Natl Cancer Inst* 86:673–680, 1994.

107. Vansteenkist JF, De Leyn PR, Deneffe GJ, et al. Clinical

prognostic factors in surgically treated stage IIIA-N2 non–small cell lung cancer: analysis of the literature. *Lung Cancer* 19:3–13, 1998.

108. Johnson DH. Treatment strategies for metastatic non-small-cell lung cancer. *Clin Lung Cancer* 1:34–41, 1999.

109. Carmichael J. Gemcitabine—a new agent in the treatment of non–small cell lung cancer. A commentary. *Lung Cancer* 25:73–75, 1999.

110. Bergqvis M, Brattsom D, Bennmaker H, et al. Irradiation of brain metastases from lung cancer: a retrospective study. *Lung Cancer* 20:57–63, 1998.

111. Kovner F, Spigel S, Rider I, et al. Radiation therapy of metastatic spinal cord compression. Multidisciplinary team diagnosis and treatment. *J Neurooncol* 42:85–92, 1999.

12

Head and Neck Cancer

■ ■ ■

Ashok R. Shaha
Snehal Patel
Daniel Shasha
Louis B. Harrison

Cancer of the head and neck constitutes approximately 4% of all cancers in the United States, and the vast majority are squamous cell carcinomas. Generally, this disease affects the elderly and is associated primarily with long-term abuse of tobacco and with alcohol consumption.

The management of head and neck tumors presents functional and esthetic problems relating to the loss of function of important structures, such as the tongue, mandible, and larynx. The results of surgery in patients with this type of cancer have been improved by such major advances as conservative or partial resections and the use of microvascular free-tissue transfer in reconstruction and by better definition of the roles of chemotherapy and radiotherapy. Despite these advances, the treatment of locoregional recurrence remains a major challenge, as success rates for salvage therapy are poor. Most patients with locoregional recurrence develop progressive disease associated with significant suffering.

Effective management of patients with head and neck cancer consists of a true multidisciplinary approach involving head and neck surgeons, medical oncologists, radiation therapists, neurosurgeons, plastic surgeons, oral surgeons, maxillofacial prosthodontists, speech therapists, nutritionists, clinical nurses, pain service, neurology service, and social workers.

TOPOGRAPHIC ANATOMY OF THE HEAD AND NECK

The major sites of the upper aerodigestive tract affected by head and neck cancer are the oral cavity, pharynx, paranasal sinuses, larynx, thyroid gland, and salivary glands (Fig. 12.1). Because they behave differently and display histologic features that are different from the other tumors in this region, tumors of the salivary glands are addressed in a separate section at the end of

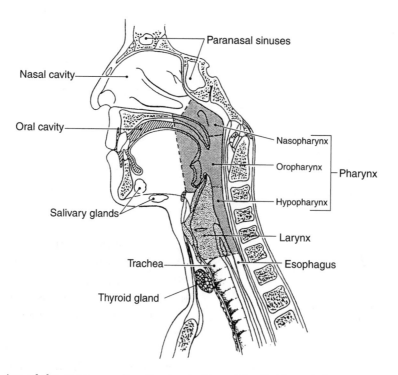

Figure 12.1   Sagittal section of the upper aerodigestive tract. (Copyright © 1993 of the Massachusetts Medical Society. All rights reserved. Reprinted with permission from EE Vokes, RR Weichselbaum, SM Lippman, WK Hong, Head and neck cancer. *N Engl J Med* 328:184–194, 1993.)

this chapter. Tumors of the thyroid gland are discussed in Chapter 27.

The oral cavity extends from the skin-vermilion junction of the lips to the junction of the hard and soft palate above and the line of the circumvallate papillae below. It is divided into specific subsites: lip, buccal mucosa, lower and upper alveolar ridges, retromolar trigone, floor of the mouth, hard palate, and anterior two-thirds of the tongue (oral tongue). Usually, lymphatic drainage from the oral cavity is orderly, and metastatic spread to the neck generally occurs in a predictable and stepwise fashion. The first-station cervical lymph nodes for anterior sites in the oral cavity are the level I nodes (submental and submaxillary), and metastasis then proceeds to levels II (upper deep cervical nodes) and III (middle deep cervical nodes). Lymphatic metastases from the tongue can involve the jugulodigastric nodes at level II or the juguloomohyoid nodes at levels III and IV directly, without involvement of the intervening levels. "Skip" metastases, however, are rare, and involvement of levels IV and V in the absence of positive nodes at more proximal levels occurs in fewer than 5% of patients [1].

The pharynx is divided into the nasopharynx, the oropharynx, and the hypopharynx (Table 12.1). The oropharynx includes the base of the tongue, vallecula, soft palate, tonsil and tonsillar fossa, and posterior pha-

ryngeal wall. The region of the nasopharynx extends from the level above the junction of the hard and soft palate to the base of the skull. The hypopharynx includes three areas: the pyriform sinus, the posterior pharyngeal wall extending from the level of the vallecula to the level of the cricoarytenoid joints, and the postcricoid area, which extends from the level of the arytenoid cartilages to the inferior border of the cricoid cartilage. The main routes of lymphatic drainage from the pharynx depend on the site of a primary tumor: The nasopharynx drains into the nodes of the upper part of the posterior triangle, the oropharynx to nodes at level II (jugulodigastric and upper deep cervical), and the hypopharynx to nodes at levels II, III (middle deep cervical), and IV (lower deep cervical). Some primary sites (e.g., the base of tongue) have a propensity to bilateral lymphatic metastasis, a tendency common also in lesions that involve or approach the midline. Tumor (T) staging of lesions at some sites (e.g., the nasopharynx and hypopharynx) takes into account the number of subsites involved in contrast to tumors of the oral cavity and oropharynx, which are staged according to the size of the lesion, mainly because of the difficulty in measuring the exact extent of lesions at these sites.

Anatomically, lesions of the larynx are classified as supraglottic, glottic, and subglottic. Primary tumors of the subglottic region are extremely rare (approximately

Table 12.1 Subsites in Head and Neck Areas

Oral cavity
  Lips (upper, lower)
  Buccal mucosa
  Floor of mouth
  Oral tongue
  Hard palate
  Gingivae (upper, lower, retromolar trigone)

Oropharynx
  Faucial arch
  Tonsillar fossa, tonsil
  Base of tongue
  Pharyngeal wall

Nasopharynx
  Posterosuperior wall
  Lateral wall

Hypopharynx
  Pyriform fossa
  Postcricoid area
  Posterior wall

Larynx
  Supraglottis
    Ventricular bands (false cords)
    Arytenoids
    Suprahyoid epiglottis (both lingual and laryngeal
      aspects)
    Infrahyoid epiglottis
  Glottis (true vocal cords, including anterior and posterior
    commissures)
  Subglottis

Source: Used with the permission of the *American Joint Committee on Cancer (AJCC®)*, Chicago. *AJCC® Cancer Staging Manual* (5th Edition), 1997. Philadelphia: Lippincott-Raven.

1% of laryngeal tumors) in contrast to the much more common occurrence of a glottic tumor extending into the subglottis. The true vocal cord (glottis) has a very sparse lymphatic network; consequently, lymphatic metastases are uncommon. However, when glottic tumors extend to involve the adjacent supraglottic or subglottic areas, they have a high propensity to metastasize to the jugular chain and tracheoesophageal groove lymph nodes. The supraglottic larynx has a rich lymphatic drainage, and tumors of this region often metastasize bilaterally.

The nasal cavity extends from the vestibule anteriorly to the nasopharynx posteriorly and from the nasal septum medially to the turbinates laterally. The middle meatus, which lies between the middle and inferior turbinates, drains the frontal, maxillary, and ethmoid sinuses. Blockage of these openings by tumor may cause symptoms of sinusitis and radiologic opacification of the sinuses.

Cancer of the maxillary sinus is the most common paranasal sinus tumor. Other sites affected in this region include the ethmoid sinuses, nasal cavity, and sphenoid sinus. Neoplasms of the sphenoid and frontal sinuses are very rare. The maxillary antrum is divided into an anteroinferior (infrastructure) and a superoposterior portion (suprastructure) by an imaginary plane—Ohngren's line—joining the medial canthus of the eye to the angle of the mandible. Infrastructure tumors generally are treated by partial maxillectomy and rehabilitation generally involves the use of prosthetic obturators. In contrast, tumors of the suprastructure are in closer proximity to the orbit and skull base, and their treatment involves additional considerations, including resection and reconstruction of the orbital floor and management of the eye itself. Approximately 15% of patients with tumors of the maxillary sinus will present with metastases to the regional lymph nodes at levels I (submandibular) and II (upper deep cervical).

The major salivary glands are the parotid, submaxillary, and sublingual. Tumors arising in the minor salivary (mucus-secreting) glands of the upper aerodigestive tract are not staged as salivary tumors but are staged according to the respective T staging of the particular site of origin.

The lymph nodes of the neck can be divided into various groups (Figs. 12.2, 12.3): preauricular and parotid group, submental and submandibular group, deep jugular lymph nodes, supraclavicular lymph nodes, lymph nodes along the accessory nerve in the posterior triangle, occipital group, and lymph nodes in the tracheoesophageal groove and superior mediastinum. The Memorial Sloan-Kettering Cancer Center classification, which groups cervical lymph nodes into five levels (Fig. 12.4), has stood the test of time and remains anatomically relevant and clinically reproducible after more than half a century of use [2, 3]. Level I includes lymph nodes in the submandibular triangle; levels II, III, and IV are the upper, middle, and lower jugular nodes; and level V includes nodes in the posterior triangle of the neck. The nodes of the anterior compartment of the neck (prelaryngeal, pretracheal, and paratracheal nodes) have been labeled as level VI, and nodes in the superior mediastinum are designated as level VII.

Over the last few decades, the management of cervical lymph node metastasis has undergone many changes. For more than the first three-fourths of this century, the classic radical neck dissection, popularized by George Crile in 1906, was commonly used. However, with improved understanding of the anatomy and patterns of cervical nodal metastasis came the realization that routine sacrifice of structures not directly invaded

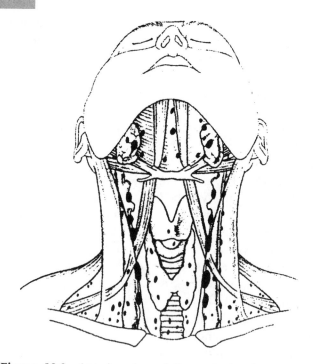

Figure 12.2 Anterior view of the neck showing regional lymph node groups. (Reprinted with permission from JP Shah, J Medina, AR Shaha, et al., Cervical lymph node metastasis. *Curr Probl Surg* 30:273–344, 1993.)

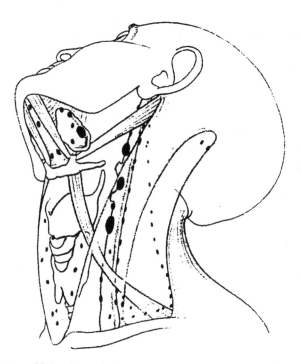

Figure 12.3 Lateral view of the neck showing regional lymph node groups. (Reprinted with permission from JP Shah, J Medina, AR Shaha, et al., Cervical lymph node metastasis. *Curr Probl Surg* 30:273–344, 1993.)

by tumor does not result in better control. In addition, the results of surgical treatment now are judged as much by survival results as by the quality of life, and the pendulum swung in favor of more conservative operations with preservation of the uninvolved accessory nerve, the sternomastoid muscle, and the internal jugular vein. It now is possible to evaluate the biology of the tumor and its spread, and a more specifically tailored surgical procedure can be performed for individual patients in most instances. The routine use of postoperative radiotherapy for positive cervical node findings also affected modified neck dissections and better regional control.

EPIDEMIOLOGIC CHARACTERISTICS AND RISK FACTORS

Head and neck tumors account for approximately 5% of the overall incidence of cancer in the United States and 2% of all cancer deaths (Figs. 12.5, 12.6) [4]. Worldwide, approximately 500,000 new cases of head and neck cancer are projected annually. Tumors of the upper aerodigestive tract occur mostly in the fifth and sixth decades of life and predominantly affect men. However, a recent rising trend in incidence has been

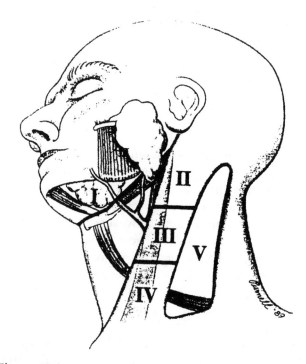

Figure 12.4 Diagram of the neck showing levels of lymph nodes. Level I, submandibular; level II, high jugular; level III, midjugular; level IV, low jugular; level V, posterior jugular. Levels VI (tracheoesophageal) and VII (superior mediastinal) not shown. (Reprinted with permission from JP Shah, J Medina, AR Shaha, et al., Cervical lymph node metastasis. *Curr Probl Surg* 30:273–344, 1993.)

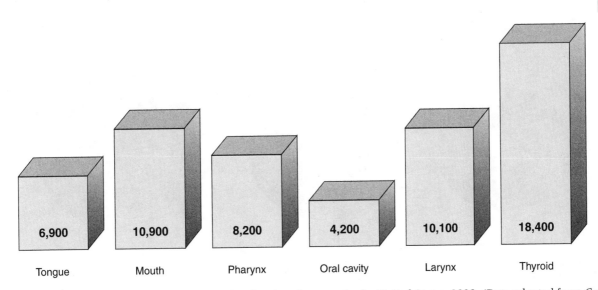

Figure 12.5   Estimated number of new cases of head and neck cancer in the United States, 1999. (Data adapted from Greenlee RT, Murray T, Bolden S, Wingo PA. Cancer statistics, 2000. *CA Cancer J Clin* 50:7–33, 2000.)

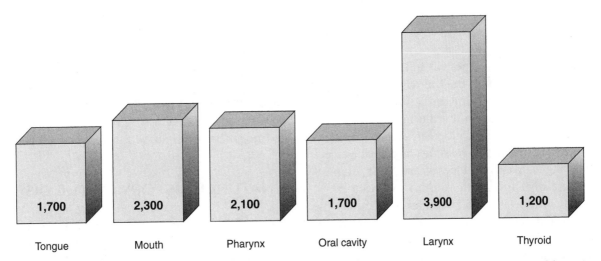

Figure 12.6   Estimated number of deaths due to head and neck cancer in the United States, 1999. (Data adapted from Greenlee RT, Murray T, Bolden S, Wingo PA. Cancer statistics, 2000. *CA Cancer J Clin* 50:7–33, 2000.)

seen among women; over the last decade, patients in their third and fourth decades have presented with head and neck cancer, especially of the tongue and oral cavity. Approximately half of all squamous cell carcinomas of the upper aerodigestive tract occur in the oral cavity. Cancers of the nasopharynx and hypopharynx are extremely common in Southeast Asia, Hong Kong, and southern China, whereas tumors of the oral cavity and base of the tongue are more common in India.

The most important risk factors for this disease are tobacco and alcohol, and approximately 80–85% of patients report a significant history of tobacco and alcohol consumption. Oral carcinogenesis has been correlated strongly with the use of smokeless tobacco. Alcohol

seems to have a synergistic effect on the carcinogenic potential of tobacco. Experimental evidence has suggested that ethanol suppresses the efficiency of DNA repair after exposure to nitrosamine compounds. In India, chewing betel nut with lime and catechu (in a quid of betel leaf called *paan*) is a common habit that has been associated with a high incidence of oral cancer, especially of the buccal mucosa. Chronic abuse of snuff and marijuana has also been linked to head and neck carcinogenesis.

Dietary factors include nutritional deficiency, especially in alcoholics. The Plummer-Vinson syndrome, which includes esophageal web, iron-deficiency anemia, and dysphagia, is associated with a high incidence

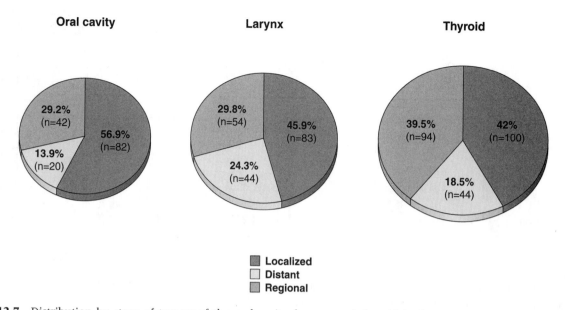

Oral cavity

Larynx

Thyroid

- Localized
- Distant
- Regional

Figure 12.7 Distribution by stage of tumors of the oral cavity, larynx, and thyroid in the United States, 1983–1987. (Data adapted from Landis SH, Murray T, Bolden S, Wingo PA. Cancer statistics, 1999. *CA Cancer J Clin* 49:8–31, 1999.)

of postcricoid carcinoma, especially in Europe. This condition is very rarely seen in the United States. Epidemiologic data suggest a protective role for dietary carotenoids and for consumption of fruits and vegetables.

Occupations associated with greater risk of head and neck cancer include nickel refining (laryngeal cancer), woodworking (cancers of the nasal cavity and paranasal sinuses), and steel and textile workers (oral cancer).

Genetic predisposition to head and neck cancer has been suggested by its sporadic occurrence in young adults and in nonusers of tobacco and alcohol. Mutagen-induced chromosomal fragility is an independent risk factor and correlates with the prospective development of second primary tumors. A subset of patients may have genetic anomalies that increase their susceptibility to tobacco- or alcohol-induced carcinogenesis [5]. Genetic instability associated with the Bloom syndrome and the Li-Fraumeni syndrome has been implicated in head and neck carcinogenesis through an increase in the susceptibility of affected individuals to environmental carcinogens.

Increasing evidence suggests a role for viruses in the development of head and neck cancer. Nasopharyngeal cancer has been linked strongly to the Epstein-Barr virus, and viral DNA has been identified in nasopharyngeal tissue, along with elevated titers of IgG and IgA antibodies in affected patients [6]. Human papillomavirus (HPV) infection also has been linked to head and neck carcinogenesis. On the basis of the most sensitive method

of detection, the polymerase chain reaction, the overall prevalence of HPV in head and neck tumors approaches 35%. HPV types 16 and 18 have been associated with a higher risk, but conclusive proof of the mechanism of carcinogenesis will require further research [7].

NATURAL HISTORY OF THE DISEASE

Although the diagnosis of most head and neck cancers is relatively easy, only one-third of affected patients present at an early disease stage (i.e., I or II). Approximately half of patients present with locally advanced disease, either at the primary site or in the cervical lymph nodes (Fig. 12.7). The pattern of lymph node metastasis from primary tumors of the head and neck is understood better as a result of the studies conducted by Shah [8] (Tables 12.2, 12.3). Generally, such a metastatic pattern is predictable on the basis of the site of the primary tumor.

The sites of distant metastasis from head and neck primaries are well recognized also. The lungs are the most common site. However, an important distinction is that a solitary pulmonary nodule in patients with head and neck cancer most likely is a second primary tumor rather than metastatic cancer. The presence of multiple pulmonary nodules, on the other hand, is suggestive of metastatic disease. Other sites of distant metastasis include the mediastinal lymph nodes, liver,

Table 12.2 Distribution and Histologic Confirmation of Metastatic Disease by Site

Primary Site	No. of Patients	No. of RNDs	Positive Nodes in Elective RNDs (%)	Positive Nodes in Therapeutic RNDs (%)
Oral cavity	501	516	34	76
Oropharynx	207	213	31	84
Hypopharynx	126	128	17	97
Larynx	247	262	37	84
Total	1,081	1,119	33	82

RND = radical neck dissection.

Note: Results for 1,081 patients undergoing 1,119 elective and therapeutic radical neck dissections.

Source: Reprinted from JP Shah, Patterns of cervical lymph node metastasis from squamous carcinoma of the upper aerodigestive tract. *Am J Surg* 160:405–409, 1990, with permission from Excerpta Medica, Inc.

brain, and bones. The incidence of distant metastasis varies with the primary site; tumors of the nasopharynx and hypopharynx are at highest risk. A direct correlation appears to exist between the bulk of cervical nodal disease and the development of distant metastasis.

Aberrant metastatic spread may occur in patients who have undergone previous treatment for head and neck cancer. Patients who have had radical neck dissection or radiotherapy are at increased risk of developing aberrant metastases to the neck and to subcutaneous and cutaneous sites. Tumors also may spread along nerves; hence, this route is an important consideration in planning therapy for certain tumors, such as those that invade the mandible and place the inferior alveolar nerve at risk. Direct invasion of other nerves (e.g., the hypoglossal, lingual, and vagus and the sympathetic chain) may occur from tumors in their vicinity. Large, high-grade parotid tumors are known to involve the facial nerve and to cause paralysis, but benign tumors, even when they are huge, rarely do so.

CLINICAL PRESENTATION

Of the several warning signs of cancer promulgated by the American Cancer Society, at least three pertain to the head and neck region: dysphagia, chronic ulcer, and lump in the neck. Despite these obvious and common complaints, two of every three patients with head and neck cancer present at an advanced stage, primarily because of neglect on the patients' part, but also often owing to delayed diagnosis. In high-risk patients who present with head and neck complaints, an extremely

important precaution is to rule out the presence of malignancy by the appropriate investigations and to seek expert opinion if necessary.

Symptoms vary from site to site. Some tumors may become symptomatic at an early stage, as happens with tumors of the vocal cords, whereas others (e.g., those of the nasopharynx or hypopharynx) may not be suspected at all. Common symptoms in patients with oral cancer include painful ulceration, slurred speech, bleeding, and an exophytic mass. Occasionally, the diagnosis of oral cancer is made on routine examination by a dentist or oral surgeon.

Patients with early nasopharyngeal cancer may present with unilateral otitis media. Tumors of the oropharynx and laryngopharynx are associated with odynophagia, dysphagia, change of voice and, occasionally, airway obstruction. Unexplained weight loss is an important finding in patients with head and neck cancer. Occasionally, affected patients may neglect change of voice or minor airway distress until they present to the emergency room with acute airway obstruction requiring emergency airway intervention.

Tumors of the nasal cavity and paranasal sinuses may remain undetected for a long time, as symptoms may be attributed mistakenly to sinusitis or allergic rhinitis. Recurrent epistaxis, malar swelling, and diplopia are common symptoms of advanced maxillary sinus tumors. These symptoms may long remain uninvestigated. Pain, a relatively late symptom in head and neck tumors, generally is mediated by the trigeminal or glossopharyngeal nerves. The glossopharyngeal and vagus nerves transmit pain from pharyngeal and laryngeal tumors as referred pain to the ear. Hypopharyngeal neoplasms or tumors of the base of the tongue may cause otalgia mediated by Arnold's nerve, the auricular branch of the vagus nerve. In advanced stages, affected patients may present with acute airway distress (as described) or with intense pain, severe dysphagia and weight loss, obvious involvement of the skin of the face and neck and, occasionally, mandibular involvement with loose teeth. Advanced cancers of the oral cavity may erode through the subcutaneous tissue and skin and present with an orocutaneous fistula.

Synchronous and Metachronous Second Primary Tumors

Patients with head and neck cancer run a substantial risk of a second primary tumor. Such factors as smoking and alcohol intake have a carcinogenic effect on the en-

Table 12.3 Percentage of Metastatic Lymph Nodes Involved in Elective and Therapeutic Radical Neck Dissections

Level of Nodes	Primary Site							
	Oral Cavity		Oropharynx		Hypopharynx		Larynx	
	E (%)	T (%)	E (%)	T (%)	E (%)	T (%)	E (%)	T (%)
I	58	61	7	17	0	10	14	8
II	51	57	80	85	75	78	52	68
III	26	44	60	50	75	75	55	70
IV	9	20	27	33	0	47	24	35
V	2	4	7	11	0	11	7	5

E = elective; T = therapeutic.
Source: Reprinted from JP Shah, Patterns of cervical lymph node metastasis from squamous carcinoma of the upper aerodigestive tract. *Am J Surg* 160:405–409, 1990, with permission from Excerpta Medica, Inc.

tire surface of the upper aerodigestive tract, and the potential for development of tumors persists even after the carcinogenic insult has ceased. Although affected patients may present at any time with one primary cancer, they face an approximate 15% incidence of a synchronous second primary tumor, including cancer of the lung or esophagus. The incidence of metachronous cancer is approximately 4% annually; principally for this reason, a patient with head and neck cancer always should remain under close observation [9].

Diagnostic Workup

The diagnostic workup in patients with head and neck cancer may include a detailed medical history and physical examination; examination under anesthesia and biopsy, including fine-needle aspiration (FNA) cytology; and imaging studies, including a panoramic x-ray film of the mandible, computed tomographic (CT) scan, ultrasonography and, occasionally, magnetic resonance imaging (MRI) as indicated. Meticulous history recording must include directed questions looking for such relevant specific symptoms as otalgia, odynophagia, malar swelling, and the like, symptoms that affected patients may not attribute to their disease. Such symptoms as hoarseness of voice and sore throat must be investigated carefully. A thorough head and neck examination includes a detailed survey of the region; palpation of the neck and thyroid; bimanual palpation of the floor of the mouth and base of the tongue (if relevant); a mirror examination; and nasopharyngolaryngoscopy using a rigid or fiberoptic scope. Some sites (e.g., scalp, nape of the neck, and gingivolabial and gingivobuccal sulci) are easily overlooked, and clinicians must set up a routine sequence of examination to avoid missing tumors in these sites. Commonly, FNA is used

in the evaluation of neck masses and cervical node, thyroid, and salivary gland tumors.

Radiologic Imaging Studies

The use of routine plain x-ray films of the head and neck no longer is practiced, and the use of CT and MRI reveals tumors in such difficult locations as the base of the skull and base of the tongue. The CT scan is very helpful also in evaluating nonpalpable cervical lymph nodes. Tumors of the parapharyngeal space and the parotid also are well defined using these techniques. Ultrasonography has been used effectively in detecting lesions and in guiding FNA of small cervical nodes [10] and in determining carotid artery invasion by tumor [11]. The role of fluorodeoxyglucose-positron emission tomography (FDG-PET) scans in head and neck cancer continues to be investigated [12].

Examination Under Anesthesia and Biopsy: Techniques

Examination under a general anesthetic is important in evaluating patients with tumors of the base of the tongue and laryngopharynx and in patients who have oral cavity tumors that present with trismus. Patients with laryngeal and pharyngeal lesions will need a detailed endoscopic examination to map out the extent of involvement and to plan treatment. Routine esophagoscopy and bronchoscopy probably is not justified in every patient undergoing examination under anesthesia, but patients with hypopharyngeal tumors should undergo cervical esophagus examination, mainly to delineate the lower limit of the lesion.

An accurate histologic diagnosis is crucial for initiating correct treatment, and although pathologists' responsibility in interpreting the biopsy material is crucial, perhaps equally important is the surgical technique of the biopsy. Commonly used techniques include punch biopsy, incisional biopsy, excisional biopsy, curettage, core-needle biopsy, and FNA biopsy.

Punch biopsy is the technique used most frequently for obtaining a mucosal biopsy in the head and neck. Various punch biopsy forceps are available, but the cup forceps is used most often. Even though the periphery of a lesion generally is the recommended site for performing a biopsy, a small portion of an exophytic lesion is satisfactory to make a diagnosis, especially for squamous cell carcinoma. Usually, local pressure for a few minutes is adequate to stop bleeding from the biopsy site, so sutures rarely are necessary. If infection or necrotic material is present, the biopsy should be performed on a fleshy, nonulcerated region of the tumor.

Small oral cavity lesions may be sampled easily by an excisional biopsy with satisfactory margins. In patients with diffuse areas of leukoplakia or erythroplakia in the oral cavity, surface staining with such vital dyes as toluidine blue may help to direct attention to a particularly suspicious site and may improve the yield of biopsy. The dye is an acidophilic, metachromatic nuclear stain that preferentially colors areas of squamous cell carcinoma.

The incisional biopsy is applied best to lesions of the skin and soft tissue or to submucosal masses in the oral cavity and oropharynx. Frozen-section confirmation can ensure adequate sampling and enhance diagnostic yield. Biopsy of irradiated tissue always is difficult because of mucosal edema and radiation changes, such as fibrosis.

Generally, biopsies of the larynx and pharynx are performed endoscopically under anesthesia. If the chest roentgenogram is normal, detection of lung lesions is unlikely via routine bronchoscopy and selective bronchial washings.

Needle biopsy has been popular in this country since the 1930 landmark article by Hayes Martin [13]. However, the fear of needle tract implantation kept it out of routine clinical use until the 1970s. FNA is now used in the evaluation of almost all head and neck masses (especially cervical lymphadenopathy [14]) and of thyroid and salivary tumors. The technique of FNA has been described extensively in the literature, and every individual dealing with head and neck tumors should be conversant with the technique (Fig. 12.8) [15].

In the evaluation of cervical lymphadenopathy, an algorithmic approach can be used in patients presenting with features of a malignant pathology (Fig. 12.9). The results of FNA cytology of cervical nodal masses can

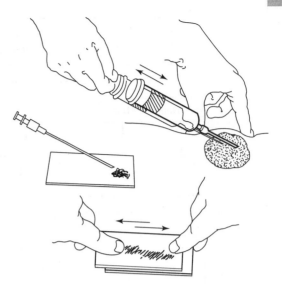

Figure 12.8 Technique of fine-needle aspiration. (Reprinted with permission from JP Shah, *Color Atlas of Head and Neck Surgery*. Copyright © 1987 by Grune & Stratton: Orlando, FL)

be interpreted as metastatic squamous cell carcinoma, metastatic adenocarcinoma, metastatic thyroid carcinoma, or suspicious of lymphoma [16]. Cells for the immunocytochemical or flow cytometric evaluation of T- and B-cell markers, or even for molecular assays of antigen receptor gene rearrangements, can often be obtained by FNA. These results, in conjunction with cytomorphology can usually distinguish reactive lymphoid processes from non-Hodgkin's lymphoma [16]. This is usually not necessary if morphologic findings suggest a lymphoma, since classification of most lymphomas will still require an open biopsy for routine histology. FNA has become the first-choice diagnostic test in the evaluation of a thyroid mass. The investigation appears to be cost-effective, and its accuracy in detecting thyroid tumors exceeds 80%. Results of FNA of the thyroid may be interpreted as malignant, suspicious, benign, or indeterminate. The diagnoses of benign follicular adenoma and follicular carcinoma cannot be based on cytologic features alone, because the entire capsule of the tumor must be evaluated after excision of the thyroid mass. FNA samples are usually processed as smears, which provide only a cytologic, rather than histologic, diagnosis. In some cases, it may be useful to place a portion of the sample into a liquid preservative solution so that cell pellets obtained by centrifugation may be embedded in paraffin and sectioned for histologic staining.

The role of FNA in salivary gland lesions is controversial, as most of these lesions can be evaluated easily in the clinic. However, in certain tumors that involve

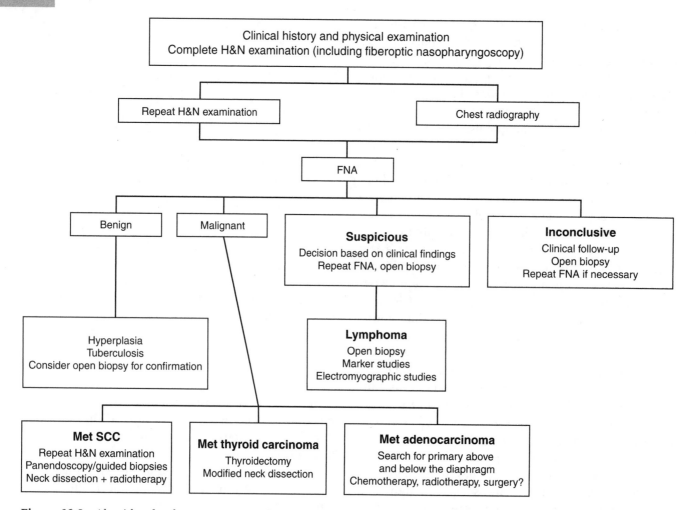

Figure 12.9   Algorithm for the management of cervical lymphadenopathy. *H&N* = head and neck; *FNA* = fine-needle aspiration; *Met* = metastatic; *SCC* = squamous cell carcinoma. (Reprinted from AR Shaha, C Webber, J Marti, Fine-needle aspiration in the diagnosis of cervical adenopathy. *Am J Surg* 152:420–423, 1986, with permission from Excerpta Medica, Inc.)

the tail of the parotid and in which a clinical diagnosis may be uncertain, FNA is very helpful in differentiating salivary from nonsalivary pathologic features. On average, the accuracy of FNA in detecting salivary lesions exceeds 80% (Table 12.4) [15].

Despite the many pitfalls of FNA biopsy of head and neck tumors, clearly it is one of the most important diagnostic tests available today. Clinical correlation must be made with the results of FNA and, in case of discrepancy, further investigation (including open biopsy) must be undertaken as appropriate.

Staging System

In 1997, the American Joint Committee on Cancer, in collaboration with the Union Internationale Contre le

Cancer, updated the TNM (*t*umor, *n*ode, *m*etastasis) staging system for cancers of the head and neck [1]. Primary tumors are classified as T1 to T4 (Table 12.5); nodal disease as N1, N2, or N3 (Table 12.6; Fig. 12.10); the presence of distant metastasis is staged as M1; and the overall stage grouping consists of stages I to IV (Table 12.7). Stage I and stage II are considered to be early cancers with a prognosis more favorable than that of advanced (stage III and stage IV) cancers.

Pathologic Classification

Because the upper aerodigestive tract is lined mainly by squamous epithelium, the most common tumors in the head and neck are squamous cell carcinomas. However, other tumors, such as adenocarcinomas, lymphomas,

Table 12.4 Effectiveness of Needle Biopsy in Detecting Salivary Lesions

Authors	Year	No. of Cases	Sensitivity (%)	Specificity (%)	Accuracy (%)
Enroth and Zlajicek	1970	690	64	95	89
Kline et al.	1981	47	100	95	96
Sismanis et al.	1981	51	85	96	92
Qizilbash et al.	1985	101	88	100	98
Lindberg and Akerman	1986	461	67	85	81
O'Dwyer et al.	1986	341	73	94	93
Layfield et al.	1987	171	91	98	92
Nettle and Orell	1989	106	80	99	94
Jayram et al.	1989	195	81	94	88
Rodriguez et al.	1989	64	85	97	93
Shaha et al.	1990	160	95	98	97

Source: Reprinted from AR Shaha, C Webber, T DiMaio, BM Jaffe, Needle aspiration biopsy in salivary gland lesions. *Am J Surg* 160:373–376, 1990, with permission from Excerpta Medica, Inc.

Table 12.5 Tumor Staging of Head and Neck Tumors

Classification	Definition
TX	Primary tumor cannot be assessed
T0	No evidence of primary tumor
Tis	Carcinoma in situ

Oral cavity and lip

T1	Tumor ≤ 2 cm in greatest dimension
T2	Tumor > 2 cm but ≤ 4 cm in greatest dimension
T3	Tumor > 4 cm in greatest dimension
T4 (lip)	Tumor invades adjacent structures (e.g., through cortical bone, inferior alveolar nerve, floor of mouth, skin of face)
T4 (oral cavity)	Tumor invades adjacent structures (e.g., through cortical bone into deep [extrinsic] muscle of tongue, maxillary sinus, skin. Superficial erosion alone of bone/tooth socket by gingival primary is not sufficient to classify as T4)

Oropharynx

T1	Tumor ≤ 2 cm in greatest dimension
T2	Tumor > 2 cm but ≤ 4 cm in greatest dimension
T3	Tumor > 4 cm in greatest dimension
T4	Tumor invades adjacent structures (e.g., pterygoid muscle[s], mandible, hard palate, deep muscle of tongue, larynx)

Nasopharynx

T1	Tumor confined to nasopharynx
T2	Tumor extends to soft tissues of oropharynx and/or nasal fossa
T2a	Without parapharyngeal extension
T2b	With parapharyngeal extension
T3	Tumor invades bony structures and/or paranasal sinuses
T4	Tumor with intracranial extension and/or involvement of cranial nerves, infratemporal fossa, hypopharynx, or orbit

Hypopharynx

T1	Tumor limited to one subsite of hypopharynx, ≤ 2 cm in greatest dimension
T2	Tumor involves more than one subsite of hypopharynx or an adjacent subsite, or measures > 2 but ≤ 4 cm in greatest dimension without fixation of hemilarynx
T3	Tumor measures > 4 cm in greatest dimension or with fixation of hemilarynx
T4	Tumor invades adjacent structures (e.g., thyroid/cricoid cartilage, carotid artery, soft tissues of neck, prevertebral fascia/muscles, thyroid and/or esophagus)

continued

Table 12.5   *(continued)*

Classification	Definition
Supraglottis	
T1	Tumor limited to one subsite of supraglottis with normal vocal cord mobility
T2	Tumor invades mucosa of more than one adjacent subsite of supraglottis or glottis or region outside supraglottis (e.g., mucosa of base of tongue, vallecula, medial wall of piriform sinus) without fixation of larynx
T3	Tumor limited to larynx with vocal cord fixation and/or invades any of the following: postcricoid area, preepiglottic tissues
T4	Tumor invades through thyroid cartilage and/or extends into soft tissues of neck, thyroid, and/or oesophagus
Glottis	
T1	Tumor limited to vocal cord(s) (may involve anterior or posterior commissure) with normal mobility
T1a	Tumor limited to one vocal cord
T1b	Tumor involves both vocal cords
T2	Tumor extends to supraglottis and/or subglottis and/or with impaired vocal cord mobility
T3	Tumor limited to larynx with vocal cord fixation
T4	Tumor invades through thyroid cartilage and/or to other tissues beyond larynx (e.g., trachea, soft tissues of neck, including thyroid, pharynx)
Subglottis	
T1	Tumor limited to subglottis
T2	Tumor extends to vocal cord(s) with normal or impaired mobility
T3	Tumor limited to larynx with vocal cord fixation
T4	Tumor invades through cricoid or thyroid cartilage and/or extends to other tissues beyond larynx (e.g., trachea, soft tissues of neck, including thyroid, esophagus)
Maxillary sinus	
T1	Tumor limited to antral mucosa with no erosion or destruction of bone
T2	Tumor causing bone erosion or destruction, except for posterior antral wall, including extension into hard palate and/or middle nasal meatus
T3	Tumor invades any of the following: bone of posterior wall of maxillary sinus, subcutaneous tissues, skin of cheek, floor or medial wall of orbit, infratemporal fossa, pterygoid plates, ethmoid sinuses
T4	Tumor invades orbital contents beyond floor or medial wall, including any of the following: orbital apex, cribriform plate, base of skull, nasopharynx, sphenoid, frontal sinuses
Ethmoid sinus	
T1	Tumor confined to ethmoid sinus with or without bone erosion
T2	Tumor extends into nasal cavity
T3	Tumor extends to anterior orbit and/or maxillary sinus
T4	Tumor with intracranial extension, orbital extension including apex, involving sphenoid and/or frontal sinus and/or skin of external nose

Source: Used with the permission of the *American Joint Committee on Cancer (AJCC®)*, Chicago. *AJCC® Cancer Staging Manual* (5th Edition), 1997. Philadelphia: Lippincott-Raven.

and melanomas, also are seen. Rare tumors include soft-tissue sarcomas (e.g., leiomyosarcoma, rhabdomyosarcoma, synovial sarcoma, Kaposi's sarcoma, and fibrosarcoma). Another important finding is that such lesions as leukoplakia and erythroplakia occur fairly frequently in patients with a history of heavy smoking and alcohol abuse. *Leukoplakia* is a clinical term used to describe a white mucosal patch; it has no histologic meaning. Generally, the lifetime incidence of squamous cell carcinoma in an existing setting of leukoplakia is quoted as approximately 2–5%, but the actual risk of malignancy depends directly on the histologic presence and grade of dysplasia in the lesion. In contrast, the incidence of squamous cell carcinoma in erythroplakia is approximately 30%. On a practical basis, an important precaution is to biopsy any suspicious lesions, especially in high-risk patients, and to keep affected patients under careful surveillance.

Verrucous carcinoma is a clinical diagnosis used to characterize an exophytic tumor of wartlike appearance. Histologically, the tumor may be so well differentiated as to cause confusion in diagnosis of malignancy.

Table 12.6 Node Staging of Head and Neck Tumors

Nasopharyngeal cancer

NX	Regional lymph nodes cannot be assessed
N0	No regional lymph node metastasis
N1	Unilateral metastasis in lymph node(s), ≤ 6 cm in greatest dimension, above the supraclavicular fossa
N2	Bilateral metastasis in lymph node(s), ≤ 6 cm in greatest dimension, above the supraclavicular fossa
N3	Metastasis in a lymph node(s)
N3a	> 6 cm in greatest dimension
N3b	Extension to the supraclavicular fossa

All other sites except the thyroid gland

NX	Regional lymph nodes cannot be assessed
N0	No regional lymph node metastasis
N1	Metastasis in a single ipsilateral lymph node, ≤ 3 cm in greatest dimension
N2	Metastasis in a single ipsilateral lymph node, > 3 cm but ≤ 6 cm in greatest dimension; or in multiple ipsilateral lymph nodes, none > 6 cm in greatest dimension; or in bilateral or contralateral lymph nodes, none > 6 cm in greatest dimension
N2a	Metastasis in a single ipsilateral lymph node > 3 cm but ≤ 6 cm in greatest dimension
N2b	Metastasis in multiple ipsilateral lymph nodes, none > 6 cm in greatest dimension
N2c	Metastasis in bilateral or contralateral lymph nodes, none > 6 cm in greatest dimension
N3	Metastasis in a lymph node > 6 cm in greatest dimension

Notes: Histologic examination of a selective neck dissection specimen should include six or more lymph nodes. A radical or modified radical neck dissection specimen should include 10 or more lymph nodes.
Source: Used with the permission of the *American Joint Committee on Cancer (AJCC®)*, Chicago. *AJCC® Cancer Staging Manual (5th Edition)*, 1997. Philadelphia: Lippincott-Raven.

Table 12.7 AJCC Stage Grouping for Head and Neck Tumors

Nasopharyngeal cancer

Stage 0	Tis	N0	M0
Stage I	T1	N0	M0
Stage IIA	T2a	N0	M0
Stage IIB	T1	N1	M0
	T2	N1	M0
	T2a	N1	M0
	T2b	N0	M0
	T2b	N1	M0
Stage III	T1	N2	M0
	T2a	N2	M0
	T2b	N2	M0
	T3	N0	M0
	T3	N1	M0
	T3	N2	M0
Stage IVA	T4	N0	M0
	T4	N1	M0
	T4	N2	M0
Stage IVB	Any T	N3	M0
Stage IVC	Any T	Any N	M1

All other head and neck cancers

Stage 0	Tis	N0	M0
Stage I	T1	N0	M0
Stage II	T2	N0	M0
Stage III	T3	N0	M0
	T1	N1	M0
	T2	N1	M0
	T3	N1	M0
Stage IVA	T4	N0	M0
	T4	N1	M0
	Any T	N2	M0
Stage IVB	Any T	N3	M0
Stage IVC	Any T	Any N	M1

AJCC = American Joint Committee on Cancer.
Source: Used with the permission of the *American Joint Committee on Cancer (AJCC®)*, Chicago. *AJCC® Cancer Staging Manual (5th Edition)*, 1997. Philadelphia: Lippincott-Raven.

Commonly, these tumors are seen in the mucosa of the cheek and the larynx. Traditionally, surgical excision has been the preferred form of treatment, but some reports cite good results with radiotherapy. Anaplastic transformation of verrucous carcinoma to a more aggressive neoplasm has been reported to occur following radiotherapy. However, recent studies indicate this is uncommon and should not prevent consideration of radiotherapy as a treatment option. Other morphologic types of squamous cancers in the head and neck include the exophytic, the ulcerating, and the infiltrating types.

As a generalization, infiltrating tumors may be associated with a prognosis worse than that of exophytic types. Lymphoepithelial carcinomas or lymphoepitheliomas are poorly differentiated squamous cell carcinomas with lymphoid stroma. These tumors are seen most commonly in the nasopharynx and tonsil and are notable for their radiosensitivity.

Prognostic factors related to the pathology of the tumor include the differentiation of the tumor; the presence of lymphatic, vascular, or perineural invasion; and the depth of invasion of the tumor. The depth of invasion has been correlated directly to the incidence of cervical nodal metastases and survival [17].

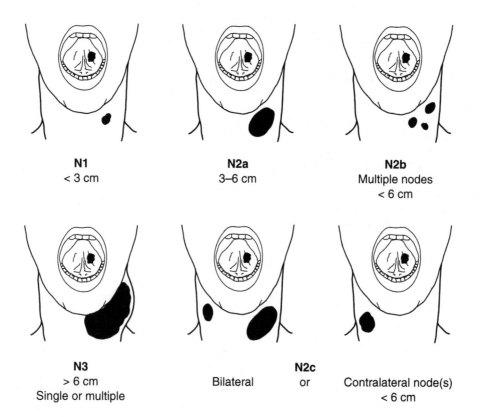

Figure 12.10   TNM staging system for cervical lymph nodes. (Reprinted with permission from JP Shah, J Medina, AR Shaha, et al., Cervical lymph node metastasis. *Curr Probl Surg* 30:273–344, 1993.)

TREATMENT

The management of head and neck cancer requires both a detailed evaluation of the extent of disease and a multidisciplinary approach. Therapeutic options include surgery, radiotherapy, chemotherapy, and immunotherapy. At present, the role of immunotherapy remains investigational. Several randomized and nonrandomized trials have evaluated chemotherapy for treatment of head and neck cancer [18], and various chemotherapeutic agents have been shown to produce response. None of these agents, in any combination, have demonstrated an improvement in survival. However, chemotherapy in conjunction with radiotherapy has been used successfully to preserve the function of important organs (e.g., the larynx in patients with advanced head and neck tumors). The main treatment modalities for head and neck cancer, therefore, remain surgery and radiotherapy. A combination of chemotherapy and radiotherapy is used commonly for patients with advanced nasopharyngeal cancers and for patients with stage III or stage IV laryngeal cancer for organ preservation. In addition, chemoradiotherapy is used for inoperable tumors and as salvage therapy for recurrent tumors.

Decisions regarding appropriate treatment are based on an overall consideration of a variety of factors (e.g., features of the tumor and patient and physician factors). Features of the tumor having an impact on treatment include the site, size, histology, depth of invasion, disease stage, previous treatment, and need for reconstructive surgery. Patient factors that merit consideration include the impact on quality of life, medical condition (including cardiopulmonary status), patient preference, treatment cost and convenience, and compliance. Last, the type of treatment delivered will depend also on the availability of the necessary expertise and multidisciplinary personnel, the preference of treating physicians, and institutional policy. When these various parameters are considered, individual patients are treated best using a tailored approach.

Early-stage disease (stage I and stage II) can be treated with either surgery or radiotherapy with equivalent control rates. For small lesions of the oral cavity, wide local excision is preferred over radiotherapy. Since any site can usually receive radiotherapy only once, one strategy is to reserve primary use of this modality for certain lesions, such as those of the larynx, in which surgery is known to produce poorer functional results [19]. For patients treated with primary surgery, radiotherapy is used if indicated in the postoperative setting, depending on the margin status and the pathologic findings.

More advanced lesions (stage III and stage IV) are treated with combined-modality therapy using surgery followed by radiotherapy. Postoperative radiotherapy is administered with the intent of sterilizing any residual disease. Advantages of postoperative irradiation include reduction in target tumor volume, clear definition of extent of tumor, and fewer wound complications in nonirradiated patients than in patients irradiated preoperatively. Adjuvant postoperative radiotherapy should be considered for all patients with locally advanced cancers and for patients who have early cancers and ominous pathologic findings. Features of tumors that mandate postoperative radiotherapy are listed in Table 12.8. Generally, postoperative irradiation is recommended to begin within six weeks of the operation. Postoperative radiotherapy improves local control and survival, as compared to surgery alone [20].

A variety of tools and techniques are available to radiation oncologists in designing a treatment plan. Depending on the disease treated and the clinical situation, *photon-beam irradiation* generally is delivered by megavoltage irradiation. Photon-beam irradiation has the advantage of relative skin sparing, as the effects of the beam are in deeper structures. For lesions in the nasopharynx, oral cavity, and oropharynx, *interstitial irradiation* applying radioisotopes (e.g., iodine, iridium, radium, or gold) may be used to augment dose locally to desired areas while maximally sparing normal tissues. Interstitial implantation or brachytherapy has shown very promising results in patients with tumors of the base of the tongue. *Electron-beam therapy* is superficially

penetrating and therefore is used as an accessory technique to boost doses to superficial regions of the head and neck (e.g., the posterior cervical nodes). On the basis of tumor size and individual clinical situations, radiation oncologists select the appropriate total and daily irradiation dose. Typically, daily doses are 180 cGy (or rads) or 200 cGy. Subclinical microscopic cancer requires at least 5,000 cGy delivered over a five-week period; small lesions (T1) require 6,000–6,600 cGy, intermediate lesions (T2) require 6,600–7,000 cGy; generally, doses in excess of 7,000 cGy are required to eradicate large (T3 and T4) tumors. However, the risk of complications increases as dose increases, especially beyond 7,000 cGy. Often, interstitial implants are used in an effort to escalate doses safely to the high levels necessary for permanent control of larger lesions. Shrinking-field techniques are applied, with dose delivered to each region corresponding to the amount of cancer present in that region at the time of presentation. This technique enables safe delivery of doses adequate to eradicate tumor. The primary site receives the higher doses, and peripheral areas (including distant lymph nodes) receive the lowest doses, but never less than 4,500 cGy in 4.5 weeks. Strict attention is paid to patient immobilization by the frequent use of customized immobilization molds to ensure that treatment is delivered accurately and reproducibly each day of therapy. Complications are reduced further by the use of customized lead-alloy blocks to minimize dose to normal structures.

The role of chemoradiotherapy in preserving laryngeal function without compromising survival was brought into focus by the Department of Veterans Affairs Laryngeal Cancer trial [21] that compared conventional treatment (surgery with postoperative irradiation) and induction chemotherapy followed by radiotherapy in patients with advanced laryngeal cancer. Survival in each arm was 68%, but as many as 64% of patients in the chemoradiation arm retained a functional larynx. The European Organization for Research and Treatment of Cancer phase III randomized trial of larynx-preserving therapy in advanced hypopharyngeal cancer further validated the use of organ-preserving chemoradiation approaches [22].

Unknown Primary Tumors

An *unknown primary tumor* is defined as the presence of metastatic cancer in the neck while the primary tumor remains undetected despite thorough physical, endoscopic, and radiologic examination by multiple examin-

---

Table 12.8   Indications for Postoperative Radiotherapy

Features of the primary tumor
  Advanced T stage (bulky tumor; involvement of bone,
    nerves, or skin)
  High histologic grade
  Positive surgical resection margins
  Lymphatic permeation
  Vascular invasion
  Perineural spread

Features of the cervical lymph nodes
  More than two pathologically involved nodes
  Involvement at more than one lymph node level in the neck
  Lymph node > 3 cm in diameter (N2 or N3 stage)
  Presence of extracapsular spread
  Microscopic or gross residual disease in the neck
  Involvement of critical levels (IV or V)

ers. Although any lymph node group may be involved, the upper jugular lymph nodes are affected most commonly, followed in frequency by midjugular and supraclavicular chains. This finding is relevant, as the location of the cervical adenopathy usually correlates with the location of the occult primary lesion. Generally, metastases to the neck from infraclavicular primaries involve the supraclavicular nodes. Two-thirds of tumors identified subsequent to definitive therapy are found to originate above the clavicles; one-third originate from the nasopharynx and oropharynx, one-third arise from the tonsil and base of tongue, and a few arise from the hypopharynx. One-third of cervical metastases are found to have their primary origin infraclavicularly, with 50% of these originating in the lungs; the breast, stomach, pancreas, and ovary account for the remainder. Generally, metastatic adenocarcinoma to the supraclavicular region presenting as Virchow's lymph node (supraclavicular or scalene node, near the lower portion of jugular vein) is considered to be a systemic disease and is treated best by chemotherapy. The role of neck dissection in the management of metastatic adenocarcinoma is extremely limited and is reserved for palliation of a fungating tumor or pressure symptoms.

The importance of a thorough evaluation of the head and neck cannot be overemphasized, and the use of fiberoptic telescopes and nasopharyngoscopes provides access to otherwise difficult areas. Such imaging studies as CT or MRI are extremely helpful and must be an early part of the diagnostic workup in suspected patients. Elevated serum Epstein-Barr virus antibody titers may indicate the presence of nasopharyngeal cancer. Examination under anesthesia is routine, and panendoscopy includes evaluation of the nasopharynx, larynx, pharynx, esophagus, and lungs. The exact extent of endoscopy depends on the location of the metastatic tumor. The role of "blind biopsies" of certain high-risk areas (e.g., nasopharynx, base of the tongue, tonsils, and pyriform sinus) is controversial because of the low diagnostic yield. On the basis of patterns of lymphatic drainage of the head and neck and the incidence of nodal metastases, directed biopsies of specific primary sites can be performed, depending on the location of the nodal metastases. Although open biopsy of a neck node has not been shown conclusively to alter prognosis [23], consideration of it is prudent only after thorough evaluation with imaging, examination under anesthesia, and FNA of the node are found to be inconclusive or are suggestive of alternative pathology (e.g., lymphoma). If open biopsy must be done, affected patients should be prepared for the possibility of a formal neck dissection on the basis of the report of frozen-section analysis.

Alternatively, if the plan involves waiting for a final histologic report, great care must be taken to place the incision so that it can be excised with the definitive resection, and dissection of tissue planes must be kept to a minimum to avoid tumor spread. Generally, the supraclavicular nodes are involved by metastatic tumors from lung, pancreas, or stomach. These nodes may be involved also in tumors of the breast, ovary, and testes.

The standard treatment of metastatic squamous cell carcinoma with an unknown primary lesion remains neck dissection followed by radiotherapy. Considerable controversy concerns whether the nasopharynx should be included in the portals for postoperative radiotherapy. If the metastatic nodal disease involves the upper neck or affected patients present with an elevated serum antibody titer to Epstein-Barr virus, the nasopharynx should be included routinely in the irradiation portals. On the other hand, patients with enlarged lymph nodes only at level III or level IV may be spared irradiation of the nasopharynx.

The role of radiotherapy in treating other potential primary mucosal sites also is controversial [24]. The rationale in withholding radiotherapy is that the primary tumor will manifest itself in only approximately 4–16% of patients on long-term follow-up, and this incidence is similar to that of second primary tumors for which no prophylactic radiotherapy is recommended. Mucosal recurrence rates after treatment range from 11% to 14%, and prognosis depends on the pathologic features of the metastatic cancer, including histologic features (squamous versus adenocarcinoma versus anaplastic), tumor grade, and the presence of extracapsular spread. The prognosis is better in patients whose primary tumor never is identified. Generally, metastatic adenocarcinoma of the neck originates in structures below the clavicle (e.g., lung, breast, stomach, pancreas, and ovary). Occasionally, a primary tumor may be located in the salivary gland [25].

Neck

Treatment of the neck is required in two situations: elective treatment for clinical N_0 disease and management of node-positive disease. For the past half century, radical neck dissection, described by George Crile [2] in 1906 and popularized by Hayes Martin [13], has been considered standard treatment for the node-positive neck. The procedure involves excision of all lymph nodes in the neck from level I to level V, with routine sacrifice of the internal jugular vein, spinal accessory nerve, and sternocleidomastoid muscle. In the mid-

Table 12.9 Complications of Radical Neck Dissection

Timing and Nature of Complication	Sequelae
Intraoperative	
Injury to nerves	
Marginal mandibular nerve	Deformity of angle of mouth
Hypoglossal and lingual nerve	Difficulty in moving the tongue
Vagus nerve	Hoarseness, aspiration
Sympathetic chain	Horner's syndrome
Phrenic nerve	Paralyzed ipsilateral diaphragm
Brachial plexus	Weakness or paralysis of limb muscles
Injury to thoracic or major lymphatic duct	Chyle leak
Injury to dome of pleura	Pneumothorax (tension)
Injury to pharynx or esophagus	Salivary fistula
Other complications	
Stimulation of carotid bulb	Bradycardia
Injury to internal carotid artery	Cerebrovascular stroke
Air embolism through major venous injury	Hypotension, mortality
Early and intermediate postoperative	
Reactionary or secondary hemorrhage	Hematoma
Carotid artery exposure and rupture	Mortality or cerebrovascular stroke
Physiologic consequences	
Spinal accessory nerve	Shoulder dysfunction
Other nerves	Anesthesia of skin flaps, ear lobe, and cheek
Internal jugular vein ligation (bilateral)	Cerebral edema, airway obstruction, blindness, edema of face and neck

1960s, Suarez [26] and Bocca [27] popularized the modified neck dissection on the basis of their contention that the morbidity of radical neck dissection (Table 12.9)—especially loss of shoulder function due to sacrifice of the spinal accessory nerve—could be minimized with no compromise in local control rates. Over the ensuing years, Richard Jesse, Allando Ballantyne, and Robert Byers popularized modified neck dissections in the United States [3]. Numerous modifications were practiced and proposed, causing considerable confusion in nomenclature. In an effort to clear the confusion, the American Academy of Otolaryngology-Head and Neck Surgery convened a special task force that published its report in 1991 [28]. This and other classification systems for neck dissections are itemized in Table 12.10 (Robbins et al. [28], Medina [29], and Spiro et al. [30]).

Simultaneous bilateral radical neck dissection is a very morbid procedure and is associated with a mortality of approximately 17% (see Table 12.9). Performing a modified neck dissection is preferable, saving the internal jugular vein on the side with lesser disease and performing radical neck dissection on the side of bulky disease. In the rare event that bilateral radical neck dissections are indicated, staging the procedures at separate operations may be a good alternative.

Management of the clinically negative neck continues to generate controversy. Elective treatment is considered on the basis of the perceived risk of micrometastases and should be undertaken if the probability of micrometastasis is more than 15–20%. Although irradiation and surgery are equally effective in controlling the N0 neck, routine radiotherapy generally is avoided because of the complications related to radiotherapy and its potential long-term sequelae. A risk of micrometastases of less than 15–20% is insufficient justification for electively irradiating the remaining 80% of patients unnecessarily, thereby subjecting them to potential complications. An exception may be made, however, when surgical resection of the primary tumor requires access to the neck and limited or selective neck dissection can be added to the procedure without additional morbidity. The supraomohyoid neck dissection, which includes removal of lymph nodes at levels I, II, and III, has become a routine staging procedure for most tumors of the oral cavity [8].

In the treatment of node-positive disease, the roles of radical neck dissection and routine sacrifice of uninvolved structures are becoming unpopular. Radical neck dissection is the standard operation for many patients with N2 or N3 disease involving, or in close proximity to, the vein, nerve, or muscle. In selected patients with N1 tumors, especially those with involvement of nodes away from the spinal accessory nerve, every effort is made to preserve the accessory nerve and its function. Almost all patients with node-positive disease require postoperative radiotherapy (see Table 12.8), a procedure that has resulted in improvement of local control rates to more than 70% for N2 and N3 disease, as compared with rates of 30–50% for surgery alone. An important note is that as many as 30% of patients with N1 disease will experience recurrent disease in the neck if treated with surgery alone, and postoperative radiotherapy should be considered (as indicated).

Radiotherapy alone (6,000 cGy) will result in sterilization of 90% of pathologically involved nodes mea-

Table 12.10   Comparison of Neck Dissection Terminology

Robbins et al [28]	Medina [29]	Spiro et al. [30]
Radical neck dissection	**Comprehensive neck dissection** (all five node levels resected) Radical neck dissection	**Radical neck dissection** (four or five node levels resected) Conventional radical neck dissection
Modified radical neck dissection (preservation of one or more nonlymphatic structures)	Modified radical neck dissection Type I (XIn preserved) Type II (XIn and IJV preserved) Type III (XIn, IJV, and sternomastoid preserved)	Modified radical neck dissection Extended radical neck dissection Modified and extended radical neck dissection
Selective neck dissection (preservation of one or more lymph node groups) Supraomohyoid neck dissection Posterolateral neck dissection Anterior compartment neck dissection Lateral neck dissection	**Selective neck dissection** (fewer than five node levels resected)	**Selective neck dissection** (three node levels resected) Supraomohyoid neck dissection Jugular dissection Any other three levels resected
Extended radical neck dissection (resection of additional lymph node groups or nonlymphatic structures)		**Limited neck dissection** (no more than two node levels resected) Paratracheal node dissection Mediastinal node dissection Any other 1 or 2 levels resected

XIn = spinal accessory nerve; IJV = internal jugular vein.

suring less than 2 cm. Doses of irradiation required for tumor eradication increase as a function of disease bulk, while at the same time overall disease control decreases with increasing bulk. Approximately 80% of nodes larger than 3 cm are controlled by doses of 7,000 cGy. Nodes larger than 3 cm rarely disappear during the course of irradiation, with the exception of primary tumors of the nasopharynx or tonsillar fossa, wherein a complete response to irradiation often occurs despite advanced nodal disease. Generally, combined surgery and irradiation should be used to treat patients with N2 and N3 disease. Typically, doses in the range of 5,000–6,000 cGy are given to involved nodes in a preoperative setting, whereas approximately 6,300 cGy is required in the postoperative setting. To minimize the risk of disease progression and treatment morbidity, no more than four to six weeks should elapse between therapies.

Nasopharynx

The World Health Organization (WHO) classifies nasopharyngeal tumors into three main classes: *WHO 1*, keratinizing squamous cell carcinoma; *WHO 2*, nonkeratinizing carcinoma; and *WHO 3*, lymphoepithelioma or poorly differentiated tumor [31]. Tumors of the nasopharynx are peculiar in that approximately 75% of affected patients will present with cervical nodal metastases. Accurate imaging using CT or MRI (or both) is crucial to determining the extent of disease, bone erosion, local extension to parapharyngeal spaces and orbit, and the presence of cervical metastases, especially the retropharyngeal nodes that are the first-station nodes. MRI seems to be more sensitive than CT in detecting skull base erosion, soft-tissue invasion outside the nasopharynx, and involvement of the retropharyngeal nodes [32]. In patients presenting with bulky nodal disease, the incidence of asymptomatic distant metastases is 40%, and all patients with nodal disease may undergo workup for distant disease (chest radiograph, liver ultrasonography, bone scan) [33]. Histologic type has a significant impact on outcome; treatment with radiotherapy and chemotherapy results in better local control and survival in patients with undifferentiated tumors (WHO 3) as compared to those with keratinizing tumors [34].

Radiotherapy is the treatment of choice for most patients, and even massive nodal disease responds well. Wide-field irradiation is mandated, with treatment portals encompassing structures from the base of the skull to clavicles to cover the primary site and all cervical lymph nodes. Typical doses in the range of 66–72 Gy are delivered to the primary site, using a shrinking-field technique to maximize dose to sites of gross disease. Persistent nodal disease after radiotherapy may be treated with neck dissection. Primary radiotherapy delivering 70–72 Gy in six weeks controls approximately 75% of early tumors [35]. Brachytherapy may be used to boost treatment in selected cases [36]. The treatment of advanced disease involves addition of cisplatin-based chemotherapy to radiotherapy. A randomized trial of neoadjuvant chemotherapy using cisplatin, epirubicin, and bleomycin followed by irradiation has shown a significant survival advantage over irradiation alone (47.1% versus 30%) [37]. Three-dimensional conformal therapy seems to target the tumor in a very precise fashion. Likewise, a large, multicenter randomized trial has demonstrated superior control and survival in patients treated with concomitant cisplatin and irradiation as compared to irradiation alone [38]. The role of surgery in treating the local site is very limited. Selected patients with small recurrences may be salvaged by surgery [39], and involved surgeons may have a role in providing access for placement of brachytherapy catheters.

Posttreatment follow-up includes careful examination, radiologic imaging, and investigation of symptoms. Laboratory testing must include monitoring of treatment-related side effects, including endocrine dysfunction of the pituitary gland.

Oral Cavity

The most common sites of tumors in the oral cavity are the tongue and the floor of the mouth. The treatment decisions depend on T stage, size, location (anterior or posterior), relation to the mandible (proximity or involvement), and incidence of gross or occult nodal metastasis. Early-stage lesions can be treated equally effectively using surgery or radiotherapy. Larger lesions are treated most effectively by combining surgery with postoperative radiotherapy. The indications for postoperative radiotherapy are listed in Table 12.8.

Small lip lesions can be excised in the fashion of a V with primary closure or local flap reconstruction. Patients with larger lesions require more complex reconstruction, such as the Abbe-Estlander or Karapandzic flaps. Surgical excision, external-beam irradiation, or temporary interstitial implant alone yields local control in more than 90% of cases. Excision of small lesions involving no more than 33% of the lower lip or 25% of

the upper lip can be performed with minimal cosmetic or functional sequelae. However, lesions involving the commissure or larger lesions should be considered for treatment with radiotherapy to minimize cosmetic or functional morbidity. Functional consequences of surgery include microstomia and oral incompetence, both of which are more common after extensive resection. For patients with early-stage (T1-T2 N0) disease, treatment should be directed only at the primary site, reserving neck treatment for more advanced lesions (T3-T4 node-positive). The five-year survival rates are 85% for patients with T1 and T2 lesions and 75% for patients with T3 and T4 disease. For patients with N0 disease, the five-year survival rate is 85%; for patients with N1 to N3 disease, the five-year survival rate drops to 65%.

Early lesions of the tongue can be excised with minimal functional consequences. Small defects can be closed primarily or can be left to heal by secondary intention. An ipsilateral supraomohyoid neck dissection is undertaken for tumors that are believed to infiltrate beyond 2–3 mm into the substance of the tongue [17]. More advanced lesions are treated with a combination of surgery and postoperative radiotherapy. Excision of a primary tumor may require a cheek flap or mandibular resection, depending on the tumor's relation to the mandible. A posterior lesion may require the mandibular swing approach for adequate exposure. Reconstruction using microvascular free-tissue transfer (e.g., radial forearm flap) produces good functional results, but the overall five-year survival rate is only 50% [40].

Small lesions of the floor of the mouth also can be excised transorally, and the defect can be closed primarily or by skin graft or may be left open to heal by secondary intention. Whenever a lesion in the anterior floor of the mouth near the opening of the submandibular salivary glands is excised, due consideration must be given to excision of the submandibular gland, owing to the risk of obstructive sialadenitis. In certain selected cases, the duct may be transposed into the adjacent normal mucosa. More extensive lesions may require marginal or segmental mandibulectomy (discussed later). The five-year survival rates for patients with stage I and stage II disease are 90% and 70%, respectively. Although surgery and irradiation provide equivalent results, the complication rates after radiotherapy are higher. The survival results drop to approximately 55–65% for advanced tumors treated with combined-modality treatment [41].

Surgery and radiotherapy give equal cure rates for early buccal lesions, but irradiation failures present at a higher stage and are more likely to require extensive surgery and reconstruction. Small lesions may be excised through the open mouth, and the defect can be left open to heal by secondary intention or may be closed by skin graft. Larger lesions and those that involve the oral commissure, the full thickness and skin of the cheek, or the mandible require more extensive surgery. Composite resection may result in a full-thickness soft-tissue defect with bone loss that may need microvascular free-tissue transfer. Approximately 50–75% of patients will be alive and free of disease five years after treatment [42]. Lesions of the alveolar ridge have a greater propensity to metastasize to cervical nodes. Surgery is the preferred modality in view of the proximity to bone, which may be managed by partial or composite resection. Usually, surgery includes neck dissection, and the overall survival rate is approximately 60%.

Oropharynx

The oropharynx sites involved most commonly are the tonsils and the base of the tongue. Other sites are the soft palate and the pharyngeal wall. Lymphatic metastasis is an early and common feature of tonsillar tumors. Treatment decisions are dictated by anatomic and tumor factors and by morbidity associated with the various therapeutic modalities. In general, early-stage disease can be treated by either radiotherapy or surgery, whereas more advanced lesions are treated by combinations of these methods. Radiotherapy is chosen more often than surgery for most early lesions because the cure rates are high and the functional outcome is better.

Early tonsillar tumors can be treated with radiotherapy, but more advanced lesions, especially those with metastatic nodes, are resected best surgically and followed up with postoperative irradiation. Irradiation treatment portals encompass both the primary site and the ipsilateral neck, including the retropharyngeal lymph nodes. Care is taken to minimize dose to the contralateral parotid gland to reduce the risk of xerostomia. Radiotherapy for T1 and T2 lesions results in local control rates of 70–90%, and salvage surgery is successful in approximately two-thirds of patients, yielding an ultimate local control of 90%. Gaining access to the larger lesions of the oropharynx through the open mouth is difficult, and resection of most tonsillar and base-of-tongue tumors requires a lower lip-splitting incision with a mandibulotomy. Most patients need a neck dissection because of the high incidence of cervical metastases. Depending on the size and location of a soft-tissue defect, closure may be attained primarily or by a pedicle or free flap.

The most common approach for locally advanced lesions is surgery followed by radiotherapy, although definitive radiotherapy with the addition of a neck dissection for node-positive patients is a reasonable alternative. Radiotherapy of advanced lesions (T3-T4) achieves local control rates in the range of 25–70%, which may be improved by twice a day fractions. Five-year T-stage-specific survival rates have been reported to be 89%, 55%, 49%, and 15% for T1 through T4, respectively. Patients who present with bulky nodal disease and a small primary tumor may be managed with bimodality therapy: neck dissection followed promptly by radiotherapy to control the primary site [43].

Primary radiotherapy is the preferred definitive treatment for most early tumors of the base of the tongue. Infiltrative or endophytic T3 or T4 lesions call for either surgery combined with postoperative radiotherapy or an organ-preserving approach using radiotherapy and chemotherapy. A number of investigators have demonstrated that the combination of external-beam irradiation and an implant boost is an effective treatment for patients with base-of-tongue cancer, which optimizes functional outcome [44]. Irradiation portals include sites of primary involvement and sites of probable extension and bilateral regional and retropharyngeal lymph node groups. Irradiation may be delivered as external-beam treatment alone or in combination with an implant. The advantage of the latter approach is relative sparing of normal surrounding tissues, with decreased treatment-related morbidity and improved local control [33–36]. One treatment approach calls for a combination of external-beam irradiation (50–54 Gy) plus an interstitial ^{192}Ir implant (20–30 Gy) to treat a primary site and external-beam irradiation combined with a neck dissection to treat cervical lymph nodes when indicated [44]. External irradiation of the neck is performed in lieu of a neck dissection in patients who present with clinically negative (N0) necks. Chemoradiation followed by implant and neck dissection may be considered in the treatment of advanced lesions that otherwise would require total laryngectomy at the time of presentation if treated surgically. The overall five-year survival rate for such patients is reported at 26%. Five-year T-stage-specific survival rates are 45% for patients with T1 and T2 disease and 10% for patients with T3 and T4 disease. Five-year N-stage-specific survival rates are 45% for patients with N0 disease and 20% for patients with N1 to N3 disease [27, 29, 37–39, 40, 45, 46].

If surgery is used, the standard surgical approach to base-of-tongue lesions includes resection of the base of the tongue by the mandibulotomy approach and ipsilat-

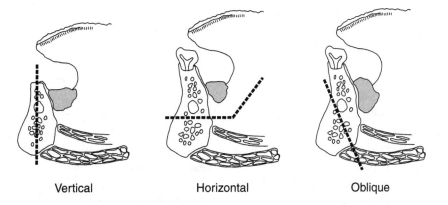

Vertical   Horizontal   Oblique

Figure 12.11 Various types of marginal mandibulectomies: vertical, horizontal, and oblique cuts. (Reprinted with permission of Wiley-Liss, Inc., a subsidiary of John Wiley & Sons, Inc., from AR Shaha, Marginal mandibulectomy for carcinoma of the floor of the mouth. *J Surg Oncol* 49:116–119, 1992.)

eral neck dissection with reconstruction. Often, a total glossectomy or a supraglottic (or even total) laryngectomy may be necessary, depending on the site and extent of primary disease. The functional consequences of resection of these tumors includes significant difficulty with speech and swallowing, both of which adversely impair ability to work, communication with others, and eating in public. The majority of patients managed surgically require postoperative irradiation because of close resection margins, nodal metastases, and advanced local disease. Small tumors of the base of the tongue may be resected by the transhyoid pharyngotomy approach.

Mandible

The mandible must be considered in the management of oral and oropharyngeal cancers, either because it may be involved by the disease or because it may limit access to the primary tumor. Preoperative evaluation of the mandible is vital to the proper management of patients with oral cavity cancer, especially those who present with lesions that are in close proximity or adherent to the medial aspect of the mandible. No definitive investigation can evaluate the status of the mandible with absolute accuracy. Clinical evaluation remains the best "test," mainly because demonstrating minimal bony invasion radiologically is difficult [47]. Imaging modalities available include dental x-ray films, panoramic x-ray films of the mandible, dentascans, and CT, MRI, and bone scans. Dental fillings lead to considerable artifacts on CT scan, and all imaging modalities have a high incidence of false-positive results. A panoramic view of the mandible may be useful to evaluate the extent of resection necessary in the event of gross destruction of bone. Although the reliability of imaging in detecting bony

involvement is low, all potential candidates for bone resection must undergo radiologic imaging for planning and preparation of templates for mandibular reconstruction.

Understanding of tumor spread to the mandible from oral cavity cancer has evolved considerably. In the past, tumors were believed to spread to cervical lymph nodes along lymphatic channels that pierce the mandibular periosteum and bone. However, it has been shown that tumors of the oral cavity spread to the mandible by direct extension along the alveolar ridge through pores on the alveolar border or through the dental socket. Clearly, the edentulous mandible is at high risk for direct invasion, as are tumors of the retromolar region. This improved understanding of the anatomy of spread has led to a trend away from routine segmental mandibulectomy, which was used for access, toward conservation of the uninvolved mandible. Minimal periosteal or bone involvement can be treated with marginal mandibulectomy, and a mandibulotomy is used if greater access is required for lesions in the posterior oral cavity or oropharynx.

Marginal mandibulectomy can be performed via a horizontal, vertical, or oblique cut (Fig. 12.11) [48]. Use of the oblique method allows retention of a strong mandibular remnant. The oblique cut has the advantage also of providing better tumor clearance, especially if a tumor invades the diaphragm of the floor of the mouth. The defect after marginal mandibulectomy can be resurfaced easily by advancement of adjacent mucosa or by a split-thickness skin graft. Selected small defects may be left open to heal by secondary intention. For larger defects, the radial forearm-free microvascular flap yields best functional results.

Mandibular swing or mandibulotomy is indicated for surgical access to tumors of the posterior oral cavity or oropharynx. Segmental resection of the uninvolved mandible purely to gain access generally is not advocated. The mandibular osteotomy may be situated in either a paramedian or a midline location; lateral mandibulotomy is not indicated routinely. A paramedian mandibulotomy is superior to a midline or lateral mandibulotomy for the following reasons: The paramedian osteotomy can be situated in the natural space between the incisor and canine teeth, avoiding the need for dental extraction; the inferior alveolar nerve and vessels are spared; genial muscles do not have to be divided; the osteotomy lies outside the portal of irradiation; and the mandibular segments can be fixed adequately using miniplates or stainless steel wires. After the osteotomy is complete, the swing is performed by incising the mucosa of the floor of the mouth along the medial aspect of the mandible posteriorly toward the region of the tumor. This approach also provides good exposure for resection of parapharyngeal tumors, including those of the deep lobe of the parotid. The cosmetic and functional results are excellent, as demonstrated by Spiro et al. [49].

Patients with advanced oral or oropharyngeal tumors that involve the mandible will require mandibular resection and reconstruction. Primary mandibular reconstruction, especially after segmental resection of the arch, now is routine practice, owing to the availability of microvascular free flaps. Commonly used flaps include the fibula, iliac crest, and scapula, but the choice of donor site depends largely on the bone stock required, the soft-tissue defect, and the choice of the individual microvascular surgeon [50]. Microvascular flaps have been shown to tolerate postoperative radiotherapy well and, after completion of therapy, cosmetic and functional results can be improved with osseointegrated dental implants. Under difficult circumstances, reconstruction with A-O plates may be performed, but success rates are limited, and the extrusion rate is high.

Treating osteonecrosis of the mandible after radiotherapy is difficult, and prophylactic measures must be instituted before commencing treatment. These include preirradiation dental evaluation and extraction of unhealthy teeth, fluoride treatment, and regular follow-up through the course of irradiation. The clinical differentiation between residual or recurrent tumor and osteoradionecrosis may be difficult, though PET scanning seems to be a useful new tool [51]. Early, limited osteoradionecrosis may be treated conservatively with débridement, long-term antibiotics, use of intensive oral irrigations and, occasionally, hyperbaric oxygen. Selected patients with more extensive necrosis may

benefit from aggressive surgical excision and immediate microvascular reconstruction [52].

Larynx

In the United States, tumors of the larynx involve the supraglottis (30%), glottis (69%), and subglottis (1%) [53]. Tumors of the glottis present early, owing to the readily apparent symptom of hoarseness, whereas tumors in the other two sites have a tendency to remain silent and present late.

Vocal cord cancers metastasize to cervical nodes less frequently, owing to sparse lymphatic supply, and therefore have a relatively better prognosis. Surgery is slightly better at controlling early (T1 and T2) lesions than is irradiation alone, but the control rates are equalized by surgical salvage of irradiation failures. Surgery may involve endoscopic excision with a CO_2 laser or, otherwise, laryngofissure with cordectomy or vertical partial laryngectomy. However, T1 and T2 tumors are treated best with irradiation because cure rates are excellent (80–90%) and resultant voice quality is better than that with hemilaryngectomy or partial laryngectomy. Irradiation fields for T1 and T2 glottic tumors encompass only the primary site, because the risk of lymph node involvement is very small. Owing to decreased local control with radiotherapy, surgery should be offered when the histologic type is relatively resistant to irradiation (i.e., verrucous, adenocarcinoma, sarcoma). Carcinoma in situ may be treated equally well with cord stripping, laser treatment, or external-beam irradiation. However, repeat stripping, frequently required for recurrence, results in a thickened cord and hoarse voice. Radiotherapy should be considered in patients who experience rapid or multiple recurrences after cord stripping or laser treatment. Laryngeal conservation is possible in approximately 70–90% of radiotherapy failures; local control rates of 60–80%, equivalent to those for total laryngectomy, can be achieved using partial laryngectomy [54, 55].

Patients with cord fixation (T3) or thyroid or cricoid cartilage invasion (T4) can be offered either total laryngectomy with postoperative irradiation, as indicated, or attempted organ preservation with chemoradiation. Generally, cartilage invasion contraindicates irradiation as a primary modality. Patients who accept the nonsurgical approach must be able to undergo frequent follow-up examinations, so that salvage laryngectomy may be performed in a timely manner if necessary.

Either supraglottic laryngectomy or external-beam

radiotherapy may be used with equal efficacy to treat patients with T1, T2, and selected T3 squamous cell carcinomas of the supraglottic larynx. Patients with more advanced disease can be treated with external-beam irradiation only in the presence of favorable factors, such as exophytic tumor and still-mobile vocal cords or limited cartilage or soft-tissue extension or base-of-tongue invasion. The risk of local failure after radiotherapy rises to 40–50% in T2 and T3 lesions in the presence of reduced cord mobility.

Generally, total laryngectomy is recommended for unfavorable T3 cancers, which include endophytic or bulky tumors that usually are bilateral and often present with vocal cord fixation or airway compromise (or both). Other issues that argue in favor of primary irradiation treatment for affected patients include major medical contraindications, inadequate pulmonary reserve, poor patient compliance, and advanced age.

Surgery for early supraglottic cancer involves supraglottic (horizontal) partial laryngectomy, which is designed to remove the entire supraglottic unit, including the epiglottis and the aryepiglottic folds down to the false vocal cords with the overlying thyroid cartilage and the intervening preepiglottic space. Only selected patients are suited for this operation, mainly because it results inevitably in some degree of aspiration that may cause postoperative pulmonary problems. The quality of voice, however, is relatively well preserved, and few patients need long-term nutritional support, as poor swallowing does not ensue. The operation is oncologically sound, and control rates of more than 90% have been reported [56, 57]. Owing to the high incidence of nodal metastasis and the associated poor outcome [58], treatment of the neck should be considered in all patients with supraglottic cancer. If primary irradiation is the treatment of choice, the portals should include the cervical lymph nodes. Alternatively, if supraglottic laryngectomy is undertaken, selective neck dissection of levels II, III, and IV is used to stage the neck disease and to select patients for postoperative irradiation.

Traditionally, advanced laryngeal cancer has been treated with total laryngectomy combined with postoperative radiotherapy. The combined use of chemotherapy and irradiation in larynx-preserving protocols, such as the Veterans Administration trial [21], now has provided another option. A common dilemma in the follow-up evaluation of patients treated with primary irradiation is the differential diagnosis between radionecrosis and residual or recurrent tumor. Four months after treatment, the FDG-PET scan seems to be superior to any imaging modality currently available for differentiating recurrent tumor from postirradiation soft-tissue changes [12]. If total laryngectomy is undertaken, a jugular node dissection for lymph nodes at levels II, III, and IV usually is included for patients with a clinically negative neck. Paratracheal groove nodes are dissected for subglottic tumors, and an ipsilateral thyroid lobectomy is performed for tumors that involve the subglottis or the pyriform sinus apex. Survival rates of approximately 50–60% have been reported for stage III and stage IV laryngeal tumors [59, 60].

Hypopharynx

Most patients with hypopharyngeal cancer present in advanced stages, and more than 50% of patients will have palpable cervical lymph nodes at presentation. Consequently, the majority of patients require combined-modality treatment. Currently, a number of trials are evaluating the role of chemoradiotherapy in organ preservation for such advanced lesions. Most often, surgery involves total laryngopharyngectomy, but selected patients may be treated with partial pharyngectomy or partial laryngopharyngectomy. Reconstruction of the pharyngeal defect after total laryngopharyngectomy depends on the extent of mucosal loss. Partial circumference defects can be repaired using a myocutaneous or microvascular free-flap patch pharyngoplasty. Ideally, full circumferential defects are reconstructed with a free jejunal graft. Total laryngopharyngoesophagectomy may be required for lesions that extend into the cervical esophagus, and the defect is reconstructed using gastric pull-up and pharyngogastrostomy. All patients routinely undergo neck dissection in conjunction with laryngopharyngectomy in view of the high incidence of nodal metastasis. Primary radiotherapy and chemoradiation have been used in an attempt to conserve the larynx, but the results are not equivalent to those for laryngeal cancer [61]. Patients with hypopharyngeal cancer also have a more than 20% incidence of distant metastases, especially in the presence of advanced neck metastases. The overall prognosis for such patients is dismal, and only approximately 25% survive five years after treatment.

Nasal Cavity and Paranasal Sinuses

Surgery for tumors of the nasal cavity and paranasal sinuses ranges from lateral rhinotomy to craniofacial resection, depending on a variety of factors that include the extent and type of the lesion. Small lesions localized to the lateral nasal wall can be excised adequately by a medial maxillectomy through a lateral rhinotomy.

Treating infrastructure maxillary lesions is easier, and functional and cosmetic results are satisfactory with good local control. Generally, such tumors can be resected by a partial maxillectomy that removes part of the hard palate along with the medial and lateral walls of the maxillary sinus. Treatment of suprastructure lesions, on the other hand, may require total maxillectomy with resection and reconstruction of the orbital floor. In addition, orbital exenteration may be necessary if a tumor extends to involve the soft tissue of the orbit. Tumors that extend up to the skull base may require a combined craniofacial approach performed by a head and neck surgeon in conjunction with a neurosurgeon.

Adequate rehabilitation of patients undergoing any form of maxillary resection depends on the active involvement of a maxillary prosthodontist. Preoperative dental impressions are taken to fabricate a temporary prosthesis, which is inserted into the defect at the end of the operation. The defect after maxillectomy may be resurfaced with a split-thickness skin graft bolstered in place by the temporary prosthesis. Affected patients may require modification of the prosthesis as the defect heals and changes shape. Ultimately, when the defect has stabilized, a final prosthesis is fashioned, and the patient can easily care for the skin-graft-lined cavity. Complex and extensive resections may necessitate more complicated reconstruction, but innovations by a prosthodontist often can produce acceptable functional and cosmetic results. Large defects may be reconstructed with microvascular free flaps; commonly, rectus abdominis flaps are used. Postoperative radiotherapy is used for the usual indications, but its delivery is complicated by the proximity of the eye, the brain, and the spinal cord.

Cervical lymph node metastasis occurs in approximately 15% of patients and predicts a dismal outcome. Radiotherapy alone (to nodes and primary tumor) has been reported to control disease in 52% of patients at five years, but treatment was complicated by unilateral blindness in one-third of such patients [62]. Although the overall five-year survival rate has been reported to range from 35% to 40% [63], more aggressive resection using the craniofacial approach has improved results [64]. Concurrent cisplatin infusion chemotherapy and hyperfractionated radiotherapy have been shown to result in a complete response rate of 92% and a three-year survival rate of 58% in a small number of patients with stage IV disease [65], but the role of chemotherapy requires further study. A study of treatment of these tumors by intraarterial high-dose platinum and radiotherapy (the RADPLAT regimen) is ongoing.

Recurrent Head and Neck Cancer

The treatment of recurrent head and neck cancer depends on the type of previous treatment and the initial extent of the disease. Tumors that recur in such locations as the anterior floor of the mouth can be treated satisfactorily with surgical resection and appropriate reconstruction. Tumors in such other locations as the skull base are not amenable to surgical salvage. Other contraindications to surgical resection include involvement of the common or internal carotid artery, invasion of the prevertebral fascia, and tumor adherence to the vertebral bodies. Resection of a recurrent tumor should encompass the entire initial extent of a primary tumor rather than encompassing the localized recurrent disease or tumor nidus. Accurate and detailed documentation of the initial extent of disease is vital in all patients undergoing nonsurgical primary treatment.

Advanced, Inoperable Cancer

In the evaluation of advanced cancer, an extremely important factor is attending surgeons' ability to distinguish operable from inoperable lesions. Such surgeons should evaluate the inoperability of the tumor and should obtain a second opinion, if necessary. The best options available under these circumstances may be investigational protocols or new approaches, such as hyperfractionated radiotherapy and chemoradiosensitizers. For many patients, however, the aim of treatment becomes satisfactory palliation, including avoidance of airway problems, maintenance of nutrition, and care of fungating tumor. Combined treatment with chemotherapy and radiotherapy may be possible in patients who have not received irradiation previously.

Table 12.11 summarizes the results of randomized trials of induction or adjuvant chemotherapy in patients with advanced head and neck tumors. Complete response rates vary from 37% to 86%, but no improvement in survival has been demonstrated. Though the consideration of surgical resection is tempting in patients who respond to treatment, equally important is the realization that surgical resection is unlikely to improve survival and at the same time places affected patients at considerable risk of morbidity and even mortality from the radical surgical procedure.

Table 12.11 Randomized Trials of Induction or Adjuvant Chemotherapy (or Both)

Study	No. of Patients	Drugs	CT Response Rate (CR)	Local Therapy	Outcome	Comments
Jacobs	443	Cisplatin, bleomycin	37% (3%)	S/RT	No significant difference in survival	Induction and adjuvant CT, survival benefit for N2 disease by subset analysis, decreased distant metastases with adjuvant CT
Shuller	158	Cisplatin, methotrexate, bleomycin, vincristine	70% (19%)	S/RT	No significant difference in survival	Induction CT, decreased distant metastases
VA larynx study	332	Cisplatin, 5-FU	86% (31%)	RT versus S/RT	No significant difference in survival	Induction CT, decreased distant metastases, larynx preservation
Laramore	448	Cisplatin, 5-FU	NA	S/RT	No significant difference in survival	CT adjuvant to surgery, decreased incidence of distant metastases

CT = chemotherapy; CR = complete response; S/RT = local therapy with surgery or radiotherapy (or both); RT = radiotherapy; VA = Veterans Administration; 5-FU = 5-fluorouracil; NA = not applicable.
Source: Reprinted with permission from EE Vokes, RR Weichselbaum, *Chemoradiotherapy for Head and Neck Cancer.* [PPO Updates, vol 7, no. 6.] Philadelphia: Lippincott, 1993.

Chemotherapy and Organ Preservation

The role of chemotherapy in the treatment of head and neck cancer has been investigated extensively over the last several decades. Currently, cisplatin and 5-fluorouracil (5-FU) are the most active agents, but newer agents (e.g., paclitaxel, docetaxel, vinorelbine, and gemcitabine) are currently being evaluated.

With most single agents, response rates range from 10% to 30% in patients with recurrent or metastatic disease, but these agents no longer are used as monotherapy. Generally, two or three non-cross-resistant agents are used in combination, cisplatin and 5-FU being used the most widely [18, 21, 66–70]. In vitro evidence demonstrates synergy between the two agents [71]: Cisplatin increases intracellular folic acid that in turn promotes the covalent binding of 5-

fluorodeoxyuridylate, an active 5-FU metabolite to its target enzyme, thymidylate synthase. Response rates with 5-FU are reported to be significantly better when it is administered over a five-day period as a continuous infusion as compared to a daily bolus injection over the same period. When this combination is used as primary treatment before surgery or irradiation (i.e., neoadjuvant or induction chemotherapy), response rates as high as 90% have been reported, with complete response rates of 40–60% [18].

Neoadjuvant chemotherapy has been found to show no overall survival benefit in randomized trials, but some conclusions can be drawn from the results of selected trials (see Table 12.11). These trials showed that response rates up to 90% can be achieved in previously untreated patients [66], that the rate of distant metastases can be reduced [67], and that this form of therapy may allow for organ preservation in selected patients [21]. Combination chemoradiotherapy also has been demonstrated to prolong survival in patients with unresectable primary disease and in those with N2 disease. With a few exceptions, however, the role of neoadjuvant chemotherapy remains restricted to the clinical trial setting.

Chemotherapy also has been used concurrently with radiotherapy on the basis of the following rationale: it acts locally and systemically outside the radiotherapy field; chemotherapy and irradiation have different cellular targets, and chemotherapy eliminates tumor cells that were damaged sublethally by radiotherapy; it acts against radioresistant hypoxic tumor cells; and certain chemotherapeutic agents (e.g., cisplatin, carboplatin, 5-FU, hydroxyurea, and paclitaxel) act as radiosensitizers. Concurrent chemoradiotherapy can be delivered in one of three ways: the classic course, which is one to three doses of single-agent chemotherapy added to an uninterrupted course of irradiation; split-course treatment, which gives simultaneous chemotherapy and irradiation with scheduled breaks to allow normal tissues to recover; and alternating chemotherapy and radiotherapy, wherein one modality immediately follows the other.

Several randomized trials have shown a statistically significant benefit in locoregional control with concurrent chemoradiotherapy [68, 69]. Some have even reported prolonged survival [45, 70].

PREVENTION

Head and neck cancer is a disease of lifestyle, and prevention includes limiting exposure to such main etiologic factors as tobacco and alcohol (see Chapter 4). Early intervention may reduce the risk of malignant progression in patients who have documented premalignant lesions or of second primary tumors in those who have been treated for malignancy. The use of vitamin A analogs and *cis*-retinoic acid has been associated with a beneficial effect but remains investigational. Retinoids have been shown to reverse leukoplakic changes in 55–100% of the patients, but the effects are short-lived, and the treatment produces substantial side effects [72].

SALIVARY TUMORS

The salivary glands can be divided into major and minor types. Major salivary glands include the parotid, submandibular, and sublingual salivary glands. Approximately 500–700 minor salivary glands are distributed throughout the mucosa of the upper aerodigestive tract, but approximately half are located on the hard palate [73]. This distribution accounts for the dictum that a lesion of the hard palate should be considered a minor salivary gland tumor unless proved otherwise. Malignant tumors of the salivary glands are rare, but the incidence of malignancy depends on the anatomic site involved (Table 12.12). The majority (75%) of parotid neoplasms are benign, and half of submandibular gland tumors are malignant. In contrast, the majority (81%) of minor salivary gland neoplasms are malignant. A tumor of the sublingual glands can be mistaken easily for a tumor of the floor of the mouth.

The parotid gland is the largest salivary gland and is also the most common site of salivary neoplasms. The facial nerve divides the gland into superficial lobes (80% of the substance) and deep lobes (20% of the substance). Most parotid tumors involve the superficial lobe; deep lobe tumors are rare. Successful surgery of the parotid gland depends on identification, dissection, and preservation of the facial nerve and its branches. The facial nerve exits the skull through the stylomastoid foramen and passes lateral to the styloid process. The main trunk of the nerve can be located at the confluence of three important anatomic structures: the posterior belly of the digastric muscle, the tip of the mastoid process, and the bony auditory canal. Then the nerve enters the substance of the gland and divides into two main divisions: the upper zygomaticotemporal division and the lower cervicomandibular division. By the time the nerve exits the gland at its anterior and superior borders, it divides into its five main branches: temporal, zygomaticoorbital, buccal, mandibular, and cervical. The orbital branch, supplying the eyelids, and the mandibular branch (ramus mandibularis), supplying the lip, are functionally the most important of the five branches. Injury to these branches during surgery can cause considerable cosmetic and functional disability.

The submandibular gland lies in the submandibular triangle on the surface of the hyoglossus muscle above

Table 12.12   Site-Wise Distribution of Salivary Tumors

Site	Percentage of all Neoplasms	Percentage Malignant
Parotid gland	65	25
Submandibular gland	8	50
Minor salivary glands	27	81

Source: Reprinted with permission from JP Shah, JK Ihde, Salivary gland tumors. *Curr Probl Surg* 27:775–883, 1990.

the digastric. The three nerves in close proximity to the submandibular gland are the lingual, hypoglossal, and ramus mandibularis. Proper evaluation of these nerves is extremely important in the management of malignant neoplasms of the submandibular gland. The submandibular salivary (Wharton's) duct runs forward from the deeper portion of the gland under the mylohyoid muscle to the floor of the mouth, where it opens just lateral to the frenulum of the tongue.

Diagnostic Workup

Most salivary gland tumors are evaluated adequately by physical examination. Palpation of the parotid gland may reveal an obviously hard, fixed malignancy. The presence of facial nerve paralysis is an extremely reliable indicator of malignancy, as benign masses almost never cause facial palsy, even when they become huge. Radiologic imaging with CT scanning or MRI is helpful in evaluating the extent of disease, especially deep-lobe parotid tumors and minor salivary gland tumors in such locations as the nasal cavity and paranasal sinuses, and in detecting previously unnoticed cervical lymphadenopathy.

FNA cytology is helpful in confirming the diagnosis of malignancy, but a negative finding cannot rule out cancer. FNA is sometimes unable to distinguish among the various types of salivary gland neoplasms. For example, a benign mixed tumor may occasionally be interpreted as an adenoid cystic carcinoma. It does, however, help to distinguish between salivary and nonsalivary (lymph node) pathology when a tumor is located in the region of the tail of the parotid. If the FNA helps to establish a preoperative diagnosis of malignancy, involved surgeons can prepare affected patients better for appropriate management of the facial nerve. FNA is a simple technique, and it may reveal valuable information if it is used with the understanding that negative results generally do not constitute a final diagnosis.

Although minor salivary gland tumor staging is similar to that used for squamous cell carcinoma arising in the same location, Tables 12.13 and 12.14 shows the American Joint Committee on Cancer staging for cancer of the major salivary glands.

Benign Parotid Tumors

Common benign lesions seen in the parotid gland include benign mixed tumor, Warthin's tumor, oncocy-

Table 12.13 TNM Staging for Cancers of the Major Salivary Glands

Classification	Definition
Primary tumor (T)	
TX	Primary tumor cannot be assessed
T0	No evidence of primary tumor
T1	Tumor $\leq$ 2 cm in greatest dimension without extraparenchymal extension
T2	Tumor > 2 cm but $\leq$ 4 cm in greatest dimension without extraparenchymal extension
T3	Tumor having extraparenchymal extension without seventh nerve involvement and/or > 4 cm but $\leq$ 6 cm in greatest dimension
T4	Tumor invades base of skull, seventh nerve, and/or > 6 cm in greatest dimension
Regional lymph nodes (N)	
NX	Regional lymph nodes cannot be assessed
N0	No regional lymph node metastasis
N1	Metastasis in a single ipsilateral lymph node, 3 cm or less in greatest dimension
N2	Metastasis in a single ipsilateral lymph node, > 3 cm but $\leq$ 6 cm in greatest dimension; or in multiple ipsilateral lymph nodes, none > 6 cm in greatest dimension; or in bilateral or contralateral lymph nodes, none > 6 cm in greatest dimension
N2a	Metastasis in a single ipsilateral lymph node > 3 cm but $\leq$ 6 cm in greatest dimension
N2b	Metastasis in multiple ipsilateral lymph nodes, none > 6 cm in greatest dimension
N2c	Metastasis in bilateral or contralateral lymph nodes, none > 6 cm in greatest dimension
N3	Metastasis in a lymph node > 6 cm in greatest dimension
Distant metastasis (M)	
MX	Distant metastasis cannot be assessed
M0	No distant metastases
M1	Distant metastasis

AJCC = American Joint Committee on Cancer.
Source: Used with the permission of the *American Joint Committee on Cancer (AJCC®)*, Chicago. AJCC® *Cancer Staging Manual* (5th Edition), 1997. Philadelphia: Lippincott-Raven.

toma, and benign lymphoepithelial lesions. Approximately 80% of benign parotid lesions are benign mixed tumors. They are classified histologically as pleomorphic adenoma owing to the diversity of myxoid, chondroid, fibroid, and epithelial components that make up the tumor. Generally, such tumors grow slowly, but an occasional patient may present with rapid growth in a

Table 12.14 AJCC Stage Grouping for Cancers of the Major Salivary Glands

Stage I	T1	N0	M0
	T2	N0	M0
Stage II	T3	N0	M0
Stage III	T1	N1	M0
	T2	N1	M0
Stage IV	T4	N0	M0
	T3	N1	M0
	T4	N1	M0
	Any T	N2	M0
	Any T	N3	M0
	Any T	Any N	M1

AJCC = American Joint Committee on Cancer.
Source: Used with the permission of the *American Joint Committee on Cancer (AJCC®)*, Chicago. *AJCC® Cancer Staging Manual* (5th Edition), 1997. Philadelphia: Lippincott-Raven.

long-standing tumor. This change may signify carcinoma developing in a benign mixed tumor (carcinoma ex pleomorphic adenoma), which occurs in 1–7% of patients. Most patients present with a solitary, well-defined mass in the superficial lobe of the parotid gland. Occasionally, the tumor may extend into the deep lobe of the gland. The most appropriate and optimal surgery for benign mixed tumors is superficial or subtotal parotidectomy with dissection and preservation of the facial nerve and its branches.

Excising tumors of the deep lobe of the parotid may be difficult, and surgery essentially will result in enucleation; however, facial nerve function can be preserved by careful dissection and separation of the nerve and its branches. Patients who have undergone inadequate local excision or enucleation are prone to local recurrence. An important reminder is that any tumor in the parotid area is considered a parotid tumor until proved otherwise. Thus, all affected patients should be brought to the operating room for appropriate surgical intervention, which consists of a standard parotid incision, identification of the facial nerve and its branches, and removal of the parotid tumor. Occasionally, for a very large deep-lobe parotid tumor, a lower-lip split incision and mandibulotomy approach may be required.

Warthin's tumor, also called *papillary cystadenoma lymphomatosum*, originates in the periparotid or intraparotid lymph nodes. It accounts for approximately 10–15% of benign parotid tumors. Ten percent of these tumors are multifocal, and 10% may be bilateral. The risk of malignant transformation is extremely small, and the diagnosis of Warthin's tumor can be made easily with FNA cytologic analysis.

Oncocytomas are rare, fleshy, slow-growing benign tumors of the parotid that constitute approximately 1% of salivary gland tumors. With the increasing incidence of the acquired immunodeficiency syndrome (AIDS) and human immunodeficiency virus infection, benign lymphoepithelial lesions are becoming more common. They are seen also in patients with AIDS-related complex. These lesions involve the periparotid and intraparotid lymph nodes. Generally, affected patients present with a large mass in the tail of the parotid, which may be cystic. The long duration of the mass (4–6 months), the history of human immunodeficiency virus positivity, and the characteristic clinical picture along with the cystic consistency of the mass render the clinical diagnosis relatively obvious. The CT scan has been used to document multiple cystic areas and bilaterality. Because the natural history of the disease is still evolving, involved physicians tend toward conservative treatment that may consist of multiple needle aspirations and close observation. However, if affected patients are symptomatic and have no obvious stigmata of AIDS, surgical excision may be considered, as it appears to produce excellent results. Radiotherapy has been used in select individuals.

Malignant Parotid Tumors

Adenoid cystic carcinoma constitutes approximately 10% of parotid malignancies. This tumor exhibits an unpredictable behavior, owing to its tendency to local extension beyond the gross lesion, its perineural involvement, and its high incidence of local recurrence. Distant metastases also are fairly common, mostly to the lung, where they may remain dormant for a long time. Characteristically, the histopathologic appearance of these tumors has been described as Swiss cheese-like.

Mucoepidermoid carcinomas are more common and constitute approximately 44% of parotid malignancies. These tumors originate in the salivary duct epithelium and are classified as low or high grade. Clinically, low-grade lesions can mimic benign mixed tumors. A standard superficial parotidectomy is adequate treatment for low-grade mucoepidermoid carcinomas, as the incidence of local recurrence and distant metastasis is small. High-grade tumors can invade the facial nerve, and the incidence of lymph node metastasis at presentation is approximately 50%.

Malignant mixed tumors, accounting for approximately 17% of parotid malignancies, may originate in slow-growing benign mixed tumors [73, 74]. Approximately 15–20% of affected patients present with regional lymph node metastases. Malignant mixed tu-

Table 12.15 Involvement of Cervical Lymph Nodes by Metastasis of Primary Carcinoma in Salivary Glands

Time of Appearance	Parotid Gland (%) (n = 623)	Submandibular Glands (%) (n = 129)	Minor Glands (%) (n = 526)
Initially	20	33	13
Subsequently	5	4	9
Total	25	37	22

Source: Data drawn from DJ Kelley, RH Spiro, Management of the neck in parotid carcinoma. *Am J Surg* 172:695–697, 1996. Reprinted with permission from JP Shah, JK Ihde, Salivary gland tumors. *Curr Probl Surg* 27:775–883, 1990.

mors are often divided into two types. The first type, also known as carcinoma ex pleomorphic adenoma, is a carcinoma (usually adenocarcinoma) that develops in a pre-existing benign mixed tumor. Commonly, such patients are characterized by a long-term history of a benign mixed tumor that suddenly shows rapid growth of recent origin with fixation to deeper structures and skin, occasionally with ulceration. The facial nerve may be involved in the malignant pathology. The second type is the true malignant mixed tumor or carcinosarcoma. These tumors have malignant epithelial and mesenchymal components. They are relatively rare, accounting for 2–5% of malignant salivary gland tumors.

Treatment

SURGICAL EXCISION

Surgical excision in combination with adjuvant postoperative radiotherapy, if indicated, is the treatment of choice for malignant salivary tumors. Enucleation of parotid tumors is condemned uniformly and must not be carried out. The minimal operation for a lesion involving the parotid gland is a superficial parotidectomy with identification and preservation of the facial nerve. Most tumors are located in the superficial lobe of the parotid gland and can be excised easily and adequately using this operation. Tumors of the deep lobe constitute a challenge, both in terms of surgical approach and in preserving the facial nerve. Generally, the nerve is wrapped around the lesion, and careful identification, dissection, and preservation of its branches is crucial. In most instances, a deep-lobe parotid tumor can be removed without injuring the branches of the facial nerve. Occasionally, though, if the bulk of the tumor is against the pharyngeal wall, a mandibulotomy approach may be necessary for better exposure of the parapharyngeal area.

In a very few instances, a fully functioning facial nerve would be sacrificed. The trend currently is toward conservatism in managing the nerve in surgery for malignant tumors. In general, if the facial nerve is not paralyzed preoperatively and no direct extension of the disease into the nerve is found at surgery, every effort is made to preserve the nerve. A nerve that adheres to tumor may be peeled off carefully, in which case postoperative radiotherapy is warranted. Immediate nerve grafting using cable interposition grafts from the greater auricular nerve, the cervical plexus, or the sural nerve may be undertaken if the main trunk or major branches are sacrificed. If the nerve is sacrificed, eye function and eye closure can be improved by implantation of a Gold Weight (Gold Eyelid Implants; MedDev, Palo Alto, CA) in the upper eyelid. This procedure avoids exposure keratitis.

The management of malignant submandibular tumors is complicated by the presence of three important nerves in its vicinity: the ramus mandibularis, the hypoglossal, and the lingual. Block dissection of the submandibular gland entails removal of the entire contents of the submandibular triangle. If the tumor adheres to the mandible, excision of the outer periosteum or even the mandible may be required. A supraomohyoid neck dissection may be carried out as part of the procedure.

The standard of management of minor salivary gland tumors remains wide local excision. Generally, tumors involving the hard palate require a full-thickness excision or infrastructure partial maxillectomy with a dental obturator.

Management of cervical lymph nodes in patients with malignant salivary tumors remains controversial. The incidence of metastases in primary carcinoma of the salivary glands is listed in Table 12.15.

High-grade mucoepidermoid and primary squamous cell carcinoma are the only subtypes with a substantial risk of nodal metastases. Elective supraomohyoid neck dissection, therefore, may be considered for treatment of high-grade, high-stage lesions. If suspicious lymph nodes are found at surgery, a modified neck dissection

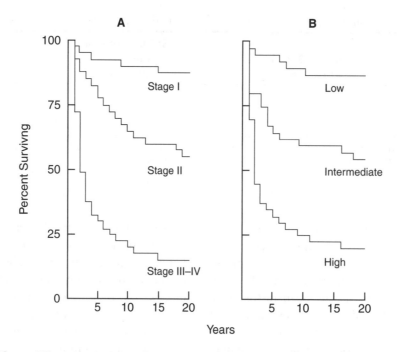

Figure 12.12   (A) Significant differences in survival were observed when previously untreated patients with salivary tumors were grouped according to the clinical stage ($p < .0001$). (B) Survival differences were similar in patients who had adenocarcinomas, mucoepidermoid carcinoma, or squamous cell carcinoma and were analyzed by histologic grade ($p < .0001$). (Reprinted with permission of Wiley-Liss, Inc., a subsidiary of John Wiley & Sons, Inc., from RH Spiro, Salivary neoplasms: overview of a 35-year experience with 2,807 patients. *Head Neck Surg* 8:177–184, 1986.)

Table 12.16   Determinate Cure Rates in Patients with Malignant Tumors

Interval (Yr)	Parotid Gland (%) (n = 623)	Submandibular Glands (%) (n = 129)	Minor Glands (%) (n = 526)
5	55	31	48
10	47	22	37
15	40	15	23
20	33	14	15

Source: Reprinted with permission of Wiley-Liss, Inc., a subsidiary of John Wiley & Sons, Inc., from RH Spiro, Salivary neoplasms: overview of a 35-year experience with 2,807 patients. *Head Neck Surg* 8:177–184, 1986.

may be completed. The presence of grossly palpable nodes at initial evaluation requires modified or radical neck dissection, as indicated. Table 12.16 shows the determinate cure rates in patients with malignant tumors of the three types of salivary glands.

RADIOTHERAPY

Indications for radiotherapy in treating salivary gland cancer include advanced inoperable cancer, high-grade, high-stage primary tumor, positive margins after surgery, deep-lobe malignant tumors, lymph node metastases, and tumor spillage at surgery. The use of fast neutrons for treating advanced salivary gland neoplasms has been under investigation and has shown much promise. Because the incidence of local recurrence in adenoid cystic carcinoma is high, postoperative radiotherapy must be considered in high-stage lesions.

Prognosis

Tumor stage remains the most important prognostic factor in salivary gland neoplasms. The overall 10-year survival rates for stages I through III are approximately 90%, 65%, and 22%, respectively (Fig. 12.12) [74]. Grade is also an important prognostic factor: The 10-year survival rate for low-grade tumors is 90% compared with 25% for high-grade tumors (see Fig. 12.12). Histologic type of the tumor also has an impact on prognosis: Acinic or low-grade mucoepidermoid tumors have a better prognosis than adenocarcinoma, malignant mixed tumor, adenoid cystic, or squamous cell carcinoma. Generally, tumors of the submandibular gland are more aggressive than are parotid tumors, as are minor salivary gland tumors in some locations (e.g., the paranasal sinuses), the examination of which is difficult.

FOLLOW-UP

Standard surveillance of patients treated for head and neck cancer includes a follow-up visit every six to eight weeks in the first year, every two to three months in the second year, every three to four months in the third year, and every 6–12 months thereafter for life. The degree to which patients undergoing routine follow-up should be investigated has been a subject of much debate. A chest radiograph probably should be performed every six months for the first two to three years and annually thereafter. An important policy is to evaluate the chest radiograph critically and to compare the films with previous radiographs for any abnormalities in the lung fields. The value of routine endoscopic evaluation of the upper aerodigestive tract is unproved; thus, endoscopic procedures should be undertaken only if affected patients have symptoms suggestive of a problem in the lungs or esophagus.

REFERENCES

1. Fleming ID, Cooper JS, Henson DE, et al. (eds). *AJCC Cancer Staging Manual* (5th ed). Philadelphia: Lippincott-Raven, 1997.
2. Shah JP. Cervical lymph node metastases: diagnostic, therapeutic and prognostic implications. *Oncology* 4:61–76, 1990.
3. Shah JP, Medina JE, Shaha AR, et al. Cervical lymph node metastasis. *Curr Probl Surg* 30:273–344, 1993.
4. Greenlee RT, Murray T, Bolden S, Wingo PA. Cancer statistics, 2000. *CA Cancer J Clin* 50:7–33, 2000.
5. Davidson BJ, Hsu TC, Schantz SP. The genetics of tobacco-induced cancer susceptibility. *Arch Otolaryngol Head Neck Surg* 119:1198–1205, 1993.
6. Liebowitz D. Nasopharyngeal carcinoma: the Epstein-Barr virus association. *Semin Oncol.* 21: 376–381, 1994.
7. McKaig RG, Baric RS, Olshan AF. Human papillomavirus and head and neck cancer: epidemiology and molecular biology. *Head Neck* 20:250–265, 1998.
8. Shah JP. Patterns of cervical lymph node metastasis from squamous carcinomas of the upper aerodigestive tract. *Am J Surg* 160:405–409, 1990.
9. Vokes EE, Weichselbaum R, Lippman SM, Hong WK. Head and neck cancer. *N Engl J Med* 328:184–194, 1993.
10. McIvor NP, Freeman JL, Salem S, et al. Ultrasonography and ultrasound-guided fine-needle aspiration biopsy of head and neck lesions: a surgical perspective. *Laryngoscope* 104:669–674, 1994.
11. Mann WJ, Beck A, Schreiber J, et al. Ultrasonography for evaluation of the carotid artery in head and neck cancer. *Laryngoscope* 104:885–888, 1994.
12. McGuirt WF, Greven K, Williams D, et al. PET scanning in head and neck oncology: a review. *Head Neck* 20:208–215, 1998.
13. Martin HE. Biopsy by needle puncture and aspiration. *Ann Surg* 92:169–181, 1930.
14. Shaha AR, Webber C, Marti J. Fine-needle aspiration in the diagnosis of cervical lymphadenopathy. *Am J Surg* 152:420–423, 1986.
15. Shaha AR, Weber C, DiMaio T, Jaffe BM. Needle aspiration biopsy in salivary gland lesions. *Am J Surg* 160:373–376, 1990.
16. Layfield LJ. Fine-needle aspiration of the head and neck. *Pathology* 4:409–438, 1996.
17. Spiro RH, Huvos AG, Wong GY, et al. Predictive value of tumor thickness in squamous carcinoma confined to the tongue and floor of the mouth. *Am J Surg* 152:345–350, 1986.
18. Forastiere AA. Randomized trials of induction chemotherapy. A critical review. *Hematol Oncol Clin North Am* 5:725–736, 1991.
19. Mendenhall WM, Parsons J, Stringer SP, et al. The role of radiation therapy in laryngeal cancer. *CA Cancer J Clin* 40:150–165, 1990.
20. Vikram B, Strong EW, Shah JP, Spiro RH. Failure at the primary site following multimodality treatment in advanced head and neck cancer. *Head Neck Surg* 6:730–733, 1984.
21. Department of Veterans Affairs Laryngeal Cancer Study Group. Induction chemotherapy plus radiation compared with surgery plus radiation in patients with advanced laryngeal cancer. *N Engl J Med* 324:1685–1690, 1991.
22. Lefebvre J, Chevalier D, Luboinski B, et al. Larynx preservation in pyriform sinus cancer: preliminary results of a European Organization for Research and Treatment of Cancer Phase III trial. *J Natl Cancer Inst* 88:890–899, 1996.
23. Parsons JT, Million R, Cassisi NJ. The influence of excisional or incisional biopsy of metastatic neck nodes on the management of head and neck cancer. *Int J Radiat Oncol Biol Phys* 11:1447–1454, 1985.
24. Freeman D, Mendenhall W, Parsons JT, Million RR. Unknown primary squamous cell carcinoma of the head and neck: Is mucosal irradiation necessary? *Int J Radiat Oncol Biol Phys* 23:889–890, 1992.
25. Lee NK, Byers RM, Abbruzzese JL, Wolf P. Metastatic adenocarcinoma to the neck from an unknown primary source. *Am J Surg* 162:306–309, 1991.
26. Suarez O. El problema de las metastasis linfaticas y alejadas del cancer de laringe y hipofaringe. *Rev Otorrinolaringol (Santiago)* 23:83–99, 1963.
27. Bocca E. Supraglottic laryngectomy and functional neck dissection. *J Laryngol* 80:831–838, 1966.
28. Robbins KT, Medina JE, Wolfe GT, et al. Standardizing neck dissection terminology. *Arch Otolaryngol Head Neck Surg* 117:601–605, 1991.
29. Medina JE. A rational classification of neck dissections. *Otolaryngol Head Neck Surg* 100:169–176, 1989.
30. Spiro RH, Strong EW, Shah JP. Classification of neck dissection: variations on a new theme. *Am J Surg* 168:415–418, 1994.

31. Percy C, van Holten VD, Muir C. *International Classification of Diseases for Oncology (ICD-O)* (2nd ed). Geneva: World Health Organization, 1990.

32. Chong VFH, Fan YF. Skull base erosion in nasopharyngeal carcinoma: detection by CT and MRI. *Clin Radiol* 51:625–631, 1996.

33. Micheau C, Boussen H, Klijanienko K, et al. Bone marrow biopsies in patients with undifferentiated carcinoma of nasopharyngeal type. *Cancer* 60:2459–2464, 1987.

34. Gallo O, Bianchi S, Gianni A, et al. Correlation between histopathological and biological findings in nasopharyngeal carcinoma and its prognostic significance. *Laryngoscope* 101:487–493 , 1991.

35. Ang KK, Peters LJ, Weber RS. Concomitant boost radiotherapy schedules in the treatment of oropharynx and nasopharynx. *Int J Radiat Oncol Biol Phys* 19:1339–1345, 1990.

36. Chang JT, See LC, Tang SG, Lee SP, et al. The role of brachytherapy in early-stage nasopharyngeal carcinoma. *Int J Rad Oncol Biol Phys* 36:1019–1024, 1996.

37. International Nasopharynx Cancer Study Group. VUMCA I trial: preliminary results of a randomized trial comparing neoadjuvant chemotherapy (cisplatin, epirubicin, bleomycin) plus radiotherapy vs radiotherapy alone in stage IV (> or = N2, M0) undifferentiated nasopharyngeal carcinoma: a positive effect on progression-free survival. *Int J Radiat Oncol Biol Phys* 35:463–469, 1996.

38. Al-Sarraf M, LeBlanc M, Giri M, et al. Chemoradiotherapy versus radiotherapy in patients with advanced nasopharyngeal cancer: phase III randomized Intergroup study 0099. *J Clin Oncol* 16:1310–1317, 1998.

39. Fee WE Jr, Robertson JB Jr, Goffinet DR. Long-term survival after surgical resection for recurrent nasopharyngeal cancer after radiotherapy failure. *Arch Otolaryngol* 117:1233–1236, 1991.

40. Franceschi D, Gupta R, Spiro RH, Shah JP. Improved survival in the treatment of squamous carcinoma of the oral tongue. *Am J Surg* 166:360–365, 1993.

41. Rodgers LW, Stringer SP, Mendenhall WM, et al. Management of squamous cell carcinoma of the floor of mouth. *Head Neck* 15:16–19, 1993.

42. Bloom ND, Spiro RH. Carcinoma of the cheek mucosa: a retrospective analysis. *Am J Surg* 149:556–559, 1980.

43. Byers RM, Clayman GL, Guillamondegui OM, et al. Resection of advanced cervical metastases prior to definitive radiotherapy for primary squamous carcinomas of the upper aerodigestive tract. *Head Neck* 14:133–138, 1992.

44. Harrison LB, Zelefsky M, Sessions RB, et al. Base-of-tongue cancer treated with external beam irradiation plus brachytherapy. *Radiology* 184:267–270, 1992.

45. Lo TC, Wiley AL Jr, Ansfield FJ, et al. Combined radiation therapy and 5-fluorouracil for advanced squamous cell carcinoma of the oral cavity and oropharynx: a randomized study. *Am J Roentgenol* 126:229–235, 1976.

46. Wendt CD, Peters LJ, Delclos L, et al. Primary radiotherapy in the treatment of stage I and II oral tongue cancers: importance of the proportion of therapy delivered with interstitial therapy. *Int J Radiat Oncol Biol Phys* 18:1287–1292, 1990.

47. Shaha AR. Preoperative evaluation of the mandible in patients with carcinoma of the floor of mouth. *Head Neck* 13:398–402, 1991.

48. Shaha AR. Marginal mandibulectomy for carcinoma of the floor of the mouth. *J Surg Oncol* 49:116–119, 1992.

49. Spiro RH, Gerold F, Shah JP, et al. Mandibulotomy approach to oropharyngeal tumors. *Am J Surg* 166:466–469, 1985.

50. Hidalgo DA, Disa J, Cordeiro PG, Hu QY. A review of 716 consecutive free flaps for oncologic surgical defects: refinement in donor-site selection and technique. *Plast Reconstr Surg* 102:722–734, 1998.

51. Minn H, Aitasalo K, Happonen RP. Detection of cancer recurrence in irradiated mandible using positron emission tomography. *Eur Arch Otorhinolaryngol* 250:312–315, 1993.

52. Shaha AR, Cordeiro PG, Hidalgo DA, et al. Resection and immediate microvascular reconstruction in the management of osteoradionecrosis of the mandible. *Head Neck* 19:406–411, 1997.

53. Shah JP, Karnell LH, Hoffman HT, et al. Patterns of care for cancer of the larynx in the United States. *Arch Otolaryngol Head Neck Surg* 123:475–483, 1997.

54. Lydiatt WM, Shah JP, Lydiatt KM. Conservation surgery for recurrent carcinoma of the glottic larynx. *Am J Surg* 172:662–664, 1996.

55. McLaughlin MP, Parsons JT, Fein DA, et al. Salvage surgery after radiotherapy failure in T1-T2 squamous cell carcinoma of the glottic larynx. *Head Neck* 18: 229–235, 1996.

56. Suarez C, Rodrigo JP, Herranz J, et al. Supraglottic laryngectomy with or without postoperative radiotherapy in supraglottic carcinomas. *Ann Otol Rhinol Laryngol* 104: 358–363, 1995.

57. Weems DH, Mendenhall WM, Parson JT, et al. Squamous cell carcinoma of the supraglottic larynx treated with surgery and/or radiation therapy. *Int J Radiat Oncol Biol Phys* 13:1483–1487, 1987.

58. Levendag P, Sessions R, Vikram B, et al. The problem of neck relapse in early stage supraglottic larynx cancer. *Cancer* 63:345–348, 1989.

59. Johnson JT, Myers EN, Hao SP, et al. Outcome of open surgical therapy for glottic carcinoma. *Ann Otol Rhinol Laryngol* 102:752–755, 1993.

60. Goepfert H, Jesse R, Fletcher GH, Hamberger A. Optimal treatment for technically resectable squamous cell carcinoma of the supraglottic larynx. *Laryngoscope* 85:14–32, 1975.

61. Kraus DH, Pfister DG, Harrison LB, et al. Larynx preservation with combined chemotherapy and radiation therapy in advanced hypopharynx cancer. *Otolaryngol Head Neck Surg* 111:31–37, 1994.

62. Parsons JT, Mendenhall W, Mancuso AA, et al. Malignant tumors of the nasal cavity and ethmoid and sphenoid sinuses. *Int J Radiat Oncol Biol Phys* 14:11–22, 1988.

63. Spiro JD, Soo KC, Spiro RH. Squamous cell carcinoma of the nasal cavity and paranasal sinuses. *Am J Surg* 158:328–332, 1989.

64. Shah JP, Kraus DH, Arbit E, et al. Craniofacial resection for tumors involving the anterior skull base. *Otolaryngol Head Neck Surg* 106:387–393, 1992.

65. Choi KN, Rotman M, Aziz H, et al. Locally advanced para-

nasal sinus and nasopharynx tumors with hyperfractionated radiation and concomitant infusion of cisplatin. *Cancer* 67:2748–2752, 1991.

66. Schuller DE, Metch B, Mattox D, McCracken JD. Prospective chemotherapy in advanced head and neck cancer: final report of the Southwest Oncology Group. *Laryngoscope* 98:1205–1211, 1988.

67. Paccagnella A, Orlando A, Marchiori C, et al. Phase III trial of initial chemotherapy in stage III or IV head and neck cancers: a study by the Gruppo di Studio sui Tumori della Testa e del Collo. *J Natl Cancer Inst* 86:265–272, 1994.

68. Bachaud JM, David JM, Boussin G, Daly N. Combined postoperative radiotherapy and weekly cisplatin infusion for locally advanced squamous cell carcinoma of the head and neck: preliminary report of a randomised trial. *Int J Radiat Oncol Biol Phys* 20:243–246, 1991.

69. Adelstein DJ, Saxton JP, Van Kirk MA, et al. Continuous course radiation therapy and concurrent combination chemotherapy for squamous cell head and neck cancer. *Am J Clin Oncol* 17:369–373, 1994.

70. Merlano M, Vitale V, Rosso R, et al. Treatment of advanced squamous cell carcinoma of the head and neck with alternating chemotherapy and radiotherapy. *N Engl J Med* 327:1115–1121, 1992.

71. Nishiyama M, Yamamoto W, Parks JS, et al. Low-dose cisplatin and 5-fluorouracil in combination can repress increased gene expression of cellular resistance determinants to themselves. *Clin Cancer Res* 5:2620–2628, 1999.

72. Hong WK, Lippmann S, Itri LM, et al. Prevention of second primary tumors with isotretinoin in squamous-cell carcinoma of the head and neck. *N Engl J Med* 323:795–801, 1990.

73. Shah JP, Ihde JK. Salivary gland tumors. *Curr Probl Surg* 27:775–883, 1990.

74. Spiro RH. Salivary neoplasms: overview of a 35-year experience with 2,807 patients. *Head Neck Surg* 8:177–184, 1986.

13

Esophageal Cancer

■ ■ ■

Elisabeth I. Heath

Richard F. Heitmiller

Arlene A. Forastiere

ESOPHAGEAL CANCER IS AN UNCOMMON BUT deadly disease. Its unique epidemiologic characteristics, high mortality, and increasing incidence have triggered significant research in many areas within various disciplines. This chapter discusses the epidemiologic and histopathologic characteristics, clinical presentation and evaluation, staging system, and treatment of localized and metastatic esophageal cancer.

EPIDEMIOLOGIC CHARACTERISTICS

Esophageal cancer is the ninth most common malignancy in the world, with the highest incidence seen in developing countries [1]. The geographic variability of this disease has led to numerous epidemiologic studies with a common objective: to identify possible causes, risk factors, and patterns that may explain these differences. High-risk areas in the world are located in parts of China; the Caspian region of Iran; South Africa; and parts of France. The age-adjusted cancer incidence in male persons in these regions is as high as 100 per 100,000 people, as compared to 4.2 per 100,000 people in areas of low incidence, such as Canada [2]. In the United States, esophageal cancer accounts for approximately 1% of all newly diagnosed cancers per year, afflicting 12,300 people and resulting in 12,100 deaths [3]. However, even within the United States, differences are seen in the rates of esophageal cancer, with one of the highest rates located in the northeast corridor. Overall, the incidence of esophageal cancer is increasing in the United States. Blot et al.[4] reported in 1991 that from 1976 to 1987, the number of men in whom adenocarcinoma of the esophagus was diagnosed increased anywhere from 4% to 10% annually. In general, male individuals are affected two to four times more often than are their female counterparts. In addition to gender differences, racial differences exist. Although the incidence of esophageal adenocarcinoma is surpassing the incidence of squamous cell carcinoma in white men, the incidence of squamous cell carcinoma in black men remains the highest.

Among the risk factors cited for esophageal cancer are the following:

- Tobacco use
- Dietary habits
- Alcohol consumption
- Obesity
- Barrett's esophagus
- Plummer-Vinson syndrome
- Caustic injury (lye)
- Chronic achalasia
- Tylosis

Risk factors that have been studied extensively include alcohol consumption, tobacco use, and dietary habits. Many studies have shown that alcohol and smoking increase the risk of squamous cell cancer of the esophagus, irrespective of geographic location. Gao et al. [5] performed a population-based study in Shanghai, China, and showed that alcohol and smoking significantly increased the risk of squamous cell esophageal cancer. More recently, in the United States, Gammon et al. [6] performed a large population-based study in New Jersey, Connecticut, and Washington. The results showed that smoking increased the risk of squamous cell esophageal cancer by five times in current smokers and by nearly three times in previous smokers, whereas the regular consumption of hard liquor increased the risk three times. However, with respect to esophageal adenocarcinoma, the relationship with smoking is slightly different. Although the risk of developing esophageal adenocarcinoma in current and previous smokers is shown to be only doubled, that risk persists for up to 30 years. One interpretation of the results is that smoking may play a significant role in the early stages of tumor development. Interestingly, consumption of beer and hard liquor does not affect the risk of esophageal adenocarcinoma, but drinking wine was reported to reduce the risk by 40%.

Another risk factor for esophageal adenocarcinoma is Barrett's esophagus [7], a condition that usually occurs in the distal esophagus. Normal squamous epithelium lining the esophagus is replaced by glandular columnar epithelium. The etiology of Barrett's esophagus still is uncertain. One well-accepted hypothesis is that of chronic persistent gastroesophageal reflux disease (GERD) causing damage to the normal esophageal squamous epithelium, with subsequent replacement by mucosa of the glandular columnar epithelial type. What does appear certain is that once a patient develops Barrett's esophagus, reversal or disappearance of the condition is unlikely. The presence of Barrett's esophagus increases the risk of development of esophageal adenocarcinoma by between 30-fold [8] and 40-fold [9].

Using the rationale that long-standing GERD may result in an increased cancer risk, a recent population-based study in the same three states (New Jersey, Connecticut, and Washington) sought to determine the association of calcium channel blockers, asthma drugs, and several other lower esophageal sphincter–relaxing drugs with esophageal adenocarcinoma [10]. No association was found in patients using calcium channel blockers, nitroglycerin, and tricyclic antidepressants. However, the data suggested an increased risk in chronic asthma patients, especially in female patients chronically taking theophylline and beta-agonists. Further studies must be performed to confirm this association.

Other studies evaluating the relationship of various medications with risk of esophageal adenocarcinoma have been performed. The most striking of these studies reports the use of nonsteroidal antiinflammatory drugs and the reduction in risk of esophageal adenocarcinoma [11]. The use of such antiinflammatory agents and aspirin at least once weekly for 6 months or more was shown to decrease by 50% the risk of squamous cell and esophageal adenocarcinoma. Unclear, however, is whether this relationship is causal in nature.

The role of nutrition also has been researched widely. Some associations have been discovered, but none are as significant as smoking or alcohol consumption. Hu et al.[12] performed a case-control study in the Heilongjiang Province in northeast China and determined several associations: High vitamin C intake was inversely proportional to the risk of esophageal cancer, high temperature of food and beverages was directly proportional, and pickled vegetables and salt-preserved foods were not associated. A recent study performed in the United States by Rogers et al. [13] demonstrated similar results. Another study showed that ingestion of moldy corn contaminated with fumonisin B_1 may play a role in an increased incidence of esophageal cancer in the counties of Cixian and Linxian in China [14].

In addition to evaluating dietary factors, researchers have evaluated obesity and its relationship to esophageal cancer. Chow et al. [15] reported that increasing obesity, measured in terms of body mass index (BMI), is associated with increasing risk of esophageal adenocarcinoma. Increased intraabdominal pressure resulting in more frequent GERD was a possible etiology. The study reported the highest increase in risk to be among younger patients (defined as younger than 50 years).

No relationship was established between obesity and squamous cell carcinoma of the esophagus.

Other associations with the development of esophageal cancers are observed in women with Plummer-Vinson syndrome (esophageal webs, iron-deficiency anemia, and glossitis) and in patients with esophageal strictures from lye injuries, chronic achalasia, or autosomal dominantly inherited tylosis [16]. Plummer-Vinson or Paterson-Kelly syndrome affects more women than men. Esophageal cancer is believed to develop in the areas of esophageal webs, but the pathophysiologic course of this process is not well delineated. Similarly, patients with esophageal strictures from caustic injury, such as lye exposure, may develop squamous cell cancer of the esophagus. The esophageal cancer resulting from this condition does not appear to be as aggressive as does esophageal cancer resulting from other predisposing conditions. The time to tumor progression is, on average, 40 years from the time of the initial caustic injury. However, patients with esophageal achalasia experience a shorter time to tumor progression (approximately 17 years). Achalasia is a condition affecting the motor function of the esophagus and resulting in aperistalsis of the organ [17]. The reason for these patients' increased risk of developing squamous cell esophageal cancer is unclear. Finally, tylosis is an autosomal dominant disease in which hyperkeratosis of the skin occurs on the palms and soles. Up to 37% of such patients will develop squamous cell cancer of the esophagus.

Esophageal cancers can occur also as second primary tumors, especially in patients with a previous primary head and neck carcinoma. In a phenomenon known as *field cancerization,* injury to the epithelium of the upper aerodigestive tract occurs as a result of various toxic carcinogens. Such diffuse injury may explain why a proportion of head and neck cancer patients develop esophageal cancer as a second primary malignancy.

HISTOPATHOLOGIC FEATURES

Squamous cell carcinoma remains the most common histologic presentation of esophageal cancer. It can arise anywhere in the esophagus but most commonly occurs in the upper two-thirds of the organ. Adenocarcinoma is the second most common histologic feature, but its incidence is rising in the United States. Most commonly, adenocarcinoma is located in the distal esophagus. Other histologic types of esophageal cancer are small-cell, primary malignant lymphoma, leiomyosarcoma, and neuroendocrine carcinoma. However, these tumors

are fairly uncommon and account for no more than 1% to 2% of all esophageal cancers.

CLINICAL PRESENTATION AND EVALUATION

Evaluation of new patients should include a physical examination and the recording of a thorough history (Fig. 13.1). The two most common clinical symptoms are dysphagia and weight loss. Dysphagia can occur with solid or liquid foods (or both) and may be accompanied by odynophagia and spontaneous vomiting. A typical esophageal cancer patient is a man who is in his midfifties, has experienced several months of dysphagia and a 5- to 10-pound unintentional weight loss, and has a long-standing history of tobacco and alcohol use. Typically, patients present at an advanced stage because usually the symptoms of odynophagia and chest pain are intermittent and vague, resulting in a delay in diagnosis. At present, no indications exist for preventive screening with upper endoscopy in this patient population. Poor prognostic signs indicating possible advanced disease include hoarseness (involvement of recurrent laryngeal nerve), chronic aspiration pneumonia (development of tracheoesophageal fistula), shortness of breath (possible malignant pleural effusion), and persistent bone pain (signaling metastatic disease). A thorough lymph node examination also should be included in the physical examination, as the discovery of supraclavicular nodes in a patient with distal esophageal tumor indicates distant metastatic disease.

In addition to a complete history and physical examination, several diagnostic procedures are available to document and stage disease:

- Barium esophagogram
- Upper endoscopy (esophagogastroduodenoscopy)
- Computed tomography scans of the chest, abdomen, pelvis
- Bronchoscopy
- Bone scan
- Endoscopic ultrasonography
- Exploratory laparotomy

Usually, a barium esophagogram will show an irregular filling defect and is helpful in localizing the disease. An esophagogastroduodenoscopy is performed to obtain histopathologic information; to describe the size, shape, and location of the tumor; and to determine the degree of obstruction. Computed tomographic (CT) scans of the chest, abdomen, and pelvis are performed to deter-

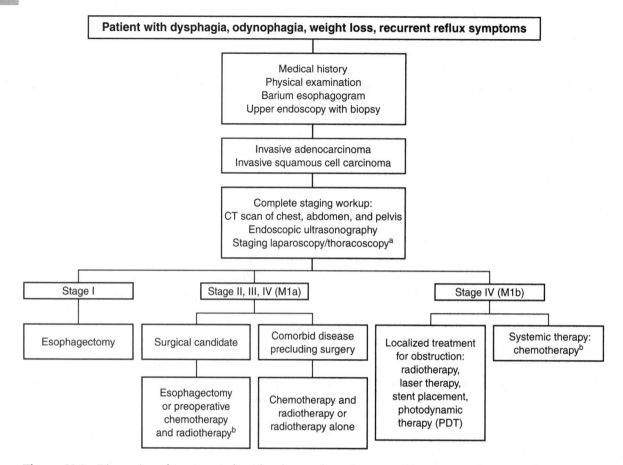

Figure 13.1   Diagnosis and treatment algorithm for esophageal cancer. *CT* = computed tomography; [a]Laparoscopy for middle to distal thoracic disease, gastroesophageal junction, cardia. Thoracoscopy for middle to upper thoracic disease; [b]Clinical trials preferred.

mine the extent of disease, such as the presence of liver or lung metastases and involvement of lymph nodes. CT scan is particularly useful for assessing invasion of surrounding structures (e.g., the aorta and pericardium), which would preclude surgery. For any suspicion of tracheoesophageal fistula either by clinical symptoms or tumor location at the carina, a bronchoscopy is indicated. A bone scan is warranted in the presence of complaints of persistent bone pain or elevated alkaline phosphatase level (or both).

Endoscopic ultrasonography (EUS) and laparoscopy are two new modalities often used to determine more accurately disease stage in esophageal cancer patients. An ultrasonographic probe is used during endoscopy to visualize at least five layers of alternating hyperechoic and hypoechoic images. In measuring appropriate time and distance, these layers correspond to the histologic features of the esophagus. When performed by a highly skilled gastroenterologist, EUS can give an accurate (90%) measurement of the depth of the tumor. Studies have shown that the accuracy of EUS in experienced

hands is superior to that of the CT scan [18, 19]. With regard to nodal staging, EUS also is more accurate than is the CT scan [20]. In addition to nodal size, EUS provides the echogenicity, shape, and border features of the nodes. To document malignancy in a small node, ultrasonographically guided fine-needle aspiration can be performed. EUS is recommended for use in conjunction with CT scans to improve the staging of esophageal cancer.

Another advance in the staging workup is diagnostic laparoscopy. Most often, laparoscopy is performed in patients with distal esophageal cancers to determine both peritoneal and liver metastasis and celiac node involvement that may be missed on CT scan. Studies have shown that patients were spared laparotomies 18% to 52% of the time by the discovery of metastatic, unresectable disease during laparoscopy [21–23].

The experience at the Johns Hopkins Oncology Center is similar to that reported in the literature. At this institution, a combination of the results of the CT scan, EUS, and staging laparoscopy has been found to be most accurate in staging patients. The importance of accurate staging should be underscored because the treatment options for localized versus metastatic disease are very different.

STAGING SYSTEM

The staging system for esophageal cancer is based on the guidelines provided by the 1998 American Joint Committee for Cancer (AJCC) and is described in Tables 13.1 and 13.2 [24]. The divisions of the esophagus are as follows: cervical (up to 18 cm from the incisors), upper thoracic (18–24 cm), midthoracic (24–32 cm), and lower thoracic (32 cm, including the gastroesophageal junction). True pathologic TNM (tumor-node-metastases) stage is determined accurately by surgery. Patients treated with a neoadjuvant approach are staged

Table 13.1 TNM Staging for Esophageal Cancer

Classification	Definition
Primary tumor (T)	
TX	Primary tumor cannot be assessed
T0	No evidence of primary tumor
Tis	Carcinoma in situ
T1	Tumor invades lamina propria or submucosa
T2	Tumor invades muscularis propria
T3	Tumor invades adventitia
T4	Tumor invades adjacent structures
Regional lymph nodes (N)	
NX	Regional lymph nodes cannot be assessed
N0	No regional lymph node metastasis
N1	Regional lymph node metastasis
Distant metastasis (M)	
MX	Distant metastasis cannot be assessed
M0	No distant metastasis
M1	Distant metastasis
Tumors of the lower thoracic esophagus	
M1a	Metastasis in celiac lymph nodes
M1b	Other distant metastasis
Tumors of the midthoracic esophagus	
M1a	Not applicable
M1b	Nonregional lymph nodes and/or other distant metastasis
Tumors of the upper thoracic esophagus	
M1a	Metastasis in cervical nodes
M1b	Other distant metastasis

Source: Used with the permission of the *American Joint Committee on Cancer (AJCC®)*, Chicago. *AJCC® Cancer Staging Manual* (5th Edition), 1997. Philadelphia: Lippincott-Raven.

Table 13.2 AJCC/UICC Stage Grouping for Esophageal Cancer

Stage 0	Tis	N0	M0
Stage I	T1	N0	M0
Stage IIA	T2	N0	M0
	T3	N0	M0
Stage IIB	T1	N1	M0
	T2	N1	M0
Stage III	T3	N1	M0
	T4	Any N	M0
Stage IV	Any T	Any N	M1
Stage IVA	Any T	Any N	M1a
Stage IVB	Any T	Any N	M1b

AJCC = American Joint Committee on Cancer; UICC = Union Internationale Contre le Cancer.
Source: Used with the permission of the *American Joint Committee on Cancer (AJCC®)*, Chicago. *AJCC® Cancer Staging Manual* (5th Edition), 1997. Philadelphia: Lippincott-Raven.

clinically by the TNM system using the modalities described previously.

The difference between the newest staging system and the 1988 AJCC TNM staging system is found only in the description of the metastatic group. Distant nodal metastases (M1) are classified further by the location of the primary tumor. For example, malignancy found in the cervical lymph nodes, when the primary tumor is located in the upper thoracic esophagus, and celiac nodes, with a primary tumor in the distal esophagus, is considered distant metastatic disease M1a. Any other distant nodes and organ metastases are considered stage M1b. The stage groupings have remained the same except for the addition of groups of stage IVA and stage IVB. Stage IVA describes any T, any N, and M1a disease, whereas stage IVB describes tumors with any T, any N, and M1b disease.

TREATMENT FOR LOCALIZED DISEASE
Single-Modality Therapy

SURGERY

Surgery remains the gold standard for the treatment of localized esophageal cancer. The goal of surgery is to provide definitive cure for the disease and to provide palliation of symptoms, such as dysphagia and odynophagia. The operative procedure, generally termed an *esophagectomy*, actually is a partial esophagogastrectomy with one-field lymphadenectomy (Fig. 13.2). As a result of esophageal anatomy and variations in tumor location, body habitus, previous surgery, and comorbidities,

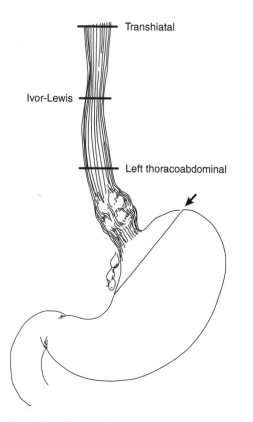

Transhiatal

Ivor-Lewis

Left thoracoabdominal

Figure 13.2 Partial esophagogastrectomy with one-field lymphadenectomy. Reprinted with permission of Mosby, Inc., from *Current Therapy in Gastroenterology,* (4th Edition).

no single incisional strategy can be used to perform esophagectomy in all patients; therefore, a number of incisional options have developed. The most common approaches are illustrated in Figure 13.3.

Historically, proponents of each incisional technique argued that their approach yielded the best results. It now is clear that the morbidity and mortality of these surgical approaches are equivalent and that survival is based on tumor staging, *not* on surgical technique. The two most common surgical approaches at present are the Ivor-Lewis esophagogastrectomy and the transhiatal esophagectomy (see Fig. 13.2).

In 1946, Dr. Ivor Lewis combined two surgical procedures: a right thoracotomy and abdominal laparotomy. This combination afforded surgeons excellent exposure of the intrathoracic esophagus and the opportunity to perform a complete regional nodal dissection. The other major surgical approach—the transhiatal esophagectomy (originally perfected by Dr. Mark Orringer)—was described first in the early 1900s but became a mainstream procedure in the 1970s. The morbidity and mortality for both surgical approaches are similar [25]. The transhiatal approach avoids a thoracotomy but often is criticized because lymph node sampling rather than a

complete lymphadenectomy is performed. Proponents of the transhiatal approach believe that because the two surgeries demonstrate no major differences in overall survival, the criticism is not pertinent.

The left thoracoabdominal approach originally was reported in 1938. This surgical technique affords excellent exposure of the lower esophagus and left upper abdomen. The radical en bloc esophagogastrectomy is a more aggressive surgical approach, first described in 1963 by Logan (as reported by Lee and Miller [26]). The objective of this surgery is to remove as much surrounding tissue and as many nodes as possible. Depending on the location of the tumor, the initial incision is either a left thoracotomy or a right thoracotomy with a laparotomy incision. Instead of the 5-cm margin used in the Ivor Lewis or transhiatal esophagectomy approach, a 10-cm margin is used, along with a three-field lymphadenectomy: cervical, mediastinal, and abdominal nodal dissection.

Overall, these surgical techniques exhibit no significant differences in morbidity and mortality and in 5-year survival rates. Generally, the leak rate at the anastomotic site is less than 2%, mortality is less than 5%, and the overall 5-year survival rates for all stages is approximately 20%. The performance status of the patient, the presence of other comorbid illness, the stage of disease, and the experience of the thoracic surgeon are more likely to contribute to the success of the operation, irrespective of the type of surgical technique.

RADIOTHERAPY

Radiotherapy given as a single modality to achieve cure produces poor results. Multiple studies have used doses ranging from 40 to 79 Gy. Five-year survival rates of 15% to 25% are reported for small early lesions only [27]. What should be noted, however, is that most of the patients referred for single-modality radiotherapy were characterized by inadequate performance status to undergo surgical resection; thus, patient selection bias may have contributed to the poor survival. No randomized trials compare radiotherapy alone with surgery. Also, three randomized trials clearly showed that radiotherapy in comparison to combined-modality treatment with irradiation and chemotherapy produced inferior results (discussed in detail later) [28–30]. Radiotherapy does relieve dysphagia with relatively few complications and thus is useful for palliation. However, the use of radiotherapy as a single, definitive treatment with curative intent for localized esophageal cancer is not recommended.

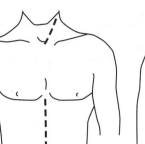

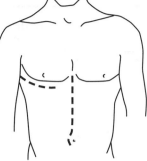

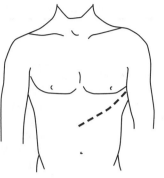

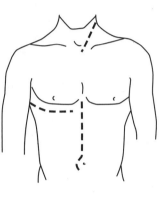

Transhiatal approach   Ivor-Lewis approach   Left thoracoabdominal approach

Three-incision approach

Figure 13.3 Various surgical techniques. Reprinted with permission of Lippincott-Raven.

Combined-Modality Therapy

RADIOTHERAPY PRIOR TO SURGERY

Radiotherapy prior to surgery was administered with the expectation of achieving improved local tumor control and increased overall survival. However, radiotherapy given as preoperative treatment does not improve survival. At least four phase III randomized trials show no impact of preoperative radiotherapy on survival; median survival is 10 to 12 postoperative months, with or without preoperative radiotherapy [31–33]. The differing doses of irradiation administered in these trials did not affect outcome. Preoperative irradiation did result in tumor shrinkage, and the addition of surgery did result in tumor removal, but these effects did not translate into prolongation of survival. Life-threatening complications from radiation were minimal. Some of the more frequent complications included esophageal strictures, irradiation pneumonitis, irradiation pericarditis, myocarditis, and myelitis. The results from the combined-modality neoadjuvant treatment approaches show greater promise of improving survival (Table 13.3). Therefore, radiotherapy alone given preoperatively is not recommended.

CHEMOTHERAPY AND RADIOTHERAPY

The rationale for using a combination of chemotherapy and radiotherapy (chemoradiotherapy) is based on the success of this treatment paradigm developed in patients with anal cancer. The same chemotherapeutic agents have antitumor activity in both diseases and can enhance irradiation sensitivity.

Definitive treatment with concurrent chemotherapy and radiotherapy is considered in several clinical situations: in patients with squamous cell carcinoma of the cervical esophagus and in patients who are poor surgical candidates because of comorbid illness or because of unresectable local disease. No randomized trials compare definitive chemoradiotherapy to surgery. However, at least eight nonrandomized trials have evaluated definitive chemotherapy and radiotherapy, and three large randomized trials compared irradiation alone to chemotherapy and irradiation. Araujo et al. [28] used irradiation alone and bleomycin and mitomy-

Table 13.3   Summary of Randomized Trials of Combined-Modality Treatment

Author	Chemotherapy	Radiation (cGy)	No. Patients	Survival Rate (%)			
				Median	1 yr	2 yr	3 yr
Chemotherapy followed by surgery							
Kelsen [38]	Cisplatin/5-FU	—	213	14.9	59	35	23
	Surgery	—	227	16.1	60	37	26
Schlag [36]	Cisplatin/5-FU	—	22	10	—	—	—
	Surgery	—	24	10	—	—	—
Roth [37]	Cisplatin/vindesine/bleomycin	—	19	9	—	—	25
	Surgery	—	20	9	—	—	5
Chemotherapy-radiotherapy followed by surgery							
Urba [46]	Cisplatin/vinblastine/5-FU	4,500	50	1.41	—	41	32
	Surgery	—	50	1.46	—	36	15
Walsh [47]	Cisplatin/5-FU	4,000	58	16	52	37	32*
	Surgery	—	55	11	44	26	6
Bossett [48]	Cisplatin/5-FU	3,700	142	18.6	—	—	38
	Surgery	—	139	18.6	—	—	38
Chemoradiotherapy as definitive treatment							
Araujo [28]	Cisplatin/MMC/5-FU	5,000	28	8	64	38	—
	Control	5,000	31	8	55	22	—
Al-Sarraf [34], Herskovic [30]	Cisplatin/5-FU	5,000	61	14.1	52	36	30*
	Control	6,400	62	9.3	34	10	0

5-FU = 5-fluorouracil; MMC = mitomycin C.
*Statistically significant.

cin concomitantly with 5,000 cGy of irradiation in patients with squamous cell carcinoma. The combined-modality arm had a better 3-year survival, although the difference was not significant (16% versus 6%, respectively). The Eastern Cooperative Oncology Group compared irradiation alone to 5-fluorouracil (5-FU) and mitomycin with 4,000 cGy of irradiation in patients with squamous cell cancer of the esophagus [29]. Survival of patients in the combined-modality arm was significantly better. Finally, a US Intergroup trial initially reported by Herskovic et al. [30] compared irradiation alone (6,400 cGy) to 5-FU, cisplatin, and concurrent irradiation (5,000 cGy) in patients with squamous cell cancer of the esophagus. A final report with long-term follow-up showed a significant difference in 5-year survival rate: 0% for patients in the irradiation-only arm versus 27% for patients receiving chemoradiotherapy [34]. Despite a significant reduction in distant and local recurrence, 44% of patients treated with combined chemoradiotherapy had persistent or recurrent disease in the esophagus at 12 months. To date, no studies have addressed such definitive combined therapy in adenocarcinoma of the esophagus. In summary, these data support the use of definitive chemoradiotherapy in patients who have medical risks that preclude esophagectomy or in patients who have extensive inoperable disease.

CHEMOTHERAPY PRIOR TO SURGERY

The pattern of failure in patients with esophageal cancer is characterized by both local and distant disease. Thus, the rationale for administering chemotherapy prior to surgery is to treat occult metastatic disease early and to achieve shrinkage of the primary tumor so as to improve local control. Multiple nonrandomized trials have suggested improved survival with preoperative cisplatin-based combination chemotherapy, but four randomized trials have failed to confirm those observations.

Preoperative chemotherapy, in general, has not increased operative morbidity and mortality. Nygaard et al. [35] reported on a four-arm study evaluating surgery alone, preoperative chemotherapy, preoperative irradiation, and preoperative chemoradiotherapy given sequentially. This study reported no difference in survival in any of the four arms. Schlag [36] and Roth et al. [37] randomly assigned smaller numbers of patients to preoperative chemotherapy (cisplatin and 5-FU) or surgery, and both trials had similar median survivals of 9 to 10 months for both treatment arms. Kelsen et al. [38] recently reported on a large intergroup trial that compared surgery alone to neoadjuvant chemotherapy with cisplatin and 5-FU followed by surgery. This trial of 440 patients with adenocarcinoma and squamous cell carcinoma showed no improvement in resectability or median or 1- or 2-year survival rates with combined treatment. The toxicities in the combined-modality arm were acceptable. Surgical mortality was 6% for the surgery-alone patients and 6% for patients in the chemotherapy group. Chemotherapy prior to surgery offers no improvement in survival and therefore remains experimental.

INDUCTION CHEMORADIATION PRIOR TO SURGERY

The use of all three modalities—chemotherapy, radiotherapy, and surgery—has the potential to increase survival by decreasing distant metastases and eliminating residual local disease with surgery after chemoradiation. Many phase II, predominantly single-institution trials have evaluated the role of preoperative chemotherapy and radiotherapy. Most of the trials report promising results [39–44], being characterized by the achievement of pathologic complete response in 25% to 30% of patients after chemoradiotherapy and of long-term survival for this group. Approximately two-thirds of patients are downstaged. Median survivals exceed 2 years, whereas 3-year and 5-year survival rates are in the 40% and 30% ranges, respectively. These results suggest improvement over the 15% to 20% 5-year survival expected from surgery alone.

Because of these encouraging phase II trial results, either at a single-institution or cooperative group level, randomized phase III trials have been performed. Three randomized trials have evaluated the role of concomitant chemotherapy and radiotherapy given prior to esophagectomy [45–49]. Urba et al. [45, 46], from the University of Michigan Medical Center, conducted a study comparing transhiatal esophagectomy alone to preoperative 5-FU, cisplatin, and vinblastine in combination with concurrent hyperfractionated irradiation (total dose, 4,500 cGy). A total of 100 patients were assigned randomly; 75 had adenocarcinoma, a reflection of the increasing incidence of this malignancy. No difference in median survival was observed (16.1 versus 16.8 months). However, a difference in the 3-year survival rate was observed: 32% of patients receiving preoperative chemoradiotherapy as compared to 15% in the surgery-only arm ($p = .07$), suggesting a trend for improved outcome with combined treatment [46].

A second randomized trial was performed by Walsh et al. [47]. All 113 patients in the trial had adenocarcinoma and were assigned randomly to either surgery alone or a regimen of 5-FU and cisplatin with concurrent irradiation (4,000 cGy) followed by surgery. This trial did demonstrate a survival benefit for the combined-treatment arm, with an improved median survival of 16 months versus 11 months and an improved 3-year survival of 32% versus 6% (data based on the intent-to-treat analysis as compared to actual treatment analysis).

The third randomized trial was performed by Bossett et al. [48] from the European Organization for Research and Treatment of Cancer Group. Patients with squamous cell carcinoma limited to stage I or II disease were assigned randomly either to esophagectomy alone or to single-agent cisplatin and concomitant irradiation (3,700 cGy total dose) followed by esophagectomy. No improvement in overall survival resulted, but disease-free survival and local control improved significantly, and a decrease occurred in cancer mortality and in the incidence of curative resection required for patients treated with preoperative chemotherapy and radiotherapy. These patients experienced an increase in operative mortality, however, which may explain the lack of significant benefit for overall survival.

Two randomized studies have evaluated the role of sequential chemotherapy and radiotherapy prior to surgery. LePrise et al. [49] compared patients with surgery alone to patients receiving cisplatin and 5-FU given before and after irradiation (2,000 cGy) followed by surgery. This trial showed no improvement in median or overall survival and was, in fact, terminated prior to achieving the final projected total patient accrual. Nygaard et al. [35] compared surgery alone to sequential preoperative bleomycin and cisplatin chemotherapy followed by radiotherapy and surgery. No survival advantage resulted for the combined treatment. However, this study has been criticized for the small number of patients enrolled in each arm and for lack of balance between treatment arms with regard to stage.

In view of the results from these five randomized trials, surgery is the current treatment recommendation for patients with resectable esophageal cancer. Preoperative combined chemotherapy and radiotherapy should not be administered outside of a clinical trial setting. However, enrollment in properly designed clinical trials is encouraged highly, as this approach to treatment holds the most promise for improving survival.

ADJUVANT CHEMOTHERAPY OR RADIOTHERAPY

No definitive trials prove a role for adjuvant chemotherapy after esophagectomy. Pouliquen et al. [50] compared cisplatin and 5-FU to observation after esophagectomy in patients with completely resected squamous cell cancer of the esophagus. No difference was seen in survival. The Eastern Cooperative Oncology Group is conducting a trial of docetaxel and cisplatin combination chemotherapy after resection in patients with stage IIB and stage III disease. At present, other than for a clinical trial, adjuvant chemotherapy cannot be recommended.

The role of adjuvant radiotherapy has been studied in several randomized phase III trials. Fok et al. [51] compared adjuvant radiotherapy (total dose, 4,900 cGy) to observation in patients with resected squamous cell carcinoma. However, the treatment was fairly toxic, and the overall survival rate in the adjuvant radiotherapy arm was worse than that in the surgery-only arm. Teniere et al. [52] treated patients with up to 5,500 cGy postoperatively and also observed no survival benefit. The only clinical situation that might warrant postoperative radiotherapy is patients with positive surgical margins, and it should be limited to that group.

Palliative Care

Patients with disease that is incurable because of locally advanced or metastatic carcinoma or those who have poor functional status and cannot tolerate potential treatment-related toxicities should be provided with symptom management. This management includes pain control and improvement in swallowing function and overall quality of life. The choice of which palliative treatment to administer relates to performance status, age, extent of tumor, degree of obstruction from the tumor, treatment history, other medical comorbid conditions, patient wishes, and estimated survival time. Because the anticipated survival time is short (< 6 months) in the majority of patients, surgical intervention for palliation of dysphagia is not recommended. Segalin et al. [53] reported 10% mortality and a 46% postoperative morbidity rate in 156 patients who had palliative esophagectomy. Some reports indicate less morbidity and mortality but, in general, effective alternative treatments are available to improve swallowing function.

Endoscopic Therapy

DILATATION THERAPY

Often, dysphagia and odynophagia can be relieved with simple dilatation therapy [54, 55]. Three common types of dilators are used: the Maloney, the Savary-Gilliard, and the balloon-type dilators. The dilators are used in different clinical settings, and success depends on the experience of gastroenterologists. For example, the Maloney dilator works best on a short, symmetric lesion, as compared to the Savary-Gilliard dilators, which work best on a long, asymmetric lesion. The advantage of this therapy is that it is inexpensive, can be performed on an outpatient basis, has a low complication rate, and is immediately effective. Other than a small risk of perforation, the main disadvantages inherent in this type of therapy are that the effects are transient and the procedure may need to be performed as frequently as every 3 to 4 weeks. Thus, patients who have a very short life expectancy and whose quality of life would be improved with temporary relief of dysphagia stand to benefit most from dilator therapy.

STENT THERAPY

The concept of relieving malignant esophageal obstruction with a "tube" is not new. The type of tubes used are either rigid plastic or expandable metal; over the years, both have been improved by various modifications. The stents are placed either during endoscopy or under fluoroscopy. Rigid plastic stents have not been used as often because the risk of perforation is as high as 10% in some series, along with such other complications as bleeding and stent migration. As plastic stents have fallen out of favor, expandable metal stents have gained popularity. Four main types of metal stents are available: the EsophaCoil, the Ultraflex, the Wallstent, and the Z-Stent. The main advantages to these stents are ease of placement, decreased rate of perforation, and decreased rate of stent migration as compared with plastic stents. The disadvantages are the higher cost, difficulty of repositioning the stent after placement, and higher rate of reocclusion due to tumor growth through the mesh spaces.

A pivotal randomized trial to determine the best type of stent was performed by Knyrim et al. [56]. Compared to plastic stents, metal stents were not associated with any treatment-related deaths or stent migration. However, trial patients had to undergo more procedures, including laser therapy and additional stent placements, to maintain patency of the esophagus. In the final analysis, metal stents had a lower overall cost. Another trial performed by De Palma et al. [57] evaluated the safety and efficacy of expandable metal stents as compared to plastic stents. The study involved a total of 39 patients with inoperable esophageal cancer. The study considered metal stents to be safer (i.e., involved less morbidity) than plastic stents.

At present, improvements have been made in the expandable metal stents, such as silicone coating to prevent tumor regrowth through the spaces in the mesh. Future trials should be conducted to determine the efficacy of these improved metal stents. These types of stents may be useful also in treating tracheoesophageal fistulas.

Nd:YAG LASER THERAPY

Laser therapy with neodymium–yttrium aluminum garnet (Nd:YAG) laser is administered through an endoscope. Laser therapy burns cancerous tissue by the absorption of light energy and its conversion to thermal energy. This form of therapy is effective in achieving relief of dysphagia in 69% to 100% of cases. Complications include perforation and bleeding. Another trial by Abdel-Wahab et al. [58] reported results of a trial with Nd:YAG laser in patients with advanced esophageal cancer. Luminal patency was achieved in 93% of affected patients, which enabled the majority of patients to eat and to gain weight.

PHOTODYNAMIC THERAPY

Photodynamic therapy (PDT) uses different principles from laser treatment to achieve patency of the esophageal lumen. Porphyrin analogs are chemical photosensitizers that, when injected intravenously in patients, are taken up by esophageal tumors. Then, light is administered at the tumor site through a cylindric diffuser located at the end of the endoscope and, eventually, necrosis occurs secondary to the development of oxygen free radicals. This effect is contrasted to Nd:YAG laser treatment, which employs heat to burn malignant tissue. Lightdale et al. [59] conducted a multicenter randomized trial comparing PDT with Nd:YAG laser therapy. The two treatment modalities had different side effects, but each was effective in palliating dysphagia. Although easier to administer and better tolerated by patients, PDT produced sunburn, nausea, and fever in more patients than did laser therapy. However, perforation occurred more often in patients in the Nd:YAG laser treatment group. Additional studies are ongoing to determine the role of PDT in palliation of dysphagia in esophageal cancer.

Radiotherapy

Radiotherapy applied either as brachytherapy or external-beam irradiation can result in significant relief of dysphagia, which usually lasts for several months. Brachytherapy involves placement of radioactive seeds via endoscopy in the tumor bed. A randomized trial performed by Low and Pagliero [60] compared brachytherapy and laser treatment. The results were similar in terms of efficacy and degree of palliation. Use of external-beam radiotherapy has been studied predominantly in squamous cell carcinoma. This method of palliation is truly noninvasive as compared to the other modalities; 50% to 70% of affected patients experience relief from dysphagia, although complications that occur include esophagitis, formation of tracheoesophageal fistulas, and irradiation fibrosis.

Chemotherapy

The role of single or combination chemotherapy has been studied well in patients with unresectable or widely metastatic esophageal cancer. At least 25 trials in the literature evaluated various agents, such as 5-FU, cisplatin, bleomycin, and mitomycin C. The response rates ranged from 10% to 30% and are brief (on the order of 2–4 months), and no data indicate survival prolongation. When measured, palliation of symptoms is short-lived. Two newer agents are showing more promise: vinorelbine and the taxanes paclitaxel and docetaxel. Vinorelbine is a semisynthetic alkaloid that inhibits microtubule assembly; it was studied by Conroy et al. [61] in a phase II trial. A 20% response rate was achieved in patients with metastatic squamous cell carcinoma of the esophagus. The taxanes (paclitaxel and docetaxel) are drugs that stabilize microtubules and also affect the cell cycle. Unlike vinorelbine, taxanes have been studied in both squamous cell carcinoma and adenocarcinoma of the esophagus. Paclitaxel administered as a 24-hour infusion has been shown by Ajani et al. [62] to produce a 32% overall response rate. Use of docetaxel is being studied at the authors' institution in patients with incurable esophageal adenocarcinoma.

Combination chemotherapy has been evaluated predominantly in patients with squamous cell cancer of the esophagus. Multiple trials of various combination chemotherapy regimens, such as cisplatin and bleomycin with or without a vinca alkaloid and the combination of cisplatin and 5-FU, have been tested. The response rates range from 11% to 50%, with a median response duration of 5 to 6 months. Recently, a phase II multicenter trial incorporated paclitaxel into the regimen of 5-FU and cisplatin. Ilson et al. [63] reported major response in 48% of the patients, with a median response duration of 5.7 months. However, this combination caused considerable toxicity, such that 48% of the patients required hospitalization. Improvement in response rates and survival will require the identification of new, more effective agents. At present, no single drug or combination of drugs effectively palliates symptoms and improves quality of life or survival time. Thus, patients should be offered the opportunity to participate in clinical trials that evaluate new and novel therapies.

REFERENCES

1. Day NE, Varghese C. Oesophageal cancer. *Cancer Surv* 19/20:43–54, 1994.

2. Blot WJ. Esophageal cancer trends and risk factors. *Semin Oncol* 21:403–410, 1994.

3. Greenlee RT, Murray T, Bolden S, Wingo PA. Cancer statistics, 2000. *CA Cancer J Clin* 50:7–33, 2000.

4. Blot WJ, Devessa SS, Kneller RW. Rising incidence of adenocarcinoma of the esophagus and gastric cardia. *JAMA* 265:1287–1289, 1991.

5. Gao YT, Mclaughlin JK, Blot WJ, et al. Risk factors for esophageal cancer in Shanghai, China: I. Role of cigarette smoking and alcohol drinking. *Int J Cancer* 58:192–196, 1994.

6. Gammon MD, Schoenberg JB, Habibul A, et al. Tobacco, alcohol, and socioeconomic status and adenocarcinomas of the esophagus and gastric cardia. *J Natl Cancer Inst* 89:1277–1284, 1997.

7. Bremner CG, Bremner RM. Barrett's esophagus. *Surg Clin North Am* 77:1115–1137, 1997.

8. Cameron AJ, Zinsmeister AR, Ballard DJ, et al. Prevalence of columnar-lined (Barrett's) esophagus. Comparison of population-based clinical and autopsy findings. *Gastroenterology* 99:918–922,1990.

9. Spechler SJ, Goyal RK. Barrett's esophagus. *N Engl J Med* 315:362–371,1986.

10. Vaughan TL, Farrow DC, Hansten PD, et al. Risk of esophageal and gastric adenocarcinomas in relation to use of calcium channel blockers, asthma drugs, and other medications that promote gastroesophageal reflux. *Cancer Epidemiol Biomarkers Prev* 7:749–757, 1998.

11. Farrow DC, Vaughan TL, Hansten PD, et al. Use of aspirin and other nonsteroidal anti-inflammatory drugs and risk of esophageal and gastric cancer. *Cancer Epidemiol Biomarkers Prev* 7:97–102, 1998.

12. Hu J, Nyren O, Wolk A, et al. Risk factors for oesophageal cancer in Northeast China. *Int J Cancer* 57:38–46, 1994.

13. Rogers MA, Vaughan TL, Davis S, et al. Consumption of nitrate, nitrite, and nitrosodimethylamine and the risk of upper aerodigestive tract cancer. *Cancer Epidemiol Biomarkers Prev* 4:29–36, 1995.

14. Chu FS, Li GY. Simultaneous occurrence of fumonisin B_1 and other mycotoxins in moldy corn collected from the People's Republic of China in regions with high incidences of esophageal cancer. *Appl Environ Microbiol* 60:847–852, 1994.

15. Chow WH, Blot WJ, Vaughan TL, et al. Body mass index and risk of adenocarcinomas of the esophagus and gastric cardia. *J Natl Cancer Inst* 90:150–155, 1998.

16. Sandler RS, Nyren O, Ekborn A, et al. The risk of esopha-

17. Loviscek LF, Cenoz MC, Badaloni AE, et al. Early cancer in achalasia. *Dis Esophagus* 11:239–247, 1998.

18. Lightdale CJ. Staging of esophageal cancer: I. Endoscopic ultrasound. *Semin Oncol* 21:438–446, 1994.

19. Botet JF, Lightdale CJ, Zuger G, et al. Preoperative staging of esophageal cancer: comparison of endoscopic US and dynamic CT. *Radiology* 181:419–425, 1991.

20. Souquet JC, Napoleon B, Pujol B, et al. Endosonography-guided treatment of esophageal carcinoma. *Endoscopy* 24:324–328, 1992.

21. van Dijkum EJ, de Wit LT, van Delden OM, et al. The efficacy of laparoscopic staging in patients with upper gastrointestinal tumors. *Cancer* 79:1315–1319, 1997.

22. Krasna MJ. Advances in staging of esophageal carcinoma. *Chest* 113:107S–111S, 1998.

23. Luketich JD, Schauer P, Landrenau R, et al. Minimally invasive surgical staging is superior to endoscopic ultrasound in detecting lymph node metastases in esophageal cancer. *J Thorac Cardiovasc Surg* 114:817–823, 1997.

24. Fleming ID, Cooper JS, Henson DE, et al. (eds). *AJCC Cancer Staging Manual* (5th ed). Philadelphia: Lippincott-Raven, 1997.

25. Pommier RF, Vetto JT, Ferris BL, et al. Relationships between operative approaches and outcomes in esophageal surgery. *Am J Surg* 175:422–425, 1998.

26. Lee RB, Miller JI. Esophagectomy for cancer. *Surg Clin North Am* 77:1169–1196, 1997.

27. Launois B, Delarue D, Campion J, et al. Preoperative radiotherapy for carcinoma of the esophagus. *Surg Gynecol Obstet* 153:690–692, 1981.

28. Araujo CM, Souhami L, Gil RA, et al. A randomized trial comparing radiation therapy versus concomitant radiation therapy and chemotherapy in carcinoma of the esophagus. *Cancer* 67:2258–2261, 1991.

29. Smith TJ, Ryan LM, Douglass HO, et al. Combined chemoradiotherapy vs radiotherapy alone for early stage squamous cell carcinoma of the esophagus: a study of the Eastern Cooperative Oncology Group. *Int J Radiat Oncol Biol Phys* 42:269–276, 1998.

30. Herskovic A, Martz K, al-Sarraf M, et al. Combined chemotherapy and radiotherapy compared with radiotherapy alone in patients with cancer of the esophagus. *N Engl J Med* 326:1593–1598, 1992.

31. Gignoux M, Roussel A, Paillot B, et al. The value of preoperative radiotherapy in esophageal cancer: results of a study of EORTC. *Recent Results Cancer Res* 110:1–13, 1988.

32. Wang M, Gu XZ, Yin WB, et al. Randomized clinical trial on the combination of preoperative irradiation and surgery in the treatment of esophageal carcinoma: a report of 206 patients. *Int J Radiat Oncol Biol Phys* 16:325–327, 1989.

33. Arnott SJ, Duncan W, Gignoux M, et al. Preoperative radiotherapy in esophageal carcinoma: a meta-analysis using individual patient data (oesophageal cancer collaborative group). *Int J Radiat Oncol Biol Phys* 41:579–583, 1998.

34. Al-Sarraf M, Martz K, Herskovic A, et al. Progress report of combined chemoradiotherapy versus radiotherapy alone in patients with esophageal cancer: an intergroup study. *J Clin Oncol* 15:277–284, 1997.

35. Nygaard K, Hagen S, Hansen HS, et al. Preoperative radio-

geal cancer in patients with achalasia. *JAMA* 374:1359–1362, 1995.

therapy prolongs survival in operable esophageal carcinoma: a randomized, multicenter study of preoperative radiotherapy and chemotherapy. The second Scandinavian trial in esophageal cancer. *World J Surg* 16:1104–1109, 1992.

36. Schlag PM. Randomized trial of preoperative chemotherapy for squamous cell cancer of the esophagus: the Chirurgische Arbeitsgemeinschaft für Onkologie der Deutschen Gesellschaft fur Chirurgie Study Group. *Arch Surg* 127:1446–1450, 1992.

37. Roth JA, Pass HI, Flanagan MM, et al. Randomized clinical trial of preoperative and postoperative adjuvant chemotherapy with cisplatin, vindesine, and bleomycin for carcinoma of the esophagus. *J Thorac Cardiovasc Surg* 96:242–248, 1988.

38. Kelsen DP, Ginsberg R, Pajak T, et al. Chemotherapy followed by surgery versus surgery alone for localized esophageal cancer. *N Engl J Med* 339:1979–1984, 1998.

39. Forastiere AA, Orringer MB, Perez-Tamayo C, et al. Concurrent chemotherapy and radiation therapy followed by transhiatal esophagectomy for local-regional cancer of the esophagus. *J Clin Oncol* 8:119–127, 1990.

40. Forastiere AA, Orringer MB, Perez-Tamayo C, et al. Preoperative chemoradiation followed by transhiatal esophagectomy for carcinoma of the esophagus: final report. *J Clin Oncol* 11:1118–1123, 1993

41. Poplin E, Fleming T, Leichman L, et al. Combined therapies for squamous-cell carcinoma of the esophagus, a Southwest Oncology Group Study (SWOG-8037). *J Clin Oncol* 5:622–628, 1987.

42. Poplin EA, Jacobson J, Herskovic A, et al. Evaluation of multimodality treatment of locoregional esophageal carcinoma by Southwest Oncology Group 9060. *Cancer* 78:1851–1856, 1996.

43. Keller SM, Ryan LM, Coia LR, et al. High dose chemoradiotherapy followed by esophagectomy for adenocarcinoma of the esophagus and gastroesophageal junction: results of a phase II study of the Eastern Cooperative Oncology Group. *Cancer* 83:1908–1916, 1998.

44. Seydel HG, Leichman L, Byhardt R, et al. Preoperative radiation and chemotherapy for localized squamous cell carcinoma of the esophagus: an RTOG study. *Int J Radiat Oncol Biol Phys* 14:33–35, 1988.

45. Urba SG, Orringer MB, Turrisi A, et al. A randomized trial comparing transhiatal esophagectomy to preoperative concurrent chemoradiation followed by esophagectomy in locoregional carcinoma. *Proc Am Soc Clin Oncol* 14:199, 1995.

46. Urba SG, Orringer MB, Turrisi A, et al. A randomized trial comparing surgery (S) to preoperative concomitant chemoradiation plus surgery in patients (pts) with resectable esophageal cancer (CA): updated analysis. *Proc Am Soc Clin Oncol* 16:983, 1997.

47. Walsh T, Noonan N, Hollywood D, et al. A comparison of multimodality therapy and surgery for esophageal adenocarcinoma. *N Engl J Med* 335:462–467, 1996.

48. Bossett JF, Gignoux M, Triboulet JP, et al. Chemoradiotherapy followed by surgery compared with surgery alone in squamous-cell cancer of the esophagus. *N Engl J Med* 337:161–167, 1997.

49. LePrise E, Etienne PL, Meunier B, et al. A randomized study of chemotherapy, radiation therapy, and surgery versus surgery for localized squamous cell carcinoma of the esophagus. *Cancer* 73:1779–1784, 1994.

50. Pouliquen X, Levard H, Hay JM, et al. 5-Fluorouracil and cisplatin therapy after palliative surgical resection of squamous cell carcinoma of the esophagus: a multicenter randomized trial. *Ann Surg* 223:127–133 1996.

51. Fok M, Sham JST, Choy D, et al. Postoperative radiotherapy for carcinoma of the esophagus: a prospective, randomized controlled study. *Surgery* 113:138–147, 1993.

52. Teniere P, Hay JM, Fingerhut A, et al. Postoperative radiation therapy does not increase survival after curative resection for squamous cell carcinoma of the middle and lower esophagus as shown by a multicenter controlled trial. *Surg Gynecol Obstet* 173:123–130, 1991.

53. Segalin A, Little AG, Ruol A, et al. Surgical and endoscopic palliation of esophageal carcinoma. *Ann Thorac Surg* 48.267–271, 1989.

54. Reed CE. Pitfalls and complications of esophageal prosthesis, laser therapy, and dilation. *Chest Surg Clin North Am* 7:623–636, 1997.

55. Lundell L, Leth R, Lind T, et al. Palliative endoscopic dilation in carcinoma of the esophagus and esophagogastric junction. *Acta Chir Scand* 155:179–184, 1989.

56. Knyrim K, Wagner HJ, Bethge N, et al. A controlled trial of an expansile metal stent for palliation of esophageal obstruction due to inoperable cancer. *N Engl J Med* 329:1302–1307, 1993.

57. De Palma GD, di Matteo E, Romano G, et al. Plastic prosthesis versus expandable metal stents for palliation of inoperable esophageal thoracic carcinoma: a controlled prospective study. *Gastrointest Endosc* 43:478–482, 1996.

58. Abdel-Wahab M, Gad-Elhak N, Denewer A, et al. Endoscopic laser treatment of progressive dysphagia in patients with advanced esophageal carcinoma. *Hepatogastroenterology* 45:1509–1515, 1998.

59. Lightdale CJ, Heier SK, Marcon NE, et al. Photodynamic therapy with porfimer sodium versus thermal ablation therapy with Nd:YAG laser for palliation of esophageal cancer: a multicenter randomized trial. *Gastrointest Endosc* 42:507–512, 1995.

60. Low DE, Pagliero KM. Prospective randomized clinical trial comparing brachytherapy and laser photoablation for palliation of esophageal cancer. *J Thorac Cardiovasc Surg* 104:173–178, 1992.

61. Conroy TC, Etienne PL, Adenis A, et al. Phase II trial of vinorelbine in metastatic squamous cell esophageal carcinoma. *J Clin Oncol* 14:164–170, 1996.

62. Ajani J, Ilson DH, Daugherty K, et al. Activity of Taxol in patients with squamous cell carcinoma and adenocarcinoma of the esophagus. *J Natl Cancer Inst* 86:1086–1091, 1994.

63. Ilson DH, Ajani J, Bhalla K, et al. Phase II trial of paclitaxel, fluorouracil and cisplatin in patients with advanced carcinoma of the esophagus. *J Clin Oncol* 16:1826–1834, 1998.

14

Gastric Cancer

■ ■ ■

Walter Lawrence, Jr.

MORE THAN 90% OF ALL GASTRIC CANCER IS adenocarcinoma. Primary non-Hodgkin's lymphoma, sarcoma, carcinoid, plasmacytoma, and even less common metastatic lesions in the stomach comprise the remainder. Although these other gastric cancers are included, the primary emphasis of this chapter is on adenocarcinoma of the stomach.

GASTRIC ADENOCARCINOMA

Incidence

In 2000, death from gastric cancer is expected to represent 2.4% of all cancer deaths in the United States, making it eighth in mortality in terms of anatomic site of cancer origin [1]. This standing represents approximately 21,500 new cases and approximately 13,000 deaths during that year. Gastric cancer is found more commonly in people between 50 and 70 years of age and is predominantly a disease of men rather than women (1.7:1 ratio) [2]. In the United States, gastric cancer is more common than cancer of the esophagus, small intestine, biliary tract, or liver but is slightly less frequent than pancreatic cancer and much less frequent than colorectal cancer.

Epidemiology and Etiology

VARIATIONS IN INCIDENCE

Two unusual observations have been made about the epidemiology of gastric cancer. The first highlights a striking decline in both incidence and mortality in the United States from 1930, when gastric cancer was the number one cause of cancer mortality and caused 38% of all cancer deaths. This decline, occurring mainly between 1930 and 1995, is shown graphically in Figure 14.1, where it is contrasted with the mortality data for

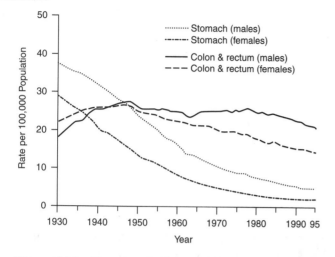

Figure 14.1 Changing death rates for gastric cancer in the United States as compared with trends for colon and rectal cancer.

cancers of the colon and rectum. Because this unique decrease in mortality occurred specifically in the United States—not in most other countries and not in association with significant alterations in diagnostic or treatment methods—some exogenous factor (or factors) affecting incidence is presumed to be responsible.

The second observation is a wide variation from country to country in death rates from gastric cancer. Gastric cancer is a relatively common cause of death in Japan, Chile, and Iceland, where the death rate is approximately five times that in the United States. A 1980 United Nations estimate of cancer incidence in 24 world areas showed that stomach cancer was the most common cancer, when combined data (incidence in both men and women) were reviewed [3, 4]. For no apparent reason, the incidence of gastric cancer appears to be greater in countries farther from the equator. Also, in most countries, people in lower socioeconomic classes tend to develop the disease more frequently than do those in the upper classes; however, no rural-urban or occupational differences are observed in incidence.

The change in methods and in quality of food preservation in the United States, with more emphasis on frozen foods over the last several decades, and an increased intake of vitamin C may play a role in the difference in frequency of gastric cancer in the United States and that in many other countries. Much study still must be performed to delineate those dietary factors that contribute to these geographic differences in incidence [5, 6].

ROLE OF ATROPHIC GASTRITIS IN ETIOLOGY

The epidemiologic findings regarding the foregoing incidence and their etiologic implications are tied closely to various cancer-associated pathologic changes that occur in the stomach [7]. Atrophic gastritis has been observed increasingly in many of the countries exhibiting a higher incidence of gastric cancer. Progression from atrophic gastritis to gastric cancer has been demonstrated on repeated biopsies in a selected group of patients [8]. Also, some data suggest a higher incidence of gastric cancer in patients with atrophic mucosal changes after a prior distal gastrectomy for benign gastric ulcer disease, particularly after a 20-year interval. Serial endoscopic studies with biopsy after partial gastrectomy support this concept of evolving neoplastic change in the remaining stomach subsequent to gastric resection. Findings of dysplasia on random biopsy indicate a greater likelihood of development of carcinoma in the remaining stomach, and this tendency identifies a subset of patients requiring more aggressive endoscopic surveillance after gastrectomy [9].

CARCINOGENS IN ETIOLOGY

What is the stimulus for the chain of pathologic events from dysplasia or atrophic gastritis to carcinoma? Nitrosamines, which produce gastric cancer in experimental animals, may be carcinogenic in humans. Nitrosamines are produced in the stomach from nitrates. The intermediate product in the synthesis of nitrosamines from nitrates is nitrites. Nitrites are produced from nitrates by bacteria in the stomach, but the bacteria with enzymes capable of catalyzing this reaction are killed by the acid environment present in the normal stomach. This capability might explain why gastric cancer develops more frequently in patients with atrophic gastritis and hypochlorhydria. Once nitrites are formed, they quickly combine with amines present in gastric juice to form nitrosamines. Both changes in methods of food preservation and the increased use of vitamin C are factors that would interfere with this proposed mechanism of carcinogenesis for gastric cancer.

Patients who have pernicious anemia, hypochlorhydria, or achlorhydria appear to develop gastric cancer more frequently than do others. As noted, atrophic gastritis and intestinal metaplasia have been thought to be the major precursor lesions. Adenomatous polyps are not considered major precursor lesions for gastric cancer, but patients with adenomatous polyps in the stomach do have an increased incidence of gastric cancer. In contrast to their occurrence in the colon, however, adenomatous polyps are uncommon in the stomach and probably are less common than gastric cancer itself.

GENETICS AND ETIOLOGY

Reports have cited a 15% to 20% increased incidence of gastric cancer in persons with blood group A, and this finding suggests a genetic relationship. A small increased incidence in gastric cancer has been noted in the direct relatives of people who have had gastric cancer. Napoleon Bonaparte's family is the best-known example of one of the few reported families that have demonstrated a remarkably high incidence of gastric cancer. One study of Japanese immigrants, however, has provided some evidence against major familial trends in gastric cancer [10]. Japanese immigrants in the United States maintain nearly the same incidence of gastric cancer as that seen in the region where they spend their first 20 years of life. In contrast, their offspring living in their adopted country have an incidence of gastric cancer that is lower and almost comparable to that of whites living nearby. These findings suggest probable exposures in early life, rather than an inherited genetic influence, as the major causative factors in gastric cancer. In one sense, all cancer is a result of genetic alterations in cells, but little evidence supports inheritance as a major causative factor in gastric cancer.

HELICOBACTER PYLORI INFECTION

In more recent years, *Helicobacter pylori* infection has received considerable attention as a potential causative factor for gastric cancer [11–15]. The relationship of possible antibiotic control of *H. pylori* to the decreasing incidence of peptic ulcers now appears likely, and a similar mechanism may be operative for the marked decrease noted in the incidence of some forms of gastric cancer over these last few decades. Chronic infection with *H. pylori* is associated with atrophic gastritis, the precancerous change most often associated with an "intestinal type" characteristic of distal gastric cancer. Inadvertent control of this organism may be linked to the shift that has been noted from distal gastric lesions to more frequent proximal lesions, because the association of *H. pylori* with the proximal diffuse type of cancers is less impressive.

Pathology

In terms of gross pathology, the first classification of adenocarcinoma of the stomach was constructed by Borrmann in 1926 and is summarized as follows:

- *Type I (polypoid carcinoma):* clearly demarcated; may be ulcerated; late metastasis; relatively good prognosis
- *Type II (ulcerating carcinoma, or "ulcerocancer"):* sharply defined margins; difficult to differentiate from benign ulcer on gross examination; requires biopsy; relatively good prognosis
- *Type III (ulcerating and infiltrating):* lacks clear-cut margins; extensive submucosal infiltration and usually extends to the serosa; most common gross type of gastric cancer; relatively poor prognosis
- *Type IV (diffuse infiltration):* early metastasis; includes linitis plastica ("leather-bottle stomach"); poorest prognosis of all gastric cancers

Both types I and II appear to be decreasing in incidence in the United States, in contrast to types III and IV. Additional gross classifications of gastric cancer include superficial spreading carcinoma (large, ulcerating, and irregular borders that are confined in the mucosa and submucosa) and "early gastric cancer" (small, usually very early lesions that do not infiltrate beyond the submucosa). These early cancers, with a favorable prognosis, constitute up to 35% of some series in Japan, but they still are fairly uncommon in the United States. Other gross classifications have been defined, but this classification is very utilitarian.

Most adenocarcinomas arise from the distal portion of the stomach and present on the lesser curvature, also a common site for benign gastric ulcer. In one large series, 45% of all malignant lesions were primarily in the distal one-third of the stomach, 33% were in the pars media, and 22% were in the proximal one-third of the stomach. However, a recent trend in the United States has been toward an increasing incidence of proximal gastric cancers [16–18]. This tendency may be related to an increase or reduction in some of the proposed etiologic factors for specific types of gastric cancer.

The cause of the shift in anatomic location of gastric cancer from the distal stomach to the proximal stomach is unclear. Recent observations about *H. pylori* may provide a partial explanation because, as noted earlier, this chronic infection is associated with atrophic gastritis, the precancerous change associated most often with the intestinal type of gastric cancer that is characteristic of distal gastric lesions. Reduction in infection by this organism may have led to this decrease in distal gastric cancer. Also, the proximal trend in anatomic site may be related, in some unexplained way, to the marked increase in incidence of adenocarcinoma of the distal esophagus, an increase observed over recent years.

Histologic Classification

The original histologic classification for gastric cancer was developed by Broder, who described four grades (I–IV) for all carcinomas on the basis of the degree of differentiation present. A later, now frequently used histologic classification was described by Lauren [19]. He described two major types of lesion: the intestinal, a well-differentiated lesion, and the diffuse, or undifferentiated, carcinoma. This histologic classification is useful because, in certain countries, atrophic gastritis is associated only with cancers of the intestinal variety. This also suggests that the intestinal and diffuse types of lesions may well have differing causes.

Because adenocarcinoma of the stomach originates from the mucosal layer of the stomach, lesions described as "early gastric cancer" are grossly and histologically limited to the mucosa or submucosa. Many or all gastric cancers initially may be confined to the mucosa or the submucosa (or both), but clinical diagnosis of gastric cancer at this stage has been fairly uncommon in the United States. In Japan, where incidence is higher and screening measures have been more vigorous, cancer limited to the mucosa has been identified increasingly. In the United States, usually gastric cancer has invaded the muscular layers of the gastric wall and frequently is present on the external serosal surface of the stomach at diagnosis.

Mechanisms of Spread

Gastric adenocarcinomas can penetrate the gastric wall and can invade contiguous anatomic structures and adjacent organs directly. These adenocarcinomas can involve the pancreas, spleen, esophagus, colon, duodenum, gallbladder, liver, or adjacent mesenteries. Local posterior extension of the cancer to the adjacent body of the pancreas and transverse mesocolon is the most frequent route of local spread. All local extensions occur after growth to and through the serosal surface of the stomach and are associated with some diminution in prognosis.

Often, gastric cancers spread to the peritoneal surface of the abdominal cavity. This type of spread produces tiny "implants," coalesced peritoneal surface masses, or a reactive ascites, all findings that have the same poor prognostic significance as hematogenous spread of the disease.

Gastric adenocarcinoma spreads via lymphatics in almost two-thirds of the patients undergoing surgical exploration. The initial regional lymphatics involved are determined by the anatomic location of the primary lesion in the stomach. Usually, the lymph nodes adjacent to the primary lesion are involved first, but eventual regional lymph node spread may be fairly extensive and can involve the lymphatic chains on both the lesser and greater curvatures of the stomach. The next level of regional lymphatic spread is along the hepatic and splenic vessels. More distant lymphatic spread, particularly that detected in the left supraclavicular nodes (Virchow's node) is a classic sign of stage IV disease, indicating that surgery is not a major primary treatment option.

Gastric adenocarcinomas may spread hematogenously through the portal circulation to the liver and, less often, to other sites. Histologic evidence of metastatic spread to the lungs has been identified in approximately 25% of patients at autopsy, whereas on clinical evaluation, hematogenous spread to the lungs and other distant sites rarely is noted.

Primary and Secondary Prevention

No established program or plan for primary prevention of gastric cancer exists, but some of the preceding material in this chapter points to certain possible strategies. Following up on the nitrosamine hypothesis of causation, consumption of foods with high levels of antioxidants and vitamin C may be beneficial. More recent information regarding *H. pylori*, and the resulting gastritis, as a causative factor leads to the concept of possibly controlling such an infection early in life in certain populations. This control may have occurred inadvertently in the United States, because most children receive antibiotics for ear or other infections, but a concerted plan to control *H. pylori* infections in all children may prove beneficial, particularly in undeveloped countries where this cancer still is a major health hazard.

In some Japanese centers, screening for gastric cancer has detected cancers that are confined to the mucosa, so-called early gastric cancer [20]. These early gastric cancers have had a much higher cure rate, and the relatively rare early gastric cancers that have been diagnosed in the United States have a comparable prognosis. However, the yield from gastric cancer screening in the United States would be far too low ever to approach cost-effectiveness. A few high-risk populations (e.g., patients with pernicious anemia and, possibly, patients who previously have undergone partial gastrectomy for benign disease) might be exceptions. Despite the lack of feasibility of gastric cancer screening in the United States, the increasing use of upper gastrointestinal en-

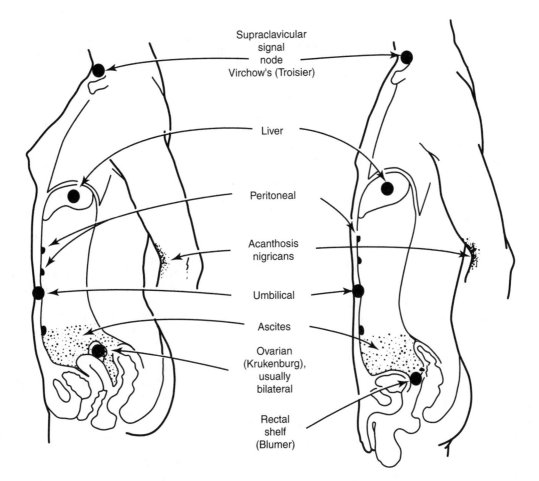

Figure 14.2 Routes of spread of gastric cancer.

doscopy over the last several decades has allowed a more precise, and possibly an earlier, diagnosis of gastric lesions.

Diagnosis

CLINICAL PRESENTATION

The symptoms of gastric cancer are nonspecific [21]. The vast majority of gastric cancer patients present with such vague gastrointestinal complaints as epigastric discomfort or indigestion, occasional vomiting, belching, or postprandial fullness or early satiety. From 5% to 10% of gastric cancer patients may have complaints fairly similar to those of patients who have peptic ulcer disease. Another 10% have nonspecific symptoms of chronic disease, such as anemia, weakness, and weight loss. A small number of patients are seen first with an acute intraabdominal problem, such as massive upper gastrointestinal bleeding, acute obstruction of the esophagus or pylorus, or gastric perforation, often re-

quiring emergency surgery. Diagnosis is difficult because most of these symptoms can be manifestations of either local or distant extensions of neoplasm or can be attributed to other acute, noncancerous diseases in the upper abdomen.

The physical examination rarely is helpful, except in identifying signs of advanced and often incurable disease (Fig. 14.2). On physical examination, the only observation that may lead to a reasonably early diagnosis of gastric cancer is a positive fecal occult blood test. Other physical signs suggest more advanced disease and include palpable ovarian masses (from metastases), liver enlargement, an abdominal or pelvic mass, ascites, jaundice, and cachexia. Although a patient with a palpable gastric cancer may be a suitable candidate for curative resection, often this physical finding is associated with a poor prognosis.

DIAGNOSTIC WORKUP

Lacking specific diagnostic symptoms or signs, physicians must evaluate any patient with persistent upper gastrointestinal symptoms, particularly individuals who are older than 40 years. The diagnosis can be established by upper gastrointestinal barium radiographic examination, upper gastrointestinal endoscopy, or a combination of the two. Radiographic study may be sufficient to allow the initiation of therapy, but upper gastrointestinal endoscopy, in conjunction with biopsy, is the standard approach, providing a precise diagnosis in 95% of patients. Additional benefits of endoscopy over radiography are the differentiation of an ulcerating neoplasm from a benign gastric ulcer and the identification of very superficial or early cancers. Multiple biopsies taken from an area of suspicious mucosa, or of any ulcerations that are noted, or from any polypoid change will establish the diagnosis of adenocarcinoma or, alternatively, the diagnosis of other malignant neoplasms. Benign biopsy specimens are presumptive but inconclusive evidence of a benign ulcer. A gastric ulcer must be proved to be benign by healing.

STAGING

Clinical staging of gastric cancer is based on the extent of disease, as shown by physical examination and the diagnostic studies described, as well as by computed tomography (CT) and by newer diagnostic tests that have become available in recent years (e.g., endoscopic ultrasonography, with or without fine-needle aspiration biopsy, and diagnostic laparoscopy). These approaches should improve our ability to stage the disease prior to treatment intervention, a particular advantage if the initial treatment chosen is to be nonsurgical.

Tables 14.1 and 14.2 outline the American Joint Committee on Cancer staging schema for categorizing gastric adenocarcinoma [22]. The prognosis may be affected by other parameters, such as carcinoembryonic antigen [23] or other tumor markers; histologic grading [24]; p53 expression [25]; cell proliferation kinetic indicators; and tumor DNA ploidy pattern [26]; but none of these parameters currently is incorporated in the TNM (tumor–regional lymph node spread–metastases) staging system. The technique for determining the TNM classification for adenocarcinoma of the stomach begins with a complete physical examination, because palpable supraclavicular lymph nodes, liver enlargement, ascites, or findings on pelvic or rectal examinations (or both) will alert clinicians to the likelihood of distant metastases. Confirmatory biopsy or cytologic examination from these sites will lead to categorization as M1 (stage IV). Liver function tests may be employed to identify patients who are likely to have liver metastases (M1), but

Table 14.1 TNM Staging for Stomach Cancer

Classification	Definition
Primary tumor (T)	
TX	Primary tumor cannot be assessed
T0	No evidence of primary tumor
Tis	Carcinoma in situ; intraepithelial tumor without invasion of lamina propria
T1	Tumor invades lamina propria or submucosa
T2	Tumor invades the muscularis propria or the subserosa
T3	Tumor penetrates the serosa (visceral peritoneum) without invasion of adjacent structures
T4	Tumor invades adjacent structures
Regional lymph nodes (N)	
NX	Regional lymph node(s) cannot be assessed
N0	No regional lymph node metastasis
N1	Metastasis in 1–6 regional nodes
N2	Metastasis in 7–15 regional nodes
N3	Metastasis in more than 15 regional lymph nodes
Distant metastasis (M)	
MX	Presence of distant metastasis cannot be assessed
M0	No distant metastasis
M1	Distant metastasis

Source: Used with the permission of the *American Joint Committee on Cancer (AJCC®)*, Chicago. *AJCC® Cancer Staging Manual* (5th Edition), 1997. Philadelphia: Lippincott-Raven.

Table 14.2 AJCC/UICC Stage Grouping

Stage 0	Tis	N0	M0
Stage IA	T1	N0	M0
Stage IB	T1	N1	M0
	T2	N0	M0
Stage II	T1	N2	M0
	T2	N1	M0
	T3	N0	M0
Stage IIIA	T2	N2	M0
	T3	N1	M0
	T4	N0	M0
Stage IIIB	T3	N2	M0
Stage IV	T4	N1	M0
	T1	N3	M0
	T2	N3	M0
	T3	N3	M0
	T4	N2	M0
	T4	N3	M0
	Any T	Any N	M1

AJCC = American Joint Committee on Cancer; UICC = Union Internationale Contre le Cancer.
Source: Used with the permission of the *American Joint Committee on Cancer (AJCC®)*, Chicago. *AJCC® Cancer Staging Manual* (5th Edition), 1997. Philadelphia: Lippincott-Raven.

metastatic disease rarely is seen on the chest roentgenogram.

CT is a valuable additional staging technique for detecting distant disease in the abdomen, and it allows both more accurate tumor classification and some estimation of the presence or absence of regional lymph node spread [27, 28]. The sensitivity, specificity, and predictive value of contrast-enhanced CT varies considerably in published reports. Helical CT assists in lymph node evaluation, and this assessment is related to the size of the lymph nodes. Of lymph nodes that are more than 14 mm in diameter, 83% prove to be positive. Of lymph nodes that are smaller than 14 mm, almost 90% are negative. Magnetic resonance imaging may be used for assessing extragastric abdominal disease, but it appears to be less accurate than is CT.

Endoscopic ultrasonography (EUS) is another staging technique that can define the depth of invasion of the primary tumor in the stomach wall, a factor of importance in tumor classification (Fig. 14.3) [29, 30]. Assessment of lymph node status by EUS, with or without fine-needle biopsy, is less precise than is tumor stage determination, but EUS does allow more precise nodal staging prior to operative intervention, an approach primarily useful for staging if nonoperative treatment is to be employed *prior* to resection. EUS depends on the degree of disruption of the normal mucosal stratification; the overall accuracy of this technique for tumor staging is in the range of 85%. For EUS evaluation of regional lymph nodes, sensitivity in various studies ranges from 58% to 80%. The addition of fine-needle aspiration biopsy to this technique is not substantiated, as yet, for improved TNM staging of gastric neoplasms, but it may increase accuracy [31]. A flow chart for diagnosis and staging is shown in Figure 14.4.

Laparoscopy is another staging approach that well may prove useful, particularly if findings on the peritoneal surfaces or in the liver will lead to a decision not to proceed with surgical exploration [32]. Both EUS and laparoscopy are particularly helpful in patients who are entered into clinical trials of nonoperative therapy instead of, or prior to, operation [33]. The most accurate staging classification for end-result reporting after surgical treatment, however, is based on the extent of disease found at the time of surgical exploration and combined with the histologic study of the surgical specimen (clinicopathologic stage).

Treatment

Currently, surgery is the only curative treatment of gastric adenocarcinoma but, despite major improvements over the years in both surgical procedures and postsurgical management, overall survival rates remain fairly low for all patients but those with early gastric cancer. All patients with gastric cancer, *except* those with evidence of peritoneal metastasis, documented liver metastasis, or other proved distant metastases (usually cervical lymph nodes), should be subjected to exploratory celiotomy to select both potentially curable patients and those who might benefit from palliative resection. If the cancer is localized regionally at exploration, adequate resection of the primary tumor and the potential regional lymphatic extension is performed.

The major options for surgical resection are distal subtotal gastric resection, proximal subtotal resection, or total gastrectomy. Usually, the choice of operation is determined by the location of the cancer in the stomach and by the extent of involvement (Fig. 14.5). Restoration of continuity of the alimentary tract is achieved by anastomosis of the small intestine to the gastric remnant (gastroenterostomy), distal stomach to the esophagus (esophagogastrostomy and pyloroplasty), or small intestine to the esophagus, with or without a jejunal reservoir. These procedures may include resection of adjacent organs affected by local extension of the cancer, such as the body and tail of the pancreas, a portion of the liver, the transverse colon or, in rare instances, the duodenum and the head of the pancreas. Inclusion of extragastric organs in the resection is an infrequent

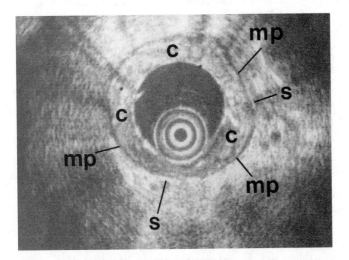

Figure 14.3 Endoscopic ultrasonographic image of gastric cancer that allows tumor staging prior to treatments. Five layers of the gastric wall have been disrupted by the cancer (*c*). The fourth hypoechoic layer, the muscularis propria (*mp*), and the fifth layer, the serosa (*s*) are visible.

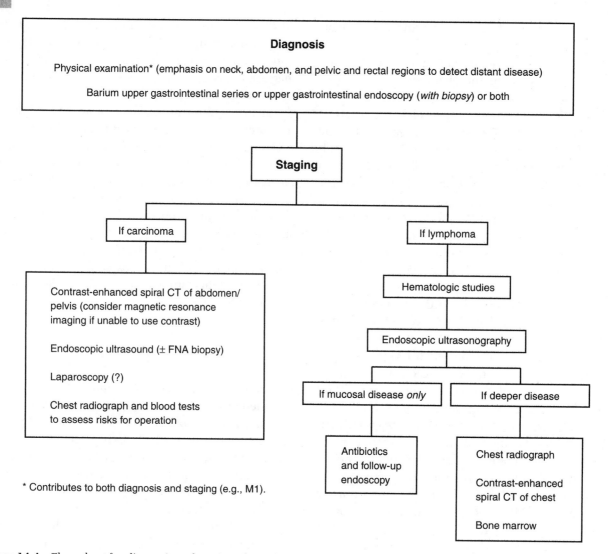

Diagnosis

Physical examination* (emphasis on neck, abdomen, and pelvic and rectal regions to detect distant disease)

Barium upper gastrointestinal series or upper gastrointestinal endoscopy (*with biopsy*) or both

Staging

If carcinoma

If lymphoma

Contrast-enhanced spiral CT of abdomen/pelvis (consider magnetic resonance imaging if unable to use contrast)

Endoscopic ultrasound (± FNA biopsy)

Laparoscopy (?)

Chest radiograph and blood tests to assess risks for operation

Hematologic studies

Endoscopic ultrasonography

If mucosal disease *only*

If deeper disease

Antibiotics and follow-up endoscopy

Chest radiograph

Contrast-enhanced spiral CT of chest

Bone marrow

* Contributes to both diagnosis and staging (e.g., M1).

Figure 14.4   Flow chart for diagnosis and staging of gastric cancer. *CT* = computed tomography; *FNA* = fine-needle aspiration.

consideration, because involvement of such organs often is accompanied by other gross signs of incurability.

Microscopic spread of the cancer beyond the gross margin of the gastric lesion renders removal of a generous margin of normal stomach around the cancer a standard principle of gastric resection. In distal gastric lesions, generous resection of the adjacent first portion of the duodenum is required; in proximal lesions, the removal of several centimeters of the distal esophagus is necessary. Failure to control a potentially curable cancer by not achieving an adequate gross margin around the primary tumor is a serious and avoidable error.

LYMPHATIC SPREAD

In designing a radical gastrectomy for patients with a potentially curable gastric cancer, the removal of regional lymph nodes must be considered. Although the incidence of regional lymphatic spread varies with different gross and histologic types of cancer, the overall incidence of lymphatic spread from carcinoma of the stomach is fairly high—higher than 60%. Palpation during surgery is not a particularly accurate way to evaluate lymph nodes. Potential areas of lymphatic spread always must be considered in the design of radical gastrectomy, because the status of the regional lymphatics can be determined with confidence only by histologic examination. The optimal extent of lymphatic removal remains controversial.

In general, surgeons in Japan and other areas in the Far East tend to perform a lymph node dissection more extended than those performed by surgeons in the Western world [34]. Because the results of treatment of gastric cancer in Japan generally are superior to results obtained in the United States and Europe, these improved results often are claimed to be due to the use

Distal   Proximal   Total

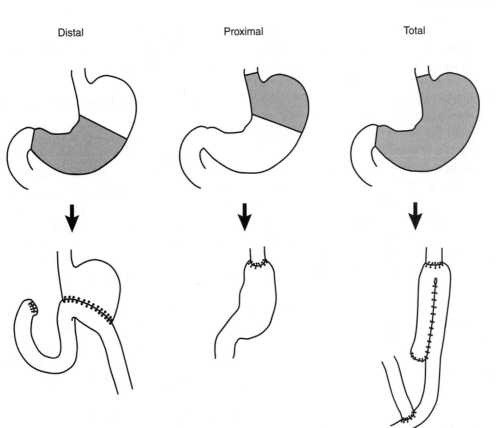

Figure 14.5 Operative resections employed for gastric cancer. (Left) Distal gastrectomy. (Middle) Proximal gastrectomy. (Right) Total gastrectomy. Methods of reconstruction are shown below each procedural diagram.

of more extensive regional lymph node resection in the Far East. Many other factors confuse this situation, however.

The possibility that differences in results are due to underlying racial or ethnic differences in gastric cancer in these various populations has been suggested, but comparisons of results of surgery on Japanese patients in Hawaii and in Japan tend to discredit this explanation [35]. Another major reason for differences in end results is the much higher proportion of early gastric cancer in Japan, cancers that always have a better survival rate after surgical therapy. Diagnostic criteria for gastric carcinoma differ greatly between Japanese and Western pathologists also, as has been shown in a recent study [36], but this in itself would not have an impact on results of surgical treatment for anything more advanced than T1a cancers. As most of the treatment data relating to the question of the optimal extent of lymphadenectomy were from nonrandomized comparisons, the question as to the importance of the extent of lymphadenectomy was unanswered until recently.

As the years have passed, a number of reports from the Western world have seemed to demonstrate im-

proved results in patient populations that had been subjected to extended lymphadenectomy for gastric cancer. These reports have come from Germany [37], Austria [38], and the United States [39]. This information further increased the suspicion around the world that extended lymphadenectomy was a better treatment option. However, recent retrospective evaluations from the United States, using a large database from the American College of Surgeons, failed to show survival benefit from the extended dissection [40]. These intriguing observations of better survival after extended lymphadenectomy in a number of retrospective series clearly led to the need for data from randomized trials to answer the question more firmly.

Four randomized clinical trials have addressed the optimal extent of lymphadenectomy; however, drawing definitive conclusions from published reports was difficult until recently. The first study, a small, completed South African trial reported by Dent et al. [41], failed to show a survival benefit from extended dissections in a comparison of such patients with those in a group undergoing standard regional lymphadenectomy. A more recent trial, reported from Hong Kong, compared subtotal gastrectomy and standard regional node dissection with extended lymphadenectomy and total gastrectomy [42]. All patients in this trial had antral cancers, and the study failed to show survival benefit in those in the extended lymphadenectomy group, while demonstrating some increase in morbidity. A much larger trial, reported recently from the Netherlands—a prospective, randomized comparison of standard lymph node dissection with extended dissection—demonstrated increased morbidity with the extended dissection [43, 44]. Recent analysis seemed to show no survival benefit from extended dissection, despite improved survival data in both arms of the study as compared with earlier results [45]. As no randomized trial data thus far support the contention that more extensive lymphatic dissection is justified for gastric cancer, the generally accepted performance of a standard regional dissection of perigastric nodes probably is appropriate as a curative procedure for gastric cancer.

ADJUVANT THERAPY

The role of external-beam irradiation as an adjunct in the "curative" surgical treatment of gastric cancer is not established clearly, but clinical trials are exploring this therapy and intraoperative irradiation for their usefulness at the time of resection [46, 47]. The obvious problem in using irradiation as adjuvant therapy is the difficulty of employing a field large enough to encompass the entire volume at risk for residual disease.

High local and distant failure rates after surgical resection cause systemic therapy to seem desirable. Many chemotherapeutic agents and combinations of agents have been employed in clinical trials of adjuvant chemotherapy with or without irradiation, but their results have been disappointing [48–50]. Another type of adjuvant systemic chemotherapy that is showing some promise and has some support in randomized trials is the combined use of chemotherapy and adjuvant immunotherapy. This approach has been explored in Japan [51], and Kim et al. [52] have reported a large, randomized Korean trial of this approach as well. In this three-arm study comparing combined postoperative immunotherapy and chemotherapy, postoperative adjuvant chemotherapy alone, and no adjuvant therapy, the 5-year survival was significantly improved in the patients in the group receiving immunochemotherapy as compared with the survival of patients in the two other groups. These data should encourage further clinical trials to attempt confirmation of these findings. Other phase II trials of chemotherapy prior to gastric resection, or both preoperatively and postoperatively,

are ongoing, but adjuvant chemotherapy, preoperatively or postoperatively (or both), cannot currently be recommended as a routine plan.

RESULTS OF OPERATIVE TREATMENT

The prognosis for patients with gastric cancer after primary surgery or combined therapy remains poor, and many patients are found to be incurable on the basis of their pretreatment evaluation at the time of initial diagnosis. For many years, the overall success rate after treatment of gastric adenocarcinoma was only 10% to 15% of all patients presenting with this problem. However, despite lack of major improvements in treatment, the more recent data from the National Cancer Database demonstrate a 20% 5-year survival of patients with this disease in the United States [2]. Results in some parts of the world, particularly Japan, are considerably better than this, but much of that outcome can be attributed to a higher proportion of patients with early-stage disease in these areas.

PALLIATIVE TREATMENT

Surgery

A significant number of patients explored surgically with hope for resection have unfavorable operative findings, such as serosal implants, liver or ovarian metastases, or metastases in lymph nodes outside the limits of an en bloc lymph node resection. These findings are less frequent than they were in the past, as CT scanning identifies some of these patients with incurable disease prior to operation. Laparoscopy preceding operative exploration has been advocated to assess curability but, because of the limited impact of nonoperative therapy on this disease, most surgeons perform a resection, if feasible, regardless of whether signs of incurability exist. The increased benefit of a palliative resection of an incurable gastric cancer over the results of bypass operations or "ostomies" has been appreciated for a long time. Resection, when feasible, achieves a higher rate of symptomatic relief and a somewhat longer survival [53, 54].

Palliative distal gastrectomy is well accepted, but total gastrectomy for palliation generally has been avoided, owing to the expectation of a much higher morbidity and mortality. Now that improved postoperative management has led to a marked decrease in morbidity and mortality after total gastrectomy, occasionally this procedure is indicated for palliation [55]. Patients receiving the most benefit are those with obstruction of the distal stomach prior to treatment or those patients in whom the only anatomic reason for incurability is distant lymphatic spread. These patients have longer survival intervals after palliative therapy than do patients whose disease is incurable because of liver or peritoneal metastases. The goal of palliative surgery for incurable gastric cancer is the restoration of patients' ability to ingest food. This goal can be accomplished in only some patients.

Radiotherapy

Although it has not been demonstrated to have a meaningful adjuvant role to other therapies, radiotherapy has been useful for palliation in patients who have a localized area of obstruction in the region of the cardia or in those experiencing a local recurrence of their carcinoma at the site of an esophageal anastomosis. A complete response is not achieved, but some regression may relieve these specific problems.

Chemotherapy

The results of single and multiple chemotherapeutic agents in advanced cancer patients have been disappointing. The standard chemotherapy combination employed for palliation has been 5-fluorouracil, doxorubicin (Adriamycin), and mitomycin C. Limited response rates and a limited survival prolongation in the palliative setting lead to a continued exploration of other drugs and drug combinations. The nonoperative approach to the advanced cancer patient is a fertile field for further investigation by clinical trials.

Rehabilitation and Follow-Up

POSTGASTRECTOMY PROBLEMS AND SOLUTIONS

Because the primary treatment of gastric cancer is surgical resection, the short-term sequelae of the surgical procedures described include those complications that follow all major abdominal operations. An additional factor always is a possibility of leakage from the anastomosis between the esophagus and the stomach or the jejunum, when either the proximal or the entire stomach is resected. The leak rate from esophageal anastomoses is less than 5% but is higher than that from other gastrointestinal anastomoses. The late sequelae of gastrectomy are more significant than are these short-term effects.

After full recovery from gastrectomy, some patients have various postprandial symptoms associated with the surgical alterations of internal anatomy. The symptom complex described most frequently is the so-called dumping syndrome. This problem may follow either partial removal of the stomach or total gastrectomy but is associated more frequently with the latter. The primary cause of such symptomatology is the loss of the pyloric mechanism that normally delays transit of foodstuff into the small intestine, but the usual physiologic explanation given is the reaction of the small bowel to hyperosmolar feedings. Among patients, great variability is exhibited in regard to the development of these symptoms, but experience has proved the wisdom of avoiding hyperosmolar feedings soon after gastric surgery until affected patients have stabilized on a reasonable diet and have recovered completely from surgery. A diet that tends to reduce symptoms when the pylorus has been removed is a six-feeding, high-protein, low-carbohydrate diet, although not all patients require the same level of attention in their dietary management. In addition, various types of substitute reservoirs constructed after total removal of the stomach tend to reduce these symptoms.

Another latent problem after gastrectomy is the development of anemia. The most frequent early cause is decreased iron absorption secondary to the gastrectomy. Inadequate absorption of vitamin B_{12}, due to the loss of intrinsic factor, is a later mechanism for anemia after total gastrectomy, but this effect does not prove to be a problem until 4 or more years after the procedure. Initially available intrinsic hepatic stores of vitamin B_{12} are the reason for the delay in the development of vitamin B_{12} deficiency and accompanying neurologic sequelae.

When employed, anticancer chemotherapy is accompanied by the common side effects of these agents. Radiotherapy causes nausea more frequently in the treatment of gastric cancer than in the treatment of cancer of other anatomic sites, possibly because the liver is included in the radiation field.

FOLLOW-UP STRATEGY AND SURVEILLANCE

Initial follow-up strategy for patients treated surgically for gastric cancer deals with dietary guidance to solve the postgastrectomy problems listed earlier. Because very limited treatments are available at this time for those patients who develop recurrent disease, the benefit of intense later surveillance is questionable. A reasonable approach, however, is to consider periodic endoscopic surveillance of those patients undergoing partial gastrectomy, as the remaining stomach is at higher risk for developing a second primary lesion [9]. This precaution is not carried out frequently, however, as the likelihood of a curable second gastric primary cancer is fairly remote.

UNCOMMON GASTRIC CANCERS
Primary Lymphoma

Malignant lymphoma can arise in and be limited to the stomach. Because the gross pathology of this lesion is so similar to the gross pathology of adenocarcinoma, the diagnosis is not made until pathologic study of a biopsy or the operative specimen is completed. Current techniques of preoperative endoscopy and biopsy of potentially neoplastic lesions of the stomach usually can identify the gastric lymphoma prior to development of a therapeutic plan.

In recent years, a new pathologic entity has been described as mucosa-associated lymphoid tissue (MALT) lymphoma. This new category includes, in addition to superficial lymphomas, those lesions previously termed *pseudolymphoma* [56]. MALT lymphoma is particularly interesting as it appears to have an association with *H. pylori* gastritis [57]. Also interesting is the fact that many of these MALT lesions regress with antibiotic therapy. The spectrum of primary gastric lymphoma ranges, then, from this superficial mucosal lesion to bulkier lesions involving the entire gastric wall and, in some instances, the regional lymph nodes.

Generally, the incidence of primary gastric lymphoma was believed to be less than 3% of all gastric cancers until the last few decades. The incidence of this entity in our population has gradually increased and now approximates 10% of all malignant gastric tumors [58, 59]. Because management of this disorder differs from that of adenocarcinoma in many respects, pretreatment endoscopic biopsy is vital to treatment planning.

Clinical Presentation

Primary gastric lymphoma may present as a gastric ulcer, similar in many ways to the "ulcerocancer" form of gastric adenocarcinoma (Borrmann II). It may present as a superficial process similar to early gastric cancer or may present as a larger ulcerating and infiltrating lesion similar to the Borrmann type III adenocarcinoma. In some instances, the lymphoma appears only as large rugae in the stomach. In most instances, the diagnosis of lymphoma is established only by histologic study of the lesion, and this then prompts various staging techniques.

Staging

When the biopsy report is non-Hodgkin's lymphoma, staging techniques should include hematologic studies; CT scans of the chest, abdomen, and pelvis; and bone marrow aspiration or biopsy. As with gastric adenocarcinoma, EUS of the primary lesion is useful for staging and, in this instance, may be fairly relevant to the choice of treatment [60]. Superficial mucosal lesions, now classified as MALT lymphomas, can be assessed by EUS, which allows selection of those patients who should receive a trial of antibiotic therapy. This staging approach is summarized and contrasted with staging of adenocarcinoma in the flow chart shown in Figure 14.4.

Treatment

A major development in terms of therapy is the use of nonoperative programs for primary lymphoma of the stomach. These modalities range from antibiotic therapeutic trials for MALT lymphomas to anticancer chemotherapy, with or without radiotherapy, for more invasive lesions. The superficial lesion limited to the mucosa (MALT lymphoma) may respond completely to antibiotic therapy directed at *H. pylori* (e.g., metronidazole, clarithromycin, and omeprazole) and may require no anticancer drugs [61].

Deep-wall extension on EUS should prompt the other staging studies (listed earlier) before a decision is made regarding the treatment approach. Some lesions still are treated by surgical resection [62, 63], but neither resection nor irradiation appear to offer any additional survival advantage when compared with chemotherapy alone in stage I and stage II gastric lymphomas [64]. Earlier concerns that a primary chemotherapy program for deeper lymphomas might lead to significant danger of gastric perforation, as occurs on occasion with primary chemotherapy of small-bowel lymphomas, have not been realized. Upper gastrointestinal bleeding may be an indication for performing primary resection *before* instituting chemotherapy in patients in this group.

For low-grade gastric lymphomas that are seen to invade the entire gastric wall on pretreatment EUS, primary resection with a standard regional node dissection probably still is an appropriate approach, but the ultimate prognosis is enhanced in all but a few groups of patients by the use of adjuvant postoperative chemotherapy programs. Postoperative radiotherapy is used infrequently. All the foregoing observations and considerations regarding management of primary gastric lymphoma emphasize the importance of multidisciplinary discussions between pathologists and clinicians from the various oncologic specialties.

OTHER MALIGNANT GASTRIC TUMORS

Other than primary gastric lymphoma, the most common cancer of mesodermal origin arising from the stomach is the gastrointestinal stromal cell tumor formerly known as *leiomyosarcoma*. Noteworthy is that the benign form of this lesion, the leiomyoma, is much more frequent than is the malignant counterpart. Though some leiomyosarcomas were infiltrative lesions on gross examination and clearly were cancerous, others were differentiated from benign leiomyomas only by the frequency of mitotic figures seen on histologic section. This problem in differentiating many of these lesions and recent thoughts on the true cell of origin have led, in recent years, to the classification of this entire group of gastric tumors as *gastrointestinal stromal tumors* [65].

Less frequent types of sarcoma that arise from the stomach are classified histogenetically as liposarcoma, fibrosarcoma, carcinosarcoma, and malignant tumors of vascular origin. These other mesodermal lesions are fairly uncommon, together representing fewer than 3% of all gastric cancers.

Another rare type of malignant gastric tumor is the carcinoid, a low-grade malignant lesion that occurs more commonly in the small intestine. Generally, carcinoids are small, firm, yellow, well-circumscribed submucosal lesions, as they are in other locations, but some present as rather large lesions that appear similar to primary adenocarcinoma of the stomach. Carcinoid tumors may spread to regional lymph nodes, and a gastric resection similar to that employed for adenocarcinoma is indicated. No adjuvant therapy has been established as being advantageous for these lesions. Carcinoids that metastasize to the liver may develop the so-called carcinoid syndrome and may necessitate use of the drug octreotide as therapy for the pharmacologic effects of the metabolic products of these hepatic lesions.

Even more uncommon than the aforementioned malignant lesions of the stomach are plasmacytomas and carcinomas metastatic to the stomach from other organs. The primary site for these unusual metastatic gastric cancers varies, but primary lung cancer and malignant melanoma are two of the more common primary sites.

SUMMARY

Adenocarcinoma is far and away the most common cancer arising from the stomach. Of all the major cancers in humans, gastric cancer (along with cervical cancer) has markedly decreased in incidence in the United States over the last 50 years. This experiment of nature may well furnish clues relating to cancer causation in general and eventually may help us to plan prevention strategies for other cancers.

The treatment of gastric adenocarcinoma has changed little in recent years, because radiotherapy and chemotherapy have less impact on this cancer than on many other human cancers. However, survival data after surgery for gastric cancer in Japan continue to be better than data from the Western world. Although many researchers have attributed this difference to the performance of more extensive nodal resections in Japan, clinical trial results now indicate that this difference in results is due in part to disease diagnosis at an earlier stage in the East. This finding should encourage us to pursue new approaches for earlier diagnosis simultaneously with the development of prevention strategies.

Of the less common gastric cancers, primary lymphoma has stimulated interest for two reasons. First, an unexplained recent increase in incidence of this gastric neoplasm has been noted in the United States. Second, relatively recent evidence points to reversal of the MALT lymphoma with antimicrobial agents. This therapeutic approach to this subgroup of patients has become feasible as techniques for the diagnosis and staging of gastric neoplasms have been refined. Such progress in pretreatment histologic classification and staging will be important also in the development of other treatment strategies for all forms of gastric cancer.

REFERENCES

1. Greenlee RT, Murray T, Bolden S, Wingo PA. Cancer statistics, 2000. *CA Cancer J Clin* 50:7–33, 2000.
2. Lawrence W Jr, Menck HR, Steele GD Jr, Winchester DP. The National Cancer Data Base report on gastric cancer. *Cancer* 75:1734–1744, 1995.
3. Parkin DM, Laara E, Muir CS. Estimates of the worldwide frequency of 16 major cancers in 1980. *Int J Cancer* 41:184–197, 1988.
4. Parkin DM, Muir CS, Whelan YT, et al. (eds). *Cancer Incidence in Five Continents*, vol VI. [IARC Sci. Pub. No. 120.] Lyon, France: International Agency for Research on Cancer, 1992:865–870.

5. Chyou PH, Nomura AM, Hankin JH, Stemmermann GN. A case-cohort study of diet and stomach cancer. *Cancer Res* 50:7501–7504, 1990.

6. Harrison LE, Zhang Z-F, Karpeh MS, et al. The role of dietary factors in the intestinal and diffuse histologic subtypes of gastric adenocarcinoma (a case-control study in the US). *Cancer* 80:1021–1028, 1997.

7. Correa P. Human gastric carcinogenesis: a multistep and multifactorial process. First ACS award lecture on cancer epidemiology and prevention. *Cancer Res* 52:6735–6740, 1992.

8. Sirula M, Varis K, Wilijasala M. Studies of patients with atrophic gastritis: a 10- to 15-year follow-up. *Scand J Gastroenterol* 1:40–48, 1966.

9. Greene FL. Management of gastric remnant carcinoma based on the results of a fifteen year endoscopic screening program. *Ann Surg* 223:701–708, 1996.

10. Haenszel WM, Kurihara M. Studies of Japanese immigrants: I. Mortality from cancer and other diseases in the United States. *J Natl Cancer Inst* 40:43–68, 1968.

11. Talley NJ, Zinsmeister AW, DiMagno EP, et al. Gastric adenocarcinoma and *Helicobacter pylori* infection. *J Natl Cancer Inst* 83:1734–1738, 1991.

12. Kuipers EJ, Uyterlinde AM, Pena AS, et al. Long-term sequelae of *Helicobacter pylori* gastritis. *Lancet* 345:1525–1528, 1995.

13. Endo S, Ohkusa T, Saito Y, et al. Detection of *Helicobacter pylori* infection in early-stage gastric cancer (a comparison between intestinal and diffuse type gastric adenocarcinomas). *Cancer* 75:2203–2208,1995.

14. Shibata T, Imoto I, Ohuchi Y, et al. *Helicobacter pylori* infection in patients with gastric carcinoma and biopsy and surgical resection specimens. *Cancer* 77:1044–1049, 1996.

15. Zhang H-M, Wakisaka N, Maeda O, Yamamoto T. Vitamin C inhibits the growth of a bacterial risk factor for gastric carcinoma: *Helicobacter pylori*. *Cancer* 80:1897–1903, 1997.

16. Meyers WC, Damiano RJ, Postlethwait RW, Rotlo F. Adenocarcinoma of the stomach (changes in pattern over the last four decades). *Ann Surg* 205:1–8, 1987.

17. Salvon-Harman JC, Cady B, Nikulasson S, et al. Shifting proportions of gastric adenocarcinomas. *Arch Surg* 129: 381–389, 1994.

18. Zheng T, Mayne ST, Holford TR, et al. The time trend in age period cohorts: effects on incidence of adenocarcinoma in the stomach in Connecticut from 1959–1989. *Cancer* 72:330–340, 1993.

19. Lauren P. The two histologic main types of gastric carcinoma: diffuse and so-called intestinal type carcinoma, an attempt at a histochemical classification. *Acta Pathol Microbiol Scand* 64:31–49, 1965.

20. Hisamichi S, Tsubono Y, Fukad A. Screening for gastric cancer: a critical appraisal of the Japanese experience. *Gastrointest Cancer* 1:87–93, 1995.

21. LaDue JS, Murison PJ, McNeer G, Pack GT. Symptomatology and diagnosis of gastric cancer. *Arch Surg* 60:305–335, 1950.

22. Fleming ID, Cooper JS, Henson DE, et al. (eds). *AJCC Cancer Staging Manual* (5th ed). Philadelphia: Lippincott-Raven, 1997.

23. Nakane Y, Okamura S, Akehira K, et al. Correlation of preoperative carcinoembryonic antigen levels and prognosis of gastric cancer patients. *Cancer* 73:2703–2708, 1994.

24. Rugge M, Sonego F, Panozzo M, et al. Pathology and ploidy in the prognosis of gastric cancer with no extranodal metastasis. *Cancer* 73:1127–1133, 1994.

25. Poremba C, Yandell DW, Huang Q, et al. Frequency and spectrum of p53 mutations in gastric cancer. *Virchows Arch* 426:447–455, 1995.

26. Ohyama S, Yonemura Y, Miyazaki I. Prognostic value of S-phase fraction and DNA ploidy studied with in vivo administration of bromodeoxyuridine on human gastric cancers. *Cancer* 65:116–121, 1990.

27. Minami M, Kawauchi N, Itai Y, et al. Gastric tumors: radiologic-pathologic correlation and accuracy of T staging with dynamic CT. *Radiology* 185:173–178, 1992.

28. Fukuya T, Hiroshi H, Hayashi T, et al. Lymph node metastases: efficacy of detection with helical CT in patients with gastric cancer. *Radiology* 197:705–711, 1995.

29. Smith JW, Brennan MF, Botet JF, et al. Preoperative endoscopic ultrasound can predict the risk of recurrence after operation for gastric carcinoma. *J Clin Oncol* 11:2380–2385, 1993.

30. Dittler HJ, Siewert JR. Role of endoscopic ultrasonography in gastric carcinoma. *Endoscopy* 25:162–166, 1993.

31. Wiersema MJ, Cochman ML, Cramer HM, et al. Endosonography-guided real-time fine-needle aspiration biopsy. *Gastrointest Endosc* 40:700–701, 1994.

32. Lowy AM, Mansfield PF, Leach SD, Ajani J. Laparoscopic staging for gastric cancer. *Surgery* 119:611–614, 1996.

33. Sendler A, Dittler HJ, Feussner H, et al. Preoperative staging of gastric cancer as precondition for multimodal treatment. *World J Surg* 19:501–508, 1995.

34. Noguchi Y, Imada T, Matsumoto A, et al. Radical surgery for gastric cancer (a review of the Japanese experience). *Cancer* 64:2053–2062, 1989.

35. Hundahl SA, Stemmermann GN, Oishi A. Racial factors cannot explain superior Japanese outcomes in stomach cancer. *Arch Surg* 131:170–175, 1996.

36. Schlemper RJ, Itabasi M, Kato Y, et al. Differences in diagnostic criteria for gastric carcinoma between Japanese and Western pathologists. *Lancet* 349:1725–1729, 1997.

37. Bollschweiler E, Boettcher K, Hoelscher AH, et al. Is the prognosis for Japanese and German patients with gastric cancer really different? *Cancer* 71:2918–2925, 1993.

38. Jatzko GR, Lisborg PH, Denk H, et al. A ten-year experience with Japanese-type radical lymph node dissection for gastric cancer outside of Japan. *Cancer* 76:1302–1312, 1995.

39. Volpe CM, Koo J, Miloro SM. The effect of the extended lymphadenectomy on survival in patients with gastric adenocarcinoma. *J Am Coll Surg* 181:56–64, 1995.

40. Wanebo HJ, Kennedy BJ, Winchester DP, et al. Gastric carcinoma: does lymph node dissection alter survival? *J Am Coll Surg* 183:616–624, 1996.

41. Dent DM, Maddes MV, Price SK. Randomized comparison of R1 and R2 gastrectomy for gastric carcinoma. *Br J Surg* 75:110–112, 1988.

42. Robertson CS, Chung SCS, Woods SDS, et al. A prospective randomized trial comparing R-1 sub-total gastrectomy with R-3 total gastrectomy for antral cancer. *Ann Surg* 220:176–182, 1994.

43. Bunt AMG, Hermans J, Boon MC, et al. Evaluation of the

extent of lymphadenectomy in a randomized trial of Western vs Japanese type surgery in gastric cancer. *J Clin Oncol* 12:4117–4122, 1994.

44. Bonnenkamp JJ, Songun I, Hermans J, et al. Randomized comparisons of morbidity after D1 and D2 dissection for gastric cancer in 996 Dutch patients. *Lancet* 345:745–748, 1995.

45. Bonenkamp JJ, Hermans J, Sasako M, Van de Velde CJH (for the Dutch Cancer Group). Extended lymph node dissection for gastric cancer. *N Engl J Med* 340:908–914, 1999.

46. Gunderson LL, Nagorney DM, Martenson JA, et al. External beam plus intra-operative irradiation for gastrointestinal cancers. *World J Surg* 19:191–197, 1995.

47. Sindelar WF, Kinsella TJ, Tepper JE. Randomized trial of intra-operative radiotherapy in carcinoma of the stomach. *Am J Surg* 165:178–187, 1993.

48. Ajani JA, Mayer RJ, Ota DM, et al. Preoperative and postoperative combination chemotherapy for potentially resectable gastric carcinoma. *J Natl Cancer Inst* 85:1839–1844, 1993.

49. MacDonald JS, Schnall SF. Adjuvant treatment of gastric cancer. *World J Surg* 19:221–225, 1995.

50. Kelson D, Karpeh M, Schwartz G, et al. Neoadjuvant therapy of high-risk cancer. *J Clin Oncol* 14:1818–1828, 1996.

51. Kyoto Research Group for Digestive Surgery. A comprehensive multi-institutional study on postoperative adjuvant immunotherapy with oral streptococcal preparation OK-432 for patients after gastric cancer surgery. *Ann Surg* 216:44–54, 1992.

52. Kim J-P, Kwon OJ, Sung T, Yang HK. Results of surgery on 6589 gastric cancer patients and immunochemosurgery as the best treatment of advanced gastric cancer. *Ann Surg* 216:269–279, 1992.

53. Lawrence W Jr, McNeer G. The effectiveness of surgery for palliation of incurable gastric cancer. *Cancer* 11:28–32, 1958.

54. Haugstvedt T, Viste A, Eide GE, et al. The survival benefit of resection in patients with advanced stomach cancer: the Norwegian multi-center experience. *World J Surg* 13:617–622, 1989.

55. Monson JRT, Donohue JH, McIlraith DC, et al. Total gastrectomy for advanced cancer—a worthwhile palliative procedure. *Cancer* 68:1863–1868, 1991.

56. Orr RK, Lininger JR, Lawrence W Jr. Gastric pseudolymphoma (a challenging clinical problem). *Ann Surg* 200:185–194, 1984.

57. Bayerdorffer E, Neubauer A, Rudolph B, et al. Regression of primary gastric lymphoma of mucosa-associated lymphoid tissue after cure of *Helicobacter pylori* infection. *Lancet* 345:1591–1594, 1995.

58. Hayes J, Dunn E. Has the incidence of primary gastric lymphoma increased? *Cancer* 63:2073–2076, 1989.

59. Severson RK, Davis S. Increasing incidence of primary gastric lymphoma. *Cancer* 66:1283–1287, 1990.

60. Shuder G, Hildebrandt U, Kreissler-Haag B, et al. Role of endosonography in the surgical management of non-Hodgkin's lymphoma of the stomach. *Endoscopy* 24:509–512, 1993.

61. Neubauer A, Thiede C, Morgner A. Cure of *Helicobacter pylori* infection and duration of remission of low-grade gastric MALT lymphoma. *J Natl Cancer Inst* 89:1350–1355, 1997.

62. Rosen CB, Van Heerden JA, Martin JK, et al. Is aggressive surgical approach to the patient with gastric lymphoma warranted? *Ann Surg* 205:634–639, 1987.

63. Shiu MH, Nisce LZ, Pinna A, et al. Recent results of multimodal surgery of gastric lymphoma. *Cancer* 58:1389–1399, 1986.

64. Major MH, Velasquez WS, Fuller LM, Sivermintz KB. Stomach conservation in stages Ie and IIe gastric non-Hodgkins lymphoma. *J Clin Oncol* 8:266–271, 1990.

65. Ludwig DJ, Traverse W. Gut stromal tumors and their clinical behavior. *Am J Surg* 173:390–394, 1997.

15

Colorectal Cancer

■ ■ ■

PAUL F. ENGSTROM

IN THE UNITED STATES, COLORECTAL CANCER accounts for 14% of cancer deaths. It is estimated that in 2000, 130,200 new cases and 56,300 deaths from colorectal cancer will occur [1]. The geographic distribution of colorectal cancer in the United States concentrates in the Mid-Atlantic states, New England, and population centers in the Midwest [1].

Colorectal cancer is predominantly a disease of people 50 years of age and older. The overall 5-year survival is 62% for white men, 62% for white women, 53% for black men, and 52% for black women [2]. The age-adjusted incidence and mortality has decreased over the last 50 years, possibly owing to better detection methods, more accurate diagnosis, and more effective treatment.

The vast majority of patients present with moderately differentiated to well-differentiated adenocarcinoma. Ten to fifteen percent of cases produce sufficient mucin to be categorized as mucinous or colloid adenocarcinomas; only approximately 3% to 5% of lesions are poorly differentiated tumors, which tend to have the worst prognosis [3]. The biological behavior of the moderately differentiated adenocarcinoma is highly unpredictable; however, molecular studies of bowel cancer indicate that when present, mutations in chromosome 18q (the *DCC* gene) confer a higher likelihood of recurrence in patients with stage II carcinoma [4].

Carcinoid tumors of the large bowel are found primarily in the appendix and rectum [5]. Metastasis rarely occurs when the primary tumor is smaller than 2 cm. The management of carcinoid tumor relies primarily on complete resection. Metastatic spread to the liver may cause the carcinoid syndrome, the symptoms of which can be alleviated with the somatostatin analog octreotide, which blocks the serotonin and other vasoactive protein secretion [6]. Anal cancers, which are primarily epidermoid or cloacogenic in type, generally are managed with sphincter-preserving chemoradiotherapy; abdominal-perineal resection and femoral lymph node dissection are reserved for patients with recurrent disease [7].

ETIOLOGY AND PATHOGENESIS

The adenomatous polyp is considered to be the precursor lesion for colon and rectal adenocarcinoma. Adenomatous polyps are premalignant and account for some two-thirds of polyps; hyperplastic polyps, mucosal tags, lipomas, and hamartomas probably have no clinical importance relative to cancer of the bowel. The incidence of colon adenomas increases from 25% at age 50 years to more than 50% by age 80 years [8]. The adenomas are distributed in the bowel in a manner similar to that of cancer, with 50% in the rectosigmoid, 18% in the descending colon, 11% in the transverse colon, and 20% in the ascending colon and cecum. High-grade dysplasia will be found in only 1% of adenomas measuring less than 5 mm but in approximately 20% of adenomas larger than 1 cm [9]. However, few adenomas develop cancer. The rate of transformation is estimated to be 2.5 polyps per 1,000 individuals per year. Estimates based on observational studies and case control studies posit that it takes an average of 10 years for an adenoma of less than 1 cm to transform into an invasive carcinoma [10].

Dietary factors are considered to be responsible for 80% to 90% of all cases of colorectal cancer. Meta-analysis of 13 case-control studies shows an inverse relation of colorectal cancer mortality and high consumption of vegetable or cereal fibers (or both) [11]. In the fat-fiber hypothesis, ingestion of large quantities of vegetables or cereal fibers (or both) increases stool bulk, bacterial fermentation, and large-bowel transit rate. On the other hand, diets high in animal fat and total energy are associated with increased colorectal cancer rates. Some have hypothesized that dietary fat, bile acids, and intestinal bacteria produce increased intraluminal diacylglycerol, an established intracellular cell growth messenger, via protein kinase C activation [12].

A number of micronutrients in the diet have been associated with reduced colorectal cancer mortality. Studies show that calcium binds bile acids and fatty acids and may reduce the exposure to potentially carcinogenic compounds. In short-term feeding studies, calcium supplements in excess of 1,250 mg/day will lower the labeling index in the bowel mucosal cells [13]. Folic acid supplements of up to 400 mg/day and ingested over periods of 10 to 15 years have been shown in case-control studies to produce a 50% reduction in colorectal cancer incidence [14].

Recently, molecular models of carcinogenesis were developed for colon and rectal cancer. The basal cells of the bowel crypts are epithelial stem cells that, when stimulated, overgrow the crypt and give rise to aberrant crypts that ultimately may cause production of adenomatous polyps [15]. Vogelstein et al. [16] postulated that a series of genetic mutations are associated with the progression of the dysplastic polyp to invasive colon carcinoma (Fig. 15.1). These changes include hypomethylation of DNA, K-*ras* mutation on chromosome

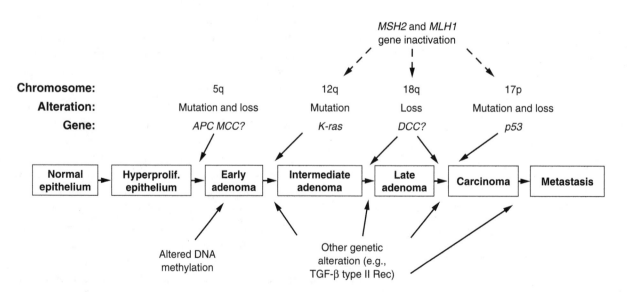

Figure 15.1 Genetic model of colorectal cancer: development of bowel cancer from hyperproliferative epithelium and associated sequential alterations in genes. The mismatch repair gene (*MSH2* and *MLHI*) inactivation accentuates or speeds up mutation accumulation in late stages of carcinogenesis. *TGF-β* = tumor necrosis factor-β; *Rec* = receptor.

12p, *DCC* loss on chromosome 18q, and *p53* loss on chromosome 17p. Specific inherited mutations are permissive or increase the likelihood of colon and rectal cancer. The mutation in the *APC* gene on chromosome 5 in the familial adenomatous polyps (FAP) syndrome results in hundreds of adenomatous polyps, some of which, because of their large number, are virtually guaranteed to result in cancer. Patients with hereditary nonpolyposis colorectal cancer (HNPCC) develop adenomatous polyps at roughly the same rate as that in the general population, but these polyps progress to cancer more often and in shorter time because of defective mismatch repair resulting in an increased mutation rate [17]. In juvenile polyposis syndrome and in ulcerative colitis, stromal proliferation stimulates carcinoma formation. This new understanding of the molecular basis for colon cancer will allow an earlier molecular diagnosis of the disease and a prediction of which individuals in a family may develop colorectal cancer and ultimately will lead to improved treatment and chemoprevention of colorectal cancer [18].

RISK FACTORS

Approximately 75% of all new cases of colorectal cancer occur in people with no known predisposing factors (Fig. 15.2). People with a family history of colorectal

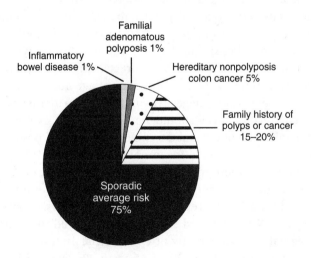

Figure 15.2 Risk factors associated with new cases of colorectal cancer. *IBD* = inflammatory bowel disease; *FAP* = familial adenomatous polyposis; *HNPCC* = hereditary nonpolyposis colon cancer; *FH* = family history of polyps or cancer; *Sporadic* = men and women aged 50 years and older with no special risk factors. (From ST Winawer, D Schottenfeld, J Flehinger, Colorectal Cancer Screening–1991. *J Natl Cancer Inst* 83:243–253, 1991. Reprinted with permission of Oxford University Press.)

cancer but no apparent defined genetic syndrome make up 15% to 20% of the high-risk group. With a family history of polyps or colorectal cancer, the first-degree relatives have a risk two times that of the general population, and the cancer is more likely to occur before age 55 [19]. HNPCC (or Lynch syndrome) may account for 5% to 10% of new cases in the United States [20]. Typically, affected patients' cancer occurs in the fourth and fifth decade and is located predominantly in the right or proximal colon. Adenomatous polyps precede the development of the cancer but do not occur in large numbers. Classic HNPCC is characterized under the Amsterdam Criteria [21] by three or more relatives with colorectal cancer (one of whom is a first-degree relative), one or more members with colorectal cancer diagnosed before 50 years, and cancer in two successive generations. HNPCC is associated with other familial cancers, including cancers that affect the endometrium, ureter, stomach, and small bowel. Cancers from HNPCC carriers can be identified by the presence of microsatellite instability or a replication error phenotype due to mutation in mismatch repair enzymes. The genetic mutations occur in *MLH1, MSH2, PMS1,* and *PMS2,* which are found on chromosomes 2, 3, and 7 [21]. Patients with proved or suspected HNPCC should undergo subtotal colectomy for treatment of adenoma or colorectal cancer. Women should be considered for elective bilateral salpingo-oophorectomy and total abdominal hysterectomy at the time of the bowel resection.

FAP accounts for perhaps 1% of annual new cases of colorectal cancer [22]. FAP is associated with the mutation in the *APC* gene located on the long arm of chromosome 5, which is inherited as an autosomal dominant syndrome. Affected individuals characteristically develop hundreds or even thousands of adenomatous polyps in the colon by age 30 and have a 100% likelihood of developing colorectal cancer by age 40. For this reason, affected individuals should have a total colectomy by age 30 years to reduce their risk of colorectal cancer. Variations of the FAP syndrome include Turcot syndrome (familial colorectal cancer and brain cancer) and Gardner syndrome (familial colorectal cancer, osteomas, and benign soft-tissue tumors or desmoid tumors).

The cancer risk for individual patients with ulcerative colitis or Crohn's disease may approach 30% after 10 years of active inflammatory bowel disease [23]. The pathogenesis of colorectal cancer in inflammatory bowel disease is unknown but probably relates to a breakdown of the normal mucosal barriers to carcinogens, the hyperstimulation of the epithelium and stroma by the inflammatory condition, and the loss of the detoxifying enzymes in the bowel. Patients with long-standing, active inflammatory bowel disease should be considered for a colectomy to prevent single or metach-ronous colon cancers.

PREVENTION OF COLORECTAL CANCER

Enough information has accumulated regarding the re-lationship of diet to colorectal cancer to warrant recom-mending that individuals who eat a typical Western diet—35% to 40% of calories from fat—and ingest low quantities of fresh fruit, vegetables, and dietary fiber would benefit from a reduction in fat consumption to less than 25% calories from fat and an increased intake of 10 g/day of wheat bran or vegetable fiber supplement [24]. The interest in chemoprevention of colorectal can-cer has increased with the understanding that nonste-roidal antiinflammatory drugs with cyclooxygenase (COX) inhibition (such as aspirin and sulindac), includ-ing selective type-2 COX inhibitors (such as Celecoxib), will arrest or inhibit polyp growth in patients with FAP [25]. In the *min*-mouse, which has a mutation of the *APC* gene and, therefore, develops spontaneous adeno-matous polyps and cancers of the large and small bowel, the condition can be reversed by the addition of a cy-clooxygenase type 2 inhibitor or sulindac sulfone, which is an apoptosis inducer [26]. Current clinical tri-als are testing the effectiveness of the cyclooxygenase inhibitors in people with FAP or HNPCC, as well as in people with a history of adenomas but no known ge-netic predisposition. Clinical trials have shown that Celecoxib can reduce adenoma formation in FAP, and Celecoxib has been approved by the Food and Drug Ad-ministration for this indication.

SCREENING

The rationale for colon cancer screening is based on sev-eral recently reported studies. The Minnesota Trial [27] randomly assigned 46,550 people aged 50 to 80 years to a fecal occult blood test (FOBT) annually, an FOBT every other year, or usual care. The 13-year cumulative mortality from colorectal cancer per 1,000 study sub-jects was 5.88 in the annually screened group, 8.33 in the biennially screened group, and 8.83 in the control group. A 33% reduction in colorectal cancer was noted in the group offered annual screening, as compared to those in the control group. The Nottingham, England

Study [28] randomly assigned 150,251 patients, aged 45 to 74 years and registered with general practitioners, to an FOBT every 2 years or to usual care. After 7.8 years of follow-up, those in the screened group exhib-ited a 15% reduction in mortality. The Danish Trial [29] randomly assigned 61,993 people aged 45 to 75 years to an FOBT every 2 years or to usual care. After 10 years, those in the screened group demonstrated an 18% reduction in colorectal cancer mortality. In all the studies, colonoscopy was used to evaluate patients with a positive FOBT. Adenomatous polyps were resected, and the patients with cancer were referred for definitive surgery. In all three trials, the cancers diagnosed in the screened group were earlier-stage lesions as compared to those in the control group.

Although flexible sigmoidoscopy or screening colon-oscopy has not been studied in a randomized, con-trolled fashion, case-control studies show that sigmoid-oscopy is associated with a 60% to 80% reduction in mortality from rectosigmoid carcinoma in patients who have had one or more studies in their lifetime [30]. Indirect evidence suggests that people who have undergone colonoscopy with polypectomy have a 40% to 50% reduction in colorectal cancer incidence [10]. Therefore, the American Cancer Society [31] and the American Gastroenterological Association [10] recom-mend that asymptomatic people at average risk and 50 years and older participate in fecal occult blood screen-ing annually. Flexible sigmoidoscopy should be per-formed every 5 years; all polyps smaller than 1 cm should undergo biopsy, and polyps larger than 1 cm should be removed colonoscopically or surgically. People with a family history of polyps or colorectal cancer should be-gin screening by total colonoscopy at age 40.

For a history suggestive of HNPCC, patients with a colorectal cancer should have the tumor evaluated for microsatellite instability phenotype and, if positive, should be considered for mutation testing for *MSH2* or *MLH1* after appropriate genetic counseling [32]. HNPCC family members should have colonoscopy beginning at age 20 to 25 years repeated every 1 to 2 years. Women in an HNPCC kindred should be considered for trans-vaginal ultrasonography or endometrial aspirate annu-ally beginning at age 25 to 35 years. Patients with an HNPCC history and presenting with an adenoma or ad-enocarcinoma should undergo a subtotal colectomy with ileorectal anastomosis.

Individuals with a history of FAP should be screened for polyps beginning at age 15 to 20 years [22]. Patients with the full syndrome should have a colectomy by age 25 years to reduce the likelihood of invasive cancer.

Presymptomatic individuals with a positive history of FAP should be considered for *APC* genetic testing. *APC*-positive individuals should undergo flexible sigmoidoscopy every 12 months beginning at puberty. *APC*-negative individuals should undergo flexible sigmoidoscopy once at age 25 and, if results are negative, routine screening should begin at age 50.

STAGING AND THERAPY FOR COLORECTAL CANCER

The staging criteria for bowel cancer depend on the pathologic examination of a completely resected colon or rectal cancer. The TNM (primary *t*umor, *n*odal involvement, and distant *m*etastasis) system has replaced the Duke's system and its Astler-Coller modification (Table 15.1) [33]. Staging is based on the natural history of the tumor, which usually starts as a polyp with in situ carcinoma and invades into the wall of the bowel (submucosa to the muscularis propria to the subserosa to the nonperitonealized pericolic or perirectal tissues to adjacent organs or structures). Generally, metastasis is to the regional lymph nodes or via the bloodstream to such distant organs as the liver, lung, bone, or brain. Because the prognosis deteriorates with advancing stage, management of colorectal cancer is based on stage of disease and performance status of affected patients.

The symptoms of colon and rectal cancer will vary depending on the area of the bowel affected by the primary tumor. Frequently, cancers arising in the left or descending colon present with symptoms of obstruction. Pain, if it is present, is colicky and made worse by ingestion of food. Usually, bleeding is intermittent and may be occult or can appear as red blood mixed with the stool. Over time, obstruction may occur and results in bouts of diarrheal stool. Cancer of the right or ascending colon is characterized by ill-defined pain located in the right midabdomen and occult bleeding contributing to chronic anemia and fatigue; obstruction occurs late in the course of the disease and is associated with tumors near or involving the ileocecal valve. Patients with cancer of the rectum may complain of tenesmus, which is caused by tumor infiltration of the stretch receptors. Bleeding causes bright red coating of the stool and all too often is mistaken for hemorrhoidal bleeding. Complete obstruction due to cancer in the rectum is rare.

Surgical Therapy

The primary therapy for colorectal cancer remains surgical [34, 35]. Adenomatous polyps with in situ or low-grade adenocarcinoma can be treated with polypectomy only if the margins indicate all cancer was resected completely. Cancerous polyps that are fragmented at polypectomy or have positive resection margins require laparotomy and sleeve resection of the colon. Invasive colon cancer should be treated with a wide surgical resection. The right colectomy, transverse colectomy, and

Table 15.1 Colorectal Cancer Stage Classification and Grouping

Pathologic Description	AJCC (1997)	Astler-Coller Modification Duke's Stage
Carcinoma in situ	Stage 0: Tis, N0, M0	Stage 0
Tumor invades submucosa	Stage 1: T1, N0, M0	Stage I-A
Tumor invades muscularis propria	Stage I: T2, N0, M0	Stage I-B1
Tumor invades through muscularis propria into subserosa or nonperitonealized perirectal tissues	Stage II: T3, N0, M0	Stage II-B2
Tumor directly invades other organs or structures or perforates visceral peritoneum (or both)	Stage II: T4, N0, M0	Stage II-B3
Any degree of bowel wall invasion with regional node metastasis, without distant metastasis	Stage III: any T, N1–3, M0	Stage III-C1, C2
Any degree of bowel wall invasion with or without nodal metastasis but with any distant metastasis	Stage IV: any T, any N, M1	Stage IV-D

Source: Used with the permission of the *American Joint Committee on Cancer (AJCC®)*, Chicago. AJCC® *Cancer Staging Manual* (5th Edition), 1997. Philadelphia: Lippincott-Raven.

left hemicolectomy are defined anatomically by the ileocolic, middle colic, and left colic vessels (Figs. 15.3–15.5) [35]. En bloc removal of regional lymph nodes is necessary to facilitate pathologic review of the pericolonic and, especially, perirectal soft tissue. At the time of laparotomy, the surgeon should visualize, palpate and, where appropriate, use intraoperative ultrasonic evaluation to determine the extent of spread, especially to the liver. Laparoscopy-assisted colon resection is being investigated to determine safety and efficacy. Unless an affected patient is participating in a clinical trial, laparoscopy-assisted resection should not be used routinely for treating invasive colon cancer [36]. Patients with T1 and T2 adenocarcinoma of the middle or distal rectum may be cured with transanal, transcoccygeal, or transsacral resections or low anterior resection with coloanal reanastomosis, thereby avoiding abdominal perineal resection with descending colostomy. Generally, patients with tumors in the rectosigmoid colon are managed with a low anterior resection, thus avoiding a colostomy. All patients with stage III lesions are candidates for adjuvant chemotherapy or radiotherapy treatment (or both).

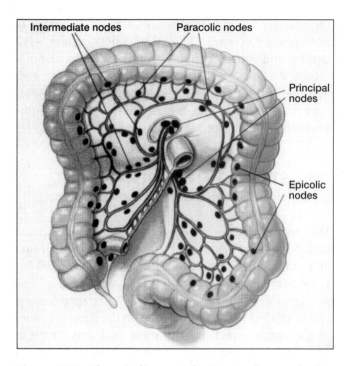

Figure 15.3   The epicolic, paracolic, intermediate, and principal lymph node groups accompanying the vessels of the colon. (Reprinted with permission of Lippincott from RS Grinnel, Lymphatic metastases of carcinoma of the colon and rectum. *Ann Surg Oncol* 131:494–506, 1950.)

Radiotherapy

Radiotherapy plays a major role in the management of rectal carcinoma. Because recurrence after rectal surgery may be to local and regional lymph nodes, postoperative radiotherapy can reduce pelvic failure significantly. Irradiation toxicity can be minimized by excluding small bowel from the pelvis (retroperitonealized pelvic floor), treating the patient prone with the bladder distended, and using small doses per fraction. The advantage of postoperative radiotherapy is that it does not delay surgery and is given after the extent of disease is defined, thus sparing patients with stage I or stage IV disease [37]. Many radiotherapists advocate preoperative irradiation because it may increase resectability, may enhance the antitumor effect because tissues are well vascularized and oxygenated, may reduce toxicity because the small bowel is mobile, and theoretically can decrease implantation of viable cancer cells during surgical manipulation [38]. Mounting evidence suggests that fluorouracil-based adjuvant chemotherapy can improve the outcome when used as a component of a multimodality approach to curative treatment of stage II and stage III rectal carcinoma [39]. However, the optimal sequence of surgery, irradiation, and chemotherapy is not known and is the subject of ongoing clinical trials.

Chemotherapy

5-Fluorouracil (5-FU) is the time-tested agent for systemic chemotherapy for recurrent or metastatic colon cancer. However, the objective response to 5-FU is 15% to 20%, with only the responding patients showing a median survival benefit of 12 to 18 months [40]. The therapeutic effect of 5-FU can be enhanced by administering the drug by continuous infusion or by combining 5-FU with leucovorin (LV). Patients with metastatic disease limited to the liver have been palliated successfully with hepatic artery continuous infusion of fluorodeoxyuridine [41]. However, hepatic artery infusion therapy requires a laparotomy and implanted pump, may cause biliary sclerosis, and has not shown survival superiority over intravenous fluorodeoxyuridine therapy. Irinotecan (Camptosar) is approved for the treatment of patients with progressive metastatic disease for which 5-FU-based therapy has failed [42] and as initial therapy for metastatic disease in combination with 5-FU and LV. In patients with stage III colon cancer, 5-FU plus LV or 5-FU plus levamisole as adjuvant treatment is recommended. Large, multicenter clinical trials show a 20% improvement in disease-free survival in patients

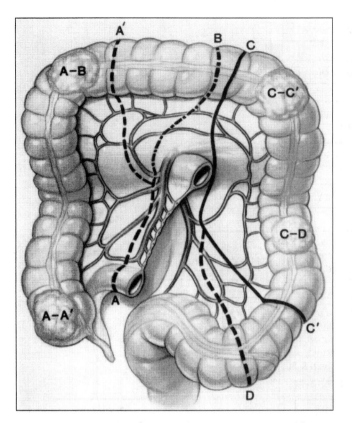

Figure 15.4 Segments of bowel and lymph node containing mesentery to be removed for carcinoma of the cecum (A-A′), hepatic flexure (A-B), splenic flexure (C-C′), and descending colon (C-D). (From G Steele Jr, RT Osteen, Surgical treatment of colon cancer. In G Steele Jr, RT Osteen [eds], *Colorectal Cancer: Current Concepts in Diagnosis and Treatment*. New York: Marcel Dekker, 1986:127–162. Reprinted by courtesy of Marcel Dekker, Inc.)

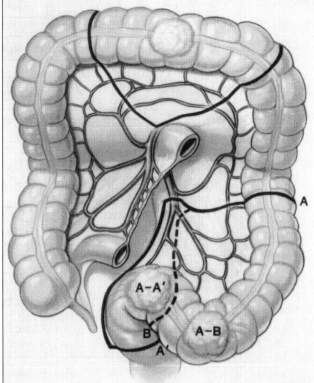

Figure 15.5 Segments of bowel and lymph node containing mesentery to be removed for carcinoma of the transverse colon, the apex of the sigmoid (A-B), and the lower sigmoid or rectosigmoid (A-A′). (From G Steele Jr, RT Osteen, Surgical treatment of colon cancer. In G Steele Jr, RT Osteen [eds], *Colorectal Cancer: Current Concepts in Diagnosis and Treatment*. New York: Marcel Dekker, 1986:127–162. Reprinted by courtesy of Marcel Dekker, Inc.)

who receive surgery plus chemotherapy as compared to surgery alone [43].

Several new agents, some with novel mechanisms of action, show promising activity in colorectal cancer [42]. In combination with 5-FU and LV, trimetrexate has produced encouraging response rates in phase II studies. Oxaliplatin, a third-generation platinum complex, appears to have synergistic effects when combined with 5-FU in treating patients who have 5-FU-resistant tumors. Capecitabine and UFT (a combination of uracil and tegafur) are orally active pro-drugs of 5-FU that may prove to have a clinical spectrum of activity similar to 5-FU but with the advantage of oral administration and prolonged continuous effect on liver metastasis. The biological agent 17–1A monoclonal antibody specifically binds to cell-surface glycoproteins that are expressed preferentially on adenocarcinomas. In randomized trials in Europe, the 17–1A monoclonal antibody

increased the survival of patients with stage III disease, as compared to survival with surgery only.

MANAGEMENT GUIDELINES FOR COLORECTAL CANCER

The management guidelines discussed here are based on deliberation by an expert panel assembled by the National Comprehensive Cancer Network of Comprehensive Cancer Centers and have been disseminated for use by physicians who treat colorectal cancer [44]. As part of the initial workup of colon cancer patients, a thorough history should note weight loss, anemia, obstruction symptoms, change in bowel size and frequency of movements, blood loss, and family history of colorectal cancer (Fig. 15.6). The physical examination should include a careful rectal examination for mass or evidence

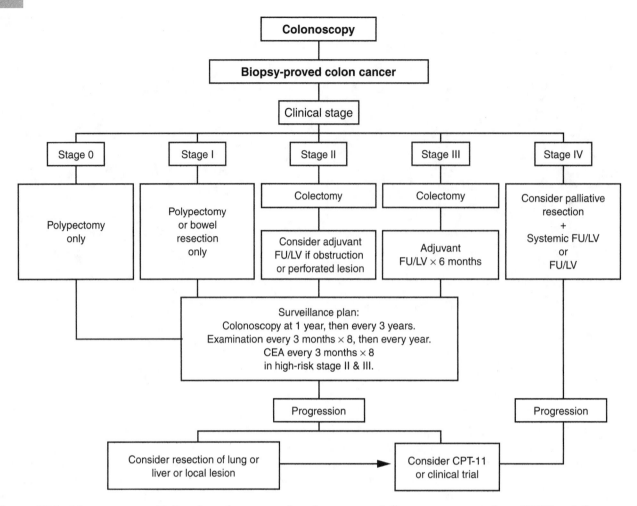

Figure 15.6 Management guideline for colon cancer based on stage of disease at presentation. *FU/LV* = 5-fluorouracil-leucovorin; *CEA* = carcinoembryonic antigen; *CPT-11* = irinotecan.

of blood loss in the stool, adenopathy in the neck, and enlarged liver. All patients should have a full colonoscopy or a flexible sigmoidoscopy and barium enema. Minimum laboratory studies include a complete blood cell count, liver function studies, a baseline carcinoembryonic antigen (CEA) level, a chest roentgenogram and, if clinically indicated, a computed tomographic scan of the abdomen and pelvis.

The initial treatment is based on clinical findings. Patients with an adenomatous polyp or villous adenoma with cancer at polypectomy should undergo full colonoscopy if it has not been performed already. The specimen should be reviewed for evidence that the polyp was resected completely because, if it is fragmented, colectomy is recommended. Ulcerating and invasive cancer on endoscopic biopsy should be treated with colectomy and en bloc removal of regional lymph nodes. Patients who present with an obstructed or perforated lesion may require a diverting colostomy with subse-

quent resection of the tumor. In patients who present with suspected or biopsy-proved liver metastasis, palliative resection of the primary tumor and, if possible, resection of a solitary liver metastasis should be accomplished at laparotomy.

Adjuvant therapy for colon cancer depends on the tumor's pathologic stage at the time of resection. Patients with stage 0 or stage I disease require no adjuvant therapy. Patients who have stage II (T3N0M0) disease and present with obstruction or perforation may benefit from 6 months of 5-FU/LV chemotherapy. All patients with stage III disease are advised to receive adjuvant chemotherapy using 5-FU/LV for 6 months or 5-FU/levamisole for 12 months [45]. Patients who have stage IV disease may be palliated with 5-FU/LV chemotherapy. If one to three small liver metastases are noted, hepatic resection followed by adjuvant 5-FU/LV chemotherapy should be considered. If patients have multiple unresectable liver metastases and the primary bowel lesion

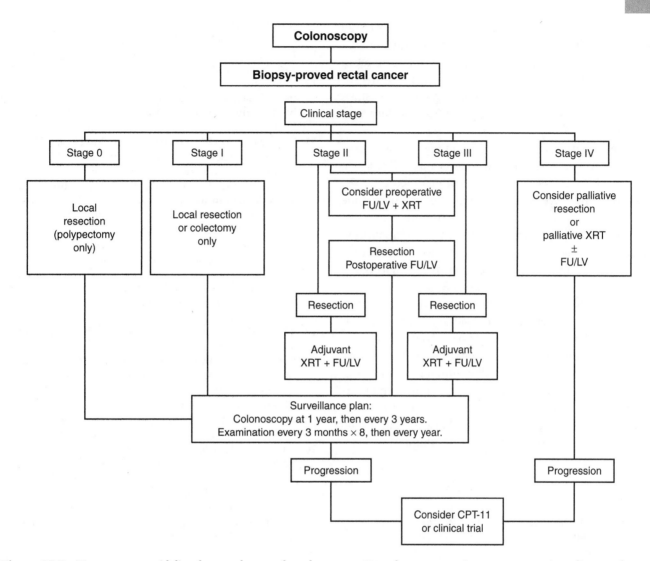

Figure 15.7 Management guideline for rectal cancer based on stage. Note that preoperative or postoperative adjuvant chemoradiotherapy should be considered for stage II or stage III disease. *FU/LV* = 5-fluorouracil-leucovorin; *XRT* = radiotherapy; *CPT-11* = irinotecan.

has been removed, continuous intrahepatic artery infusion therapy with fluorodeoxyuridine can be considered [41]. Depending on the extent of disease and the performance status of the patient, clinical trial or observation with symptomatic management may be appropriate for stage IV disease.

The National Comprehensive Cancer Network guidelines recommend the following monitoring surveillance program in patients who have had definitive therapy of stage 0, stage I, stage II, or stage III cancers. Clinicians should perform a physical examination, including digital rectal examination and a stool analysis for occult blood, every 3 months for 2 years, then every 6 months until 5 years, and then annually. Colonoscopy should be performed at 1 year and should be repeated annually

if results are abnormal or every 3 to 5 years if the examination results are normal. The use of CEA as a follow-up test should be considered, particularly if the CEA level was elevated preoperatively and if the patient is a candidate for aggressive resection of metastatic lesions [46]. In this situation, the CEA test should be repeated every 3 months for 2 years.

Patients who develop recurrent or metastatic cancer after successful treatment of the primary cancer should be considered for aggressive treatment with surgical resection in the presence of an isolated lesion in the liver, lung, or ovaries [47]. Generally, patients who develop bowel obstruction will benefit from bypass surgery. Patients with widespread recurrence in liver, lung, or abdomen may be considered for palliative chemotherapy.

In the absence of prior chemotherapy, 5-FU/LV should be considered. If patients have progressed on 5-FU/LV therapy, they should be considered for irinotecan second-line treatment or should participate in investigational protocol therapy. Patients with bone metastasis or local pelvic metastasis may benefit from palliative radiotherapy.

Patients with rectal cancer are managed in a fashion similar to that for patients with colon cancer (Fig. 15.7). If a superficial rectal polypoid carcinoma measures less than 3 cm and is well differentiated, the options include full-thickness rectal resection by the transanal or transcoccygeal route, endocavitary irradiation, or fulguration in highly selected cases [36]. In patients with invasive carcinoma of more than 6 cm from the anal verge, a low anterior resection with a 2- to 3-cm distal margin is recommended. Patients who have suspected cancer adherent to or invasion of the bladder, prostate, presacrum, or pelvic side walls should be considered for preoperative chemotherapy and radiotherapy to decrease tumor volume so as to allow abdominal perineal resection followed by further radiotherapy and chemotherapy [39]. Adjuvant therapy for rectal cancer is used for all patients with stage II and stage III disease and should include radiotherapy plus 5-FU chemotherapy.

REFERENCES

1. Greenlee RT, Murray T, Bolden S, Wingo PA. Cancer statistics, 2000. *CA Cancer J Clin* 50:7–33, 2000.
2. SEER. *Cancer Statistics Review, 1973–1997.* Bethesda, MD: National Cancer Institute, National Institutes of Health, 1998.
3. Cooper, HS, Slemmer JR. Surgical pathology of carcinoma of colon and rectum. *Semin Oncol* 18:367–380, 1991.
4. Jen J, Kim H, Piantadosi S, et al. Allelic loss of chromosome 18q and prognosis in colorectal cancer. *N Engl J Med* 331:213–221, 1994.
5. Kulke MH, Mayer RJ. Medical progress: carcinoid tumors. *N Engl J Med* 340:858–868, 1999.
6. Kvols LK, Moertel CG, O'Connell MJ, et al. Treatment of the malignant carcinoid syndrome: evaluation of a long-acting somatostatin analog. *N Engl J Med* 315:663–666, 1986.
7. Cummings BJ. The role of radiation therapy with 5-fluorouracil in anal canal cancer. *Semin Radiat Oncol* 7:306–312, 1997.
8. Williams AR, Balasooriya BAW, Day DW. Polyps and cancer of the large bowel: a new necropsy study in Liverpool. *Gut* 123:835–842, 1982.
9. O'Brien MS, Winawer SJ, Zauber AG, et al. The National Polyp Study: patient and polyp characteristics associated with high-grade dysplasia in colorectal adenomas. *Gastroenterology* 98:371–379, 1990.
10. Winawer SJ, Fletcher RH, Miller L, et al. Colorectal cancer screening: clinical guidelines and rationale. *Gastroenterology* 112:594–642, 1997.
11. Potter JD. Colorectal cancer: molecules and populations. *J Natl Cancer Inst* 91:916–932, 1999.
12. Morotomi M, Guillem J, Logerfo P, Weinstein IB. Production of diacylglycerol an activator of protein kinase C, by human intestinal microflora. *Cancer Res* 50:3595–3599, 1990.
13. Buset M, Lipkin M, Winawer S, et al. Inhibition of human colonic epithelial cell proliferation in vivo and in vitro by calcium. *Cancer Res* 46:5426–5430, 1986.
14. Giovannucci E, Stampfer MJ, Colditz GA, Hunter DJ, et al. Multivitamin use, folate, and colon cancer in women in the Nurses' Health Study. *Ann Intern Med* 129:517–524, 1998.
15. Pretlow TP, Banow BJ, Ashton WS, et al. Aberrant crypts: putative preneoplastic foci in human colonic mucosa. *Cancer Res* 51:1564–1567, 1991.
16. Vogelstein B, Fearon ER, Hamilton SR, et al. Genetic alterations during colorectal tumor development. *N Engl J Med* 319:525–532, 1988.
17. Kinzler KW, Vogelstein B. Landscaping the cancer terrain. *Science* 280:1036–1037, 1998.
18. Garay CA, Engstrom PF. Chemoprevention of colorectal cancer: dietary and pharmacologic approaches. *Oncology* 13:89–98, 1999.
19. Ahsan H, Neugut AI, Garbowski GC, et al. Family history of colorectal adenomatous polyps and increased risk for colorectal cancer. *Ann Intern Med* 128:900–905, 1998.
20. Aaltonen LA, Salovaana R, Kristo P, et al. Incidence of hereditary nonpolyposis colorectal cancer and the feasibility of molecular screening for the disease. *N Engl J Med* 338:1481–1487, 1998.
21. Wignen JT, Vasen HFA, Khan PM, et al. Clinical findings with implications for genetic testing in families with clustering of colorectal cancer. *N Engl J Med* 339:511–518, 1998.
22. Giardiello FM, Brensinger JD, Petersen GM, et al. Use and interpretation of commercial APC gene testing for familial adenomatous polyposis. *N Engl J Med* 336:823–827, 1997.
23. Lennard-Jones JE. Prevention of cancer mortality in inflammatory bowel disease. In Young GP, Rozen P, Levin B (eds), *Prevention and Early Detection of Colorectal Cancer.* London: Saunders, 1996:217–238.
24. Vargas PA, Alberts DS. Primary prevention of colorectal cancer through dietary modification. *Cancer* 70:1229–1235, 1992.
25. Waddell WR, Gariser GF, Cerise EJ, Loughry RW. Sulindac for polyposis of the colon. *Am J Surg* 157:175–178, 1989.
26. Subbaramaiah K, Zakin D, Weksler BB, Dannenberg AJ. Inhibition of cyclooxygenase: a novel approach to cancer prevention. *Proc Soc Exp Biol Med* 216:201–210, 1997.
27. Mandel JS, Church TR, Ederer F, Bond JH. Colorectal cancer mortality: effectiveness of biennial screening for fecal occult blood. *J Natl Cancer Inst* 91:434–437, 1999.
28. Handcastle JD, Chamberlain JO, Robinson MH, et al. Randomized controlled trial of fecal occult blood screening for colorectal cancer. *Lancet* 348:1472–1477, 1996.
29. Kronberg O, Fenger C, Olsen J, et al. Randomized study of screening for colorectal cancer with fecal-occult blood test. *Lancet* 348:1467–1471, 1996.

30. Selby JV, Friedman GD, Quisenberry CP, et al. A case control study of screening sigmoidoscopy and mortality from colorectal cancer. *N Engl J Med* 326:653–657, 1992.

31. Byers T, Levin B, Rothenberger D, et al. American Cancer Society guidelines for screening and surveillance for early detection of colorectal polyps and cancer: update 1997. *CA Cancer J Clin* 47:154–160, 1997.

32. Burke W, Petersen G, Lynch P, et al. Recommendations for follow-up care of individuals with an inherited predisposition to cancer: hereditary nonpolyposis colon cancer. *JAMA* 277:915–919, 1997.

33. American Joint Committee on Cancer. Colon and rectum. In Fleming ID, Cooper JS, Henson DE, et al. (eds), *AJCC Cancer Staging Manual* (5th ed). Philadelphia: Lippincott-Raven, 1997:83–90.

34. Steele G Jr, Osteen RT. Surgical treatment of colon cancer. In Steele G Jr, Osteen RT (eds), *Colorectal Cancer: Current Concepts in Diagnosis and Treatment*. New York: Marcel Dekker, 1986:127–162.

35. Zaheer S, Pemberton JH, Farouk R, et al. Surgical treatment of adenocarcinoma of the rectum. *Ann Surg* 227:800–811, 1998.

36. Fleshman JW, Nelson H, Peters WR, et al. Early results of laparoscopic surgery for colorectal cancer: retrospective analysis of 372 patients treated by clinical outcomes of surgical therapy (COST) study group. *Dis Colon Rectum* 10:S53–S58, 1996.

37. Medical Research Council Rectal Cancer Working Party. Randomized trial of surgery alone versus surgery followed by radiotherapy for mobile cancer of the rectum. *Lancet* 348:1610–1614, 1996.

38. Swedish Rectal Cancer Trial. Improved survival with preoperative radiotherapy in resectable rectal cancer. *N Engl J Med* 336:980–987, 1997.

39. O'Connell MS, Martensen JA, Wiland HS, et al. Improving adjuvant therapy for rectal cancer by combining protracted-infusion fluorouracil with radiation therapy after curative surgery. *N Engl J Med* 331:502–507, 1994.

40. Moertel CG. Chemotherapy for colorectal cancer. *N Engl J Med* 330:1136–1142, 1994.

41. Meta-Analysis Group in Cancer. Reappraisal of hepatic arterial infusion in the treatment of non-resectable liver metastases from colorectal cancer. *J Natl Cancer Inst* 88:252–258, 1996.

42. Punt CJA. New drugs in the treatment of colorectal carcinoma. *Cancer* 83:679–689, 1998.

43. Moertel CG, Fleming TR, Macdonald JS, et al. Fluorouracil + levamisole as effective adjuvant therapy after resection of stage III colon carcinoma—a final report. *Ann Intern Med* 122:321–326, 1995.

44. Engstrom PF, Benson AB, Cohen A, et al. NCCN colorectal cancer practice guidelines. *Oncology* 10(suppl 11):140–175, 1996.

45. Haller DG, Catalano, PJ, MacDonald JS, Mayer RJ. Fluorouracil, leucovorin and levamisole adjuvant therapy for colon cancer: five-year final report of INT–0089. *Am Soc Clin Oncol Prog Proc* 17:256a, 1998.

46. American Society of Clinical Oncology. Clinical practice guidelines for the use of tumor markers in breast and colorectal cancer. *J Clin Oncol* 14:2843–2877, 1996.

47. Goldberg RM, Fleming TR, Tangen CM, et al. Surgery for recurrent colon cancer: strategies for identifying resectable recurrence and success rates after resection. *Ann Intern Med* 129:27–35, 1998.

16

Tumors of the Pancreas, Gallbladder, and Bile Ducts

■ ■ ■

PHILIP N. REDLICH
STEVEN A. AHRENDT
HENRY A. PITT

PANCREATIC CANCER

Tumors of the Exocrine Pancreas

Cancer of the exocrine pancreas is a common neoplasm of the gastrointestinal tract, second in incidence only to colorectal carcinoma. An estimated 28,300 new cases of pancreatic cancer will occur in 2000, resulting in a similar number of deaths and representing nearly 22% of all deaths due to cancer of the digestive system [1]. Overall, pancreatic cancer is the fourth leading cause of cancer death in both men and women [1].

The ability to diagnosis this disease and to improve cure rates is hindered by the retroperitoneal location of the pancreas and the usual late presentation in the course of the disease. Nevertheless, improvements in outcome have been achieved over the last decade, primarily on the basis of improved imaging, operative techniques, and overall patient management. Practice guidelines for the diagnosis and management of pancreatic cancer have been developed by a multidisciplinary committee composed of physicians from member institutions of the National Comprehensive Cancer Network (NCCN). These guidelines can be accessed through the NCCN Web site at www.nccn.org.

BIOLOGICAL FEATURES

Though the etiology of pancreatic cancer is unknown, much has been written about risk factors and genetic alterations pertaining to this disease. The incidence of pancreatic cancer increases steadily with age; the majority of cases occur between ages 60 and 80 years. In the United States, a difference exists with respect to race, with higher incidence rates and mortality in blacks of both genders as compared to their white counterparts [2]. Pancreatic cancer occurs more frequently in men than in women, but the incidence and mortality rates have decreased in men while they have increased in women over the last 20 years. Other risk factors associated with pancreatic cancer include Jewish origin, lower socioeconomic status, and habitation of industrialized societies.

Various identified host and environmental factors have been associated with an increased risk for pancreatic cancer. An association between diabetes and pancreatic cancer has been described, though the finding is not consistent [2]. An association between chronic pancreatitis and pancreatic cancer is suspected, though a precise relationship thus far has not been identified. An increased incidence of pancreatic cancer in patients with pernicious anemia has been reported. Cigarette smoking is considered a risk factor for pancreatic cancer on the basis of a number of case-control studies. Furthermore, pancreatic cancer can be induced in animals by the long-term administration of tobacco-specific carcinogens [3]. Dietary factors have been studied, but no consistent relationships have been demonstrated. Many clinical studies have suggested an elevated risk with increased carbohydrate or meat intake and a decreased risk with intake of fiber, fruit, or vegetables. Studies of the relationship of coffee ingestion to pancreatic cancer have not demonstrated consistent findings, suggesting that a relationship between coffee and pancreatic cancer is either nonexistent or very weak. A number of occupations have been linked to pancreatic cancer, affecting such people as chemists and coal gas workers, those in the metal, leather-tanning, and textile industries, and those chronically exposed to dichlorodiphenyltrichloroethane (known commonly as *DDT*).

MOLECULAR PATHOGENESIS

Like other malignancies, pancreatic cancer is a disease of inherited and acquired genetic mutations [4]. It is associated with multiple tumor suppressor genes and the activation of an oncogene, *K-ras*. Evidence for genetic alterations in pancreatic cancer have been obtained from karyotyping, comparative genomic hybridization, and allelotyping (Table 16.1) [4]. These studies have identified high frequencies of loss of chromosomal arms 1p, 9p (*p16*), 17p (*p53*), and 18q (*DPC4*). A number of known tumor suppressor genes located at these chromosomal sites have been identified as inactivated or mutated in pancreatic cancer. Specifically, the *p53* tumor suppressor gene, located on chromosomal arm 17p, is inactivated in 50% to 75% of pancreatic carcinomas. This inactivation leads to loss of important controls of cell growth involved in the regulation of proliferation and induction of cell death (apoptosis). The *p16* (or

MTS1) tumor suppressor gene located on chromosomal arm 9p is inactivated in up to 90% of pancreatic cancers. The *p16* gene product plays an important role in the control of the cell cycle, and its loss suggests that regulation of the cell is compromised. The *DPC4* tumor suppressor gene, residing on chromosomal arm 18q, is inactivated in approximately 50% of pancreatic cancers. *DPC4* may play a role in signal transduction. In contrast to the *p53* and *p16* genes, *DPC4* may be relatively specific to pancreatic cancer. Co-inactivation of different tumor suppressor genes has been observed at the time of resection, demonstrating the accumulation of numerous mutations in the same cancer by the time of diagnosis.

The *K-ras* oncogene is the gene mutated most commonly in pancreatic cancer. Point mutations in *K-ras* impair gene function, resulting in a protein that is constitutively activated in signal transduction. From 80% to 100% of pancreatic cancers have been reported to have *K-ras* point mutations, most commonly in codon 12. Detecting *K-ras* mutations in clinical samples is relatively easy (e.g., the identification of mutant *K-ras* in stool samples of patients with pancreatic cancer) [5]. The potential for gene-based testing for pancreatic cancer has been raised by such findings, but further study is required.

Several familial genetic syndromes that have been identified are associated with an increased risk of pancreatic cancer (see Table 16.1). Hereditary nonpolyposis colorectal cancer is caused by germline mutations in one of the DNA mismatch repair genes. The development of pancreatic cancer in several kindreds with hereditary nonpolyposis colorectal cancer has been re-

Table 16.1 Genetic Alterations and Related Syndromes Associated with Pancreatic Cancer

Sporadic alterations
  Oncogenes
    K-ras
  Tumor suppressor genes
    p53
    p16
    DPC4
    BRCA2

Familial syndromes
  Hereditary nonpolyposis colon cancer (HNPCC)
  Breast cancer (*BRCA2* gene)
  Hereditary pancreatitis
  Ataxia-telangiectasia
  Peutz-Jeghers syndrome
  Familial atypical multiple mole–melanoma syndrome
    (FAMMM)

Table 16.2 Characteristics of Solid Nonendocrine Neoplasms of the Pancreas

Neoplasm	Peak Incidence	Characteristics and Comments
Ductal adenocarcinoma	Seventh decade	Most common neoplasm; male predominance; 60% arising in head; metastasizes widely
Adenosquamous carcinoma	Seventh decade	Rare variant of ductal adenocarcinoma; history of prior chemotherapy or radiotherapy; relatively poor prognosis
Acinar-cell carcinoma	Elderly; rare reports in children	One percent of pancreatic malignancies; lipase release; equal distribution throughout pancreas
Giant-cell carcinoma	Seventh decade	Five percent of pancreatic malignancies; equal frequency throughout the pancreas; poor prognosis
Pancreatoblastoma	First, second decades	Rare; prognosis better than for infiltrating ductal carcinoma

ported. However, defective mismatch repair is present in only 2% to 3% of pancreatic cancers. Germline mutations of *BRCA2*, associated with an increased risk of breast and ovarian cancer, are associated also with the development of pancreatic cancer. Germline mutations in the *BRCA2* gene may be responsible for a small but significant fraction of all pancreatic cancers, and a strong family history of breast or ovarian cancer may be absent. Increased risk of pancreatic cancer has been identified in such other syndromes as Peutz-Jeghers, ataxia-telangiectasia, and familial atypical multiple mole–melanoma syndromes. Individuals with hereditary pancreatitis, a rare disease, also are at an increased risk for developing pancreatic cancer.

Cases of familial pancreatic cancer (two or more first-degree relatives with pancreatic cancer) occur outside of the known genetic syndromes, suggesting a genetic basis for this disease. In many such cases, the genetic basis of the inherited susceptibility to pancreatic cancer remains unknown. A further understanding of the genetic basis of the disease may lead to gene-based screening tests and novel therapies.

PATHOLOGIC FEATURES

Pancreatic malignancies can be subclassified by histologic type into epithelial tumors (carcinomas) and mesenchymal tumors (sarcomas); a further subdivision divides the epithelial neoplasms into solid and cystic tumors. The most common primary malignancy of the exocrine pancreas is ductal adenocarcinoma, which accounts for nearly 95% of pancreatic primary malignancies (Table 16.2) [6]. Sixty percent of ductal adenocarcinomas arise in the head of the pancreas, and the remainder originate in the body and tail or diffusely involve the entire gland. Microscopy reveals infiltrating glands surrounded by dense reactive fibrous tissue. Sites of metastases include the liver, peritoneum, lungs, pleura, and adrenal glands. Precursor ductal lesions have been identified and are termed *pancreatic intraepithelial neoplasia*. Several lines of evidence suggest that these ductal lesions progress to infiltrating ductal adenocarcinoma [7]. Less common solid neoplasms include adenosquamous carcinoma, acinar cell carcinoma, giant-cell carcinoma, and pancreatoblastoma.

Cystic neoplasms of the pancreas should be distinguished from their solid counterparts because of their different behavior and outcome (Table 16.3). Serous cystoadenomas are more common in women than in men. Often, affected patients present in the seventh decade of life with abdominal pain, weight loss, and a palpable mass. Most serous cystic neoplasms are benign, but malignant behavior (serous cystadenocarcinoma) has been reported. In contrast, mucinous cystic neoplasms demonstrate malignant potential and must be treated differently from serous lesions. Mucinous cystic neoplasms are more common in women, with the mean age of diagnosis in the fifth decade. Complete resection is required for treatment, and the expected five-year survival is 40% to 50%, markedly different from that of infiltrating ductal adenocarcinoma. Other less common cystic neoplasms include intraductal papillary-mucinous and solid and cystic papillary neoplasms.

Mesenchymal tumors are extremely rare and consist of such tumors as schwannoma, leiomyosarcoma, liposarcoma, and malignant fibrous histiocytoma. The pancreas can be a site also for metastatic disease and for involvement by leukemia and lymphoma.

Table 16.3   Characteristics of Cystic Neoplasms of the Pancreas

Neoplasm	Peak Incidence	Characteristics and Comments
Serous cystic neoplasm	Seventh decade	Female predominance; most benign; few reports of malignant behavior
Mucinous cystic neoplasm	Fifth, sixth decades	Female predominance; malignant potential; complete resection recommended; good prognosis
Intraductal papillary-mucinous neoplasm	Seventh decade	Equal frequency in both genders; communication with pancreatic duct
Solid and cystic papillary neoplasm	Third decade	Female predominance; complete resection recommended

DIAGNOSIS AND STAGING

Often, the clinical diagnosis of pancreatic cancer is made late in the course of the disease. The most common signs of this disease include jaundice (which may be present in up to 50% of affected patients), weight loss, and abdominal pain. Jaundice may occur early if the tumor is located adjacent to the common duct, leading to obstruction while the tumor is small. Pain may be due to tumor invasion of the celiac or mesenteric plexus. Secondary signs of pancreatic cancer include anorexia, pruritus, alterations in bowel habits (e.g., steatorrhea due to exocrine insufficiency from obstruction of the pancreatic duct), thrombophlebitis, and depression. Glucose intolerance is present in most patients with pancreatic cancer.

Except for jaundice, the signs and symptoms of pancreatic cancer are nonspecific and require a heightened awareness by clinicians so that appropriate diagnostic tests are undertaken. The location of the tumor has an influence on signs and symptoms. As noted, a tumor involving the head of the pancreas may cause obstruction of the pancreatic and common bile ducts, potentially leading to an earlier diagnosis. A tumor growing in the body and tail may become very large and can invade local structures prior to producing symptoms warranting investigation.

The initial diagnostic test for the evaluation of symptoms suggestive of pancreatic cancer is computed tomography (CT) scanning. Advances in this imaging modality with helical techniques have improved its diagnostic accuracy, and it allows for establishment of resectability criteria. The CT scan identifies small tumors that are most amenable to resection, identifies major vessels adjacent to the pancreas and assesses invasion or thrombosis, and visualizes peripancreatic tissues and identifies metastases in the liver. Optimal scanning requires thin slices through the pancreas and helical scanning such that the entire procedure can be performed in 20 to 30 seconds with one breath-hold and can retain the potential for three-dimensional reconstruction. CT scanning is reported to be more than 90% accurate in the staging of patients with pancreatic cancer [8]. CT findings of pancreatic cancer include a mass (identified in 96% of cases); dilatation of the bile and pancreatic ducts (double-duct sign) suggesting a pancreatic head location; dilatation of the pancreatic duct proximal to the tumor; and atrophy of the pancreas distal to a tumor (Fig. 16.1A, B). Signs of nonresectable disease include vascular encasement or occlusion of the celiac axis or splenic, hepatic, or superior mesenteric arteries. Encasement of the portal vein or superior mesenteric vein is, likewise, a contraindication to resection (see Fig. 16.1C). However, adherence of the tumor to a segment of these veins may allow resection with venous reconstruction. Identification of metastases to the liver precludes resection (see Fig. 16.1D). Spiral CT scanning allows three-dimensional reconstruction of arterial anatomy, thereby increasing surgeons' knowledge regarding vessel anomalies and proximity to the tumor (see Fig. 16.1E). CT scans are useful in following up affected patients for local recurrence and for distant metastases (see Fig. 16.1F).

Magnetic resonance imaging (MRI) may be useful in diagnosing pancreatic cancer if CT scanning is indeterminate or contraindicated [8]. Both T_1- and T_2-weighted images may be useful in identifying the tumor. Gadolinium enhancement aids in the detection of small pancreatic tumors. MRI cholangiopancreatography may identify obstructed common bile ducts and pancreatic ducts, which may be traced to an obstructing tumor.

Endoscopy plays a major role in the evaluation and diagnosis of pancreatic masses. Endoscopic retrograde cholangiopancreatography (ERCP) is used for visualizing the common and pancreatic ducts and to obtain tissue biopsy or cytologic samples from duct brushings.

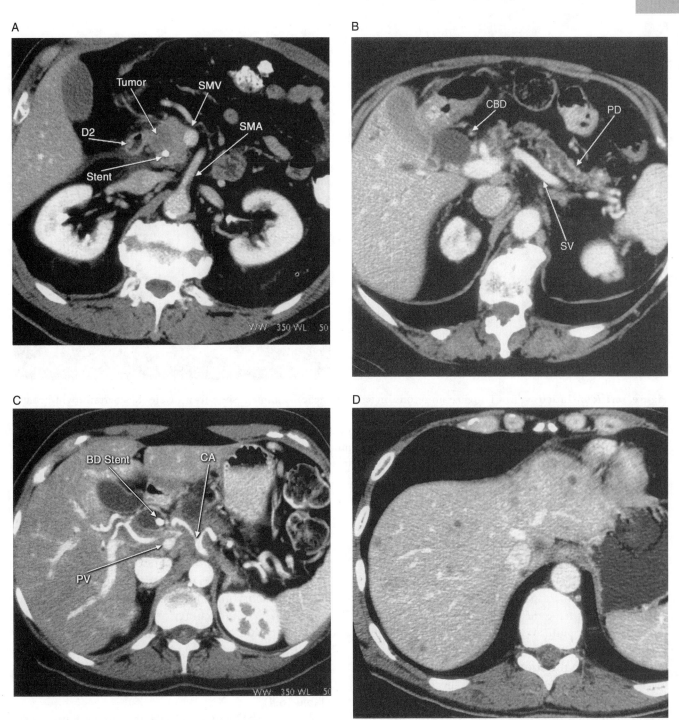

Figure 16.1 (A) Computed tomography (CT) scan demonstrating resectable carcinoma of the head of the pancreas. The tumor and indwelling common bile duct stent are identified by arrows. A margin of normal enhancing pancreatic tissue is shown between the superior mesenteric vein and the tumor, indicating its resectability. *D2* = duodenum; *SMV* = superior mesenteric vein; *SMA* = superior mesenteric artery. (B) CT scan demonstrating markedly dilated common bile duct (*CBD*) and dilated pancreatic duct (*PD*). This image demonstrates the double-duct sign in the case of pancreatic carcinoma. *SV* = splenic vein. (C) CT scan of a patient with unresectable carcinoma of the pancreas. This image demonstrates encasement of the celiac artery (*CA*) and its branches by tumor. Also noted is a dilated bile duct with an indwelling stent (*BD Stent*). *PV* = portal vein. (D) Thin-section CT image of a patient with pancreatic cancer. Demonstrated are multiple small hepatic metastases throughout the liver.

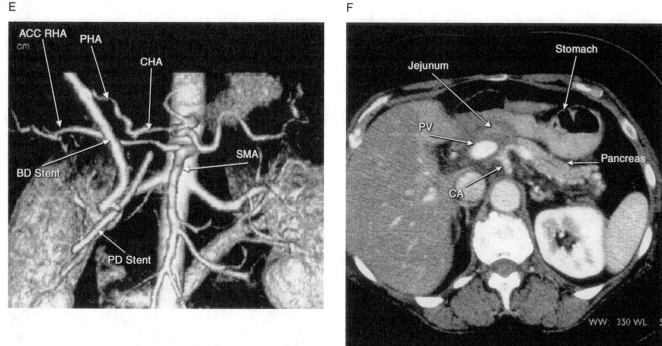

Figure 16.1 (continued)   (E) CT angiogram reconstructed from helical scanning (see part C). Note the aberrant right hepatic artery (*ACC RHA*), common hepatic artery (*CHA*), and proper hepatic artery (*PHA*). Note also narrowing of the ACC RHA and CHA due to encasement by tumor. *SMA* = superior mesenteric artery; *PD Stent* = pancreatic duct stent; *BD Stent* = bile duct stent. (F) CT scan of a patient who has undergone a Whipple procedure. Demonstrated is the distal pancreas adjacent to a limb of jejunum. *PV* = portal vein; *CA* = celiac artery. (CT scan images courtesy of W. Dennis Foley, MD, Professor of Radiology [Digital Imaging], Medical College of Wisconsin.)

Placement of stents may permit preoperative decompression of an obstructed common bile duct or may be useful in a palliative fashion for nonoperative therapy. Endoscopic ultrasonography (EUS) has been used as a method to evaluate pancreatic masses and to detect tumors. Studies have demonstrated sensitivities in the range of 90% or better [9]. However, the success of EUS may vary as it is operator-dependent. EUS may be helpful in identifying the size of the tumor and in assessing for local invasion. EUS-guided fine-needle aspiration has been described for diagnosing pancreatic lesions and lymph nodes, but its clinical utility has yet to be determined.

Percutaneous needle biopsy under either CT or ultrasonographic guidance demonstrates high sensitivity and specificity in the diagnosis of pancreatic cancer [9]. Percutaneous needle biopsy should be performed only in patients for whom surgery is not indicated. Percutaneous fine-needle aspiration has the potential of causing tumor spread, and caution should be used in its performance in patients with potentially resectable disease.

Adjunct laboratory tests may be useful in the evaluation of pancreatic masses. Liver function tests may iden-

tify an obstructive component. An elevated amylase level may identify underlying pancreatitis. The tumor marker most useful in the diagnosis of pancreatic cancer is CA-19-9. CA-19-9 is superior to other markers, such as carcinoembryonic antigen, in the diagnosis of pancreatic cancer. The accuracy of CA-19-9 is related to the reference value chosen: A value of greater than 100 units/ml should be used [10]. The utility of CA-19-9 in the diagnosis of pancreatic cancer is increased when its value is interpreted in conjunction with CT scanning (Table 16.4).

CA-19-9 has been used in determining the prognosis for patients with pancreatic cancer. In recent reports, patients with resectable disease were determined to have a better prognosis if their preoperative CA-19-9 levels were below 100 units/ml [10]. Longer survival times correlate with normalization of levels after resection. Additionally, the application of CA-19-9 in monitoring the response to combined-modality treatments has been reported [10], though more studies are required to determine its utility in this regard.

Staging of pancreatic cancer is performed best using the TNM (*t*umor, *n*ode, *m*etastasis) staging system of the

Table 16.4 Utility of CA-19-9 for Pancreatic Cancer

Use	Comments
Diagnosis	Combines with computed tomographic imaging to yield a positive predictive value > 99% when a CA-19-9 value of > 100 units/ml occurs in non-icteric patients.
Prognosis	Elevated levels are associated with poorer prognosis; longer survival with quickly declining values to normal range after resection.
Monitoring	Elevated posttreatment levels are associated with local extension or metastatic disease; in advanced disease, decreasing levels with chemotherapy are associated with longer survival.

Table 16.5 TNM Staging for Cancer of the Exocrine Pancreas

Classification	Definition
Primary tumor (T)	
TX	Primary tumor cannot be assessed
T0	No evidence of primary tumor
Tis	In situ carcinoma
T1	Tumor limited to the pancreas ≤ 2 cm in greatest dimension
T2	Tumor limited to the pancreas > 2 cm in greatest dimension
T3	Tumor extends directly into any of the following: duodenum, bile duct, peripancreatic tissues
T4	Tumor extends directly into any of the following: stomach, spleen, colon, adjacent large vessels
Regional lymph nodes (N)	
NX	Regional lymph nodes cannot be assessed
N0	No regional lymph node metastasis
N1	Regional lymph node metastasis
pN1a	Metastasis in a single regional lymph node
pN1b	Metastasis in multiple regional lymph nodes
Distant metastasis (M)	
MX	Distant metastasis cannot be assessed
M0	No distant metastasis
M1	Distant metastasis

Source: Used with permission of the American Joint Committee on Cancer (AJCC), Chicago, Illinois. Reprinted from ID Fleming, JS Cooper, DE Henson, et al. (eds), *AJCC Cancer Staging Manual* (5th ed). Philadelphia: Lippincott-Raven, 1997:121–126.

American Joint Committee on Cancer (Tables 16.5, 16.6) [11]. Staging based on the known histologic status of the tumor and nodes is optimal, but clinical staging is acceptable for patients with unresectable disease. The primary tumor is assessed by CT scan for size and direct extension. Patients with stage I disease have tumors that do not extend into adjacent structures and who may benefit most from operative therapy. Laparoscopy has been recommended by some experts to identify peritoneal implants or metastases on the liver surface that are not visualized well by CT scanning [12]. The major advantages of laparoscopy are the avoidance of laparotomy in those patients who have metastatic disease and facilitation of appropriate referrals of patients with nonmetastatic disease to centers of expertise. The prevalence of liver or peritoneal involvement identified by laparoscopy is 24% in recent series [12].

Assessment of the peritoneal washings for cytologic evidence of tumor has an impact on prognosis and is an extension of standard staging criteria [13]. Washings for cytology are collected during laparoscopy or laparotomy. Positive cytologic findings correlate with peritoneal or liver metastases [13]. Furthermore, an increased incidence of positive cytologic findings has been reported in patients who have undergone percutaneous needle biopsy [14]. To enhance the detection of malignant cells in peritoneal cytologic samples, the use of immunohistochemistry or polymerase chain reaction in the search for *K-ras* mutations is being explored.

TREATMENT OF RESECTABLE DISEASE

Surgical resection offers the only chance for cure of a pancreatic malignancy. However, only 10% to 20% of patients with pancreatic cancer are candidates for surgical resection. Physiologic preparation for surgery is required and includes adequate hydration, correction of electrolyte deficits, parenteral vitamin K as indicated, and decompression of the obstructed biliary tree by stenting (as appropriate) to optimize liver function. Often, endoscopic or percutaneous drainage of the biliary tree is performed, although preoperative biliary decompression has not been proven to reduce operative morbidity or mortality. Cardiovascular monitoring during surgery is mandatory, as is perioperative antibiotic administration. Nutritional repletion may be considered in

Table 16.6   AJCC Stage Grouping for Cancer of the Exocrine Pancreas

Stage 0	Tis	N0	M0
Stage I	T1	N0	M0
	T2	N0	M0
Stage II	T3	N0	M0
Stage III	T1	N1	M0
	T2	N1	M0
	T3	N1	M0
Stage IVA	T4	Any N	M0
Stage IVB	Any T	Any N	M1

AJCC = American Joint Committee on Cancer.
Source: Used with permission of the American Joint Committee on Cancer (AJCC), Chicago, Illinois. Reprinted from ID Fleming, JS Cooper, DE Henson, et al. (eds), *AJCC Cancer Staging Manual* (5th ed). Philadelphia: Lippincott-Raven, 1997:121–126.

selective patients who are candidates for resection but manifest severe nutritional deficits. A poor physiologic condition, rather than age, may be a contraindication to resection.

The Whipple procedure (i.e., pancreaticoduodenectomy) was reported in 1935 as a procedure in which the entire duodenum was removed because of ampullary carcinoma [15]. Several variations of this procedure exist; the most common type is the pylorus-preserving pancreatoduodenectomy (depicted in Fig. 16.2). In this operation, the duodenum is divided approximately 2 cm distal to the pylorus, the distal biliary tree is resected with the gallbladder, the jejunum is resected distal to the ligament of Treitz, and the pancreas is resected at its neck.

Several methods of restoring intestinal continuity exist, particularly with respect to the management of the pancreatic remnant. One example is shown in Figure 16.3. Aside from a pancreatoduodenostomy, a pancreaticogastrostomy may be used with an expected similar outcome [16]. The pylorus-preserving pancreatoduodenectomy is preferred, owing to improved maintenance of nutrition without compromising the oncologic operation, as compared to the classic Whipple procedure in which the gastric antrum and pylorus are resected. Reasons for sacrificing the pylorus include ischemia of the duodenal cuff after resection, tumor involvement of the first portion of the duodenum, or prior surgery involving the proximal duodenum [17]. Total pancreatectomy may be required if multifocal tumor is found to involve the entire gland and negative margins of the pancreatic resection cannot be achieved. In such cases, however, an insulin-dependent diabetic state is created.

Historically, involvement of the portal vein pre-

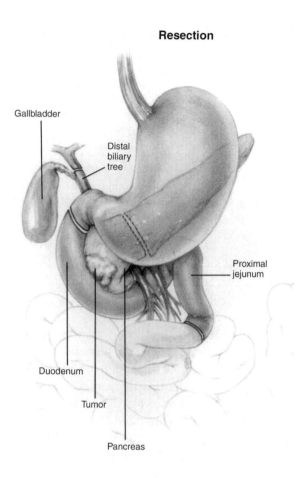

Resection

Figure 16.2   Upper gastrointestinal tract with tumor in the head of the pancreas. Demonstrated are the resection lines for a pylorus-preserving Whipple operation. An en bloc resection is performed to include the following: a portion of the first part and all of the second, third, and fourth parts of the duodenum; proximal jejunum; neck, head, and uncinate process of the pancreas; gallbladder; and distal biliary tree. (Reprinted with permission from JL Cameron, GB Bulkley, TR Gadacz, et al., *Atlas of Surgery,* vol I. St. Louis, Mosby, 1990.)

cluded pancreatic resection. However, a number of authors have demonstrated that limited portal vein resection can be accomplished for patients with focal tumor involvement of the portal vein. For patients who undergo portal vein resection, the results suggest a prognosis that is no different from that achieved by patients who undergo standard pancreatic resection [18].

Complications

Over the last two decades, the complication rate from a Whipple procedure has diminished markedly. Overall, mortality from a pancreatoduodenectomy now is being reported to be less than 4%, and a recent series of 650 operations demonstrated a 30-day mortality of 1.4%

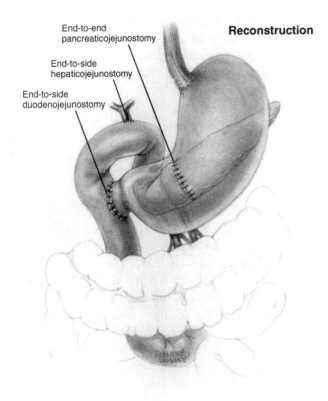

End-to-end pancreaticojejunostomy

End-to-side hepaticojejunostomy

End-to-side duodenojejunostomy

Reconstruction

Figure 16.3 One example of reconstruction by which intestinal continuity is restored by pancreaticojejunostomy, hepaticojejunostomy, and duodenojejunostomy. (Reprinted with permission from JL Cameron, GB Bulkley, TR Gadacz, et al., *Atlas of Surgery,* vol I. St. Louis, Mosby, 1990.)

[19]. The improved mortality is related to improved general management, surgeon expertise, and higher volume of procedures being performed in a hospital [20].

Overall, the complication rate varies and is up to 41% in some series [19]. In the series from the Johns Hopkins Hospital, the most common complications included delayed gastric emptying, pancreatic fistula, and wound infection. Complications occurring in 5% or fewer of the cases included intraabdominal abscess, cholangitis, bile leak, and marginal ulcer. The most lethal complication is a leak from the pancreatic anastomosis. Delayed gastric emptying is the most common complication, though improvement in this outcome has been achieved by using erythromycin as a promotility agent [21].

Outcome

Survival after pancreatoduodenectomy for cancer of the pancreas is poor. A review of multiple series published in the 1980s reveals a five-year survival rate of approxi-

mately 5% [22]. Centers with extensive experience, however, have reported improving results over the last two decades. In an analysis of pancreatoduodenectomy for cancer of the head of the pancreas performed in 201 patients between 1970 and 1994, the actuarial five-year survival was 21% [23]. When analyzed by decades, survival clearly improved from the 1970s to the 1990s (Fig. 16.4). Strongest predictors of long-term survival included diploid tumor, tumor diameter less than 3 cm, negative nodal status, and negative resection margins.

Adjuvant Chemotherapy and Radiotherapy

Adjuvant therapy has been studied by a limited number of groups. Data from the Gastrointestinal Tumor Study Group (GITSG) suggested that chemoradiation after pancreatic resection significantly improved median and long-term survival [24, 25]. More recently, a prospective single-institution experience also suggested improved survival with postoperative adjuvant chemoradiation. The use of such treatment improved the immediate survival from 13.5 months without therapy to 19.5 months with treatment [26]. Interestingly, a group receiving more intensive chemoradiation did not show an improved survival advantage over the standard chemoradiation group. Another report from the Medi-

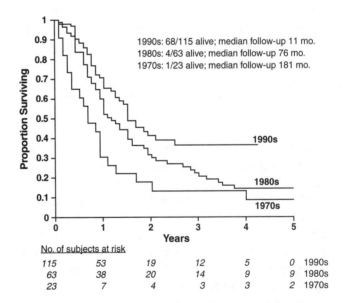

1990s: 68/115 alive; median follow-up 11 mo.
1980s: 4/63 alive; median follow-up 76 mo.
1970s: 1/23 alive; median follow-up 181 mo.

No. of subjects at risk

115	53	19	12	5	0	1990s
63	38	20	14	9	9	1980s
23	7	4	3	3	2	1970s

Figure 16.4 The actuarial survival curves for 201 patients undergoing pancreaticoduodenectomy for pancreatic carcinoma by decade. A significant improvement ($p=.002$) in survival has occurred from the 1970s (N = 23) to the 1980s (N = 63) to the 1990s (N = 115). Median follow-up is given for survivors. (Reprinted with permission of Lippincott-Raven from CJ Yeo, JL Cameron, KD Lillemoe, et al., Pancreaticoduodenectomy for cancer of the head of the pancreas: 201 patients. *Ann Surg* 221:721–733, 1995.)

cal College of Wisconsin evaluating 61 patients in a retrospective fashion also demonstrated improved survival with adjuvant chemoradiation [27]. The advantage in survival, however, was noted for only stage I patients and was not observed in patients with stage III disease. The conclusions of these studies strongly suggest the consideration of adjuvant chemoradiation in patients who are rendered free of gross disease postoperatively.

TREATMENT OF UNRESECTABLE DISEASE

Because only a minority of patients will undergo resection for cure of pancreatic cancer, the palliation of symptoms is of primary importance in most patients to improve their quality of life. The primary symptoms of pancreatic cancer are obstructive jaundice, duodenal obstruction, and pain [28]. Both operative and nonoperative techniques are available for palliation of these symptoms so that patient management can be tailored to the specific presentation of such symptoms and patients' prognosis.

Obstructive jaundice is the most common presenting symptom and occurs in approximately 70% of affected patients. Progressive liver dysfunction and early death occur if jaundice is untreated. In addition, symptoms of pruritus, anorexia, nausea, and malnutrition are associated with jaundice. Therefore, relief of the obstruction improves the quality of life in such patients. The approach used most often is a nonoperative technique of stenting the obstructed common duct. The two approaches are percutaneous and endoscopic placement of a stent. Different types of stents have been used; often, they are plastic, but these stents are characterized by limited length of patency. More recently, self-expanding metallic stents have been used, with early reports suggesting an increase in the length of patency. Most often, surgical management includes either cholecystojejunostomy or hepaticojejunostomy, with the latter bypass preferred, owing to longer patency. Surgical and nonoperative techniques are equally effective in short-term relief of jaundice, but recurrent jaundice occurs in up to 38% of patients in the nonoperative group, and duodenal obstruction is not addressed by nonoperative techniques [28].

In the course of pancreatic cancer, duodenal obstruction occurs in 13% to 21% of patients as unresectable disease progresses [28]. A number of reviews have addressed the issue of whether patients should undergo prophylactic gastrojejunostomy to avoid subsequent duodenal obstruction requiring a second operative procedure. On the basis of these collected reviews, prophylactic gastroduodenostomy has been advocated in pa-

tients who undergo laparotomy and are found to have unresectable disease. In addition, a recent prospective, randomized trial from the Johns Hopkins Hospital also suggests that prophylactic gastrojejunostomy should be performed routinely [29].

The most disturbing symptom of pancreatic cancer is pain. Though pain is reported in only 30% to 40% of patients at presentation, most patients with unresected disease experience significant pain at the time of death. To address this issue, the value of intraoperative chemical splanchnicectomy has been studied in a prospective randomized trial. Either 20 ml of 50% alcohol or a saline placebo was injected on each side of the aorta at the level of the celiac axis to accomplish the chemical splanchnicectomy [30]. The results showed a significant reduction or prevention of pain in patients in the alcohol-injected group, leading the authors to conclude that chemical splanchnicectomy should be routine in patients who undergo laparotomy for unresectable pancreatic cancer. For patients who do not undergo laparotomy, oral agents are used routinely. Long-acting narcotics are preferred, reserving short-acting agents for breakthrough pain.

Pancreatoduodenectomy has been evaluated for the palliation of pancreatic cancer in a retrospective analysis comparing the outcome to a group of patients with unresectable disease, 87% of whom underwent combined biliary and gastric bypass [31]. Though the postoperative stay was longer after pancreatoduodenectomy, the mortality was identical in both groups (1.6%), and the overall actuarial survival was improved significantly in patients who underwent resection. In the setting of low operative morbidity and mortality, the authors suggest that pancreatoduodenectomy with gross or microscopic disease at the surgical resection margin may be advantageous in selected patients.

Tumors of the Endocrine Pancreas

Endocrine tumors of the pancreas are rare, with a reported prevalence of 10 per one million population. These tumors are considered to be neuroendocrine neoplasms and are classified as *APUDomas* (tumors composed of *a*mine *p*recursor *u*ptake and *d*ecarboxylation cells). Endocrine pancreatic tumors are categorized according to their function and are named according to the specific hormone released and the associated clinical syndrome. Of all pancreatic endocrine tumors, 15% to 30% are reported to be nonfunctional. Insulinoma is the most common of the pancreatic endocrine tumors, followed by gastrinoma. VIPomas (tumors that produce *v*asoactive *i*ntestinal *p*eptide), glucagonomas, and somatostatinomas are very rare.

A hallmark of endocrine tumors is the impossibility of distinguishing benign from malignant behavior on the basis of histologic appearance alone. The diagnosis of malignancy is established by evidence of metastatic spread. Once the clinical syndrome and type of tumor are identified, localization using a variety of radiologic procedures is the next step in management. When it is localized, the tumor is staged on the basis of evidence of any regional or distant spread, and treatment is initiated. Treatment varies from simple enucleation for benign insulinomas to debulking procedures for malignant tumors. Such debulking procedures are palliative, but surgery remains the mainstay of treatment, providing relief of symptoms and allowing improved quality of survival, given the indolent course of many of these endocrine tumors [32].

INSULINOMA

Insulinoma is the most common tumor of the endocrine pancreas [33]. The clinical symptoms of insulinoma are due to hypoglycemia and are characterized by Whipple's triad, consisting of (1) symptoms of hypoglycemia during prolonged fasting, (2) documentation of a blood glucose level of less than 50 mg/dl, and (3) relief of symptoms after administration of glucose. The average age at presentation is in the middle of one's fifth decade, with a range between 20 and 75 years. In most series, women predominate. Most symptoms of insulinomas are categorized as either neuroglycopenic (e.g., visual disturbances, confusion, altered consciousness, and weakness) or cardiovascular secondary to catecholamine release (e.g., palpitations, tremulousness, and sweating). The diagnosis is confirmed by simultaneous measurement of glucose and insulin levels during a prolonged fast. An insulin-glucose ratio of less than 0.4 is normal, whereas ratios greater than 0.4 correlate with the diagnosis of insulinoma. By 72 hours of a fasting test, virtually all patients with insulinomas will achieve a diagnostic insulin-glucose ratio. Other conditions may be associated with fasting hypoglycemia and must be differentiated from insulinoma (Table 16.7). Additional tests that are helpful in this regard include plasma determination of pro-insulin, C-peptide levels, and antibodies to insulin. In patients with surreptitious use of exogenous insulin, the pro-insulin and C-peptide levels are diagnostic, the pro-insulin level being either normal or decreased and the C-peptide level being low. Both these levels would be elevated in a patient with insulinoma.

Table 16.7 Differential Diagnosis of Insulinoma

Factitious hypoglycemia
Sulfonylurea ingestion
Autoantibodies to insulin
Autoantibodies to the insulin receptor
Pancreatic islet disease (diffuse β-cell adenomatosis, nesidioblastosis)
Alcohol abuse
Extrapancreatic tumors that secrete insulinlike growth factors

Insulinomas tend to be small tumors, with 90% smaller than 2 cm. These tumors are distributed evenly throughout the gland, with one-third located in the head, one-third in the body, and one-third in the tail of the pancreas. The malignancy rate of insulinomas is perhaps 10% and is determined by the presence of metastatic disease. Multiple tumors occur approximately 10% of the time; in such cases, multiple endocrine neoplasia type 1 (MEN1) should be suspected. Owing to the small size of these tumors, their occurrence throughout the pancreas, and the potential for multiplicity, localization studies are extremely useful prior to operation. Dynamic CT scanning may be helpful but is limited because of these tumors' small size; however, liver metastases can be identified by this modality. A few studies have demonstrated usefulness of MRI in localization, but additional studies are necessary for confirmation.

Because most insulinomas are highly vascular, angiography has been very useful in preoperative localization in up to 80% of cases. More recently, EUS has been reported to be the most useful test in preoperative localization. Percutaneous transhepatic portal venous sampling is one of the most sensitive methods for localization but should be reserved for problem cases. Blood samples are taken from the splenic and superior mesentery veins along the major pancreatic draining veins, and insulin levels are measured. This test can localize the tumor to an area of the pancreas but does not identify a specific site. By taking advantage of the fact that calcium is a potent stimulant of insulin release from the insulinoma, arterial stimulation with calcium infusion and venous sampling from the hepatic veins has successfully localized these lesions. The advantages of arterial stimulation and venous sampling over portal venous sampling include less morbidity and less time consumption. A localization rate of 88% has been reported [34]. Recently, octreotide scintigraphy generated some interest as a localizing modality, but more evaluation of this method is warranted. Finally, intraoperative ultrasonography has proved to be a very sensitive technique for localization of the pancreatic tumor and, when combined with palpation, may increase the sensitivity to almost 100%.

All patients who have insulinomas but no evidence of metastatic disease should undergo surgery for removal of the tumor. The entire pancreas must be mobilized and explored, owing to the 10% incidence of multifocality. For small solitary tumors, enucleation should be performed. In the head of the pancreas, careful dissection is required to avoid damage to the main pancreatic duct. Usually, distal pancreatectomy is performed for multiple lesions in the body or tail or if a lesion is large and malignancy is suspected. A pancreatoduodenectomy should be performed for large malignant tumors in the pancreatic head. If an insulinoma cannot be found, options include a blind distal resection or performance of additional postoperative localization procedures to allow specific tumor localization and appropriate surgical excision at a second operation.

Tumor debulking may be helpful in treating patients with distant metastases. Resection of limited metastases to the liver may lead to symptomatic improvement and prolonged survival and should be considered in selected patients [32]. In patients in whom resection is not undertaken, medical therapy with diazoxide or octreotide has been reported [32]. Diazoxide reduces insulin secretion by acting directly on the beta cells. Octreotide may control the symptoms of hypoglycemia in some patients, but its use requires further evaluation.

GASTRINOMA

In 1955, Zollinger and Ellison described a clinical syndrome of extreme hypersecretion of gastric acid with associated ulcer disease [35, 36]. The Zollinger-Ellison syndrome is known to be caused by gastrinomas, an endocrine tumor that elaborates the hormone gastrin. Gastrinomas are slightly more common in male individuals (60%) than in female individuals (40%). The mean age at diagnosis is in the fifth to sixth decade. Patients with gastrinomas should be classified as having either sporadic or familial disease, with 20% to 25% having MEN1. The most common clinical symptoms include abdominal pain, diarrhea, and esophageal reflux. Many patients present with diarrhea as their only symptom. In recent series, most patients present with atypical duodenal ulcers, but up to 25% have no ulcer at the time of diagnosis [32]. A delay of three to six years between the onset of symptoms and diagnosis is typical.

Gastrinomas are suspected on the basis of the clinical presentation and are established by documentation of gastric acid hypersecretion and fasting hypergastri-

nemia. A basal acid output greater than 15 mEq/hr in patients without previous acid-reducing operations and a fasting serum gastrin greater than 1,000 pg/ml are diagnostic. If the fasting serum gastrin is normal or equivocal, a secretin-provocative test may be required to establish the diagnosis.

Recent reports documenting the malignancy rate in gastrinomas have suggested that 50% to 60% are malignant, as compared to early studies suggesting that 60% to 90% were malignant. Usually, metastases occur in two sites: parapancreatic lymph nodes and the liver. Malignancy cannot be established by histologic features alone but requires the presence of metastatic disease. Tumor size has been shown to be an important prognostic factor for liver metastases but not for lymph node metastases. As compared to patients with sporadic gastrinoma, patients with MEN1 are younger, and their tumors almost always are multiple and frequently small.

Initially, gastrinomas were thought to occur most commonly in the pancreas. Recent studies suggest that approximately 50% of tumors occur in the duodenum and in lymph nodes near the pancreatic head. Most gastrinomas are found to the right of the superior mesenteric vessels in an area called the *gastrinoma triangle,* the apices of which are the cystic duct–common bile duct junction, the border of the second and third portion of the duodenum, and the junction of the neck and body of the pancreas (Fig. 16.5) [37]. Also, recent reports suggest that many of these tumors originate in the duodenal wall.

Because gastrinomas frequently are multiple and extrapancreatic, tumor localization is extremely important prior to definitive surgical therapy. A number of techniques have been reported for localization of gastrinomas. A CT scan may be helpful for the detection of the primary lesion and is valuable in evaluating for metastatic disease to the liver. Selective angiography has been reported, as has MRI. EUS has been reported to be successful by some authors but may be operator-dependent. Recently, scanning with radiolabeled octreotide has capitalized on the presence of somatostatin receptors on gastrinomas as well as on other pancreatic endocrine tumors. Some authors suggest that somatostatin-receptor scanning should be the initial procedure of choice [32].

The observation of the paradoxical release of gastrin with intravenous secretin has led to development of localization procedures. The selective injection of secretin in one of three parapancreatic arteries (gastroduodenal, superior mesenteric, or splenic) with sampling of gastrin from the hepatic vein has been suggested as a very sensitive localizing procedure as compared to the more

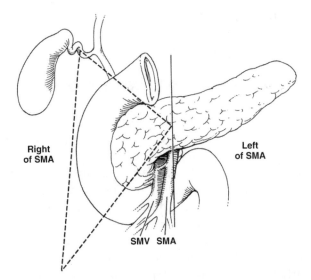

Right
of SMA

Left
of SMA

SMV SMA

Figure 16.5 Retroperitoneal structures, including the pancreas, duodenum, extrahepatic biliary system, superior mesenteric artery (*SMA*), and superior mesenteric vein (*SMV*). Anatomic areas are separated to the right and left of the SMA (*solid vertical line*). The gastrinoma triangle (*dashed lines*) is located to the right of the SMA. (Reprinted with permission of Lippincott-Raven from TJ Howard, M Sawicki, KJ Lewin, et al., Pancreatic polypeptide immunoreactivity in sporadic gastrinoma: relationship to intraabdominal location. *Pancreas* 11:350–356, 1995.)

technically difficult portal vein–sampling procedure. Intraoperative ultrasonography and endoscopy have been used as operative adjuncts with considerable success.

Treatment is twofold. First, gastric acid hypersecretion most often is controlled pharmacologically with proton pump inhibitors. Second, all patients with gastrinomas should undergo imaging studies for localization of the primary tumor and assessment of metastatic disease. Laparotomy with resection of the tumor is recommended for patients with sporadic-type gastrinoma. The rationale for this approach is based on reported cases of long-term cures in patients undergoing surgery as compared to medical management alone [38]. Because symptoms can be controlled with antisecretory agents, all patients should undergo localization procedures prior to surgery. Primary tumors that are small and well encapsulated can be enucleated carefully. Multiple lymph node biopsies, with emphasis on excision of paraduodenal and pancreatic nodules, are very important. Finally, the routine use of duodenotomy and of intraoperative endoscopy with transillumination has increased the detection rate of gastrinomas to more than 90% in patients so treated.

Gastrinomas in the body and tail of the pancreas are managed best by distal pancreatectomy. Total gastrectomy has not been recommended in the recent litera-

ture because of the success of proton pump inhibitors. However, it may be indicated in special situations (e.g., patients who are noncompliant and have recurrent ulcer complications). In patients with MEN1, surgical management is less clear. Such patients should undergo surgical management of the parathyroid disease first, as hyperparathyroidism may exacerbate gastric acid hypersecretion. Controversies exist as to whether MEN1 patients can be cured by resection of their gastrinomas, as invariably the lesions are multiple and localizing them preoperatively is difficult. Overall, of those patients who have sporadic disease and undergo complete resections, up to 70% are considered cured. In patients with unresectable or metastatic gastrinoma, chemotherapy with streptozocin may be helpful. Cytoreductive surgery may be helpful in selected cases.

GLUCAGONOMA

The most common findings in patients with glucagonoma are dermatitis, stomatitis, weight loss, malnutrition, anemia, diabetes, and thromboembolic disease [36, 39]. The dermatitis, termed *necrolytic migratory erythema*, is pathognomonic of glucagonoma. The diagnosis is suspected from the clinical picture and from biopsy of the skin lesion and is confirmed by documentation of elevated fasting glucagon levels. Glucagonomas occur in the sixth to seventh decades, usually as a 5- to 10-cm tumor located mostly in the body and tail of the pancreas. Usually, these lesions are large and solitary. CT scanning is used for localization.

Treatment is focused at correcting the metabolic abnormalities. This approach includes initiation of total parenteral nutrition to reverse the malnutrition and administration of octreotide to reduce circulating glucagon levels and to allow an improved response to total parenteral nutrition. Surgical treatment consists of distal pancreatectomy. In patients with metastases, which are found in 50% to 80% of cases at the time of initial diagnosis, a safe debulking procedure may be warranted and may allow an extended symptom-free interval for such patients. In patients with widely metastatic disease, such chemotherapeutic agents as streptozocin have been used. Octreotide can be helpful in controlling hyperglycemia and the dermatitis associated with unresectable disease.

VIPOMA

Initially, Verner and Morrison [39] described VIPoma in 1958 as a syndrome characterized by severe diarrhea and hypokalemia associated with an islet-cell tumor of the pancreas. Other names include the *WDHA* (*watery diarrhea, hypokalemia,* and *achlorhydria*) *syndrome* and *pancreatic cholera syndrome.* Among the major symptoms are intermittent, severe, large-volume, watery diarrhea with associated metabolic abnormalities, including hypokalemia, hypochlorhydria, and hyperglycemia. Additional symptoms are weakness, lethargy, and abdominal cramping pain. The mean age for adults with this disease is approximately 50 years. The disease exhibits a female predominance and can occur in children as well.

The diagnosis of VIPoma requires demonstration of an elevated plasma concentration of VIP and the presence of large-volume, watery diarrhea. Most tumors are located in the pancreas, but 10% may be extrapancreatic. Usually, these tumors are large and solitary; 40% to 70% reveal metastasis at the time of diagnosis. CT scanning is used to localize the tumor. If disease is not seen in the abdomen, a thoracic CT is indicated. Most tumors are present in the distal pancreas.

Treatment is initiated by correction of the dehydration and electrolyte abnormalities. In addition to intravenous fluids and potassium, octreotide can control the diarrhea in more than 80% of patients. After the tumor's location is identified, patients without metastatic disease should undergo surgical excision for cure. In those patients with metastatic disease, safe debulking operations may help to control symptoms. Approximately 30% of patients were cured with complete resection in a number of series [32]. Partial responses to chemotherapy, including streptozocin, have been reported.

SOMATOSTATINOMA

Somatostatinomas are the least common pancreatic endocrine tumor [39]. Symptoms of this disease are nonspecific and include abdominal pain and diarrhea. Characteristically, patients have diabetes, gallbladder disease, diarrhea, weight loss, steatorrhea, and hypochlorhydria. An elevated plasma somatostatin level confirms the diagnosis. The mean age at diagnosis is approximately 50. Tumors occur in the pancreas in approximately 75% of cases, and the remainder occur in the upper small intestine. Most tumors within the pancreas are found in the head and are solitary, with 80% to 90% of affected patients having metastatic disease at presentation.

CT scanning is indicated for localization of such tumors. Treatment consists of the control of hyperglycemia, nutritional support, and surgical resection. Cholecystectomy is indicated even in the absence of documented gallstones. Because a high proportion of

these tumors are malignant and reveal metastatic disease at diagnosis, cytotoxic therapy has been used, though with a varying degree of success.

NONFUNCTIONING ISLET-CELL TUMORS

Up to one-third of patients with tumors of the endocrine pancreas demonstrate no defined clinical syndrome. Such patients are considered to have nonfunctional endocrine neoplasms. Symptoms include abdominal pain, weight loss, and obstructive jaundice, similar in presentation to ductal adenocarcinoma of the pancreas. Pancreatic polypeptide may be elevated in these tumors but does not cause a clinical syndrome. Elevated levels of pancreatic polypeptide may be particularly useful as a marker for recurrence of disease after surgery or for monitoring the response to nonsurgical therapy. Mostly, these tumors are found in the head, neck, and uncinate process of the pancreas. Approximately 50% to 90% of tumors are malignant. These tumors tend to grow in an indolent fashion and are associated with longer survival than is adenocarcinoma of the pancreas. Localization studies include CT scanning, which also evaluates for hepatic metastases (Fig. 16.6).

Treatment is dictated by the location of the tumor,

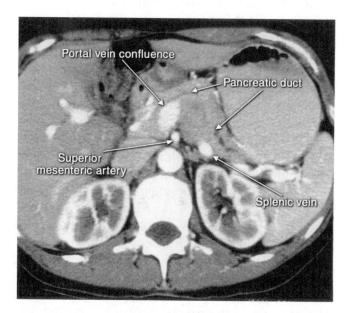

Figure 16.6 Computed tomography scan of a patient performed during a workup for steatorrhea. Shown are a mass in the body of the pancreas, dilatation of the pancreatic duct in the tail, and a normal-caliber duct in the head. The mass was resected with uninvolved surgical margins, revealing a nonfunctioning islet-cell tumor. (CT scan images courtesy of W. Dennis Foley, MD, Professor of Radiology [Digital Imaging], Medical College of Wisconsin.)

but local excision usually is not performed. Either pancreaticoduodenectomy or distal pancreatectomy may be required for resection. The overall five-year survival is approximately 50%. In patients with unresectable disease, combination chemotherapy with streptozocin and doxorubicin has been associated with a significant survival advantage [36].

GALLBLADDER CANCER

Cancer of the gallbladder is an aggressive malignancy that occurs predominantly in the elderly. With the exception of cases detected incidentally during cholecystectomy for gallstone disease, the prognosis for most patients is poor. Gallbladder cancer is the fifth most common gastrointestinal malignancy and is two to three times more common in women than in men [40]. Approximately 5,000 new cases are diagnosed annually in the United States. The incidence of gallbladder cancer varies with both ethnic background and geographic location. In the United States, gallbladder cancer is more common in Native Americans, whereas worldwide, the incidence is particularly high in Chile [41].

A strong association has long been noted between gallbladder cancer and cholelithiasis, which is present in 75% to 90% of cases [42]. The risk of gallbladder cancer is seven times higher in people with gallstones, and the risk is higher in patients with symptomatic gallstones than in patients with asymptomatic gallstones [41]. Approximately 1% of all elective cholecystectomies performed for cholelithiasis will harbor an occult gallbladder cancer [40]. In addition, an anomalous pancreatic duct–biliary duct junction and porcelain gallbladder have been associated with gallbladder cancer. Practice guidelines for gallbladder cancer can be accessed through the NCCN Web site at www.nccn.org.

Pathologic Features

Ninety percent of gallbladder cancers are classified as adenocarcinomas [42]. Six percent of gallbladder cancers demonstrate papillary features on histopathologic workup; commonly, such tumors are diagnosed while localized to the gallbladder and are associated also with an improved overall survival [42]. At diagnosis, 25% of cancers are localized to the gallbladder wall, 35% have associated metastases to regional lymph nodes or extension into adjacent organs, and 40% already have metastasized to distant sites [42].

Lymphatic drainage from the gallbladder occurs in a predictable fashion and correlates with the pattern of lymph node metastases seen in gallbladder cancer [43]. Initially, the cystic duct and pericholedochal nodes are involved, followed by more distant metastases to nodes posterior to the head of the pancreas and then to inter-aortocaval lymph nodes. Secondary routes of lymphatic drainage include the retroportal and right celiac lymph nodes. Commonly, gallbladder cancer also extends directly into the liver and porta hepatis, resulting in narrowing or obstruction of the common hepatic or right hepatic duct.

Clinical Presentation

Most often, gallbladder cancer patients present with right-upper-quadrant abdominal pain often mimicking acute or chronic cholecystitis [40, 41]. Weight loss, jaundice, and an abdominal mass are less common presenting symptoms. The preoperative diagnosis of gallbladder cancer is difficult. In a recent series, carcinoma of the gallbladder was correctly diagnosed preoperatively in only 8% of 53 patients [44]. The most common misdiagnoses included chronic cholecystitis (28%), pancreatic cancer (13%), acute cholecystitis (9%), choledocholithiasis (8%), and gallbladder hydrops (8%) [44].

Diagnosis and Staging

Ultrasonography is often the first diagnostic modality used in evaluating patients with right-upper-quadrant abdominal pain. Common ultrasonographic features of gallbladder cancer are a heterogeneous mass replacing the gallbladder lumen and an irregular gallbladder wall. The sensitivity of ultrasonography in the detection of gallbladder cancer ranges from 70% to 100% [45]. Usually, CT reveals a mass replacing the gallbladder or extending into adjacent organs (Fig. 16.7). Spiral CT also shows the adjacent vascular anatomy. With newer MRI techniques, gallbladder cancers may be differentiated from the adjacent liver and biliary obstruction, or encasement of the portal vein may be visualized easily [41].

Cholangiography also may be helpful in diagnosing gallbladder cancer in jaundiced patients. The typical cholangiographic finding in gallbladder cancer is a long stricture of the common hepatic duct. Angiography, spiral CT, or MRI may identify encasement of the portal vein or hepatic artery. If radiologic studies suggest that the tumor is unresectable (liver or peritoneal metastases, portal vein encasement, or extensive hepatic inva-

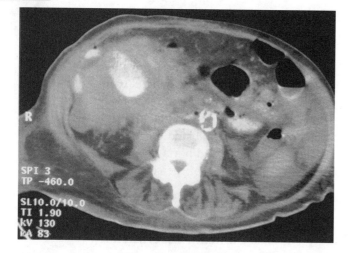

Figure 16.7 Computed tomography scan of a patient demonstrating a porcelain gallbladder encompassed by a mass invading the liver and surrounding structures.

sion), a biopsy of the tumor is warranted and can be performed under ultrasonographic or CT guidance.

Carcinoma of the gallbladder is staged according to the depth of invasion and extent of spread, using the American Joint Committee on Cancer TNM classification (Tables 16.8, 16.9) [46]. Stage I and II tumors are confined to the gallbladder but are differentiated by depth of invasion. Stage III tumors penetrate the serosa, extend less than 2 cm into the liver or into another adjacent organ, or involve first-order lymph nodes. Stage IV tumors exhibit extensive liver invasion, metastatic spread to second-order lymph nodes, or distant metastases.

Management

The appropriate operative procedure for patients with localized gallbladder cancer is determined by the pathologic stage. Usually, patients with tumors confined to the gallbladder mucosa or submucosa (T1a) are identified after cholecystectomy for gallstone disease; they have an overall five-year survival approaching 100% [47]. Recurrent cancer at port sites and peritoneal carcinomatosis have been reported after laparoscopic cholecystectomy, even for patients with in situ disease. Thus, patients with suspected gallbladder cancer preoperatively should undergo open cholecystectomy to minimize the chance of bile spillage and tumor dissemination [41].

Cancer of the gallbladder with invasion into the gallbladder muscularis (T1b) or beyond (stages II–IVA) is associated with an increasing incidence of regional

Table 16.8 TNM System for Gallbladder Cancer

Classification	Definition
Primary tumor (T)	
TX	Primary tumor cannot be assessed
T0	No evidence of primary tumor
Tis	Carcinoma in situ
T1	Tumor invades lamina propria or muscle layer
T1a	Tumor invades lamina propria
T1b	Tumor invades muscle layer
T2	Tumor invades perimuscular connective tissue; no extension beyond serosa or into liver
T3	Tumor perforates the serosa or directly invades one adjacent organ or both (extends ≤ 2 cm or less into liver)
T4	Tumor extends > 2 cm into liver, and/or into two or more adjacent organs
Regional lymph nodes (N)	
NX	Regional lymph nodes cannot be assessed
N0	No regional lymph node metastasis
N1	Metastasis in cystic duct, pericholedochal, and/or hilar lymph nodes (i.e., in the hepatoduodenal ligament)
N2	Metastasis in peripancreatic (head only), periduodenal, periportal, celiac, and/or superior mesenteric lymph nodes
Distant metastasis (M)	
MX	Distant metastasis cannot be assessed
M0	No distant metastasis
M1	Distant metastasis

Source: Used with permission of the American Joint Committee on Cancer (AJCC), Chicago, Illinois. Reprinted from ID Fleming, JS Cooper, DE Henson, et al. (eds), *AJCC Cancer Staging Manual* (5th ed). Philadelphia: Lippincott-Raven, 1997:103–108.

lymph node metastases and should be managed with an extended lymphadenectomy, including the cystic duct, pericholedochal, portal, right celiac, and posterior pancreatoduodenal lymph nodes [41, 48]. Extension into the hepatic parenchyma is common, and extended cholecystectomy should incorporate at least a 2-cm margin beyond the palpable or ultrasonographic extent of the tumor. For smaller tumors, this goal can be achieved with a wedge resection of the liver. For larger tumors, an anatomic liver resection may be required to achieve a histologically negative margin.

The major goal of therapy for gallbladder cancer is

palliative. If a tissue diagnosis can be established in patients with an unresectable tumor, nonoperative palliation should be considered. Many such patients have obstructive jaundice that can be managed with either an endoscopic or percutaneously placed biliary stent. Pain is another problem that should be treated aggressively to improve quality of life. Percutaneous celiac ganglion nerve block may reduce the need for narcotics.

The results of chemotherapy in the treatment of patients with gallbladder cancer have been fairly poor. Re-

Table 16.9 AJCC Stage Grouping for Gallbladder Cancer

Stage 0	Tis	N0	M0
Stage I	T1	N0	M0
Stage II	T2	N0	M0
Stage III	T1	N1	M0
	T2	N1	M0
	T3	N0	M0
	T3	N1	M0
Stage IVA	T4	N0	M0
	T4	N1	M0
Stage IVB	Any T	N2	M0
	Any T	Any N	M1

AJCC = American Joint Committee on Cancer.
Source: Used with permission of the American Joint Committee on Cancer (AJCC), Chicago, Illinois. Reprinted from ID Fleming, JS Cooper, DE Henson, et al. (eds), *AJCC Cancer Staging Manual* (5th ed). Philadelphia: Lippincott-Raven, 1997:103–108.

cently, the combination of intravenous 5-fluorouracil, high-dose levofolinic acid, and oral hydroxyurea has achieved a partial response rate of 30%, with a median survival of eight months in patients with unresectable gallbladder cancer [49]. Both external-beam and intraoperative radiotherapy have been used in the management of patients with gallbladder cancer. However, no randomized data have demonstrated improved survival with either technique.

Survival in patients with gallbladder cancer is influenced strongly by the pathologic stage of the disease at presentation. Patients with cancer limited to the gallbladder mucosa and submucosa (T1a) have a uniformly excellent prognosis [49]. Invasion into the muscular wall of the gallbladder increases the risk of recurrence; reported five-year survivals for patients with T1b gallbladder cancer range from 20% to 100% [41, 48, 50]. Invasion into the muscularis or into the subserosa increases the risk of regional lymph node metastases to 15% and 50%, respectively [41]. Recently, several groups reported five-year overall survival of 40% to 63% and 19% to 25%, respectively, for patients with stage III and stage IV gallbladder cancer who underwent resection (Fig. 16.8) [51, 52]. However, most patients with gallbladder cancer have advanced, unresectable disease at the time of presentation. As a result, fewer than 15% of all patients with gallbladder cancer are

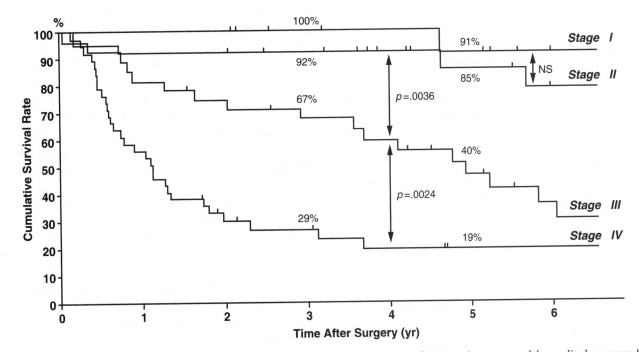

Figure 16.8 Kaplan-Meier survival curves according to stage (TNM system) of 106 patients treated by radical surgery for carcinoma of the gallbladder. The number of patients in each stage are as follows: stage I, 15; stage II, 24; stage III, 28; stage IV, 39. *NS* = not significant. (Reprinted with permission of Mosby, Inc. from K Tsukada, K Hatakeyama, I Kurosaki, et al., Outcome of radical surgery for carcinoma of the gallbladder according to the TNM stage. *Surgery* 120:816–822, 1996.)

alive after five years [42]. The median survival for stage IV patients at the time of presentation is only one to three months.

CHOLANGIOCARCINOMA

Biliary tract cancers may occur anywhere along the intrahepatic or extrahepatic biliary tree. The hepatic duct bifurcation is the site involved most frequently, and approximately 60% to 80% of cholangiocarcinomas encountered at tertiary referral centers are found in the perihilar region. Distal tumors are the second most common type, whereas purely intrahepatic cholangiocarcinomas occur with the lowest frequency. Approximately 3,000 new cases of cholangiocarcinoma are diagnosed annually in the United States, and these tumors occur with similar frequency in men and women. Practice guidelines for cholangiocarcinoma can be accessed through the NCCN Web site at www.nccn.org.

A number of diseases and environmental agents have been linked to cholangiocarcinoma, including primary sclerosing cholangitis, choledochal cysts, and hepatolithiasis. Factors common to a number of these etiologic factors include bile duct stones, biliary stasis, and infection. Multiple other risk factors for cholangiocarcinoma have been identified, including liver flukes, Thorotrast, dietary nitrosamines, and exposure to dioxin [40, 41].

Classification

Cholangiocarcinoma is classified best into three broad groups: intrahepatic, perihilar, and distal (Fig. 16.9) [45]. This classification correlates with anatomic distribution and implies the preferred treatment for each site. Intrahepatic tumors, like hepatocellular carcinoma, are treated with hepatectomy, when possible. Distal tumors are managed with pancreatoduodenectomy, as are other periampullary malignancies. The perihilar tumors make up the largest group and are managed with resection of the bile duct with or without hepatic resection.

Diagnosis and Staging

More than 90% of patients with perihilar or distal tumors present with jaundice. Intrahepatic cholangiocarcinomas, by definition, do not involve the major bile ducts, and patients are not jaundiced until late in the course of the disease. Less common presenting clinical

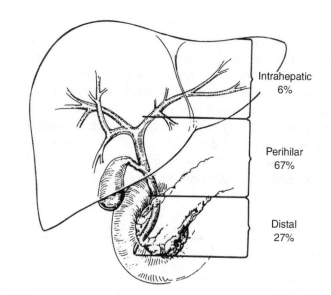

Figure 16.9 Distribution of 294 cholangiocarcinomas into intrahepatic, perihilar, and distal subgroups. (Reprinted with permission of Lippincott-Raven from A Nakeeb, HA Pitt, TA Sohn, et al., Cholangiocarcinoma: a spectrum of intrahepatic, perihilar, and distal tumors. *Ann Surg* 224:463–475, 1996.)

features include pruritus, fever, mild abdominal pain, fatigue, anorexia, and weight loss [40]. Cholangitis is not a frequent presenting finding but most commonly develops after cholangiography or placement of an endoscopic or percutaneous stent.

The initial radiographic evaluation in patients suspected of having a biliary tract cancer consists of either abdominal ultrasonography or CT scan. Intrahepatic cholangiocarcinomas are visualized easily on CT scans; however, visualizing perihilar tumors with standard CT scans often is difficult. A scan of a hilar cholangiocarcinoma will show a dilated intrahepatic biliary tree, a normal or collapsed gallbladder and extrahepatic biliary tree, and a normal pancreas. Distal tumors will lead to dilation of the gallbladder and both the intrahepatic and extrahepatic biliary tree [41].

After documentation of bile duct dilation, biliary anatomy has been defined traditionally by cholangiography variously through the percutaneous, transhepatic, or endoscopic retrograde routes. In patients with perihilar tumors, the most proximal extent of the tumor is the most important feature in determining resectability. Percutaneous cholangiography defines the proximal extent of tumor involvement most reliably [40]. Usually, ERCP demonstrates an obstructing lesion in the distal common bile duct and a normal pancreatic duct in patients with a distal cholangiocarcinoma. Recently, magnetic resonance cholangiopancreatography has documented diagnostic accuracy comparable to percutaneous and endoscopic cholangiography. The sensitivity, specificity, and overall accuracy of magnetic resonance cholangiopancreatography at determining the level of biliary obstruction and detecting the presence of a benign or malignant lesion are similar to that achieved with ERCP. MRI angiography, spiral CT, and conventional angiography all are useful for evaluating vascular involvement prior to planned resection. Prolonged efforts to establish a preoperative tissue diagnosis are not indicated unless affected patients are not surgical candidates.

Intrahepatic cholangiocarcinoma is staged according to the TNM staging system, liver being the primary site [53]. The stage classification depends on the size of the tumor (2 cm being the discriminating limit), number of tumors, lobar involvement, vascular invasion, invasion of adjacent organs, nodal involvement, and distant spread. The TNM staging system is used also for *extrahepatic* cholangiocarcinoma (Tables 16.10, 16.11) [54]. According to this system, stage I tumors are limited to the bile duct mucosa or muscular layer, whereas stage II tumors invade periductal tissues. Stage III tumors are associated with regional lymph node metastases, whereas stage IV tumors either invade adjacent structures (stage IVA) or involve distant metastases (stage IVB).

Management

Curative treatment of patients with cholangiocarcinoma is possible only with complete resection. The operative approach depends on the site and extent of the tumor. For patients with anatomically resectable intrahepatic cholangiocarcinoma and without advanced cirrhosis, partial hepatectomy is the procedure of choice [55]. Patients with perihilar tumors that involve the bifurcation or proximal common hepatic duct and have no vascular invasion are candidates for local tumor excision. Biliary-enteric continuity is restored with bilateral hepaticojejunostomies [40, 41, 56]. If preoperative evaluation suggests involvement of the right or left hepatic duct, right or left hepatic lobectomy, respectively, should be planned [56–58]. To achieve negative margins, resection of the adjacent caudate lobe may be required. For patients with resectable distal cholangiocarcinoma, pancreatoduodenectomy is the optimal procedure. This pylorus-preserving procedure can be performed safely, is an adequate cancer operation, and provides better quality of life than do more radical operations.

Surgical exploration should be undertaken in "low-risk" patients without evidence of metastatic or locally unresectable disease; however, intraoperatively, more

Table 16.10 TNM Staging for Cancer of the Extrahepatic Bile Ducts

Classification	Definition
Primary tumor (T)	
TX	Primary tumor cannot be assessed
T0	No evidence of primary tumor
Tis	Carcinoma in situ
T1	Tumor invades subepithelial connective tissue or fibromuscular layer
T1a	Tumor invades subepithelial connective tissue
T1b	Tumor invades fibromuscular layer
T2	Tumor invades perifibromuscular connective tissue
T3	Tumor invades adjacent structures: liver, pancreas, duodenum, gallbladder, colon, stomach
Regional lymph nodes (N)	
NX	Regional lymph nodes cannot be assessed
N0	No regional lymph node metastasis
N1	Metastasis in cystic duct, pericholedochal, and/or hilar lymph nodes (i.e., in the hepatoduodenal ligament)
N2	Metastasis in peripancreatic (head only), periduodenal, periportal, celiac, and/or superior mesenteric and/or posterior pancreaticoduodenal lymph nodes
Distant metastasis (M)	
MX	Distant metastasis cannot be assessed
M0	No distant metastasis
M1	Distant metastasis

Source: Used with permission of the American Joint Committee on Cancer (AJCC), Chicago, Illinois. Reprinted from ID Fleming, JS Cooper, DE Henson, et al. (eds), *AJCC Cancer Staging Manual* (5th ed). Philadelphia: Lippincott-Raven, 1997:109–113.

than half of such patients are found to have either peritoneal or hepatic metastases or, more likely, locally unresectable disease [40, 45]. In patients with locally advanced unresectable perihilar tumors, several operative approaches are available for palliation, including a Roux-en-Y choledochojejunostomy with intraoperative placement of Silastic biliary catheters or a segment III or V cholangiojejunostomy [41, 59]. Most distal bile duct tumors are resectable; if resection is not possible owing to vascular encasement, cholecystectomy, Roux-en-Y hepaticojejunostomy proximal to the tumor, and a gastrojejunostomy to prevent gastric outlet obstruction should be performed.

Patients with unequivocal evidence of unresectable cholangiocarcinoma at initial evaluation should receive nonoperative palliative care. Nonoperative palliation can be achieved both endoscopically and percutaneously. Percutaneous biliary drainage has several advantages over endoscopic management in patients with perihilar cholangiocarcinoma, whereas endoscopic palliation is the preferred approach in patients with distal cholangiocarcinoma [41]. More recently, metallic stents have been used to provide palliation in patients with malignant biliary obstruction. These stents remain patent longer than do plastic stents and require fewer subsequent manipulations [41].

Numerous reports have suggested that radiotherapy improves survival for patients with cholangiocarcinoma, especially when resection is impossible. External-beam radiotherapy has been delivered using a variety of innovative techniques, including intraoperative radiotherapy and brachytherapy with ^{192}Ir via percutaneous or endoscopic stents [40]. However, no prospective, randomized trials have been reported. A recent well-controlled but not randomized trial from the Johns Hopkins University reported no benefit for postoperative adjuvant radiotherapy (Fig. 16.10) [60]. Also, chemotherapy has not been shown to improve survival in patients with either resected or unresected cholangiocarcinoma. Given the potential radiosensitization effect of 5-fluorouracil, the combination of irradiation and chemotherapy may be more effective than either therapeutic modality is alone.

Table 16.11 AJCC Stage Grouping for Cancer of the Extrahepatic Bile Ducts

Stage 0	Tis	N0	M0
Stage I	T1	N0	M0
Stage II	T2	N0	M0
Stage III	T1	N1	M0
	T1	N2	M0
	T2	N1	M0
	T2	N2	M0
Stage IVA	T3	Any N	M0
Stage IVB	Any T	Any N	M1

AJCC = American Joint Committee on Cancer.
Source: Used with permission of the American Joint Committee on Cancer (AJCC), Chicago, Illinois. Reprinted from ID Fleming, JS Cooper, DE Henson, et al. (eds), *AJCC Cancer Staging Manual* (5th ed). Philadelphia: Lippincott-Raven, 1997:109–113.

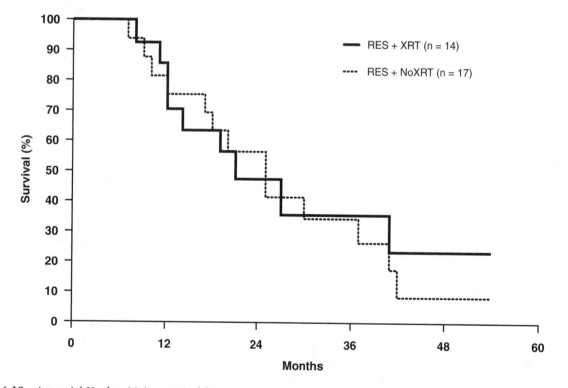

Figure 16.10 Actuarial Kaplan-Meier survival for patients who underwent resection (RES) for perihilar cholangiocarcinoma and did (*solid line;* n = 14) or did not (*dotted line;* n = 17) receive postoperative radiotherapy (XRT). (Reprinted with permission of Lippincott-Raven from HA Pitt, A Nakeeb, RA Abrams, et al. Perihilar cholangiocarcinoma: postoperative radiotherapy does not improve survival. *Ann Surg* 221:788–798, 1995.)

Long-term survival in patients with cholangiocarcinoma depends largely on the stage of disease at presentation and on whether such patients are treated by a palliative procedure or by complete tumor resection. For resectable intrahepatic cholangiocarcinoma, overall five-year survival ranges from 30% to 40% [41, 55]. In comparison, overall five-year survival for patients with resectable perihilar tumors has been only 10% to 20%, though it may be as high as 33% to 46% in patients with negative margins on microscopy [56–58]. Patients with distal bile duct cancer have the highest rate of resection. Those with resectable distal bile duct cancer experience a median survival of 32 to 38 months and a five-year survival rate of 28% to 45% [45]. Even with multimodality adjuvant therapy, median survival for unresectable intrahepatic tumors has been only six to seven months. Similarly, median survival for patients with unresectable perihilar tumors varies between five and eight months [59].

REFERENCES

1. Greenlee RT, Murray T, Bolden S, Wingo PA. Cancer statistics, 2000. *CA Cancer J Clin* 50:7–33, 2000.
2. Gold EB, Goldin S. Epidemiology of and risk factors for pancreatic cancer. *Surg Oncol Clin North Am* 7:67–91, 1998.
3. Evans DB, Abbruzzese JL, Rich TA. Cancer of the pancreas. In DeVita VT Jr, Hellman S, Rosenberg SA (eds), *Cancer: Principles and Practice of Oncology* (5th ed). Philadelphia: Lippincott-Raven, 1997:1054–1087.
4. Hruban RH, Petersen GM, Ha PK, Kern SE. Genetics of pancreatic cancer: from genes to families. *Surg Clin Oncol North Am* 7:1–23, 1998.
5. Caldas C, Hahn SA, Hruban RH, et al. Detection of *K-ras* mutations in the stool of patients with pancreatic adenocarcinoma and pancreatic ductal hyperplasia. *Cancer Res* 54:3568–3573, 1994.
6. Wilantz RE, Hruban RH. Pathology of cancer of the pancreas. *Surg Clin Oncol North Am* 7:43–65, 1998.
7. Brat DJ, Lillemoe KD, Yeo CJ, et al. Progression of pancreatic intraductal neoplasias to infiltrating adenocarcinoma of the pancreas. *Am J Surg Pathol* 22:163–169, 1998.
8. Bluemke DA, Fishman EK. CT and MR evaluation of pancreatic cancer. *Surg Clin Oncol North Am* 7:103–124, 1998.
9. Stevens PD, Lightdale CJ. The role of endosonography in the diagnosis and management of pancreatic cancer. *Surg Clin Oncol North Am* 7:125–133, 1998.
10. Ritts RE, Pitt HA. CA 19–9 in pancreatic cancer. *Surg Clin Oncol North Am* 7:93–101, 1998.
11. American Joint Committee on Cancer. Exocrine pancreas. In Fleming ID, Cooper JS, Henson DE, et al. (eds), *AJCC Cancer Staging Manual* (5th ed). Philadelphia: Lippincott-Raven, 1997:121–126.
12. Fernández-del Castillo C, Rattner DW, Warshaw AL. Further experience with laparoscopy and peritoneal cytology in staging for pancreatic cancer. *Br J Surg* 82:1127–1129, 1995.
13. Fernández-del Castillo C, Warshaw AL. Laparoscopic staging and peritoneal cytology. *Surg Clin Oncol North Am* 7:135–142, 1998.
14. Warshaw AL. Implications of peritoneal cytology for staging of early pancreatic cancer. *Am J Surg* 161:26–30, 1991.
15. Whipple AO, Parsons WB, Mullins S. Treatment of carcinoma of the ampulla of Vater. *Ann Surg* 102:763–779, 1935.
16. Yeo CJ, Cameron JL, Maher MM, et al. A prospective randomized trial of pancreaticogastrostomy versus pancreaticojejunostomy after pancreaticoduodenectomy. *Ann Surg* 222:580–592, 1995.
17. Yeo CJ. Pylorus-preserving pancreaticoduodenectomy. *Surg Clin Oncol North Am* 7:143–156, 1998.
18. Harrison LE, Brennan MF. Portal vein resection for pancreatic adenocarcinoma. *Surg Clin Oncol North Am* 7:165–181, 1998.
19. Yeo CJ, Cameron JL, Sohn TA, et al. Six hundred fifty consecutive pancreaticoduodenectomies in the 1990s. *Ann Surg* 226:248–260, 1997.
20. Leibermann MD, Kilburn H, Lindsey M, Brennan MF. Relation of perioperative deaths to hospital volumes among patients undergoing pancreatic resection for malignancy. *Ann Surg* 222:638–645, 1995.
21. Yeo CJ, Barry MK, Sauter PK, et al. Erythromycin accelerates gastric emptying after pancreaticoduodenectomy: a prospective, randomized, placebo-controlled trial. *Ann Surg* 218:229–238, 1993.
22. Bell RH Jr. Neoplasms of the endocrine pancreas. In Greenfield LJ, Mulholland M, Oldham KT, et al. (eds), *Surgery: Scientific Principles and Practice.* Philadelphia: Lippincott-Raven, 1997:901–918.
23. Yeo CJ, Cameron JL, Lillemoe KD, et al. Pancreaticoduodenectomy for cancer of the head of the pancreas: 201 patients. *Ann Surg* 221:721–733, 1995.
24. Kalser MH, Ellenberg SS. Pancreatic cancer. Adjuvant combined radiation and chemotherapy following curative resection of pancreatic cancer. *Arch Surg* 120:889–903, 1985.
25. Gastrointestinal Tumor Study Group. Further evidence of effective adjuvant combined radiation and chemotherapy following curative resection of pancreatic cancer. *Cancer* 59:2006–2010, 1987.
26. Yeo CJ, Abrams RA, Grochow LB, et al. Pancreaticoduodenectomy for pancreatic adenocarcinoma: postoperative adjuvant chemoradiation improves survival. *Ann Surg* 225:621–636, 1997.
27. Demeure MD, Doffek KM, Komorowski RA, et al. Molecular metastases in stage I pancreatic cancer: improved survival with adjuvant chemoradiation. *Surgery* 124:663–669, 1998.
28. Lillemoe KD. Palliative therapy for pancreatic cancer. *Surg Clin Oncol North Am* 7:199–216, 1998.
29. Lillemoe KD, Cameron JL, Hardacre JM, et al. Is prophylactic gastrojejunostomy indicated for unresectable periampullary cancer? A prospective randomized trial. *Ann Surg* 230:322–328, 1999.
30. Lillemoe KD, Cameron JL, Kaufmann HS, et al. Chemical

splanchnicectomy in patients with unresectable pancreatic cancer: a prospective randomized trial. *Ann Surg* 217:447–457, 1993.

31. Lillemoe KD, Cameron JL, Yeo CJ, et al. Pancreaticoduodenectomy: Does it have a role in the palliation of pancreatic cancer? *Ann Surg* 223:718–728, 1996.

32. Fraker DL, Jensen RT. Pancreatic endocrine tumors. In DeVita VT Jr, Hellman S, Rosenberg SA (eds), *Cancer: Principles and Practice of Oncology*. Philadelphia: Lippincott-Raven, 1997:1678–1704.

33. Wayne JD, Tanaka R, Kaplan EL. Insulinomas. In Clark OH, Duh QY (eds), *Textbook of Endocrine Surgery*. Philadelphia: Saunders, 1997:577–591.

34. Doppman JL, Chang R, Fraker DL, et al. Localization of insulinomas to regions of the pancreas by intra-arterial stimulation with calcium. *Ann Intern Med* 123:269–273, 1995.

35. Wilson SD. Gastrinoma. In Clark OH, Duh QY (eds), *Textbook of Endocrine Surgery*. Philadelphia: Saunders, 1997: 607–618.

36. Yeo CJ. Neoplasms of the endocrine pancreas. In Greenfield LJ, Mulholland M, Oldham KT, et al. (eds), *Surgery: Scientific Principles and Practice* (2nd ed). Philadelphia: Lippincott-Raven, 1997:918–929.

37. Passaro E Jr, Howard TJ, Sawicki MP, et al. The origin of sporadic gastrinomas within the gastrinoma triangle. *Arch Surg* 133:13–16, 1998.

38. Fraker DL, Norton JA, Alexander HR, et al. Surgery in Zollinger-Ellison syndrome alters the natural history of gastrinoma. *Ann Surg* 220:320–330, 1994.

39. Norton JA. Somatostatinoma and rare pancreatic endocrine tumors. In Clark OH, Duh QY (eds), *Textbook of Endocrine Surgery*. Philadelphia: Saunders, 1997:626–633.

40. Pitt HA, Dooley WC, Yeo CJ, Cameron JC. Malignancies of the biliary tree. *Curr Probl Surg* 32:1–90,1995.

41. Ahrendt SA, Pitt HA. Malignant diseases of the biliary tract. In Morris PJ, Wood WC (eds), *Oxford Textbook of Surgery*. Oxford: Oxford University Press, 2001. (In press).

42. Carriaga MT, Henson DE. Liver, gallbladder, extrahepatic bile ducts, and pancreas. *Cancer* 75:171–190, 1995.

43. Shirai Y, Yoshida K, Tsukada K, et al. Identification of the regional lymphatic system of the gallbladder by vital staining. *Br J Surg* 79:659–662, 1992.

44. White K, Kraybill WG, Lopez MJ. Primary carcinoma of the gallbladder: TNM staging and prognosis. *J Surg Oncol* 39:251–255, 1988.

45. Nakeeb A, Pitt HA, Sohn TA, et al. Cholangiocarcinoma: a spectrum of intrahepatic, perihilar, and distal tumors. *Ann Surg* 224:463–475, 1996.

46. American Joint Committee on Cancer. Gallbladder. In Fleming ID, Cooper JS, Henson DE, et al. (eds), *AJCC Cancer Staging Manual* (5th ed). Philadelphia: Lippincott-Raven, 1997:103–108.

47. Shirai Y, Yoshida K, Tsukada K, Muto T. Inapparent carcinoma of the gallbladder: an appraisal of a radical second operation after simple cholecystectomy. *Ann Surg* 215: 326–331, 1992.

48. Ogura Y, Mizumoto R, Isaji S, et al. Radical operations for carcinoma of the gallbladder: present status in Japan. *World J Surg* 15:337–343, 1991.

49. Gebbia V, Majello E, Testa A, et al. Treatment of advanced adenocarcinomas of the exocrine pancreas and the gallbladder with 5-fluorouracil, high-dose levofolinic acid and oral hydroxyurea on a weekly schedule. *Cancer* 78: 1300–1307, 1996.

50. Donohue JH, Stewart AK, Menck HR. The National Cancer Data Base report on carcinoma of the gallbladder, 1989–1995. *Cancer* 83:2618–2628, 1998.

51. Tsukada K, Hatakeyama K, Kurosaki I, et al. Outcome of radical surgery for carcinoma of the gallbladder according to the TNM stage. *Surgery* 120:816–822, 1996.

52. Bartlett DL, Fong Y, Fortner JG, et al. Long-term results after resection for gallbladder cancer: implications for staging and management. *Ann Surg* 224:639–646, 1996.

53. American Joint Committee on Cancer. Liver (including intrahepatic bile ducts). In Fleming ID, Cooper JS, Henson DE, et al. (eds), *AJCC Cancer Staging Manual* (5th ed). Philadelphia: Lippincott-Raven, 1997:97–101.

54. American Joint Committee on Cancer. Extrahepatic bile ducts. In Fleming ID, Cooper JS, Henson DE, et al. (eds), *AJCC Cancer Staging Manual* (5th ed). Philadelphia: Lippincott-Raven, 1997:109–113.

55. Casavilla FA, Marsh JW, Iwatsuki S, et al. Hepatic resection and transplantation for peripheral cholangiocarcinoma. *J Am Coll Surg* 185:429–436, 1997.

56. Ahrendt SA, Cameron JL, Pitt HA. Current management of patients with perihilar cholangiocarcinoma. *Adv Surg* 30:427–452, 1996.

57. Sugiura Y, Nakamura S, Iida S, et al. Extensive resection of the bile ducts combined with liver resection for cancer of the main hepatic duct junction: a cooperative study of the Keio Bile Duct Cancer Study Group. *Surgery* 115:445–451, 1994.

58. Klempnauer J, Ridder GJ, von Wasielewski R, et al. Resectional surgery of hilar cholangiocarcinoma: a multivariate analysis of prognostic factors. *J Clin Oncol* 15:947–954, 1997.

59. Nordback IH, Pitt HA, Coleman JA, et al. Unresectable hilar cholangiocarcinoma: percutaneous versus operative palliation. *Surgery* 115:597–603, 1994.

60. Pitt HA, Nakeeb A, Abrams RA, et al. Perihilar cholangiocarcinoma: postoperative radiotherapy does not improve survival. *Ann Surg* 221:788–798, 1995.

17

Liver Cancer

■ ■ ■

Rohan J. H. Hammett
John L. Gollan

PRIMARY MALIGNANT TUMORS OF THE LIVER are relatively rare in North America and western Europe, although they are common in areas of the world where hepatitis viral infection is endemic (e.g., Africa and Asia). Indeed, primary liver cancer is the fifth most common cancer worldwide, accounting for 5.4% of new cancer cases each year [1]. In contrast, hepatic metastases are much more common, arising most commonly from carcinomas of the breast, lung, and gastrointestinal tract.

The initial aim in evaluating hepatic neoplasms is to distinguish among a primary malignant tumor of the liver, a primary benign tumor, and metastatic disease. Although a number of other tumors can arise within the liver (e.g., cholangiocarcinoma, hemangiosarcoma), this chapter concentrates on hepatocellular carcinoma (HCC) and the common metastatic carcinomas, particularly those responsive to treatment.

HEPATOCELLULAR CARCINOMA
Incidence

In the United States, an estimated 7,000 new cases of primary liver cancer occur annually [2]. This incidence equates to 3.23 cases per 100,000 population, a figure significantly higher in the developing world. In China, for example, the incidence is as high as 35.84 cases per 100,000; in Central Africa, it is 28.38 cases per 100,000 [1, 2]. The prevalence as determined at autopsy varies from 0.15% to 0.69% in the United States but is substantially higher in sub-Saharan Africa and parts of Asia. The incidence at autopsy is 1.8% in Uganda but as high as 20% in Ethiopia. In these countries, primary carcinoma of the liver may account for 10% to 50% of all malignancies. This wide geographic variation probably reflects the relative prevalence of chronic hepatitis B and C infections, acquired either through vertical transmission (mother to newborn) or during the early neonatal period.

Though the incidence of HCC rises steadily with age, primary carcinoma of the liver affects a greater proportion of young persons than do most other carcinomas. In the United States, Asia, and western Europe, HCC typically occurs in middle age or later. In Africa, the disease is seen predominantly among young adults and persons in early middle age.

Etiologic Factors

CHRONIC HEPATITIS B INFECTION

Epidemiologic studies have established a close association between chronic hepatitis B virus (HBV) infection and HCC. Indeed, this virus may be the primary carcinogen in up to 80% of patients with the tumor worldwide. One prospective study in Taiwan found that among chronic carriers of HBV, the risk for HCC was 200 times that of noncarriers and that their long-term risk for development of HCC was approximately 50% [3]. Several large, prospective case-control studies have demonstrated a high relative risk of HCC in patients positive for the hepatitis B surface antigen. Although the mechanism by which chronic HBV infection leads to carcinoma of the liver is still unclear, viral DNA has been found integrated into the host genome in tumor and nontumor tissues in patients with HCC.

CHRONIC HEPATITIS C INFECTION

The ability to detect antibodies to hepatitis C virus (HCV) has enabled researchers to study the role of HCV infection in liver diseases, including HCC. Case studies, cohort studies, and case-control studies support an epidemiologic relationship between HCV infection and HCC [4, 5]. The degree of association varies, depending on the geographic area; the highest association is found in such locations as western Europe and Japan, where the prevalence of HBV is relatively low and the rates of HCV infection are high. The mechanism by which HCV causes HCC also is unclear, but it probably differs from that of HBV, because HCV is an RNA virus and thus cannot be integrated into the host genome. Some researchers have proposed that HCV is associated with carcinoma of the liver in the setting of cirrhosis, a disease that is common in patients with HCV infection and HCC. What should be noted, however, is that HCC has been demonstrated in noncirrhotic patients with HCV.

CIRRHOSIS

Cirrhosis is an independent risk factor for development of HCC. Between 60% and 90% of patients with HCC also have cirrhosis, the level of risk depending on the degree of hepatic fibrosis and the underlying etiology of the cirrhosis. Eventually, primary liver cell carcinoma develops in 2% to 3% of patients with alcoholic cirrhosis and in an estimated 3% to 10% of patients with the macronodular (posthepatic) cirrhosis due to chronic HBV infection. On average, the risk for HCC is approximately 40 times greater in persons with cirrhosis than in those whose liver is normal.

Cirrhosis due to alpha$_1$-antitrypsin deficiency and other inborn errors of metabolism (e.g., tyrosinemia) also is associated with an increased incidence of HCC. HCC occurs in 10% to 22% of patients with hemochromatosis and cirrhosis, even in those treated with phlebotomy, and has been reported in patients without cirrhosis [6]. Earlier recognition of hemochromatosis and prevention of HCC are anticipated as a result of the recent discovery of the gene responsible for hemochromatosis and the availability of definitive genetic testing. Interestingly, carcinoma of the liver is relatively rare in patients with cirrhosis associated with Wilson's disease.

CARCINOGENS

Many environmental carcinogens have been implicated in the development of HCC. Aflatoxins, nitrosamines, azo-compounds (aminoazotoluene, paradimethyl aminoazobenzene), methylcholanthrene, acetyl aminofluorene, senecio alkaloids, and cycasin variously have been shown to cause this type of carcinoma in experimental animals. Aflatoxin B is the most potent of the known hepatocarcinogens and, unlike the other compounds mentioned, its presence in foodstuffs may cause human HCC in some areas in which the disease is endemic (e.g., Africa, China). The radiographic contrast agent Thorotrast has been associated with the development of hepatic angiosarcoma, although not with the development of HCC. Such hormones as androgens have also been implicated in tumorigenesis. Though the synthetic hormones used in oral contraceptives have been associated with benign liver tumors (e.g., focal nodular hyperplasia and hepatic adenoma), no association with HCC has been proved. Usually, the benign neoplasms associated with the use of these hormones regress on withdrawal of the hormonal agent.

Table 17.1 TNM Staging for Liver Cancer

Classification	Definition
Primary tumor (T)	
TX	Primary tumor cannot be assessed
T0	No evidence of primary tumor
T1	Solitary tumor ≤ 2 cm in greatest dimension without vascular invasion
T2	Solitary tumor ≤ 2 cm in greatest dimension without vascular invasion, or multiple tumors limited to one lobe, none > 2 cm in greatest dimension without vascular invasion, or a solitary tumor > 2 cm in greatest dimension without vascular invasion
T3	Solitary tumor > 2 cm in greatest dimension with vascular invasion, or multiple tumors limited to one lobe, none > 2 cm in greatest dimension, with vascular invasion, or multiple tumors limited to one lobe, any > 2 cm in greatest dimension, with or without vascular invasion
T4	Multiple tumors in more than one lobe or tumor(s) involve(s) a major branch of the portal or hepatic vein(s) or invasion of adjacent organs other than the gallbladder or perforation of the visceral peritoneum
Regional lymph nodes (N)	
NX	Regional lymph nodes cannot be assessed
N0	No regional lymph node metastasis
N1	Regional lymph node metastasis
Distant metastasis (M)	
MX	Distant metastasis cannot be assessed
M0	No distant metastasis
M1	Distant metastasis

Source: Used with permission of the American Joint Committee on Cancer (AJCC), Chicago, Illinois. Reprinted from ID Fleming, JS Cooper, DE Henson, et al. (eds), *AJCC Cancer Staging Manual* (5th ed). Philadelphia: Lippincott-Raven, 1997:97–99.

Pathologic Features

The major types of primary carcinoma in the liver are HCC and cholangiocarcinoma, which occur in a ratio of approximately 12:1. Fibrolamellar HCC, a recently described subtype that occurs in younger noncirrhotic patients, is associated with a survival rate higher than that of the other types of HCC. Hepatoblastoma, seen in infancy and childhood, has distinct pathologic and clinical characteristics. When diagnosed early, this tumor usually is unifocal, resectable, and highly curable. The presence of large-cell dysplasia in liver biopsy and surgical specimens has been shown to be predictive of development of HCC in some series.

Diagnosis and Staging

STAGING

The American Joint Committee on Cancer has classified HCC according to the TNM (*t*umor, *n*ode, *m*etastasis) staging system (Tables 17.1, 17.2) [7].

Table 17.2 AJCC Stage Grouping for Liver Cancer

Stage	T	N	M
Stage I	T1	N0	M0
Stage II	T2	N0	M0
Stage IIIA	T3	N0	M0
Stage IIIB	T1	N1	M0
	T2	N1	M0
	T3	N1	M0
Stage IVA	T4	Any N	M0
Stage IVB	Any T	Any N	M1

AJCC = American Joint Committee on Cancer.
Source: Used with permission of the American Joint Committee on Cancer (AJCC), Chicago, Illinois. Reprinted from ID Fleming, JS Cooper, DE Henson, et al. (eds), *AJCC Cancer Staging Manual* (5th ed). Philadelphia: Lippincott-Raven, 1997:96–99.

DIFFERENTIAL DIAGNOSIS

A mass in the liver may be a benign or a malignant primary tumor, a metastatic tumor, or a cyst. Metastatic tumors are by far the most common and are confirmed best by the identification of a tumor at the primary site. Benign tumors are not uncommon and have been recognized much more frequently since the advent of routine ultrasonography and scanning procedures. Cysts, either developmental or parasitic in origin, are diagnosed readily by ultrasonography or computed tomography (CT).

Hamartomas of the bile duct seldom are larger than 2 cm, may be multiple, and present few problems except that they are understandably mistaken for metastatic disease when the liver is examined during laparotomy. Hepatic adenomas, which occur most often in young women who take oral contraceptives, are rare. Usually, they are solitary and may present as a mass lesion or may be seen in conjunction with intraperitoneal hemorrhage. Although such tumors may require resection, smaller adenomas in patients on oral contraceptives usually will regress once these drugs are discontinued. Occasionally, multiple adenomas are found, raising the possibility of metastatic disease or a multicentric HCC. A potential, albeit low-grade, risk of malignant transformation of large adenomas exists, and surgical resection often is indicated in this setting.

Focal nodular hyperplasia is relatively common and is observed in both genders and over a wide age range. This condition is associated less strongly with the use of oral contraceptives than are hepatic adenomas. Hyperplastic lesions, which seldom bleed spontaneously and do not become malignant, have a characteristic angiographic pattern and often are highly vascular and poorly demarcated. Surgery rarely is indicated for focal nodular hyperplasia unless operative biopsy is required to make the diagnosis.

CLINICAL FEATURES

In more than 80% of patients, HCC is symptomatic at the time of diagnosis. The most common symptoms are right upper abdominal pain, weight loss, anorexia, and malaise. Sometimes, fever of unknown origin is noted. A sudden deterioration in liver function or clinical status (i.e., increased ascites or abdominal pain) occurs in 30% of cirrhotic patients with superimposed HCC. Occasionally, the presentation is dramatic, with severe abdominal pain and life-threatening hypotension when the tumor ruptures through the liver capsule, resulting in hemoperitoneum. Rarely, patients present with evidence of metastatic disease, including pulmonary changes, bone pain, or bleeding from the gastrointestinal tract. In approximately 10% of patients, HCC remains undetected and is an incidental finding at autopsy.

PHYSICAL EXAMINATION

Frequently, some or all of the usual peripheral stigmata of chronic liver disease (jaundice, palmar erythema,

Dupuytren's contractures, parotid enlargement, spider nevi, gynecomastia, splenomegaly, and testicular atrophy) occur in the majority of HCC patients. However, the most striking physical finding heralding the development of HCC in patients with known chronic liver disease is that of tender hepatomegaly or a palpable discrete hepatic mass. One or both of these signs are evident in 30% to 40% of patients with HCC. The signs of portal hypertension secondary to portal vein obstruction (ascites, caput medusa, and splenomegaly) may be the presenting features but more usually appear late in the course of the disease. Ascites is unusual in patients with noncirrhotic HCC.

LABORATORY INVESTIGATIONS

The goals in the initial laboratory evaluation are (1) to distinguish primary liver cell cancer from a benign liver tumor or metastatic carcinoma, (2) to assess the extent of the tumor, and (3) to assess the residual liver function. Diagnosis is based on a careful history and physical examination, together with laboratory findings, radiologic investigation, and pathologic confirmation. Most patients with advanced disease are anemic, but polycythemia occasionally is seen. Usually, liver function tests show a mixed pattern: elevation of serum levels of bilirubin, alkaline phosphatase, and aspartate aminotransferase. Leukocytosis, erythrocytosis, hypercalcemia, and hypoglycemia are common, but nonspecific, findings.

Serum alpha-fetoprotein (AFP) is elevated in 30% to 40% of patients with primary carcinoma of the liver, but it may be elevated also in low titer in the presence of testicular, ovarian, gastric, pancreatic, and pulmonary malignant tumors, especially when the liver contains a large metastatic tumor. Although AFP levels are high also during pregnancy and in cirrhosis (indicative of regeneration), levels in excess of 500 ng/dl in adults strongly suggest the presence of HCC.

RADIOLOGIC STUDIES

Ultrasonography and intravenous contrast–enhanced CT have been the main imaging modalities for the diagnosis of lesions of the liver. Spiral CT, which allows rapid acquisition of images after the injection of a bolus of iodinated contrast medium, achieves a sensitivity of 90% in detecting lesions of the liver. It has the advantage of being less operator-dependent than ultrasonography but is not as effective at evaluating portal venous involvement. Currently, therefore, ultrasonography is the diagnostic procedure of choice for screening hepatic tumors. Recent advances in magnetic resonance imaging (MRI) have rendered it the diagnostic tool of choice in centers with access to sufficiently sophisticated equipment and software. It has been shown to be more sensitive than helical CT in small series published to date [8, 9].

Differentiation among HCC, benign liver tumors, and metastatic lesions may require the use of a combination of CT, MRI, arteriography, and nuclear medicine scans. The use of these modalities relies on the fact that most primary liver neoplasms are hypervascular, whereas most metastatic lesions are relatively hypovascular. Lipiodol, an iodinated contrast agent containing poppy seed oil, also is useful in identifying small tumor nodules on CT, because it is retained selectively by tumor vessels over time.

Radiography of the chest, CT of the chest, abdomen, and pelvis, portal venography, and bone scanning are performed selectively (as indicated) to assess the extent of local disease and possible distant metastases. Preoperative percutaneous biopsy to establish the pathologic diagnosis is not advised for patients with a resectable hepatic tumor for which surgery is planned, as bleeding complications and seeding of the biopsy tract with tumor cells have been reported [10]. In patients who are not surgical candidates or who are thought to have focal nodular hyperplasia, percutaneous biopsy of the liver lesion may be indicated when the pathologic diagnosis would change the management approach.

Screening

Screening for primary carcinoma of the liver presents a difficult problem. In the United States, because the tumor is uncommon and seldom produces early symptoms, the yield of widespread screening programs is likely to be very low. However, in many parts of the world with a high incidence of HCC, current resources are insufficient to offer generalized screening programs.

Researchers had hoped that serum testing for AFP or other tumor markers would provide a relatively inexpensive, accurate screening test for HCC. AFP may be present in the serum of patients with primary carcinoma of the liver up to 18 months before symptoms develop; however, in the United States and Europe, only approximately 30% of patients with HCC have elevated AFP levels. In contrast, in parts of Africa, AFP levels are elevated in up to 75% of patients with HCC. Serum AFP is possibly the cheapest and most readily available screening tool available for use in the developing world, but it has substantial limitations. In the

United States, serum AFP levels are more useful as a surveillance tool in select patients at high risk for HCC or as an indicator of recurrence after surgical resection.

In addition to AFP, ultrasonography may be useful in diagnosing asymptomatic HCC in populations at risk. However, equipment costs and operator variability have limited the widespread application of this modality in the developing world.

Current clinical practice, which notably is not rooted in an evidence-based approach, is to use ultrasonography and serum AFP every 4 to 12 months to screen patients at higher-than-average risk for tumor development. Candidates for this approach include patients with cirrhosis from chronic HBV or HCV infection or hemochromatosis. The use of CT, MRI, or hepatic angiography has been reported in screening programs in high-risk patient populations. To date, no data suggest that any of these methods of screening alters rates of mortality from HCC.

Treatment

SURGICAL EXPLORATION AND RESECTION

Only 15% to 30% of patients with HCC are candidates for surgery. After a thorough diagnostic workup, patients who have limited primary carcinoma of the liver, adequate liver function, and no obvious metastases should undergo surgical exploration. Surgical exploration is the most definitive means of determining resectability. Conditions that render carcinoma of the liver unresectable are extensive disease within the organ itself and distant intraabdominal and extraabdominal metastases. Large tumor size, bilobar involvement, and the presence of cirrhosis do not necessarily preclude resection but do adversely affect operative mortality and prognosis. In noncirrhotic patients, adequate liver function can be maintained as long as one-fifth of the liver remains after resection. In the United States, resection generally is limited to patients with small peripheral lesions and preserved hepatic function, with transplantation as an option in patients with unresectable disease but no distant metastases and in those with well-established cirrhosis.

The presence or absence of cirrhosis is the main determinant of morbidity and mortality after hepatic resection [11]. In Western countries, more than 60% of patients with HCC do not have underlying cirrhosis. Cirrhotic patients should be evaluated carefully to assess liver reserve preoperatively, using a combination of liver histology, laboratory measures of hepatic synthetic function, and dynamic nuclear medicine studies that estimate hepatic metabolic function. If reserve is adequate, resection can be performed safely, and as much liver as possible should be retained. With earlier detection of small-sized tumors, less extensive segmental and subsegmental resections can be performed. Preoperative chemoembolization may be used in patients with larger tumors to allow resection.

Overall, the reported five-year cure rate for all HCC patients who have undergone hepatic resection is approximately 30%, although some centers have reported higher survival rates with combination therapy in small series of patients [12]. Operative mortality is approximately 1% for noncirrhotic patients and 10% for those with cirrhosis. When resection is not possible, palliative treatment is in order, including hepatic artery ligation or embolization in combination with radiotherapy, chemotherapy, or both (modalities discussed in further detail later).

The role of liver transplantation in patients with HCC remains controversial. Although liver transplantation has been performed in patients with unresectable HCC confined to the liver, malignant tumor usually recurs in transplanted livers within 6 to 24 months. In general, patients with tumors larger than 3 cm or with more than three nodules of tumor in the liver do poorly after transplantation. Orthotopic liver transplantation has demonstrated a survival benefit in selected patients and is advocated as first-line therapy by some groups. A role for adjuvant therapy remains to be established for patients undergoing liver transplantation. The generally poor long-term results and the lack of availability of donor livers has limited the use of transplantation for HCC in the last decade [13].

LOCAL ABLATIVE THERAPY

Recent years have seen the emergence of local ablative therapy as a primary treatment modality in patients with poor hepatic reserve. In particular, percutaneous ethanol injection (PEI) and transhepatic arterial chemoembolization have emerged as realistic alternatives to surgery in selected patients. The fact that HCCs derive their blood supply from the hepatic artery has led to the use of intraarterial devices aimed at delivering drugs directly to the tumor, with the purpose of reducing systemic toxicity. Hepatic artery infusion of 5-fluorouracil (5-FU) and fluorodeoxyuridine (FUDR) with or without doxorubicin and methotrexate has been used most frequently. This combination can be administered either directly via a surgically placed catheter or through a percutaneous catheter via the left brachial artery. Mitomycin C and interferon-α also have been used. The intraarterial catheter is attached to a portable pumping device that infuses any agent continuously; in some instances, an implanted pump or reservoir has been employed.

A recent advance in local ablative therapy has been the suspension of chemotherapeutic agents in lipidol to promote selective, prolonged retention by tumor tissue. Response rates have ranged from 50% to 70%; median survival time is 12 to 16 months in patients who responded to treatment. However, serious side effects of FUDR—including cirrhosis, narrowing of the bile duct (resembling primary sclerosing cholangitis), progressive liver atrophy, and hepatic failure—may occur with this mode of therapy. In addition, postembolization syndrome—characterized by abdominal pain, vomiting, and fever—occurs after almost every procedure, limiting patient tolerance. Three randomized trials have failed to confirm the survival benefits from chemoembolization reported in early nonrandomized trials. Regional infusions of new drugs used in combination with other treatment modalities (e.g., Gelfoam embolization, internal radiotherapy, or hepatic artery ligation) may be useful [14]. Additional clinical studies are required to improve patient selection and delivery techniques to evaluate fully the safety and efficacy of these approaches.

PEI has been shown to have response rates similar to those of surgical resection in patients with small tumors (< 5 cm) and is advocated as first-line therapy in patients who have small lesions and are not good operative candidates. Advances in radiologic techniques have made this a favored, minimally invasive therapeutic option. It is safer than surgery (0% mortality), is cheaper, and results in equivalent long-term survival. The other advantage it has over surgery is that it can be used repeatedly to treat intrahepatic recurrence without increasing patient risk. It has fewer side effects than those of chemoembolization and, although no direct comparative studies have been performed, is reported to be more efficacious. PEI has been used as primary therapy or as part of a combination treatment regimen involving chemotherapy and surgery. A recent study has shown that percutaneous injection of acetic acid may be even more effective than is ethanol, although these data require confirmation [15]. The five-year survival rate for patients who have HCC smaller than 5 cm and are undergoing PEI approaches 50% [16].

PEI, cryosurgery, isolated hepatic artery perfusion, interstitial radiofrequency ablation, and radioimmunotherapy variously have been used with limited success for palliation [17]. Studies already under way are aimed at further defining the role of these therapies in specific stages of HCC.

RADIOTHERAPY

Usually, the value of radiotherapy is limited in treating HCC, because the liver normally can tolerate only 2,500 or 3,000 cGy of irradiation. However, irradiation of the liver, either alone or combined with chemotherapy, occasionally can provide palliation of pain for six to eight months. Brachytherapy has been shown to be useful in palliation of selected patients who have cholangiocarcinoma with biliary obstruction, but no survival benefit has been proved [18].

SYSTEMIC CHEMOTHERAPY

Although systemic chemotherapy is palliative, patients who respond to systemic chemotherapy occasionally will survive 9 to 12 months longer than would be expected. Use of chemotherapy is limited by affected patients' underlying hepatic function. A number of trials have been conducted to establish effective chemotherapy for patients with HCC. With regard to single agents, doxorubicin was found to be most effective (response rate, 19%). Many studies have evaluated the effects of antimetabolites (e.g., 5-FU, FUDR, and methotrexate). 5-FU has yielded response rates of 0% to 15% when used in a manner similar to that for gastrointestinal malignancies. Other agents, including cisplatin, mitomycin C, etoposide, and ifosfamide, appear to lack significant antitumor activity. Combination chemotherapy has not been proved to be more effective than single agents.

The median survival for patients receiving systemic chemotherapy is approximately five months (1- and 2-year survival rates = 27% and 8%, respectively). Owing to the poor results of chemotherapy, a number of authors have advocated including in phase II trials of newer agents all patients undergoing chemotherapy, in the hope that a useful regimen will be identified. No definitive recommendation regarding the optimal drug regimen can be made from the data currently available, and clinical practice will vary with local expertise.

HORMONAL THERAPY

The presence of male and female sex hormone receptors on HCC cells and evidence of hormone respon-

siveness in experimental tumor growth have prompted investigations of hormonal manipulation for palliation in HCC patients. Estrogen receptors are present in approximately 30% of patients; however, to date several small studies have provided conflicting data regarding the effects of antiestrogens such as tamoxifen on survival in HCC. A meta-analysis of tamoxifen use in HCC showed a survival benefit, although the two largest randomized trials showed no such benefits [19]. Further studies to define the role of tamoxifen are nearing completion. Antiandrogenic compounds, progestins, and luteinizing hormone–releasing hormone agonists have been shown to be ineffective in treating HCC.

IMMUNOMODULATION

The definition of the roles of immunity and immune modification in the treatment of disease continues. In the treatment of HCC, preliminary studies have reported the use of lymphokine-activated killer cells, interleukin-2, interferon-α, and antibody-targeted radioisotopes. The therapeutic value, cost-effectiveness, and feasibility of these treatments are under investigation, although early results do not appear promising.

Prognosis

Cure and long-term survival are possible only when tumors can be resected completely. Resectability rates associated with HCC have been reported to be approximately 30% in adults and 40% in children, whereas 80% of hepatoblastomas in children are resectable. Currently available radiologic and laboratory investigative techniques should contribute to earlier detection of small-sized tumors; in turn, such early detection might contribute to a higher resectability rate and better overall prognosis. This theory remains to be proved in controlled trials.

Typically, median survival for patients with unresected tumors is three to four months. Progression of the disease is characterized by cachexia, gastrointestinal or intraperitoneal bleeding, and hepatic coma. Some one-third of patients show direct extension of the tumor into the extrahepatic portal vein, accompanied by thrombosis, portal hypertension, varices, and gastrointestinal bleeding. Less often, patients have hepatic vein thrombosis with the clinical features of the Budd-Chiari syndrome (ascites, hepatomegaly, and right-upper-quadrant tenderness). Metastases are primarily to the lung but may involve also the regional lymph nodes, adrenal glands, bone, kidneys, heart, pancreas, and stomach.

Posttreatment Monitoring

Because approximately 70% of patients with resected tumors will have pulmonary metastases later, radiography of the chest at regular intervals may be used to reveal such spread. The other common site of recurrence is the liver, and periodic CT or MRI should permit early detection of hepatic metastases. Liver failure or the development of a new mass constitutes obvious evidence of a recurrence; a more subtle sign is an elevated serum AFP, although normal levels after surgery do not necessarily preclude metastasis. The optimal treatment for recurrent lesions has not yet been determined.

METASTATIC CARCINOMA OF THE LIVER

A metastatic neoplasm is the most common malignant disease of the liver in the United States. Most hepatic metastases derive from primary malignant neoplasms of the colon, pancreas, breast, ovaries, rectum, and stomach. Metastases reach the liver by four routes: portal vein, lymphatic channels, hepatic artery, and direct extension. Usually, liver metastases are found either at diagnosis of the primary lesion or within the following two years. The extent of liver involvement is an important factor in affected patients' prognosis. The mean survival of patients with minimal disease is perhaps 16 months, as compared with three months for patients with advanced disease.

Diagnosis

Hepatic metastases may be discovered in asymptomatic patients during surgical resection of a primary lesion or during staging for curative surgery. Usually, symptomatic patients present with constitutional symptoms (malaise, fever, weight loss, and anorexia), a palpable mass, or pain in the right upper abdominal quadrant (often dull, constant, and not well localized). Although jaundice usually appears late in the disease, it may occur early if hilar ductal obstruction occurs.

Serologic testing may reveal elevated levels of serum alkaline phosphatase and aspartate aminotransferase. Often, arteriography or magnetic resonance angiogra-

phy (currently used to define the vascular anatomy for hepatic resection or catheter placement for regional infusion treatment) fails to detect small metastases. Ultrasonography, CT, and MRI are the procedures most useful for detecting liver metastasis. Over the last five years, new imaging modalities have increased to 85% to 90% the sensitivity of screening for hepatic tumors. These modalities include sequential dynamic bolus CT, delayed iodine CT, CT angiography, CT arterial portography, magnetic resonance cholangiopancreatography, and intraoperative ultrasonography.

Treatment

SURGERY

Surgical resection of liver metastases may be beneficial in treating tumors of colorectal origin and selected other primary sites, including sarcoma, Wilms' tumor, ocular melanoma, and neuroendocrine tumors of the gastrointestinal tract. In general, resection should be undertaken only when all hepatic lesions can be removed with tumor-free margins and when no demonstrable extrahepatic disease is present. One notable exception to this rule is liver metastases from neuroendocrine tumors, for which debulking without complete excision may be performed for palliation of symptoms. Hepatic lobectomy is unnecessary when metastases can be excised by wedge resection. The operative mortality associated with hepatic resection for metastases is approximately 1% to 2%. The reported five-year disease-free survival rate is approximately 25% to 35%. In the case of metastases from colorectal cancer, approximately one-third of affected patients will be found at operation to have extrahepatic disease or anatomically unresectable liver metastasis, despite normal results on chest radiography, barium study, colonoscopy, and abdominal CT during the preoperative workup.

Patients with one to three metastatic lesions in one or both lobes of the liver may benefit from resection of these lesions. Survival prospects after surgical resection are best in patients with a single metastatic lesion in one lobe of the liver (25–40% being disease-free at five years). Studies of patients who underwent hepatic resection for colorectal metastases have shown that the extent of hepatic and intraabdominal metastases and the characteristics of the primary cancer are important prognostic determinants, whereas patient age, gender, and the time of occurrence of metastases (synchronous versus metachronous) have little prognostic significance. Adjuvant chemotherapy for patients after complete resection of hepatic metastasis has not proved beneficial.

HEPATIC ARTERY INFUSION CHEMOTHERAPY

Objective rates of response to regional chemotherapy have varied from 50% to 80%, with a median survival time of 8 to 27 months among patients who respond. A recent prospective, randomized trial of patients with colorectal carcinoma metastases showed a survival benefit at two years in patients treated with a hepatic artery infusion in addition to systemic chemotherapy, as compared to the outcome in those treated with systemic chemotherapy alone [20]. Hepatic artery infusion pump insertion and chemotherapy delivery are associated with a mortality of some 4%. Complications from using this therapy include gastric and duodenal ulcers, occlusion of the hepatic artery, and migration of the catheter into the bile ducts. Sclerosing cholangitis induced by FUDR has been reported in approximately 25% of patients on a rigid-dose schedule.

OTHER REGIONAL THERAPY

The following treatments of metastatic carcinoma of the liver have been associated with some response: hepatic artery embolization or chemoembolization; hepatic artery ligation alone or with chemotherapy; cryosurgery; PEI; interstitial laser hyperthermia; and interstitial radiotherapy. To date, none of these methods has yielded response or survival rates better than those achieved with arterial infusion alone.

SYSTEMIC CHEMOTHERAPY

Modest response rates have been achieved with systemic chemotherapy using drugs similar to those used to treat primary carcinoma of the liver. Other agents showing activity include methotrexate; combinations of 5-FU and levamisole; 5-FU or FUDR with mitomycin C; and such new drugs as irinotecan (CPT-11, a topoisomerase inhibitor) and raltitrexed (Tomudex, a thymidylate synthase inhibitor). Continuous intravenous therapy using 5-FU or FUDR may achieve results better than those obtained from either intermittent or bolus chemotherapy. For many asymptomatic patients with unresectable metastatic carcinoma involving the liver, observation without therapy is a reasonable option, because chemotherapy confers only a limited survival advantage in such patients.

RADIOTHERAPY

Radiotherapy to the liver is limited by the sensitivity of normal hepatocytes to irradiation. Doses higher than 2,500 to 3,000 cGy can cause hyperemia, resulting in hepatic cell loss and obliteration of the hepatic veins. Usually, children are less able than are adults to tolerate radiotherapy to the liver. Some researchers have suggested that pediatric patients should receive doses no higher than 1,200 to 1,500 cGy, particularly when radiotherapy is combined with actinomycin D (dactinomycin), partial hepatic resection, or both.

In several studies of radiotherapy for extensive liver metastases, pain was relieved for the remainder of affected patients' lives, but significant treatment-related morbidity was observed. Recent studies showed an increased median survival of 20 months resulting from three-dimensional radiotherapy in combination with hepatic artery chemotherapy using FUDR as an irradiation sensitizer [21]. More potent sensitizers, such as bromodeoxyuridine, are being investigated.

SUMMARY

Many cases of HCC may be avoided by preventing alcoholic cirrhosis and, more importantly, by eradicating HBV infections through the use of vaccines or the timely use of antiviral therapy for hepatitis B or hepatitis C. Early detection of hemochromatosis and the use of phlebotomy before cirrhosis develops can reduce greatly the risk of subsequent HCC associated with this disorder. In addition, reduction of exposure to aflatoxins and other carcinogens may help to prevent primary carcinoma of the liver.

Surgical resection remains the only opportunity for cure in HCC patients who have a resectable lesion. A variety of palliative measures are available, and some are being investigated for patients who have unresectable disease on presentation. Resection is offered to selected patients with hepatic metastases. Such innovative treatment strategies as combination therapy and the use of biological response modifiers or growth factor modulators are being evaluated with a view toward improving the prospects of patients with HCC.

REFERENCES

1. Parkin DM, Pisani P, Ferlay J. Global cancer statistics. *CA Cancer J Clin* 49:33–64, 1999.

2. Schafer DF, Sorrell MF. Hepatocellular carcinoma. *Lancet* 353:1253–1257, 1999.

3. Beasley RP, Hwang LY, Lin CC, Chein CS. Hepatocellular carcinoma and hepatitis B virus: a prospective study of 22,707 men in Taiwan. *Lancet* 2:1129–1133, 1981.

4. Bruix J, Barrera JM, Calvet X, et al. Prevalence of antibodies to hepatitis C virus in Spanish patients with hepatocellular carcinoma and hepatic cirrhosis. *Lancet* 2:1004–1006, 1989.

5. Colombo M, Rumi MG, Donato MF, et al. Hepatitis C antibody in patients with chronic liver disease and hepatocellular carcinoma. *Dig Dis Sci* 36:1130–1133, 1991.

6. Goh J, Callagy G, McEntee G, et al. Hepatocellular carcinoma arising in the absence of cirrhosis in genetic haemochromatosis: three case reports and a review of literature. *Eur J Gastroenterol Hepatol* 11:915–919, 1999.

7. Fleming ID, Cooper JS, Henson DE, et al. (eds). *AJCC Cancer Staging Manual* (5th ed). Philadelphia: Lippincott-Raven, 1997:97–102.

8. Muller RD, Vogel K, Neumann K, et al. SPIO-MR imaging versus double-phase spiral CT in detecting malignant lesions of the liver. *Acta Radiol* 40:628–635, 1999.

9. Solbiati L, Cova L, Ierace T, et al. Liver cancer imaging: the need for accurate detection of intrahepatic disease spread. *J Comput Assist Tomogr* 23(suppl 1):S29–S37, 1999.

10. Chapoutot C, Perney P, Fabre D, et al. Needle-tract seeding after ultrasound-guided puncture of hepatocellular carcinoma. A study of 150 patients. *Gastroenterol Clin Biol* 23:552–556, 1999.

11. Figueras J, Ramos E, Ibanez L, et al. Surgical treatment of hepatocellular carcinoma in cirrhotic and non-cirrhotic patients. *Transplant Proc* 31:2455–2456, 1999.

12. Yamamoto J, Iwatsuki S, Kosuge T, et al. Should hepatomas be treated with hepatic resection or transplantation? *Cancer* 86:1151–1158, 1999.

13. Bismuth H, Majno PE, Adam R. Liver transplantation for hepatocellular carcinoma. *Semin Liver Dis* 19:311–322, 1999.

14. Raoul JL, Boucher E, Kerbrat P. Nonsurgical treatment of hepatocellular carcinoma. *Bull Cancer* 86:537–543, 1999.

15. Ohnishi K. Comparison of percutaneous acetic acid injection and percutaneous ethanol injection for small hepatocellular carcinoma. *Hepatogastroenterology* 45(suppl 3):1254–1258, 1998.

16. Okada S. Local ablation therapy for hepatocellular carcinoma. *Semin Liver Dis* 19:323–328, 1999.

17. Buscarini L, Rossi S. Technology for radiofrequency thermal ablation of liver tumors. *Semin Laparosc Surg* 4:96–101, 1997.

18. Gunderson LL, Haddock MG, Foo ML, et al. Conformal irradiation for hepatobiliary malignancies. *Ann Oncol* 10(suppl 4):221–225, 1999.

19. Mathurin P, Rixe O, Carbonell N, et al. Review article: overview of medical treatments in unresectable hepatocellular carcinoma—an impossible meta-analysis? *Aliment Pharmacol Ther* 12:111–126, 1998.

20. Kemeny N, Huang Y, Cohen AM, et al. Hepatic arterial infusion of chemotherapy after resection of hepatic metastases from colorectal cancer. *N Engl J Med* 341:2039–2048, 1999.

21. Robertson JM, Lawrence TS, Walker S, et al. The treatment of colorectal liver metastases with conformal radiation therapy and regional chemotherapy. *Int J Radiat Oncol Biol Phys* 32:445–450, 1995.

SELECTED READINGS

Adam R, Akpinar E, Johann M, et al. Place of cryosurgery in the treatment of liver tumors. *Ann Surg* 225:38–39, 1997.

Blum HE: Does hepatitis C virus cause hepatocellular carcinoma? *Hepatology* 19:251–255, 1994.

Bosch FX. Global epidemiology of hepatocellular carcinoma. In Okuda K, Tabor E (eds), *Liver Cancer*. New York: Churchill Livingstone, 1997:13–28.

Dmitrewski J, El-Gazzaz G, McMaster P. Hepatocellular cancer: resection or transplantation. *J Hepatobil Pancreat Surg* 5:18–23, 1998.

Ganne-Carrie N, Chastang C, Chapel F, et al. Predictive score for the development of hepatocellular carcinoma and additional value of liver large cell dysplasia in western patients with cirrhosis. *Hepatology* 23:1112–1118, 1996.

Ingold JA, Reed GB, Kaplan HS, Bagshaw MA. Radiation hepatitis. *Am J Roentgenol* 93:200–208, 1965.

Kemeny NE, Conti JA, Bertino JR. Chemotherapy for colorectal cancer (letter). *N Engl J Med* 331:680–681, 1994.

Kew MC. Hepatitis B and C viruses and hepatocellular carcinoma. *Clin Lab Med* 16:395–406, 1996.

Mazzaferro V, Regalia E, Doci R, et al. Liver transplantation for the treatment of small hepatocellular carcinomas in patients with cirrhosis. *N Engl J Med* 334:693–699, 1996.

Mor E, Kaspa RT, Sheiner P, Schwartz M. Treatment of hepatocellular carcinoma associated with cirrhosis in the era of liver transplantation. *Ann Intern Med* 129:643–653, 1998.

Ohnishi K, Yoshioka H, Ito S, Fujiwara K. Prospective randomized controlled trial comparing percutaneous acetic acid injection and percutaneous ethanol injection for small hepatocellular carcinoma. *Hepatology* 27:67–72, 1998.

Pompili M, Rapaccini GL, de Luca F, et al. Risk factors for intrahepatic recurrence of hepatocellular carcinoma in cirrhotic patients treated by percutaneous ethanol injection. *Cancer* 79:1501–1508, 1997.

Riordan SM, Williams R. Preoperative investigation and indication for operation in hepatocellular carcinoma. *J Hepatobil Pancreat Surg* 5:1–6, 1998.

Rossi S, Di Stasi M, Buscarini E, et al. Percutaneous RF interstitial thermal ablation in the treatment of hepatic cancer. *Am J Roentgenol* 167:759–768, 1996.

Rougier P, Mitry E, Clavero-Fabri MC. Chemotherapy and medical treatment of hepatocellular carcinoma. *Hepatogastroenterology* 45(suppl 3):1264–1266, 1998.

Sherlock S. Viruses and hepatocellular carcinoma. *Gut* 35:828–832, 1994.

Takano S, Yokosuka O, Imazeki F, et al. Incidence of hepatocellular carcinoma in chronic hepatitis B and C: a prospective study of 251 patients. *Hepatology* 21:650–655, 1995.

Tsao JI, Loftus JP, Nagomey DM, et al. Trends in morbidity and mortality of hepatic resection for malignancy: a matched comparative analysis. *Ann Surg* 220:199–205, 1994.

Tsukuma H, Hiyama T, Tanaka S, et al. Risk factors for hepatocellular carcinoma among patients with chronic liver disease. *N Engl J Med* 328:1797–1801, 1993.

van Thiel DH, Carr B, Iwatsuki S, et al. The 10 year Pittsburgh experience with liver transplantation for hepatocellular carcinoma: 1981–1991. *J Surg Oncol* 3(suppl 1):78–82, 1993.

Venook AP. Treatment of hepatocellular carcinoma: too many options? *J Clin Oncol* 12:1323–1334, 1994.

Wands JR, Blum HE. Primary hepatocellular carcinoma (editorial). *N Engl J Med* 325:729–731, 1991.

18

Urologic and Male Genital Cancer

A. Introduction

■ ■ ■

Gerald P. Murphy

The diagnosis and treatment of urologic cancers has undergone significant change over the last decade. The authors of the sections of this chapter have contributed an in-depth description of all aspects of each of these cancers in both men and women.

First to be discussed is bladder cancer. New molecular information that is now available regarding the pathogenesis of this disease and the molecular modifications that underlie it contribute to improved diagnosis. Although the treatment of superficial bladder cancer has not changed dramatically over the last five years, combined therapeutic and chemotherapeutic approaches have been modified slightly. Though the enthusiasm that was expressed initially for some forms of multiagent chemotherapy has dwindled, newer drug combinations will continue to be evaluated in terms of both their toxicity and their benefit.

The next section of this chapter addresses the management of renal cell carcinoma. The author uses information presented in recent workshops (sponsored by the Union Internationale Contre le Cancer) on both diagnosis and staging to provide readers with current recommendations regarding kidney cancer. The field of immunotherapy, including such regimens as dendritic cell treatment, represents perhaps the most important new trend, as it offers a unique avenue of therapeutic management.

The section on testicular cancer reflects a major change in the staging of this cancer and the use of tumor markers as prognostic factors. Therapeutic alternatives are discussed, and some long-term chemotherapy results that now are available may alter the enthusiasm that initially was evident for this treatment modality in testicular cancer patients.

The section that addresses prostate cancer has been updated to reflect the dynamic changes in our thinking about both diagnosis and treatment of this disease. The application of prostate-specific antigen as a monitoring tool for treatment results and for diagnosis is being rapidly refined. Equally impressive is the presentation of molecular information on pathogenesis that was not available five years ago. Widespread use of new screening methods has resulted in a significant trend toward earlier stage of disease at diagnosis and detection of cancer in patients at a younger age. The use of nerve-sparing surgery is being implemented as the standard of care, and our treatment options are widening with the availability of more precise external-beam radiotherapy and brachytherapy. Follow-up data on both surgical and radiotherapeutic management, using prostate-specific antigen results reported from studies begun in 1985, are provided in this chapter. Innovative treatment methods for relapsed disease also are presented.

Finally, cancers of the penis and urethra are comprehensively reviewed. Although in North America few cases are seen in any single institution, these cancers are a significant cause of morbidity and mortality in Central and Latin America and in developing countries worldwide.

From these sections on the major organ sites of urologic and male genital cancer, one can conclude that our knowledge of the biology of these cancers is expanding rapidly and is being applied to improve both diagnosis and treatment. In this chapter, we have focused on improvements in the precision of our screening tests and staging and on our treatment strategies. The urologic malignancies remain in the forefront of the application of new knowledge to the management of cancer.

B. Bladder Cancer

■ ■ ■

DONALD L. LAMM
LEROY J. KORB
MARY ANN SENS

Worldwide, an estimated 261,000 new cases of bladder cancer occur annually, with 53,200 of those occurring in the United States in 2000 [1, 2]. Bladder cancer is the

fourth most prevalent noncutaneous malignancy in the United States [3]. The incidence of bladder cancer continues to increase, but the mortality has been fairly stable for at least two decades.

Bladder cancer is divided into superficial and invasive disease, owing to the significant differences in its natural history, treatments, and prognosis. Three-fourths of patients present with superficial disease that is amenable to complete transurethral surgical resection, the treatment of choice, but as many as 90% of patients will have tumor recurrence if additional treatment is not given [4]. Improvements in surgical techniques, including bladder substitution and the combination of radiotherapy and chemotherapy, have provided improvements in the quality of life for patients with invasive bladder cancer. Advances in intravesical therapy and in the treatment of advanced disease with combination chemotherapy are coincident with a reduction in the percentage of mortality of bladder cancer over the last two decades.

ETIOLOGIC FEATURES

Since bladder cancer is one of the first malignancies associated with industrialization, not surprisingly, the incidence continues to rise, particularly in western Europe and the United States. Estimates maintain that as many as one-fourth of bladder cancer cases in men in the United States are associated with occupational exposure. In addition to aromatic amines used in the dye industry and first associated with bladder cancer in 1895, increased incidence of bladder cancer has been reported in workers in the manufacture of rubber, textiles, leather, paint, chemicals, and petroleum. Identified carcinogens include alpha- and beta-naphthylamine, 4-aminobiphenyl, benzidine, chlornaphazine, 4-chloro-*o*-toluidine, *o*-toluidine, 4,4'-methylene *bis*-(2-chloro-aniline), methylene dianiline, benzidine-derived azo dyes, and phenacetin.

Exposure to the aforementioned listed organic chemicals increase the risk for bladder cancer by as much as 60-fold, but exposure to a less potent carcinogen—cigarette smoke—accounts for a greater number of bladder cancers. Cigarette smoking increases the risk of bladder cancer approximately threefold, but it is estimated to cause as many as 60% of the cases of bladder cancer. Other forms of tobacco exposure, including cigar and pipe smoking, use of chewing tobacco, and second-hand smoke, also are implicated as risk factors for bladder cancer. The average interval between carcinogen exposure and bladder tumor diagnosis is approximately 20 years. For that reason, proving that smoking cessation reduces the risk for bladder tumor recurrence and progression has been difficult; however recent research has confirmed this benefit [5].

Other causes of bladder cancer include schistosomiasis, chronic bladder infection, Balkan nephropathy, and arsenic exposure. In some geographic areas, presumably owing to pesticide usage or industrial contamination, increased water intake has been associated with an increased risk of bladder cancer. However, in a large study of physicians in the United States, the risk for bladder cancer was increased in those with the least fluid intake [6]. Therefore, unless a water supply is contaminated with carcinogens, a generous fluid intake (including water) is recommended to dilute and wash out bladder carcinogens that are concentrated in the urine and otherwise would remain in contact with the bladder for extended periods.

EPIDEMIOLOGIC CONSIDERATIONS

The risk for bladder cancer increases with age, and the most frequent age of onset is the mid-sixties. Men are affected three times as often as are women in the United States and five times more frequently worldwide. Black men and women have an incidence of bladder cancer that is nearly half that of nonblacks; however, blacks more commonly present with more advanced disease and have reduced survival [7]. In the United States in 2000, an estimated 53,200 new cases will occur, and 12,200 patients will die of the disease [2].

MOLECULAR BIOLOGICAL FEATURES

Studies of X-chromosome inactivation suggest that bladder cancers, though frequently appearing at different times and at different sites in the bladder, actually originate from a single transformed cell [8]. The transformation of this single cell presumably induces a growth advantage that results in the successive replacement of nontransformed cells. With accumulation of genetic defects, transformed cells become overtly malignant and present as individual tumors. Numerous genetic abnormalities are seen in bladder cancers, including expression of such recognized oncogenes as *ras* and c-*myc*, but these oncogenes are present in only a minority of bladder tumors. Approximately 60% of bladder tumors have abnormalities of chromosome 9, with deletion of regulators of cell proliferation *p15* or *p16*. These abnormalities are seen primarily in low-grade, papillary

tumors. In high-grade tumors, abnormal expression of *p53* is common. Because *p53* serves to remove cells with abnormal DNA, gene alteration is associated with a significant increase in the risk of disease progression [9].

The retinoblastoma gene *RB* also is seen with increased frequency in high-grade bladder tumors, and it too appears to be associated with an increased risk of disease progression. Alterations in protooncogenes, tumor suppressor genes, and genes regulating cell growth are common in bladder cancer. In the future, detection of these genes may result in improved treatment strategies.

PATHOLOGIC CHARACTERISTICS
Transitional Cell Carcinoma

Transitional cell carcinoma is the most common variety of bladder cancer, causing 90% of cases or more in the United States. However, in countries where schistosomiasis is endemic, squamous cell carcinoma occurs most frequently. In the United States, 3–5% of cases are squamous cell carcinoma, 2% or fewer are adenocarcinoma, and 1% or fewer are rhabdomyosarcoma. Squamous cell carcinoma, adenocarcinoma, and rhabdomyosarcoma are highly malignant tumors that typically present at a more advanced stage than that of transitional cell carcinoma and generally are less responsive to systemic chemotherapy.

The prognosis of transitional cell carcinoma of the bladder clearly is related to tumor grade and stage. Both the grading and staging systems for bladder cancer were revised in 1998. The current staging system and examples of the various grades are presented in Figure 18.1 and Color Plate 18.1. What formerly was termed *bladder papilloma* by some and *grade 1, stage Ta transitional cell carcinoma* by others now is termed *papilloma*. *Papillary carcinoma of low malignant potential* is the new term for many lesions formerly classified as grade 1 transitional cell carcinoma. *Papillary carcinoma, low-grade* is the current term that encompasses many papillary carcinomas previously classified as grade 1 to grade 2 tumors. *High-grade urothelial carcinoma* is the current term for grade 2 to grade 3 tumors.

Tumors invading the lamina propria or detrusor muscles are termed *invasive neoplasia* (see Fig. 18.1). Tumors not invading the lamina propria of the bladder are termed *stage Ta*, whereas those invading the lamina propria are termed *stage T1*. The risk for subsequent invasion or metastasis is 9% for stage Ta tumors and 29% for stage T1 tumors [10]. Tumors that invade the detrusor muscle are termed *T2: T2a* if the inner, more superficial half of the detrusor is invaded, and *T2b* if deep muscle

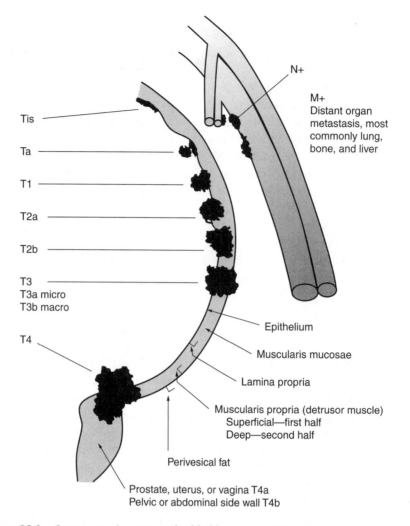

Tis

Ta

T1

T2a

T2b

T3
T3a micro
T3b macro

T4

N+

M+
Distant organ
metastasis, most
commonly lung,
bone, and liver

Epithelium

Muscularis mucosae

Lamina propria

Muscularis propria (detrusor muscle)
Superficial—first half
Deep—second half

Perivesical fat

Prostate, uterus, or vagina T4a
Pelvic or abdominal side wall T4b

Figure 18.1   Current staging system for bladder cancer. TIS (CIS) = carcinoma in situ.

is invaded. Once invasion of the detrusor muscle occurs, tumors cannot be reliably resected transurethrally, metastasis is much more frequent, and cystectomy is generally recommended. Even with such aggressive treatment as cystectomy, mortality from bladder cancer increases to the range of 50% with muscle invasion. Stage T3 tumors extend to the perivesical fat: The extension of T3a tumors can be visualized microscopically, whereas that of T3b tumors is macroscopic. Stage T4 tumors invade adjacent structures: T4a tumors invade the prostate, uterus, or vagina, whereas T4b lesions invade the pelvic or abdominal side wall.

Carcinoma In Situ

Unlike most papillary urothelial tumors, carcinoma in situ (CIS) of the bladder is a highly malignant, aggressive neoplasm that requires special attention. First de-

scribed by Melicow and Hollowell [11] in 1952, CIS is a diffuse, heterogeneous disease that can extend from the renal calyx to the fossa navicularis of the glans penis. Its pathologic appearance is that of a flat, anaplastic, intraepithelial neoplasm that typically involves multiple sites in the bladder. Prior to the advent of bacillus Calmette-Guérin (BCG) immunotherapy, in 54% of patients with CIS the disease would progress to muscle-invasive or metastatic disease within five years [12]. CIS may occur simultaneously with papillary tumors of the bladder and, when present, increases the risk for recurrence, progression, and extension of disease to the ureters and urethra.

CLINICAL FEATURES AND DIAGNOSIS

The most frequent presenting feature of bladder cancer is hematuria, which is present in approximately 80%

of patients. Hematuria may be gross or microscopic and commonly is painless and intermittent. The intermittent nature of the bleeding is problematic, because that characteristic can lull patients and physicians into the belief that resolution of bleeding, whether spontaneous or after antibiotic treatment, is an indication that the symptom is unimportant. All too often, patients present with advanced disease that could have been treated effectively if a workup for previous hematuria had been done.

Symptoms of urinary frequency or urgency or dysuria are present in up to one-third of patients. These symptoms are suggestive of cystitis or prostatitis and occur commonly with high-grade bladder cancer, particularly CIS. However, these tumors typically express positive results on urine cytology, which is a useful screen for bladder cancer in these patients. Symptoms of advanced disease, including weight loss, abdominal mass, suprapubic or flank pain, and lymphedema, are uncommon.

Cystoscopic examination is the primary diagnostic procedure for bladder cancer, because urinary cytologic testing and imaging studies have relatively low sensitivity in bladder cancer. During cystoscopy, the entire bladder should be visualized. Typically, tumors appear as papillary projections into the bladder lumen, but high-grade tumors may appear solid and smooth, and CIS may have the appearance of inflamed or even normal urothelium. Cytologic workup is an important adjunct to cystoscopy because diagnosis of low-grade tumors typically is easy by cytoscopy and difficult by cytology, whereas poorly visualized high-grade tumors generally demonstrate positive results on urinary cytology.

Intravenous urography is the mainstay of radiographic evaluation for hematuria because, unlike ultrasonography or computed axial tomography, intravenous urography provides detailed visualization of the calyces, renal pelvis, and ureters. Visualization of the bladder, however, often is inadequate for small or flat bladder tumors. Only 2–3% of patients with bladder cancer have upper-tract tumors, but half of patients with ureteral tumors will develop transitional cell carcinoma of the bladder. The wise precaution, therefore, is to perform at least a baseline intravenous urogram or retrograde pyelogram in patients with bladder cancer. For patients with noninvasive bladder cancer, computed tomography or magnetic resonance imaging is neither necessary nor cost-effective, though these studies are of some value in staging tumors in patients with invasive disease. The standard workup for hematuria is intravenous urography, cystoscopy and, if an obvious source of bleeding is not found, urinary cytology.

New urinary markers, including tests for bladder tumor-associated antigens, fibrinogen degradation products, and nuclear matrix protein, are more sensitive but less specific than is cytology for bladder cancer. The clinical role of these markers remains to be defined, but they may be useful in screening high-risk populations or in reducing the frequency of follow-up cystoscopic examinations.

TREATMENT

Superficial Bladder Cancer

PRIMARY DISEASE

The primary treatment of superficial bladder cancer, which accounts for approximately 80% of cases, is transurethral resection. Under spinal or general anesthesia—or even local anesthesia in stoic patients with small tumors—transurethral resection or biopsy and laser or electrocautery fulguration accomplishes the most important diagnostic and therapeutic steps simultaneously. Under anesthesia, a careful bimanual examination is performed at the same time to detect residual palpable tumor within or beyond the bladder wall. Using the resectoscope loop, the tumor is resected, and effort is made to remove a margin of uninvolved bladder at the edges and depth of the resection. Muscle should be included in the resection so that the presence of muscle invasion can be ascertained. Areas suspicious for CIS are cauterized. In patients with potentially aggressive tumors, random biopsies and biopsy of the prostatic urethra are performed to assess further the extent of disease and to formulate to a treatment plan.

RECURRENT OR PROGRESSIVE DISEASE

Solitary, low-grade tumors are at low risk for disease progression but frequently do recur. Surgical resection alone is considered to be adequate treatment, but several studies have demonstrated that recurrence can be reduced by 10–20% with a single instillation of chemotherapy at the conclusion of the resection [13]. Table 18.1 lists the intravesical chemotherapeutic regimens that are used currently, the appropriate doses, and the expected short-term benefit in terms of reduction in tumor recurrence and complete response in papillary and in situ transitional cell carcinoma. In contrast to its short-term benefits, intravesical chemotherapy reduces the long-term risk of tumor recurrence (> 5 years) by only 7% compared with surgery alone and has no demonstrable effect on the risk of disease progression [14].

Patients who are at risk for disease progression are

Table 18.1 Results of Intravesical Therapy in Bladder Cancer

Treatment	Standard Dose	No. of Controlled Trials[a]	Average Decrease in Recurrence[b] (%)	Complete Response Rate[c] (%) Papillary	CIS
Thiotepa	30 mg/30 ml	7/11	15	34	38
Doxorubicin	50 mg/50 ml	3/6	16	42	48
Mitomycin C	20–40 mg/20 ml	3/6	20	47	53
Epodyl	1 g/dl	1/1	31		
Epirubicin	50 mg/50 ml	2/2	14		
BCG	50–81 mg/50 ml	7/7	44	62	72

CIS = carcinoma in situ; BCG = bacillus Calmette-Guérin.
[a]Statistically significant ($p < .05$) advantage for treatment/total number of trials.
[b]Reduction in recurrence with treatment as compared with no treatment in prophylaxis studies.
[c]Reported complete response percentages in papillary and carcinoma in situ.
Source: Modified from DL Lamm, F Torti, Bladder cancer, 1996. *CA Cancer J Clin* 46(2):103–112, 1996.

candidates for immunotherapy with BCG. This agent provides improved protection from tumor recurrence (see Table 18.1) but, more important, has been found to reduce disease progression significantly [15, 16].

Some would argue that BCG is appropriate for patients with low risk of progression; however, owing to the increased risk of systemic side effects from BCG [17], intravesical chemotherapy generally is preferred initially. Generally, patients with high-grade transitional cell carcinoma, lamina propria invasion, or CIS are treated best with intravesical BCG immunotherapy.

This treatment, unlike chemotherapy, never should be initiated immediately after tumor resection. To reduce the risk of systemic BCG dissemination, installations are begun two weeks after tumor resection. Connaught (81 mg) or Tice (50 mg) BCG is diluted in 50 ml of saline and is instilled by gravity flow into the bladder through a small catheter. If the catheterization is traumatic (as evidenced by bleeding), instillation should be postponed for a week. Patients are asked to lie on their abdomen for 15 minutes to displace the bubble of air that enters the bladder ahead of the suspension and then are requested to retain the BCG for up to two hours. Treatments are repeated weekly for an additional five weeks. The standard six-week BCG treatment schedule provides long-term protection from tumor recurrence and progression, but the immune stimulation induced by BCG wanes with time. By 15 years, the benefit of BCG therapy is lost [15].

MAINTENANCE INTRAVESICAL THERAPY

Previous attempts to extend the benefit of BCG by using maintenance schedules of single instillations monthly or quarterly and by using repeated six-week installa-

tions at six-month intervals failed to reduce tumor recurrence in controlled trials. In a Southwest Oncology Group trial [18], however, highly significant further reduction in tumor recurrence and disease worsening was documented using a series of three instillations once weekly at 3, 6, 12, 18, 24, 30, and 36 months. In patients with CIS, the complete response rate increased from 68% to 84% with maintenance BCG and, in patients with Ta or T1 tumors, the recurrence rate at eight years was reduced from the expected 52% with induction BCG to only 25% with three-week maintenance doses of BCG [18].

In contrast to immunotherapy, wherein maintenance clearly is superior to induction therapy, on the basis of both biological principles and statistically significant randomized trials, maintenance chemotherapy has not proved to be effective. To date, studies have failed to demonstrate that multiple treatments or maintenance chemotherapy is superior to a single instillation of chemotherapy given at the time of tumor resection. The concept of prophylactic intravesical chemotherapy is theoretically unsound. Cytotoxic chemotherapy kills by coming into direct contact with rapidly dividing cells. It can be effective only if malignant or transformed cells are present at the time of administration. Cytotoxic chemotherapy is mutagenic and, in the absence of malignancy, may be counterproductive. Repeated instillation of thiotepa, doxorubicin, or mitomycin into normal rodent bladders can induce hyperplasia, dysplasia, CIS, and even invasive transitional cell carcinoma.

FOLLOW-UP

Patients with superficial bladder cancer are at highest risk for tumor recurrence within three months of tumor resection. Recurrence of tumor at three months increases the risk for subsequent recurrence and progression, but patients remain at risk for recurrence indefinitely. Patients with low-grade tumors have a low risk for progression and therefore require cystoscopic surveillance less frequently than do patients with high-grade tumors.

Schedules for cystoscopy vary, but patients with low-grade tumors can be followed up safely at three months, then at six-month intervals for two years, and then annually. Typically, patients with high-grade tumors are followed at three-month intervals for two years, six-month intervals for two years, and then annually. Patients with CIS or high-grade carcinoma (formerly termed *grade 3 carcinoma*) require annual assessment of the upper tracts and prostatic urethra to reduce the chance for progression at those sites.

Muscle-Invasive and Locally Advanced Bladder Cancer

Once invasion of the detrusor muscle occurs, the treatment and prognosis of bladder cancer changes markedly. Frequently, stage Ta and stage T1 bladder cancer can be resected completely transurethrally, but once muscle invasion occurs, complete resection is infrequent, and the risk of lymph node and distant metastasis increases dramatically. The overall five-year survival of patients with Ta or T1 bladder cancer is similar to that of the unaffected population; however, even with cystectomy (the recommended treatment for patients with muscle-invasive bladder cancer), approximately one-third of patients with high-grade tumors die from their malignancy.

Though generally not useful in patients with superficial bladder cancer [19], radiotherapy may play a role in patients who have muscle-invasive bladder cancer but are not candidates for cystectomy. Primary radiotherapy, instead of surgery, is an uncommon treatment in medically fit patients the United States, but it is common in Europe and Canada. Most bladder cancer patients in the United States so treated are those who are unable to tolerate surgery, refuse surgery, or have disease too advanced for surgery. However, in Great Britain and Canada, cystectomy generally is reserved for those patients in whom irradiation fails. Bladder preservation using combinations of chemotherapy (cisplatin or 5-fluorouracil) and irradiation have been evaluated and appear to result in response rates higher than those obtained with radiotherapy alone. Two studies using 5-fluorouracil and irradiation resulted in complete response rates of 60% [20, 21]. Another controlled, randomized study showed an increase from 45% to 67% in two-year freedom from local relapse by adding cisplatin to irradiation [22]. Other combination irradiation and chemotherapy trials have shown similar encouraging results [23].

The ideal candidates for irradiation should have adequate bladder capacity and minimal voiding symptoms. Though some researchers suggest the use of preoperative radiotherapy in both T2 and T3 lesions [24], controlled trials have failed to confirm an advantage [25, 26]. Usually, external irradiation is given through multiple fields, each precisely shaped to treat only the areas of concern. Other forms of radiotherapy include temporary implantation of radioisotopes into the tumor, a central balloon containing an irradiation source, intraoperative electron-beam treatments, and neutron therapy.

In North America, the treatment of choice for muscle-invasive bladder cancer is radical cystectomy with pelvic lymphadenectomy, which may be partly responsible for the current increased five-year survival in North America. The estimated five-year survival figures for bladder cancer are 56% worldwide, 57% in northwestern Europe, and 80% in North America [27]. Radical cystectomy includes removal of the pelvic lymph nodes and bladder along with the prostate in men and removal of the urethra, anterior vagina, and uterus in women. Five-year survivals have increased over the years, and recent series report five-year survivals as high as 80% for stage T2a and stage T2b disease and 61% for stage T3 disease.

Efforts have been made to improve the survival of patients undergoing cystectomy for invasive bladder cancer by using adjuvant or neoadjuvant chemotherapy. Despite significant improvements in combination chemotherapy for transitional cell carcinoma, the improvement in survival with chemotherapy in patients undergoing cystectomy is limited. The results of studies to date are inconsistent, so neoadjuvant or adjuvant chemotherapy cannot be recommended routinely.

The standard Bricker procedure is an effective urinary diversion that has served patients well for many decades. The advent of continent urinary diversion and orthotopic bladder substitution represents a major advance in surgical management of bladder cancer and has increased the acceptance of cystectomy greatly. Continent urinary diversions allow patients to avoid external collection devices. A common continent diversion, the Indiana pouch (Fig. 18.2), uses the detubularized right colon as an internal reservoir. The reservoir is emptied by catheterization through the narrowed distal ilium; this intussusception maintains continence. The distal ileum is brought up to the umbilicus.

Orthotopic bladder substitution using ilium or colon provides the best approximation of normal function. An example of the Studer neoilial bladder is depicted in Figure 18.3. By permitting urethral voiding, orthotopic neobladders provide both protection from infection and an improved body image. Originally, creation of orthotopic neobladders was performed only in men, but several centers now have performed the procedure successfully in women as well.

Metastatic Bladder Cancer

The combination of methotrexate, vinblastine, doxorubicin (Adriamycin), and cisplatin (MVAC) [28] or the three-drug combination exclusive of doxorubicin [29] has improved significantly the treatment of metastatic bladder cancer. MVAC has been demonstrated to be superior both to cisplatin (39% versus 12% response; median survival = 12.5 versus 8.2 months) [30] and to combination chemotherapy with cyclophosphamide, doxorubicin, and cisplatin (response rate = 65% versus 46%; median survival = 11.1 months versus 8.3 months; p = .004) [31]. These randomized studies demonstrate that survival of patients with metastatic bladder cancer can be improved significantly using this aggressive combination. Recent studies suggest that comparable response rates can be achieved with cisplatin combined with taxol or gemcitabine or with both taxol and gemcitabine. The results of these preliminary studies will have to be compared to those of MVAC, but experience suggests that newer combinations are less toxic than is MVAC. Radiotherapy may offer excellent results when one is attempting to control the symptoms of advanced or metastatic disease. Bleeding, pain in the bladder or bone, and obstruction variously may benefit from a short course of treatment.

SUMMARY

Bladder cancer is a common malignancy, and its incidence continues to increase, a trend that will not be reversed without a reduction in tobacco use and exposure to environmental carcinogens. Prompt and appropriate diagnosis of the source of hematuria can reduce the stage of disease at diagnosis and can result in improved patient survival. Treatment with surgical resection, intravesical therapy (particularly BCG immunotherapy),

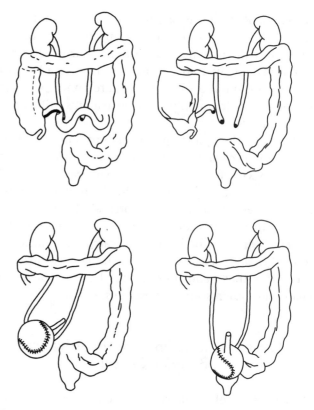

Figure 18.2 A common continent diversion, the Indiana pouch.

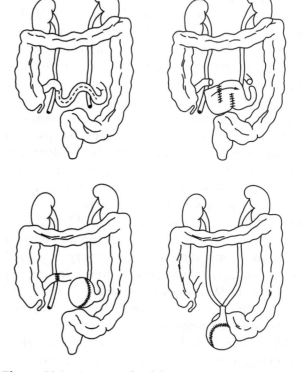

Figure 18.3 An example of the Studer neoilial bladder.

and close follow-up is highly effective in early-stage disease.

Currently, muscle-invasive bladder cancer is treated in the United States with radical cystectomy. Improvement in surgical techniques with continent reservoirs and orthotopic bladder substitution has improved the acceptance of this surgery. The survival of patients with advanced bladder cancer has been improved with cisplatin and methotrexate-based combination chemotherapy, and new chemotherapeutic agents (including paclitaxel [Taxol®] and gemcitabine) hold promise for further improvement. More effective chemotherapy combinations or combined chemotherapy and radiotherapy may reduce the need for radical surgery in the future.

C. Renal Cell Carcinoma

■ ■ ■

DAVID G. BOSTWICK

EPIDEMIOLOGIC CONSIDERATIONS

The incidence of renal cell carcinoma is 31,200 cases per year [2], representing 2–3% of new cancers. Men are affected approximately twice as often as are women, and the mean age at diagnosis is approximately 60 years. Some 4,500 patients died of renal cancer in 1998.

ETIOLOGIC FEATURES

Little is known about the causes of renal cancer. Risk factors that have been proved or implicated include smoking, obesity, analgesic abuse, and occupational exposure to cadmium or aromatic hydrocarbons. Approximately 1% of renal cancers cluster in families, most of whose members have abnormalities on the short arm of chromosome 3 and on the *p53* gene on chromosome 17. Features suggestive of familial renal cell cancer include a history of two or more first-degree relatives with the same cancer, multicentric cancer, bilateral cancer, and early-onset cancer. Patients with acquired renal cystic disease are nearly 100 times more likely to develop renal cell carcinoma than is the general population, and

the risk is particularly high in men who have large kidneys and are receiving hemodialysis.

More than 80% of patients with von Hippel-Lindau (VHL) disease have an inactivated *VHL* gene (chromosome 3p25), and renal cancer is the most common cause of death. VHL disease is an autosomal dominant disease characterized by retinal angiomas, nervous system hemangioblastomas, pheochromocytomas, pancreatic tumors, and clear-cell renal carcinomas that are bilateral and multicentric and have early onset. Accepted and proposed precursor lesions of renal cancer are shown in Table 18.2.

DETECTION AND DIAGNOSIS
Prevention and Early Detection

Screening for sporadic renal cancer is not practical, owing to its low incidence in the general adult population. However, it may be useful in high-risk patients, such as those with VHL disease, dialysis-dependent acquired renal cystic disease, autosomal dominant polycystic kidney disease, tuberous sclerosis, familial renal

Table 18.2 Accepted and Proposed Precursor Lesions in Renal Cell Carcinoma

Potential Precursor Lesion or Clinical Setting	Description
Renal cysts with clear cells in von Hippel-Lindau disease patients	Accepted precursor lesion
Acquired renal cysts with a nodular epithelial proliferation of clear cells	Should be considered cystic pattern of renal cell carcinoma if more than two clear cells thick [35]
Intratubular epithelial dysplasia	Uncertain significance; unknown relationship with renal cell carcinoma
Papillary renal adenoma	Lesions < 5 mm and no clear cells considered benign; for larger lesions, and associated higher likelihood of aggressive behavior

cell cancer, and symptoms suggestive of cancer. Genetic counseling also is indicated for many of the individuals in these groups.

Clinical Diagnosis

Renal cell carcinoma is asymptomatic when it is small, producing symptoms only when it has reached sufficient size to displace other organs. Advances in imaging techniques, including ultrasonography and abdominal computed tomography (CT), have greatly increased the early detection of clinically unsuspected cancer. The classic triad of hematuria, flank pain, and mass occurs in fewer than 10% of patients and usually is associated with advanced cancer. Approximately 45% of patients have gross hematuria.

As one of the great "mimics" in medicine, renal cancer may present with one of a wide array of symptoms and signs. Up to 40% of patients have a paraneoplastic syndrome, indicating production of specific hormones by cancer cells or an immune response to the cancer. Hormones produced include parathyroid-like hormone, erythropoietin, an adrenocorticotropic hormone-like substance, gonadotropins, insulin, human chorionic gonadotropin, renin, and placental lactogen. These syndromes produce anemia (in up to 40% of cases), fatigue and weight loss (in 33%), fever (in 30%), hypertension (in 24%), hypercalcemia (in 10–15%), amyloidosis (in 5%), erythrocytosis (in 4%), enteropathy (in 3%), and neuromyopathy (in 3%) [32]. Stauffer's syndrome, present in up to 6% of cases, is a reversible hepatorenal condition associated with abnormal liver function tests in the absence of liver metastases; it does not imply metastatic cancer. Cytokines, including interleukin-6, also may be elevated with renal cancer.

Approximately 30% of patients have metastases at the time of diagnosis. The frequency of appearance of metastases at various sites is as follows: lung, 50–60%; bone, lymph nodes, and liver, each 30–40%; adrenal gland, 20%; opposite kidney, 10%; and brain, 5%.

Specific Diagnostic Tests and Markers

Diagnostic imaging of the kidneys includes plain-film radiography, ultrasonography, CT, magnetic resonance imaging (MRI), angiography, and nuclear medicine scanning. Use of the three most popular modalities for renal tumors—urography, ultrasonography, and CT scanning—is responsible for the detection, and thus the increased incidence, of asymptomatic renal masses, ac-

counting for 6%, 68%, and 22% of such cases, respectively [33]. An ultrasonographic screening study of 45,905 Japanese adults revealed 469 renal tumors, including 19 asymptomatic and 16 symptomatic cases of renal cell carcinoma [34]. The likelihood of renal cancer in sonographically detected lesions was 7.5%, 5.4%, and 21.6% for asymptomatic patients, asymptomatic patients with microscopic hematuria, and symptomatic patients, respectively [34]. The accuracy of imaging techniques varies in detecting extrarenal cancer and pathologic stage.

Histopathologic Characteristics

The histologic classification of renal cortical epithelial neoplasms is accepted internationally [35]. This classification was based chiefly on light-microscopical tumor appearance but is consistent with the prevailing genetic understanding of tumors.

Conventional (clear-cell) renal carcinoma is the most common cancer of the renal cortex, accounting for approximately 70% of cases. Rare cases demonstrate a predominance of material in chromosome 3p, and half show somatic mutations in the VHL gene. Up to 20% of others show inactivation of the VHL gene by hypermethylation. Nearly 5% of cases exhibit sarcomatoid change.

Papillary renal cell carcinoma accounts for approximately 15% of renal cell cancers. Characteristic genetic changes include trisomies of chromosomes 3q, 7, 12, 16, 17, and 20 and loss of the Y chromosome. The term papillary carcinoma is appropriate when these genetic changes are present, even if papillae are not prominent.

Chromophobe renal carcinoma accounts for 5% or so of cases of renal cell carcinoma. The cytoplasm contains numerous microvesicles that appear blue with Hale's colloidal iron stain. Often, a halo surrounds the nucleus, owing to cytoplasmic condensation near the chromatinic rim. Genetic changes include monosomy of chromosomes 1, 2, 6, 10, 13, 17, and 21, and hypodiploidy.

Collecting-duct carcinoma is a rare renal cell carcinoma, representing fewer than 1% of cases. Features that contribute to its recognition remain somewhat controversial; typically, the tumor is described as containing irregular channels lined by highly atypical epithelium, often with a hobnail-cell appearance. A recently described, highly aggressive variant—medullary carcinoma—arises from the collecting ducts of the renal medulla and is associated with sickle cell trait. Collecting-duct origin for these tumors is based on iden-

Table 18.3 Current Prognostic Factors in Renal Cell Carcinoma

Patient-related factors
  Symptomatic patient presentation
  Weight loss > 10% body weight
  ECOG performance status 2–3
  ESR > 30
  Anemia < 10 g/dl (female); < 12 g/dl (male)
  Hypercalcemia
  Elevated alkaline phosphatase

Tumor-related factors
  Cancer size
  Macroscopic positive surgical margins
  Solitary unresectable or multiple metastases
  Liver and lung metastases
  Primary tumor stage (according to TNM system)
  Grade
  Histologic type
  Sarcomatoid architecture

ECOG = Eastern Cooperative Oncology Group; ESR = erythrocyte sedimentation rate; TNM = tumor, node, metastasis.
Note: These factors are well supported by the literature and generally are used in patient management.

tification of dysplastic changes in collecting ducts and affinity for *Ulex europaeus* lectin. Genetic abnormalities are not well understood.

Designation as unclassified renal cell carcinoma is reserved for cases that do not fulfill the criteria for the foregoing cancers. These tumors are morphologically and genetically variable and often are high-grade.

Grading

Numerous nuclear grading systems are in use throughout the world, and no optimal consensus system exists [36]. Grading is an important prognostic factor for patients with clear-cell and papillary renal cell carcinoma, but the utility of grading other less common histologic types is uncertain. A variety of additional prognostic factors are used regularly for patient management (Table 18.3) [37, 38].

Staging

The recommended testing sequence to establish clinical staging is (1) ultrasonography; (2) abdominal CT scan with and without intravenous contrast; (3) radiologic metastatic survey, including chest radiography (bone scan being unnecessary unless serum alkaline phospha-

tase concentration is elevated); and (4) complete blood count and blood chemistry tests, including liver function tests. Excretory urography may be valuable for investigating hematuria or function of the contralateral kidney. A nuclear renal scan may be of value to patients at risk for renal insufficiency and dialysis after nephrectomy. MRI is useful for evaluating venous thrombus. Lymphangiography is inaccurate for evaluation of high paraaortic and pericaval lymph nodes.

The TNM (*t*umor, *n*ode, *m*etastasis) classification of renal cell carcinoma was revised in 1997 (Tables 18.4, 18.5) [39, 40]. Significant changes from the previous revision included both the introduction of a cut point of 7.0 cm to separate T1 and T2 cancer and the compression of the regional lymph node descriptions to include N1 (metastasis to a single regional lymph node) and N2 (metastasis to more than one node).

PRIMARY TREATMENT
Surgery

Surgery is the preferred treatment for resectable renal cancer (Fig. 18.4). Radical nephrectomy consists of removal of the kidney, perinephric fat, Gerota's capsule, and lymph nodes and is useful for localized cancer and for palliation of intractable bleeding and pain. Most surgeons prefer an open approach to nephrectomy, but several investigators have advocated laparoscopic nephrectomy for cancers measuring less than 6 cm in diameter [41]. Partial nephrectomy, also known as *nephron-sparing surgery,* is increasingly popular, owing to improved surgical methods and outcome. Partial nephrectomy is adequate treatment for small localized cancer and also offers some value for bilateral synchronous cancer, cancer in a functionally or anatomically solitary kidney, cancer in a patient with compromised renal function, and cancer in a patient with VHL disease. Bench surgery is a variation of partial nephrectomy and consists of removal of the kidney, resection of the tumor or tumors, and autotransplantation of the residual kidney.

Cancer-specific survival after nephrectomy varies by stage and grade. Five-year survival rates are 60–80%, 50–80%, 15–35%, and less than 15% for stages I, II, III, and IV, respectively. Solitary metastases also are cured occasionally by resection, especially in such soft tissues as the lung. Venous invasion can be treated successfully with surgery in some cases; five-year cancer-specific survival rates were 50–60% and 3–50% for renal vein and vena caval involvement, respectively. Embolectomy may be useful for management of disease

Table 18.4   TNM Staging for Renal Cell Carcinoma

Classification	Definition
Primary tumor (T)	
TX	Primary tumor cannot be assessed
T0	No evidence of primary tumor
T1	Tumor ≤ 7.0 cm or less in greatest dimension, limited to the kidney
T2	Tumor > 7.0 cm in greatest dimension, limited to the kidney
T3	Tumor extending into major veins or invading adrenal gland or perinephric tissues but not beyond Gerota fascia
T3a	Tumor invades adrenal gland or perinephric tissues but not beyond Gerota fascia
T3b	Tumor grossly extending into renal vein or vena cava below diaphragm
T3c	Tumor grossly extending into vena cava above diaphragm
T4	Tumor invading beyond Gerota fascia
Regional lymph nodes (N)[a]	
NX	Regional lymph nodes cannot be assessed
N0	No regional lymph node metastasis
N1	Metastasis in a single regional lymph node
N2	Metastasis in more than one regional lymph node
Distant metastasis (M)	
MX	Distant metastasis cannot be assessed
M0	No distant metastasis
M1	Distant metastasis
Pathologic classification (pTNM)[b]	
Histopathologic grading (G)	
GX	Grade of differentiation cannot be assessed
G1	Well differentiated
G2	Moderately differentiated
G3–4	Poorly differentiated or undifferentiated

[a]The regional lymph nodes are the hilar, abdominal, paraaortic, and pericaval nodes. Laterality does not affect the *N* categories.
[b]The pT, pN, and pM categories correspond to the T, N, and M categories.
Note: The classification applies only to renal cell carcinoma. The disease should be confirmed histologically. The procedures for assessing the *T, N,* and *M* categories are physical examination and imaging.
Source: Reprinted from LH Sobin, CH Wittekind (eds), *TNM Classification of Malignant Tumors* (5th ed). This material is used with permission of Wiley-Liss, Inc., a subsidiary of John Wiley & Sons, Inc.

in some patients, despite massive pulmonary involvement [42].

Radiotherapy

The propensity for irradiation nephritis precludes routine use of radiotherapy for primary treatment of renal

Table 18.5   Stage Grouping for Renal Cell Carcinoma

Stage I	T1	N0	M0
Stage II	T2	N0	M0
Stage III	T1	N1	M0
	T2	N1	M0
	T3	N0, N1	M0
Stage IV	T4	N0, N1	M0
	Any T	N2	M0
	Any T	Any N	M1

Source: Reprinted from LH Sobin, CH Wittekind (eds), *TNM Classification of Malignant Tumors* (5th ed). This material is used with permission of Wiley-Liss, Inc., a subsidiary of John Wiley & Sons, Inc.

cancer. Sometimes, postoperative irradiation is used and may be useful for patients with residual local cancer, extension of cancer into perinephric fat, regional lymph node involvement, renal vein invasion, and cancer spillage or transection during surgery. It is used also after surgical excision of metastases. Palliative radiotherapy for metastatic renal cancer is particularly effective for bone pain, with a response rate of up to 86% [43].

Chemotherapy

Single-agent and combination cytotoxic therapies have shown response rates of 10% or less. These modalities play no significant role in current routine treatment of primary or metastatic renal cancer [44].

Hormonal Therapy

Progesterone has been used for treatment of metastatic cancer. However, its efficacy has not been proved.

Immunotherapy

Biological therapy or immunotherapy that exploits the host immune system has generated considerable interest in recent years, owing to preliminary favorable results with cytokines for patients with metastatic renal cancer. The results with interferon-α now are considered generally modest, and this agent as monotherapy has little long-term efficacy for treatment of metastases. Interleukin-2 augments natural killer cell function, and monotherapy has resulted in complete or partial responses in up to 70% of patients; however, severe renal, cardiopulmonary, and other toxicities are limiting [45].

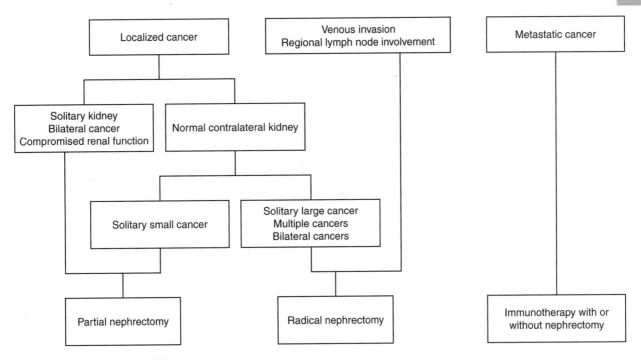

Figure 18.4   Surgical management algorithm for renal cell carcinoma.

Combination therapy consisting of interleukin-2 and tumor-infiltrating lymphocytes or interferon-α has provided promising results, and trials continue to optimize this therapy. Autolymphocyte therapy, consisting of re-infusing autologous lymphocytes after activation in culture and irradiation to inactivate suppressor T lymphocytes, has shown definitive responses in previously refractory disease [46].

The future of immunotherapy rests on cancer vaccines, gene therapy, and adoptive immunotherapy. Approaches under investigation include combinations of cytokine therapy, use of new cytokines, combinations of cytokine modulation and autologous cancer vaccination, and use of genetically engineered cancer cells to augment endogenous immune system responses. Activation of cytotoxic T lymphocytes may be the common mechanism of action of many of these disparate treatments, including gene therapy. Adoptive immunotherapy that exploits dendritic cells as effectors is actively being investigated [47].

RELAPSE AND PALLIATION

Usually, relapses of renal cell carcinoma result from widespread metastases to bone, lung, liver, brain, or lymph nodes.

INVESTIGATIONAL ACTIVITIES

A recent international workshop defined clinical and basic scientific investigational priorities in renal cell carcinoma (Table 18.6) [48]. As stated previously, renal cell carcinoma is an attractive target for gene therapy and cancer vaccines.

D. Testicular Cancer

■ ■ ■

PAUL M. DODD

WILLIAM K. KELLY

EPIDEMIOLOGIC CONSIDERATIONS

Testicular cancers are an uncommon and histologically diverse group of neoplasms. Most are of germ-cell origin, although lymphoma is the most common testicular neoplasm among patients older than 50 years. Frequently, germ-cell tumors are limited in extent to the

Table 18.6 Future Research Recommendations in Renal Cell Carcinoma

Determine the clinical utility of periodic routine ultrasonography as a tool for early diagnosis of renal cell carcinoma.

Develop a diagnostic test using urine or blood to detect early-stage and occult renal carcinoma.

Develop a genetic assay to determine malignant potential in kidney lesions.

Evaluate the clinical utility of microsatellite DNA analysis in renal neoplasms.

Identify factors that predict response to immunotherapy and gene therapy.

Further define the genotype of specific histologic types of renal cell carcinoma, particularly in association with family history.

Evaluate the significance of multidrug resistance in renal cell carcinoma.

Establish a national or international database and working group for renal cell carcinoma.

Critically and systematically determine the utility of immunotherapy in renal cell carcinoma.

Critically and systematically determine the role of vaccine therapy and gene therapy in renal cell carcinoma.

Undertake chemoprevention trials of renal cell carcinoma, including short-term trials to determine the efficacy of surrogate end-point biomarkers.

Define the combination of patient factors that could be used for prediction of individual outcome using neural networkbased technology.

testicle of origin but may metastasize both through predictable lymphatic drainage routes and hematogenously. A small proportion of germ-cell tumors arises in extragonadal sites. The management of testicular cancer is truly multidisciplinary, with surgery, radiotherapy, and chemotherapy all being important components of therapy. The development of cisplatin-based chemotherapeutic regimens produced marked improvement in the management of testicular cancer, and curative therapy exists for all stages of disease [49]. However, appropriate selection of therapy based on risk stratification is essential to minimize toxicity without compromising the opportunity for curative outcome.

Testicular cancers represent only approximately 1% of tumors occurring in men, but germ-cell tumors are the most common cancer in male persons between ages 15 and 34. Approximately 6,900 new cases will occur in 2000, and approximately 300 patients will die of the disease in this year [2]. The incidence is greatest in northern Europe and North America and, for uncertain reasons, has increased slowly during the last 40 years.

The incidence in blacks is approximately one-fifth that in whites.

The great majority of testicular cancers are sporadic in origin. The primary epidemiologic risk factor for testicular cancer is cryptorchidism, with an abdominal cryptorchid testis being at greater risk of malignant degeneration than is an inguinal cryptorchid testis. Orchiopexy, which should be performed prior to puberty, decreases the risk of subsequent malignant transformation. Persons with Klinefelter's syndrome are at a higher risk for developing mediastinal germ-cell tumor.

BIOLOGICAL CHARACTERISTICS

The etiology of germ-cell tumors is understood partially. Most germ-cell tumors are hyperdiploid, triploid, or tetraploid and have at least one X and one Y chromosome [50]. Because separation of X and Y chromosomes occurs in anaphase I of meiosis, genetic events critical to malignant transformation must occur in the pre-anaphase I spermatogonia. Despite a hyperdiploid state, widespread allelic loss has been noted in germ-cell tumors of all stages, suggesting that this genetic loss is another early event contributing to transformation. The presence of an excess copy number of the short arm of chromosome 12 (isochromosome 12p) is an abnormality specific to germ-cell tumors [51]. It has been found in approximately 80% of germ-cell tumors of all histologic types and in preinvasive carcinoma in situ. The presence of isochromosome 12p may be useful in diagnosis of poorly differentiated mediastinal germ-cell tumors.

HISTOLOGIC ELEMENTS

Commonly, germ-cell tumors arise from intratubular germ-cell neoplasia (carcinoma in situ), which is found in virtually all patients. A unique feature of germ-cell tumors is the capacity to differentiate into any immature or mature tissue phenotype; therefore, these tumors may be composed of multiple histologic elements. The germ-cell tumors can be subdivided into two major histologic groups, seminomas and nonseminomas, each of which constitute approximately 50% of cases. The pathologic differentiation of seminoma from nonseminoma is critical, as therapy and prognosis for each are significantly different.

Seminomas

Most commonly, seminomas present in the fourth decade of life and are defined by the absence of other germ-cell elements (pure seminoma). Trophoblastic giant cells, which are capable of producing human chorionic gonadotropin (HCG), are present in a minority of otherwise pure seminomas and do not change the classification. Tumors with other nonseminomatous elements or elevation of alpha-fetoprotein (AFP), a marker of nonseminomatous elements, are classified as nonseminomas. Seminomas have a relatively low propensity for metastasis, and approximately 75% are localized to the testis (stage I) at diagnosis. Approximately 20% have spread to the retroperitoneal lymph nodes (stage II). Spread of tumor to nonregional lymph nodes or to visceral organ sites occurs in approximately 5% (stage III).

Nonseminomas

Typically, nonseminomas present in the third decade of life. Such tumors may be composed of several histologic elements that are similar to normal human tissues. This feature reflects the potential of germ cells to differentiate into any other human cell type. Examples of specific histologic elements of germ-cell tumors and the normal tissue to which they bear resemblance are as follows:

Embryonal cell carcinoma	Embryo
Yolk sac tumor	Yolk sac
Choriocarcinoma	Placenta
Immature teratoma	Fetal tissue
Mature teratoma	Mature adult tissue

Immature and mature teratoma may resemble fetal and adult tissue of any type, respectively, including bone, cartilage, epidermis, or neural tissue. Nonseminoma germ-cell tumors also may contain seminomatous tumor elements but, by definition, may not be pure seminoma. Nonseminomas may be composed of only one or any combination of the aforementioned histologic types. Tumors composed of more than one histologic type are termed *mixed germ-cell tumors.*

Yolk-sac elements produce AFP, and choriocarcinomatous elements synthesize HCG, tumor markers that are useful for evaluating response to treatment or relapse. In general, nonseminomas have a propensity to metastasize that is higher than that of pure seminomas. At diagnosis, approximately one-third of the tumors are stage I, one-third are stage II, and one-third are stage III. A subset of patients with nonseminomas has metastases in liver, bone, or brain or greatly elevated tumor markers, features that portend a markedly poorer prognosis [52].

CLINICAL PRESENTATION

The most common presentation of testicular cancer is the development of a focal testicular mass or diffuse testicular enlargement over a period of days to months. Testicular masses may be painless, though frequently a sense of testicular heaviness or discomfort is reported. Hemorrhage into a testicular tumor or epididymitis may cause significant pain. The differential diagnosis of a testicular mass includes epididymitis, hydrocele, spermatocele, orchitis, infarction, or trauma. Less frequently, the initial symptoms of germ-cell tumors relate to metastatic disease. Back pain may occur in the setting of extensive retroperitoneal lymphadenopathy. Pulmonary metastases may manifest as dyspnea, cough, or chest pain.

Key elements of the physical examination include careful palpation of both testes, examination for the presence of a palpable abdominal mass due to retroperitoneal lymphadenopathy, and evaluation for extraregional lymphadenopathy.

DIAGNOSTIC EVALUATION

If the cause of testicular swelling or pain is uncertain, often a brief trial of antibiotic therapy or observation is reasonable. Failure of a testicular abnormality to resolve over a period of two to four weeks demands prompt diagnostic evaluation. Transscrotal ultrasonography is useful in characterizing testicular abnormalities to permit distinguishing solid masses from nonsolid abnormalities. Typically, testicular tumors appear as one or more hypoechoic masses within the testicular parenchyma. If a testicular cancer is suspected, a radical inguinal orchiectomy should be performed for confirmation of the diagnosis and to determine the histologic type.

An evaluation to determine the extent of disease should include a computed tomography (CT) scan of the chest, abdomen, and pelvis. CT scan of the abdomen is moderately sensitive and specific for identifying metastases to retroperitoneal lymph nodes. However, a normal abdominal CT scan does not preclude the possibility of retroperitoneal nodal metastasis. For evaluation of the thorax, chest CT scanning is more sensitive than is plain radiography. Because the presence of disease above the diaphragm may alter subsequent treatment dramatically, chest CT scanning is the preferred diagnostic modality. Lymphangiography occasionally is useful. Patient symptoms or laboratory abnormalities should guide additional diagnostic evaluation.

TUMOR MARKERS

Tumor markers AFP, HCG, and lactate dehydrogenase (LDH) have independent prognostic significance in germ-cell tumors and are valuable in assessing tumor status. AFP is produced by yolk-sac components of non-seminomas. The half-life of AFP is 5–7 days. HCG is produced by choriocarcinomatous elements of a nonseminoma. Trophoblastic giant cells cause a mild elevation of HCG in 10–25% of patients with pure seminoma. Unlike elevation of AFP, mild elevation of HCG does not alter the classification or prognosis of otherwise pure seminoma. The half-life of HCG is 18–36 hours. LDH is a less specific tumor marker that reflects tumor bulk.

In all patients, levels of AFP, HCG, and LDH should be determined before orchiectomy is performed. Subsequently, periodic determination of tumor marker levels is helpful in assessing response to postorchiectomy therapy and in evaluating for relapse. In patients who have elevated tumor markers and are receiving therapy for metastatic disease, AFP and HCG should decline according to their serum half-lives. A slower rate of decline of these markers potentially indicates the development of drug resistance and subsequent treatment failure [53].

STAGING OF GERM-CELL TUMORS

The pathologic findings at radical orchiectomy, physical examination, radiographic evaluation, and serum tumor marker levels are the essential components of the current TNM (*t*umor, *n*ode, *m*etastasis) staging system (Tables 18.7–18.9) [54]. Stage I reflects disease limited to the testis, stage II disease is confined to the retroperitoneum, and stage III represents more advanced disease. A new category, stage IS, was added for patients with persistently elevated AFP or HCG concentrations in the absence of clinically or radiographically evident disease.

The International Germ-Cell Consensus Classifica-

tion divides stage III patients into three risk groups depending on primary site of the tumor, sites of metastatic disease, and levels of serum tumor markers (see Table 18.8) [52]. For nonseminomas, presence of a mediastinal primary site, a nonpulmonary visceral metastasis, or a profound elevation of tumor markers imparts a particularly poor prognosis. Note that no poor-risk category exists for seminomas.

TREATMENT

Early-Stage Disease

CLINICAL STAGE I SEMINOMA

Irradiation of retroperitoneal, bilateral common iliac and ipsilateral, external iliac lymph nodes remains the standard postoperative treatment of clinical stage I seminoma. Usually, 2,500–3,000 cGy is administered in fractions of 125–180 cGy/day. The remaining testicle should be shielded to preserve fertility. After adequate radiotherapy, relapse rates are less than 5% [55]. Observation without postoperative irradiation is under investigation for stage I seminoma. Relapse rates approximate 10%, and most relapses subsequently are cured with radiotherapy or chemotherapy. Though most relapses occur within three years, late relapses have been noted, necessitating close surveillance of patients for longer than five years [56]. Therefore, observation alone remains investigational.

CLINICAL STAGE I NONSEMINOMA

The standard postorchiectomy treatment of clinical stage I nonseminoma is a "nerve-sparing" modified retroperitoneal lymph node dissection (RPLND) [57]. For many years, complete bilateral RPLND, which included the pericaval, precaval, interaortocaval, preaortic, para-aortic, and bilateral common iliac lymph nodes, was standard. Mortality from this procedure is less than 1%, and significant morbidity is unusual. However, infertility secondary to disruption of sympathetic fibers that mediate ejaculation occurs in approximately 90% of patients after full bilateral RPLND. On the basis of pathologic studies, modified nerve-sparing lymph node dissections have become common for patients with clinical stage I or IIA disease [58]. These procedures produce similar outcomes but spare the sympathetic fibers and preserve potency in 60–90% of patients. Modified RPLND takes one of two general forms: nerve dissecting, in which the sympathetic fibers specifically are

Table 18.7   TNM Staging for Testicular Cancer

Classification	Definition
Primary tumor (pT)	
pTX	Primary tumor cannot be assessed (if no radical orchiectomy has been performed, TX is used.)
pT0	No evidence of primary tumor (e.g., histologic scar in testis)
pTis	Intratubular germ-cell neoplasia (carcinoma in situ)
pT1	Tumor limited to the testis and epididymis without vascular/lymphatic invasion; tumor may invade into the tunica albuginea but not the tunica vaginalis
pT2	Tumor limited to the testis and epididymis with vascular/lymphatic invasion, or tumor extending through the tunica albuginea with involvement of the tunica vaginalis
pT3	Tumor invades the spermatic cord with or without vascular/lymphatic invasion
pT4	Tumor invades the scrotum with or without vascular/lymphatic invasion
Regional lymph nodes (N)	
Clinical	
NX	Regional lymph nodes cannot be assessed
N0	No regional lymph node metastasis
N1	Metastasis with a lymph node mass ≤ 2 cm in greatest dimension; or multiple lymph nodes, none > 2 cm in greatest dimension
N2	Metastasis with a lymph node mass > 2 cm but < 5 cm in greatest dimension; or multiple lymph nodes; any one mass > 2 cm but ≤ 5 cm in greatest dimension
N3	Metastasis with a lymph node mass > 5 cm in greatest dimension
Pathologic involvement (pN)	
pNX	Regional lymph nodes cannot be assessed
pN0	No regional lymph node metastasis
pN1	Metastasis with a lymph node mass ≤ 2 cm in greatest dimension, and ≤ 5 nodes positive, none > 2 cm in greatest dimension
pN2	Metastasis with a lymph node mass > 2 cm but ≤ 5 cm in greatest dimension; or > 5 nodes positive, none > 5 cm; or evidence of extranodal extension
pN3	Metastasis with a lymph node mass > 5 cm in greatest dimension
Distant metastases (M)	
MX	Distant metastasis cannot be assessed
M0	No distant metastasis
M1	Distant metastasis
M1a	Nonregional nodal or pulmonary metastasis
M1b	Distant metastasis other than to nonregional lymph nodes and lungs

Source: Used with permission of the American Joint Committee on Cancer (AJCC), Chicago, Illinois. Reprinted from ID Fleming, JS Cooper, DE Henson, et al. (eds), *AJCC Cancer Staging Manual* (5th ed). Philadelphia: Lippincott-Raven, 1997:226–227.

Table 18.8   Serum Tumor Markers

Serum Level Designation	LDH	HCG (mIU/ml)	AFP (ng/ml)
SX	Marker studies not available or not performed		
S0	Marker study levels within normal limits		
S1	$< 1.5 \times N$	$< 5,000$	$< 1,000$
S2	$1.5–10.0 \times N$	$5,000–50,000$	$1,000–10,000$
S3	$> 10.0 \times N$	$> 50,000$	$> 10,000$

LDH = lactate dehydrogenase; HCG = human chorionic gonadotropin; AFP = alpha-fetoprotein; N = upper limit of normal for the LDH assay.
Source: Used with permission of the American Joint Committee on Cancer (AJCC), Chicago, Illinois. Reprinted from ID Fleming, JS Cooper, DE Henson, et al. (eds), *AJCC Cancer Staging Manual* (5th ed). Philadelphia: Lippincott-Raven, 1997:227.

Table 18.9   AJCC Stage Grouping for Testicular Cancer

Stage IA	T1	N0	M0	S0
Stage IB	T2–4	N0	M0	S0
Stage IS	Any T	N0	M0	S1
Stage IIA	Any T	N1	M0	S0–1
Stage IIB	Any T	N2	M0	S0–1
Stage IIC	Any T	N3	M0	S0–1
Stage IIIA	Any T	Any N	M1	S0–1
Stage IIIB	Any T	Any N	M0–1	S2
Stage IIIC	Any T	Any N	M0–1	S3
	Any T	Any N	M2	Any S

Source: Used with permission of the American Joint Committee on Cancer (AJCC), Chicago, Illinois. Reprinted from ID Fleming, JS Cooper, DE Henson, et al. (eds), *AJCC Cancer Staging Handbook*. Philadelphia: Lippincott-Raven, 1998.

identified and preserved, and nerve avoiding, in which the dissection below the inferior mesenteric artery is ipsilateral to the tumor and, therefore, spares the sympathetic fibers contralaterally. With nerve-sparing modified RPLND, relapse will occur in approximately 10% of patients with pathologically negative lymph nodes and in approximately 25% of those found at surgery to have N1 disease. Almost all patients who experience relapse will be cured successfully with chemotherapy, so overall survival is in excess of 95% [57].

Because of the efficacy of chemotherapy for patients with relapsed nonseminomatous germ-cell tumors, studies have examined the role of observation without routine RPLND in clinical stage I patients [59]. In approximately 25–30% of patients managed with observation, disease relapse will occur, almost always within the first two years. Usually, relapsing patients require chemotherapy plus RPLND. Despite this combination, overall survival is similar to that for clinical stage I nonseminomas managed with immediate RPLND, and the majority of patients who are closely observed will be spared an unnecessary RPLND. Currently, either observation, including serial CT scan of the abdomen and pelvis, or immediate RPLND is considered reasonable treatment for patients with clinical stage I disease, T1 tumors without vascular invasion, and declining marker levels [59].

CLINICAL STAGE II SEMINOMA

For patients with stage IIA or IIB seminoma (nodes < 5 cm), radiotherapy to approximately 2,500–3,000 cGy (as in clinical stage I seminoma) represents standard therapy. Areas of gross nodal involvement are treated to a total dose of 3,500–4,000 cGy. Relapse rates for nonbulky clinical stage II seminoma are approximately 5%, and most relapsing patients are cured effectively with chemotherapy [55]. Mediastinal irradiation does not improve outcome, adds toxicity, and limits subsequent delivery of chemotherapy to relapsing patients [55].

In contrast, for patients with stage IIC seminoma (> 5 cm) radiotherapy is insufficient. This subset of stage II patients should be treated with chemotherapy.

CLINICAL STAGE II NONSEMINOMA

For patients with stage IIA disease and for some patients with stage IIB disease, standard therapy consists of RPLND [60]. Nerve-sparing approaches may be relevant, depending on the extent of disease. Patients having fewer than six involved lymph nodes at RPLND, with no lymph node larger than 2 cm, generally do not require adjuvant chemotherapy. In contrast, patients with more than six nodes involved by tumor or with any lymph node larger than 2 cm experience a higher frequency of relapse [61]. Therefore, two cycles of adjuvant cisplatin-based chemotherapy generally are recommended. Patients not receiving adjuvant therapy must be observed diligently, as they will require a full course of chemotherapy if relapse occurs [61].

Many patients with clinical stage IIB disease (lymph node masses 2–5 cm in maximum dimension) are found to have unresectable disease at RPLND. Therefore, most of these patients are managed with primary chemotherapy followed by RPLND. All patients with stage IIC disease are managed with primary chemotherapy [61].

Advanced Disease

Advanced seminoma or nonseminoma consists of stage IIC disease (retroperitoneal lymph node > 5 cm) and stage III disease (supradiaphragmatic lymph nodes or visceral involvement). For patients with advanced disease, classification into risk groups is essential (Table 18.10).

RELATIVELY GOOD-RISK PATIENTS

Appropriate treatment of stage IIC and good-risk stage III patients has been defined in a series of well-controlled trials. Patients should receive three cycles of bleomycin, etoposide, and cisplatin (BEP) or four cycles of etoposide and cisplatin (EP) (Table 18.11). Each of these regimens has been associated with five-year overall survival of approximately 90% [49,62].

POOR-RISK PATIENTS

The standard treatment of poor-risk stage III patients consists of four cycles of BEP, which results in five-year survival for 30–50% of patients [63]. A series of trials has demonstrated that higher doses of cisplatin or substitution of other agents (e.g., ifosfamide) does not improve the outcome for this group of patients [64]. The efficacy of high-dose chemotherapy with autologous bone marrow transplantation in the setting of relapsed or refractory germ-cell tumors led to its investigation in the front-line treatment of poor-risk germ-cell tumors [65, 66]. Currently, a large randomized trial is comparing four cycles of BEP to two cycles of BEP followed by two cycles of cyclophosphamide, etoposide, and carboplatin with autologous bone marrow transplantation for poor-risk patients.

Table 18.10   Germ-Cell Consensus Classification

Seminoma

Good risk (90% of seminomas; 5-year PFS, 82%; 5-year overall survival, 86%)
  Any primary site
  No nonpulmonary visceral metastases
  Normal AFP, any HCG, any LDH
Intermediate risk (10% of seminomas; 5-year PFS, 67%; 5-year overall survival, 72%)
  Any primary site
  Presence of nonpulmonary visceral metastases
  Normal AFP, any HCG, any LDH
Poor (high) risk (no pure seminomas classified as high-risk)

Nonseminoma

Good risk (56% of nonseminomas; 5-year PFS, 89%; 5-year overall survival, 92%)
  Testis-retroperitoneal primary site
  No nonpulmonary visceral metastases
  Good markers: all of AFP < 1,000 ng/ml; HCG < 5,000 mIU/ml; LDH < 1.5 × upper limit of normal)
Intermediate risk (28% of nonseminomas; 5-year PFS, 75%; 5-year overall survival, 80%)
  Testis-retroperitoneal primary site
  No nonpulmonary visceral metastases
  Intermediate markers: any of AFP ≥ 1,000 and ≤ 10,000 ng/ml; HCG ≥ 5,000 and ≤ 50,000 mIU/ml; LDH ≥ 1.5 ×
    normal and ≤ 10 × normal)
Poor (high) risk (16% of nonseminomas; 5-year PFS, 41%; 5-year overall survival, 48%)
  Mediastinal primary
  Nonpulmonary visceral metastases
  Poor risk markers: any of AFP > 10,000 ng/ml; HCG > 50,000 mIU/ml; LDH > 10 × upper limit of normal)

PFS = progression-free survival; AFP = alpha-fetoprotein; HCG = human chorionic gonadotropin; LDH = lactate dehydrogenase.

Table 18.11   Chemotherapeutic Regimens for Germ-Cell Tumors

Common Abbreviation	Agent	Dosage	Schedule	Notes
For untreated patients				
PEB	Cisplatin	20 mg/m²/day	Days 1–5	3 cycles for good-risk disease, 4 cycles for poor-risk disease*
	Etoposide	100 mg/m²/day	Days 1–5	
	Bleomycin	30 units/wk	Days 2, 9, 16	
EP	Cisplatin	20 mg/m²/day	Days 1–5	4 cycles for good-risk disease*
	Etoposide	100 mg/m²/day	Days 1–5	
For pretreated patients				
VIP	Etoposide (VP16), ifosfamide, cisplatin			
	or			
VeIP	Vinblastine, ifosfamide, cisplatin			
	or			
HDC	High-dose chemotherapy with autologous bone marrow–stem cell transplantation			

POSTCHEMOTHERAPY SURGERY

Postchemotherapy surgery is a critical adjunct to the chemotherapeutic treatment of patients with advanced seminoma or nonseminoma. Patients with residual viable germ-cell tumor at surgery should receive two cycles of adjuvant BEP, after which a 30–50% risk of relapse exists. Patients without viable tumor at surgery are observed.

For nonseminomas, any residual abnormality in the retroperitoneum requires bilateral RPLND [67, 68]. Occasional patients will be candidates for nerve-sparing procedures. Pathologic findings will include viable germ-cell cancer elements in 15–20% of patients, teratoma in 30%, and necrotic debris in 50%. For patients with normal abdominal CT scans after chemotherapy, consideration may be given to observation or RPLND. Despite normal CT examination, a small proportion of these patients will have residual cancer at surgery and will suffer relapse without therapy. No satisfactory criteria exist to identify such patients and thus obviate RPLND.

For patients with seminoma, extensive desmoplastic reaction may make RPLND impossible, in which case large masses should be resected and multiple biopsies should be taken of unresectable abnormalities [69]. For patients with seminoma, residual masses measuring less than 3 cm do not require resection, as viable cancer is rare in this subset of patients. Regardless of the tumor's histology, residual abnormalities at other sites (mediastinum, liver, bone) always should be resected.

Relapsed Disease

Standard therapy fails in 20–30% of patients with advanced germ-cell tumors and in a small number of patients with localized tumors. For those patients not treated previously with chemotherapy, generally four cycles of BEP are required at the time of relapse. For patients who have advanced disease and experience relapse after BEP, two main treatment options exist (see Table 18.11) [70, 71]. Standard-dose salvage chemotherapy—commonly vinblastine (Velban®), ifosfamide, and cisplatin (VeIP)—effects cure in approximately 25% of patients who achieved a prior complete response. The combination of etoposide (VP16), ifosfamide, and cisplatin (VIP) has demonstrated similar efficacy.

High-dose chemotherapy with autologous bone marrow transplantation initially was studied in patients in whom two previous chemotherapy regimens had failed. Once efficacy had been demonstrated in this set-ting, high-dose chemotherapy was examined for patients in whom one prior regimen had failed. Currently, patients not achieving a complete response to the initial cisplatin-containing regimen are considered for high-dose chemotherapy. Patients who achieve an initial complete response to front-line therapy are reasonable candidates for conventional-dose salvage therapy, high-dose chemotherapy being reserved for third-line treatment [72]. Approximately 25% of patients will achieve cure through the use of high-dose chemotherapy. The morbidity and mortality associated with high-dose chemotherapy has decreased substantially because of the current ability to collect peripheral blood stem cells, increased familiarity with potential complications, and the shifting of high-dose chemotherapy to patients who have undergone less prior treatment.

Toxicity of Therapy

In addition to acute effects, several late sequelae arise from the treatment of germ-cell tumors. Commonly, RPLND results in infertility, especially in patients for whom nerve-sparing approaches are not applicable. Occasionally, radiotherapy and chemotherapy are associated with permanent infertility. Sperm banking should be offered to all patients prior to treatment, to preserve fertility options. Patients treated for germ-cell tumors have a 2–3% lifetime risk of developing a second primary germ-cell tumor in the contralateral testis. Additionally, the use of etoposide chemotherapy has been associated with a small but definite risk (< 0.5%) of secondary acute leukemia. This treatment-induced leukemia is characterized by translocations involving chromosome 11. Prognosis is extremely poor. Patients treated with radiotherapy have an increased risk of secondary gastrointestinal malignancy [73].

OTHER TESTICULAR TUMORS

Occasionally, testicular tumors that are not of germ-cell origin arise or the testicle is involved by metastatic disease. Testicular stromal tumors, including Leydig cell tumors and Sertoli cell tumors, account for 2–3% of all testicular tumors. Generally, these tumors present as a painless mass and are diagnosed at inguinal orchiectomy. They generally behave in a benign manner, and metastases are the only reliable indicator of malignancy [74, 75]. Lymphoma is the most common testicular tumor in men older than age 50. A small subset of patients having primary testicular lymphomas are cured by inguinal orchiectomy, but most patients have systemic disease. Rarely, the testicle may be involved with other metastatic tumors [76].

E. Prostate Cancer

■ ■ ■

William K. Kelly
Paul M. Dodd

Excluding skin cancer, adenocarcinoma of the prostate is the cancer diagnosed most commonly in men and is the second leading cause of cancer-related mortality in men. The availability of prostate-specific antigen (PSA) screening coupled with increased awareness of the disease has led to marked changes in the incidence, presentation, and management of prostate cancer [77]. PSA screening has resulted in a profound stage migration of this disease, defined as an increase in the proportion of cancers diagnosed at an early stage in which they are potentially curable. Prostate cancer is a biologically heterogeneous tumor, with some patients suffering rapid debilitation and death and others never developing clinical manifestations of the disease [78]. Selection of the appropriate curative modality for those with localized disease remains dependent on many factors, including tumor characteristics, comorbid disease, and patient preference. Likewise, treatment of patients with advanced disease requires consideration of both tumor and patient characteristics. This section provides an overview of current concepts of prostate cancer biology, diagnosis, and management.

EPIDEMIOLOGIC CONSIDERATIONS

The projected incidence of adenocarcinoma of the prostate is 180,400 new cases in 2000, and the disease is expected to result in 31,900 deaths [2]. The incidence of prostate cancer was in excess of 300,000 cases per year during the early 1990s, mainly because of an increase in screening for the disease [77]. Generally, prostate cancer is considered a disease of the elderly, with a median age at diagnosis of 65 years. Many patients with diagnosed prostate cancer will have comorbid conditions and will die of causes other than the cancer [78].

A number of risk factors for prostate cancer have been identified, age being the most important [79]. The prevalence of clinical and histologic prostate cancer increases dramatically with age. Autopsy data demonstrate that 15–30% of men older than age 50 have histologic evidence of prostate cancer, compared with 60–70% of men at age 80. In general, clinically evident prostate cancer is most common in western European nations and in the United States [80]. Persons emigrating from an area of low risk to one of high risk gradually assume the higher risk of the adopted region. Blacks have a higher incidence of prostate cancer at all ages than do whites of similar socioeconomic class and education [81]. Also, stage-corrected survival rates are uniformly shortened for blacks.

A number of studies suggest that prostate cancer risk is increased two- to fivefold in relatives of patients with prostate cancer. Environmental factors, including total and saturated fat intake, also may contribute to prostate cancer risk [82]. Cigarette smoking, alcohol use, obesity, the presence of benign prostatic hypertrophy (BPH), and previous vasectomy have not been linked convincingly to prostate cancer incidence.

ANATOMY OF THE PROSTATE GLAND

The normal prostate gland consists of a transitional zone, a central zone, and a peripheral zone. It is oriented with the broad base superiorly, the midsection, and the narrow apex inferiorly. The gland is surrounded almost completely by the prostatic capsule. The prostate is bordered by the bladder superiorly, the rectum posteriorly, and the dorsal vein complex anteriorly. Two neurovascular bundles are located immediately posterior to the prostatic capsule and provide autonomic innervation that is critical for erection. Posterolateral to the prostate are the paired seminal vesicles. The pelvic side walls are in proximity laterally. Both the neurovascular bundles and the seminal vesicles are common early sites of extraprostatic spread of prostate cancers. Primary lymph node drainage from the prostate is to the obturator hypogastric nodes. Secondary drainage is to the iliac and inguinal nodes.

HISTOLOGIC FEATURES OF PROSTATIC NEOPLASIA

Almost all prostate cancers are adenocarcinomas. The earliest recognizable prostatic lesion is prostatic intraepithelial neoplasia (PIN). PIN is characterized by proliferation within the prostatic ducts of cells with anaplastic morphology and nuclei. PIN may be characterized as low-grade or high-grade. Usually, PIN precedes the development of prostate cancer by years, and not all patients with PIN will develop cancer. Both PIN and prostate adenocarcinoma commonly originate in the peripheral zone. In contrast, BPH, which probably is not a precursor to prostate cancer, commonly involves the transitional zone.

Histologic grade of prostate cancer has been correlated with outcome, and the grading system used most commonly is that of Gleason [83]. This system assigns a grade of 1 to 5 to both the predominant and secondary growth patterns of the tumor, with higher numbers representing poorer differentiation. The two grades are added to obtain a total Gleason score between 2 and 10. Tumors with a higher Gleason score are correlated with increased likelihood of metastasis and mortality [83, 84].

MOLECULAR BIOLOGICAL FEATURES OF PROSTATIC NEOPLASIA

At a genetic level, the process of prostatic carcinogenesis is complex, with multiple genetic lesions implicated in the progression from PIN to localized cancer, locally advanced cancer, and metastatic cancer [85]. The processes of carcinogenesis and the progression of prostate cancer are regulated by both activation of tumor-promoting genes (oncogenes) and inactivation of tumor-inhibiting genes (tumor suppressor genes). Of note, mutation of *p53* probably is a late event, rarely being found in localized prostate cancer but detected in up to 50% of metastatic prostate cancers [86].

The development of androgen independence by prostate cancers is associated with hormone resistance and poor survival of patients. The normal prostate is an androgen-dependent gland, the effects of androgens being mediated by the androgen receptor (AR). Androgen stimulation is important in the development of the malignant phenotype, and most prostate cancers initially demonstrate sensitivity to androgen deprivation. After a variable period, clones resistant to the effects of androgen deprivation predominate. Amplification of the *AR* gene [87] or development of *AR* point mutations that alter its spectrum of hormone sensitivity have been reported as possible means of androgen resistance [88, 89].

SCREENING FOR PROSTATE CANCER

The availability of PSA as a diagnostic tool, coupled with increased awareness of the disease, has produced a marked increase in the number of new cases diagnosed [77, 90]. Disease detected by elevated PSA in the setting of a palpably normal gland (T1c disease) now is the most common presentation of prostate cancer [91]. Important considerations in prostate cancer screening include whether cancers detected by PSA elevation alone are biologically important and, if important, whether early screening affects survival. Several retrospective analyses have shown that cancers detected through screening share histologic features with clinically detected tumors and are significant [92, 93]. Prospective randomized studies have not evaluated adequately whether screening is associated with a decrease in overall or prostate cancer-specific mortality. The American Cancer Society [94] and the American Urological Association [95] have made formal recommendations regarding screening of men for prostate cancer [94]:

> The American Cancer Society recommends that the PSA test and the digital rectal exam should be offered annually, beginning at age 50, to men who have at least a 10-year life expectancy and to younger men who are at high risk. Information should be provided to men regarding potential risks and benefits of screening.

These guidelines for asymptomatic individuals are concerned with early detection and are not intended to recommend screening for mass populations. Other preventive health care organizations, including the United States Preventive Services Task Force, do not recommend screening.

CLINICAL PRESENTATION
Common Symptoms and Signs

Before the availability and frequent application of PSA determinations, the most common presentation of prostate cancer was with symptoms of urinary obstruction or bony pain. Most prostate cancers arise in the periphery of the gland and do not produce local symptoms until they are bulky. Cancers arising in the transitional zone of the gland may produce earlier symptoms of urinary frequency, nocturia, hesitancy, decreased force of the urinary stream, and urge incontinence. Less commonly, these symptoms may progress to complete obstruction before the patient presents for diagnosis. These symptoms are indistinguishable from those produced by benign prostatic pathology, particularly BPH. Common symptoms in advanced disease include bone pain, fatigue, and anorexia. Spinal cord compression is uncommon at diagnosis. The widespread application of

PSA screening heralded a change in the presentation of prostate cancer, with the majority of patients being asymptomatic at the time of diagnosis.

Digital Rectal Examination

Digital rectal examination (DRE), an essential component of evaluation for prostate cancer, typically reveals a hardened nodule, although either diffuse induration of the gland or a normal gland may be present. Palpable tumor may extend to the seminal vesicles or pelvic side wall. Patients with elevated PSA on screening examination frequently have a normal DRE, even if the gland contains cancer.

Prostate-Specific Antigen

PSA is relatively specific to prostatic tissues and has been highly useful for diagnosing and following up the clinical course of prostate cancer. DRE does not significantly affect the results of PSA determination, but prostate biopsy does result in an elevation of PSA. Therefore, PSA determination should not be performed for four to six weeks after biopsy. The additive value of acid phosphatase determination, once widely used to guide management of prostate cancer, currently is uncertain.

INTERPRETING PSA TEST RESULTS

Interpretation of the PSA determination must include both the degree of elevation and the results of other examinations, particularly findings of the DRE. In most cases, a PSA level greater than 4.0 ng/ml is considered abnormal. In one analysis, a PSA level greater than 4 ng/ml was associated with a 32% likelihood of detection of cancer on subsequent prostatic biopsy [96]. Consideration of the results of DRE markedly influenced the predictive value of the PSA. If the DRE was abnormal, cancer was detected in 48% of patients with a PSA level greater than 4 ng/ml, whereas if DRE was normal, cancer was found in only 24%. The degree of PSA elevation has been correlated strongly with the likelihood of localized cancer and five-year survival [92, 97].

INCREASING THE SPECIFICITY AND SENSITIVITY OF PSA TESTING

Fewer than 50% of patients with a PSA between 4 and 10 ng/ml will prove to have prostate cancer on subse-

quent biopsy. Additionally, a fraction of patients with prostate cancer will have a normal DRE and a PSA level of less than 4.0 ng/ml. Identification of persons having prostate cancer and a PSA level lower than 10 ng/ml is important, because the probability of localized prostate cancer is high. However, the unnecessary cost and discomfort accruing to men without prostate cancer is considerable.

A variety of approaches to improving the specificity or sensitivity of the PSA test have been examined. The use of age-specific PSA or PSA velocity have been proposed as potential means to improve specificity, but their utility has not been confirmed. PSA circulates in free and complexed forms in the serum, with the majority of PSA being complexed with protease inhibitors. Numerous reports have correlated a decreased percentage of free to total PSA with an increased risk of prostate cancer, whereas a normal percentage suggests a benign etiology for an elevated PSA [98–100]. A multicenter prospective clinical trial recently confirmed that, for patients having a PSA level of 4–10 ng/ml, use of percentage of free PSA could reduce unnecessary biopsies, with a minimal decrease in sensitivity [98].

DIAGNOSIS

The diagnostic procedure of choice for localized prostate cancer is transrectal biopsy, often directed by transrectal ultrasonography (TRUS). Indications for biopsy include elevated PSA, abnormal DRE, or the presence of suspicious symptoms. The use of a decreased ratio of free to total PSA also appears useful in the selection of patients for biopsy. Typically, six core needle biopsy specimens are taken, including the left and right base, midportion, and apex of the gland. Additional biopsy of palpable or TRUS-detected abnormalities may be performed. Transitional zone biopsy specimens sometimes are obtained, particularly if previous biopsy of the peripheral zone is nondiagnostic and the suspicion of prostate cancer is high.

TNM Staging Classification

The American Joint Committee on Cancer TNM (*t*umor, *n*ode, *m*etastasis) staging system is used to classify prostate cancer (Tables 18.12, 18.13) [101]. Critical issues in the staging of prostate cancer include determination of whether a tumor is organ-confined (T2b) or has extracapsular extension (T3) and whether nodal or distant metastatic spread exists.

Table 18.12 TNM Staging for Prostate Cancer

Classification	Definition
Histopathologic grade (G)	
GX	Grade cannot be assessed
G1	Well differentiated (slight anaplasia)
G2	Moderately differentiated (moderate anaplasia)
G3	Poorly differentiated or undifferentiated (marked anaplasia)
Primary tumor (T)	
TX	Primary tumor cannot be assessed
T0	No evidence of primary tumor
T1	Clinically inapparent tumor not palpable nor visible by imaging
T1a	Tumor incidental histologic finding in 5% or less of tissue resected
T1b	Tumor incidental histologic finding in more than 5% of tissue resected
T1c	Tumor identified by needle biopsy (e.g., because of elevated PSA level)
T2	Tumor confined within prostate[a]
T2a	Tumor involves one lobe
T2b	Tumor involves both lobes
T3	Tumor extends through the prostate capsule[b]
T3a	Extracapsular extension (unilateral or bilateral)
T3b	Tumor invades seminal vesicle(s)
T4	Tumor is fixed or invades adjacent structures other than seminal vesicles: bladder neck, external sphincter, rectum, levator muscles, and/or pelvic wall
Regional lymph nodes (N)	
NX	Regional lymph nodes cannot be assessed
N0	No regional lymph node metastasis
N1	Metastasis in regional lymph node or nodes
Distant metastasis (M)	
MX	Distant metastasis cannot be assessed
M0	No distant metastasis
M1	Distant metastasis
M1a	Nonregional lymph node(s)
M1b	Bone(s)
M1c	Other site(s)

PSA = prostate-specific antigen.

[a]Tumor found in one or both lobes by needle biopsy but not palpable or reliably visible by imaging is classified as T1c.

[b]Invasion into the prostatic apex or into (but not beyond) the prostatic capsule is not classified as T3 but as T2.

Source: Used with permission of the American Joint Committee on Cancer (AJCC), Chicago, Illinois. Reprinted from ID Fleming, JS Cooper, DE Henson, et al. (eds), *AJCC Cancer Staging Manual*, Philadelphia: Lippincott-Raven, 1997.

Table 18.13 Stage Grouping for Prostate Cancer

Stage I	T1a	N0	M0	G1
Stage II	T1a	N0	M0	G2–4
	T1b	N0	M0	Any G
	T1c	N0	M0	Any G
	T2	N0	M0	Any G
Stage III	T3	N0	M0	Any G
Stage IV	T4	N0	M0	Any G
	Any T	N1	M0	Any G
	Any T	Any N	M1	Any G

Source: Used with permission of the American Joint Committee on Cancer (AJCC), Chicago, Illinois. Reprinted from ID Fleming, JS Cooper, DE Henson, et al. (eds), *AJCC Cancer Staging Manual*, Philadelphia: Lippincott-Raven, 1997.

Assessment of Risk for Extracapsular Spread

Extracapsular spread of prostate cancer affects the choice of local treatment modality and has a negative impact on prognosis. As individual modalities, DRE, PSA, and TRUS are inadequate to assess the local extent of prostate cancer. Magnetic resonance imaging (MRI) with an endorectal coil has been used to assess extracapsular spread of cancer but is not sensitive for detection of microscopic extracapsular extension [102, 103].

On the basis of the results of PSA, DRE, and histologic grade of the tumor, several groups have developed nomograms that predict the likelihood of extracapsular extension of tumor [97, 104, 105]. Using data from 4,133 patients, Partin et al. [104] performed a multinomial logistic regression analysis correlating PSA, clinical stage, and Gleason grade with likelihood of organ-confined disease, isolated capsular penetration, seminal vesicle involvement, and pelvic lymph node involvement. Using data from 983 patients with clinically localized prostate cancer, Kattan et al. [105] developed a nomogram that allows prediction of disease recurrence based on pretreatment PSA, clinical stage, and Gleason score (Fig. 18.5).

Assessment of Lymph Node or Distant Metastasis

Most commonly, prostate cancer spreads to bone or pelvic lymph nodes. Frequently, the pattern of bony metastasis is blastic and is visualized readily by bone scintigraphy. If the etiology of bone scan abnormalities is uncertain, routine radiography or MRI can be useful for clarification. Generally, the distribution of bony metas-

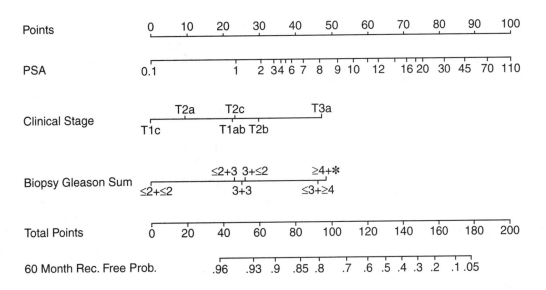

Instructions for Physician: Locate the patient's PSA on the PSA axis. Draw a line straight upward to the Points axis to determine how many points toward recurrence the patient receives for his PSA. Repeat this process for the Clinical Stage and Biopsy Gleason Sum axes, each time drawing straight upward to the points axis. Sum the points acheived for each predictor and locate this sum on the Total Points axis. Draw a line straight down to find the patient's probability of remaining recurrence-free for 60 months, assuming he does not die of another cause first.

Note: *This nomogram is not applicable to a man who is not otherwise a candidate for radical prostatectomy. You can use this only on a man who has already selected radical prostatectomy as treatment for his prostate cancer.*

Instruction to patient: "Mr. X, if we had 100 men exactly like you, we would expect between (predicted percentage from nomogram – 10%) and (predicted percentage + 10%) to remain free of their disease at 5 years following radical prostatectomy, and recurrence after 5 years is very rare."

© 1997   Michael W. Kattan and Peter T. Scardino
Scott Department of Urology

Figure 18.5 Preoperative nomogram for prostate cancer recurrence. PSA = prostate-specific antigen. Rec. = recurrence; Prob. = probability. (Reprinted with permission of Oxford University Press from MW Kattan, JA Eastham, AMF Stapleton, et al., A preoperative nomogram for disease recurrence following radical prostatectomy for prostate cancer. *J Natl Cancer Inst* 90:766–771, 1998.)

tasis mimics the distribution of bone marrow in adults, with metastases found most commonly in the spine, pelvis, femur, skull, and ribs. Assessment of regional lymph nodes is important in the treatment of both metastatic disease and apparently localized disease. Computed tomography (CT) scanning or MRI of the abdomen and pelvis can be used to assess the presence of metastasis to regional lymph nodes. Assessment of pelvic lymph nodes is particularly important in patients who have clinically localized disease and in whom lymph node metastasis precludes cure by local means alone. The utility of CT and MRI in this setting remains uncertain because of suboptimal sensitivity and specificity [105, 106]. Several studies have suggested that ^{111}In-labeled capromab pendetide (ProstaScint) scanning can assist in determining extent of disease in pa-

tients who have an increasing PSA level after prostatectomy [106, 107].

TREATMENT
Localized Disease

The principle goal of therapy for localized prostate cancer is cure. Several curative options exist, but lack of randomized comparisons among them complicates selection of the appropriate treatment for any given patient. In particular, radical prostatectomy and external-beam radiotherapy have not been compared in randomized trials. Ultimately, selection of appropriate therapy depends on tumor and patient characteristics and on patient preference.

OBSERVATION

Many patients with diagnosed localized prostate cancer are elderly and have comorbid conditions. Because the rate of progression of localized prostate cancers is slow, a policy of observation is appropriate for some patients, generally those with a life expectancy of less than 10 years and low-grade tumors [108].

RADICAL PROSTATECTOMY

Usually, radical prostatectomy is reserved for patients who have T1 or T2 disease and are suitable candidates for major surgery. The operation may be performed using either a retropubic or a perineal approach. Using either approach, the prostate, seminal vesicles, and a cuff of bladder neck are removed en bloc, and a vesicourethral reanastomosis is performed. When the retropubic approach is used, a bilateral pelvic lymph node dissection may be performed in patients at risk for lymph node metastasis. Perineal prostatectomy does not facilitate lymph node dissection and, therefore, generally is considered in patients at low risk of lymph node spread. Enhanced understanding of the anatomy of the pelvic plexus has enabled preservation of sexual function in selected patients through "nerve-sparing" prostatectomy. Depending on the extent of disease at surgery, either one or both neurovascular bundles may be spared without compromising cancer control [109].

PSA level is being used to assess outcome and should remain undetectable after radical prostatectomy. Recent series have used PSA relapse to assess outcome [110]. PSA relapse-free survival for patients with T1 or T2 tumors ranges from 71% to 85%, whereas substantially fewer patients with capsular penetration were PSA relapse-free [111–113]. Generally, patients with lymph node metastases are incurable with surgery alone [111, 112].

Early complications of radical prostatectomy include occasional rectal injury, myocardial infarction, and deep venous thrombosis or pulmonary embolus. The operation is associated with a mortality less than 1%. Bladder neck contracture, urinary incontinence, and impotence are long-term complications. Often, reports of the prevalence of long-term complications have used nonstandardized data collection instruments and techniques, often in selected patient populations [114]. In several recent series, reported rates of urinary incontinence ranged from 6% to 35% [115–117]. Before the development of nerve-sparing prostatectomy, impotence was an almost universal complication of the procedure [109]. Approximately 60% of selected patients treated with nerve-sparing prostatectomy, including up to 90% of patients younger than 50 years, may preserve potency [116, 118]. However, other studies suggest that the incidence of postprostatectomy impotence is as high as 95% [114].

RADIOTHERAPY

External-beam radiotherapy is a second curative modality for localized prostate cancer. The development of three-dimensional conformal radiotherapy has allowed precise control of irradiation delivery to the entire tumor and a rim of surrounding normal tissue. Generally, the prostate is treated to a total dose of 6,500–7,000 cGy, but with conformal techniques, this dose can be increased substantially.

Often, radiotherapy series include patients with more extensive local disease than do surgical series, rendering problematic comparison of the outcome and complications of therapy. Additionally, chronic toxicity of radiotherapy generally develops over the 1–2-year period after completion of therapy. Acute toxicities of radiotherapy, including urinary frequency, dysuria, diarrhea and, occasionally, rectal bleeding, occur in up to 50% of the patients [119]. Generally, resolution of acute toxicities occurs within one month. Long-term complications include bladder neck contraction, sexual dysfunction, and urinary incontinence. In one study, 3 and 12 months after radiotherapy, 58% and 67% of patients, respectively, reported erections insufficient for intercourse [114]. The incidence of urinary incontinence, measured by the necessity for wearing pads in underwear, was approximately 5%. Evaluation of PSA relapse after radiotherapy is problematic, because the PSA level does not reach a nadir until 12–24 months after completion of therapy and usually does not become undetectable. Overall, survival rates from older irradiation series appear comparable to those for patients treated with prostatectomy.

Preliminary assessment of the efficacy of three-dimensional conformal radiotherapy recently was reported from the University of Michigan. Researchers there noted a PSA relapse rate of 15% for patients with favorable disease characteristics [120].

INTERSTITIAL BRACHYTHERAPY

Radioactive seed implantation using ^{125}I or ^{103}Pd is another promising treatment option for patients with localized prostate cancer. Improvements in technology allow for better planning and irradiation dose distribution than was possible previously. CT or TRUS are used to design a treatment plan that provides adequate irradiation to the entire target volume. Using spinal anesthesia, seeds are inserted through the perineum under radiographic guidance. Wallner et al. [121] reported four-year PSA-determined relapse-free survival of 63%, but longer follow-up is required. Acute toxicity of treatment was minimal and included urinary retention, dysuria, and urgency. Late toxicities included rectal ulceration, which was noted in five of 92 patients, and persistent urinary obstructive symptoms. Preservation of sexual function was clearly related to status before treatment. Among patients with potency prior to treatment, only 14% developed impotence at three years. Although more data and longer follow-up are needed, interstitial irradiation may lead to better preservation of sexual function.

CRYOSURGERY

Cryosurgical ablation of the prostate involves use of cooling probes that cause necrosis of prostatic tissue through freezing. Results are preliminary, and the procedure remains investigational. Whether the efficacy will equal that of radical prostatectomy remains unclear. Complications include urinary retention, perineal pain, impotence, and rectal fistulas [122].

Metastatic Prostate Cancer

Metastatic prostate cancer is considered incurable. Control of tumor growth, palliation of symptoms, and maintenance of quality of life are important goals of therapy. The most common presentation of metastatic disease is a rising PSA after primary therapy without other signs or symptoms. However, PSA-determined relapse portends the eventual development of overt metastatic disease. Although prostate cancer most commonly metastasizes to bone, lymph nodes, lung, liver, pleura, adrenal glands, and other sites also may be involved.

The prognosis for patients with metastatic prostate cancer is variable, but prognostic factors associated with poor outcome have been identified. A National Cancer Institute Intergroup Trial [123, 124] stratified patients based on extent of disease (minimal or severe) and performance status. Median survival for the group with minimal disease (defined as lymph node and axial bone metastases only) and favorable performance status was 53 months, significantly better than that for patients with severe disease, whose median survival approximated 30 months. Anemia, anorexia, pain, and elevated alkaline phosphatase also have been found to have prognostic significance in some studies [125].

Androgen deprivation forms the cornerstone for the management of metastatic prostate cancer. Androgen deprivation may be achieved medically or surgically. The most common medical approaches to achieve testicular androgen deprivation include luteinizing hormone-releasing hormone (LHRH) agonists with or without antiandrogens. Orchiectomy and LHRH agonist therapy are equally effective as initial treatment of metastatic prostate cancer and are standard treatment options.

Serial PSA determination is important in evaluating response, and radiographic imaging is useful for following up patients with visible metastatic disease. Because of its widespread use, a rising PSA level is the only manifestation of metastatic disease in a large number of patients. Failure to normalize the PSA level has been recognized as a poor prognostic feature in patients treated with androgen deprivation therapy. A large, recent multicenter trial reported normalization of PSA (< 4 ng/ml) in approximately 75% of patients [126]. Response proportions measured by radiographic assessment are somewhat lower, perhaps reflecting bulk of the disease [127, 128]. The median duration of response is approximately 18 months [129].

ORCHIECTOMY

Orchiectomy removes the major source of male testosterone production. It was the original means of androgen deprivation and has the advantage of permanency without repeated injections or oral medications.

LHRH AGONISTS

LHRH agonists cause castrate levels of testosterone by decreasing its production. Initially, LHRH agonists bind to LHRH receptors in the pituitary, resulting in stimulation of luteinizing hormone (LH) secretion and consequent increase in testosterone production. Subsequently, a down-regulation of LH receptors on the pituitary gland occurs, leading to decreased LH secretion and to castrate levels of testosterone. During the initial phase of LHRH agonist administration, increased testosterone can cause a "flare" reaction, in which clinical worsening may occur. For this reason, commonly an antiandrogen is administered for one week before initiation of LHRH agonist therapy, to antagonize the effect of increased testosterone. Two LHRH agonists—goserelin acetate and leuprolide acetate—are available. Each is available as monthly, three-monthly, or four-monthly injections. The main side effects are hot flashes, loss of libido and potency, and eventual decrease in muscle mass. LHRH agonists and orchiectomy have demonstrated equivalent efficacy in randomized trials, so LHRH analogs are acceptable monotherapy [126]. Recent investigations suggest that intermittent hormonal deprivation may provide benefits equal to those of continuous androgen deprivation, but this approach remains investigational [130].

ANTIANDROGENS

Antiandrogens competitively inhibit binding of testosterone to the androgen receptor. Because they act at the intracellular level, libido and potency are spared in some patients. Increased LH production results from antiandrogen use, which ultimately results in elevation of the testosterone level. Three nonsteroidal antiandrogens—bicalutamide, flutamide, and nilutamide—are available in the United States. The major side effects are fatigue, nausea, diarrhea, elevation of hepatic transaminases, and delayed adjustment to night vision. Mixed results have emerged from trials comparing antiandrogens to orchiectomy so, at present, antiandrogen monotherapy cannot be considered a standard first-line treatment option [131]. Antiandrogen monotherapy can, however, be considered for patients to whom potency is very important and who understand the risks.

COMBINED ANDROGEN BLOCKADE

Monotherapy using orchiectomy or LHRH agonists does not block adrenal androgens, which can bypass the effects of testicular hormone deprivation. The adrenal gland accounts for 10–15% of circulating androgens. Using an antiandrogen in combination with either orchiectomy or an LHRH agonist offers the benefit of blockage of both testicular and adrenal androgen effects.

Studies examining combined androgen blockade (CAB) have reached divergent results. Some randomized trials have reported survival benefits [123], but other trials reached the opposite conclusion. Two meta-analyses also reached divergent conclusions [132, 133]. A recent National Cancer Institute Intergroup Trial in 1,387 patients did not show a survival benefit to CAB [126]. Currently, the benefit of CAB relative to monotherapy for first-line treatment of metastatic prostate cancer is unclear. CAB is significantly more expensive, and antiandrogen therapy adds toxicity. Some studies suggest that patients with minimal disease gain significant benefit, and CAB may be reasonable in this subset of patients [124].

Relapsed Disease

Almost all patients with metastatic disease will progress at a variable interval after the initiation of primary hormonal treatment. Usually, this progress signifies the development of androgen-independent disease in which the tumor proliferates despite castrate levels of testosterone. Documentation of a low level of testosterone is important prior to concluding that progression has occurred. Usually, progression is manifested by a rising PSA level in the absence of symptoms or by progression at prior sites of disease. Options for second-line treatment include antiandrogen withdrawal, secondary hormonal therapy, chemotherapy, or the use of novel investigational agents. The median survival of patients after progression is approximately one year, and no second-line therapy has been shown to improve survival.

ANTIANDROGEN WITHDRAWAL

Since responses to flutamide withdrawal were recognized in 1993, a number of retrospective series have documented that approximately 35% of patients respond to flutamide or bicalutamide withdrawal, with a median response duration of four months [134]. Because of the lack of associated toxicity, antiandrogen withdrawal should be attempted in most patients before more toxic therapies are initiated.

SECONDARY HORMONAL THERAPIES

Secondary hormonal maneuvers benefit a subset of patients [129]. In patients treated with LHRH agonists or orchiectomy, an initial trial of an antiandrogen is reasonable and has been associated with a clinical benefit in 20–40% of patients. A few patients respond to high-dose bicalutamide even after progression on flutamide [135]. In addition to stimulating appetite, high-dose megestrol acetate produces occasional objective or subjective responses. Ketoconazole is an inhibitor of adrenal steroidogenesis and recently was evaluated for patients after flutamide withdrawal [136]. Among 50 patients, the PSA response proportion was 62.5%, and the median duration of response was 3.5 months. Several studies have noted improvements in quality of life using corticosteroids alone or in combination with other agents [137].

CYTOTOXIC CHEMOTHERAPY

The role of cytotoxic chemotherapy for patients after progression on androgen blockade is being re-evaluated, but recent studies suggest that significant palliation may be derived and objective responses can be obtained. Tannock et al. [138] conducted a randomized, multi-institutional comparison of mitoxantrone plus prednisone versus prednisone alone in symptomatic patients with hormone-refractory disease. A significant advantage in palliation, as measured by decrease in pain without an increase in requirements for analgesic medications, was noted for the combination (29% versus 12%). The duration of palliation also was longer in the combined therapy arm (43 versus 18 weeks). Therapy was very well tolerated [138].

Most patients with disease relapse have osseous disease only, which renders response assessment difficult. However, more than 90% of such patients have an elevated PSA level at the time of relapse, and posttherapy changes in this tumor marker have been associated with improved survival. In particular, a posttherapy PSA decline of 50%, achieved within 12 weeks of the initiation of treatment, has been shown to correlate with prolongation of survival [139].

Trials using posttherapy PSA decline as an end point have identified several active agents that are undergoing further testing. In particular, the combination of estramustine with vinblastine, etoposide, docetaxel, or paclitaxel has resulted in significant PSA decline in 30–70% of patients and measurable disease regression in 30–50% of cases [140–142].

INVESTIGATIONAL APPROACHES

Because no curative therapy for metastatic prostate cancer exists, the need for better treatment is urgent. An array of novel approaches to therapy is under investigation. These approaches include differentiating agents, angiogenesis inhibitors, antibodies to growth factor receptors, and antimetastatic agents. Immunologic therapy is being studied in patients with low-volume disease (with an elevated PSA level only). Selection of end points for trials using noncytotoxic approaches is an evolving science. Traditional end points, such as PSA decline and tumor shrinkage, may not be suitable.

F. Penile and Urethral Cancer

■ ■ ■

CURTIS A. PETTAWAY
COLIN P. N. DINNEY

PENILE CANCER
Incidence and Epidemiologic Considerations

Penile carcinoma is a rare malignancy in Western countries, accounting for less than 1% of all cancers in men [143, 144]. In developing countries, however, the incidence is substantial, approaching 10–20% of cancers in men in Asia, Africa, and South America [145–148].

The most common etiologic factor among men with penile carcinoma is the presence of a foreskin. In male persons who are circumcised early in infancy, the incidence of penile cancer is virtually nonexistent [144, 149]. Yet, this protective effect does not appear to exist if the patient is circumcised later in childhood or in adulthood [149]. Factors related to the presence of the foreskin and the development of cancer may be the presence of a closed preputial environment, with accompanying inflammation allowing for metaplastic transformation. Phimosis has been correlated strongly with penile cancer, occurring in up to 50% of patients [144, 150, 151]. The association between phimosis and penile cancer may result from a carcinogenic agent (bacteria, virus, etc.) within the closed preputial cavity and lack of proper hygiene. Smegma, the debris of desquamating epithelial cells on the inner surface of the prepuce, has been proposed as a potential carcinogen [147, 152]. *Mycobacterium smegmatis* may act primarily or secondarily as a carcinogen by direct effect or by converting smegma sterols into carcinogenic sterols. This hypothesis has not been proved definitively [153, 154].

The role of human papillomavirus (HPV) has now come to the forefront as an etiologic agent in squamous penile cancer. Epidemiologic data provided the first clues of this association by demonstrating that the wives or ex-wives of men with penile cancer had a threefold higher risk of cervical carcinoma [155]. Further investigation revealed that the male partners of women with cervical intraepithelial neoplasia had a significantly higher incidence of penile intraepithelial neoplasia [156]. These same male patients also were found to have a greater incidence of HPV.

Advanced molecular biological techniques, such as polymerase chain reaction and in situ hybridization, have provided increased evidence for an etiologic role for HPV by identifying specific DNA sequences from different HPV types in primary penile lesions (malignant and benign) but not in normal foreskins [157, 158]. HPV types 6 and 11 are associated most commonly with nondysplastic lesions, such as genital warts, but these are noted also in nonmetastatic verrucous carcinomas. In contrast, HPV types 16, 18, 31, and 33 are associated with in situ and invasive carcinomas [159]. HPV16 appears to be the type detected most frequently in primary carcinomas and has been detected also in metastatic lesions [157, 159]. The HPV genome encodes oncoprotein E6, which binds the tumor suppressor protein p53 [160], and oncoprotein E7, which binds the retinoblastoma protein [161]. Although HPV infection may be an important factor in the development of penile cancer, its presence is not invariable; 31% to 63% of patients with penile carcinomas test positive [159], indicating that additional factors also may be involved in the development of the disease.

Ultraviolet radiation also appears to be a carcinogen in squamous cell carcinoma (SCC) of the penis. This possibility is demonstrated best by the increased incidence of penile carcinoma in patients who have psoriasis and are treated with ultraviolet A phototherapy [162].

Finally, recent epidemiologic evidence has linked cigarette smoking to penile cancer [149]. Occupational hazards, other venereal diseases (i.e., gonorrhea, syphilis, herpesvirus), and marijuana or alcohol intake have not been shown to be associated with a higher incidence of penile cancer [149].

Although the disorder is a disease of older men, patient age at diagnosis ranges from 22 to 90 years [163, 164]. Data regarding race and penile carcinoma are conflicting and suggest either no difference or a significant increase in incidence of penile cancer for black versus white men [165, 166]. However, this divergence may reflect a difference in neonatal circumcision practices or other confounding variables rather than a genetic predisposition. In the United States, 22% of the patients were younger than 40 years, and 7% were younger than 30 years. Furthermore, penile cancer has been reported in children [163].

Presentation, Clinical Manifestations, and Natural History

In its early stages, penile cancer often follows an indolent course, beginning as a small lesion producing local symptoms (mass, ulceration, irritation, bleeding, pain, and discharge) of varying duration prior to presentation and histologic confirmation. For multiple reasons, including denial, ignorance, and embarrassment, delayed presentation of patients with penile cancer is common. More than half of all patients with penile cancer will delay seeking medical attention for at least six months after the appearance of symptoms, with one-third of patients waiting more than one year [167]. Commonly, patients seeking medical attention will be treated with antimicrobials for a presumed infectious etiology. For all these reasons, tumors having metastasized beyond the primary site at the time of presentation are not uncommon. Tumor spread occurs via penile and regional lymphatic vessels [168]. Metastatic deposits enlarge in the inguinal nodal areas, eventually producing ulceration and infection. Often, death results from sepsis or, less commonly, from hemorrhage after erosion of the tumor into the femoral vessels [144]. Although fewer than 10% of patients have distant metastases at presentation, advanced regional disease often is a harbinger of metastatic disease development, which can occur in several organs, including lung, liver, bone, and brain [144, 169].

Pathologic Characteristics and Differential Diagnosis

BENIGN LESIONS

Because the gross appearance of the primary lesion in penile cancer varies widely—from an exophytic papillary mass to a scaly plaque or a frank ulcerative lesion—it can be confused with benign conditions involving the penis. Nonmalignant lesions of the penis are relatively rare, with the exception of condylomata acuminata. Condylomata are caused by HPV (types 6 and 11) and grossly appear as either painless sessile or papillary exophytic lesions on the penile shaft or glans [159]. Occasionally, condylomata occur within the urethra. These lesions are treated with topical podophyllin, freezing, or laser ablation.

Other benign lesions of the penis include herpes genitalis, caused by herpes simplex virus type 2 and manifesting as a small, painful ulcerated lesion, and balanitis xerotica obliterans (lichen sclerosis et atrophicus), characterized by white epidermal plaques often involving the glans or prepuce. Distinction of these benign lesions from penile cancer can be made definitively only by histologic examination of a biopsy specimen.

When malignancy is suspected, small lesions are managed best by excisional biopsy rather than by incisional or punch dermatologic biopsy. Most often, lesions involving the prepuce are treated by circumcision. No disfiguring procedure should be considered without first establishing a histologic diagnosis of cancer. Skin tests, serology, culture, and special stains may be used to rule out an infectious etiology if biopsy is negative for carcinoma. Careful follow-up with a low threshold for repeat biopsy should be maintained for nonhealing penile lesions.

CARCINOMA IN SITU

Premalignant lesions of the penis include erythroplasia of Queyrat and Bowen's disease [170, 171]. Erythroplasia of Queyrat appears as a shiny, red, velvety elevated plaque involving the prepuce or glans, most commonly occurring in uncircumcised men in the fifth or sixth decade of life. Bowen's disease appears as a scaly plaque on the shaft of the penis without erythematous discoloration and typically arises one decade earlier than erythroplasia of Queyrat. Although originally described separately, owing to their slightly differing clinical presentations, these two entities are best classified together as penile carcinoma in situ [170, 171]. Although carcinoma in situ was believed to be associated with a higher incidence of internal malignancy, case-control studies have shown no such association [172]. Thus, patients with carcinoma in situ do not need to be screened routinely for internal malignancies [172, 173]. These intraepithelial neoplasms progress to invasive SCC in approximately 10% of cases [174]. Histologically, these lesions demonstrate proliferation of large atypical cells, multinucleated cells, loss of polarity, and numerous mitoses, but these findings are restricted to the epithelium. In contrast, *bowenoid papulosis* is a term describing a similar condition that occurs in younger men but that may be multicentric, follows an indolent course, and does not progress to invasive carcinoma.

INVASIVE SQUAMOUS PENILE CANCER

SCC of the penis is histologically identical to that in other areas of the body and most often is graded by degree of differentiation according to the Broder's system used for cutaneous SCC [175]. Well-differentiated penile SCC consists of hyperkeratotic epidermis giving rise to fingerlike projections of atypical squamous cells with associated keratin pearls. With progression to higher grades, keratin pearls are lost, and nuclear pleomorphism and mitotic figures are more prominent.

Verrucous carcinoma, also known as *giant condyloma of Buschke-Lowenstein*, is a variant of penile SCC and presents as a large fungating, often ulcerated mass, arising most commonly from the coronal sulcus. Histologically, this lesion is a well-differentiated SCC with an exophytic papillary growth pattern, and it may represent malignant degeneration of HPV condylomata. Clinically, these tumors extend locally by burrowing into normal tissue but do not metastasize.

NONSQUAMOUS MALIGNANCIES OF THE PENIS

Nonsquamous malignancies account for only 5% of penile cancers. These tumors include a variety of sarcomas, basal cell carcinoma, and melanoma [174]. The incidence of Kaposi's sarcoma of the penis has increased dramatically, secondary to the rise in the acquired immunodeficiency syndrome, and is the presenting sign in up to 3% of patients afflicted with that disorder [174]. These lesions can be managed by local excision or radiotherapy.

METASTATIC TUMORS

Metastases to the penis are rare and usually represent a late manifestation of systemic metastasis. Usually, the metastasis is seen clinically in a patient who has a known cancer and presents with new-onset priapism or an unusual penile lesion [176]. The most common primary site for penile metastasis is the prostate, followed by the bladder, the rectosigmoid colon, and the kidney [176]. The prognosis is poor, and treatment should be supportive and systemic. Rarely, partial or total penectomy for localized lesions offers good palliation when negative margins can be achieved [177].

Staging and Prognostic Factors

Two staging systems currently used to evaluate the extent of disease in patients with penile cancer are the Jackson staging system (Table 18.14) [178] and the American Joint Committee on Cancer's (AJCC's) TNM (*tumor*, *node*, *metastasis*) staging system (Table 18.15) [179]. Using the Jackson system is simple, and it correlates with survival. However, it has been replaced largely by the TNM system, which provides improved stratification of the depth of invasion of the primary tumor and nodal involvement. Because prognosis and

Table 18.14   Jackson System of Staging Penile Squamous Carcinoma

Stage	Definition
I	Lesions confined to the glans or prepuce (or both)
II	Lesions extending onto the shaft of the penis
III	Lesions associated with operable malignant inguinal lymph nodes
IV	Lesions extending off the shaft of the penis or inoperable inguinal metastases or distant metastasis

Source: Reprinted with permission of Blackwell Science from SM Jackson, The treatment of carcinoma of the penis. *Br J Surg* 53:33,1966.

Table 18.15   TNM Staging for Penile Squamous Cancer

Classification	Definition
Primary tumor (T)	
TX	Primary tumor cannot be assessed
T0	No evidence of primary tumor
Tis	Carcinoma in situ
Ta	Noninvasive verrucous carcinoma
T1	Tumor invades subepithelial connective tissue
T2	Tumor invades corpus spongiosum or cavernosum
T3	Tumor invades urethra or prostate
T4	Tumor invades other adjacent structures
Regional lymph nodes (N)	
NX	Regional lymph nodes cannot be assessed
N0	No regional lymph node metastasis
N1	Metastasis in a single superficial, inguinal lymph node
N2	Metastasis in multiple or bilateral superficial inguinal lymph nodes
N3	Metastasis in deep inguinal or pelvic lymph node(s), unilateral or bilateral
Distant metastasis (M)	
MX	Distant metastasis cannot be assessed
M0	No distant metastasis
M1	Distant metastasis

Source: Used with permission of the American Joint Committee on Cancer (AJCC), Chicago, Illinois. Reprinted from ID Fleming, JS Cooper, DE Henson, et al. (eds), *AJCC Cancer Staging Manual* (5th ed). Philadelphia: Lippincott-Raven, 1997:215–217.

therapeutic determinations depend on cancer stage at presentation, particularly the depth of invasion in low-stage disease, an accurate assessment of the extent of disease is mandatory.

Staging studies begin with a physical examination of the primary lesion and the inguinal region, tumor biopsy, chest roentgenography, and computed tomography (CT) of the abdomen and pelvis. However, non-invasive staging of regional disease long has been considered highly inaccurate because only 35–60% of palpable adenopathy actually is caused by nodal metastasis, with the remainder resulting from inflammation or infection. Conversely, up to 66% of patients with palpably normal findings subsequently will have nodal metastasis [180, 181]. This distinction is crucial, because 95% of patients with proved nodal metastasis treated conservatively die within three years of diagnosis, as compared with a five-year survival rate of 77% for patients with nonmetastatic disease [181, 182].

Depth of invasion of the primary lesion is the most prognostically useful indicator of lymph node involvement. Tumors limited to the prepuce and subepithelium of the glans (AJCC stage T1) are associated with nodal metastasis in only 5–11% of cases [183]. Recent studies suggest that this classification can be subdivided further: On the basis of the pathologic stage and grade of the primary tumor, subsets of patients with a very low risk of metastasis now can be defined. Patients with primary tumors of pathologic stages Tis, Ta, and T1 (and grade 1) exhibit an incidence rate of nodal metastasis of 0–2% [184, 185]. Similarly, Hall et al. [186] found that patients with stage T_1 tumors invading not more than 0.5 cm in depth remained without recurrence at a median follow-up of 10 years. In contrast, in patients with corporal invasion (Jackson stage II and AJCC stages T2, T3, and T4), the incidence of nodal involvement rises to 47–68% [185]. DNA flow cytometric studies of the penile tumor have not proved useful in predicting lymph node metastases [186].

The prognosis for patients with penile carcinoma depends greatly on stage, particularly on regional nodal involvement. Five-year survival falls sharply, from 66% to 90% for patients with Jackson stage I disease to 20–24% and 0–5% for patients with Jackson stages III and IV, respectively [149, 183]. Furthermore, the extent of nodal involvement adversely affects survival. In a study by Ravi [187] of 201 patients, five-year survival declined from 95% for patients without nodal disease to 81% and 50% when one to three or more than three inguinal lymph nodes were positive, respectively. No patient with pelvic nodal disease survived to five years [187].

Ilioinguinal lymphadenectomy, a surgical procedure with both therapeutic and diagnostic advantages, remains the most reliable staging technique to assess regional nodal status. However, because of its invasive nature and attendant morbidity [188], other less invasive strategies have been evaluated and include (1) needle aspiration (with or without lymphangiography) [189], (2) sentinel lymph node biopsy (via the Cabanas technique) [190], and (3) extended sentinel lymph node dissection [191]. However, these techniques have failed to predict the presence of metastatic disease in some cases, owing either to sampling error within the inguinal field or to the presence of anatomic variation in lymphatic distribution. Thus, lymphadenectomy for patients with invasive tumors (AJCC stage T2 or greater), high-grade tumors, or tumors exhibiting vascular invasion is a reasonable approach even when the nodes are clinically negative [180, 192, 193]. Whether a more limited complete dissection or intraoperative lymphatic mapping (used in breast cancer and melanoma) will decrease the morbidity of surgical staging while maintaining efficacy requires further study [194, 195].

Treatment

PRIMARY TUMOR STAGE TIS, TA, OR T1

Surgery remains the mainstay of therapy for penile cancer. However, less invasive techniques have been recognized as suitable for the treatment of patients with low-stage disease. In considering therapeutic options for such patients, urologic surgeons weigh the benefit of functional organ preservation using minimally invasive therapy (e.g., topical chemotherapy, radiotherapy, circumcision, laser ablation, Mohs' micrographic surgery) against the risk of recurrent or persistent disease [196, 197].

Topical chemotherapy is an effective alternative for the treatment of carcinoma in situ. Data from several case reports suggest that a treatment duration of three to seven weeks with 5-fluorouracil (5%) is necessary to prevent recurrence [170, 198]. Potential drawbacks include inadequate treatment because of poor patient compliance or severe local skin irritation.

Radiotherapy may be delivered as external-beam therapy or with brachytherapeutic techniques. Radiotherapy may be used to treat selected patients with distal penile lesions (Jackson stage I or AJCC stage T1), with control rates in several series ranging from 78% to 90% [199–202]. However, complications are common and include stricture, fistula formation, and distal penile or skin necrosis in 17–40% of treated patients. Approximately 20% of patients with low-stage lesions require subsequent amputation after radiotherapy as a result of recurrent disease or iatrogenic complications [200]. For these reasons, radiotherapy should be reserved for patients who have low-stage lesions and refuse surgical therapy.

More recently, microscopically controlled tumor excision (Mohs' micrographic surgery) [196, 197] and laser tumor ablation [203] have become popular therapeutic options for low-stage disease. Mohs' micrographic surgery involves fixation of the tumor with a topical solution followed by layer-by-layer tumor excision until a negative surgical margin is obtained. In one series, local tumor control in 35 patients was 94% at five years, with survival rates of 86% and 62% for clinical stage I and stage II disease, respectively [197]. A potential drawback of the Mohs' technique is that it requires a trained Mohs dermatologic surgeon and specialized equipment and personnel, resources that might not be readily available at all centers.

When organ preservation is appropriate, laser ablation of small-volume penile cancer has become a popular technique. Overall, local control in four early series of patients (AJCC stages Tis, T1, and T2) using the neodymium-yttrium aluminum garnet (Nd:YAG) laser ranged from 68% to 100% (mean follow-up = 17–60 months) [203–206]. Local failure commonly occurs when invasive lesions (AJCC stage T2 or greater) are treated with this modality [207]. Usually, laser ablation is accomplished in one outpatient session and does not carry the morbid complications of radiotherapy. In general, healing occurs over approximately six weeks, with excellent cosmesis and sexual function at three months [204]. A potential drawback of laser therapy is that the specimen is not available for pathologic review.

STAGE T2, T3, T4, OR BULKY TA

Verrucous carcinoma, although classically noninvasive, may present as a bulky mass replacing the glans penis [208]. These lesions, in addition to invasive SCC, require either partial or total penectomy. Partial penectomy is the option of choice when the primary tumor can be removed with a 2-cm disease-free margin and the remaining corpus is sufficient to allow the patient to stand and direct the urine stream during voiding. If these requirements cannot be met, a total penectomy with creation of a perineal urethrostomy is the only remaining option. In either case, a confirmation of negative surgical margins by frozen section is imperative. Local recurrence rates after partial and total penectomy are similarly low, ranging from 0% to 6% [181, 209]. An algorithm for the management of the primary penile tumor is presented in Figure 18.6.

REGIONAL LYMPH NODES (N0–N2)

For patients exhibiting invasive primary lesions and proved inguinal metastasis, a complete ilioinguinal dis-

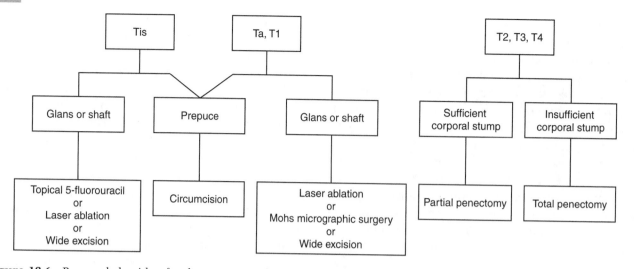

Figure 18.6   Proposed algorithm for the treatment of primary squamous cell carcinoma of the penis. (Reprinted with permission from MD Abeloff, JO Armitage, AS Lichter [eds], *Clinical Oncology* [2nd ed]. London: Churchill Livingstone, 1999:1894–1895.)

section is performed with sartorius muscle flap transposition to cover the femoral vessels. (The reader is referred to several other sources for a review of surgical techniques for lymphadenectomy [185, 210].) Patients with ulcerated inguinal masses are admitted several days prior to surgery for optimization of wound care by intravenous antibiotics, dressing changes, whirlpool baths, and local antisepsis. Plans for wound closure (skin graft or flap coverage) are anticipated in patients requiring wide resection of the skin. If necessary, plastic surgery consultation is obtained preoperatively.

The role of inguinal lymphadenectomy is becoming clearer in patients who lack palpable adenopathy at presentation. The dilemma involves the excess morbidity of performing routine lymphadenectomy in all patients versus the excess mortality in those patients who subsequently develop positive nodes and are not cured with surgery [181]. Considering the limits of surgical curability, diagnosis of metastatic disease at its earliest time point is advantageous. Thus, a risk-adapted approach should be used, based on the stage and grade of the primary tumor and the presence of vascular invasion (Figs. 18.7, 18.8) [180, 187, 192, 193].

The necessity and timing of inguinal lymph node dissection is complicated by the fact that 40–60% of patients with penile cancer have palpable adenopathy at presentation. Of these patients, only 30–60% will exhibit histologic evidence of cancer in the lymph nodes. The remaining patients show evidence of inflammatory adenopathy. Because of the need to separate patients

with inflammation from those with cancer, the initial treatment of patients with penile carcinoma and palpable inguinal adenopathy has been to excise the primary tumor and to initiate a course of antibiotic therapy to differentiate cancerous nodes from inflammatory nodes. If no response to antibiotics is achieved, the adenopathy is considered to represent lymphatic metastasis, and ilioinguinal lymphadenectomy is performed. This strategy remains a reasonable approach in those patients at low risk for metastases (Tis, Ta, T1, grade 1) (see Fig. 18.7). However, in patients exhibiting tumors of high pathologic stage (T2 or greater) or grade (III) or vascular invasion, the incidence of nodal metastases is greater than 50%, and lymphadenectomy (regardless of physical examination findings) probably is warranted (see Fig. 18.8) [180, 192, 193]. Lymphadenectomy clearly benefits select patients. However, cure with surgery alone is achieved best in the setting of unilateral inguinal metastases (fewer than two or three involved nodes), with no accompanying extranodal extension of cancer or pelvic lymph node metastasis [187].

Radiotherapy plays a limited role in the management of regional disease. When given as prophylaxis in the setting of clinically negative regional lymphatics, the rate of subsequent development of symptomatic nodal metastasis approaches 25%, similar to that of untreated patients [211]. As monotherapy for clinically involved lymph nodes, radiotherapy is inferior to surgery [212, 213]. External-beam therapy may be most useful for palliation of inoperable fungating nodal metastases.

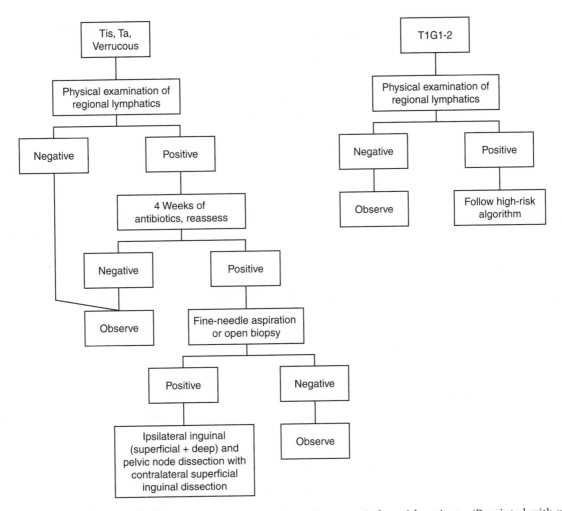

Figure 18.7 Proposed algorithm for the treatment of regional penile cancer in low-risk patients. (Reprinted with permission from MD Abeloff, JO Armitage, AS Lichter [eds], *Clinical Oncology* [2nd ed]. London: Churchill Livingstone, 1999:1894–1895.)

UNRESECTABLE OR DISTANT METASTASIS (N3, M1)

The development of effective systemic therapy for patients with advanced squamous penile cancer is imperative. Cisplatin, bleomycin, and methotrexate have been used as monotherapy with response rates between 20% and 60% [214, 215]. However, responses often are partial and of short duration. Combination chemotherapy regimens have been modestly successful in controlling advanced disease. A prospective phase II study of combination methotrexate, cisplatin, and bleomycin for advanced genitourinary SCC at the MD Anderson Cancer Center achieved an objective response rate of 55%, with a median survival of 17 months for responders [216]. More importantly, however, in patients rendered disease-free with chemotherapy alone or with chemotherapy followed by surgical resection or radiotherapy

(one case), the median survival was 34 months [216]. A similar approach using a weekly chemotherapeutic regimen in combination with surgery recently was reported by Pizzocaro and Piva [217] to provide enhanced survival. Thus, we believe an aggressive multimodal approach to achieve disease-free status may be important in advanced penile cancer. Future studies will emphasize the integration of chemotherapy and surgical management to achieve greater duration of disease-free status.

Disease will progress in approximately 40% of patients with advanced penile carcinoma, despite aggressive lymph node dissection. Typically, recurrent disease is seen in the inguinal nodes and eventually may progress to distant sites, such as the liver, lung, bone, or brain. In the absence of treatment, usually such patients die in less than two years [218]. Almost all patients who die from carcinoma of the penis first experience relapse

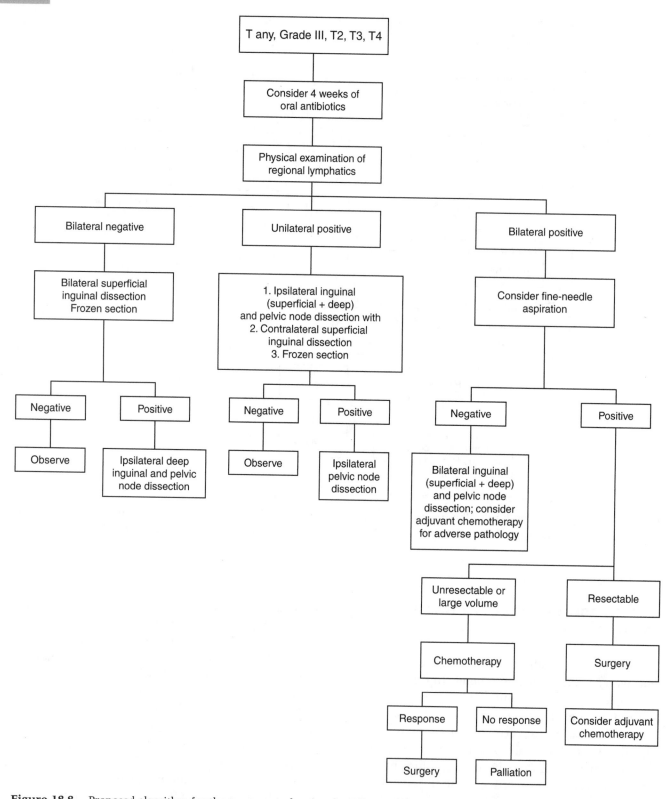

Figure 18.8. Proposed algorithm for the treatment of regional penile cancer in high-risk patients. (Reprinted with permission from MD Abeloff, JO Armitage, AS Lichter [eds], *Clinical Oncology* [2nd ed]. London: Churchill Livingstone, 1999:1894–1895.)

in the regional lymphatics [219]. The causes of death include inanition, arterial erosion, and severe local infection with subsequent sepsis.

Cure of distant metastases is rare, and palliative measures are often used. Although unlikely to achieve a cure, radiotherapy has been used for palliation [220]. For patients with advanced ulcerated or infiltrating tumors and poor performance status, radiotherapy may provide temporary tumor regression and may decrease pain and bleeding. Chemotherapy in patients with a reasonably good performance status may facilitate a palliative surgical resection (as noted) [216, 217]. Since prognostic factors for elapse after inguinal lymphadenectomy now are appreciated (more than two or three nodes positive for metastasis, extranodal extension of cancer, and positive pelvic lymph nodes), the roles of neoadjuvant or adjuvant chemotherapy and radiotherapy must be explored further in multiinstitutional trials.

URETHRAL CANCER

Urethral cancer is the only urologic malignancy with a higher incidence in women than in men. The median age at diagnosis ranges between 55 and 60 years, with no recognized racial predisposition. As in penile cancer, development of urethral cancer has been associated with chronic inflammation and HPV infection [221], and urethral cancer frequently is noted in men at a site of previous stricture formation. In distinction to that from penile cancer, death from urethral cancer often results from failure of local control of the primary tumor.

Anatomic and Histologic Characteristics

The male urethra has three anatomic segments: the prostatic, the membranous, and the penile urethra. The prostatic urethra is lined with transitional epithelium, whereas the membranous and penile urethra (excluding the fossa navicularis) are lined by stratified and pseudostratified columnar epithelium. The fossa navicularis is lined by stratified squamous epithelium. Anatomically, the penile urethra consists of the bulbar urethra, the pendulous urethra, and the fossa navicularis, but male urethral carcinomas commonly are termed *anterior* or *posterior urethral carcinoma*. In this context, bulbar urethral carcinomas are considered, along with carcinomas of the membranous and prostatic urethra, as posterior urethral carcinomas because of similarities with respect to clinical presentation, management, and prognosis. Anterior urethral carcinomas include lesions within the pendulous penile urethra and the fossa navicularis. Carcinoma of the urethra may originate from any of the lining epithelial cell types or from associated glands. Sixty percent of urethral carcinomas arise within the bulbar and membranous portions of the urethra. Another 30–35% arise within the anterior urethra, and only 5–10% arise within the prostatic urethra [222]. Most of these carcinomas (70–80%) are SCC, although 20% are transitional cell carcinomas (TCC), and 5% are adenocarcinomas.

The female urethra is between 2 and 4 cm long. The mucosa is composed of stratified squamous epithelium distally (anterior urethra) and of stratified or pseudostratified columnar epithelium proximally (posterior urethra). The mucosa at the bladder neck is predominantly transitional cell.

SCC is the most common histologic type, found in more than 50% of all cases. Adenocarcinoma and TCC types occur with equal frequency (10–15%); melanoma, undifferentiated carcinoma, and others are less common. A small percentage of urethral cancers in both genders are classified as undifferentiated and, rarely, sarcomas and melanomas are encountered.

Presentation, Diagnosis, and Staging

The onset of urethral cancer is insidious, and symptoms often are attributed to a stricture or inflammatory lesion. This condition results in a significant delay from the onset of symptoms to presentation and diagnosis [223, 224]. Consequently, patients often present with locally or regionally advanced disease, especially if the tumor arises in the posterior urethra. The presenting signs and symptoms in male patients vary with the anatomic location of the lesion. Commonly, tumors in the penile urethra present with irritative or obstructive voiding symptoms. Often, these tumors arise at the site of a presumed urethral stricture so that the diagnosis of urethral carcinoma should be considered when management of a "benign" stricture becomes difficult. Anterior lesions may produce a palpable mass, whereas those arising from the posterior urethra may present as a perineal mass [223]. Lesions in the prostatic or bulbomembranous urethra and advanced lesions of the penile urethra present with decreased force and caliber of urinary stream, obstruction, or overflow incontinence and may produce a filling defect on retrograde urethrography. Hematuria or purulent discharge may accompany a lesion at any site. In female patients, urethral or vaginal bleeding is the most common presenting symptom, and a mass or ulceration may be de-

Table 18.16   Clinical Staging Systems for Urethral Cancer

Stage	Female Urethral Cancer: Grabstald System [228]	Male Urethral Cancer: Ray System [229]
0	Carcinoma in situ	Confined to mucosa
A	Submucosal extension	Invasion into but not beyond the lamina propria
B	Invasion of periurethral muscle	Invasion into but not beyond the corpus spongiosum
C	Periurethral extension	Direct extension into tissues beyond the corpus spongiosum (corpus cavernosa, muscle, fat, fascia, skin, bone) or beyond the prostatic capsule
C1	Invasion of muscular wall of vagina	
C2	Invasion of muscular wall of vagina with invasion of vaginal mucosa	
C3	Invasion of adjacent structures (bladder, labia, clitoris)	
D	Metastasis	Metastasis
D1	Inguinal lymphatics	Regional, including inguinal or pelvic lymph nodes
D2	Pelvic lymphatics below the aortic bifurcation	Lymph nodes above the aortic bifurcation or distant metastasis
D3	Pelvic lymphatics above the aortic bifurcation	
D4	Distant metastasis	

Source: Reprinted with permission from MD Abeloff, JO Armitage, AS Lichter (eds), *Clinical Oncology* (2nd ed). London: Churchill Livingstone, 1999:1899.

tected on physical examination. Histologic confirmation is necessary to distinguish a cancer from benign lesions, such as urethral caruncles, condylomata, or diverticula.

Characteristically, urethral carcinomas invade adjacent structures relatively early in their natural history. Despite the rich vasculature surrounding the urethra, hematogenous spread is rare. Usually, metastases occur by lymphatic embolization to regional nodes. The lymphatics of the anterior urethra drain into the superficial and deep inguinal lymph nodes and, occasionally, into the external iliac lymph nodes. The lymphatics of the posterior urethra drain preferentially to the pelvic lymph nodes. Frequent exceptions occur, and up to 30% of posterior urethral tumors metastasize to the inguinal lymph nodes. Overall, between 15% and 30% of patients have lymph node metastasis at the time they present. Distant metastases are rare; Kaplan et al. [224] reported distant metastasis in only 29 of 232 patients, most often accompanying posterior lesions. As indicated previously, the lungs, liver, and bones are the most common sites for metastasis. Twenty-eight patients in the Kaplan group series received only palliative or no therapy, and the average survival was only three months. Death was a result of a chronic infection, sepsis, or hemorrhage.

Likewise, female urethral cancers spread predominantly by local extension into adjacent organs, then by lymphatic and, finally, by hematogenous metastases. Lymph node metastases are clinically apparent in 20–

50% of all patients. Grabstald et al. [225] reported that pathologic examination of these palpable enlarged nodes confirmed the presence of cancer in 22 of 25 patients (88%). In the same series, 13 of 26 patients undergoing pelvic lymphadenectomy had positive nodes. Only three of 65 patients presented with distant metastases, which occur most commonly in the lungs, liver, bone, and brain. No correlation exists between lymph node metastases and distant metastases. Distant metastases are uncommon even in patients dying from their cancer. A higher incidence of distant metastasis is seen in patients with adenocarcinoma. Untreated patients die within 12–18 months, and patients whose disease progresses despite therapy rarely survive for more than two years. Usually, death results from progressive incapacitation caused by regional spread, inanition, and sepsis.

Diagnosis is made by urethroscopic biopsy, although very distal lesions may be amenable to direct visual biopsy, especially in female patients. Several staging systems have been proposed for defining the extent of disease in male and female patients with urethral carcinoma. The Grabstald staging system [225] for female urethral cancer and the Ray staging system [226] for male urethral cancer are shown in Table 18.16. Though these clinical staging systems are simple, the TNM staging system of the Union Internationale Contre le Cancer [227], shown in Table 18.17, emphasizes tumor invasion, extent of regional node involvement, and distant metastasis.

Table 18.17 UICC TNM Staging for Urethral Cancer

Classification	Definition
Primary tumor (T)	
TX	Primary tumor cannot be assessed
T0	No evidence of primary tumor
Ta	Noninvasive papillary, polypoid, or verrucous carcinoma
Tis	Carcinoma in situ
T1	Tumor invades subepithelial connective tissue
T2	Tumor invades periurethral musculature (corpus spongiosum or prostate)
T3	Tumor invades anterior vagina or bladder neck (corpus cavernosum or beyond prostate or bladder neck)
T4	Tumor invades other adjacent structures
Regional lymph nodes (N)	
NX	Regional lymph nodes cannot be assessed
N0	No regional lymph node metastasis
N1	Metastasis in a single superficial inguinal lymph node, ≤ 2 cm in greatest dimension
N2	Metastasis in a single lymph node > 2 cm but < 5 cm in greatest dimension, or multiple nodes involved, none > 5 cm
N3	Metastasis to a lymph node > 5 cm in greatest dimension
Distant metastasis (M)	
MX	Presence of distant metastasis cannot be assessed
M0	No distant metastasis
M1	Distant metastasis

UICC = Union Internationale Contre le Cancer.
Source: Reprinted with permission from MD Abeloff, JO Armitage, AS Lichter (eds), *Clinical Oncology* (2nd ed). London: Churchill Livingstone, 1999:1900.

A thorough bimanual examination under anesthesia, with attention to the anus, rectum, urogenital diaphragm, and vagina, defines the local extent of disease and should be performed at the time of urethroscopy and biopsy. Simultaneously, a careful inguinal examination should be performed to detect inguinal adenopathy. Because patients with urethral carcinoma often present with advanced disease, chest roentgenography and serum chemistries are indicated for staging purposes. A CT scan of the abdomen and pelvis also should be performed to identify pelvic or retroperitoneal metastases. Fine-needle aspiration of suspicious lymph nodes detected by palpation or CT scan is recommended. Magnetic resonance imaging of the pelvis may be valuable prior to surgery for defining the extent of soft tissue or bony involvement by a locally invasive lesion.

Therapy

FEMALE URETHRAL CARCINOMA

Anterior Urethra

In women, small tumors confined to the mucosa of the anterior urethra can be treated effectively by transurethral resection, laser fulguration, or distal urethrectomy. Stages Tis, T1, and T2 anterior urethral tumors are amenable to distal urethrectomy if negative margins can be confirmed by frozen section. Urinary continence should be maintained in patients after resection of the distal one-third of the urethra. However, equally good results have been reported with interstitial irradiation [228, 229], often supplemented with external-beam or intracavitary irradiation [230, 231]; five-year disease-free survival for these patients ranges from 30% to 100%.

Consequently, adequate surgical resection and carefully planned radiotherapy appear to be equally effective for the management of low-stage anterior urethral carcinoma. However, the complications of radiotherapy are substantial. Bracken et al. [232] reported a 42% incidence of complications, which included incontinence in 30%, and local necrosis, fistula, stricture, abscess, cystitis, cellulitis, and osteomyelitis. For lesions of a more advanced stage, more aggressive therapy is necessary. These advanced lesions are unlikely to remain confined to the anterior urethra, and therapy is the same as that appropriate for advanced lesions involving the posterior (or entire) urethra.

Posterior Urethra

Rarely does a carcinoma of the posterior urethra *not* involve the bulk of the urethra. Low-stage lesions (stages Ta, T1) may be treated successfully by transurethral resection, laser fulguration, local excision, or interstitial irradiation. Certain small, stage T2 carcinomas can be treated also by interstitial irradiation with or without local excision. These lesions are exceptionally rare. Often, patients with advanced carcinoma of the urethra demonstrate extension to the bladder and vagina. Such patients require an aggressive therapeutic approach.

The results of anterior exenteration alone for advanced urethral carcinomas are poor, with five-year survival ranging between 10% and 20%. Local recurrence is documented in 60–100% in patients after surgery alone. Radiotherapy as a single-therapy modality for advanced urethral cancer is associated with a five-year survival of between 0% and 57%. More recently, radiotherapy has been used in combination with anterior exenteration. Grigsby and Herr [233] described four female patients with advanced proximal urethral cancer treated by preoperative radiotherapy with anterior exenteration, resection of the genitourinary diaphragm, partial symphysiectomy, and lymphadenectomy. Two were cured, but two died after local and distant failure within five months of surgery [233]. Narayan and Konety [234] reviewed the results of four small series of 34 patients treated with preoperative radiotherapy and surgery and noted an average five-year survival rate of 55%. Bracken et al. [232] documented a more favorable prognosis for advanced urethral carcinoma (five-year survival of between 50% and 60%) with preoperative irradiation and anterior exenteration. These investigators reported local recurrence in 22% of patients treated with both modalities, as compared with 64% of those treated with surgery alone and 46% of those treated with irradiation alone.

MALE URETHRAL CARCINOMA

Anterior Urethra (Fossa Navicularis, Penile Urethra)

Recognizing the aggressive natural history of carcinoma of the male urethra, the most rational approach to therapy is wide surgical excision. However, for certain patients, organ preservation is possible. For the rare patient who presents early with a stage Ta or T1 lesion, local excision may suffice. In the literature, reports cite 20 patients managed with local excision of a small primary tumor, none of whom have suffered a local recurrence. Usually, more advanced carcinomas of the fossa navicularis or pendulous penile urethra can be managed by a partial penectomy, 2 cm proximal to visible or palpable tumor or induration. Partial penectomy is an effective surgical procedure for achieving local control, and collectively in six contemporary series [235] no local recurrences were seen in 44 patients, and only one death occurred owing to urethral carcinoma.

Radical penectomy is performed for more extensive cancers not amenable to partial penectomy. A cystoprostatectomy with total penectomy, urethrectomy, and scrotectomy is indicated to minimize local recurrence in the presence of extensive scrotal involvement from a distal lesion. In general, the results of radical penectomy are inferior to those obtained with partial penectomy, owing to the advanced stage and grade of the carcinomas treated in this manner. In the compilation of six series just cited, at least six local recurrences were seen in 51 patients undergoing total penectomy, and 12 patients died from their carcinoma [235]. In our recent series, a radical penectomy was necessary in one patient to secure locoregional control. This patient is alive without recurrence. An additional patient required radical

cystoprostatectomy, total penectomy, urethrectomy, and scrotectomy, but died with local recurrence.

In a series of 23 male patients with anterior urethral cancer treated at MD Anderson Cancer Center, all four patients with tumors located in the fossa navicularis were disease-free at a mean follow-up of 93 months, and six of 11 patients with penile urethral tumors were disease-free at a mean of 48 months [236]. No local recurrences were noted in the four patients with fossa navicularis primary lesions. Furthermore, eight of nine patients who had penile urethral tumors and in whom local control was attempted were free of local recurrence. Adjuvant chemotherapy in combination with partial or total penectomy may improve local control for locally advanced tumors.

Posterior Urethra (Bulbous, Membranous, and Prostatic Urethra)

The rare superficial lesions (Ta, Tis, T1) occurring within the posterior urethra can be managed with transurethral resection [235]. Aggressive transurethral resection can assist in staging and may have therapeutic benefit in some cases. Invasion into and beyond the periurethral smooth muscle, prostatic ducts and, most important, the prostatic stroma is more ominous and requires more extensive surgical resection to achieve locoregional control. This goal may involve radical en bloc excision of the penis, scrotum, prostate, and bladder, with pelvic lymphadenectomy and excision of the pubic ramus for suspected invasion. Despite this aggressive surgical approach, the five-year survival rate has been poor (20%) owing to a failure of local control and distant metastases. Two small series suggested that an incremental benefit in local control and survival may be achieved by the integration of chemotherapy or radiotherapy with surgery [234, 236].

Management of Inguinal Lymph Nodes

The benefit of prophylactic inguinal dissection in men with urethral carcinoma has not been documented. Because of the morbidity of lymphadenectomy, current recommendations for therapy include surveillance by physical examination every three months for patients with no palpable adenopathy. Groin dissection is reserved for those patients with proved inguinal lymph node metastases. In an attempt to decrease morbidity, Dinney et al. [236] have described the use of a limited sentinel lymph node dissection in nine patients with urethral carcinoma. In two patients, the sentinel lymph node was the only positive node, and both these patients were treated with radical groin dissection and subsequent chemotherapy. Both patients achieved durable long-term survival, although in one patient disease subsequently recurred, with distant metastasis at 46 months.

Prognosis

The prognosis for men with urethral carcinoma depends on both the stage and the site of the tumor. No significant difference in prognosis is noted among patients with lesions of different histologic types. In the series of Ray et al. [226], the five-year disease-free survival was 43% for those with anterior urethral tumors and 14% for those with posterior urethral tumors. The five-year disease-free survival rate was 100% for those with stage T1, 80% for those with stage T2, 17% for those with stage T3, and 20% for those with nodal metastasis. Our recent experience is similar to that reported by Ray et al., with the exception that the survival for patients with stage T3 or TX node-positive carcinoma has improved. The prognosis for patients with posterior carcinomas is worse, with only 25% having a long-term disease-free survival. In most series, the reason for the poor survival of patients with posterior urethral carcinoma has been the advanced stage at diagnosis. In our experience, the most common explanation has been difficulty in achieving locoregional control.

The prognosis of female urethral carcinoma also depends on the location and stage at diagnosis and is unrelated to the cell type or histologic grade. Bracken et al. [232] reported an overall five-year survival rate of 32% in 81 patients. Correlation existed between tumor size and prognosis; patients with tumors measuring less than 2 cm had the best prognosis, whereas patients with tumors larger than 5 cm in diameter had the least favorable prognosis. Patients with tumors of the anterior urethra have a better overall survival rate (47%; range = 32–100%) than those with disease involving the entire urethra (11%; range = 0–21%). Survival rates reported by Bracken et al. [232], according to stage for tumors of all sites, were 100% for stage Ta or T1 disease, 41% for stage T2 disease, 26% for stage T3 disease, and 18% for patients with metastatic carcinoma.

Investigational Therapy

Clearly, failure to achieve local control or the subsequent development of distant metastasis in patients with invasive urethral carcinomas has a dismal outcome. In most advanced cases of cancer, surgical procedures alone have failed to affect the natural history of the disease. The suggestion that incremental improvements in local control and survival could be achieved with the combination of chemotherapy or radiotherapy (or both) with surgery have led to attempts to integrate these modalities [233, 234, 236].

At the Memorial Sloan-Kettering Cancer Center, 11 patients with stages T2 to T4 tumors of the posterior urethra without evidence of nodal disease or distant metastases were treated with neoadjuvant methotrexate, vinblastine, doxorubicin (Adriamycin), and cisplatin (MVAC) chemotherapy [233]. Disease in four of 10 evaluable patients was downstaged to stage T0. Three of five patients with TCC achieved a complete remission. Complete remissions were not achieved in patients with mixed or nontransitional histology with this regimen.

At the MD Anderson Cancer Center, we have initiated multimodal therapeutic regimens for patients with locally advanced urethral carcinoma (T2–4,N0 or T1–4,N1–3,M0) that combine aggressive and systemic local therapy as determined by the chemotherapeutic sensitivity and radiosensitivity of the primary tumor. For patients with TCC of the urethra, neoadjuvant MVAC chemotherapy is combined with surgical resection in an attempt to achieve local and systemic control of the malignancy. SCCs are sensitive to cisplatin-containing chemotherapeutic regimens in combination with radiotherapy [237]. Thus, patients exhibiting this histologic type will receive neoadjuvant radiotherapy (50 cGy) with concomitant cisplatin and 5-fluorouracil chemotherapy, again followed by aggressive surgical resection. Adenocarcinoma is relatively resistant to radiotherapy and responds poorly to standard chemotherapy. Accumulating evidence indicates that the combination of paclitaxel (Taxol®) and cisplatin (or carboplatin) is active in a variety of adenocarcinomas, including breast, prostate, lung, bladder, gastrointestinal, ovarian, and endometrial cancers [238–242]. At our institution, patients with primary adenocarcinoma of the urethra receive five cycles of Taxol®, methotrexate, and cisplatin and subsequently undergo surgical consolidation to achieve control of their malignancy.

Despite tenuous evidence, we believe that the prognosis for patients with urethral carcinoma has improved. In 1980, Bracken et al. [232] reported a median survival duration of only 22 months and that only 33% of patients were alive without evidence of disease at a median follow-up of 29 months. In a more recent series from the same institution, median survival has not been reached yet despite a longer follow-up, and currently 55% of patients are alive and free from recurrence. This improvement in the survival for patients with urethral carcinoma may be the result of earlier intervention in the disease process, improvements in surgery, the use of adjuvant chemotherapy, or other unrecognized selection factors.

References

1. Parkin MD, Pisani P, Ferlay J. Global cancer statistics. *CA Cancer J Clin* 49:33–64, 1999.

2. Greenlee RT, Murray T, Bolden S, Wingo PA. Cancer statistics, 2000. *CA Cancer J Clin* 50:7–33, 2000.

3. Feldman AR, Kessler L, Myers MH, Naughton MD. The prevalence of cancer: estimates based on the Connecticut Tumor Registry. *N Engl J Med* 315:1394–1397, 1986.

4. Lamm DL, Griffith JG. The place of intravesical chemotherapy as defined by results of prospective randomized studies (substances and treatment schemes). *Prog Clin Biol Res* 378:43–53, 1992.

5. Fleshner N, Moadel A, Herr H, et al. Influence of smoking status on the disease-related outcomes in patients with tobacco-associated superficial transitional cell carcinoma of the bladder. *Cancer* 86:2337–2345, 1999.

6. Michaud DS, Spiegelman D, Clinton SK, et al. Fluid intake and the risk of bladder cancer in men. *N Engl J Med* 340:1390–1397, 1999.

7. Lynch HT, Cohen MB. Urinary system. *Cancer* 75 (suppl):316–324, 1995.

8. Sidransky D, Frost P, von Eschenbach A, et al. Clonal origin of bladder cancer. *N Engl J Med* 326:737–740, 1992.

9. Cordon-Cardo C, Sheinfeld J, Dalbagni G. Genetic studies and molecular markers of bladder cancer. *Semin Surg Oncol* 13:319–327, 1997.

10. Bostwick DG. Natural history of early bladder cancer. *J Cell Biochem* 161:31–38, 1992.

11. Melicow MM, Hollowell JW. Intra-urothelial cancer—carcinoma in situ, Bowen's disease of the urinary system: discussion of thirty cases. *J Urol* 68:763–772, 1952.

12. Lamm DL. Carcinoma in situ. *Urol Clin North Am* 19:499–508, 1992.

13. Oosterlinck W, Kurth KH, Schröder F, et al. A prospective European Organization for Research and Treatment of Cancer genitourinary group randomized trial comparing transurethral resection followed by a single intravesical instillation of epirubicin or water in single state Ta, T1 papillary carcinoma of the bladder. *J Urol* 149:749–752, 1993.

14. Pawinsky A, Sylvester R, Kurth KH, et al. A combined analysis of European Organization for Research and Treatment of Cancer and the Medical Research Council randomized clinical trials for the prophylactic treatment of stage TaT1 bladder cancer. *J Urol* 156:1934–1941, 1996.

15. Herr HW, Laudone VP, Badalment RA, et al. Bacillus Calmette-Guérin therapy alters the progression of superficial bladder cancer. *J Clin Oncol* 6:1450–1455, 1988.

16. Lamm DL. Preventing progression and improving survival with BCG maintenance. *Eur Urol* 37 (suppl 1):9–15, 2000.

17. Lamm DL, van der Meijden PM, Morales A, et al. Incidence and treatment of complications of bacillus Calmette-Guérin intravesical therapy in superficial bladder cancer. *J Urol* 147:596–600, 1992.

18. Lamm DL, Blumenstein BA, Crissman JD, et al. Maintenance bacillus Calmette-Guerin immunotherapy for recurrent Ta, T1 and carcinoma in situ transitional cell carcinoma of the bladder: a randomized Southwest Oncology Group study. *J Urol* 163:1124–1129, 2000.

19. Waples MJ, Messing EM. The management of T1, grade 3 transitional cell carcinoma of the bladder. *Adv Urol* 5:33, 1992.

20. Rotman M, Macchia R, Silverstein M, et al. Treatment of advanced bladder carcinoma with irradiation and concomitant 5-fluorouracil infusion. *Cancer* 59:710–714, 1987.

21. Russell KJ, Boileau MA, Ireton RC, et al. Transitional cell carcinoma of the urinary bladder: histologic clearance with combined 5-FU and radiation therapy. Preliminary results of a bladder-preservation study. *Radiology* 167:845–848, 1988.

22. Coppin C, Gospodarowicz M, Dixon P, et al. Improved local control of invasive bladder cancer by concurrent cisplatin and pre-operative or radical radiation (abstract). *Proc Am Soc Clin Oncol* 11:607A, 1992.

23. Shipley WU, Kaufman DS, Henry NM, et al. An update of combined modality therapy for patients with muscle invading bladder cancer using selective bladder preservation or cystectomy. *J Urol* 162:445–450, 1999.

24. Parsons J, Million R. Role of planned preoperative irradiation in the management of clinical stage B2-C (T3) bladder cancer in the 1980s. *Semin Surg Oncol* 5:255–265, 1989.

25. Smith JA Jr, Crawford ED, Paradelo JC, et al. Treatment of advanced bladder cancer with combined preoperative irradiation and radical cystectomy versus radical cystectomy alone: a phase III intergroup study. *J Urol* 157:805–808, 1997.

26. Huncharek M, Muscat J, Geschwind JF. Planned preoperative radiation therapy in muscle-invasive bladder cancer: results of a meta-analysis. *Anticancer Res* 18:1931–1934, 1998.

27. Stein JP, Freeman JA, Boyd SD, et al. Radical cystectomy in the treatment of invasive bladder cancer: long-term results in a large group of patients. *J Urol* 159:213, 1998.

28. Sternberg CN, Yagoda A, Scher HI, et al. Preliminary results of M-VAC (methotrexate, vinblastine, doxorubicin, and cisplatin) for transitional cell carcinoma of the urothelium. *J Urol* 133:403–407, 1985.

29. Harker WG, Meyer FJ, Freiha FS, et al. Cisplatin, methotrexate, and vinblastine (CMV)—an effective chemotherapy regimen for metastatic transitional cell carcinoma of the urinary tract: a Northern California Oncology Group study. *J Clin Oncol* 3:1463–1470, 1985.

30. Loehrer PJ Sr, Einhorn LH, Elson PJ, et al. A randomized

comparison of cisplatin alone or in combination with methotrexate, vinblastine, and doxorubicin in patients with metastatic urothelial carcinoma: a comparative group study. *J Clin Oncol* 10:1066–1073, 1992.

31. Logothetis CJ, Dexeus FH, Finn L, et al. A prospective randomized trial comparing MVAC and CISCA chemotherapy for patients with metastatic urothelial tumors. *J Clin Oncol* 8:1050–1055, 1990.

32. McDougal WS, Garnick MB. Clinical signs and symptoms of renal cell carcinoma. In Vogelzang NJ, Scardino PT, Shipley WU, Coffey DS (eds), *Comprehensive Textbook of Genitourinary Oncology.* Baltimore: Williams & Wilkins, 1996:154–159.

33. Bostwick DG, Eble JN, Murphy GP. Conference summary: diagnosis and prognosis of renal cell carcinoma: 1997 workshop. *Cancer* 80:975–976, 1997.

34. Medeiros LJ, Jones ED, Aizawa S, et al. Grading of renal cell carcinoma: workgroup no. 2. *Cancer* 80:990–991, 1997.

35. Guinan P, Sobin, LH, Algaba F, et al. TNM staging of renal cell carcinoma: workgroup no. 3. *Cancer* 80:992–993, 1997.

36. Sobin LH, Wittekind CH (eds), *TNM Classification of Malignant Tumors* (5th ed). New York: Wiley, 1997:108–112.

37. Aso Y, Homma Y. A survey of incidental renal cell carcinoma in Japan. *Urology* 147:340–343, 1992.

38. Sawczuk IS. Autolymphocyte therapy in the treatment of metastatic renal cell carcinoma. *Urol Clin North Am* 20:297–301, 1993.

39. Srigley JR, Hutter RVP, Gelb AB, et al. Current prognostic factors—renal cell carcinoma: workgroup no. 4. *Cancer* 80:994–996, 1997.

40. Swanson DA, Rothenberg HJ, Boynton AL, et al. Future prognostic factors for renal cell carcinoma: workgroup no. 5. *Cancer* 80:997–998, 1997.

41. Novick AC. A comparison of recipient renal outcomes with laparoscopic versus live donor nephrectomy. *J Urol* 162:969–964, 1999.

42. Kubota H, Furuse A, Kotsuka Y, et al. Successful management of massive pulmonary tumor embolism from renal cell carcinoma. *Ann Thorac Surg* 61:708–710, 1996.

43. DiBiase SJ, Valicenti RK, Schultz D, et al. Palliative irradiation for focally symptomatic metastatic renal cell carcinoma: support for dose escalation based on a biological model. *J Urol* 158:746–749, 1997.

44. Hartmann JT, Bokemeyer C. Chemotherapy for renal cell carcinoma. *Anticancer Res* 19(2C):1541–1543, 1999.

45. Huland E, Heinzer H, Huland H. Treatment of pulmonary metastatic renal-cell carcinoma in 116 patients using inhaled interleukin-2 (IL-2). *Anticancer Res* 19(4A):2679–2683, 1999.

46. Hanash KA, Aquilina JW, Barrett DM, et al. Clinical research priorities in renal cell carcinoma. Renal cell carcinoma chemoprevention strategies including target populations, proposed agents, and clinical trial designs—workgroup no. 6. *Cancer* 80:999–1001, 1997.

47. Tosaka A, Ohya K, Yamada K, et al. Incidence and properties of renal masses and asymptomatic renal cell carcinoma detected by abdominal ultrasonography. *J Urol* 144:1097–1101, 1990.

48. Simons JW, Marshall FF. Future directions in renal cell carcinoma. In Ernstoff MS, Heaney JA, Peschel RE (eds), *Urologic Cancer.* Cambridge, MA: Blackwell Science, 1997:492–496.

49. Bosl GJ, Motzer RJ. Testicular germ-cell cancer. *N Engl J Med* 337:242–253, 1997.

50. Murty VVVS, Chaganti RSK. A genetic perspective of male germ cell tumors. *Semin Oncol* 25:133–144, 1998.

51. Bosl GJ, Ilson DH, Rodriguez E, et al. Clinical relevance of the i(12p) marker chromosome in germ cell tumors. *J Natl Cancer Inst* 86:349–355, 1994.

52. International Germ Cell Collaborative Group. International germ cell consensus classification: a prognostic factor-based staging system for metastatic germ cell cancers. *J Clin Oncol* 15:594–603, 1997.

53. Gerl A, Lamerz R, Clemm C, et al. Does serum tumor marker half-life complement pretreatment risk stratification in metastatic nonseminomatous germ cell tumors. *Clin Cancer Res* 2:1565–1570, 1996.

54. Fleming ID, Cooper JS, Henson DE, et al. (eds). *AJCC Cancer Staging Manual* (5th ed). Philadelphia: Lippincott-Raven, 1997:225–228.

55. Gospodarowicz MK, Warde PR, Panzarella T, et al. The Princess Margaret Hospital experience in the management of stage I and II seminoma—1981 to 1991. In Jones WG, Harnden P, Appleyard I (eds), *Germ Cell Tumors III.* Oxford: Pergamon, 1994:177–185.

56. Warde P, Gospodarowicz MK, Panzarella T, et al. Stage I testicular seminoma: results of adjuvant irradiation and surveillance. *J Clin Oncol* 13:2255–2262, 1995.

57. Sternberg CN. The management of stage I testis cancer. *Urol Clin North Am* 25:435–451, 1998.

58. Donohue JP, Zachary JM, Maynard BR. Distribution of nodal metastases in nonseminomatous testis cancer. *J Urol* 128:315–319, 1982.

59. Foster RS, Roth BJ. Clinical stage I nonseminoma: surgery versus surveillance. *Semin Oncol* 25:145–153, 1998.

60. Motzer RJ. Adjuvant chemotherapy for stage II nonseminomatous testicular cancer: what is its role? *Semin Urol Oncol* 14:30–33, 1996.

61. Williams SD, Stablein DM, Einhorn LH, et al. Immediate adjuvant chemotherapy versus observation with treatment at relapse in pathological stage II testicular cancer. *N Engl J Med* 317:1433–1438, 1987.

62. Bajorin DF, McCaffrey JA. Therapy for good-risk germ cell tumors. *Semin Oncol* 25:186–193, 1998.

63. Williams SD, Birch R, Einhorn LH, et al. Treatment of disseminated germ-cell tumors with cisplatin, bleomycin, and either vinblastine or etoposide. *N Engl J Med* 316:1435–1440, 1987.

64. Dodd PM, Motzer RJ, Bajorin DF. Poor-risk germ cell tumors: recent developments. *Urol Clin North Am* 25:485–493, 1998.

65. Motzer RJ, Mazumdar M, Bajorin DF, et al. High-dose carboplatin, etoposide, and cyclophosphamide with autologous bone marrow transplantation in first-line therapy for patients with poor-risk germ cell tumors. *J Clin Oncol* 15:2546–2552, 1997.

66. Siegert W, Beyer J. Germ cell tumors: dose-intensive therapy. *Semin Oncol* 25:215–223, 1998.

67. Toner GC, Panicek DM, Heelan RT, et al. Adjunctive surgery after chemotherapy for nonseminomatous germ

cell tumors: recommendations for patient selection. *J Clin Oncol* 8:1683–1694, 1990.

68. Debono DJ, Heilman DK, Einhorn LH, Donohue JP. Decision analysis for avoiding postchemotherapy surgery in patients with disseminated nonseminomatous germ cell tumors. *J Clin Oncol* 15:1455–1464, 1997.

69. Puc HS, Heelan R, Mazumdar M, et al. Management of residual mass in advanced seminoma: results and recommendations from the Memorial Sloan-Kettering Cancer Center. *J Clin Oncol* 14:454–460, 1996.

70. Murphy BA, Motzer RJ, Bosl GJ. Chemotherapy for cisplatin-resistant germ cell tumors. *Probl Urol* 8:127–140, 1994.

71. Nichols CR, Saxman S. Primary salvage treatment of recurrent germ cell tumors: experience at Indiana University. *Semin Oncol* 25:210–214, 1998.

72. Motzer RJ, Mazumdar M, Bosl GJ, et al. High-dose carboplatin, etoposide, and cyclophosphamide for patients with refractory germ cell tumors: treatment results and prognostic factors for survival and toxicity. *J Clin Oncol* 14:1098–1105, 1996.

73. Hoff Wanderas E, Fossa SD, Tretli S. Risk of subsequent non-germ cell cancer after treatment of germ cell cancer in 2006 Norwegian male patients. *Eur J Cancer* 33:253–262, 1997.

74. Young RH, Koelliker DD, Scully RE. Sertoli cell tumors of the testis, not otherwise specified: a clinicopathologic analysis of 60 cases. *Am J Surg Pathol* 22:709–721, 1998.

75. Pagano SA, Meazza A, Marzorati G, Gregorio P. Review of the literature. Tumor of interstitial Leydig cells. Apropos of a cure. *J Urol* 86:219–221, 1980.

76. Duncan PR, Checa F, Gowing NF, et al. Extranodal non-Hodgkin's lymphoma presenting in the testicle: a clinical and pathologic study of 24 cases. *Cancer* 45:1578–1584, 1980.

77. Mettlin CJ, Murphy GP, Rosenthal DS, Menck HR. The National Cancer Data Base report on prostate carcinoma after the peak in incidence rates in the U.S. *Cancer* 83:1679–1684, 1998.

78. Satariano WA, Ragland KE, Van Den Eeden SK. Cause of death in men diagnosed with prostate carcinoma. *Cancer* 83:1180–1188, 1998.

79. Pienta KJ, Esper PS. Risk factors for prostate cancer. *Ann Intern Med* 118:793–803, 1993.

80. Landis SH, Murray T, Bolden S, Wingo PA. Cancer statistics, 1998. *CA Cancer J Clin* 48:6–29, 1998.

81. Bacquet CR, Horm JW, Gibbs T, Greenwald P. Socioeconomic factors and cancer incidence among blacks and whites. *J Natl Cancer Inst* 83:551–557, 1991.

82. Wittemore AS, Kolonel LN, Wu AH, et al. Prostate cancer in relation to diet, physical activity, and body size in blacks, whites, and Asians in the United States and Canada. *J Natl Cancer Inst* 87:652–660, 1995.

83. Gleason DF. Classification of prostatic carcinomas. *Cancer Chemother Rep* 50:125–137, 1966.

84. Gleason DF. Histologic grading of prostate cancer: a perspective. *Hum Pathol* 23:273–279, 1992.

85. Dong J-T, Isaacs WB, Isaacs JT. Molecular advances in prostate cancer. *Curr Opin Oncol* 9:101–107, 1997.

86. Cohen RJ, Cooper K, Haffejee Z, et al. Immunohistochemical detection of oncogene proteins and neuroendocrine differentiation in different stages of prostate cancer. *Pathology* 27:229–232, 1995.

87. Koivisto P, Visakorpi T, Kallioniemi O-P. Androgen receptor gene amplification: a novel molecular mechanism for endocrine therapy resistance in human prostate cancer. *Scand J Clin Lab Invest* 56 (suppl 226):57–64, 1996.

88. Tilley WD, Buchanan G, Hickey TE, Bentel J. Mutations in the androgen receptor gene are associated with progression of human prostate cancer to androgen independence. *Clin Cancer Res* 2:277–285, 1996.

89. Taplin M-E, Bubley GJ, Shuster TD, et al. Mutation of the androgen-receptor gene in metastatic androgen-independent prostate cancer. *N Engl J Med* 332:1393–1398, 1995.

90. Mettlin CJ, Murphy GP, Ho R, Menck HR. The National Cancer Data Base report on longitudinal observations on prostate cancer. *Cancer* 77:2162–2166, 1996.

91. Catalona WJ, Richie JP, Ahmann FR, et al. Comparison of digital rectal examination and serum prostate specific antigen in the early detection of prostate cancer: results of a multicenter clinical trial of 6,630 men. *J Urol* 151:1283–1290, 1994.

92. Lerner SE, Seay TM, Blute ML, et al. Prostate specific antigen detected prostate cancer (clinical stage T1c): an interim analysis. *J Urol* 155:821–826, 1996.

93. Orohi M, Wheeler TM, Dunn JK, et al. The pathologic features and prognosis of prostate cancers detectable with current diagnostic tests. *J Urol* 152:1714–1720, 1994.

94. von Eschenbach A, Ho R, Murphy GP, et al. American Cancer Society guidelines for the early detection of prostate cancer. *Cancer* 80:1805–1807, 1997.

95. American Urological Association. Early detection of prostate cancer and use of transrectal ultrasound. In *American Urological Association 1992 Policy Statement Book*, vol 4. Baltimore: American Urological Association, 1992:20.

96. Orohi M, Scardino PT. Early detection of prostate cancer: the nature of cancers detected with current diagnostic tests. *Semin Oncol* 21:522–526, 1994.

97. Partin AW, Yoo J, Carter HB, et al. The use of prostate specific antigen, clinical stage and Gleason score to predict pathological stage in men with localized prostate cancer. *J Urol* 150:110–114, 1993.

98. Catalona WJ, Partin AW, Slawin KM, et al. Use of the percentage of free prostate-specific antigen to enhance differentiation of prostate cancer from benign prostatic disease. *JAMA* 279:1542–1547, 1998.

99. Catalona WJ, Smith DS, Wolfert RL, et al. Evaluation of percentage of free serum prostate-specific antigen to improve specificity of prostate cancer screening. *JAMA* 274:1214–1220, 1998.

100. Demura T, Shinohara N, Tanaka M, et al. The proportion of free to total prostate specific antigen: a method of detecting prostate carcinoma. *Cancer* 77:1137–1143, 1996.

101. Fleming ID, Cooper JS, Henson DE, et al. (eds), *AJCC Cancer Staging Handbook*. Philadelphia: Lippincott-Raven, 1998.

102. D'Amico AV, Whittington R, Malkowicz SB, et al. Critical analysis of the ability of the endorectal coil magnetic resonance imaging scan to predict pathologic stage, margin status, and postoperative prostate-specific antigen failure

in patients with clinically organ-confined cancer. *J Clin Oncol* 14:1770–1777, 1996.

103. Perrotti M, Kaufman RP Jr, Jennings TA, et al. Endorectal coil magnetic resonance imaging in clinically localized prostate cancer: Is it accurate? *J Urol* 156:106–109, 1996.

104. Partin AW, Kattan MW, Subong ENP, et al. Combination of prostate-specific antigen, clinical stage, and Gleason score to predict pathological stage of localized prostate cancer. A multi-institutional update. *JAMA* 277:1445–1451, 1997.

105. Kattan MW, Eastham JA, Stapleton AMF, et al. A preoperative nomogram for disease recurrence following radical prostatectomy for prostate cancer. *J Natl Cancer Inst* 90:766–771, 1998.

106. Kahn D, Williams RD, Manyak MJ, et al. [111]Indium-capromab pendetide in the evaluation of patients with residual or recurrent prostate cancer after radical prostatectomy. The ProstaScint Study Group. *J Urol* 159:2041–2047, 1998.

107. Kahn D, Williams RD, Haseman MK, et al. Radioimmunoscintigraphy with In-111-labeled capromab pendetide predicts prostate cancer response to salvage radiotherapy after failed radical prostatectomy. *J Clin Oncol* 16:284–289, 1998.

108. Albertsen PC. Early-stage prostate cancer. *Hematol Oncol Clin North Am* 10:611–625, 1996.

109. Walsh PC. Radical prostatectomy: a procedure in evolution. *Semin Oncol* 21:662–671, 1994.

110. Nadler RB, Andriole GL. Who is best benefited by radical prostatectomy? *Hematol Oncol Clin North Am* 10:581–593, 1996.

111. Catalona WJ, Smith DS. 5-Year recurrence rates after anatomic radical retropubic prostatectomy for prostate cancer. *J Urol* 152:1837–1842, 1994.

112. Walsh PC, Partin AW, Epstein JI. Cancer control and quality of life following anatomical radical retropubic prostatectomy: results at 10 years. *J Urol* 152:1831–1836, 1994.

113. Zincke H, Oesterling JE, Blute ML, et al. Long-term (15 years) results after radical prostatectomy for clinically localized (stage 2c or lower) prostate cancer. *J Urol* 152:1850–1857, 1994.

114. Talcott JA, Rieker P, Clark JA, et al. Patient-reported symptoms after primary therapy for early prostate cancer: results of a prospective cohort study. *J Clin Oncol* 16:275–283, 1998.

115. Steiner MS, Morton RA, Walsh PC. Impact of anatomical radical prostatectomy on urinary continence. *J Urol* 145:512–515, 1991.

116. Catalona WJ, Basler JW. Return of erections and urinary continence following nerve-sparing radical retropubic prostatectomy. *J Urol* 150:905–907, 1993.

117. Leandri P, Rossignol G, Gautier J-R, Ramon J. Radical retropubic prostatectomy: morbidity and quality of life. Experience with 620 consecutive cases. *J Urol* 147:883–887, 1992.

118. Quinlan DM, Epstein JI, Carter BS, Walsh PC. Sexual function following radical prostatectomy: influence of preservation of neurovascular bundles. *J Urol* 145:998–1002, 1991.

119. Hartford AC, Zietman AL. Prostate cancer: Who is best benefited by external beam radiation therapy. *Hematol Oncol Clin North Am* 10:595–610, 1996.

120. Sandler HM, Hayman JA, Sullivan MA, et al. Results of 3D conformal radiation therapy for patients potentially suitable for radical prostatectomy. *Proc Am Soc Clin Oncol* 17:307a, 1998.

121. Wallner K, Roy J, Harrison L. Tumor control and morbidity following transperineal Iodine 125 implantation for stage T1/T2 prostate carcinoma. *J Clin Oncol* 14:449–453, 1996.

122. Schmidt JD, Doyle J, Larison S. Prostate cryoablaton: update 1998. *CA Cancer J Clin* 48:239–253, 1998.

123. Crawford ED, Eisenberger MA, McLeod DG, et al. A controlled trial of leuprolide with and without flutamide in prostatic carcinoma. *N Engl J Med* 321:419–424, 1989.

124. Eisenberger MA, Crawford ED, Wolf M, et al. Prognostic factors in stage D2 prostate cancer—important implications for future trials: results of a Cooperative Intergroup Study [INT.0036]. *Semin Oncol* 21:613–619, 1994.

125. Robson M, Dawson N. How is androgen-dependent metastatic prostate cancer best treated. *Hematol Oncol Clin North Am* 10:727–747, 1996.

126. Eisenberger MA, Blumenstein BA, Crawford ED, et al. Bilateral orchiectomy with or without flutamide for metastatic prostate cancer. *N Engl J Med* 339:1036–1042, 1998.

127. Denis LJ, Whelan P, Carneiro de Moura JL, et al. Goserelin acetate and flutamide versus bilateral orchiectomy: a phase III EORTC trial (30853). *Urology* 42:119–130, 1993.

128. Denis JL, Keuppens F, Smith PH, et al. Maximal androgen blockade: final analysis of EORTC Phase III Trial 30853. *Eur Urol* 33:144–151, 1998.

129. Small EJ, Vogelzang NJ. Second-line hormonal therapy for advanced prostate cancer: a shifting paradigm. *J Clin Oncol* 15:382–388, 1997.

130. Oliver RTD, Williams G, Paris AMI, Blandy JP. Intermittent androgen deprivation after PSA-complete response as a strategy to reduce induction of hormone-resistant prostate cancer. *Urology* 49:79–82, 1997.

131. Chodak G, Sharifi R, Kasimis B, et al. Single-agent therapy with bicalutamide: a comparison with medical or surgical castration in the treatment of advanced prostate carcinoma. *Urology* 46:849–855, 1995.

132. Prostate Cancer Trialists' Collaborative Group. Maximum androgen blockade in advanced prostate cancer: an overview of 22 randomised trials with 3283 deaths in 5710 patients. *Lancet* 346:265–269, 1995.

133. Cauber J-F, Tosteson TD, Dong EW, et al. Maximum androgen blockade in advanced prostate cancer: a meta-analysis of published randomized controlled trials using nonsteroidal antiandrogens. *Urology* 49:71–78, 1997.

134. Kelly WK, Slovin S, Scher HI. Steroid hormone withdrawal syndromes. *Urol Clin North Am* 24:421–431, 1997.

135. Liebertz C, Kelly W, Theodoulou M, et al. High-dose Casodex for prostate cancer (PC): PSA declines in patients (PTS) with flutamide withdrawal responses. *Proc Am Soc Clin Oncol* 14:232a, 1995.

136. Trump DL, Havlin KH, Messing EM, et al. High-dose ketoconazole in advanced hormone-refractory prostate

cancer: endocrinologic and clinical effects. *J Clin Oncol* 7:1093–1098, 1989.

137. Tannock I, Gospodarowicz M, Meakin W, et al. Treatment of metastatic prostate cancer with low-dose prednisone: evaluation of pain and quality of life as pragmatic indices of response. *J Clin Oncol* 7:590–597, 1989.

138. Tannock IF, Osoba D, Stockler MR, et al. Chemotherapy with mitoxantrone plus prednisone or prednisone alone for symptomatic hormone-resistant prostate cancer: a Canadian randomized trial with palliative end points. *J Clin Oncol* 14:1756–1764, 1996.

139. Scher HI, Kelly WK, Zhang Z-F, et al. Post-therapy serum prostate-specific antigen level and survival in patients with androgen-independent prostate cancer. *J Natl Cancer Inst* 91:244–251, 1999.

140. Seidman A, Scher HI, Petrylak D, et al. Estramustine and vinblastine: use of prostate specific antigen as a clinical trial end point for hormone refractory prostate cancer. *J Urol* 147:931–934, 1992.

141. Hudes GR, Greenberg R, Krigel RL, et al. Phase II study of estramustine and vinblastine, two microtubule inhibitors, in hormone-refractory prostate cancer. *J Clin Oncol* 10:1754–1761, 1992.

142. Hudes GR, Nathan F, Khater C, et al. Phase II trial of 96-hour paclitaxel plus oral estramustine phosphate in metastatic hormone-refractory prostate cancer. *J Clin Oncol* 15:3156–3163, 1997.

143. Walton GR, Olsson CA. Localized squamous cell carcinoma of the penis. In Resnick MI, Kursh ED (eds), *Current Therapy in Genitourinary Surgery* (2nd ed). St Louis: Mosby-Year Book, 1992:138.

144. Schellhammer PF, Jordan GH, Schlossberg SM. Tumors of the penis. In Walsh PC, Retik AB, Stamey TA, Vaughan ED (eds), *Campbell's Urology* (6th ed). Philadelphia: Saunders, 1992:1264.

145. Raju GC, Naraynsingh V, Venu PS. Carcinoma of the penis in the West Indies: a Trinidad study. *Trop Geogr Med* 37:334–336, 1985.

146. Riveros M, Lebron RF. Geographic pathology of cancer of the penis. *Cancer* 16:798, 1963.

147. Shabad AL. Some aspects of etiology and prevention of penile cancer. *J Urol* 92:696, 1964.

148. Dodge OG, Linsell CA. Carcinoma of the penis in Uganda and Kenya Africans. *Cancer* 16:1255, 1963.

149. Maden C, Sherman KJ, Beckman AM, et al. History of circumcision, medical conditions, and sexual activity and risk of penile cancer. *J Natl Cancer Inst* 85:19–24, 1993.

150. Sufrin G, Huber R. Benign and malignant lesions of the penis. In Gillenwater JY, Grayhack JT, Howards SS, Duckett JW (eds), *Adult and Pediatric Urology*. St Louis: Mosby-Year Book, 1991:1643.

151. Brinton LA, Jun-Yao L, Shou-De R, et al. Risk factors for penile cancer: results from a case-control study in China. *Int J Cancer* 47:504, 1991.

152. Shabad AL. The experimental production of the penis tumours. *Neoplasma* 12:635, 1965.

153. Fishman M, Friedman HF, Stewart HL. Local effect of repeated application of 3,4-benzpyrene and of human smegma to the vagina and cervix of mice. *J Natl Cancer Inst* 2:361, 1942.

154. Pratt-Thomas HR, Heins HC, Latham E, et al. The carcin-

ogenic effect of human smegma: an experimental study. *Cancer* 9:671, 1956.

155. Graham S, Priore R, Graham M, et al. Genital cancer in wives of penile cancer patients. *Cancer* 44:1870–1874, 1979.

156. Barrasso R, De Brux J, Croissant O, et al. High prevalence of papillomavirus-associated penile intraepithelial neoplasia in sexual partners of women with cervical intraepithelial neoplasia. *N Engl J Med* 317:916–923, 1987.

157. Varma VA, Sanchez-Lanier M, Unger ER, et al. Association of human papillomavirus with penile carcinoma: a study using polymerase chain reaction and in situ hybridization. *Hum Pathol* 22:908–913, 1991.

158. Iwasawa A, Kumamoto Y, Fujinaga K. Detection of human papillomavirus deoxyribonucleic acid in penile carcinoma by polymerase chain reaction and in situ hybridization. *J Urol* 149:59–63, 1993.

159. Wiener JS, Walther PJ. The association of oncogenic human papillomaviruses with urologic malignancy. The controversies and clinical implications. *Surg Oncol Clin North Am* 4:257–276, 1995.

160. Barbosa MS, Vass, WC, Lowy DR, et al. In vitro biological activities of the *E6* and *E7* genes vary among the HPVs' different oncogenic potential. *J Virol* 65:292–298, 1991.

161. Munger K, Phelps WC, Bubb V, et al. The *E6* and *E7* genes of the human papillomavirus type 16 together are necessary and sufficient for transformation of primary human keratinocytes. *J Virol* 63:4417–4421, 1989.

162. Stern RS. Genital tumors among men with psoriasis exposed to psoralens and ultraviolet A radiation (PUVA) and ultraviolet B radiation. The Photochemotherapy Follow-up Study. *N Engl J Med* 322:1093–1097, 1990.

163. Burgers JK, Badalament RA, Drago JR. Penile cancer: clinical presentation, diagnosis, and staging. *Urol Clin North Am* 19:247–256, 1992.

164. Derrick FC Jr, Lynch KM Jr, Kretkowski RC, Yarbrough W. Epidermoid carcinoma of the penis: computer analysis of 87 cases. *J Urol* 110:303–305, 1973.

165. Beggs JH, Spratt JS. Epidermoid carcinoma of the penis. *J Urol* 91:166, 1961.

166. Muir CS, Nectoux J. Epidemiology of cancer of the testis and penis. *Natl Cancer Inst Monogr* 53:157–164, 1979.

167. Narayana AS, Olney LE, Loening SA, et al. Carcinoma of the penis: analysis of 219 cases. *Cancer* 49:2185–2191, 1982.

168. Ekstrom T, Edsmyr F. Cancer of the penis: a clinical study of 229 cases. *Acta Chir Scand* 115:25, 1958.

169. Staubitz WJ, Lent MH, Oberkircher DJ. Carcinoma of the penis. *Cancer* 8:371, 1955.

170. Gerber GS. Carcinoma in situ of the penis. *J Urol* 151:829–833, 1991.

171. Kaye V, Zhang G, Dehner LP, Fraley EE. Carcinoma in situ of the penis: Is distinction between erythroplasia of Queyrat and Bowen's disease relevant? *Urology* 36:479–482, 1990.

172. Epstein E. Association of Bowen's disease with visceral cancer. *Arch Dermatol* 82:349, 1960.

173. Lynch DF, Schellhammer PF. Tumors of the penis. In Walsh PC, Retik AB, Vaughn ED, Wein AJ (eds), *Campbell's Urology* (7th ed). Philadelphia: Saunders, 1998:2453.

174. Ayala AG, Ro JT. Pathology of penile cancer. In Raghavan D, Scher H, Leibel SA, Lange PH (eds), *Principles and Practice of Genitourinary Oncology.* Philadelphia: Lippincott-Raven, 1997.

175. Broders A. Squamous cell epithelioma of the skin. *Ann Surg* 73:141, 1928.

176. Abeshouse BS, Abeshouse GA. Metastatic tumors of the penis: a review of the literature and a report of two cases. *J Urol* 86:99, 1961.

177. Mukamel E, Farrer J, Smith RB, de Kernion JB. Metastatic carcinoma to penis: When is total penectomy indicated? *Urology* 29:15–18, 1987.

178. Jackson SM. The treatment of carcinoma of the penis. *Br J Surg* 53:33–35, 1966.

179. ID Fleming, JS Cooper, DE Henson, et al. (eds), *AJCC Cancer Staging Manual* (5th ed). Philadelphia: Lippincott-Raven, 1997:215–217.

180. Theodorescu D, Russo P, Zhang Z, et al. Outcomes of initial surveillance of node-negative invasive squamous cell carcinoma of the penis. *J Urol* 155:1626–1631, 1996.

181. McDougal WS, Kirchner FK, Edwards RH, et al. Treatment of carcinoma of the penis: the case for primary lymphadenectomy. *J Urol* 136:38–41, 1986.

182. Fraley EE, Zhang G, Samma R, et al. Cancer of the penis: prognosis and treatment plans. *Cancer* 55:1618–1624, 1985.

183. Mukamel E, de Kernion JB. Early versus delayed lymph node dissection versus no lymph node dissection in carcinoma of the penis. *Urol Clin North Am* 14:707–711, 1987.

184. Solsona E, Iborra I, Ricos JV, et al. Corpus cavernosum invasion and tumor grade in the prediction of lymph node condition in penile carcinoma. *Eur Urol* 22:115–118, 1992.

185. Pettaway CA, von Eschenbach AC. Surgery of penile carcinoma. In Bland KI, Karakousis CP, Copeland EM (eds), *Atlas of Surgical Oncology.* Philadelphia: Saunders, 1995:615.

186. Hall C, Sanders JR, Vuitch F, et al. Deoxyribonucleic flow cytometry and traditional pathologic variables in invasive penile carcinoma: assessment of prognostic significance. *Urology* 52:111–116, 1998.

187. Ravi R. Correlation between the extent of nodal involvement and survival following groin dissection for carcinoma of the penis. *Br J Urol* 72:817–819, 1993.

188. Johnson DE, Lo RK. Complications of groin dissection in penile cancer: experience with 101 lymphadenectomies. *Urology* 14:312–314, 1984.

189. Scappini P, Piscioli F, Pusiol T, et al. Penile cancer. Aspiration biopsy cytology for staging. *Cancer* 58:1526–1533, 1986.

190. Cabanas RM. An approach for the treatment of penile carcinoma. *Cancer* 39:456–466, 1977.

191. Pettaway CA, Pisters LL, Dinney CPN, et al. Sentinel lymph node dissection for penile carcinoma: the M. D. Anderson Cancer Center experience. *J Urol* 1544:1999–2003, 1995.

192. McDougal WS. Carcinoma of the penis: improved survival by early regional lymphadenectomy based on the histological grade and depth of invasion of the primary lesion. *J Urol* 154:1364–1366, 1995.

193. Lopes A, Hidalgo GS, Kowalski LP, et al. Prognostic factors in carcinoma of the penis: multivariate analysis of 145 patients treated with amputation and lymphadenectomy. *J Urol* 156:1637–1642, 1996.

194. Colberg JW, Andriole GL, Catalona WJ. Long-term follow-up of men undergoing modified inguinal lymphadenectomy for carcinoma of the penis. *Br J Urol* 79:54–57, 1997.

195. Pettaway CA, Jularbal FA, Babaian RJ, et al. Intraoperative lymphatic mapping to detect metastaases in penile carcinoma: results of a pilot study. *J Urol* 161:612A, 199.

196. Mohs FE, Snow SN, Messing EM, et al. Microscopically controlled surgery in the treatment of carcinoma of the penis. *J Urol* 133:961–966, 1985.

197. Mohs FE, Snow SN, Larson PO. Mohs micrographic surgery for penile tumors. *Urol Clin North Am* 19:291–304, 1992.

198. Goette DK, Canon TE. Erythroplasia of Queyrat: treatment with topical 5-fluorouracil. *Cancer* 38:1498–1502, 1976.

199. El-Demiry MI, Oliver RT, Hope-Stone HF, et al. Reappraisal of the role of radiotherapy and surgery in the management of carcinoma of the penis. *Br J Urol* 56:724–728, 1984.

200. Haile K, Delclos L. The place of radiation therapy in the treatment of carcinoma of the distal end of the penis. *Cancer* 45:1980–1984, 1980.

201. Grabstald H, Kelley CD. Radiation therapy of penile cancer. Six to ten year follow-up. *Urology* 15:575–576, 1980.

202. Duncan W, Jackson SM. The treatment of early cancer of the penis with megavoltage x-rays. *Clin Radiol* 23:246–248, 1972.

203. Malloy TR, Zderic SA, Curpiniello VL. External genital lesions. In Smith JA Jr, Stein BS, Benson RC Jr (eds), *Lasers in Urological Surgery* (2nd ed). Chicago: Year Book, 1989:23–34.

204. von Eschenbach AC, Johnson DE, Wishnow KI, et al. Results of laser therapy for carcinoma of the penis. Organ preservation. *Prog Clin Biol Res* 370:407–412, 1991.

205. Boon TA. Sapphire probe laser surgery for localized carcinoma of the penis. *Eur J Surg Oncol* 14:193–195, 1988.

206. Rothenberger KH. Value of the neodymium:YAG laser in the therapy of penile carcinoma. *Eur Urol* 12:34–36, 1986.

207. Malek RS. Laser treatment of premalignant and malignant squamous cell lesions of the penis. *Lasers Surg Med* 12:246–253, 1992.

208. Johnson DE, Lo RK, Srigley J, et al. Verrucous carcinoma of the penis. *J Urol* 133:216–218, 1985.

209. Persky L, de Kernion J. Carcinoma of the penis. *CA Cancer J Clin* 6:258–273, 1986.

210. Ames FC, Johnson DE. Groin dissection. In Johnson DE, Ames FC (eds), *Groin Dissection.* Chicago: Year Book, 1985:37.

211. Jones WG, Elwell CM. Radiation therapy for penile cancer. In Vogelzang NJ, Scardino PT, Shipley WU, Coffey DS (eds), *Comprehensive Textbook of Genitourinary Oncology.* Baltimore: Williams & Wilkins, 1996:1109–1114.

212. Horenblas S, van Tinteren H, Delemarre JFM, et al. Squamous cell carcinoma of the penis: II. Treatment of the primary tumor. *J Urol* 147:1533–1538. 1992.

213. Newaishy GA, Deeley TJ. Radiotherapy in the treatment of carcinoma of the penis. *Br J Radiol* 41:519–522, 1968.

214. Stadler W. Chemotherapy for penile cancer. In Vogelzang NJ, Scardino PT, Shipley WU, Coffey DS (eds), *Comprehensive Textbook of Genitourinary Oncology*. Baltimore: Williams & Wilkins, 1996:1114–1116.

215. Connell CF, Berger NA. Management of advanced squamous cell carcinoma of the penis. *Urol Clin North Am* 4:745–756, 1994.

216. Corral DA, Sella A, Pettaway CA, et al. Combination chemotherapy for metastatic or locally advanced genitourinary squamous cell carcinoma: a phase II study of methotrexate, cisplatin and bleomycin (MPB). *J Urol* 160:1770–1774, 1998.

217. Pizzocaro G, Piva L. Adjuvant and neoadjuvant vincristine, bleomycin, and methotrexate for inguinal metastases from squamous cell carcinoma of the penis. *Acta Oncol* 27:823–824, 1988.

218. Hardner GJ, Bhanalaph T, Murphy GP, et al. Carcinoma of the penis: analysis of therapy in 100 consecutive cases. *J Urol* 108:428–430, 1972

219. Srinivas V, Morse MJ, Herr HW, et al. Penile cancer. Relation of extent of nodal metastasis to survival. *J Urol* 137:880–882, 1987.

220. Ravi R, Chaturvedi HK, Sastry DVLN. Role of radiation therapy in the treatment of carcinoma of the penis. *Br J Urol* 74:646–651, 1994.

221. Weiner JS, Liu ET, Walther PJ. Oncogenic human papillomavirus type 16 is associated with squamous cell cancer of the male urethra. *Cancer Res* 52:5018–5023, 1992.

222. Terry PJ, Cookson MS, Sarosdy MF. Carcinoma of the urethra and scrotum. In Raghavan D, Scher HI, Leibel SA, Lange PH (eds), *Principles and Practice of Genitourinary Oncology*. Philadelphia: Lippincott-Raven, 1997:347–354.

223. Mostofi FK, Davis CJ, Sesterhenn IA. Carcinoma of the male and female urethra. *Urol Clin North Am* 19:347–358, 1992.

224. Kaplan GW, Bulkley GJ, Grayhack JT. Carcinoma in the male urethra. *J Urol* 98:365, 1967.

225. Grabstald H, Hilaris B, Henschke U, Whitmore WF Jr. Cancer of the female urethra. *JAMA* 197:835–842, 1966.

226. Ray B, Canto SR, Whitmore WF Jr. Experience with primary carcinoma of the male urethra. *J Urol* 117:591–594, 1977.

227. Beahrs OH, Henson DE, Hutter RVP, et al. (eds). *Manual for Staging of Cancer* (3rd ed). Philadelphia: Lippincott, 1988:210.

228. Garden AS, Zagars GK, Delclos L. Primary carcinoma of the female urethra: results of radiation therapy. *Cancer* 71:3102–3108, 1998.

229. Sailer SL, Shipley VW, Wang CC. Carcinoma of the female urethra: a review of results with radiation therapy. *J Urol* 140:1–5, 1988.

230. Weghaupt K, Gerstner GJ, Kucera H. Radiation therapy for primary carcinoma of the female urethra: a survey over 25 years. *Gynecol Oncol* 17:58–63, 1984.

231. Forman JD, Lichter AS. The role of radiation therapy in the management of carcinoma of the male and female urethra. *Urol Clin North Am* 19:383–389, 1992.

232. Bracken RB, Johnson DE, Miller LS, et al. Primary carcinoma of the female urethra. *J Urol* 116:188–192, 1976.

233. Grigsby PW, Herr HW. Urethral tumors. In Vogelzang N, Scardino PTS, Shipley WU, Coffey DS (eds), *Comprehensive Textbook of Genitourinary Oncology*. Baltimore: Williams & Wilkins, 1996:1117–1123.

234. Narayan P, Konety B. Surgical techniques of female urethral cancer. *Urol Clin North Am* 19:373–382, 1992.

235. Zeidman EJ, Desmond P, Thompson IM. Surgical treatment of carcinoma of the male urethra. *Urol Clin North Am* 19:359–372, 1992.

236. Dinney CPN, Johnson DE, Swanson DA, et al. Therapy and prognosis for male anterior urethral carcinoma: an update. *Urology* 43:506–514, 1994.

237. Hussein AM, Benedetto P, Sridhar KS. Chemotherapy with cisplatin and 5-fluorouracil for penile and urethral squamous cell carcinomas. *Cancer* 65:433–438, 1990.

238. Ajani JA, Ilson DH, Kelson DP. Paclitaxel in the treatment of patients with upper gastrointestinal carcinomas. *Semin Oncol* 23:55–58, 1996.

239. Pienta KJ, Smith DC. Paclitaxel, estramustine and etoposide in the treatment of hormone-refractory prostate cancer. *Semin Oncol* 24:72–77, 1997.

240. Price FV, Edwards RP, Kelley JL, et al. A trial of outpatient paclitaxel and carboplatin for advanced recurrent, and histologic high-risk endometrial carcinoma: preliminary report. *Semin Oncol* 24:78–82, 1997.

241. Roth BJ. Preliminary experience with paclitaxel in advanced bladder cancer. *Semin Oncol* 22:1–5, 1995.

242. Abu-Rustum NR, Aghajanian C, Barakat RR, et al. Salvage weekly paclitaxel in recurrent ovarian cancer. *Semin Oncol* 24:62–67, 1997.

19

Gynecologic Cancer

■ ■ ■

Abbie L. Fields
Joan G. Jones
Gillian M. Thomas
Carolyn D. Runowicz

Tumors of the female reproductive tract include cancers of the vulva, vagina, cervix, uterus, fallopian tubes, and ovaries. These lesions represent 13.4% of all cancers affecting women and account for 10% of their cancer deaths. Table 19.1 lists the estimated 2000 incidence and mortality rates for gynecologic malignancies in the United States.

Because a clear correlation has been established between early diagnosis and survival in gynecologic malignancies, an essential practice for all primary-care physicians is to be knowledgeable in the pathophysiologic characteristics of cancers of the reproductive tract, so as to facilitate early diagnosis (Table 19.2). Primary-care providers must educate patients about screening and prevention strategies and should initiate appropriate consultation and referral to involved gynecologists or gynecologic oncologists for patients with malignant or premalignant conditions of the female genital tract.

CERVICAL CANCER

Cervical cancer is the third most common female genital tract malignancy, with an annual incidence of 12,800 cases and 4,600 deaths per year [1]. Age distribution is bimodal, with peaks at 35 to 39 years and 60 to 64 years. With the introduction of the Papanicolaou (Pap) smear to evaluate cervical cytology, the 5-year survival among white women has increased from 58% (1960–1963) to 72% (1989–1996). The trend in black women, however, showed an initial improvement from 47% (1960–1963) to 64% (1974–1976), followed by a subsequent decline to 59% (1989–1996). Invasive cervical malignancies could be eradicated almost completely with regular screening programs available to all patients, regardless of race, age, or socioeconomic status.

Table 19.1 Gynecologic Malignancies: United States, 2000

Site	Estimated Incidence (%)	Estimated Mortality (%)
Uterus	36,100 (46)	6,500 (25)
Ovary	23,100 (30)	14,000 (53)
Cervix	12,800 (17)	4,600 (17)
Vulva	3,400 (4)	800 (3)
Vagina	2,100 (3)	600 (2)

Source: Date adapted from Greenlee RT, Murray T, Bolden S, Wingo PA. Cancer statistics, 2000. *CA Cancer J Clin* 50:7–33, 2000.

Table 19.2 Presenting Stage and Survival of Gynecologic Malignancies

Site	Stage	Presenting Stage (%)	5-Year Survival (%)
Cervix	I	45	A1 95–98
			A2 95–96
			B 80–83
	II	29	A 66–70
			B 61–63
	III	22	30–35
	IV	4	13–14
Vulva	I	49	70–95
	II	30	61–85
	III	16	44–74
	IV	5	15–31
Vagina	I	26	62–76
	II	34	44–55
	III	25	22–35
	IV	15	15–30
Uterus	I	73	81–91
	II	11	67–77
	III	13	32–60
	IV	3	5–20
Ovary	I	23	71–91
	II	13	51–69
	III	48	21–41
	IV	16	5–14

Source: Data adapted from S Pecorelli (ed), The annual report on the results of treatment of gynecological cancer. *J Epidemiol Biostat* 3:5–127, 1998.

Biological Considerations

The risk factors associated with cervical cancer (Table 19.3) suggest that a sexually transmitted agent is involved in the pathogenesis of the disease. Although herpes simplex virus (HSV) appeared to be a likely candidate, as portions of the HSV genome could be identified in cervical cancer cells when evaluated by HSV DNA hybridization techniques, more recent data implicate it as a cofactor [2]. During the last decade, the human papil-

Table 19.3 Cervical Cancer Risk Factors

Nutritional deficiencies	Carotene, folic acid, vitamin C, vitamin E
Viral or infectious factors	Human papillomavirus (> 70 types; low-risk [types 6, 11]; high-risk [types 16, 18, 31, 33, others]); herpes simplex virus; Chlamydia
Immunologic factors	Human immunodeficiency virus
Epidemiologic factors	Low socioeconomic status, young age at first coitus, number of sex partners, high-risk male partner
Cofactors	Tobacco use, oral contraceptive use

lomavirus (HPV) has become the most likely infectious agent associated with the malignant transformation of normal cells to cancer. Now, strong evidence suggests that the viral proteins E6 and E7 produced by high-risk HPV subtypes encode oncoproteins that interfere with the regulatory functions of p53 and RB tumor suppressor proteins [3, 4]. Subsequently, malignant transformation can occur as DNA-damaged cells are allowed to continue through the cell cycle rather than undergoing cell cycle arrest or apoptosis, as would occur with a functional p53 system.

Presently, more than 70 types of papillomavirus have been identified in humans, of which more than 20 types are associated with anogenital tract lesions. HPV DNA can be identified in more than 90% of preinvasive and invasive lesions, with HPV types 16, 18, 31, and 33 found primarily in invasive lesions and types 6 and 11 found in benign condylomatous lesions [5, 6]. However, 25% to 30% of women with normal Pap smear results also are identified as carrying HPV. Due to the high prevalence of HPV infection and lack of specificity between HPV typing and clinical outcome, HPV testing is not recommended as a useful screening tool for cervical neoplasia.

Historically, cigarette smoking was considered an independent etiologic agent for cervical cancer. Data from recent studies that control for HPV subtypes suggest tobacco functions as a cofactor to HPV-infected cells, facilitating neoplastic progression [7]. HPV oncoproteins impair host tumor suppressor genes [8]. Tobacco use leads to carcinogen-DNA adduct formation in cervical epithelium, causing DNA misreplication and mutation [9]. Together, carcinogen-induced genomic damage may allow cervical carcinogenesis to occur in HPV-infected cells. Evidence also substantiates that nicotine may induce cellular immortality by inhibiting apoptosis [10].

Prevention and Early Detection

Cervical carcinoma represents the final step in a continuum that begins with cervical intraepithelial neoplasia (CIN), a preinvasive process, detectable by cervical cytologic screening. According to guidelines from the American Cancer Society and the American College of Obstetricians and Gynecologists, performing Pap smear screening is recommended in all women who have reached the age of 18 or in women who are or have been sexually active [6, 11]. After three or more consecutive, satisfactory, normal Pap smear evaluations, the frequency may be reduced to every 2 to 3 years, depending on patients' particular risk factors. Because delineating which patients are at high risk for cervical cancer and compliance issues often is difficult, most practitioners recommend that all women undergo annual Pap smear screening.

The reliability of Pap smear results depends on appropriate sampling technique and on laboratory quality control (proper staining and pathologic interpretation). Samples should include cells from the squamocolumnar junction (transformation zone), where a metaplastic process normally occurs and dysplasia may develop. The endocervix should be sampled first, with an endocervical brush or moistened cotton-tipped applicator. The ectocervix should be sampled next, with a bifid-tipped wooden (Ayer) spatula. Alternatively, a cervical broom may be used to sample both sites simultaneously. Both specimens should be spread thinly across glass slides and should be fixed immediately with cytologic fixative solution.

False-negative rates vary from 10% to 25%, and false-positive rates are reported in 15% to 20% of patients. Cervical adenocarcinomas are identified less frequently with Pap smear screening for any of various reasons: The tumor is relatively inaccessible, it is localized predominantly at the base of the glands or high in the endocervix, or the cytologic abnormalities are minimal. Other gynecologic malignancies may be identified incidentally on cervicovaginal cytology. However, the Pap smear is not designed to screen for all gynecologic malignancies, a common misconception among the general population.

Recent technologic advances are being investigated to improve both sensitivity and specificity of Pap smear diagnoses specifically by addressing the weaknesses and limitations of the conventional Pap smear. The thin-layer, liquid-based Pap smear (e.g., ThinPrep [Automated Cytyc Corp., Boxborough, MA] or Cytorich [AutoCyte, Burlington, NC]) suspends the cells in a preservative so that a predetermined number of cells can be transferred to a slide for interpretation in an attempt to limit the possibility of an unsatisfactory collection technique. To diminish errors of specimen interpretation, automated computer-assisted rescreening systems (e.g., Papnet [Neuromedical Systems, Inc., Upper Saddle River, NJ] and AutoPap [NeoPath, Inc., Redmond, WA]) have been approved as rescreening devices to decrease the incidence of false-negative Pap smear results. AutoPap has been approved also for primary screening.

In 1988, the National Cancer Institute (NCI) introduced the Bethesda System of Classification of Cervical and Vaginal Cytology. This system was revised in 1991 and defines specific criteria for specimen adequacy. The Bethesda System (Fig. 19.1) classifies cells as being (1) within normal limits, (2) benign cellular changes, (3) atypical squamous cells of undetermined significance (ASCUS) or glandular cells of undetermined significance (AGUS), (4) low-grade squamous intraepithelial lesions, (5) high-grade squamous intraepithelial lesions, and (6) squamous cell or adenocarcinoma or suggestion of other malignant neoplasm.

Currently, management of an ASCUS Pap smear is controversial. Many clinicians refer patients immediately for colposcopically directed biopsy after an ASCUS Pap smear. We know already that moderate CIN or cancer will be identified in 5.0% and 0.001% of biopsies, respectively, after a single ASCUS Pap smear, rising to 10% to 28% and 0.2%, respectively, with a persistent ASCUS Pap smear [12, 13]. For this reason, in compliant patients, the preferred management for an ASCUS cytologic outcome would be a repeat Pap smear at 3- to 6-month intervals, followed by colposcopy if abnormalities persist. AGUS should be considered a more significant finding, particularly in postmenopausal patients. Because of the increased incidence of ectocervical, endocervical, and endometrial malignancies identified with this lesion, colposcopically directed biopsies, endocervical curettage, and an endometrial sampling is the minimum workup required for an AGUS Pap smear finding.

Frequently, low-grade squamous intraepithelial lesions are associated with the cellular changes of HPV (koilocytosis). Although 60% of these lesions will regress spontaneously, approximately 15% will progress to a high-grade abnormality. For this reason, most clinicians will perform colposcopy to assess the extent of the lesion adequately and then will manage affected pa-

The Bethesda System Terminology	General Descriptive	Within normal limits	Benign cellular changes Infection or Reactive/Repair	Epithelial cell abnormalities						
				ASCUS or AGUS	LGSIL		HGSIL			Invasive carcinoma
Dysplasia					HPV	Mild dysplasia	Moderate dysplasia	Severe dysplasia	Carcinoma in situ	
CIN					HPV	CIN1	CIN2	CIN3		
Papanicolaou classification		I	II	III					IV	V

Figure 19.1   Relationship of the Bethesda system to previous classification systems. *ASCUS* = atypical squamous cells of undetermined significance; *AGUS* = atypical glandular cells of undetermined significance; *LGSIL* = low-grade squamous intraepithelial lesion; *HGSIL* = high-grade squamous intraepithelial lesion; *HPV* = human papillomavirus; *CIS* = carcinoma in situ; *CIN* = cervical intraepithelial neoplasia. (Reprinted with permission of Lippincott-Raven from HM Shingleton, RL Patrick, WW Johnston, RA Smith, The current status of the Papanicolaou smear. *CA Cancer J Clin* 45:305–320, 1995.)

tients either expectantly or by ablative therapies, based on the reproductive stage and compliance of the patient. If patients and physicians select expectant management, a repeat examination should be performed in 3 to 6 months.

The finding of high-grade squamous intraepithelial lesion requires colposcopically directed biopsies to assess the extent of the lesion and to plan treatment. Cervical biopsies are reported as cervical intraepithelial neoplasia grade 1 (CIN1; mild dysplasia, koilocytosis); cervical intraepithelial neoplasia grade 2 (CIN2; moderate dysplasia), or cervical intraepithelial neoplasia grade 3 (CIN3; severe dysplasia, carcinoma in situ), depending on whether abnormalities (loss of maturation and mitotic activity) are confined to the lower one-third, to the lower two-thirds, or to more than two-thirds of the thickness of the epithelium. Most clinicians will manage CIN1 expectantly, as the majority spontaneously revert to normal within 1 year. Some clinicians will treat this lesion with cryotherapy. Usually, CIN2 and CIN3 are treated by ablation or excisional therapies. The utility of excisional cone biopsy for adenocarcinoma in situ is less clear. Despite negative margins, persistent disease has been identified at subsequent hysterectomy or cone biopsy in up to 40% of patients [14]. An essential step is that the patient be informed adequately of the risk of residual disease prior to selection of a treatment option.

For a colposcopic examination to be adequate, the entire transformation zone and the borders of all abnormal areas must be visualized clearly. If the examination is not adequate, a cone biopsy would be indicated to assess the transformation zone adequately. Other indications for cone biopsy include an abnormal endocervical curettage, lack of correlation between cytologic and histologic findings, and evaluation of depth of invasion. The cone biopsy can be performed by laser, a loop electrosurgical excision procedure (LEEP), or scalpel (cold-knife) excision, depending on physician preference and skill.

Ablative therapy in patients not requiring cone biopsy has become the most common method of treating higher-grade dysplasia. The results of electrosurgical excision are comparable to that of laser vaporization, which has become less popular due to its cost, more difficult technique, and lack of residual specimen for histopathologic evaluation. Cryosurgery, which is inexpensive and learned easily, was primarily a treatment for CIN1, which can now, alternatively, be managed expectantly.

Diagnosis

CLINICAL PRESENTATION

Frequently, patients with cervical carcinoma present with abnormal vaginal bleeding, spotting, or discharge. Although bleeding occurrence may assume any pattern, it is reported most commonly after coitus. Patients with more advanced disease may present with pelvic or back pain that may radiate down the leg, hematuria, fistulas (rectovaginal or vesicovaginal), or with evidence of metastatic disease to the supraclavicular or inguinal lymph node areas. If an obvious cervical lesion is identified on physical examination, a tissue biopsy is done to confirm the diagnosis.

DIAGNOSTIC EVALUATION

All patients require a thorough history and physical examination, with emphasis on reproductive and sexual history, Pap smear intervals and findings, and tobacco use. Cervical cancer is a clinically staged disease, and meticulous attention must be given to the cervix, vagina, parametria, pelvic side walls, and inguinal-supraclavicular lymph node regions. Required investigative tools include chest roentgenography, to rule out pulmonary metastasis, and intravenous pyelogram (IVP), to assess ureteral obstruction and implied side-wall involvement. Cystoscopy and proctosigmoidoscopy are necessary in patients with advanced disease or in those who are symptomatic, to rule out either bladder or rectal involvement. Although not part of the clinical staging, computed tomography (CT) with contrast and magnetic resonance imaging may be useful in assessing the extent of disease. If a CT scan with contrast is performed, the IVP can be eliminated. Lymphangiography is used less commonly to evaluate lymph node status. If noninvasive radiographic studies suggest suspicious lymph nodes, a fine-needle aspiration is required to confirm metastatic involvement histologically. Additionally, a complete blood count and standard blood chemistry tests should be obtained, to evaluate the patient for anemia and renal and hepatic abnormalities.

PATHOLOGIC FEATURES

Squamous cell carcinomas of the cervix are the most common tumors, accounting for 60% to 80% of cases, followed by adenocarcinomas, in order of frequency. Often, both arise at the squamocolumnar junction or transformation zone. Squamous cell carcinomas (especially the keratinizing subtype) can arise elsewhere on the ectocervix, whereas adenocarcinomas can develop deeper in the canal. Typically, squamous cell carcinomas form exophytic masses. Adenocarcinomas also may be exophytic, but a more distinctive gross appearance, seen in approximately 15% of adenocarcinomas, is the so-called barrel-shaped cervix. No gross lesion can be visualized in approximately 15% of patients.

It is generally accepted that invasive squamous cell carcinomas develop from CIN (Fig. 19.2). Microscopically, these tumors may be graded according to degree and extent of keratinization, nuclear grade, and mitotic activity, but no convincing evidence suggests that grading reliably predicts prognosis. The spectrum of preinvasive glandular lesions in the cervix is not as well defined. Microscopically, invasive adenocarcinomas may show a variety of histologic features. Those producing

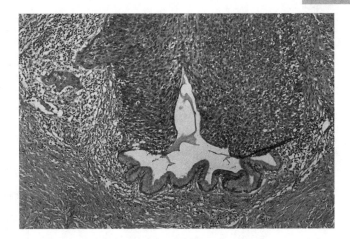

Figure 19.2 Cervix. The earliest evidence of invasion in squamous cell carcinoma of the cervix is microinvasion. Here, a small nest of cells (left) has invaded from an endocervical gland partially involved by carcinoma in situ.

mucin may have an endocervical or intestinal appearance. The endometrioid subtype has a histologic appearance that is morphologically indistinguishable from its uterine corpus counterpart. Subtypes encountered less frequently include clear-cell carcinomas, serous carcinoma, the deceptively bland minimal-deviation adenocarcinoma, and the aggressive glassy-cell carcinoma, a form of adenosquamous carcinoma. Neuroendocrine features also may occur, as in pure small-cell carcinomas, or as elements in combination with squamous cell or glandular features.

STAGING

Cervical carcinoma is staged clinically in accordance with the International Federation of Gynecology and Obstetrics (FIGO) guidelines (Table 19.4). This malignancy spreads primarily by direct extension to adjacent tissues and by lymphatic dissemination. Less frequently, hematogenous spread to lungs, liver, and bone occurs. Given the propensity for lymph node involvement in patients with extensive local disease, surgical evaluation of commonly affected lymph node groups (obturator, pelvic, paraaortic nodes) is of significant benefit in treatment planning. When imaging studies raise no suspicion of lymph node involvement, some clinicians think that affected patients may benefit from surgical lymph node exploration, either via the extraperitoneal approach or, more recently, by operative laparoscopy. Information gained from surgical staging (lymph node metastasis) can be used only to optimize treatment (e.g., extended-field irradiation or chemoradiotherapy),

Table 19.4   Clinical Staging of Carcinoma of the Uterine Cervix

FIGO	Stage	TNM	Classification	Description
I				Cervical carcinoma strictly confined to the cervix
IA				Invasive cancer identified only microscopically; all gross lesions, even with superficial invasion, are stage IB cancers; invasion limited to measured stromal invasion (maximum depth, 5.0 mm; no wider than 7.0*)
IA1	T1a1	N0	M0	Measured invasion of stroma no deeper than 3.0 mm, no wider than 7.0 mm
IA2	T1a2	N0	M0	Measured invasion of stroma > 3 mm and ≤ 5 mm, no wider than 7 mm
IB				Clinical lesions confined to the cervix or preclinical lesions > stage IA.
IB1	T1b1	N0	M0	Clinical lesions < 4 cm
IB2	T1b2	N0	M0	Clinical lesions > 4 cm
II				Cervical carcinoma invading beyond uterus but not to pelvic wall or to lower one-third of vagina
IIA	T2a	N0	M0	Without parametrial invasion; involving the upper one-third of vagina
IIB	T2b	N0	M0	With parametrial invasion
III				Cervical carcinoma extending to pelvic wall or involving lower one-third of vagina or causing hydronephrosis or nonfunctioning kidney
IIIA	T3a	N0	M0	Without pelvic wall involvement; involving lower one-third of vagina
IIIB	T1	N1	M0	Tumor extending to pelvic wall or causing hydronephrosis or nonfunctioning kidney
	T2	N1	M0	
	T3a	N1	M0	
	T3b	any N	M0	
IV				Tumor invading mucosa of bladder or rectum (IVA) or extending beyond true pelvis (IVB).
IVa	T4	any N	M0	
IVb	any T	any N	M1	

T = tumor description (equivalent to FIGO); N = regional lymph node involvement; N0 = no metastasis; N1 = regional metastasis; M = metastasis; M0 = no distant metastasis; M1 = any distant metastasis.

*The depth of invasion should not be more than 5 mm taken from the base of the epithelium, either surface or glandular, from which it originates. Vascular space involvement, either venous or lymphatic, should not alter the staging.

Source: Modified from the International Federation of Gynecology and Obstetrics, Annual report on the results of treatment in gynecological cancer. *J Epidemiol Biostat* 3:35–61, 1998.

but it will not alter such patients' disease stage. Whether surgical staging has a favorable impact on survival by altering treatment has yet to be determined.

Primary Treatment

Recommendations for treatment are based on the clinical stage of disease, on age, and on performance status of affected patients. Other factors that influence the treatment plan are known prognostic factors, such as tumor size, lymph node involvement, depth of invasion, and lymph–vascular space involvement.

Because women with stage IA1 disease have an incidence of lymph node metastasis of less than 1%, they may be treated by an extrafascial (type I) hysterectomy or, if childbearing has not been completed, a cone biopsy. The decision to offer conservative therapy, however, must be made in consultation with a gynecologic oncologist and should occur after review of the pathology to confirm depth of invasion, cell type, adequacy of margins, and absence of lymph-vascular invasion. Patient compliance must be evaluated before finalizing a treatment plan.

Patients with stage IA2, IB1, or IIA disease can be treated by radical surgery or by radiotherapy with equal

Table 19.5 Types of Abdominal Hysterectomy

| Anatomic Site | Type of Surgery | | | |
	Intrafascial	Extrafascial Type I	Modified Radical Type II	Radical Type III
Cervical fascia	Partially removed	Completely removed	Completely removed	Completely removed
Vaginal cuff removal	None	Small rim removed	Proximal 1–2 cm removed	Upper one-third to one-half removed
Bladder	Partially mobilized	Partially mobilized	Partially mobilized	Mobilized
Rectum	Not mobilized	R-V septum partially mobilized	R-V septum partially mobilized	Mobilized
Ureters	Not mobilized	Not mobilized	Unroofed in ureteral tunnel	Completely dissected to bladder entry
Cardinal ligaments	Resected medial to ureters	Resected medial to ureters	Resected at level of ureter	Resected at pelvic side wall
Uterosacral ligaments	Resected at level of cervix	Resected at level of cervix	Partially resected	Resected at postpelvic insertion
Uterus	Removed	Removed	Removed	Removed
Cervix	Partially removed	Completely removed	Completely removed	Completely removed

R-V = rectovaginal.
Type IV, extended radical hysterectomy (partial removal of bladder or ureter), in addition to Type III.
Source: Reprinted with permission from CA Perez, Uterine cervix. In CA Perez, LW Brady, eds, *Principles and Practice of Radiation Oncology* (2nd ed). Philadelphia: Lippincott, 1992.

efficacy. Surgical therapy is advised in younger patients so that ovarian and vaginal function remain unaltered. Surgery is the preferred method of treatment also in patients with diverticular disease, tubal, ovarian, or appendiceal abscesses, or pelvic kidneys. Postoperative radiotherapy is recommended in patients incidentally found to have invasive cervical cancer in the pathologic workup of a hysterectomy specimen or in patients with known cervical cancer with microscopically positive parametria, surgical margins, or lymph node metastases. Patients with bulky cervical lesions greater than 4 cm in diameter (stage IB2) have a 60% incidence of lymph node involvement. For this reason, such patients and those with stage IIB disease or greater are not treated surgically but rather with combination chemoradiotherapy in an attempt to extend the disease-free interval and survival.

SURGERY

Classically, a radical abdominal hysterectomy with total pelvic and selective paraaortic lymphadenectomy is termed a *Wertheim-Meigs hysterectomy* or a *type III hysterectomy*. The differences distinguishing a simple, extrafascial (type I) hysterectomy, a modified radical (type II) hysterectomy, and a radical (type III) hysterectomy are illustrated in Table 19.5.

As laparoscopic technique and procedures have advanced over the last decade, several investigators have explored the role of laparoscopic pelvic and selective paraaortic lymphadenectomy with a radical vaginal hysterectomy (a Schauta procedure) for patients with stage IA2 or IB1 disease [15]. Other investigators are evaluating the role of radical vaginal trachelectomy (cervical removal) with laparoscopic pelvic and selective paraaortic lymphadenectomy for early cervical carcinomas in young women who wish to preserve reproductive potential [16]. Currently, these procedures are considered investigational, with very short follow-up intervals, small sample sizes, and inconclusive evaluations of efficacy and survival. Table 19.6 summarizes the treatment options for patients with cervical cancer.

RADIOTHERAPY

In the primary treatment of cervical carcinoma, the radiation field and dose are determined by stage, volume of disease, and lymph node involvement. A combination of external teletherapy (pelvic) to treat paracervical or side-wall disease and to shrink the central tumor, followed by intracavitary brachytherapy directed toward the primary tumor, is used. Generally, the external irradiation dose is lower, and the intracavitary dose is higher in early-stage disease, as compared with more

Table 19.6 Treatment Options for Cervical Cancer

Stage	Options	Remarks
IA1 (no lymph vascular space invasion)	Conization *or* Total hysterectomy	Depth of invasion ≤ 3 mm; margins of cone biopsy must be negative for tumor
IA1 (with lymph vascular space invasion)	Total hysterectomy *or* Internal irradiation *or* Radical hysterectomy and node dissection *or* External and internal radiation	As the significance of lymph vascular involvement in stage IA1 carcinoma is controversial, many gynecologic and radiation oncologists suggest radical surgery or radiation Ovarian and vaginal function may be preserved by selecting surgery in young and medically fit women
IA2	Radical hysterectomy and node dissection *or* External and internal radiation	Internal radiation alone in selected patients Ovarian and vaginal function may be preserved by selecting surgery in young and medically fit women
IB1 (≤ 4 cm in size)	Radical hysterectomy and node dissection *or* External and internal radiation	Ovarian and vaginal function may be preserved by selecting surgery in young and medically fit women Postoperative radiation may be considered, depending on the characteristics of the tumor
IB2 (> 4 cm in size)	External and internal radiation *or* Radical hysterectomy and node dissection *or* Surgery in combination with radiation (selected patients)	Extended-field radiotherapy may be considered Neoadjuvant and concurrent chemotherapy are under clinical investigation Postoperative radiotherapy and/or chemotherapy may be considered based on the tumor characteristics
IIA	Radical hysterectomy and node dissection *or* External and internal radiation	Extended-field radiotherapy may be considered Neoadjuvant and concurrent chemotherapy are under clinical investigation Postoperative radiotherapy and/or chemotherapy may be considered based on the tumor characteristics
IIB	External and internal chemoradiotherapy	Extended-field radiotherapy may be considered Neoadjuvant chemotherapy is under clinical investigation
IIIA, IIIB	External and internal chemoradiotherapy	Neoadjuvant chemotherapy is under clinical investigation
IVA	Primary exenterative surgery in rare instances	Investigational therapies
IVB Metastatic	Short course of radiotherapy for palliation of symptoms or central disease or distant metastases *or* Palliative care only	Investigational therapies

advanced stages. This difference reflects the higher degree of side-wall and lymph node involvement in stage III and stage IV disease. Usually, dosages of irradiation delivered will be 70 to 80 Gy to point A (2 cm lateral and 2 cm above the cervical os) and 60 Gy to point B (pelvic side walls). Delivering extended-field irradiation to the lower paraaortic chain (45 Gy) also has been shown to improve survival not only in patients with documented positive paraaortic lymph nodes but when given prophylactically in patients with high risk of paraaortic node metastasis (IB2 or IIB lesions) [17].

In an attempt to decrease pelvic recurrence after a radical surgical procedure, 45 to 50 Gy has been recommended for patients with pelvic lymph node involvement, positive parametrial or vaginal margins, or very deep cervical stromal invasion. An improved recurrence-free survival at 2 years in those patients treated with postoperative pelvic radiotherapy was revealed in a preliminary evaluation of a prospective study of patients with surgically treated stage I disease at high risk for recurrence due to stromal invasion, size of primary tumor, and lymph–vascular space involvement [18].

CHEMOTHERAPY

Chemotherapy is not used in primary therapy. However, investigators have used chemotherapy prior to definitive surgery or radiotherapy (neoadjuvant). The presently available data have not confirmed a survival advantage with use of neoadjuvant chemotherapy followed by irradiation, despite favorable initial response rates [19, 20]. The use of neoadjuvant chemotherapy followed by surgery appears somewhat more promising, although owing to small numbers of reported cases, its use requires confirmation from a larger, randomized clinical trial [19, 20].

A different approach to multimodality therapy is the use of chemotherapy (single-agent or in combination) administered concomitantly with radiotherapy. The chemotherapy may function as a radiosensitizer to potentiate the effect of radiotherapy or as a cytotoxic agent, or as both. Small prospective trials have suggested a benefit in both local control and disease-free survival [21, 22]. Two recently completed randomized trials have been sufficiently promising to prompt the NCI to encourage the incorporation of concomitant cisplatin-based chemotherapy with irradiation in cervical cancer patients requiring radiotherapy. The Gynecologic Oncology Group trial demonstrated an improved progression-free interval in patients treated with cisplatin-containing regimens as compared to those treated with hydroxyurea [23]. The Radiation Therapy Oncology Group confirmed improved local control and a survival advantage in patients treated with concurrent cisplatin-containing chemotherapy with pelvic irradiation as compared to pelvic and paraaortic irradiation alone [24]. These data demonstrate the shifting trend that multimodality therapy has brought to the management of advanced cervical cancer.

Posttreatment Surveillance

Because 75% of recurrences are detected within the first 2 years after treatment, evaluation of disease status generally is recommended at 3-month intervals for the first 2 years. At these visits, a complete physical examination should be performed and should include a careful evaluation of lymph node areas (supraclavicular, inguinal), cervicovaginal cytology, and a bimanual, rectovaginal examination with palpation of the parametria and cardinal and uterosacral ligaments. Any suspicious lesions noted on cervicovaginal examination should be subjected to biopsy, and suspicious lymph nodes must be evaluated by fine-needle aspiration for cytologic confirmation. No standard recommendation is available for obtaining imaging procedures, such as chest roentgenography, CT scans, or IVP. Many investigators obtain a CT scan of the abdomen and pelvis with contrast after the first, second, and fifth years, with other evaluations requested as indicated. Because up to 50% of cases can be cured with pelvic exenteration, an important factor is to identify patients with an early isolated pelvic recurrence.

Relapse and Palliation

Patients with persistent or recurrent cervical cancer have a 5-year survival of less than 5%. This poor survival is attributable to the fact that the majority of recurrences have a distant component of disease. Patients with locally recurrent disease after primary surgical therapy may be treated with pelvic radiotherapy, which improves pelvic control and prolongs survival in approximately 40% [25]. Patients with persistent or recurrent disease after radiotherapy may be offered exploration for total pelvic exenteration, which includes removal of cervix, uterus, tubes, ovaries, bladder, rectum, and vagina. Rarely will less radical surgery be curative. With advances in surgical technique, a successful surgical outcome offers the patient 50% to 60% 5-year survival, with restoration of an adequate quality of life both personally and sexually [26].

Pelvic exenteration is offered only to patients with a resectable central recurrence. Frequently, the clinical triad of unilateral leg edema, sciatic nerve pain, and ureteral obstruction indicates unresectable side-wall disease. Evaluation to exclude distant metastases is essential prior to performing exenterative surgery. The workup should include recording a history and performing a physical examination; CT scan of chest, abdomen, and pelvis; and bone scan and possible renal scan. Because of the difficulty in distinguishing fibrosis from side-wall tumor involvement by clinical and radiographic evaluation, an exploratory laparotomy with parametrial and side-wall biopsies may be necessary to assess the resectability of disease.

The procedure of a pelvic exenteration requires an adequate surgical margin surrounding the residual tumor. The close anatomic proximity that the cervix bears to both bladder and rectum frequently necessitates their removal to obtain disease-free margins. Occasionally, an experienced gynecologic oncologist will assess the extent of the lesion and will conclude that a more tailored procedure—either anterior exenteration (rectum remaining) or posterior exenteration (bladder remaining)—will resect the recurrent disease adequately. Selected patients also may have transection of the rectosigmoid above the level of the levator muscle (supralevator), which allows the remaining rectal stump to be re-anastomosed to the sigmoid colon, thus avoiding a sigmoid colostomy. If obtaining an adequate surgical margin is not possible by performing a supralevator resection, the rectosigmoid must be excised below the levator muscle, resulting in a colostomy. The reconstructive phase of the operation includes creation of a urinary diverting mechanism that may be either a continent pouch (Koch, Miami, IN), which does not require affected patients to wear a urostomy bag, or an incontinent conduit (ileal, transverse colon). Vaginal reconstruction with myocutaneous flaps (rectus abdominus, bulbocavernosus, gracilis) allows creation of a normal-appearing, functional neovagina, which may be beneficial in maintaining the patient's sexual function.

The use of chemotherapy in the management of recurrent or persistent cervical cancer is palliative. Multiple agents have been evaluated; however, cisplatin alone or in combination has the most significant activity. When combination cisplatin-based chemotherapy is compared to single-agent cisplatin therapy, although the combination regimens have a higher response rate, they also are more toxic and are associated with survival equivalent to that of single-agent cisplatin therapy [27]. Other agents with activity in advanced or recurrent cervical cancer include paclitaxel, ifosfamide, bleomycin, and vinorelbine. Ongoing phase II trials are designed to evaluate efficacy of more novel agents, such as gemcitabine, topotecan, irinotecanan, and pyrazoloacridine.

Cervical Cancer and Pregnancy

Approximately 3% of patients with cervical cancer require alteration of treatment planning due to pregnancy [28]. Little evidence suggests that pregnancy independently results in a poor prognosis. Because most squamous cell carcinomas of the cervix are comparatively slow-growing, a "planned delay" to therapy is a possibility if affected patients desire to maintain the pregnancy and are in the middle or late trimester. Essential, however, is that such patients seek consultation from a gynecologic oncologist to be counseled adequately regarding risk of disease progression and metastasis based on stage, tumor volume, and length of treatment delay. If patients have early-stage disease with a very small cervical lesion, a vaginal delivery is not contraindicated. The risk to vaginal delivery is related more to bleeding than to an increased risk of disease dissemination.

If affected patients do not wish to maintain their pregnancy and are at less than 20 weeks' gestation, definitive surgery or radiotherapy can be planned. If the lesion is to be treated by irradiation, external-beam irradiation to the entire pelvis is initiated, with a spontaneous abortion usually occurring by the fourth week. If the fetus has not aborted spontaneously by completion of external-beam radiotherapy, a uterine evacuation can be performed at the time of brachytherapy insertion. Alternatively, if the patient is a surgical candidate (stage IB or IIA disease), a radical hysterectomy with pelvic and paraaortic lymphadenectomy can be performed. When the diagnosis of cervical cancer is made in the third trimester of pregnancy, the fetus can be delivered via cesarean section once fetal pulmonary maturity is confirmed. That can be followed by either surgery or radiotherapy, depending on the patient's stage of disease.

VULVAR AND VAGINAL CANCER

Invasive malignancies of the vulva and vagina occur much less frequently than do other gynecologic cancers, with vulvar and vaginal malignancies demonstrating incidences of 3,400 and 2,100, accounting for only 4% and 3%, respectively, of all gynecologic malignancies [1]. The majority of patients with invasive vulvar or vaginal disease tend to be postmenopausal, with a median age of 65 and 62 years, respectively. Because these diseases can be identified easily by a thorough gynecologic examination, all patients, including those who are beyond reproductive age or ability and in whom a hysterectomy has been performed, should be encouraged to continue with their routine annual gynecologic evaluations.

Biological Considerations

Although the majority of vulvar and vaginal malignancies are squamous cell carcinomas and may be associated with high-risk HPV types, the exact role of HPV in vulvar and vaginal oncogenesis has not been established clearly. The origin of such malignancies probably is multifactorial, HPV infection being one contributing factor.

In utero exposure to diethylstilbestrol (DES) is responsible for the development of clear-cell adenocarcinoma of the vagina [29]. DES was administered in the 1950s to women at risk for spontaneous abortions. Once the association among in utero DES exposure, vaginal adenosis, clear-cell carcinoma, and other benign cervicovaginal anomalies was made, the drug was withdrawn from the market. The risk that a DES-exposed woman will develop clear-cell carcinoma is approximately 1 in 1,000. The age at diagnosis ranges from 7 to 42 years (median age, 19 years). A history of DES exposure can be documented in 70% to 80% of patients with clear-cell adenocarcinoma, but 20% to 25% will develop clear-cell disease in the absence of documented DES exposure. The majority of DES-exposed clear-cell carcinomas are identified in the upper one-third of the anterior wall of the vagina or on the ectocervix. Patients affected thus have a better prognosis than do those with clear-cell disease who are not exposed to DES.

Benign changes are noted also in women exposed to DES in utero. Vaginal adenosis, large metaplastic cervical transformation zones, cervical collars, vaginal septa, pseudopolyps, and uterine anomalies, leading to miscarriage and preterm delivery, have been identified. DES exposure has been reported also to increase the risk of developing breast cancer in the mothers [30].

Prevention and Early Detection

Preinvasive disease of the vulva and vagina are of increasing prevalence. Both vaginal intraepithelial neo-plasia (VAIN) and vulvar intraepithelial neoplasia (VIN) are associated with HPV infection. Malignant transformations from VAIN or VIN have been observed, and the premalignant nature of these lesions remains well established.

Both VAIN and VIN are evaluated by visual inspection and colposcopy. Both appear as whitish, keratotic, roughened plaques that may be macular or papular on gross observation. Frequently, VIN appears as red, gray, or brown lesions reflecting vascular or melanocytic overactivity. Colposcopic evaluation may disclose acetowhite epithelium with punctation or mosaicism (or both).

The propensity for multifocal disease renders treatment of these disease processes difficult. Treatment options remain controversial and include surgical excision (for localized lesions or to exclude invasion), laser vaporization, or topical 5-fluorouracil therapy. The likelihood of successful treatment is influenced by the size, number, and accessibility of lesions requiring treatment.

Diagnosis

CLINICAL PRESENTATION

Frequently, patients with vulvar carcinomas present with the complaint of chronic pruritus unresponsive to local therapy. The lesion may be associated with pain, burning, bleeding, or discharge. Clinically, these lesions appear as raised, fleshy nodules (red, pink, or white) that may or may not have an ulcerated surface. Punch biopsy of any suspicious lesion identified is necessary for appropriate diagnosis.

Generally, vaginal carcinomas present with abnormal bleeding or discharge, although 20% may be asymptomatic. Patients with advanced disease may have symptoms consistent with involvement of adjacent structures, such as dysuria, hematuria, constipation, and pelvic or back pain. The majority of vaginal cancers are squamous cell types, which present in the upper one-third of the posterior wall of the vagina. This tendency stands in contrast to clear-cell lesions, which more commonly involve the anterior vaginal wall.

DIAGNOSTIC EVALUATION

Evaluation of patients with vulvar and vaginal malignancies begins with recording a thorough history and performing a physical examination. With vulvar cancer, careful attention should be paid to surrounding external genitalia to detect multifocal lesions. Speculum examination and Pap smear are necessary to rule out concurrent upper-tract disease. The lesion size and proximity to clitoris, urethra, anus, and other structures should be noted. Inguinal areas should be inspected for evidence of enlarged or fixed lymph nodes. Any suspicious node should be subjected to biopsy or aspirated. Vulvar cancer is staged surgically; therefore, women with small lesions and clinically negative nodes require no further preoperative testing other than that required for surgical clearance. Women with more advanced disease or suspected metastases may benefit from cystoscopy, proctoscopy, CT, or magnetic resonance imaging on the basis of clinical indications.

Vaginal cancer is staged clinically. The speculum must be rotated during the examination so that the anterior, posterior, and lateral walls may be visualized adequately. As with the evaluation for cervical carcinoma, chest roentgenography and IVP (or CT with intravenous contrast) are necessary to assess the extent of disease. Cystoscopy and proctoscopy may be beneficial in patients with advanced disease.

PATHOLOGIC FEATURES

The vulva includes structures that constitute the external genitalia and the vestibule, where Skene's and Bartholin's gland orifices are located. The types of tumors that arise differ according to the anatomic site. Squamous epithelium covers the entire surface of the vulva, and squamous cell carcinomas are the most common primary vulvar malignancies. Malignant melanoma ranks as the second most common vulvar malignancy. Identification of junctional activity of the epidermal melanocytes is necessary to confirm a primary lesion conclusively, but ulceration of benign epithelium overlying the tumor may prevent recognition of this feature.

Other malignancies, such as basal cell carcinoma and neoplasms of dermal adnexal structures, also may occur. Paget's disease is a form of intraepidermal vulvar adenocarcinoma that, in contrast to Paget's disease of the breast, is not associated invariably with an underlying invasive malignancy. Paget cells are large and round, with pale cytoplasm that stains positively for mucin and carcinoembryonic antigen (CEA). These cells aggregate as nests at the dermoepidermal junction, streaming upward in the epithelium as single cells (pagetoid spread; Fig. 19.3). A very wide excision is necessary to obtain negative margins, as the Paget's disease usually extends well beyond the grossly visualized lesion.

Adenocarcinomas of the vulva arise most commonly in Bartholin's glands, although Skene's glands or sweat

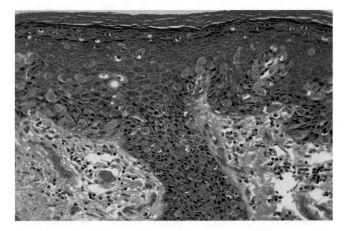

Figure 19.3   Paget's disease. Paget's cells are seen at the dermoepidermal junction and at various levels of the epidermis.

gland carcinomas may occur. Criteria for establishing a diagnosis of primary Bartholin's gland carcinoma include proper anatomic location, transition from benign to malignant Bartholin's gland elements, and lack of other known primaries with similar histologic appearance. The histologic appearance of these tumors may vary.

Primary carcinomas of the vagina are infrequent. Of these, more than 90% are squamous cell carcinomas arising from intraepithelial neoplasia in the surface squamous epithelium. Adenocarcinomas, melanomas, and sarcomas account for the remainder of primary vaginal malignancies. Because cervical and vulvar carcinomas are much more common, confirmation of the diagnosis of primary squamous cell carcinoma of the vagina requires ruling out direct extension from these adjacent anatomic sites. Squamous cell carcinomas arising at any of these sites may have the same histologic appearance.

STAGING

Owing to the anatomic proximity of the urethra or rectum, spread by direct extension may create a complicated surgical management issue. In addition to direct extension, vulvar cancer may spread by lymphatic embolization to inguinal, femoral, and pelvic node groups. Hematogenous dissemination to distant sites (bone, lung, liver) also can occur but with relative infrequency. Vulvar carcinoma is staged surgically (Table 19.7).

Vaginal cancers are staged clinically, also in accordance with FIGO guidelines (Table 19.8). These tumors spread primarily by direct extension to adjacent organs and by lymphatic dissemination. Hematogenous spread

Table 19.7   Staging of Vulvar Carcinoma

FIGO	Stage	TNM	Classification	Description
0	Tis	N0	M0	Carcinoma in situ; intraepithelial carcinoma
I	T1	N0	M0	
IA				Lesions ≤ 2 cm confined to the vulva or perineum and with stromal invasion ≤ 1.0 mm* (no nodal metastasis)
IB				Lesions ≤ 2 cm confined to the vulva or perineum, stromal invasion > 1.0 mm; no nodal metastasis
II	T2	N0	M0	Tumor confined to the vulva or perineum; greatest dimension > 2 cm; negative nodes
III	T1	N1	M0	Tumor of any size with the following:
	T2	N1	M0	(1) Adjacent spread to the lower urethra or the vagina, or the anus, *or*
	T3	N0	M0	(2) Unilateral regional lymph node metastasis
	T3	N1	M0	
IVA	T1	N2	M0	Tumor invasion of any of the following: Upper urethra,
	T2	N2	M0	bladder mucosa, rectal mucosa, pelvic bone, or bilateral
	T3	N2	M0	regional node metastasis
	T4	any N	M0	
IVB	Any T	any N	M1	Any distant metastasis including pelvic lymph nodes

T = tumor description (equivalent to FIGO); N = regional lymph node involvement; N0 = no metastasis; N1 = regional lymph node metastasis; N2 = bilateral regional lymph node metastasis; M = metastasis; M0 = no metastasis; M1 = any distant metastasis (including pelvic lymph node metastasis).

*The depth of invasion is defined as the measurement of the tumor from the epithelial-stromal junction of the adjacent, most superficial dermal papilla to the deepest point of invasion.

Source: Modified from the International Federation of Gynecology and Obstetrics. Annual report on the results of treatment in gynecological cancer. *J Epidemiol Biostat* 3(23):111–127, 1998.

Table 19.8   Staging of Vaginal Carcinoma

FIGO	Stage	TNM	Classification	Description
0	Tis	N0	M0	Carcinoma in situ; intraepithelial carcinoma
I	T1	N0	M0	Carcinoma limited to vaginal mucosa (wall)
II	T2	N0	M0	Subvaginal infiltration into parametrium, not extending to the pelvic wall
III	T1	N1	M0	Carcinoma extended to the pelvic wall
	T2	N1	M0	
	T3	N0	M0	
	T3	N1	M0	
IV				Carcinoma extended beyond the true pelvis or involves mucosa of bladder or rectum
IVA	T4,	Any N,	M0	Carcinoma spread to adjacent organs or direct extension beyond the true pelvis
IVB	Any T,	Any N,	M0	Carcinoma spread to distant organs

T = tumor description (equivalent to FIGO); N0 = no regional node metastasis; N1 = pelvic node metastasis if lesion in upper two-thirds of vagina; N1 = unilateral inguinal node metastasis if lesion in lower one-third of vagina; N2 = bilateral inguinal node metastasis; M0 = no distant metastasis; M1 = any distant metastasis.

Source: Modified from the International Federation of Gynecology and Obstetrics, Annual report on the results of treatment in gynecological cancer. *J Epidemiol Biostat* 3(23):103–109, 1998.

(lung, liver, bone) occurs much less frequently. Lesions of the upper vagina mimic cervical cancer spread patterns (pelvic, paraaortic node involvement), whereas lower vaginal lesions reflect vulvar spread patterns to inguinal and femoral nodes, with pelvic node involvement occurring secondarily.

Primary Treatment

VULVA

Surgery

Historically, vulvar carcinomas were treated by en bloc radical vulvectomy with bilateral inguinal-femoral node dissections through a single "butterfly" incision. This operation was associated with significant morbidity, including primary wound separation, suture line necrosis, and complications of myocutaneous flaps, which often were necessary primarily to reapproximate the incision. Currently, a more conservative approach is employed and has reduced operative morbidity significantly while allowing less altered body image without compromising long-term outcome.

Individualized treatment is based on prognostic factors, including lesion size, depth of invasion, lymph node status, and location of lesion. Patients with stage IA disease (lesion < 2 cm in diameter with no more than 1 mm of stromal invasion) that is well differentiated and without lymphatic space involvement, infiltrating tumor component, or confluence have a negligible risk of lymph node metastasis. Disease in such women may be managed with radical wide local excision and no formal lymph node dissection. Disease in patients with IB unifocal lateralized lesions (< 2 cm in diameter, > 1 mm stromal invasion) is managed best by radical hemivulvectomy or radical wide local excision, as long as negative lateral and deep margins of at least 1 cm can be obtained. Generally, these lesions require only ipsilateral inguinal-femoral groin dissection if the groin nodes do not contain evidence of metastasis. All other lesions of greater size or those centrally located (encroaching on the clitoris, urethra, anus) require that the primary lesion be managed by either hemivulvectomy or complete radical vulvectomy with appropriate margins or bilateral inguinal-femoral lymph node dissections.

The transition from the en bloc single incision to the triple-incision technique has decreased morbidity significantly at the site of the wound. At present, postoperative mortality is approximately 5% and is attributable primarily to the advanced age of the affected population. Affected geriatric patients require meticulous perioperative management for successful medical and cosmetic outcomes. Recognized complications after radical vulvectomy with groin dissection include lymphedema, lymphocysts, lymphangitis, and groin wound breakdown or infection. With the triple-incision technique, a primary closure of the perineal defect usually can be accomplished. In instances of insufficient skin to reapproximate the primary defect, transposition flaps (rhomboid, Z-plasty) may be of assistance. Rarely are myocutaneous flaps (gracilis, gluteus maximus, tensor fascia lata) necessary. The alternative of lymphatic mapping and identification of the sentinel lymph node via lymphoscintigraphy is under investigation [31, 32]. If it is determined to be efficacious, sentinel node biopsy would allow inguinofemoral nodal metastases to be detected in a minimally invasive fashion with decreased morbidity. Patients with advanced lesions, which would necessitate a pelvic exenterative procedure for adequate excision, currently are being offered preoperative chemoradiotherapy to reduce the volume of disease, followed by less radical surgery [33, 34].

Radiotherapy

Observational and randomized studies over the last decade have demonstrated that squamous cell carcinoma of the vulva is highly sensitive to radiotherapy [33]. As a result, irradiation now plays a definitive role in those with advanced disease and plays a significant role in palliation when cure is not possible. Integrated multimodality therapy includes surgery, irradiation, and (often) concurrent chemotherapy. The nature and extent of treatment is tailored to individual patients and to the severity of their cancer and takes into account the activity, efficacy, and toxicity of each available treatment modality alone and in combination. Management of primary vulvar lesions and of inguinal nodal regions must be considered separately.

Multiple studies in the literature demonstrate that various combinations of concurrent 5-fluorouracil, cisplatin, and mitomycin with irradiation for patients with advanced disease has resulted in maintaining 76% of patients alive and disease-free, with nearly 90% spared radical surgery or exenteration [33, 34]. A more recent study has demonstrated that even when a modest dose of radiation in combination with chemotherapy is used in a planned preoperative setting, the combination is highly effective in reducing and controlling advanced disease. Only 7% of patients (5 of 71) with T3 and T4 primaries required exenteration or had unresectable disease [35].

Bilateral node dissection remains the standard management for regional nodes except when they are fixed or ulcerating. For those with two or more involved inguinal nodes, postoperative groin and pelvic irradiation significantly improves survival (68% versus 54%) as compared to surgical resection of pelvic nodes [36]. The improvement in survival is attributable to the reduction in recurrence in the inguinal node regions (5% versus 24%). In addition to even larger benefits in those with two or more involved nodes is a suggestion from two other studies that patients with macroscopic involvement of a single node or extracapsular extension of disease may have a prognosis similar to those with two or more nodes and should be considered also for adjuvant nodal irradiation.

VAGINA

Treatment of vaginal squamous carcinomas depends on lesion size and on involvement of adjacent structures. Patients with small, early, stage I lesions may be offered surgical therapy. Patients with proximal lesions require radical hysterectomy, pelvic lymphadenectomy, and partial or complete vaginectomy, whereas distal vaginal lesions are treated by radical vaginectomy-vulvectomy with inguinal-femoral lymph node dissection.

Women with larger, more advanced lesions or with lesions of the midvagina require radiotherapy. Combination external-beam irradiation (teletherapy) followed by intracavitary or interstitial brachytherapy is planned to deliver a total dose of 75 to 80 Gy to the vaginal lesion and 65 Gy to the parametria and paravaginal tissues.

Specific Malignancies

NONSQUAMOUS AND VERRUCOUS VULVAR MALIGNANCIES

Malignant melanoma accounts for 5% to 10% of vulvar malignancies affecting postmenopausal women (median age, 57 years). Up to 80% of these melanomas originate in the labia minora and clitoris. Malignant melanomas may develop from preexisting junctional nevi, compound nevi, or de novo lesions. Subtypes include nodular, superficial spreading, and acral lentiginous melanomas. Commonly, vulvar melanomas appear as pigmented, ulcerated growths with an inflammatory margin.

Vulvar melanoma is staged by measured tumor thickness (Breslow staging) or by level of invasion relative to skin layers (Clark's system). Prognosis has been correlated with tumor thickness and level of invasion, tumor volume, lymph-vascular involvement, mitotic rate, and ploidy. Generally, vulvar melanomas are treated with radical local excision [37]. Inguinal-femoral lymph node dissection is performed in patients with high-risk tumor characteristics suggestive of nodal metastases.

Verrucous carcinomas are locally invasive squamous malignancies resembling a giant venereal wart. HPV type 6 has been found in association with this lesion. Usually, radical wide local excision is adequate, as lymph node metastases are rare. Irradiation is contraindicated, as it may induce anaplastic transformation of the tumor, leading to a more aggressive metastatic process.

Basal cell carcinomas of the vulva are indolent, locally invasive tumors accounting for 2% to 4% of vulvar malignancies. Commonly, these lesions appear on the labia majora as a sessile growth, with surface ulceration and rolled edges. Their histologic appearance is identical to that of basal cell carcinomas elsewhere on the skin. Radical wide local excision is a treatment of choice for both primary and recurrent lesions. Lymph node metastases are infrequent.

Vulvar adenocarcinomas develop from Bartholin's gland and account for 5% of vulvar malignancies. A history of chronic vulvar inflammation or recurrent Bartholin's abscess often is noted. Delay in diagnosis is common, resulting in advanced lesions at initial diagnosis. The deep origin of Bartholin's gland may contribute to diagnostic delays and early spread to adjacent pelvic structures. Recommended treatment is radical vulvectomy and bilateral groin lymphadenectomy.

Typically, Paget's disease occurs in elderly white women and causes chronic vulvar pain and pruritus. The lesion may appear red or white, eczematoid, and well demarcated. Unlike Paget's disease of the breast, only 10% to 15% of vulvar Paget's disease is associated with an occult adenocarcinoma, usually of the rectum, bladder, urethra, Bartholin's gland, or apocrine glands. Treatment is by wide local excision, but total vulvectomy may be necessary to excise more extensive lesions adequately. Recurrence is common and is expected in perhaps one-third of cases. Although invasion is rare, when it is identified, a radical vulvectomy and groin lymphadenectomy is indicated.

NONSQUAMOUS VAGINAL MALIGNANCIES

Primary adenocarcinomas of the vagina are so rare that the possibility of a metastatic lesion must be excluded (endometrium, ovary, endocervix, breast, colon). The most frequent histologic subtype is clear-cell carcinoma, the majority of which cases occur in young women with a history of in utero exposure to DES (Fig. 19.4).

Treatment for small stage I tumors includes a radical, wide local excision with bilateral pelvic and paraaortic lymph node dissection and radiotherapy. This conservative option allows preservation of reproductive and vaginal function in this typically young group of women. Other patients with stage I disease may be treated with radical hysterectomy, upper vaginectomy, and bilateral pelvic lymphadenectomy. Ovarian preservation is permissible in the absence of evidence of metastatic disease. Larger and more advanced stages require treatment by radiotherapy.

Vaginal sarcomas are an extremely rare but clinically striking diagnosis. Embryonal rhabdomyosarcomas (sarcoma botryoides) are identified almost exclusively in

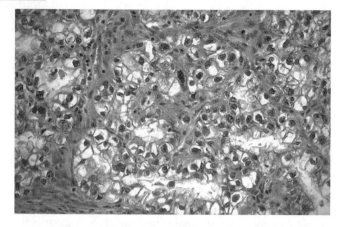

Figure 19.4 Clear-cell carcinoma. The clear appearance of the cytoplasm is attributable to glycogen. Clear-cell carcinomas also occur in the uterus and ovary.

children younger than age 5 and present as grapelike clusters protruding from the vagina, with vaginal bleeding and discharge.

Historically, such children were treated with radical pelvic surgery, representing poor survival. Presently, treatment is less surgically aggressive and is used in conjunction with preoperative or postoperative chemotherapy (vincristine, dactinomycin, cyclophosphamide) and postoperative irradiation [38]. This more conservative, multimodality approach to managing this highly malignant tumor has resulted in significantly improved survival.

Posttreatment Surveillance

Usually, patients with vulvar or vaginal carcinomas are evaluated at 3-month intervals for the first 1 to 2 years and then every 6 months for the next 3 years. At these examinations, a thorough physical evaluation should be performed. A meticulous pelvic examination should focus on close inspection of the vulva and vagina. Whether cervicovaginal cytology is necessary at every office visit in patients with vulvar cancer is debated, with most clinicians performing evaluations at 6-month intervals. In patients with vaginal carcinomas, however, a Pap smear is performed at every office visit. Owing to the propensity for lymph node metastasis in these malignancies, careful inspection of the supraclavicular and inguinal-femoral regions should be performed. Recommendation for radiographic evaluation is not standardized and remains at the physician's discretion, based on patient compliance, physical findings, and stage of disease.

UTERINE CORPUS CANCER
Endometrial Carcinoma

The uterus is a site for epithelial, stromal, and mixed glandular-stromal malignancies. Endometrial carcinoma is the most common female genital cancer, ranked fourth in incidence behind breast, lung, and colorectal cancers. Approximately 36,100 new cases and 6,500 deaths associated with this cancer are expected to occur in 2000 [1]. Endometrial cancer affects primarily postmenopausal women (median age, 58 years); however, 25% of cases occur in premenopausal women, and 5% of patients are younger than 40 years.

Two distinct phenotypes are associated with endometrial carcinomas. The first is estrogen-dependent, either from an endogenous or exogenous source. Frequently, patients afflicted with this disorder are obese, nulliparous, diabetic, and hypertensive, with late-onset menopause. This phenotype is associated with a fivefold increased risk of developing endometrial carcinoma, which generally is a well-differentiated, superficially invasive lesion arising in a background of hyperplasia and is associated with good outcome and long-term survival. The second phenotype is non-estrogen-dependent, characterized by multiparous, thin women. Frequently, such patients have poorly differentiated, deeply invasive lesions that carry a worse prognosis.

BIOLOGICAL CONSIDERATIONS

Although the exact cause of endometrial cancer is unknown, estrogen appears to play a critical role. Medical conditions associated with excess estrogen production are associated with an increased risk of endometrial cancer, such as chronic anovulation, and with estrogen-producing tumors, such as granulosa cell tumors of the ovary. Due to the peripheral conversion of androstenedione to estrone in adipose tissue, obesity is a risk factor because of this increase in endogenous estrogen production. The use of exogenous estrogen replacement (unopposed) accounted for a dramatic rise in the incidence of endometrial cancer in the United States in the early 1970s. The addition of progesterone decreased this risk by approximately 50% [39]. The use of combination estrogen-progesterone oral contraceptive pills, particularly in women with chronic anovulation, confers protection against endometrial hyperplasia and subsequent cancer development.

Tamoxifen, used in the treatment and prevention of breast cancer, has been associated with a threefold increase in uterine cancers. Tamoxifen functions as an estrogen-agonist and antagonist, depending on the specific end organ involved. It appears that in the uterus, tamoxifen acts as an estrogen agonist. Despite the increased risk of developing endometrial cancer associated with tamoxifen treatment, this drug significantly improves disease-free survival (28% reduction in treatment failure) and reduces by 37% the incidence of contralateral breast cancers [40]. Clearly, the benefit of tamoxifen therapy for breast cancer patients outweighs the potential risk of developing a secondary uterine cancer. An essential precaution for tamoxifen-treated patients is that they maintain the appropriate awareness and undergo annual gynecologic examinations.

DIAGNOSIS

Clinical Presentation

Ninety percent of patients with endometrial carcinoma present with irregular or postmenopausal bleeding. Because prompt evaluation of symptomatic patients results in early diagnosis (75% being stage I), routine screening of the general, asymptomatic population is not recommended. Any postmenopausal patient with bleeding, spotting, or brownish staining; perimenopausal patients with intermenstrual bleeding or increasingly heavy menses; and premenopausal patients (particularly if anovulatory) with abnormal bleeding require evaluation and biopsy to exclude an endometrial malignancy. Affected patients may complain also of pelvic pain and a foul or purulent vaginal discharge secondary to a pyometra. Advanced disease may present with ascites, abdominal-pelvic mass, altered bowel habits, or distant metastases. Occasionally (in 2–5% of patients), suspicion of malignancy will be raised by the presence of endometrial cells (in samples not taken during menses), histiocytes, or atypical glandular cells on a routine Pap smear in an otherwise asymptomatic patient.

Diagnostic Evaluation

The workup of postmenopausal bleeding begins with endometrial sampling, with or without transvaginal ultrasonography. In experienced hands, transvaginal ultrasonography allows an accurate evaluation of endometrial thickness. Controversy remains, however, over the extent of endometrial thickening (3 mm, 5 mm, 8 mm) sufficient to cause concern in menopausal patients. In patients taking tamoxifen, the endometrial stripe may be thickened. Most commonly, this thickening appears to represent subendometrial cystic spaces or endometrial polyps rather than signaling an increase in the endometrial lining per se. The introduction of saline instillation sonohysterography has improved the accuracy of evaluating a thickened endometrium. Injection of a small amount of saline into the uterine cavity allows one to distinguish an endometrial polyp from a thickened endometrial lining, submucosal fibroid, or subendometrial cystic changes. Hysteroscopy evaluates the endometrium by direct observation. The accuracy of hysteroscopic examination is operator-dependent and, therefore, is used in conjunction with endometrial sampling.

Endometrial biopsy is the most reliable and accurate method of detecting endometrial carcinoma and its precursor lesions. Office endometrial sampling is safe and cost-effective and provides an accurate diagnosis in 90% of the cases. If the office sampling is negative, inconclusive, or could not be performed and the patient continues to be symptomatic, a dilatation and curettage with or without hysteroscopy should be performed. The benefit of hysteroscopy is in the detection of endometrial polyps and submucosal fibroids.

All patients with a diagnosis of endometrial carcinoma should undergo a complete physical examination and a careful recording of history, with careful inspection of the external genitalia, particularly the distal vagina and suburethral areas. A fractional dilatation and curettage, required when endometrial cancer was staged clinically (before 1988), no longer is necessary. On suspicion of distant metastasis, the patient may undergo CT scanning; however, this procedure is not advocated on a routine basis. Serum tumor markers, such as CA125 and CA19–9, may be evaluated along with the standard preoperative blood work (complete blood count, serum chemistry, coagulation profile), as elevations of these markers are noted to correlate with extra-uterine disease and poor prognosis [41, 42]. If these elements are elevated prior to surgery, appropriate consultation with a gynecologic oncologist can be made to ensure that the proper surgery is performed.

Pathologic Features

The most common type of endometrial cancer is endometrioid (Fig. 19.5). The histologically more aggressive subtypes of endometrial cancers are papillary serous and clear-cell cancers. Serous carcinomas are composed of complex branching papillae lined by pleomorphic cells containing high-grade nuclei. Tumor cell tufts are common, and psammoma bodies may be present. Their histologic makeup is similar to that of ovarian serous carcinomas. Regardless of the depth of myometrial invasion, these tumors typically show widespread lymphatic permeation. Clear-cell carcinomas of the uterus have the same appearance as in other primary sites. The

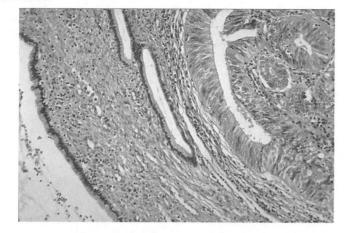

Figure 19.5 Endometrial carcinoma. The neoplastic glands in a well-differentiated endometrioid carcinoma closely resemble normal or hyperplastic endometrium. In this example, the tumor (right) has invaded the endocervix (left).

pattern may be solid, papillary, tubular, or cystic. A periodic acid–Schiff stain will highlight the glycogen that gives the tumor cells their clear cytoplasm. The cells often have a "hobnail" appearance, with nuclei in their apical, rather than basal, portions. Generally, the nuclear grade is high, and the biological behavior is aggressive. Frequently, the estrogenic (type I) carcinomas arise in a background of endometrial hyperplasia. Endometrial hyperplasia is classified as architecturally simple or complex, based on the degree of crowding and complexity of the glands, with or without cytologic atypia. The complex atypical hyperplasias are the most likely to progress. Carcinomas arising in this milieu are biologically low-grade and histologically show endometrioid or mucinous differentiation.

Staging

Endometrial carcinoma spreads by hematogenous dissemination (lung-liver-bone) and lymphatic dissemination (primarily pelvic and paraaortic lymph node chains) and to contiguous organs. Carcinomas from the lower and middle portions of the uterus drain into the parametrial, paracervical, hypogastric, and obturator lymph nodes. Fundal lesions empty primarily into the common iliac and paraaortic nodes. Invasion of the round ligament can lead to inguinal lymphadenopathy, and peritoneal implants may result from transtubal spillage or by direct extension.

From 1971 until 1988, endometrial carcinoma was a clinically staged disease. In 1988, FIGO accepted a surgical staging system, which was further modified in 1994

(Table 19.9). Surgical staging begins by obtaining peritoneal cytology immediately on entering the abdominal cavity. A thorough exploration of all pelvic, intraabdominal, and retroperitoneal structures then is performed, with appropriate biopsies as needed. The next step is a total abdominal hysterectomy and bilateral salpingo-oophorectomy, with selective pelvic and paraaortic lymph node sampling. Although surgical staging does not require a complete lymphadenectomy, adequately sampling the lymph nodes is essential, as microscopic metastasis is common. Lymph node involvement cannot be identified reliably by clinical enlargement or by palpation.

An alternate approach for surgically staging patients with suspected stage I disease is a laparoscopically assisted vaginal hysterectomy with laparoscopic selective lymph node sampling. Although this approach is feasible and decreases the mean hospital stay from 5.9 days for laparotomy to 2.7 days for laparoscopy, the laparoscopic lymph node evaluation becomes increasingly more difficult in proportion to the patient's weight [43, 44]. Laparoscopic exploration of the retroperitoneum is especially difficult in patients exceeding 180 pounds, a weight frequently surpassed in patients with endometrial carcinoma. A randomized trial now under way seeks to evaluate the role of laparoscopy as compared with laparotomy in the surgical management of such patients.

PRIMARY TREATMENT

Not all patients with endometrial hyperplasia may require surgery. Often, simple or complex hyperplasia without atypia is managed successfully with progestational therapy. Complex hyperplasia with atypia diagnosed on office biopsy should be followed by a thorough curettage if an affected patient does not wish to be treated by hysterectomy. Up to one-third of such patients are found to have a coexistent adenocarcinoma. Even if carcinoma is not identified initially, nearly one-third of such women will develop endometrial cancer in the future; therefore, hysterectomy continues to be the recommended treatment, particularly in postmenopausal patients.

Surgery

Invasive endometrial carcinoma is primarily a surgically treated disease. Medically inoperable patients may be offered radiotherapy alone or high-dose progestational therapy [45]. With alternate treatment modalities, the outcome is less favorable than with standard surgical

Table 19.9 Staging for Carcinoma of the Corpus Uteri

FIGO	Stage	TNM	Classification	Description
IA G1,2,3	T1a	N0	M0	Tumor limited to endometrium
IB G1,2,3	T1b	N0	M0	Invasion to less than one-half of the myometrium
IC G1,2,3	T1c	N0	M0	Invasion to more than one-half of the myometrium
IIA G1,2,3	T2a	N0	M0	Endocervical glandular involvement only
IIB G1,2,3	T2b	N0	M0	Cervical stromal invasion
IIIA G1,2,3	T3a	N0	M0	Tumor invading serosa or adnexa, or positive peritoneal cytology
IIIB G1,2,3	T3b	N0	M0	Vaginal metastasis
IIIC G1,2,3	T1	N1	M0	Metastases to pelvic or paraaortic lymph nodes
	T2	N1	M0	
	T3a	N1	M0	
	T3b	N1	M0	
IVA G1,2,3	T4,	Any N	M0	Tumor invasion of bladder or bowel mucosa
IVB	Any T,	Any N,	M1	Distant metastases including intraabdominal or inguinal lymph nodes

T = tumor description (equivalent to FIGO); N = regional lymph nodes; N0 = no metastasis;
N1 = regional metastasis; M = metastasis; M0 = no distant metastasis; M1 = any distant metastasis.

Notes: Histopathologic grading (degree of differentiation): Cases of carcinoma of the corpus should be classified (or graded) according to the degree of histologic differentiation (G1, ≤ 5% or less of a nonsquamous or nonmorular solid growth pattern; G2, 6–50% of a nonsquamous or nonmorular solid growth pattern; G3, > 50% of a nonsquamous or nonmorular solid growth pattern.

Pathologic grading: Notable nuclear atypia, inappropriate for the architectural grade, raises a grade 1 or grade 2 tumor by 1. In serous adenocarcinomas, clear-cell adenocarcinomas, and squamous cell carcinomas, nuclear grading takes precedence. Adenocarcinomas with benign squamous differentiation are graded according to the nuclear grade of the glandular component.

Rules related to staging: Because corpus cancer now is staged surgically, procedures previously used for determination of stages no longer are applicable (e.g., the findings from fractional dilation and curettage) to differentiate between stage I and stage II. A small number of patients who have corpus cancer will be treated primarily with radiotherapy. If that is the case, the clinical staging adopted by FIGO in 1971 still would apply, but designation of that staging system would be noted. Ideally, width of the myometrium should be measured along with the width of tumor invasion.

Source: Modified from the International Federation of Gynecology and Obstetrics, Annual report on the results of treatment in gynecologic cancer. *J Epidemiol Biostat* 3(23):35–61, 1998.

therapy. Recommendation for adjuvant postoperative pelvic radiotherapy depends on various prognostic factors, which include cell type, tumor grade, depth of myometrial invasion, vascular space invasion, and cervical extension. Poorly differentiated tumors are associated with a higher incidence of deep myometrial invasion, pelvic and paraaortic node metastasis, and an overall poor prognosis. Depth of myometrial invasion is identified consistently as the most important determinant of extrauterine spread, treatment failure, and tumor recurrence [46]. Cervical or isthmic involvement doubles the risk of pelvic nodal metastases and carries a higher relapse rate. Evidence of vascular space invasion increases the likelihood of pelvic and paraaortic node metastasis.

Extrauterine factors portending poor prognosis include adnexal involvement, abdominal spread, positive cytology, and pelvic and paraaortic node metastases. Several investigators have demonstrated a poor outcome for patients with positive cytology; however, the significance of positive cytology in the absence of extrauterine disease or other risk factors is unclear [47].

Other prognostic factors that have been identified but are not used in the routine management of endometrial carcinoma are DNA ploidy analysis, S-phase fraction, and hormone receptor status.

For patients with grade 1 or 2 lesions and no myometrial invasion (stage IA, grade 1, 2), surgery alone is adequate treatment. Patients who are at intermediate and high risk for recurrence require adjuvant pelvic radiotherapy, with or without intracavitary irradiation to the vaginal vault. In some instances, the irradiation field may be extended to include the paraaortic node chain. The role of adjuvant chemotherapy for high-risk patients remains investigational.

Radiotherapy

Radiotherapy has been shown to improve pelvic control when administered as adjuvant treatment in the management of endometrial carcinoma. Adjuvant radiotherapy has not, however, demonstrated a survival advantage [48]. Radiotherapy can be administered either to the entire pelvis (40–50 Gy over 5 weeks) or as vaginal cuff brachytherapy with a surface dose of 50 to 70

Gy in two to three applications. Findings were reported recently from a study to evaluate the difference between recurrence rates and survival in clinical stage I endometrial carcinomas treated with either vaginal brachytherapy or pelvic irradiation [49]. Although the study showed no difference in overall survival, it did show a survival benefit in a subset of patients with more than 50% myometrial invasion treated with pelvic irradiation. This study also demonstrated a decreased pelvic recurrence rate among patients treated with pelvic irradiation as compared to those treated with vaginal brachytherapy alone.

Patients with documented paraaortic node metastasis have a 5-year survival of approximately 25%. Administration of extended-field irradiation to the lower paraaortic node chain in patients with paraaortic node metastases has improved 5-year survival to nearly 40% [48, 50]. Given these findings, both patients with known paraaortic metastasis and those at significantly increased risk for paraaortic node metastasis (macroscopic pelvic node involvement, multiple positive pelvic nodes, macroscopic adnexal metastasis, or deep myometrial invasion) should be offered extended-field irradiation [50]. The treatment algorithm for uterine cancer is outlined in Figure 19.6.

Chemotherapy

Many cytotoxic agents have been investigated in the management of advanced or recurrent endometrial carcinoma. Until recently, doxorubicin had been the most active agent. Combination doxorubicin-cisplatin therapy increased the overall response rate to 45%, with a complete response rate of 22% as compared to single-agent doxorubicin, with overall and complete response rates of 27% and 8%, respectively [51]. Clinical trials investigating paclitaxel have demonstrated an overall response rate of 36%, with a complete response rate of 14% [52]. Despite improved response rates, survival remains unchanged.

Hormonal Therapy

Usually, estrogen receptor and progesterone receptor (PR) levels correlate with the degree of differentiation of the tumor. Several investigators believe that receptor status is an independent prognostic variable. Often, hormonal therapy is used in recurrent disease, as generally it is well tolerated, even by debilitated patients with a restricted performance status. An overall response rate of 68% has been observed in patients with PR-positive tumors in comparison to 10% for patients with PR-negative tumors [53]. Tamoxifen has been used also in the treatment of recurrent endometrial cancer, with response rates of up to 50% [54]. The use of aromatase inhibitors and of the antiprogestogen mifepristone and other selective estrogen receptor modulators are being investigated in the management of advanced or recurrent endometrial carcinoma.

POSTTREATMENT SURVEILLANCE

Careful surveillance is necessary during the first 2 to 3 years after therapy, when approximately 75% of recurrences take place. Routine follow-up should include recording a detailed history, noting in particular any new complaints and assessment of the abdominal and pelvic cavities, with special attention to lymph node areas. Patients are seen routinely and are examined every 3 to 6 months for the first 3 years and semiannually thereafter. Most clinicians perform a Pap smear of the vaginal apex at each office visit, although the sensitivity of Pap smear is low (7%) in detecting recurrence in patients who are otherwise asymptomatic [54]. No evidence substantiates that routine radiographic procedures (chest roentgenography, CT scan) afford earlier diagnosis or improved survival. For this reason, usually radiographic testing is performed on the basis of individual patients' symptoms or physical findings or at a physician's discretion. Although elevation of CA125 has been documented in patients with advanced and recurrent endometrial carcinoma, the value of serial CA125 evaluations in patients who are otherwise asymptomatic is limited and so these are best reserved for patients in whom the CA125 level was elevated at time of diagnosis.

RELAPSE AND PALLIATION

Recurrences occur locally in the majority of patients (50%), with 28% recurring at isolated distant sites and 21% in both the local and distant sites. When the recurrence is isolated to the vaginal apex, pelvic radiotherapy is successful. When disease recurs beyond the vaginal apex, with extension into the pelvis or to distant metastatic sites, radiotherapy is less effective, and systemic chemotherapy or hormonal therapy is the preferred management plan.

REHABILITATION AND ESTROGEN REPLACEMENT THERAPY

Historically, estrogen replacement therapy has been contraindicated in patients with hormone-sensitive tumors, such as endometrial carcinoma. However, no sci-

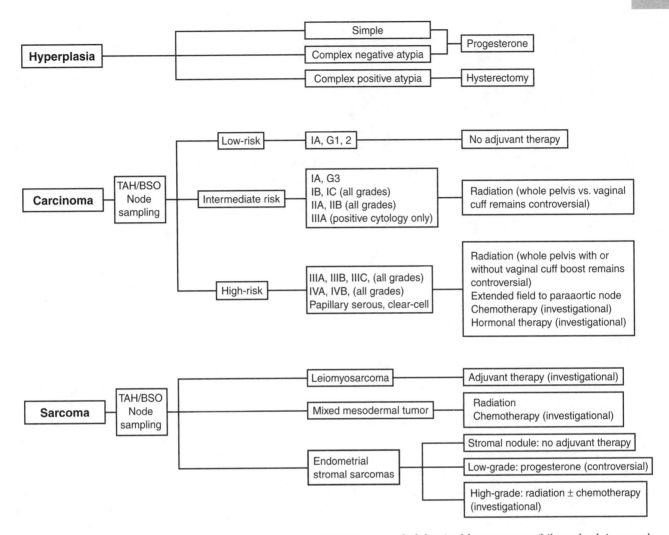

Figure 19.6 Treatment algorithm for uterine neoplasms. *TAH/BSO* = total abdominal hysterectomy/bilateral salpingooophorectomy.

entific prospective data demonstrate that estrogen replacement increases the risk of recurrence or decreases survival in these patients. Recent retrospective studies evaluating estrogen replacement in surgical stage I and II cancer survivors report no increase in recurrence or death due to carcinoma in those in the estrogen-treated group [55, 56]. However, these reports are flawed methodologically by investigator bias, as noted by patient selection, duration of therapy, short follow-up periods, and variable treatment regimens. The American College of Obstetricians and Gynecologists stated that hormone replacement therapy may be offered to such patients as long as selection is based on appropriate prognostic indicators and affected patients are willing to assume the risk of a possible recurrence due to the estrogen therapy [57]. Because the majority of patients with endometrial carcinoma have a favorable long-term outlook, it is particularly important to afford them the same benefits (e.g., decreased risk of cardiovascular disease and osteoporosis) as are made available to women without endometrial carcinoma. These patients also must be made aware of nonhormonal alternatives available to decrease heart disease and osteoporosis associated with menopause. The definitive answer as to the safety of hormone replacement therapy in this group of patients will be determined when results of an ongoing prospective randomized trial become known.

Uterine Sarcomas and Mixed Tumors

Uterine sarcomas and mixed tumors constitute 3% to 5% of all uterine cancers. Malignancies of endometrial stroma and myometrium give rise to endometrial

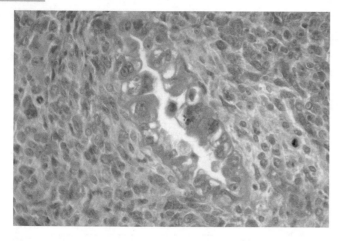

Figure 19.7 Malignant mixed mesodermal tumor. Such tumors (carcinosarcomas) exhibit both a malignant epithelial and a stromal component.

stromal sarcomas and leiomyosarcomas, respectively. Mixed tumors contain both epithelial and stromal elements. In adenosarcoma, the glands are benign, and the stroma is malignant. In mixed mesodermal tumors (carcinosarcoma), both the glands and the stroma are malignant.

Mixed mesodermal tumors (MMTs) of the uterus occur most commonly in postmenopausal women, with a median age of 62 years. Pelvic examination reveals an enlarged, soft uterus with tissue fragments protruding from the cervical os. Grossly, the uterine cavity is filled with a polypoid, fungating tumor with hemorrhage and necrosis. Distant metastases to the lungs, upper abdomen, and retroperitoneal lymph nodes are common.

Homologous and heterologous variants have been described, depending on whether the morphology of their sarcomatous component indicates differentiation toward mesenchymal tissues of the uterus (endometrial stroma or smooth muscle) or elsewhere (e.g., cartilage, striated muscle, fat), respectively (Fig. 19.7). The appearance of the sarcoma has minimal or no value in predicting the course of these uniformly aggressive neoplasms. Many investigators now consider these tumors to be metaplastic carcinomas in which a poorly differentiated subpopulation of carcinoma cells have dedifferentiated and now display a sarcomatous morphology [58]. Biologically, these tumors behave more as carcinomas, metastasizing to lymph nodes where the epithelial component predominates.

Standard therapy is a total abdominal hysterectomy and bilateral salpingo-oophorectomy. The use of adjuvant pelvic radiotherapy is beneficial to decrease pelvic recurrence but has not been shown to improve survival.

A recent study using adjuvant ifosfamide and cisplatin in patients with uterine MMTs has shown some decrease in the incidence of distant recurrence [59]. The use of combination adjuvant radiotherapy and chemotherapy is under investigation and shows encouraging preliminary results [60]. Overall, 5-year survival for patients with stage I uterine MMTs is less than 50%, with nearly 85% of patients having some element of distant recurrence. For patients with metastatic disease, systemic cytotoxic therapy is the treatment of choice; single-agent ifosfamide producing a 32% response rate, cisplatin producing a 19% rate, and combination ifosfamide-cisplatin producing a 54% rate [61, 62].

Patients with uterine leiomyosarcomas present at an average age of 53, with complaints of postmenopausal bleeding. Uterine enlargement can lead to lower abdominal pain, abdominal pressure, constipation, or urinary frequency. Most cases are diagnosed incidentally during surgery for presumed leiomyomas. The tumors are distinguished from variants of leiomyomas by mitotic activity, cytologic atypia, and coagulative tumor cell necrosis (Fig. 19.8). A diagnosis of leiomyosarcoma requires at least 10 mitoses per 10 high-power fields or, if cellular atypism is present, 5 to 9 mitoses per 10 high-power fields. However, predicting biological behavior of tumors in the latter category is difficult, and some pathologists designate them as smooth-muscle tumors of undetermined malignant potential rather than as sarcomas. Five-year survival for patients with stage I disease ranges from 40% to 75%. The addition of adjuvant radiotherapy decreases pelvic recurrence but does not have an impact on overall survival. Chemotherapy seems to offer little benefit to either recurrence rate or

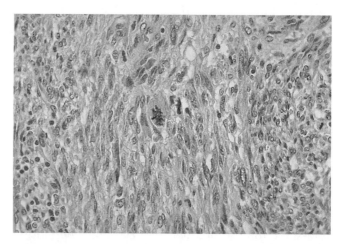

Figure 19.8 Leiomyosarcoma. This malignant smooth-muscle neoplasm is composed of fascicles of moderately pleomorphic spindle cells. At the center is an abnormal mitosis.

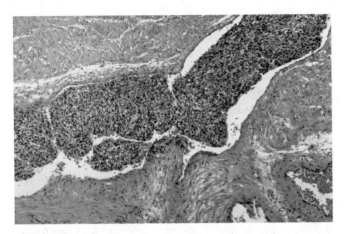

Figure 19.9 Low-grade stromal sarcoma. A plug of tumor cells fills a dilated lymphatic channel.

survival and remains investigational in the adjuvant setting. Patients with advanced or recurrent disease can be offered treatment with doxorubicin, with reported response rates of up to 25% [63].

Endometrial stromal tumors are purely homologous and are classified into three distinct entities: the stromal nodule, the low-grade stromal sarcoma (endolymphatic stromal myosis), and the high-grade stromal sarcoma. These tumors account for approximately 10% of all uterine sarcomas. The stromal nodule is composed of uniform small cells, resembling stromal cells within normal proliferative endometrium. These nodules tend to be well circumscribed, with pushing but not infiltrating margins, and they are benign. The low-grade stromal sarcomas occur mostly in premenopausal women. Uterine curettage may show stromal hyperplasia. The diagnosis can be made intraoperatively by observing characteristic wormlike structures infiltrating the broad ligament from an enlarged uterus. Histologically, this tumor is characterized by clusters of small uniform cells infiltrating the myometrium and filling distended lymphatic channels (Fig. 19.9). Usually, the mitotic count is less than 10 per 10 high-power fields, with minimal cytologic atypia. Usually, its clinical course is indolent, with long-term survival expected. Because of the tendency to invade adjacent pelvic tissues after surgical excision, adjuvant progestational therapy may be beneficial, owing to the hormonal sensitivity of this tumor and the presence of PR.

In contrast, high-grade stromal sarcomas are very aggressive, affecting primarily postmenopausal women. The mitotic count is greater than 10 per 10 high-power fields, with significant cytologic atypia. The majority of these tumors are found to have spread beyond the uterus at the time of diagnosis. A 5-year survival rate of 25% to 50% has been reported for early-stage disease. Standard treatment for high-grade stromal sarcoma is total abdominal hysterectomy and bilateral salpingo-oophorectomy with adjuvant pelvic radiotherapy to decrease pelvic recurrence. The role of systemic chemotherapy to control advanced disease in the adjuvant setting is investigational.

OVARIAN AND FALLOPIAN TUBE CANCERS
Epithelial Tumors

Ovarian neoplasms are classified according to their cell of origin: epithelial, sex cord–stromal, or germ cell. Overall, epithelial tumors account for nearly 85% of ovarian cancers, whereas germ-cell and sex cord-stromal tumors account for 10% and 5%, respectively. Usually, germ-cell tumors occur in children and in women younger than age 20, whereas epithelial ovarian cancer is a disease predominantly in postmenopausal women. The lifetime risk of a woman developing ovarian cancer is 1% to 2%. The incidence of this cancer varies with age and increases from 1.4 per 100,000 in women younger than 40 years to 38 per 100,000 in women older than 60 years.

Ovarian cancer is the fifth most common cancer diagnosed in women in the United States, with an annual incidence of 23,100 [1]. Of these women, it is estimated that 14,000 will die of their disease, accounting for 53% of all deaths from gynecologic cancers. The morbidity associated with ovarian carcinoma is partially attributable to the fact that two-thirds of patients present with advanced-stage disease (stage III or IV) at the time of diagnosis. Although multiple techniques have been developed for screening asymptomatic women to achieve an earlier stage at diagnosis, these techniques have been insufficiently sensitive and specific to meet these goals and, therefore, have not resulted in a shift toward earlier diagnosis and improved survival.

Primary carcinomas of the fallopian tube represent a rare clinical entity. These tumors have a propensity for widespread intraperitoneal dissemination, with clinical and histopathologic characteristics similar to those of ovarian carcinomas. These similarities contribute to the difficulty in distinguishing these tumors accurately from one another. Fallopian tube carcinomas display earlier symptomatology than do ovarian tumors, allowing for earlier diagnosis (66% stage I or II; 34% stage III or IV) [64]. Management and prognosis are, however, similar.

BIOLOGICAL CONSIDERATIONS

Although the specific etiology of ovarian cancer is not known, several risk factors have been identified. The risk factors are subdivided into three main groupings: reproductive, environmental, and genetic. The reproductive factors are associated with conditions of incessant ovulation, such as nulliparity, low parity, and infertility. The use of ovulation-induction agents has been reported to be increased among women with ovarian cancer. However, the indication for use of these agents—infertility itself—is associated with an increased ovarian cancer risk. Given the methodologic limitations of these studies, more research is needed before these agents should be implicated. The environmental risk factors include obese patients or those with diets high in fat or lactose and in perineal talc exposure. Conversely, the use of oral contraceptives is found to confer protection. A reduction in risk of up to 60% is reported for women who use oral contraceptives for 5 years or more, with the protective effect appearing to be long-term [65].

Of all the risk factors, the most significant appears to be that of family history. Approximately 7% to 10% of ovarian cancers are due to inherited susceptibility genes, with the remaining 90% of cases being sporadic [66]. Of the inherited cases, 65% to 75% are linked to the breast-ovarian cancer syndrome; 10% to 15% are linked to the site-specific ovarian cancer syndrome; and 10% to 15% are linked to the hereditary nonpolyposis colon cancer syndrome (or Lynch II). Fewer than 1% are attributable to very rare cancer syndromes, such as Cowden's disease and to Li-Fraumeni syndrome or ataxia-telangiectasia [67]. On the basis of the current literature, the majority of breast-ovarian and site-specific ovarian cancer syndromes are believed to be linked to mutations in the tumor suppressor genes known as *BRCA1*, located on chromosome 17, and *BRCA2*, on chromosome 13. Additionally, likely a third *BRCA* gene is suspected of being on chromosome 8; however, this gene and the clinical features associated with its mutation have not been identified yet. These genes are inherited in an autosomal dominant pattern with variable penetrance. In the Ashkenazi population, most recent estimates find that mutations carriers have a 56% lifetime risk (by age 70) of developing a breast cancer and a 16.5% risk of developing ovarian cancer [68]. In other populations, higher estimates have been reported. Because these cancer syndromes can affect organs other than breast and ovary, such as colon, endometrium, prostate, upper gastrointestinal tract, and neurologic system, obtaining a complete family history from patients is prudent; it should include all malignancies known to them on both maternal and paternal sides of the family, preferably going back for at least three generations and paying particular attention to the age of onset of disease.

PREVENTION AND EARLY DETECTION

The goal of identifying a particular group of patients who may be at particular risk for developing a malignancy is to allow for early detection, which should translate into better treatment outcome and improved survival. However, ovarian cancer eludes this goal. State-of-the-art molecular genetics has allowed us to identify groups of patients who may be at risk for having inherited a *BRCA1* or *BRCA2* mutation. Even the ability to perform mutational analysis of identified founder mutations is possible, as is full gene sequencing in patients with previously identified deleterious non-founder mutations. Our knowledge, however, continues to evolve in regard to the adequate interpretation of many of these results.

In 1996, the American Society of Clinical Oncologists developed a set of guidelines for genetic testing for cancer susceptibility genes [69]. The guidelines were based on the belief that patients with a strong family history and early-onset disease should be targeted for evaluation. Such patients primarily include those with breast and ovarian cancer within the same family, particularly if found within the same woman or if male breast cancer occurred; those with multiple cases of early-onset disease; or those with bilateral breast cancers. The Society's committee concluded that patients should have at least a 10% probability of carrying a mutation, derived from various statistical modeling systems, before genetic testing is recommended.

Once a high-risk family has been identified, a more informative approach is to test living affected members for the mutations identified most commonly (185delAG, 5382insC in *BRCA1*, or 6174delT in *BRCA2*). If these mutations are not identified, the affected members may be offered the considerably more costly and time-consuming full gene sequencing, with the awareness that the results may not be fully interpretable. Once the affected members have been tested and have an identifiable and interpretable mutation, unaffected family members may be offered testing. If the unaffected members test positive for the previously identified mutation, they are likely at increased risk of developing a malignancy. If, however, the unaffected members test negative for the known mutation identified in an affected member, their risk reverts to that of the normal population. If a family appears to be at significant risk of a hereditary cancer syndrome but tests negative for deleterious mutations based on current knowledge, likely that family should continue to be considered at high risk.

What must be understood, however, is that knowledge of cancer genetics is expanding rapidly. Thus, now known is that approximately 2.5% of Ashkenazi Jews have a *BRCA1* mutation at 185delAG or 5382insC or *BRCA2* at 6174delT [68, 70]. In an unselected white population, these same mutations would be identified in only 0.1%. Also known is that although approximately 50% of Ashkenazi Jews with ovarian cancer have these mutations, owing to the variable penetrance of this mutation, the lifetime risk of ovarian cancer in unaffected Jewish women without a family history of malignancy may be as low as 10%.

Once high-risk individuals have been identified, the dilemma arises as to how clinicians reliably can reduce such patients' risk of developing an ovarian malignancy. In 1997, a task force was convened by the Cancer Genetics Study Consortium of the National Human Genome Research Institute, which issued recommended surveillance strategies for *BRCA1/2* and hereditary nonpolyposis colon cancer carriers [71]. The ovarian cancer surveillance strategy was recommended as being a pelvic examination, transvaginal sonogram with color Doppler capability, and serum CA125 to be performed either annually or semiannually, beginning at the age of 25 to 35. This surveillance strategy is based on expert opinion only, as these screening strategies have not been shown to reduce mortality.

The rectovaginal bimanual examination, although easily performed and cost-effective, detects only 5% of ovarian cancers at a curable stage. Nearly 10,000 pelvic examinations must be performed to detect one early ovarian cancer. Transvaginal ultrasonography is more sensitive than is physical examination, yet it still lacks specificity. Advances in ultrasonographic technology (e.g., the addition of Doppler flow to assess blood flow and the application of such varied morphologic indices as tumor volume, wall thickness and septal structures) have improved specificity. However, the efficacy of this method in reducing cancer mortality remains unproved. In one large study that screened the general population by transabdominal ultrasonography, 65 exploratory laparotomies had to be performed to detect one case of ovarian cancer [72]. In a similar study using transvaginal ultrasonography in patients with a family

history of ovarian cancer, of 1,601 patients screened, 61 underwent operations, and two stage I invasive ovarian malignancies were identified along with three ovarian malignancies of low malignant potential [73]. The addition of CA125 to the surveillance regimen improves the specificity of transvaginal ultrasonography. When serial longitudinal values disclose a rising trend in CA125, the procedure is thought to be a more reliable predictor of malignancy.

Owing to the limitations of presently available surveillance techniques, many high-risk women consider the option of prophylactic oophorectomy. It is well-known that a small percentage of patients who have undergone oophorectomy for a significant family history of ovarian cancer subsequently have developed an intraabdominal papillary serous carcinomatosis indistinguishable from ovarian cancer, despite the absence of residual ovarian tissue [74, 75]. Although only preliminary results are available, they suggest that in women who have breast and "ovarian" cancer, nearly one-third have a papillary serous malignancy of the peritoneum [76]. Of the high-risk patients identified as having a papillary serous malignancy of the peritoneum, at least 43% were found to carry deleterious mutations in *BRCA1* [77]. Ongoing studies are evaluating these issues further and assessing the benefit of prophylactic oophorectomy in certain subsets of high-risk women. Recently, a statistical decisional analysis was published to estimate the improved life expectancy in mutation-positive patients who undergo elective surgical procedures [78]. Patients undergoing prophylactic mastectomy had an estimated 3- to 5-year gain in life expectancy, whereas those having prophylactic oophorectomy increased life expectancy by only 0.3 to 1.7 years.

DIAGNOSIS

Clinical Presentation

Patients with epithelial ovarian carcinomas present with symptoms (e.g., abdominal pain, swelling, bloating, dyspepsia, pelvic pressure, and leg pain) often attributed to other disease entities and conditions. Fifty percent of patients present with ascites or a palpable abdominal or pelvic mass. In early stages, pain may be due to the stretching of the ovarian capsule, tumor hemorrhage, necrosis, torsion, or rupture. Patients with very advanced disease may present with anorexia, weight loss, nausea, vomiting, and constipation. The presence of ascites is a strong indication of malignancy; however, a huge ovarian cyst that fills the abdomen and pelvis may elicit a fluid wave similar to ascites. Tumor infiltration to the skin through the umbilicus (Sister Mary Joseph nodule) is indicative of widespread intraabdominal carcinomatosis. Often, pelvic examination discloses bilateral ovarian masses, and a rectovaginal examination may detect a "Blummer shelf" (tumor extending from pelvic side wall to side wall).

Patients with fallopian tube carcinomas may present with the classic triad of vaginal bleeding or watery discharge; abdominal pain; and an adnexal mass (hydrops tubae profluens). The colicky abdominal pain and adnexal mass are due to fimbrial obstruction by tumor, with subsequent tubal distension. Up to 20% of patients with fallopian tube carcinoma have been found to have adenocarcinoma cells on a routine Pap smear. In this setting, if colposcopic examination and dilatation and curettage fail to reveal pathology, a sonogram, CT scan, or diagnostic laparoscopy is indicated.

Diagnostic Evaluation

The diagnostic workup should be tailored to affected patients' age, symptoms, and physical findings. Reproductive-age patients who have persistent ovarian masses or premenarchal or postmenopausal women with palpably enlarged ovaries or masses should undergo transvaginal ultrasonography. Findings of a unilateral, mobile, simple cyst, without evidence of septation or papillation and measuring less than 8 cm, frequently can be managed expectantly with repeat examinations in 4 to 6 weeks. If the masses are bilateral, fixed, solid, or complex-cystic with septa or papillations greater than 8 cm and persist over two to three menstrual cycles (in reproductive-age women) or display evidence of symptoms or advanced disease, affected patients require further evaluation and eventual surgical exploration.

When malignancy is suspected, a chest roentgenography should be ordered routinely to assess for pulmonary metastasis and possible pleural effusions. Depending on the gastrointestinal symptoms and physical examination, a barium enema or upper gastrointestinal tract series may be indicated. CT scan of the abdomen and pelvis is performed routinely in patients suspected of having an ovarian malignancy, as it allows a more complete evaluation for intrahepatic metastases and retroperitoneal lymphadenopathy. These assessments can provide helpful information for assessing the patient preoperatively.

Routine blood chemistry and albumin, calcium, magnesium, renal, and liver function tests are essential to complete the evaluation. Serum CA125 is a valuable marker for serous ovarian carcinoma. Elevations (> 35

units/ml) are identified in 80% to 85% of ovarian cancers but in fewer than 1% of normal, healthy, nonpregnant women [79]. The CA125 may be elevated by many benign and nongynecologic diseases (e.g., endometriosis, uterine leiomyomas, pelvic inflammatory disease, ectopic pregnancy, pancreatitis, cirrhosis, peritonitis, and peritoneal tuberculosis-sarcoidosis), in addition to malignancies of the pancreas, lung, breast, and colon. When germ-cell or stromal tumors are suspected, levels of such tumor markers as lactate dehydrogenase (LDH), human chorionic gonadotropin (HCG), alphafetoprotein (AFP), and serum inhibin should be assessed.

Paracentesis of ascitic fluid is not recommended unless it is deemed necessary to relieve respiratory distress prior to an operative procedure or if the diagnosis of ovarian cancer is in question. If pleural effusions are identified, a thoracentesis with cytologic evaluation is necessary, as a positive result would necessitate reclassification to stage IV.

Pathologic Features

The surface epithelial tumors of the ovary are derived from the coelomic or müllerian epithelium of the female genital tract, the same epithelium that gives rise to the epithelium of the fallopian tube, the endometrium, and the endocervix. Serous carcinomas are the most common. In advanced stages, epithelial ovarian carcinomas involve both ovaries and may involve peritoneal surfaces as well. The ovarian masses are either solid or cystic, with papillary projections found lining cyst walls. Microscopically, well-differentiated areas are composed of easily recognizable papillae, and psammoma bodies often are present (Fig. 19.10). In more solid, less-differentiated areas, the cells grow in sheets, and the tumor cells exhibit marked anaplasia and pleomorphism, including bizarre and multinucleate forms. Papillary serous carcinoma of the peritoneum (primary peritoneal carcinoma) is histologically indistinguishable from its ovarian counterpart. Macroscopically, the ovaries are of normal size or are enlarged minimally.

Given the müllerian derivation of these epithelial tumors, other histologic patterns also occur. Endometrioid differentiation is the second most common, accounting for 20% of all epithelial ovarian malignancies. In up to 30% of patients, endometriosis has been noted in the same ovary or elsewhere in the pelvis. In addition, a synchronous endometrial adenocarcinoma has been seen in 20% of patients. The gross appearance is either cystic or solid. Microscopically, endometrioid carcinoma of the ovary and of the endometrium are indistinguishable. Well-differentiated tumors will be composed of

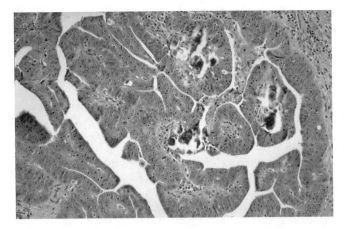

Figure 19.10 Serous carcinoma. High-grade tumor cells line papillae. Psammoma bodies are present. The same histologic findings may be seen in carcinoma arising in the uterus.

glands lined by crowded or stratified columnar cells with elongate nuclei. Foci of squamous differentiation are common and usually appear benign. As the tumors become less differentiated, the growth pattern becomes more solid. Clear-cell carcinoma is another subtype frequently associated with endometriosis. The tumor cells may be clear, containing glycogen, and may have a hobnail appearance. The cells may form sheets, line papillae, or small cysts. The nuclei may be bland or pleomorphic. The biological behavior is high-grade.

Mucinous carcinoma represents 5% to 10% of all epithelial ovarian malignancies. These tumors tend to be larger than serous carcinomas but less frequently are bilateral and in an advanced stage. The tumors are multilocated, solid, and cystic and contain thick, viscous mucin. Though the benign category of this neoplasm may be lined by epithelium typical of the endocervix or the intestine, typically the malignant tumors resemble mucin-secreting adenocarcinomas of colonic origin. Tubal carcinomas show the same histologic patterns as those of their ovarian counterparts.

Staging

Both ovarian and tubal carcinomas are characterized by transcoelomic dissemination of disease, resulting in widespread intraperitoneal metastasis. Other recognized routes of spread are via local extension, lymphatic invasion, hematogenous metastasis (liver, lungs), and transdiaphragmatic passage. The staging of both malignancies is based on surgicopathologic findings. The FIGO staging system is the staging system employed most commonly for both ovarian and tubal carcinomas (Tables 19.10, 19.11). Not until 1992, however, did FIGO establish an independent staging system for tubal cancers. Until that period, a modification of the surgical staging for ovarian cancer had been used.

PRIMARY TREATMENT

Surgery

Management of patients with ovarian carcinoma begins with surgical therapy. Prognosis depends on surgical stage, histologic subtype and grade, and extent of residual disease postoperatively. The primary goal of the surgery, therefore, is to remove as much cancer as is possible without compromising affected patients' safety. If such patients are premenopausal and have a mass that requires surgical exploration, a laparoscopic procedure is possible as long as good judgment is exercised. Any suspicious mass that cannot be removed unruptured, whether in a laparoscopically retrievable bag, via the cul de sac, or by a minilaparotomy, should be removed by laparotomy. Laparoscopic oophorectomy of a suspicious mass should be performed only by surgeons adept at oncologic laparoscopic procedures and able to complete laparoscopic staging or convert to a staging laparotomy, should that be necessary. Postmenopausal patients with a suspicious mass likely will require laparotomy.

The staging laparotomy begins with a generous incision to allow full exploration and evaluation of the upper abdominal organs. On entrance to the abdomen, any ascites is aspirated or peritoneal lavage of the right and left paracolic gutters, pelvis, and right and left hemidiaphragm is obtained for cytologic evaluation. Assessment then is made as to whether the tumor can be cytoreduced optimally (reduced to < 1 cm). Conditions that preclude optimal cytoreduction are multiple intraparenchymal hepatic metastases, involvement of the porta hepatis, or tumor infiltration to the root of the small-bowel mesentery. A total abdominal hysterectomy, bilateral salpingo-oophorectomy, omentectomy, appendectomy, pelvic and paraaortic lymph node sampling, random peritoneal biopsies, and sampling of intraabdominal adhesions are performed in patients with disease confined to the ovaries. In advanced stages, lymph node sampling is performed only if it contributes to reducing tumor volume. In some instances, intestinal resections, splenectomy, cholecystectomy, partial diaphragmatic resection, or partial liver resection may be necessary to achieve optimal cytoreduction. Supraclavicular lymphadenopathy, pleural effusions, and intraparenchymal hepatic metastasis require fine-needle aspiration to confirm disease histopathologically and to classify it as stage IV.

Table 19.10   Staging for Carcinoma of the Ovary

FIGO	Stage	TNM	Classification	Description
I				Growth limited to the ovaries
IA	T1a	N0	M0	Growth limited to one ovary; no ascites containing malignant cells; no tumor on the external surface; capsule intact
IB	T1b	N0	M0	Growth limited to both ovaries; no ascites containing malignant cells; no tumor on the external surfaces; capsules intact
IC*	T1c	N0	M0	Tumor classified as either stage IA or IB but with tumor on the surface of one or both ovaries, or with ruptured capsules, or with ascites containing malignant cells, or with positive peritoneal washings
II				Growth involving one or both ovaries, with pelvic extension
IIA	T2a	N0	M0	Extension or metastases to the uterus or tubes (or both)
IIB	T2b	N0	M0	Extension to other pelvic tissues
IIC*	T2c	N0	M0	Tumor either stage IIA or IIB but with tumor on the surface of one or both ovaries, or with capsule ruptured, or with ascites containing malignant cells, or with positive peritoneal washings
III				Tumor involving one or both ovaries with peritoneal implants outside the pelvis or positive retroperitoneal or inguinal nodes; superficial liver metastasis equal to stage III; tumor limited to the true pelvis but with histologically proved malignant extension to small bowel or omentum
IIIA	T3a	N0	M0	Tumor grossly limited to the true pelvis, with negative nodes but with histologically proved microscopic seeding of abdominal peritoneal surfaces
IIIB	T3b	N0	M0	Tumor involving one or both ovaries; histologically proved implants of abdominal peritoneal surfaces (none exceeding 2 cm in diameter); negative nodes
IIIC	T3c	N0	M0	Abdominal implants > 2 cm in diameter or positive retroperitoneal or inguinal nodes
	Any T,	N1,	M0	
IV	Any T,	Any N,	M1	Growth involving one or both ovaries, with distant metastases; for pleural effusion present, positive cytologic findings required for assignment to stage IV; parenchymal liver metastasis equal to stage IV

T = tumor description (equivalent to FIGO); N = regional lymph nodes; N0 = no nodal metastasis; N1 = regional nodal metastasis; M = metastasis; M0 = no distant metastasis; M1 = any distant metastasis (excluding peritoneal cavity).

*To evaluate the impact on prognosis of the different criteria for assigning cases to stage IC or IIC, a valuable factor would be knowledge of whether the rupture of the capsule was spontaneous or was caused by the surgeon and whether the source of malignant cells detected was peritoneal washings or ascites.

Note: Staging of ovarian carcinoma is based on findings at clinical examination and on surgical exploration. The histologic findings are to be considered in the staging, as are the cytologic findings as regards effusions. Ideally, a biopsy is taken from suspicious areas outside the pelvis.

Source: Modified from the International Federation of Gynecology and Obstetrics, Annual report on the results of treatment in gynecologic cancer. *J Epidemiol Biostat* 3(23):75–102, 1998.

Tumor cytoreductive surgery is thought to be essential in the management of ovarian cancer. The amount of residual tumor correlates closely with response to chemotherapy and survival, as demonstrated by a 39-month survival for patients without visible residual disease, 29 months for those with tumors less than 0.5 cm in diameter, 18 months for patients with tumors between 0.6 and 1.5 cm, and 11 months for patients with residual tumors greater than 1.5 cm [80]. Approximately three-fourths of all patients are found to have advanced disease (FIGO stage III and IV) after careful staging. Clinicians should not be deceived by gross inspection of the abdominal cavity, as one-third of patients thought to have stage I or II disease at initial laparotomy have been shown to have stage III and stage IV disease after subsequent staging.

Second-Look Laparotomy

Second-look surgeries are procedures offered to patients who have completed six cycles of chemotherapy and who are determined to be in a complete clinical remission by physical examination, CT scan, and a CA125 level of less than 35 units/ml. Fifty-percent of clinically complete responders will have residual disease at second look. Although there is no evidence that any surgical procedure performed following initial chemo-

Table 19.11 Staging for Fallopian Tube Carcinoma

FIGO	Stage	TNM	Classification	Description
0	Tis	N	M	Carcinoma in situ (limited to tubal mucosa)
I				Growth limited to fallopian tubes
IA	T1a	N0	M0	Growth limited to one tube; extension into submucosa or muscularis but not penetrating serosal surface; no ascites
IB	T1b	N0	M0	Growth limited to both tubes; extension into submucosa or muscularis but not penetrating serosal surface; no ascites
IC	T1c	N0	M0	Tumor either stage IA or stage IB; extension through or onto tubal serosa, or with ascites containing malignant cells, or with positive peritoneal washings
II				Growth involving one or both fallopian tubes with pelvic extension
IIA	T2a	N0	M0	Extension or metastasis to uterus or ovaries
IIB	T2b	N0	M0	Extension to other pelvic tissues
IIC	T2c	N0	M0	Tumor either stage IIA or stage IIB; ascites containing malignant cells, or with positive peritoneal washings
III				Tumor involving one or both fallopian tubes; peritoneal implants outside pelvis or positive retroperitoneal or inguinal nodes; superficial liver metastasis equal to stage III; tumor apparently limited to true pelvis but with histologically proved malignant extension to small bowel or omentum
IIIA	T3a	N0	M0	Tumor grossly limited to true pelvis; negative nodes but with histologically confirmed microscopic seeding of abdominal peritoneal surfaces
IIIB	T3b	N0	M0	Tumor involving one or both tubes; histologically confirmed implants of abdominal peritoneal surfaces (none exceeding 2 cm in diameter); negative lymph nodes
IIIC	T3c	N0	M0	Abdominal implants > 2 cm in diameter or positive retroperitoneal or inguinal nodes
	Any T,	N1,	M0	
IV	Any T,	any N,	M1	Growth involving one or both fallopian tubes, with distant metastases; for pleural effusion, positive cytologic fluid required for designating malignant cells as stage IV; parenchymal liver metastasis equal to stage IV

T = tumor description (equivalent to FIGO); N = regional lymph nodes; N0 = no nodal metastasis; N1 = regional nodal metastasis; M = metastasis; M0 = no distant metastasis; M1 = any distant metastasis (excluding peritoneal cavity).
Note: Staging for fallopian tube carcinoma is determined by the surgical pathologic system. Operative findings defining stage are determined before tumor debulking.
Source: Modified from International Federation of Gynecology and Obstetrics, Annual report on the results of treatment in gynecologic cancer. *J Epidemiol Biostat* 3(23):63–74, 1998.

therapy will prolong survival, second-look procedures continue to be offered in order to assess results of therapy accurately in the setting of a clinical trial, as well as to offer other treatment options to patients who have residual disease.

Palliative Surgery

Patients with end-stage ovarian cancer may develop recurrent intestinal obstruction. Small bowel accounts for 44% of obstructions and large bowel for 33%, while both large and small bowel are obstructed in 22%. In nearly 80% of patients, a palliative bowel resection to relieve the obstruction could be successfully performed with restoration of gastrointestinal tract function and a subsequent survival of 6.8 months [81]. Although af-

fected patients should be informed that the purpose of this procedure would be purely palliative for symptoms, it would improve the patient's quality of life significantly and would avoid the alternative of continuous nasogastric tube drainage or percutaneous gastrostomy tube placement.

Chemotherapy

Initially, single-agent melphalan or chlorambucil were the agents used in the management of ovarian carcinoma. Overall response rates to these agents were 45% to 55%, producing complete clinical response rates of 15% to 20% [82]. With the introduction of cisplatin combination chemotherapy in the late 1970s, an overall response rate of 70% to 80% was achieved, with complete clinical response rates of approximately 50% [83]. Combination platinum-cyclophosphamide chemotherapy remained the gold-standard regimen until the 1990s, when paclitaxel was introduced. Paclitaxel-cisplatin became standard first-line treatment of ovarian cancer after results from a randomized phase III trial demonstrated improved response and survival as compared to cisplatin-cyclophosphamide (cisplatin-Cytoxan) [84]. Presently, several clinical trials are seeking to identify the optimal dose and duration of paclitaxel and are evaluating the substitution of carboplatin for cisplatin.

On the basis of the widespread intraperitoneal distribution of metastatic ovarian carcinoma, the intraperitoneal route of administering chemotherapy always has been intriguing. Studies comparing drug concentrations with systemic versus intraperitoneal administration confirm a pharmacokinetic advantage for the intraperitoneal route. Direct penetration into the tissue is limited to 1 to 3 mm. Therefore, administration is restricted to patients with minimal residual disease (< 1.0 cm). Multiple phase II trials have been performed, confirming the feasibility of intraperitoneal chemotherapy, mostly after first- or second-line chemotherapy. A recently reported study in previously untreated stage III ovarian cancer (546 patients) randomly assigned patients to intraperitoneal cisplatin versus intravenous cisplatin. The study found an improved median survival of 49 months (95% confidence interval, 42–56 months) in the intraperitoneal arm versus 41 months (95% confidence interval, 34–47 months) in the intravenous arm [85]. This study has renewed interest in the intraperitoneal route of chemotherapy administration, particularly in patients with microscopic or very-small-volume residual disease.

A small percentage of patients (usually < 20%) may have progressive tumor during their initial chemotherapy treatments. This disorder is defined as *refractory disease*. Residual disease (as judged by CT scan or elevated CA125 or at second-look surgical assessment) is called *persistent disease*. Patients who have a clinical or surgical complete response to therapy but in whom disease recurs in less than 6 months from the time the chemotherapy was completed are said to have *resistant disease*.

Investigational agents that continue to be introduced exhibit promising response rates. The topoisomerase-1 inhibitors disrupt RNA and DNA synthesis, halting cellular replication. Three topoisomerase-1 inhibitors are used in the treatment of ovarian cancer: topotecan, 9-amino-camptothecin, and irinotecan. Presently, topotecan has been approved by the US Food and Drug

Administration for use in patients with ovarian cancer after failure of initial or subsequent therapy. Other agents of interest are liposomal doxorubicin (Doxil), gemcitabine (Gemzar), and vinorelbine tartrate (Navelbine), all with response rates ranging from 15% to 40% [86]. Other active agents include cyclophosphamide, ifosfamide, hexamethylmelamine, and tamoxifen. The use of monoclonal antibodies, gene therapy, and drugs to induce cellular apoptosis and to inhibit angiogenesis are under investigation.

Radiotherapy

The role of irradiation treatment remains controversial despite two decades of use and data supporting its curative potential in appropriately selected patients. As the primary postoperative treatment for some patients with epithelial ovarian cancer, it has been replaced largely by chemotherapy. A number of cooperative groups in the United States, Canada, and Italy have been unable to complete randomized studies. No firm data support a preference for chemotherapy over radiotherapy in patient subgroups identified as appropriately treated with irradiation. If radiotherapy is selected for use, available data can guide appropriate patient selection, technique, and irradiation dosage that can be delivered safely.

A detailed and validated prognostic classification has incorporated the identified independent prognostic factors, tumor stage, grade, and residual disease. Defined as intermediate-risk patients are those in a group who are within stages I to III and have no apparent or small residual pelvic disease (< 1 cm); for such patients, abdominopelvic radiotherapy is justified as primary postoperative therapy (Table 19.12) [87, 88].

Several retrospective series using whole abdominopelvic irradiation as primary adjuvant therapy have demonstrated 5- and 10-year survival rates and median survivals at least equivalent to those obtained with modern systemic agents in similarly selected patients [87, 89]. Thus, irradiation remains a modality to be considered in the treatment of such intermediate-risk patients.

Given the recognized transperitoneal route of dissemination, definitive radiotherapy must encompass the entire peritoneal cavity. The use of intraperitoneal radiocolloids (^{32}P) has intuitive appeal, because it offers the possibility of delivering high doses of irradiation to peritoneal surfaces. However, a therapeutic value for this modality has not been established. Often, the irradiation dose distributions are variable and unpredictable, and a negligible dose is delivered to retroperitoneal nodes. Two randomized studies have compared ^{32}P with

Table 19.12 Percentage of Five-Year Relapse-Free Rates ($\pm$ Standard Deviation) in "Good Prognosis" Patients According to Stage, Residuum, and Grade

Stage	Residuum	Grade 1	Grade 2	Grade 3
I	0	96 $\pm$ 2[a] (80)	78 $\pm$ 5[b] (71)	62 $\pm$ 8[b] (39)
II	0	91 $\pm$ 4[b] (45)	73 $\pm$ 7[b] (46)	52 $\pm$ 7[b] (47)
II	< 2	No relapses[b] (5)	78 $\pm$ 14[b] (9)	21 $\pm$ 11[c] (14)
III	0	63 $\pm$ 14[b] (15)	26 $\pm$ 14[c] (12)	29 $\pm$ 11[c] (20)
III	< 2	88 $\pm$ 12[b] (8)	45 $\pm$ 11[c] (20)	39 $\pm$ 10[c] (27)

Note: Numbers in parentheses indicate the numbers of patients in each cell.
[a]High-risk patients.
[b]Intermediate-risk patients.
[c]Low-risk patients.

cisplatin. Neither showed a survival difference, although relapse rates appear lower with cisplatin [90, 91].

Whole abdominopelvic irradiation must include all peritoneal surfaces. A total dose to the abdomen of 23 to 28 Gy and a dose to the pelvis of 45 Gy are accompanied by an acceptable late complication rate. Generally, the acute effects of fatigue, diarrhea, and nausea subside within 2 to 4 weeks of completing therapy. Persistent bloating or diarrhea may be experienced by 10% to 15% of patients. The frequency of major bowel complications with abdominopelvic radiotherapy is low, if appropriate fields and blocking techniques are used. Bowel complication rates are related to the total dose of irradiation, the dose per fraction, and the extent of previous surgery (particularly lymph node sampling) [92].

POSTTREATMENT SURVEILLANCE

Women with ovarian cancer have a high incidence of recurrence (75%) within the first 2 years. The recommendation for these patients is to be examined and evaluated at 3-month intervals for the first 2 years by following CA125 levels and by complete history and physical examination that includes rectovaginal, bimanual examinations. If such patients are without evidence of disease at the end of 2 years, they may be seen at 6-month intervals for the remaining 3 years. No standard recommendation governs the use of CT scan surveillance; however, most clinicians will request a CT scan with evidence of a rising CA125 or with disease-related symptoms.

Atypically Proliferating Epithelial Ovarian Neoplasms

Atypically proliferating neoplasms (formerly called *borderline tumors* or *tumors of low malignant potential*) account for 10% to 15% of epithelial ovarian cancers (median age at diagnosis = 53). Compared to invasive ovarian malignancies, 80% to 85% of atypically proliferative tumors are diagnosed as stage I disease, with excellent long-term survival of approximately 90%.

Atypically proliferating tumors have been described for all epithelial ovarian subtypes, the most common being serous and mucinous tumors. Microscopically, these tumors show greater epithelial proliferation than that seen in benign cystadenomas; by definition, however, they are noninvasive within the ovary (Fig. 19.11) [93]. These tumors may or may not be accompanied by peritoneal implants; the implants may be noninvasive or invasive. A recent review found that if atypically proliferating tumors were seen in association with "noninvasive" implants, the 5- and 10-year survival rates were greater than 98%; hence the impetus to take these tumors out of the low-malignant-potential category [94]. In the context of "invasive" implants—in which a destructive infiltrative pattern of growth is demonstrated—atypically proliferating tumors display a clinical behavior and survival similar to that of invasive primary epithelial ovarian carcinoma. Appropriate staging and management, then, depend on careful pathologic assessment.

Management of disease in women with these ovarian tumors begins with a complete surgical staging,

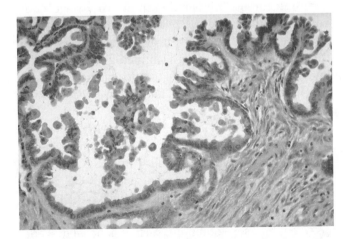

Figure 19.11 Ovary. Atypically proliferating serous tumors (borderline tumors) exhibit proliferation of the lining cells, with tufting but minimal cytologic atypia and no invasion.

including a total abdominal hysterectomy, bilateral salpingo-oophorectomy, omentectomy, appendectomy, pelvic and peritoneal lymph node sampling, and peritoneal biopsies. More conservative surgical options exist for women wishing to retain their childbearing potential. In these women, a unilateral salpingo-oophorectomy and surgical staging procedure (with inspection of the contralateral ovary, owing to a high incidence of bilaterality) may be performed. Recently, consideration has been given to substituting unilateral ovarian cystectomy for salpingo-oophorectomy in this population. Although the sample size is small and follow-up is short, the preliminary results have not revealed an increase in recurrence rates [95]. For patients with advanced-stage disease, tumor cytoreduction is indicated. In patients with mucinous, atypically proliferating tumors, appendectomy is particularly important because of the association with synchronous appendiceal primary lesions. The use of adjuvant chemotherapy or radiotherapy in patients with advanced or recurrent disease has not demonstrated a survival benefit.

Germ-Cell Tumors

Germ-cell tumors occur mainly in young women (median age, 19). These tumors are accompanied by abdominal pain, and nearly 10% will present with an acute abdomen secondary to torsion, hemorrhage, or tumor rupture with peritonitis. Malignant ovarian germ-cell tumors occur in the following order of frequency: dysgerminoma, immature teratoma, endodermal sinus tumor, embryonal carcinoma, and (rarely) choriocarcinoma. Approximately 50% to 75% of malignant germ-cell tumors are detected in an early stage. Most germ-cell tumors are not bilateral, though dysgerminomas are bilateral in up to 15% of patients. Several serum tumor markers have been identified as being elevated in association with germ-cell tumors and are helpful in the diagnosis, management, and follow-up care (Table 19.13).

Nearly 75% of dysgerminomas develop in women younger than 35 years, with 5% to 10% found in prepubertal girls. Histologically, this tumor is composed of clusters of large vesicular cells separated by delicate septa, often infiltrated by mature lymphocytes. In some cases, HCG-secreting syncytiotrophoblast cells may be detected. Intersex conditions, such as gonadal dysgenesis and androgen insensitivity syndrome, are predisposing factors. Dysgerminomas are the most irradiation-sensitive of the germ-cell tumors, although irradiation rarely is used to treat them.

Table 19.13 Serum Markers in Malignant Germ Cell Tumors of the Ovary

Malignant Germ-Cell Tumor	Serum Marker			
	AFP	β-HCG	LDH	CA125
Endodermal sinus tumor	+	−	±	±
Embryonal carcinoma	+	+	±	±
Choriocarcinoma	−	+	±	±
Immature teratoma	±	−	±	±
Dysgerminoma	−	±	±	±
Mixed germ-cell tumor	±*	±*	±*	±*

AFP = alpha-fetoprotein; β-HCG = beta subunit of human chorionic gonadotropin; LDH = lactate dehydrogenase.
*Marker depends on type of germ-cell tumors present.
Source: Reprinted with permission of the American College of Obstetricians and Gynecologists, © ACOG, 1998, from WJ Hoskins, Cancer of the ovary and uterine tube. In GB Holtzman, RD Rinehart, PJ DiSaia (eds), *Precis (Oncology)—An Update in Obstetrics and Gynecology.* Washington, DC: American College of Obstetricians and Gynecologists, 1998:48.

Immature teratomas may contain immature elements from any or all of three germ layers and can appear either in pure form or as mixed germ-cell tumors. Immature teratomas may be associated with a contralateral benign dermoid cyst. Typically, these tumors grow to an average diameter of 18 cm and appear bosselated, with solid and cystic components. In addition to stage, grade, and extent of tumor, the prognosis is influenced also by the relative amounts of immature tissue and by the degree of immaturity, which is predictive of metastatic potential. The immature element observed most frequently is primitive neuroepithelium.

Endodermal sinus tumors or *yolk-sac tumors* are the most malignant of the germ-cell tumors and mainly affect children and women younger than 20 years. Intraperitoneal dissemination is more frequent than is lymphatic spread. Frequently, it occurs as part of a mixed germ-cell tumor, with an additional component of dysgerminoma, immature teratoma, or choriocarcinoma. Pure endodermal sinus tumors can rupture and present as abdominal pain with hemorrhagic ascites. Microscopically, endodermal sinus tumors are characterized by a reticular growth pattern with Schiller-Duval bodies and AFP-containing hyaline droplets (Fig. 19.12). Serum AFP levels serve as a marker that correlates closely with extent of disease and response to chemotherapy.

Both embryonal carcinoma and choriocarcinoma are rare forms of germ-cell tumors, usually diagnosed in women younger than age 20 and in premenarchal girls who may display isosexual precocious puberty. Embryonal carcinomas secrete AFP and HCG, whereas choriocarcinomas present with HCG elevation. In both

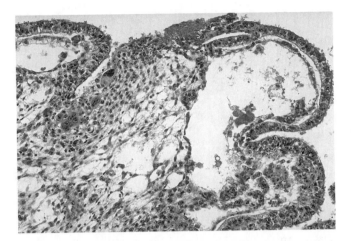

Figure 19.12 Ovary. This mixed germ-cell tumor shows yolk sac differentiation on the right, with alpha-fetoprotein-containing globules found within a vesicle, and multinucleate syncytiotrophoblast on the left.

cases, tumor markers are useful for monitoring disease outcome.

Most patients presenting with germ-cell tumors are young and exhibit unilateral ovarian involvement. Conservative surgery is appropriate to preserve such patients' fertility. Surgical therapy requires a unilateral salpingo-oophorectomy with necessary staging (cytology, omentectomy, appendectomy, pelvic and paraaortic lymph node sampling, and peritoneal and diaphragmatic evaluations). Any suspicious lesions noted in the abdomen or pelvis should be subjected to biopsy. All germ-cell tumors—with the exception of stage IA grade 1 immature teratomas and stage I pure dysgerminomas—require adjuvant chemotherapy. Chemotherapy involves a platinum-based, multidrug regimen—usually bleomycin, etoposide, and platinum—resulting in cure rates ranging from 85% to 90% [96]. Germ-cell tumors seemingly do not demonstrate a role for second-look laparotomy, except possibly in incompletely resected immature teratomas.

Sex Cord–Stromal Tumors

Sex cord–stormal tumors account for 5% to 8% of ovarian malignancies and include those tumors derived from the sex cords (granulosa and Sertoli cells) and from the gonadal stroma (theca and Leydig cells). Approximately 15% of these tumors are hormonally active. In general, sex cord–stromal tumors are indolent, slow-growing tumors. Because the embryonic gonad is sexually bipotential, the sex cord neoplasms may re-

semble male or female sex cord elements. Similarly, the stromal tumors that are functional, producing steroid hormones, may resemble tumors in another steroidogenic organ (the adrenal gland). Reports have cited hormonal production disparate from cell phenotype (i.e., female cell elements produce androgen). The sex cord–stromal tumors fall into two major classifications: granulosa–stromal cell tumors (granulosa cell and fibrothecoma) and the androblastomas or Sertoli-Leydig cell tumors.

Granulosa cell tumors are the most common sex cord neoplasms. These tumors are found in all age groups, with 5% occurring in prepubertal girls. Frequently, such tumors are associated with excess endogenous estrogen production resulting in precocious puberty, menstrual irregularity, endometrial hyperplasia (25–50%), or endometrial carcinoma (5%). Defeminization or virilization from androgen excess also can occur. Microscopically, a classic pattern of growth appears as clusters of cells surrounding small cystic cavities resembling a developing follicle known as *Call-Exner bodies* (Fig. 19.13). Other common patterns are macrofollicular, trabecular, and diffuse. Granulosa cell tumors can grow fairly large and then rupture, presenting as an acute abdomen with hemoperitoneum. The majority of patients are at stage I at diagnosis, with estimated 5-year survival of 95%, as compared to 55% and 25% in stages II and III, respectively. Late recurrence can occur up to 30 years from the original diagnosis. Serum inhibin levels are considered to be a useful marker of disease.

Fibrothecomas constitute the vast majority of stromal neoplasms and consist of thecal cells and fibroblasts. When the fibroblasts dominate, the tumor contains abundant collagen and is called a *fibroma*. When thecal cells are the major component, the tumor is clas-

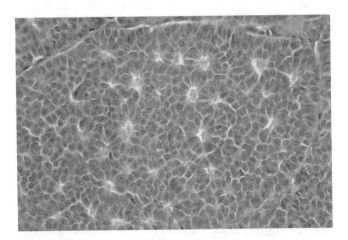

Figure 19.13 Ovary. This granulosa cell tumor contains numerous Call-Exner bodies.

sified as a *thecoma*. Meigs' syndrome (ovarian fibroma, ascites, and right hydrothorax) is present in only 1 in 150 cases. Because thecomas are estrogen-producing tumors, patients may present with postmenopausal bleeding or irregular menses. Owing to unopposed estrogen production, the risks of endometrial hyperplasia and endometrial carcinoma are similar to those of granulosa cell tumors.

Sertoli-Leydig cell tumors constitute fewer than 0.5% of ovarian neoplasms, with 75% of these tumors diagnosed in women younger than 40. Androgen excess leading to defeminization and virilization is noted in up to 85% of patients, with estrogenization reported only rarely. Heterologous elements, such as cartilage, mucinous epithelium, or skeletal muscle, occur in approximately 20% of Sertoli-Leydig cell tumors, most of which otherwise are of intermediate differentiation. Reinke crystalloids also may be seen. When heterologous elements are identified in poorly differentiated neoplasms, the tumor is clinically malignant. In general, such tumors are low-grade and rarely bilateral, with a 5-year survival of 70% to 90% and rare recurrences.

Primary treatment is conservative surgery with unilateral salpingo-oophorectomy and surgical staging being performed in young woman. Additionally, the uterus, tubes, and ovaries are removed in postmenopausal women who no longer are concerned about fertility. No data support the use of adjuvant chemotherapy or irradiation in these tumors.

GESTATIONAL TROPHOBLASTIC DISEASE

The term *gestational trophoblastic disease* includes four distinct disease entities. The hydatidiform mole is a virtually benign process. The trophoblastic neoplasias, including invasive mole, placental-site trophoblastic disease, and choriocarcinoma, represent the more malignant forms of the disease.

Hydatidiform Mole (Molar Pregnancy)

The incidence of hydatidiform mole varies widely in different parts of the world. For women in the United States and Europe, molar pregnancies occur with an incidence of 0.6 to 1.1 per 1,000 pregnancies. Asian women have a significantly higher incidence of 2 to 10 per 1,000 pregnancies. Differences in genetic makeup, rather than environmental factors, appear to account for the diverse incidence rate between racial groups

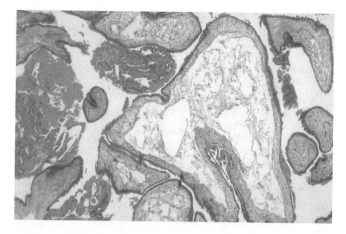

Figure 19.14 Complete mole. The chorionic villi are markedly enlarged and hydropic, showing central cistern formation. This example shows minimal trophoblast hyperplasia. Partial moles demonstrate a second population of smaller, more normal-appearing villi.

(e.g., Asian women born and raised in Hawaii sharing the same incidence as those born in Asia). Hydatidiform moles have a bimodal age distribution, with peaks at opposite ends of the reproductive spectrum (< 20 years and > 40 years). The extremes in age may reflect a higher incidence of defective gametogenesis in these age groups. A history of previous molar gestation confers a 20- to 40-fold increase in risk of having another molar gestation. Women with prior miscarriages appear to be at two to three times the normal risk.

BIOLOGICAL CONSIDERATIONS

Hydatidiform moles can be classified as complete or partial; they occur with an incidence of 1:1,200 pregnancies and 1:750 pregnancies, respectively. Both are abnormally formed placentas characterized by edematous, vesicular chorionic villi and a variable degree of trophoblast proliferation. The subclassification is based on differences in morphologic, cytogenetic, and clinicopathologic characteristics. In complete moles, the villi are edematous and avascular, trophoblast proliferation typically is present, and evidence of fetal development is lacking (Fig. 19.14). In partial moles, only a subpopulation of villi show the edematous or molar change. Other villi appear normal, vessels are present, trophoblast proliferation generally is less prominent, and fetal development may be evident. Partial moles are associated with a lower frequency of post–molar gestational trophoblastic neoplasia (5–10% versus 15–20%), and metastases are rare.

Karyotype analysis reveals that complete moles occur when normal sperm fertilize an ovum lacking maternal chromosomes. Approximately 95% of complete moles have a 46,XX composition, and 5% have 46,XY. It has been shown that the 46,XX complete moles result from duplication of a single haploid sperm (23X), whereas the 46,XY karyotype is the result of a dispermic fertilization (23X and 23Y). Approximately 80% to 95% of partial moles have a triploid karyotype, usually 69,XXY (two sets of paternal and one set of maternal chromosomes) [97]. The triploid fetus rarely will develop or survive to term.

DIAGNOSIS

Clinical Presentation

Commonly, molar gestations present with vaginal bleeding during the first 16 weeks of pregnancy. Nearly one-third of patients present with uterine size exceeding the dates of gestation, and disease may be associated with hyperemesis (less than 10%) and pregnancy-induced hypertension in the first or second trimester (1%). On occasion, patients will complain of passing grapelike tissues from the vagina. Once this sign occurs, active vaginal bleeding will ensue and may lead to significant blood loss and hypovolemic shock. Owing to an elevated HCG level, the shared alpha-subunit with thyroid-stimulating hormone may result in an elevation of total T_4 and free T_4 values (25–50%); clinical hyperthyroidism, manifested by congestive heart failure or pulmonary edema, is rare. Owing to the high levels of HCG (> 100,000 mIU/ml), the shared alpha-subunit with follicle-stimulating hormone results in ovarian hyperstimulation with theca-lutein cyst formation in nearly one-third of patients.

The described symptoms are observed most commonly in patients with a complete mole. Patients with partial moles may present with these symptoms but to a lesser extent. More frequently, partial moles will present with abnormal vaginal bleeding more consistent with signs and symptoms of a spontaneous abortion (incomplete or missed), with a definitive diagnosis being made at histopathologic review of the dilatation and curettage.

Diagnostic Evaluation

The presence of HCG-producing trophoblastic cells is the hallmark of these tumors, with HCG levels serving as a reliable index of disease status. Ultrasonography should be performed on all pregnant patients who complain of vaginal bleeding. With a complete mole, the uterus will be larger than the stated gestational age, and no fetus will be detected by sonography. A classic snow-storm pattern is pathognomonic for complete mole.

A preevacuation workup includes a physical examination and recording of a complete history; chest roentgenography; serum chemistry; complete blood cell count; coagulation profile, type, and cross-match; thyroid function tests; and urinalysis.

PRIMARY TREATMENT

In patients wishing to maintain their fertility, hydatidiform moles can be evacuated by suction followed by sharp curettage to ensure total absence of residual trophoblastic tissue. The curettage should be thorough yet gentle, to prevent uterine perforation, scarring, or adhesions. An oxytocic agent should be infused intravenously toward the end of the evacuation and for several hours thereafter, to assist with uterine contractility and decreased blood loss. Given the potential for massive blood loss, fluid resuscitation and blood component replacement should be available. Repletion of intravascular volume should be achieved with appropriate caution to decrease the possibility of subsequent pulmonary edema. A total abdominal hysterectomy is reserved for patients who have completed childbearing and desire sterilization. Hysterectomy reduces to approximately 5% the risk of post–molar trophoblastic disease but does not eliminate the need to obtain follow-up HCG levels. Trophoblast expresses CDE (Rh) factor. Patients who are Rh-negative require administration of anti-D immune globulin (RhoGAM) to prevent Rh sensitization problems with future pregnancies.

POSTTREATMENT SURVEILLANCE

Evacuation itself is curative in 80% to 85% of patients with a hydatidiform mole. The remaining 15% to 20% will develop post–molar trophoblastic neoplasia (10–17% invasive mole, 2–3% choriocarcinoma) and will require additional chemotherapy. Serum HCG titers should be followed weekly, until three successive normal values (< 5 mIU/ml) are obtained. The majority of patients will require 9 to 11 weeks' postevacuation before the HCG level has normalized. Thereafter, monthly evaluations are necessary for another 6 months. During this period, an essential requirement for the patient is to exercise appropriate contraception, as pregnancy would interfere with the HCG surveillance of this disease. Most clinicians recommend either oral contraceptives or medroxyprogesterone (Depo-Provera) injections for improved compliance.

Indications for concern of post–molar trophoblastic disease after evacuation would be a plateau in HCG levels over three consecutive weekly determinations, a rising HCG over two consecutive determinations, an HCG greater than 20,000 mIU/ml more than 4 weeks after evacuation, or patients presenting with persistently elevated HCG levels 6 months after evacuation. Identification of metastatic disease at the time of evacuation or a histopathologic diagnosis of choriocarcinoma or invasive mole in the dilatation and curettage specimen also would indicate a more aggressive management plan.

Gestational Trophoblastic Neoplasia

Gestational trophoblastic neoplasia encompasses three distinct entities: invasive mole, choriocarcinoma, and placental-site trophoblastic tumor. Although collectively called *gestational trophoblastic neoplasia,* the specific diagnosis or decision to treat often occurs without knowledge of the disorder's precise histologic makeup. The overall cure rate for these tumors exceeds 90%. Owing to the invasive nature of these tumors and their propensity for distant metastases, a delay in diagnosis or in the immediate initiation of treatment can result in significant morbidity and even death. Invasive moles constitute 70% to 90% of gestational trophoblastic neoplasia, with an overall incidence of 1:15,000 pregnancies. Owing to the invasive nature of this trophoblastic tissue, deep invasion frequently occurs through the myometrium, with extension into venous channels. Distant metastases (most often vaginal) occur in some 15% of cases and commonly present as hemorrhage. Choriocarcinomas contribute the other 10% to 30% of gestational trophoblastic neoplasia, accounting for 1:40,000 pregnancies. Approximately 50% of choriocarcinomas develop after a molar gestation, with the other 50% developing after normal pregnancy (25%) or abortion or ectopic gestation (25%). Placental-site trophoblastic tumors are extremely rare [97, 98].

BIOLOGICAL CONSIDERATIONS

The invasive mole is a hydatidiform mole in which hydropic villi have invaded the myometrium or blood vessels, with potential spread to extrauterine sites. The highly malignant choriocarcinoma is characterized by biphasic proliferation of malignant syncytiotrophoblast and cytotrophoblast, with extensive hemorrhage, necrosis, and an absence of chorionic villi (Fig. 19.15). Choriocarcinoma spreads both by direct invasion of the myometrium and through vascular channels to distant sites, most commonly the lungs, vagina or pelvis, brain,

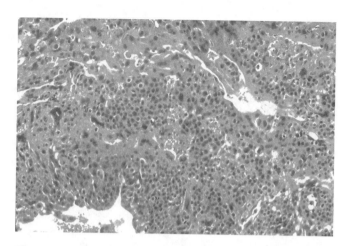

Figure 19.15 Choriocarcinoma. The tumor is composed of malignant cytotrophoblast and syncytiotrophoblast. Villi are not present.

and liver. Placental site trophoblastic tumor is extremely rare. This neoplasm is derived from intermediate trophoblast, the type normally responsible for establishing a placental implantation site. Typically, these tumors form nodular masses within the myometrium. Placental-site trophoblastic tumors differ histologically from choriocarcinoma in the absence of syncytiotrophoblast or cytotrophoblast and differ from invasive moles by the absence of chorionic villi.

Diagnosis

Most frequently, gestational trophoblastic neoplasia will be diagnosed after evacuation of a molar pregnancy, if the HCG plateaus or rises. Occasionally, the diagnosis will be made on pathologic evaluation of the specimens obtained at curettage, hysterectomy, mature placenta, or (rarely) by biopsy of metastatic lesions.

Half of the choriocarcinomas develop after a normal pregnancy or after abortion or ectopic gestation. For this reason, patients with continued complaints of vaginal bleeding must be evaluated thoroughly, with a diagnosis of trophoblastic disease in mind. Owing to the invasive nature of the trophoblast and its propensity for distant hematogenous spread, trophoblastic disease can masquerade as other diseases, depending on the organ involved. Fairly commonly, patients can present with hemoptysis, pleuritic chest pain, vaginal bleeding, seizures, neurologic deficit, abdominal pain, hemoperitoneum, or gastrointestinal tract bleeding due to metastatic disease.

Evaluation of a woman with atypical symptoms would begin with a serum β-HCG. Once an elevated level is obtained, pelvic ultrasonography is necessary to rule out a normal intrauterine pregnancy and may be useful also in detecting extensive intrauterine disease. Diagnosis of gestational trophoblastic neoplasia necessitates proceeding with evaluation for metastatic disease.

Table 19.14 National Cancer Institute's Clinical Classification of Gestational Trophoblastic Tumors

Nonmetastatic gestational trophoblastic tumor
Metastatic gestational trophoblastic tumor
Low risk
   HCG < 100,000 IU per 24-hr urine or < 40,000 mIU per milliliter of serum
   Symptoms present < 4 months
   No brain or liver metastases
   No prior chemotherapy
   Pregnancy event is not term delivery (i.e., mole, ectopic, spontaneous abortion)
High risk
   HCG > 100,000 IU per 24-hr urine or > 40,000 mIU per milliliter of serum
   Symptoms present > 4 months
   Brain or liver metastases
   Prior chemotherapeutic failure
   Antecedent term pregnancy

HCG = human chorionic gonadotropin.
Source: Modified from CB Hammond, LG Borchert, L Tyrey et al., Treatment of metastatic trophoblastic disease: good and poor prognosis. *Am J Obstet Gynecol* 115:451, 1973.

Physical examination, recording a thorough history, chest roentgenography, and CT scanning of abdomen and pelvis is recommended. In the presence of concern for cerebral metastases, a CT scan of the head should be obtained. On the rare occasion in which central nervous system involvement is suspected despite a negative head CT scan result, measurement of cerebrospinal fluid HCG may be informative.

Patients with placental site trophoblastic tumors will display a serum HCG level lower than that from patients with choriocarcinoma or invasive moles. These tumors also express human placental lactogen, which may be of diagnostic assistance. The propensity for distant metastasis with placental-site tumors is significantly less common.

STAGING

Several classification systems are used to group patients with trophoblastic tumors. The most widely used system (a clinical system) is that described by the NCI (Table 19.14) to determine treatment and report results. The World Health Organization (WHO) adopted a prognostic scoring system based on a variety of risk factors (Table 19.15), and the FIGO Cancer Committee described an anatomic staging system similar to that used for other malignancies (Table 19.16).

Table 19.15 World Health Organization Scoring System Based on Prognostic Factors for Gestational Trophoblastic Tumors

	Score			
Risk Factor	0	1	2	4
Age (yr)	≤ 39	> 39		
Antecedent pregnancy	Hydatidiform mole	Abortion	Term	
Pregnancy event–to–treatment interval (mo)	< 4	4–6	7–12	> 12
Human chorionic gonadotropin (IU/liter)	< 10^3	10^3–10^4	10^4–10^5	> 10^5
ABO blood groups (female × male)		O × A	B	
		A × O	AB	
No. of metastases		1–4	4–8	> 8
Site of metastases		Spleen	Gastrointestinal tract	Brain
		Kidney	Liver	
Largest tumor mass, including uterine (cm)		3–5	> 5	
Prior chemotherapy			Single drug	Two or more drugs

Note: The total score for a patient is obtained by adding the individual scores for each prognostic factor. Total score ≤ 4 = low risk; 5–7 = middle risk; ≥ 8 = high risk.
Source: Reprinted with permission from the World Health Organization Scientific Group, *Gestational Trophoblastic Disease.* [Tech. Rep. Ser. 692.] Geneva: World Health Organization, 1983.

Table 19.16 FIGO Staging System for Gestational Trophoblastic Tumors

Stage	Definition
I	Disease confined to uterus
IA	Disease confined to uterus; no risk factors
IB	Disease confined to uterus; one risk factor
IC	Disease confined to uterus; two risk factors
II	Gestational trophoblastic tumor extending outside uterus; limited to genital structures (adnexa, vagina, broad ligament)
IIA	Gestational trophoblastic tumor involving genital structures; no risk factors
IIB	Gestational trophoblastic tumor extending outside uterus; limited to genital structures; one risk factor
IIC	Gestational trophoblastic tumor extending outside uterus; limited to genital structures; two risk factors
III	Gestational trophoblastic tumor extending to lungs, with or without known genital tract involvement
IIIA	Gestational trophoblastic tumor extending to lungs, with or without genital tract involvement; no risk factors
IIIB	Gestational trophoblastic tumor extending to lungs, with or without genital tract involvement; one risk factor
IIIC	Gestational trophoblastic tumor extending to lungs, with or without genital tract involvement; two risk factors
IV	Including all other metastatic sites
IVA	Including all other metastatic sites; no risk factors
IVB	Including all other metastatic sites; one risk factor
IVC	Including all other metastatic sites; two risk factors

Note: Risk factors affecting staging include the following: (1) serum human chorionic gonadotropin > 100,000 mIU/ml and (2) duration of disease > 6 mo from termination of antecedent pregnancy. The following factors should be considered and noted in reporting: (1) Prior chemotherapy has been given for known gestational trophoblastic tumor; (2) placental site tumors should be reported separately; and (3) histologic verification of disease is not required.
Source: Modified from the International Federation of Gynecology and Obstetrics. Annual report on the results of treatment in gynecologic cancer. *J Epidemiol Biostat* 3(23):129–135, 1998.

PRIMARY TREATMENT

Of patients with nonmetastatic (NCI), stage I (FIGO), or WHO score 4 disease, the majority can be treated with single-agent chemotherapy (methotrexate or dactinomycin). If the HCG fails to decrease significantly after the first two cycles of therapy, the alternate drug may be used. In general, a 10-fold drop in HCG after each course is satisfactory. Once the HCG normalizes, two additional courses of chemotherapy are given to ensure complete resolution of tumor. The cure rate for nonmetastatic trophoblastic disease is nearly 100%, with 85% to 90% being cured with their initial chemotherapeutic regimen. Generally, the remaining patients are cured by alternative single-agent chemotherapy or multiagent chemotherapy. Fewer than 5% of patients will require hysterectomy for cure. Patients with metastatic low-risk disease (NCI), stage IIA or IIIA (FIGO), or WHO scores of 5 to 7 can begin treatment with single-agent chemotherapy. An alternative treatment, likely in the form of multiagent chemotherapy, will be necessary in approximately 20%.

Patients with high-risk disease (NCI), stages IIB or C, IIIB or C, and IV disease (FIGO), or a WHO score of no less than 8 require aggressive combination chemotherapy. Etoposide is a highly effective agent in gestational trophoblastic tumors and should be included in any first-line combination regimen. Presently, the regimen used most commonly is EMA-CO (etoposide, methotrexate, dactinomycin [actinomycin D], cyclophosphamide, and vincristine [Oncovin]), with cure rates in the range of 90% [99]. A modification of the EMA-CO regimen substitutes cisplatin and etoposide for cyclophosphamide and vincristine. This regimen may be used in patients unresponsive to EMA-CO therapy [98]. Continuing treatment with chemotherapy is necessary until three consecutively normal HCG levels have been reached (two additional chemotherapy cycles after the first normal HCG level). To obtain a satisfactory outcome, a swift diagnosis is imperative, and aggressive chemotherapy must be initiated immediately. Adjuvant surgical procedures (e.g., thoracotomy, laparotomy, or hysterectomy) may be necessary initially to control significant hemorrhage or in the face of persistent disease, to remove isolated foci of chemotherapy-resistant disease. Generally, surgical therapy is not recommended in the management of trophoblastic disease. Brain metastases pose a particularly difficult management problem. The blood-brain barrier significantly decreases the efficacy of chemotherapy to the central nervous system. The addition of whole-brain radiotherapy to EMA-CO therapy has increased cure rates in patients with central nervous system involvement to more than 50% [97]. Because of the risk of cerebral edema and hemorrhage, dexamethasone should be administered during whole-brain irradiation. The decision algorithm for trophoblastic disease is shown in Figure 19.16.

POSTTREATMENT SURVEILLANCE

Serum HCG levels should be followed up every 1 to 2 weeks for 3 months and then at monthly intervals to complete a 12-month period. Physical examination should be performed at 6-month intervals to complete

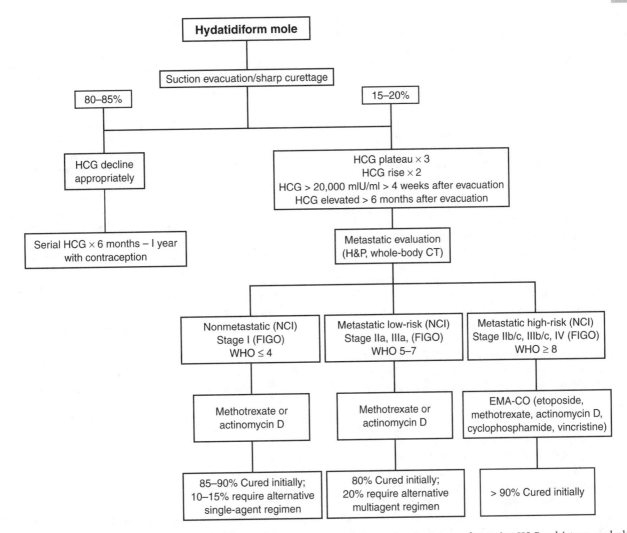

Figure 19.16   Treatment algorithm for trophoblastic disease. *HCG* = human chorionic gonadotropin; *H&P* = history and physical examination; *CT* = computed tomography; *NCI* = National Cancer Institute; *FIGO* = International Federation of Gynecology and Obstetrics; *WHO* = World Health Organization; *EMA-CO* = etoposide, methotrexate, dactinomycin (actinomycin D), cyclophosphamide, vincristine (Oncovin).

the first year and annually thereafter. Radiographic testing is performed only as indicated. Effective contraception must be encouraged in affected patients, as subsequent pregnancy could delay the diagnosis and treatment of recurrent disease. At the completion of the first disease-free year, pregnancy is allowed.

Subsequent Pregnancies

Patients who have had a prior diagnosis of trophoblastic disease are at increased risk with subsequent pregnancies. For this reason, patients with a history of trophoblastic disease require early first-trimester ultrasonography to confirm the presence of a normal intrauterine pregnancy. Additionally, any product of conception or

term placenta delivered with future pregnancies requires careful histopathologic evaluation.

REFERENCES

1. Greenlee RT, Murray T, Bolden S, Wingo PA. Cancer statistics, 2000. *CA Cancer J Clin* 50:7–33, 2000.
2. Yamakawa Y, Forslund O, Chua KL, et al. Detection of the BC 24 transforming fragment of the herpes simplex virus type 2 (HSV-2) DNA in cervical carcinoma tissue by polymerase chain reaction (PCR). *Acta Pathol Microbiol Immunol Scand* 102:401–406, 1994.
3. Scheffner M, Werness BA, Huibregtse JM, et al. The E6 oncoprotein encoded by human papillomavirus types 16 and 18 promotes the degradation of *p53*. *Cell* 63:1129–1136, 1990.

4. Heck DV, Yee CL, Howley PM, Munger K. Efficiency of binding to the retinoblastoma protein correlates with the transforming capacity of the E7 oncoproteins of the human papillomaviruses. *Proc Natl Acad Sci USA* 89:4442–4446, 1992.

5. Cannistra SA, Niloff JM. Cancer of the uterine cervix. *N Engl J Med* 334:1030–1038, 1996.

6. National Institutes of Health Consensus Panel. Cervical cancer. *NIH Consensus Statement* 14:1–38, 1996.

7. Ho GYF, Kadish AS, Burk RD, et al. HPV 16 and cigarette smoking as risk factors for high-grade cervical intraepithelial neoplasia. *Int J Cancer* 78:281–285, 1998.

8. Palefsky JM, Holly EA. Molecular virology and epidemiology of human papillomavirus and cervical cancer. *Cancer Epidemiol Biomarkers Prev* 4:415–428, 1995.

9. Simons AM, van Herckenrode CM, Rodriguez JA, et al. Demonstration of smoking-related DNA damage in cervical epithelium and correlation with human papillomavirus type 16, using exfoliated cervical cells. *Br J Cancer* 71:246–249, 1995.

10. Maneckjee R, Minna JD. Opioids induce while nicotine suppresses apoptosis in human lung cancer cells. *Cell Growth Differ* 5:1033–1040,1994.

11. American College of Obstetricians and Gynecologists. *Routine Cancer Screening.* [ACOG Committee Opinion 185.] Washington, DC: American College of Obstetricians and Gynecologists, 1997.

12. Gundersen JH, Rooney BL, Virata RL, Bobenmeyer S. Review of outcomes of atypical squamous cells of undetermined significance Papanicolaou smears for 1991 and 1992, with follow-up through 1995. *J Lower Gen Tract Dis* 1:126–131, 1997.

13. Abramowicz JS, Benson JT, Clarke-Pearson DL, et al. Gynecology: diagnostic and surgical procedures. In Visscher HC, Rinehart RD, Thiede HA (eds), *Precis V—An Update in Obstetrics and Gynecology.* Washington, DC: American College of Obstetricians and Gynecologists, 1994:210–224.

14. Im DD, Duska LR, Rosenshein NB. Adequacy of conization margins in adenocarcinoma in situ of the cervix as a predictor of residual disease. *Gynecol Oncol* 59:179–182, 1995.

15. Dargent D, Matheuet P. Schauta's vaginal hysterectomy combined with laparoscopic lymphadenectomy. *Baillieres Clin Obstet Gynecol* 9:691–705, 1995.

16. Roy ML, Plante ML. Pregnancies after radical trachelectomy for the treatment of early stage cervical cancer. *Am J Obstet Gynecol* 179:1491–1496, 1998.

17. Rotman M, Pajak TF, Choi K, et al. Prophylactic extended-field irradiation of para-aortic lymph nodes in stages IIB and bulky IB and IIA cervical carcinomas: ten-year treatment results of RTOG 79–20. *JAMA* 274(5):387–393, 1995.

18. Sedlis A, Bundy BN, Rotman M, et al. Treatment of selected patients (pts.) with Stage IB carcinoma of the cervix after radical hysterectomy and pelvic lymphadenectomy: pelvic radiation therapy (Rt) versus no further therapy (NFT) [abstr. 133]. (A GOG Study.) *Gynecol Oncol* 68:105, 1998.

19. Runowicz CD, Smith HO, Goldberg GL. Multimodality therapy in locally advanced cervical cancer. *Curr Opin Obstet Gynecol* 5:92–98, 1993.

20. Comerci JT, Fields AL, Runowicz CD, et al. The role of multimodality therapy in locally advanced cervical cancer. *Isr J Obstet Gynecol* 7:37–43, 1996.

21. Fields AL, Anderson PS, Goldberg GL, et al. Mature results of a phase II trial of concomitant cisplatin/pelvic radiotherapy for locally advanced squamous cell carcinoma of the cervix. *Gynecol Oncol* 61:416–422, 1996.

22. Pearcey RG, Stuart GCE, MacLean GD, et al. Phase II study to evaluate the toxicity and efficacy of concurrent cisplatin and radiation therapy in treatment of patients with locally advanced squamous cell carcinoma of the cervix. *Gynecol Oncol* 58:34–41, 1995.

23. Rose PG, Bundy BN, Watkins EB, et al. Concurrent cisplatin-based radiotherapy and chemotherapy for locally advanced cervical cancer. *N Engl J Med* 340:1144–1153, 1999.

24. Morris M, Eifel PJ, Lu J, et al. Pelvic radiation with concurrent chemotherapy compared with pelvic and para-aortic radiation for high-risk cervical cancer. *N Engl J Med* 340:1137–1143, 1999.

25. Jobsen JJ, Lee JEH, Cleton FJ, Hermans J. Treatment of loco-regional recurrence of carcinoma of the cervix by radiotherapy after primary surgery. *Gynecol Oncol* 33:368–371, 1989.

26. Morley GW, Hopkins MP, Lindenauer SM, Roberts JA. Pelvic exenteration, University of Michigan: 100 patients at 5 years. *Obstet Gynecol* 74:934–943, 1989.

27. Vermorken JB. The role of chemotherapy in squamous cell carcinoma of the uterine cervix: a review. *Int J Gynecol Cancer* 3:129, 1993.

28. Nevin J, Soeters R, Dehaaeck T, et al. Cervical carcinoma associated with pregnancy. *Obstet Gynecol Surv* 50:228–239, 1995.

29. Herbst Al, Cole P, Norusis MJ, et al. Epidemiologic aspects and factors related to survival in 384 registry cases of clear cell adenocarcinoma of the vagina and cervix. *Am J Obstet Gynecol* 135:876–886, 1979.

30. Colton T, Greenberg ER, Noller K, et al. Breast cancer in mothers prescribed diethylstilbestrol in pregnancy. Further follow-up. *JAMA* 269:2096–2100, 1993.

31. DeCesare SL, Fiorica JV, Roberts WS, et al. A pilot study utilizing intraoperative lymphoscintigraphy for identification of the sentinel lymph nodes in vulvar cancer. *Gynecol Oncol* 66:425–428, 1997.

32. Ansink AC, Sie-Go DM, van der Velden J, et al. Identification of sentinel lymph nodes in vulvar carcinoma patients with the aid of a patent blue V injection: a multicenter study. *Cancer* 86:652–656, 1999.

33. Thomas G, Dembo A, DePetrillo A, et al. Concurrent radiation and chemotherapy in vulvar carcinoma. *Gynecol Oncol* 34:263–267, 1989.

34. Berek JS, Heaps JM, Fu YS, et al. Concurrent cisplatin and 5-fluorouracil chemotherapy and radiotherapy for advanced-stage squamous carcinoma of the vulva. *Gynecol Oncol* 42:197–201, 1991.

35. Moore DH, Thomas GM, Montana GS, et al. Preoperative chemoradiation for advanced vulvar cancer: a Phase II study of the Gynecologic Oncology Group. *Int J Radiat Oncol Biol Phys* 42:79–85, 1998.

36. Homesley HD, Bundy BN, Sedlis A, et al. Prognostic factors for groin node metastases in squamous cell carcinoma

of the vulva (a Gynecologic Oncology Group Study). *Gynecol Oncol* 49:279–283, 1993.

37. Trimble EL. Melanomas of the vulvar and vagina. *Oncology (Huntingt)* 10:1017–1023; 1996.

38. Friedman M, Peretz BA, Nissenbaum M, Paldi E. Modern treatment of vaginal embryonal rhabdomyosarcoma. *Obstet Gynecol Surv* 41:614–618, 1986.

39. Comerci JT, Fields A, Runowicz CD, Goldberg GL. Continuous low-dose combined hormone replacement therapy and the risk of endometrial cancer. *Gynecol Oncol* 64:425–430, 1997.

40. Fisher B, Dignam J, Bryant J, et al. Five versus more than five years of tamoxifen therapy for breast cancer patients with negative lymph nodes and estrogen receptor-positive tumors. *J Natl Cancer Inst* 88:1529–1542, 1996.

41. Goldberg GL, Drubetsky Z, Smith HO, et al. Evaluation of CA19–9 in patients with gynecologic disease. *Gynecol Oncol* 49:163, 1993.

42. Rose PG, Sommers RM, Reale FR, et al. Serial serum CA125 measurements for evaluation of recurrence in patients with endometrial carcinoma. *Obstet Gynecol* 84:12–16, 1994.

43. Childers JM, Brzechffa PR, Hatch KD, et al. Laparoscopically assisted surgical staging (LASS) of endometrial cancer. *Gynecol Oncol* 51:33–38, 1993.

44. Boike G, Lurain J, Burke J. A comparison of laparoscopic management of endometrial cancer with a traditional laparotomy. *Gynecol Oncol* 52:A105, 1994.

45. Thornton JG, Brown LA, Wells M, Scott JS. Primary treatment of endometrial cancer with progestagen alone (letter). *Lancet* 2:207–208, 1985.

46. Morrow CP, Bundy BN, Kurman RJ, et al. Relationship between surgical-pathological risk factors of the endometrium. A Gynecologic Oncology Group Study. *Gynecol Oncol* 40:55–65, 1991.

47. Sutton GP. The significance of positive peritoneal cytology in endometrial cancer. *Oncology (Huntingt)* 4:21–26, 1990.

48. Roberts JA, Brunetto VL, Keys HM, et al. A phase III randomized study of surgery vs. surgery plus adjunctive radiation therapy in intermediate risk endometrial carcinoma (99). *Proc Soc Gynecol Oncol* 29:A70, 1998.

49. Irwin C, Levin W, Fyles A, et al. The role of adjuvant radiotherapy in carcinoma of the endometrium—results in 550 patients with pathologic stage I disease. *Gynecol Oncol* 70:1–8, 1998.

50. Potish RA, Twiggs LB, Adcock LL, et al. Paraaortic lymph node radiotherapy in cancer of the uterine corpus. *Obstet Gynecol* 65:251–256, 1985.

51. Thigpen T, Blessing J, Homesley H, et al. Phase III trial of doxorubicin +/- cisplatin in advanced or recurrent endometrial carcinoma: a Gynecologic Oncology Group (GOG) study. *Proc Am Soc Clin Oncol* 12:A261, 1993.

52. Ball H, Blessing JA, Lentz S, et al. A phase II trial of paclitaxel in patients with advanced or recurrent adenocarcinoma of the endometrium: a Gynecologic Oncology Group (GOG) study. *Gynecol Oncol* 62:278–281, 1996.

53. Deppe G. Chemotherapy for endometrial cancer. In Deppe G (ed), *Chemotherapy of Gynecologic Cancer*. New York: Wiley-Liss, 1990:155–174.

54. Barakat RR. Contemporary issues in the management of endometrial cancer. *CA Cancer J Clin* 48(5):299–314, 1998.

55. Lee RB, Burke TW, Park RC. Estrogen replacement therapy following treatment for stage I endometrial carcinoma. *Gynecol Oncol* 36:189–191, 1990.

56. Chapman JA, DiSaia PJ, Osann K, et al. Estrogen replacement in surgical stage I and II endometrial cancer survivors. *Am J Obstet Gynecol* 175:1195–1200, 1996.

57. American College of Obstetricians and Gynecologists. *Estrogen Replacement Therapy and Endometrial Cancer.* [ACOG Committee Opinion 126.] Washington, DC: American College of Obstetricians and Gynecologists, 1993.

58. Silverberg SG, Major FJ, Blessing JA, et al. Carcinosarcoma (malignant mixed mesodermal tumor) of the uterus. A Gynecologic Oncology Group pathologic study of 203 cases. *Int J Gynecol Pathol* 9:1–19, 1990.

59. Sutton GP, Blessing JA, Carson LF, et al. Adjuvant ifosfamide, mesna, and cisplatin in patients with completely resected stage I or II carcinosarcoma of the uterus: a study of the Gynecologic Oncology Group. *Proc Am Soc Clin Oncol* 16:1288A, 1997.

60. Fields AL, Hammerman R, Runowicz CD, et al. Survival and recurrence patterns in patients with completely resected mixed mesodermal tumors (MMT) of the uterus receiving adjuvant radiotherapy and chemotherapy vs. radiotherapy alone. *Proc Am Radium Soc* 49A:49, 1998.

61. Sutton GP, Brunetto V, Kilgore L, et al. A phase iii trial of ifosfamide alone or in combination with cisplatin in the treatment of patients with advanced, persistent, or recurrent carcinosarcoma of the uterus: a Gynecologic Oncology Group study (abstr. 266). *Gynecol Oncol* 68:137, 1998.

62. Thigpen JT, Blessing JA, Beecham J, et al. Phase II trial of cisplatin as first line chemotherapy in patients with advanced or recurrent uterine sarcomas: a Gynecologic Oncology Group study. *J Clin Oncol* 9:1962–1966, 1991.

63. Omura GA, Major FJ, Blessing JA, et al. A randomized study of Adriamycin with and without dimethyl triazenoimidazole carboxamide in advanced uterine sarcomas. *Cancer* 52:626–632, 1983.

64. Markman M, Zaino R, Fleming P, Barakat R. Carcinoma of the fallopian tube. In Hoskins WJ, Perez CA, Young RC (eds), *Principles and Practice of Gynecologic Oncology*. Philadelphia: Lippincott-Raven, 1997:1025–1038.

65. Narod SA, Risch H, Moslehi R, et al. Oral contraceptives and the risk of hereditary ovarian cancer. *N Engl J Med* 339:424–428, 1998.

66. Frank TS, Manley SA, Olopade OI, et al. Sequence analysis of BRCA1 and BRCA2: correlation of mutations with family history and ovarian cancer risk. *J Clin Oncol* 16:2417–2425, 1998.

67. Boyd J, Rubin SC. Hereditary ovarian cancer: molecular genetics and clinical implications. *Gynecol Oncol* 64:196–206, 1997.

68. Struewing JP, Hartge P, Wacholder S, et al. The risk of cancer associated with specific mutations of BRCA1 and BRCA2 among Ashkenazi Jews. *N Engl J Med* 336:1401–1408, 1997.

69. Statement of the American Society of Clinical Oncology: Genetic testing for cancer susceptibility. *J Clin Oncol* 14:1730–1736, 1996.

70. Beller U, Halle D, Catane R, et al. High frequency of BRCA1 and BRCA2 germline mutations in Ashkenazi

Jewish ovarian cancer patients, regardless of family history. *Gynecol Oncol* 67:123–126, 1997.

71. Burke W, Daly M, Garber J, et al. Recommendations for follow-up care of individuals with an inherited predisposition to cancer: II. BRCA1 and BRCA2. Cancer Genetics Studies Consortium. *JAMA* 277:997–1003, 1997.

72. Campbell S, Bhan V, Royston P, et al. Transabdominal ultrasound screening for early ovarian cancer. *Br Med J* 299:1363–1367, 1989.

73. Bourne TH, Campbell S, Reynolds KM, et al. Screening for early familial ovarian cancer with transvaginal ultrasonography and colour blood flow imaging. *Br Med J* 306: 1025–1029, 1993.

74. Tobacman JK, Greene MH, Tucker MA, et al. Intra-abdominal carcinomatosis after prophylactic oophorectomy in ovarian cancer–prone families. *Lancet* 2:795–797, 1982.

75. Piver MS, Jishi MF, Tsukada Y, Nava G. Primary peritoneal carcinoma after prophylactic oophorectomy in women with a family history of ovarian cancer. A report of the Gilda Radner Familial Ovarian Cancer Registry. *Cancer* 71:2751–2755, 1993.

76. Fields A, Jones J, Sampayo E, et al. The incidence of primary peritoneal carcinoma among patients with both breast and ovarian carcinoma. *Proc Am Soc Clin Oncol* 16:1286A, 1997.

77. Karlan BY, Baldwin RL, Lopez-Luevanos E, et al. Peritoneal serous papillary carcinoma, a phenotypic variant of familial ovarian cancer: implications for ovarian cancer screening. *Am Gynecol Obstet Soc* 17:46A, 1998.

78. Schrag D, Kuntz KM, Garber JE, Weeks JC. Decision analysis—effects of prophylactic mastectomy and oophorectomy on life expectancy among women with BRCA1 or BRCA2 mutations. *N Engl J Med* 336(20):1465–1471, 1997.

79. Bast RC Jr, Klug TL, St John E, et al. A radioimmunoassay using a monoclonal antibody to monitor the course of epithelial ovarian cancer. *N Engl J Med* 309:883–887, 1983.

80. Griffiths CT. Surgical resection of tumor bulk in the primary treatment of ovarian carcinoma. *Natl Cancer Inst Monogr* 42:101–104, 1975.

81. Rubin SC, Hoskins WJ, Benjamin I, Lewis JL. Palliative surgery for intestinal obstruction in advanced ovarian cancer. *Gynecol Oncol* 34:16–19, 1989.

82. Thigpen JT. Single agent chemotherapy in the management of ovarian carcinoma. In Alberts DS, Surwit EA (eds), *Ovarian Cancer*. Boston: Martinus Nijhoff, 1985: 115–146.

83. Thigpen JT, Blessing JA, Bance RB, et al. Chemotherapy in ovarian carcinoma: present role and future prospects. *Semin Oncol* 167:58–65, 1989.

84. McGuire WP, Hoskins WJ, Brady MF, et al. Cyclophosphamide and cisplatin compared with paclitaxel and cisplatin in patients with Stage III and IV ovarian cancer: a Gynecologic Oncology Group study. *N Engl J Med* 334:1–6, 1996.

85. Albert DS, Liu PY, Hannigan EV, et al. Intraperitoneal cisplatin plus intravenous cyclophosphamide vs. intravenous cisplatin plus intravenous cyclophosphamide for Stage III ovarian cancer. *N Engl J Med* 335:1950–1955, 1996.

86. Sabbatini P, Spriggs D. Salvage therapy for ovarian cancer. *Oncology (Huntingt)* 12(6):833–843, 1998.

87. Dembo AJ. Abdominopelvic radiotherapy in ovarian cancer: a 10-year experience. *Cancer* 55:2285–2290, 1984.

88. Carey M, Dembo AJ, Fyles AW, Simm J. Testing the validity of a prognostic classification in patients with surgically optimal ovarian carcinoma: a 15-year review. *Int J Gynecol Cancer* 3:24, 1993.

89. Hammond R, Bull C, Houghton CRS, et al. Primary adjunctive whole abdominal radiotherapy in epithelial ovarian cancer: results of 10-years experience. *Aust N Z J Obstet Gynaecol* 32:267–269, 1992.

90. Bolis G. Colombo N, Pecorelli S, et al. Adjuvant treatment for early epithelial ovarian cancer: results of two randomised clinical trials comparing cisplatin to no further treatment or chromic phosphate (32P). *Ann Oncol* 6:887–893, 1995.

91. Vergote IB, Vergote-De Vos LN, et al. Randomized trial comparing cisplatin with radioactive phosphorus or whole abdomen irradiation as adjuvant treatment of ovarian cancer. *Cancer* 69:741–749, 1992.

92. Randall ME, Thomas GM. The role of radiation therapy in the management of ovarian cancer. In Gershenson DM, McGuire WP (eds), *Controversies in the Management of Ovarian Cancer*. New York: Churchill Livingstone, 1996.

93. Seidman JD, Kurman RJ. Subclassification of serous borderline tumors of the ovary into benign and malignant types. *Am J Surg Pathol* 20(11):1331–1345, 1996.

94. Kurman RJ, Trimble CL. The behavior of serous tumors of low malignant potential: Are they every malignant? *Int J Gynecol Pathol* 12:120–127, 1993.

95. Gotlieb WH, Flikker S, Davidson B, et al. Borderline tumors of the ovary: fertility treatment, conservative management, and pregnancy outcome. *Cancer* 82(1):141–146, 1998.

96. Loehrer PJ Sr, Johnson D, Elson P, et al. Importance of bleomycin in favorable-prognosis disseminated germ cell tumors: an Eastern Cooperative Oncology Group trial. *J Clin Oncol* 13:470–476, 1995.

97. Berkowitz RS, Goldstein DP. Chorionic tumors. *N Engl J Med* 335:1740–1748, 1996.

98. Hancock BW, Newlands ES, Berkowitz RS (eds). *Gestational Trophoblastic Disease*. London: Chapman & Hall Medical, 1997.

99. Soper JT, Evans AC, Clarke-Pearson DL, et al. Alternating weekly chemotherapy with etoposide-methotrexate-dactinomycin/cyclophosphamide-vincristine for high-risk gestational trophoblastic disease. *Obstet Gynecol* 83:113–117, 1994.

20

Hodgkin's Disease and the Non-Hodgkin's Lymphomas

■ ■ ■

Bruce D. Cheson

DIFFERENTIAL DIAGNOSIS

The malignant lymphomas, Hodgkin's disease (HD) or non-Hodgkin's lymphomas (NHLs), should be considered in the differential diagnosis of persistent, unexplained lymphadenopathy. The size of a normal node varies somewhat with location, but, in general, is about 1 cm in the longest axis [1–5]. After other causes, such as infection or inflammation are ruled out, a biopsy is often needed to exclude the possibility of a malignancy, such as lymphoma. Additional symptoms that might suggest the presence of lymphoma include fevers, chills, night sweats, unexplained weight loss and, particularly in Hodgkin's disease, pruritus, or ethanol-induced pain in the nodal area.

HODGKIN'S DISEASE
Clinical Presentation

HD is distinguished from NHL on the basis of its epidemiology, pathology, orderly anatomic progression of nodal involvement, response to therapy, and outcome. It generally presents as painless lymphadenopathy. Accompanying constitutional symptoms may include fevers, night sweats, chills, and weight loss, as well as pruritus and pain in a lymph node bearing area associated with the consumption of alcohol. Laboratory findings tend to be non-specific such as a mild lymphocytosis, eosinophilia, and an elevated erythrocyte sedimentation rate (ESR).

Epidemiology

HD accounts for 14% of lymphomas, with an estimated 7,400 new cases predicted in 2000 [6]. The etiology of HD is not known. There are no clear relationships with environmental exposures, although an increase has been reported in wood workers, farmers, and meat workers. The inflammatory appearance of the pathology has suggested an infectious origin, but no specific pathogen has been identified. The best candidate is Epstein-Barr virus (EBV). People with a history of infectious mononucleosis have a threefold chance of developing HD and approximately half of all HD nodes show evidence of EBV DNA in the genome of the Reed-Sternberg (R-S) cell. However, many patients with HD do not show any evidence of EBV incorporation or evidence of having had infectious mononucleosis. There appears to be an increased frequency in patients with acquired immunodeficiency syndrome (AIDS) and following bone marrow transplantation (BMT) [7–10]. In patients with human immunodeficiency virus (HIV)/AIDS, the HD tends to involve extra nodal sites and to exhibit an aggressive clinical course with a poor outcome.

Diagnosis

An excisional biopsy is required to make the pathologic diagnosis of HD. A needle aspiration or core biopsy may be useful to document recurrent disease, but may give false-negative information due to sampling error. The distinctive cell in HD is the classic R-S cell, a multinucleate giant cell characterized by abundant eosinophilic cytoplasm and large blue nucleoli, giving an "owl eye" appearance. In patients with coexisting HD and NHL, not only have immunoglobulin heavy chain gene rearrangements been demonstrated in the R-S cells, but the same monoclonal gene rearrangement was found in both lymphomas. Thus, the cells from both tumors appear to be derived from a common precursor B-cell [11, 12].

Classification

From 1965 to 1994 HD was classified according to the Rye classification. The Revised European American Lymphoma (REAL) Classification retained the four distinct histologic subtypes of the Rye Classification, along with a provisional category of lymphocyte-rich classical HD, and another for unclassifiable cases. The World Health Organization (WHO) classification recommended changing the name to Hodgkin's lymphoma and proposed the following categories: nodular lymphocyte predominant Hodgkin's lymphoma and Classical Hodgkin's lymphoma [13] (Table 20.1). The latter is

Table 20.1 Proposed World Health Organization Classification of Hodgkin's Disease (Lymphoma)

Nodular lymphocyte-predominant Hodgkin's lymphoma

Classical Hodgkin's lymphoma
Nodular sclerosis Hodgkin's lymphoma (grades 1 and 2)
Lymphocyte-rich classical Hodgkin's lymphoma
Mixed cellularity Hodgkin's lymphoma
Lymphocyte depletion Hodgkin's lymphoma

subdivided into nodular sclerosis (NS) HD, lymphocyte-rich classical (LRC) HD, mixed cellularity (MC) HD, and lymphocyte depletion (LD) HD.

Nodular lymphocyte predominant (LP) HD accounts for only 3–8% of cases of HD. It generally exhibits a nodular growth pattern, with or without diffuse areas, and R-S cells are rare. The atypical lymphocytic and histiocytic cells are often numerous, and are called "popcorn" cells. These cells express B-cell antigens such as CD20, and rarely CD15 or CD30, and are negative for soluble immunoglobulin and CD45. LPHD is more common in adults than children, with more males than females, with a young median age (34 years). It is clinically distinct from the other histologies [14]. LPHD is more often localized than disseminated at diagnosis (> 70% stages I or II), exhibits a slowly progressive course, and has an extremely favorable outcome. Mediastinal masses are noted in fewer than 20% of cases. Although survival tends to be long, late relapses are more common than in other histologies, and may progress to a large B-cell NHL in 3% of patients.

The findings with LRCHD are similar to LPHD except for a slightly older age at presentation (40 years) and more frequent mediastinal mass. Late relapses are less common, but more often fatal. Some investigators have recommended a "watch and wait" policy for the approach to these patients. However, because of the young median age of the patients, others have suggested early intervention, and careful selection of treatment to reduce late complications.

More than 60% of patients present with the NS subtype, which is most common in females, adolescents, and young adults. They characteristically present with a mediastinal mass that may be symptomatic. The histologic pattern of NS is at least partially nodular with fibrous bands; diffuse areas may be present as well as necrosis. The characteristic R-S cell in NSHD is the lacunar variant, a giant cell with a multilobulated nucleus, but with less prominent nucleoli than the "classical" R-S cell. Following fixations of these cells with formalin, there is a contraction of the cytoplasm so that the cell is surrounded by a clear space, which gives the impression that the cell is within a lacuna. The tumor cells are CD30+, CD15+/-, and CD45-.

MCHD is less common than NSHD, occurring in 20–40% of cases, and more often in males. The histologic appearance is of a diffuse or vaguely nodular infiltrate. R-S cells are primarily of the classical variety. The cells are CD30+, CD15+/-, and CD45-. Unlike the other histologic subtypes, EBV genomic DNA is detectable in 60–70%. The clinical course may be aggressive, but still curable, and the outcome is comparable to that of NSHD.

Lymphocyte depletion HD accounts for 3% of cases of HD, making it the least common histologic type. It occurs more often in older males, those who are HIV+, and in nonindustrialized countries. Patients present with abdominal adenopathy, but with less peripheral adenopathy. Hepatosplenomegaly may be prominent, and the bone marrow is often infiltrated. The histologic appearance of the lymph nodes is characterized by a diffuse infiltrate that may appear hypocellular. R-S cells are plentiful and may have a bizarre, malignant appearance. They are CD30+, CD15+/-, and CD45-. The clinical course appears similar to the other types.

Staging

The four-stage clinical and pathologic Ann Arbor system has been most widely used for more than 25 years (Table 20.2). The stages fall into two groups with respect to survival; a favorable group that includes stages I, II, and IIIA, and a less favorable group of stages IIIB and IV. The disease-specific survival at 15 years is 96% for the former and 80% for the latter, with overall survival rates of 80% and 60%, respectively.

In 1989, the Cotswolds staging system was developed to emphasize the unfavorable prognostic impact of tumor bulk (> 10 cm or a mediastinal mass > 1/3 the transverse diameter of the chest at T5,6), which was recognized with the designation "X" [15].

To determine the extent of involvement, staging should include a chest radiograph, chest, abdominal, and pelvic computed tomography (CT) scans, and a single photon emission (SPECT) gallium scan. Although bipedal lymphangiograms may provide valuable information about lymph node architecture, this radiographic procedure is being done less frequently and too few radiologists are sufficiently expert with their interpretation to recommend this test for general use. In ad-

Table 20.2 Ann Arbor Staging System for Hodgkin's Lymphoma

Stage	Substage	Definition
I	I	Single node region
	IE	Single extralymphatic site or involvement by direct extension
II	II	Two or more node regions on same side of diaphragm
	IIE	Single node region plus single localized extranodal site
	IIS	Spleen
	IIES	Extralymphatic site plus spleen
III	III	Involvement on both sides of diaphragm
IV	IV	Diffuse extralymphatic involvement
A		No constitutional symptoms
B		Fevers, chills, night sweats, or weight loss

dition, positron emission tomography (PET) scans are being widely studied and compared with magnetic resonance imaging (MRI) and CT scans to define abnormal lymph nodes for staging. A bone marrow biopsy can be reserved for patients with CSIII-IV or stage II with adverse features such as fever, weight loss > 10%, and night sweats. However, the presence or absence of bone marrow involvement in a patient who otherwise has stage IV disease does not further affect prognosis. Staging laparotomy with splenectomy is usually not indicated in the current management of patients with HD, particularly if systemic therapy is planned or if the proposed treatment program will not be changed as the result of laparotomy findings. However, if laparotomy is being considered, vaccination with polyvalent pneumococcal vaccine should be administered about two weeks prior to the procedure because the absence of the spleen increases the risk of infections with encapsulated bacteria [16]. The efficacy of vaccination is reduced in the setting of subsequent chemotherapy for the disease [17].

An international prognostic system has recently been published that identified seven risk factors that could be used to predict outcome [18]: albumin < 4 g/liter, hemoglobin < 10.5 g/liter, male gender, age ≥ 45 years, stage IV disease, leukocytosis ≥ 15,000 × 10^9/liter, and lymphocytopenia < 0.6 × 10^9/liter or < 8% of the leukocyte count. The expected five-year survival correlated with the number of factors: 84% with none, 77% with one, 67% with two, 60% with three, 51% with four, and 42% with five or more.

Treatment

HD represents one of the major success stories of modern oncology. Most patients, even those with advanced stage disease, are curable with standard or intensive therapy.

EARLY STAGE DISEASE

Radiation therapy (RT) has been the standard approach for patients with non-bulky IA/IIA. RT achieves complete remissions (CRs) in more than 95% of patients with limited disease, and the failure-free survival and overall survival rates beyond 20 years are 75% and greater than 90%, respectively. For those patients with a very favorable presentation (e.g., stage IA, females less than 26 years of age with IIA, high neck nodes only, LP or NS histology, an ESR < 40 mm/hr, no bulky or extra nodal disease), a mantle field may be sufficient (Figure 1) [19]. Approximately 30–50% of those with pathologic stage (PS) IB or PS IIB disease treated with RT will relapse; however, 50–80% of those who relapse will subsequently achieve a durable CR with chemotherapy. Chemotherapy appears to be required for patients with additional unfavorable clinical features (e.g., B symptoms, III$_1$A, massive disease, ≥ 4 sites of involvement, extra nodal disease).

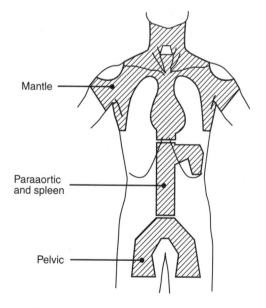

Figure 20.1. Diagram of the mantle and inverted-Y fields used in total lymphoid irradiation of Hodgkin's disease. (Reprinted with permission of the BMJ publishing group from *Calif Med* 113:23–38, 1970.

Because of the complications of staging laparotomy (surgical morbidity and mortality, post-splenectomy sepsis), and long-term toxicities from RT, the approach to limited-stage patients is currently being reassessed. There is an increasing tendency to eliminate surgery and treat with RT and/or chemotherapy in early stage patients. Newer, more effective, and less toxic chemotherapy regimens may be associated with a lower risk of sterility by reducing the cumulative doses of alkylating agents and avoiding unnecessary radiation to the pelvis. In lower risk patients, total lymphoid irradiation is being compared with attenuated courses of chemotherapy combined with involved field radiation. In higher risk patients, particularly those with bulky disease, doxorubicin (Adriamycin®), bleomycin, vinblastine, dacarbazine (ABVD) has been compared with the Stanford V regimen [20], followed by irradiation to sites of bulky disease.

The presence of bulky mediastinal or retroperitoneal tumor predicts a poor outcome following single modality therapy, even in patients with limited stage disease. For example, patients with stage IIX HD have a 50–75% chance of relapsing after RT alone and 40% following CT alone. Uncontrolled trials suggest that salvage with chemotherapy in radiation therapy failures is successful in only 50–80% of cases. Studies evaluating the combination of RT with the regimen of nitrogen mustard (Mustargen®), vincristine (Oncovin®), procarbazine, and prednisone (MOPP) demonstrated a disease-free survival of 75% at 10 years, which is longer than expected with either therapy alone; however, overall survival was compromised because of the occurrence of late complications related to MOPP such as acute myelocytic leukemia (AML) [21]. In an Italian study [22], patients were randomized to receive three cycles of either MOPP or ABVD followed by extended field RT, followed by three additional courses of chemotherapy. The CR rate, freedom from progression, relapse-free survival, and overall survival favored ABVD; moreover, only gonadal dysfunction and AML occurred in MOPP-treated patients. Anthracycline-based regimens have replaced MOPP, and the risks of secondary malignancies from the combined modality approach are minimal. However, the risk of cardiotoxicity is greater in the setting of mediastinal irradiation. Combined modality therapy is considered the standard approach for patients with massive mediastinal disease.

Approximately 80% of patients with bulky mediastinal or retroperitoneal disease who respond to therapy have a persistent radiographic abnormality that may remain beyond a year in half of those cases, without evidence of disease progression. The residual mass generally represents fibrotic tumor since these patients tend to do as well as those with a clinical CR. Patients are classified as having an unconfirmed complete remission (CR$_u$) if they have a stable residual mass persisting longer than one month following completion of radiation therapy, or more than two courses beyond maximum response to chemotherapy. A gallium scan may be useful to discriminate between fibrosis and active disease in patients whose tumor was gallium avid prior to treatment. These patients should not receive additional therapy until clear evidence of active disease. In some patients, notably those < 25 years of age, a mediastinal radiographic density may actually increase within six months following therapy. This finding may represent regenerating thymus and can be confused with progressing disease. This tissue binds gallium and, therefore, presents a diagnostic dilemma. These patients should be observed carefully with chest radiographs, but without intervention. Confirmatory re-biopsy and therapy may be indicated if the mass continues to enlarge or if disease becomes apparent outside of the radiated field. A positive PET scan may also provide evidence to differentiate residual tumor from fibrosis [23].

The optimal treatment for patients with stage IIIA disease remains controversial. Options include subtotal nodal or total nodal irradiation, or chemotherapy with a regimen such as ABVD followed by RT to previous sites of bulky disease. Combined modality appears to achieve improved relapse-free survival compared with RT alone, although whether it is superior to chemotherapy alone has not been determined.

CHEMOTHERAPY FOR ADVANCED DISEASE

Patients with stage IIIB-IV disease require combination chemotherapy for possible cure. MOPP was the standard regimen for two decades with CR rates ranging from 69% to 80% and almost half of patients relapse-free at eight years [24, 25]. Because MOPP was associated with major complications (e.g., sterility, secondary malignancies), and since most patients were not cured with this regimen, other programs were developed. The first such regimen to become popular was MOPP/ABVD, which was subsequently followed by a series of other anthracycline-based regimens (e.g., ABVD, MOPP/ABV hybrid) [26, 27]. Each of these induced CRs in 81–89% of patients with a disease-free survival of 75–80% at eight years. In several large randomized trials of untreated patients with advanced disease, ABVD-derived regimens (ABVD, MOPP/ABVD, MOPP/ABV

hybrid) induced a higher CR rate than MOPP, with longer disease-free survival, overall survival, and freedom from tumor mortality [28]. ABVD was subsequently compared with MOPP/ABV. Response rates were comparable, but toxicity, notably secondary malignancies, occurred less often with ABVD. Therefore, ABVD is now considered the standard regimen for advanced HD [29] Promising results have been reported with a standard or escalated bleomycin, etoposide, doxorubicin, cyclophosphamide, vincristine, procarbazine, and prednisone (BEACOPP) program, which showed improved failure free survival compared with cyclophosphamide, vincristine, procarbazine, and prednisone (COPP)/ABVD [30] (Table 20.3).

Radiotherapy to sites of residual disease can convert most partial responders to CRs. When used as consolidation to prior bulky disease, this approach may prolong disease-free survival in those sites, however it may not impact on the overall survival of patients with stage IV disease.

Table 20.3   Chemotherapy Regimens for Hodgkin's Disease

ABVD

Doxorubicin	25 mg/m² iv days 1 and 15
Bleomycin	10 mg/m² iv days 1 and 15
Vinblastine	6 mg/m² iv days 1 and 15
Dacarbazine	375 mg/m² days 1 and 15
Six 28-day cycles	

Stanford V

Doxorubicin	25 mg/m² iv days 1 and 15
Vinblastine	6 mg/m² iv days 1 and 15
Mechlorethamine	6 mg/m² iv day 1
Vincristine	1.4 mg/m² (maximum 2.0 mg) iv days 8 and 22
Bleomycin	5 U/m² iv days 8 and 22
Etoposide	60 mg/m² iv days 15 and 16
Prednisone	40 mg/m² po qid
Three 28-day cycles	

BEACOPP

Bleomycin	10 mg/m² iv day 8
Etoposide	100 (200) mg/m² iv days 1–3
Doxorubicin	25 (35) mg/m² iv day 1
Cyclophosphamide	650 (1,200) mg/m² iv day 1
Vincristine	1.4 mg/m² (maximum 2 mg) iv day 8
Procarbazine	100 mg/m² po days 1–7
Prednisone	100 mg/m² po days 1–7
Eight 21-day cycles	

Numbers in parentheses are escalated BEACOPP that is supported by granulocytecolony-stimulating factor. iv = intravenous; po = per os (orally); qid = four times a day.

RELAPSED/REFRACTORY DISEASE

Although HD is a relatively curable disease, 20–30% of patients never achieve a complete or partial remission (PR), and another 20–30% relapse following an initial CR. The type of initial therapy and the duration of the initial response play a major role in determining the appropriate second-line program. Patients who relapse following RT can anticipate a 50–80% likelihood of long-term disease-free survival when treated with ABVD.

Late relapses (> 12 months) from a CR or a durable PR may be successfully treated with combination chemotherapy; about 15% remain in remission at five years. Unfortunately, the outcome for patients with an early relapse from CR following MOPP, ABVD, or MOPP/ABVD is poor.

Patients who relapse but remain chemotherapy-sensitive should be considered for high-dose therapy with autologous bone marrow or peripheral blood stem cell support. This approach has been associated with a 20–40% five-year relapse-free survival. Treatment outcome will vary with prognostic factors such as performance status, number of prior chemotherapy regimens, and tumor bulk. The role of high-dose chemotherapy with autologous stem cell support as part of initial treatment in high-risk patients is being evaluated.

Data from the International Bone Marrow Transplant Registry showed that the use of allogeneic BMT in refractory patients was associated with a poor outcome and excessive treatment-related morbidity and mortality [31].

Single-agent vinblastine has proven to be an effective palliative agent for patients with relapsed HD, even after failing an autologous stem cell transplant. Gemcitabine has produced a high response rate in a small series of patients with relapsed or refractory disease and is under further study.

COMPLICATIONS OF THERAPY

Toxicities from chemotherapy depend on the specific drugs used. MOPP produces infertility that is almost universal in men, and occurs in at least 80% of women over the age of 25. This toxicity may be reversible after up to three courses of therapy. The risk of infertility is markedly lower with the newer, non-alkylating agent-containing regimens. Nevertheless, sperm banking should be considered in appropriate men prior to treatment. Pregnancies occurring in patients or their partners do not appear to be associated with an increase in complications, spontaneous abortions, or congenital abnormalities.

MOPP has also been associated with secondary AML and myelodysplasia in 3–10% of patients as early as two years following treatment, and the risk exists until approximately 11 years, after which new cases are uncommon. The risk of AML appears to be related to the cumulative dose of alkylating agents and may be enhanced by RT. RT alone is generally not associated with secondary leukemia. AML does not appear to complicate ABVD or similar regimens. Diffuse aggressive NHLs occur with a cumulative risk of 4–5% at 10 years. The frequency of solid tumors increases from 2% at 10 years to 13% at 19 years, with RT, with or without chemotherapy the major contributor to cancers in the irradiated field (e.g., lung cancer, breast cancer, soft-tissue sarcomas, melanomas). These breast cancers are more often bilateral than in women with primary breast cancer. Regular breast examination and mammography starting at an early age are recommended as part of routine management following therapy for HD [32, 33].

More than two-thirds of patients who undergo mantle irradiation will develop thyroid disease, including hypothyroidism, Graves' disease, silent thyrotoxicosis, and nodules, with a 2% risk of cancer. Myelosuppression as a result of radiation therapy correlates with the amount of irradiated bone marrow. Regimens such as vinblastine, bleomycin, and methotrexate (VBM) and Stanford V are associated with an increased risk of pulmonary and cardiac complications. The addition of mantle field irradiation adds to the risk of cardiac toxicity.

NON-HODGKIN'S LYMPHOMAS
Epidemiology

NHLs represent the fifth most common tumor type diagnosed in men in the U.S. each year and the sixth in women, with approximately 54,900 new cases predicted in the U.S. in 2000 [6], and is the fifth and sixth leading cause of cancer deaths in men and women, respectively. The frequency of NHL increased at an epidemic rate of almost 7% a year during the last two decades, for reasons that have yet to be identified. Most recently, this rate of rise has become level or decreased. This increased incidence is most striking in elderly persons and is primarily in the diffuse, large B-cell histology.

The median age for the lymphomas varies with the histologic subtype; e.g., 65 years for small lymphocytic lymphoma, 64 years for diffuse large B-cell lymphoma, 59 years for follicular NHL, 35 years for primary mediastinal large B-cell lymphoma, 31 years for Burkitt's lymphoma, and 28 years for lymphoblastic lymphoma [34].

Etiology

For most patients with NHL, the etiology is unknown. However, there is a striking increase in the frequency of aggressive NHL in patients who are taking long-term immunosuppressive agents, following allogeneic BMT, with inherited immune defects, rheumatoid arthritis, or with HIV/AIDS. There is also an association between a variety of infectious agents and the occurrence of lymphomas: human herpes virus-8 with body cavity lymphoma and multiple myeloma; hepatitis C and immunocytoma; human T-cell lymphotropic virus-1 (HTLV-1) and adult T-cell leukemia/lymphoma; *Helicobacter pylori* and gastric mucosa-associated lymphoid tissue (MALT) lymphomas; intestinal bacterial pathogens and Mediterranean lymphomas [35–44]. However, these disorders represent only a small fraction of lymphomas. Reports of an association with environmental factors such as pesticides and agricultural chemicals, exercise, smoking, and hair dyes, and others are not conclusively associated since their use is not increasing in conjunction with the increasing frequency of lymphomas [45–54].

Pathogenesis

Research into the molecular biology of NHL has identified clues as to the pathogenesis of these disorders. For example, the t(14;18) is detectable in 80–90% of patients with follicular NHL, and the BCL2 gene has been cloned at that breakpoint. Overexpression of this gene prevents apoptosis, or programmed cell death. Even when this translocation cannot be identified, the gene is overexpressed through unclear mechanisms [55]. The BCL1 gene is overexpressed in patients with mantle cell lymphoma, with overproduction of cyclin D1, which has been implicated in the development of this specific lymphoma (Table 20.4).

Diagnosis

Most patients with NHL present with signs or symptoms referable to lymphadenopathy. However, there are numerous infectious and inflammatory causes of enlarged nodes, as well as non-lymphomatous tumors. The initial diagnosis of NHL usually requires an excisional lymph node biopsy for precise classification. Problems with needle biopsies can be anticipated in distinguishing nodular versus diffuse histologies, in lesions with substantial fibrosis or sclerosis, in cases of T-cell NHL or T-

Table 20.4 Chromosome Translocations: Mechanism of Oncogene Activation in B-Cell Malignancies

Oncogene	Translocation	Protein	Disease
bcl-1	t(11;14)	Cyclin D1	Mantle cell lymphoma
bcl-2	t(14;18)	bcl-2	Follicular NHL (some diffuse)
bcl-3	t(14;19)	Rel/NF kappa B inhibitor	CLL/SLL
bcl-6	t(3;14)	Zinc-finger transcription factor	Diffuse large B-cell (some follicular)
bcl-10	t(1;14)	CARD	MALT
ALK	t(2;5)	ALK	Anaplastic large cell

NHL = non-Hodgkin's lymphoma; CLL = chronic lymphocytic leukemia; SLL = small lymphocytic leukemia; CARD = caspase recruitment domain; MALT = mucosa-associated lymphoid tissue; ALK = anaplastic lymphoma kinase.

cell-rich B-cell NHL, or in lymph nodes only partially involved with lymphoma. An aspirate or core needle biopsy may be sufficient to confirm a suspected recurrence in patients with previously diagnosed disease. With the increased use of flow cytometry, cytogenetics, and molecular genetic studies, information obtained from analysis of a core needle and (in some instances) fine-needle biopsies can make the diagnosis when dealing with a lymphoma in the mediastinal, retroperitoneal, or other inaccessible locations.

Classification

There have been several attempts at classifying the malignant lymphomas during the past century. In 1982, the National Cancer Institute (NCI) Working Formulation was adopted to facilitate communication among investigators, although the Kiel classification was still widely used in Europe. Unfortunately, there were a number of problems with the Working Formulation: first, it was not clinically useful. Second, although the various histologies were divided into low-, intermediate-, and high-grade tumors, several lymphomas were in inappropriate categories. Furthermore, a number of important, newly recognized entities did not fit into this classification, and, importantly, the Working Formulation was not designed to incorporate what was being learned about the immunology and genetics of these disorders.

The first recent major advance in the classification of the lymphomas was published in 1994 by the International Lymphoma Study Group as the REAL Classification [56]. The REAL classification attempted to use morphology, immunophenotype, and genetic as well as clinical features to distinguish the various entities. After three years of experience using the REAL classification, the WHO Classification was developed [13], making minor modifications in nomenclature, division of categories, and adoption of entities that had been considered provisional (Table 20.5).

Clinical Staging

The Ann Arbor staging (Table 20.2) is also used for the NHLs, but is less relevant than in HD since the NHLs tend to exhibit hematogenous spread and are more often advanced at presentation. Staging for the NHLs requires a chest radiograph, chest, abdominal and pelvic CT scans, and an adequate (> 2 cm) bone marrow biopsy and aspirate. A number of other studies may be useful, but are not yet recommended for routine practice (e.g. MRI scans, molecular and cytogenetic studies). SPECT gallium scanning may be valuable in assessing response in aggressive NHL, but has limited value in the indolent tumors. Laparotomy is not part of routine staging for NHL.

Treatment

The current approach to the treatment of NHL varies with the stage and histologic subtype.

INDOLENT NHL

The indolent histologies include small lymphocytic leukemia (SLL), follicular grades I (formerly follicular small cleaved cell) and grade II (formerly follicular mixed), and the marginal zone NHL.

LIMITED STAGE DISEASE

Only about 10–15% of patients with grade I or II follicular NHL present with limited disease (stage I or non-bulky stage II disease). Radiation therapy can produce a 10-year failure-free survival of 50–60%, with an overall survival of 60–80%. However, whether even limited stage disease can be curable by radiation therapy with or without chemotherapy is unclear. Patients at Stanford University with stage I and II follicular NHL were

Table 20.5 Proposed World Health Organization Classification of Lymphoid Lymphomas

B-cell neoplasms
  Precursor B-cell neoplasm
    Precursor B-lymphoblastic leukemia/lymphoma
      (precursor B-cell acute lymphoblastic leukemia)
  Mature (peripheral) B-cell neoplasms
    B-cell chronic lymphocytic leukemia/small lymphocytic lymphoma
    B-cell prolymphocytic leukemia
    Lymphoplasmacytic lymphoma
    Splenic marginal zone B-cell lymphoma ± villous lymphocytes)
    Hairy cell leukemia
    Plasma cell myeloma/plasmacytoma
    Extranodal marginal zone B-cell lymphoma of MALT type
    Nodal marginal zone B-cell lymphoma (± monocytoid B cells)
    Follicular lymphoma
    Mantle-cell lymphoma
    Diffuse large B-cell lymphoma
      Mediastinal large B-cell lymphoma
      Primary effusion lymphoma
    Burkitt's lymphoma/Burkitt cell leukemia

T-cell and NK-cell neoplasms
  Precursor T-cell neoplasm
    Precursor T-lymphoblastic lymphoma/leukemia
      (precursor T-cell acute lymphoblastic leukemia)
  Mature (peripheral) T-cell neoplasms
    T-cell prolymphocytic leukemia
    T-cell granular lymphocytic leukemia
    Aggressive NK-cell leukemia
    Adult T-cell lymphoma/leukemia (HTLV-1+)
    Extranodal NK/T-cell lymphoma, nasal type
    Enteropathy-type T-cell lymphoma
    Hepatosplenic gamma-delta T-cell lymphoma
    Subcutaneous panniculitis-like T-cell lymphoma
    Mycosis fungoides/Sezary syndrome
    Anaplastic large-cell lymphoma, T/null cell, primary cutaneous type
    Peripheral T-cell lymphoma, not otherwise characterized
    Angioimmunoblastic T-cell lymphoma
    Anaplastic large-cell lymphoma, T/null cell, primary systemic type

MALT = mucosa-associated lymphoid tissue; NK = natural killer; HTLV = human T-cell lymphotropic virus.

treated with radiotherapy and followed for a median of 7.7 years (the longest being 31 years) [57]. The median survival was 13.8 years; however, more than 10% of patients relapsed after 10 or more years in remission.

ADVANCED STAGE DISEASE

The remaining 80–90% of patients with follicular small cleaved or follicular mixed (follicular grade I and II)

Table 20.6 Therapeutic Options for Treatment of Non-Hodgkin's Lymphoma

"Watch and Wait"
Single Alkylating Agent
Combination of Alkylating Agent-based Chemotherapy ± anthracycline
Radiation Therapy
Purine analogs or combinations
Stem Cell Transplant
Biological Approaches
    Monoclonal antibodies
    Interferon
    Antisense

present with advanced stage disease (bulky stage II, stages III and IV). The median time to progression of these patients is 4–6 years, with an overall survival of 6–10 years. Unfortunately, despite this relatively long natural history, these patients are incurable [58–60]. Using the International Prognostic Index (IPI) initially developed for aggressive NHL [61], the indolent NHLs can be divided into risk groups with markedly differing outcomes based on age, stage, performance status, serum levels of lactate dehydrogenase (LDH), and number of extra nodal sites [62]. However, there is no evidence that the IPI risk group can be used to effectively direct therapy. Other factors suggested to have prognostic importance include cytogenetics and p53 mutations.

Early intervention does not appear to prolong the survival of asymptomatic patients [63, 64]. Therefore, "watch and wait" is the conventional approach until therapy is indicated by the presence of increasing adenopathy, disease-related symptoms, organ compromise, or bone marrow failure.

Since patients with low-grade NHL are not curable, yet therapies are associated with toxicities, an important question is when to initiate treatment. Several studies looked at the role of early intervention in patients who are asymptomatic from their follicular NHL, but failed to detect any benefit [64, 65]. Since there is no apparent advantage to early intervention in patients with advanced stage disease, the decision to treat is generally based on the presence of increasing adenopathy, organ compromise, bone marrow failure, or constitutional symptoms.

When treatment is required, there are numerous standard therapeutic options including a single agent (alkylating agents such as cyclophosphamide or chlorambucil; fludarabine), alkylating agent-based combinations (e.g., cyclophosphamide, vincristine, prednisone [CVP]), more aggressive approaches (e.g., cyclophos-

phamide, doxorubicin, vincristine, prednisone [CHOP]), radiation therapy, or biological agents, with no clear evidence for a survival advantage of one treatment over the others (Table 20.6). The frequency of CRs with the same or different programs varies widely among series, reflecting differences in patient selection, and staging and evaluation techniques. Response assessment for the NHLs has recently been standardized to ensure comparability among studies [5]. Other intensive regimens have failed to demonstrate benefit over less intensive programs [58, 60, 66].

RELAPSED/REFRACTORY DISEASE

Patients with low grade NHL invariably relapse. Subsequent responses can often be achieved with the same or a similar regimen, but the quality and duration of response is poorer each time [59]. The median survival following relapse after an initial remission correlates with the quality of the original response: survival after relapse from a complete remissions of a year or longer lasts 5.9 years; 4.2 years after a PR of at least a year, but only 2.4 years for an initial response shorter than a year [67]. Whereas most patients recur with a similar histology, there is a constant risk for undergoing a transformation to a high grade NHL, which is generally considered an ominous event. However, if diagnosed and treated early, a small proportion of patients with transformed NHL may experience prolonged disease-free survival. A variety of aggressive combination regimens have been used to treat relapsed or refractory patients, with no evidence for a major advantage from any of them [68–70].

NEW APPROACHES

Over the past few years, two new classes of drugs, the purine analogs and monoclonal antibodies, have resulted in major shifts in the treatment paradigm for patients with indolent NHL. Of the purine analogs fludarabine, cladribine (2-chlorodeoxyadenosine [CdA]), and pentostatin (2'-deoxycoformycin [DCF]) (Table 20.7), fludarabine is the most widely used (Table 20.8). Responses to fludarabine occur in about half of patients with relapsed or refractory indolent NHL, including 10–15% complete remissions [71, 72]. Complete remissions occur in about 40% of patients initially treated with fludarabine, with an overall response rate of about 70% [73]. Single-agent response rates with cladribine appear comparable but less durable, and the data with pentostatin are limited [74–76].

Table 20.7 Summary of Purine Analog Therapy for Treatment of Indolent Non-Hodgkins Lymphoma

Agent	Patients	Prior Therapy	CR, % (range)	RR, % (range)
Fludarabine	279	Yes	12 (0–33)	45 (31–62)
	267	No	39 (38–39)	69 (66–76)
Cladribine	299	Yes	17 (13–38)	49 (43–76)
	156	No	21 (7–37)	72 (71–100)
Pentostatin	42	Yes	1 (0–29)	26 (17–42)

CR = complete remission; RR = response rate (CR plus partial response).

Table 20.8 Fludarabine Combinations for Follicular Non-Hodgkin's Lymphoma

FND Regimen

Fludarabine	25 mg/m²/day for 3 days
Mitoxantrone	10 mg/m² day 1
Dexamethasone	20 mg days 1–5
Trimethoprim	2 double-strength tablets
sulfamethoxazole	twice a week

Fludarabine-Cyclophosphamide

Fludarabine	20 mg/m² for 5 days
Cyclophosphamide	1,000 mg/m²/day

Several randomized studies have shown a higher response rates and longer responses with fludarabine compared with alkylating agents, although with no difference in overall survival [77, 78]. Another study suggested a survival advantage for an aggressive chemotherapy regimen including interferon instead of single-agent fludarabine; however, fludarabine was better tolerated [79].

Fludarabine exhibits an oral bioavailability of 55–60% and an oral formulation is currently in clinical trials [80]. Despite the high CR rate with fludarabine, relapse is inevitable, which has led to the development of combination regimens. One of the most effective is fludarabine, mitoxantrone, and dexamethasone (FND) [81], and this has produced an overall response rate of 94% including 47% complete remissions, in patients who have failed previous chemotherapy regimens, with the complete responses lasting a median of 21 months. Fludarabine plus mitoxantrone when used as initial treatment resulted in an overall response rate of 91% with 43% complete remissions; however, the disease-free survival was comparable to prior experience with CHOP and prednisone, methotrexate, doxorubicin, cyclophosphamide, and epipodophyllotoxin VP-16 (ProMACE)/MOPP [82]. In a study from the Eastern Cooperative Oncology Group (ECOG), cyclophosphamide and fludarabine resulted in 89% complete remissions and an overall response rate of 100% in patients without prior therapy [83]. The purine analogs have also shown impressive activity against Waldenström's macroglobulinemia [84–87].

Major side effects of fludarabine, CdA, and DCF include moderate myelosuppression, profound immunosuppression, and neurotoxicity [88, 89]. Febrile neutropenia occurs in about 20% of patients treated with fludarabine, and 30–50% of those treated with CdA. Primarily affected are CD4 cells, which decrease to levels encountered in patients with AIDS and may remain depressed for a year or longer following fludarabine and perhaps even longer following CdA or pentostatin. A consequence is an increased risk of opportunistic infections, which is worsened with concurrent steroids. Neither prophylactic antimicrobial therapy nor intravenous immunoglobulins are recommended as standard therapy because they are costly, potentially toxic, and cannot cover the range of possible organisms.

Other common side effects include tumor lysis syndrome [90]. Despite the prolonged immunosuppression, there does not appear to be an increased risk of secondary malignancies [91]. Nausea, vomiting, or alopecia are uncommon and generally not severe.

New drugs in clinical trials include the nucleoside analogs gemcitabine and compound 506U, the pro-drug for ara-G, protein kinase C inhibitors such as bryostatin, and the cyclin inhibitors flavopiridol and UCN-01.

BIOLOGICAL AGENTS

Monoclonal Antibodies

A new generation of monoclonal antibodies have markedly changed the current thinking about patients with follicular/low-grade NHL. Antibodies currently in clinical use or research studies are primarily unconjugated or linked to a radioisotope (Table 20.9). The first monoclonal antibody to be approved by the Food and Drug Administration for the treatment of a human malignancy is rituximab, which is chimeric and directed against CD20. In the pivotal trial including 166 patients who had failed prior treatment, four weekly infusions of rituximab were administered at a dose of 375 mg/m². The response rate was 48% with 6% CRs and a median time to progression of about a year [92]. The best results are in patients with a follicular histology; only 12% of patients with SLL respond with this regimen. Based on these results, rituximab has become a standard agent to treat patients with follicular low-grade NHL failing previous therapy. When used as the initial treatment,

Table 20.9 Monoclonal Antibodies for the Treatment of Indolent B-cell Non-Hodgkin's Lymphoma

Antibody Conjugate	Conjugate	Antigen
Rituximab (IDEC C2B8; Rituxan)*	None	CD20
CAMPATH-1H	None	CD52
Tositumomab (BEXXAR)	I-131	CD20
Ibritumomab (Y2B8; Zevalin)	Y-90	CD20
Epratuzumab	None, I-131, Y-90	CD22
Lym1	I-131	HLA-DR
Hu-1D10	None	HLA-DR

*Commercially available.

the response rate to rituximab has been reported to be 69% with 32% complete remissions [93]. Forty percent of patients who initially respond to the antibody but subsequently relapse may achieve a second durable response [94].

Promising results have been encountered incorporating this agent into chemotherapy combinations. In one study of CHOP plus rituximab including primarily untreated patients, the response rate was 100% including 63% complete remissions, most of which were durable [95]. These results have led to several national randomized trials looking at CHOP with and without the antibody in untreated patients to determine if there is, indeed, additive benefit from such combinations.

Rituximab is generally well tolerated with the major side effects being fevers and chills, although rare patients may experience a cytokine-release syndrome that can be life-threatening, but does not recur with subsequent doses of the drug. Rare fatalities have been encountered. Patients with high numbers of circulating malignant cells have been reported to experience a rapid tumor clearance syndrome.

CAMPATH-1H is an unconjugated anti-CD52 antibody with impressive activity in patients with chronic lymphocytic leukemia (CLL) and prolymphocytic leukemia; however, initial findings were not as encouraging in NHL [96].

Monoclonal antibodies conjugated to isotopes such as ^{131}I and ^{90}Y have provided promising results. Response rates with an ^{131}I anti-CD20 (tositumomab; BEXXAR) in patients with a relapsed or refractory indolent NHL have been greater than 70%, with about 30% complete remissions [97, 98] lasting a median of approximately nine months. This antibody has also been used at myeloablative doses with stem cell support [99]. An antibody conjugated with [90]Y (ibritumomab; Zevalin) has shown response rates greater than 80% in relapsed and refractory indolent NHL with 26% complete remissions [100]. The relative role of conjugated and unconjugated antibodies is under investigation.

Interferon (IFN)

Despite extensive study, the role for IFN in the treatment of indolent NHL remains unclear. Nine randomized trials were included in a meta-analysis of 1,756 newly diagnosed patients [101]. In studies using alkylating agent-based regimens, there was a lower response rate with IFN, a longer time to progression, but no improvement in survival. The four trials that included either an anthracycline or mitoxantrone showed no clear role for IFN in improving the response rate, but there was a 14% survival advantage with IFN at five years and 19% at eight years, although limited to CRs or PRs. However, a large Southwest Oncology Group (SWOG) study was not included in this analysis [102] in which 571 patients received ProMACE-MOPP, with involved field radiation to convert PRs to CRs, and responders were randomized to receive IFN or observation. There was no difference in progression-free survival (PFS) or overall survival. The explanation for this discrepancy is not clear but may reflect differences in prognostic factors or other factors.

OTHER BIOLOGICAL THERAPIES

New promising biological approaches in development include anti-idiotype vaccines [103, 104] and BCL-2 anti-sense oligonucleotide therapy [105].

Stem Cell Transplantation (SCT)

There are limited data available on the use of allogeneic BMT in indolent NHL because of the low likelihood of a donor, the greater morbidity and mortality from allogeneic compared with autologous SCT, and the relatively long natural history of the disease. In an analysis of the data from the International Bone Marrow Transplant Registry [106], there were 81 patients transplanted at a median age of 41 years; 56% had never achieved a complete remission. The projected survival at three years was 46%, with a 43% disease-free survival. The median follow-up time was only 23 months. However, the transplant-related mortality was 44%. Chemosensitivity prior to transplant was the strongest predictor of outcome.

The experience with autologous stem cell transplantation (ASCT) for low-grade NHL has generally been disappointing with little indication for a major impact on survival [107–109]. The most favorable results have been reported in highly selected cases [109]. This

Table 20.10   Outcome of Patients with Intermediate Grade Non-Hodgkin's Lymphoma According to the International Index Risk Group; International Index (n = 2,031)

Risk Group	Risk factors	Survival (%)		Patients (%)	CR Rate (%)	Relapse-free survival (%)	
		2-yr	5-yr			2-yr	5-yr
Low	0 or 1	84	73	35	87	79	70
Low intermediate		66	51	27	67	66	50
High intermediate		54	43	22	55	59	49
High	4 or 5	34	26	16	44	58	40

CR = complete remission.

therapy should only be performed on a clinical research trial.

Short-term and long-range complications of ASCT include treatment-related mortality, prolonged anemia or thrombocytopenia, and a markedly increased rate of secondary myelodysplasia and AML that ranges from 6.8% to 19% [110].

When BMT and ASCT are compared, the long-term survival figures are relatively comparable; ASCT is accompanied by a greater likelihood of dying from disease recurrence, whereas BMT results in a high frequency of death from graft-versus-host disease (GVHD), infection, and veno-occlusive disease. On the other hand, there may be some benefit from a moderate amount of GVHD in the form of graft-versus-lymphoma effect.

MARGINAL ZONE LYMPHOMAS

Marginal zone NHL (MZL) consists of mucosa-associated lymphoid tissue (MALT) NHL, monocytoid B-cell NHL, and primary splenic lymphoma with villous lymphocytes. These tumors are CD5-, CD10-, CD23-, and CD11c+/−. Trisomy 3 and t(11;18) have been reported in 60% of extra nodal cases. Other cytogenetic abnormalities have included translocations and abnormalities of 1p or 7. The MALT lymphomas are extra nodal tumors that affect the gastrointestinal and respiratory tracts, salivary glands, kidney, prostate, and other organs. Many patients have an associated autoimmune disease, such as Sjögren's syndrome or Hashimoto's thyroiditis. Unlike most indolent NHL, most patients with MZL present with stage I or II disease, although dissemination eventually occurs in one-third of patients, often to other extra nodal sites.

MALTomas account for about 80% of the indolent NHLs of the stomach, the majority of which occur in association with infection with *H. pylori*. MALTomas of the stomach are highly responsive to double or triple antibiotic therapy (e.g., omeprazole plus amoxicillin, or omeprazole, metronidazole, and clarithromycin) and prolonged remissions are common in more than 60% of patients. However, the MALTomas arising from or involving other sites appear to require systemic chemotherapy. Histologic follow-up of gastric MALTomas appears superior to analysis by the polymerase chain reaction.

The monocytoid B-cell NHLs are the nodal counterpart of the MALTomas. Dissemination may occur in extra nodal sites and may represent the nodal spread of MALT lymphomas.

Cells from splenic lymphoma with villous lymphocytes share phenotypic features of the other marginal zone NHLs; however, the cells have a distinct histologic appearance with cytoplasmic projections such that they are confused with hairy cell leukemia cells. Patients typically have peripheral blood and bone marrow involvement, and a massively enlarged spleen. Splenectomy may be accompanied by a prolonged clinical remission; however, systemic chemotherapy is eventually required in most patients. Anecdotal reports suggest activity with fludarabine and rituximab.

AGGRESSIVE LYMPHOMAS
Prognosis

The IPI is widely used to distinguish patients with an intermediate grade NHL into low, intermediate, high intermediate, and high risk groups [61] (Table 20.10). The parameters that were identified included an age more than 60 years, serum LDH levels greater than 1× normal, a performance status greater than 2, more than one extra nodal site, and tumor stage III/IV.

Other factors associated with a poor outcome include extensive bone marrow involvement, increased cellular expression of Ki-67, expression of the adhesion molecule CD44, chromosome abnormalities, and overexpression of BCL-2. Rearrangements of the BCL-6 gene are often associated with extranodal involvement and may be associated with a better outcome [111].

Therapy for Limited Disease

Approximately 20% of patients with an intermediate grade NHL present with limited disease (stage I and non-bulky stage II). Patients with clinical stage I disease have greater than an 80% likelihood of cure with either involved field or extended field irradiation radiation therapy. However, between one-third and half of those with stage II disease treated with RT alone eventually relapse. Several nonrandomized studies suggested that combining fewer courses of chemotherapy with radiation therapy could reduce toxicity with at least comparable efficacy. SWOG investigators randomized 401 patients to either eight courses of CHOP or three courses of CHOP followed by 4,000 cGy to all sites of initial disease, with a 5,500 cGy boost to sites of residual disease [112]. Overall survival was longer in the combination arm (five-year estimate of 82% versus 72%). There was no difference in PFS, which reflects, in part, an increased number of deaths (primarily cardiac) on the CHOP alone arm. The combined modality arm was also less toxic.

Therapy for Advanced Stage Disease

The first major progress in the treatment of advanced stage intermediate grade NHL came in the 1970s when doxorubicin was incorporated into combinations with other drugs to form regimens such as BACOP and CHOP. These programs induced complete remissions in 50–70% of patients with a projected plateau on the disease-free survival curve at about 30%. A number of second- and third-generation regimens were subsequently developed in an attempt to improve on the activity of CHOP (e.g., cyclophosphamide, doxorubicin, vincristine, bleomycin, dexamethasone, methotrexate, and leucovorin [m-BACOD]; methotrexate, leucovorin, doxorubicin, cyclophosphamide, vincristine, bleomycin, and prednisone [MACOP-B]; ProMACE-MOPP; and cyclophosphamide, doxorubicin, etoposide, prednisone, cytarabine, bleomycin, vincristine, methotrexate, and leucovorin [ProMACE-CytaBOM]) [113–116]. These combinations incorporated a number of additional agents; however, with a requisite reduction in the deliverable dose of the cyclophosphamide and doxorubicin [117]. Nevertheless, exciting preliminary results

with these regimens stimulated the conduct of several large randomized studies to compare the relative efficacy and toxicity of these regimens with CHOP. Fisher and his SWOG collaborators accrued more than a thousand patients with intermediate grade NHL to a trial that randomized patients to receive either CHOP, m-BACOD, ProMACE/CytaBOM, or MACOP-B [118]. There were no differences in CR rates, event-free or overall survival among the treatment arms, even when the various IPI subsets were examined. At three years, 44% of all patients were alive and free of disease (41% with CHOP and MACOP-B and 46% with ProMACE/CytaBOM and m-BACOD). Moreover, toxic deaths occurred in 1% of patients who received CHOP, 3% of those who received ProMACE/CytaBOM, 5% of those who received m-BACOD, and 6% of those who received MACOP-B. CHOP was both the least toxic and expensive of the combinations, and remains the standard chemotherapy regimen.

ANAPLASTIC LARGE CELL LYMPHOMA

Anaplastic large cell lymphoma (ALCL) (Ki-1, CD30+) is an aggressive lymphoma not included in the original Working Formulation. Because of its morphologic appearance, it has been confused with HD, anaplastic carcinoma, or melanoma. However, there are several distinct features of this tumor that facilitate classification. Most ALCL are of T-cell or null cell origin, with expression of CD30. The characteristic cytogenetic abnormality, t(2;5)(p23;q35) is associated with expression of a nucleoplasmin-anaplastic lymphoma kinase (NPM-ALK) protein. Expression of this protein has been associated with a favorable outcome [119]. ALCL is one of the more favorable histologies of the aggressive NHL. Combination chemotherapy regimens such as CHOP induce CRs in more than 70% of patients, and almost half are alive and free of disease at five years [120, 121].

MANTLE CELL LYMPHOMA

Mantle cell NHL (MCL) was not included as an independent category within the Working Formulation, but was spread out among the small lymphocytic, follicular small cleaved cell, and comprised most of the diffuse small cleaved cell NHLs. MCLs exhibit the worst features of lymphoma; like the indolent NHLs, they are not curable, yet they may have an aggressive clinical course. MCL comprises about 4–6% of NHL. The characteristic phenotype is that of a B cell, which, like CLL, coexpresses CD5. However, MCL does not express CD23, which is a feature of CLL, nor CD10, but soluble immunoglobulin is strongly expressed. MCLs are usually associated with t(11;14)(q13;q32), and overexpression of the cyclin D1 gene. MCL may present with diffuse bowel involvement (lymphomatous polyposis); transformation to large cell NHL does not appear to occur. Central nervous system involvement has been noted in almost 20% of the cases, but is generally asymptomatic. Complete remissions can be achieved in more than half of patients using aggressive combination chemotherapy, but responses are transient with a median survival of 2.5–3 years. Recent data with aggressive acute leukemia-like regimens with transplant have shown promising results [122].

RELAPSED/REFRACTORY DISEASE

Only 40% or fewer of CHOP-treated patients are cured. Of note is that 75–80% of recurrences occur within two years. Because patients who experience a late recurrence do so with a low-grade histology 10–25% of the time [123, 124], re-biopsy is necessary to plan appropriate treatment.

Unfortunately, the therapy of patients with relapsed/refractory disease remains inadequate. A number of combination salvage regimens have been studied, all with comparable results given differences in patient selection [69, 70, 125].

High-Dose Therapy with Stem Cell Support

High-dose chemotherapy (HDCT) with autologous stem cell support was first studied in patients with relapsed or refractory disease. Philip et al [126] reported that patients who received high-dose therapy at a time of sensitive relapse had a 36% likelihood of prolonged disease-free survival, compared with 15% of those in resistant relapse; no patients with primary refractory disease experienced benefit and all died within a year. These results were subsequently confirmed by the PARMA study [127] in which 215 patients in first or second relapse were treated with two courses of dexamethasone/high-dose cytarabine/cisplatin (DHAP) chemotherapy. The 109 who were sensitive were randomized to receive either four additional courses of DHAP chemotherapy followed by radiotherapy, or a course of DHAP followed by high-dose chemotherapy and stem cell support with or without involved field RT. Both PFS and overall survival were longer in the high-dose che-

motherapy arm. Thus, ASCT has become a standard approach for patients in sensitive relapse. The use of hematopoietic growth factors and peripheral blood progenitor cells has reduced the treatment-related morbidity and mortality.

HDCT has also been used to consolidate successful induction therapy. The French Groupe d'Etudes des Lymphomes de l'Adulte (GELA) group randomized 464 patients with at least one adverse prognostic factor by the IPI and who were in complete remission following aggressive primary chemotherapy to either high-dose chemotherapy or to a more conventional dose program. There was no difference in disease-free survival or overall survival. However, in a retrospective subset analysis, there was a prolongation of PFS and a trend toward a survival advantage for patients in the high and high intermediate risk groups by the IPI [128]. The outlook is poor for patients who relapse after autologous transplantation [129]. Compared with bone marrow-harvested stem cells, autologous peripheral blood stem cells reduce the number of platelet transfusions, time of platelet recovery, with a shorter duration of hospitalization, and are more cost-effective.

An international consensus conference reviewed the available data to determine the role of HDCT in various clinical situations [130]. They concluded that this approach was warranted in patients in first or subsequent relapse who were still chemosensitive, those with primary refractory disease (based on very limited data), and those in first remission who were IPI high-intermediate/high risk (but not the other IPI categories). They noted that the data did not support high-dose therapy in patients with untested or chemorefractory relapse. There were insufficient data to determine the value of the procedure in other situations.

Allogeneic BMT

Data on allogeneic BMT are quite limited in patients with refractory NHL and there are no data using this procedure as part of the initial approach to these patients. When autologous and allogeneic stem cell transplantation are compared, the long-term survival figures are relatively comparable; ASCT is accompanied be a greater likelihood of dying from disease recurrence, whereas BMT results in a high frequency of death from GVHD, infection, and veno-occlusive disease. On the other hand, there may be some benefit from a moderate amount of graft-versus-lymphoma effect.

Adoptive immunotherapy with donor leukocyte infusions may induce remissions in patients with chronic myelogenous leukemia, acute myelogenous leukemia, myelodysplasia, and multiple myeloma who have failed an allogenic BMT, although the role of this approach in NHL is not yet defined [131].

Biological Therapies

Responses have been observed in 32% of patients with large cell NHL using rituximab [132]. I^{131}-conjugated anti-CD20 antibody (BEXXAR) has also induced durable responses [99].

LYMPHOBLASTIC LYMPHOMAS

Lymphoblastic lymphomas (LLs) generally present with symptoms referable to a mediastinal mass. The distinction between LL and acute lymphoblastic leukemia is based on an arbitrary number of bone marrow lymphoblasts (generally with a 23–30% threshold). LDH, bone marrow, and central nervous system involvement have been used to separate patients into low- and high-risk populations [133]. Complete remissions can be achieved in more than 90% of patients with low-risk disease using an aggressive, multi-agent chemotherapy regimen, with more than 80% cured; relapses rarely occurring after a year. In contrast, whereas CRs can be achieved in the majority of patients with high-risk disease, the five-year survival rate is only 20%, and these patients are suitable candidates for investigational therapy. Results with ASCT in second CR are better than with other salvage approaches; however, only 15% experience long-term survival if transplanted with resistant disease, compared with 63% in first CR and 31% second CR. The role of high-dose therapy in first CR remains to be demonstrated.

BURKITT'S LYMPHOMA AND BURKITT'S-LIKE LYMPHOMA

Diffuse small non-cleaved cell NHL, Burkitt's and non-Burkitt's types, account for less than 3% of diffuse lymphomas in adults in North America. They are generally considered to be a highly aggressive tumor. Although there are differences in morphology, biology, immunology, and molecular genetics between the Burkitt's and non-Burkitt's types, they respond to treatment in a similar fashion. Treatment usually involves intensive acute lymphocytic leukemia (ALL)-like therapy with central nervous system prophylaxis. The CR

rate is 85–95%, with 47% failure-free survival at five years. Involvement of the central nervous system and/or bone marrow is largely responsible for the poor outlook of this patient group. Adults treated on a series of aggressive chemotherapy, consolidation, and maintenance, as well as central nervous system prophylaxis, showed three-year survival rates of 74%; 100% for stages I and II, 80% for stage III, and 57% for stage IV or with ALL [134].

These lymphomas are characterized by a rapid growth rate and treatment may be associated with the potentially fatal complication of tumor lysis syndrome, with renal failure, hyperuricemia, and hyperkalemia. All biochemical abnormalities should be corrected rapidly (within 1–2 days) prior to treatment, and patients should receive allopurinol, hydration, and an alkaline diuresis.

For patients who relapse after initial therapy, high-dose chemotherapy with stem cell support appears to be associated with a superior outcome compared with standard regimens, especially when transplanted in chemosensitive relapse.

PERIPHERAL T-CELL NHL

The term PTCL encompasses a diverse group of post-thymic T-cell tumors that have in common a mature T cell phenotype [135]. They comprise fewer than 10% of NHL in the United States. These entities primarily include PTCL otherwise unspecified, which accounts for more than half the cases, ALCL, angioimmunoblastic T-cell lymphoma, angiocentric lymphoma, adult T-cell leukemia/lymphoma, and a few less common entities. These patients generally present with advanced stage disease and B symptoms. The prognosis for patients with PTCL is inferior to their B-cell counterparts. Patients tend to have higher IPI scores, B symptoms, advanced stage, and high serum levels of β2-microglobulin. In general, patients with PTCL are treated with aggressive multi-agent chemotherapy (e.g., CHOP), similar to the aggressive B cell malignancies. However, they exhibit a poor response to treatment and a high rate of relapse, with no sustained remissions.

REFERENCES

1. Glazer GM, Gross BH, et al. Normal mediastinal lymph nodes: number and size according to American Thoracic Society mapping. *AJR Am J Roentgenol* 144:261–265, 1985.

2. Dorfman RE, Alpern MB, Gross BH, Sandler MA. Upper abdominal lymph nodes: criteria for normal size determined with CT. *Radiology* 180:319–322, 1991.

3. Einstein DM, Singer AA, Chilcote WA, Desai RK. Abdominal lymphadenopathy: spectrum of CT findings. *Radiographics* 11:457–472, 1991.

4. Hopper KD, Kasales CJ, Van Slyke MA, et al. Analysis of interobserver and intraobserver variability in CT tumor measurements. *AJR Am J Roentgenol* 187:851–854, 1996.

5. Cheson BD, Horning SJ, Coiffier B, et al. Report of an International Workshop to standardize response criteria for non-Hodgkin's lymphomas. *J Clin Oncol* 17:1244–1253, 1999.

6. Greenlee RT, Murray T, Bolden S, Wingo PA. Cancer statistics, 2000. *CA Cancer J Clin* 50:7–33, 2000.

7. McCunney RJ. Hodgkin's disease, work, and the environment. A review. *J Occup Environ Med* 41:36–46, 1999.

8. Khuder SA, Mutgi AB, Schaub EA, Tano BD. Meta-analysis of Hodgkin's disease among farmers. *Scand J Work Environ Health* 25:436–441, 1999.

9. Spina M, Sandri S, Tirelli U. Hodgkin's disease in HIV-infected individuals. *Curr Opin Oncol* 11:522–526, 1999.

10. Rowlings PA, Curtis RE, Passweg JR, et al. Increased incidence of Hodgkin's disease after allogeneic bone marrow transplantation. *J Clin Oncol* 17:3122–3127, 1999.

11. Brauninger A, Hansmann ML, Strickler JG, et al. Identification of common germinal- center B-cell precursors in two patients with both Hodgkin's disease and non-Hodgkin's lymphoma. *New Engl J Med* 340:1239–1247, 1999.

12. Marafioti T, Hummel M, Anagnostopoulos I, et al, Classical Hodgkin's disease and follicular lymphoma originating from the same germinal center B cell. *J Clin Oncol* 17:3804–3809, 1999.

13. Harris NL, Jaffe ES, Diebold J, et al. World Health Organization classification of neoplastic diseases of the hematopoietic and lymphoid tissues: report of the clinical advisory committee meeting—Airlie House, Virginia. *J Clin Oncol* 17:3835–3849, 1999.

14. Diehl V, Sextro M, Franklin J, et al. Clinical presentation, course, and prognostic factors in lymphocyte-predominant Hodgkin's disease and lymphocyte-rich classical Hodgkin's disease: report from the European Task Force on Lymphoma Project on Lymphocyte-Predominant Hodgkin's Disease. *J Clin Oncol* 17:776–783, 1999.

15. Lister TA, Crowther D, Sutcliffe SB, et al. Report of a committee convened to discuss the evaluation and staging of patients with Hodgkin's disease: Cotswolds Meeting. *J Clin Oncol* 7:1630–1636, 1989.

16. Foss Abrahamsen A, Hoiby EA, Hannisdal E, et al. Systemic pneumococcal disease after staging splenectomy for Hodgkin's disease 1969–1980 without pneumococcal vaccine protection: a follow-up study 1994. *Eur J Haematol* 58:73–77, 1997.

17. Molrine DC, George S, Tarbell N, et al. Antibody responses to polysaccharide and polysaccharide-conjugate vaccines after treatment of Hodgkin's disease. *Ann Intern Med* 123:828–834, 1995.

18. Hasenclever D, Diehl V. A prognostic score for advanced Hodgkin's disease. International Prognostic Factors Project on advanced Hodgkin's disease. *N Engl J Med* 339:1506–1514, 1998.

19. Kaplan HS. In: *Hodgkin's Disease* (2nd ed). Cambridge, MA: Harvard University Press, 1980:376.

20. Horning SJ, Hoppe RT, Mason J, et al. Stanford-Kaiser Permanente G1 study for clinical stage I to IIA Hodgkin's disease: subtotal lymphoid irradiation versus vinblastine, methotrexate, and bleomycin chemotherapy and regional irradiation. *J Clin Oncol* 15:1736–1744, 1997.

21. Longo DL, Glatstein E, Duffey PL, et al. Radiation therapy versus combination chemotherapy in the treatment of early-stage Hodgkin's disease: Seven-year results of a prospective randomized trial. *J Clin Oncol* 9:906–917, 1991.

22. Santoro A, Bonadonna G, Valagussa P, et al. Long-term results of combined chemotherapy-radiotherapy approach in Hodgkin's disease: Superiority of ABVD plus radiotherapy versus MOPP plus radiotherapy. *J Clin Oncol* 5:27–37, 1987.

23. Mikhaeel NG, Timothy AR, Hain SF, O'Doherty MJ. 18-FDG-PET for the assessment of residual masses on CT following treatment of lymphomas. *Ann Oncol* 11 (suppl 1):147–150, 2000.

24. DeVita VT Jr, Serpick AA. Combination chemotherapy in the treatment of advanced Hodgkin's disease. *Ann Intern Med* 73:881–895, 1970.

25. Longo DL, Young RC, Wesley M, et al. Twenty years of MOPP therapy for Hodgkin's disease. *J Clin Oncol* 4:1295–1306, 1986.

26. Bonadonna G, Valagussa P, Santoro A. Alternating non-cross-resistant combination chemotherapy or MOPP in stage IV Hodgkin's disease. *Ann Intern Med* 104:739–746, 1986.

27. Klimo P, Connors JM. MOPP/ABV hybrid program: Combination chemotherapy based on early introduction of seven effective drugs for advanced Hodgkin's disease. *J Clin Oncol* 3:1174–1182, 1985.

28. Canellos GP, Anderson JR, Propert KJ, et al. Chemotherapy of advanced Hodgkin's disease with MOPP, ABVD, or MOPP alternating with ABVD. *N Engl J Med* 327:1478–1484, 1992.

29. Duggan D, Petroni J, Johnson J, et al. MOPP/ABV versus ABVD for advanced Hodgkin's disease—a preliminary report of CALGB 8952 (with SWOG, ECOG, NCIC). Proc ASCO 1997;16:12a (abstract 43).

30. Diehl V, Franklin J, Hasenclever D, et al. BEACOPP, a new dose-escalated and accelerated regimen, is at least as effective as COPP/ABVD in patients with advanced-stage Hodgkin's lymphoma: interim report from a trial of the German Hodgkin's lymphoma study group. *J Clin Oncol* 16: 3810–3821, 1998.

31. Gajewski JL, Phillips GL, Sobocinski KA, et al. Bone marrow transplantation from HLA-identical siblings in advanced Hodgkin's disease. *J Clin Oncol* 14:572–578, 1996.

32. Salloum E, Doria R, Schubert W, et al. Second solid tumors in patients with Hodgkin's disease cured after radiation or chemotherapy plus adjuvant low-dose radiation. *J Clin Oncol* 14:2435–2443, 1996.

33. Yahalom J, Petrek JA, Biddinger PW, et al. Breast cancer in patients irradiated for Hodgkin's disease: A clinical and

pathologic analysis of 45 events in 37 patients. *J Clin Oncol* 10:1674–1681, 1992.

34. Armitage JO, Weisenburger DD. New approach to classifying non-Hodgkin's lymphomas: clinical features of the major histologic subtypes. *J Clin Oncol* 16:2780–2795, 1998.

35. Silvestri F, Pipan C, Barillari G, et al. Prevalence of hepatitis C virus infection in patients with lymphoproliferative disorders. *Blood* 87:4296–4301, 1996.

36. Silvestri F, Barillari G, Fanin R, et al. Impact of hepatitis C virus infection on clinical features, quality of life and survival of patients with lymphoplasmacytoid lymphoma/immunocytoma. *Ann Oncol* 9:499–504, 1998.

37. Wotherspoon AC, Ortiz-Hidalgo C, Falzon MR, Isaacson PG. *Helicobacter pylori*-associated gastritis and primary B-cell gastric lymphoma. *Lancet* 338:1175–1176, 1993.

38. Wotherspoon AC, Doglioni C, Diss TC, et al. Regression of primary low-grade B-cell gastric lymphoma of mucosa-associated lymphoid tissue type after eradication of *Helicobacter pylori*. *Lancet* 342:575–577, 1993.

39. Roggero E, Zucca E, Pinotti G, et al. Eradication of *Helicobacter pylori* infection in primary low-grade gastric lymphoma of mucosa-associated lymphoid tissue. *Ann Intern Med* 122:767–769, 1995.

40. Parsonnet J, Hansen S, Rodriguez L, et al. *Helicobacter pylori* infection and gastric lymphoma. *N Engl J Med* 330:1267–1271, 1994.

41. Rettig MB, Ma HJ, Vescio RA, et al. Kaposi's sarcoma-associated herpesvirus infection of bone marrow dendritic cells from multiple myeloma patients. *Science* 276:1851–1854, 1997.

42. Said W, Chien K, Takeuchi S, et al. Kaposi's sarcoma-associated herpesvirus (KSVH or HHV8) in primary effusion lymphoma: ultrastructural demonstration of herpesvirus in lymphoma cells. *Blood* 87:4937–4943, 1996.

43. Cesarman E, Nador RG, Aozasa K, et al. Kaposi's sarcoma-associated herpesvirus in non-AIDS related lymphomas occurring in body cavities. *Am J Pathol* 49:53–57, 1996.

44. Paya CV, Fung JJ, Nalesnik MA, et al. Epstein-Barr virus-associated posttransplant lymphoproliferative disorders. ASTS/ASTP EBV-PTLD Task Force and the Mayo Clinic organized international consensus development meeting. *Transplantation* 68:1517–1525, 1999.

45. Pearce NE, Smith AH, Fisher DO. Malignant lymphoma and multiple myeloma linked with agricultural occupations in a New Zealand Cancer Registry-based study. *Am J Epidemiol* 121:225–237, 1985.

46. Pearce N, Smith AH, Reif JS. Increased risk of soft tissue sarcoma, malignant lymphoma, and acute myeloid leukemia in abattoir workers. *Am J Ind Med* 14:63–72, 1988.

47. Blair A, Zahm SH, Pearce NE, et al. Clues to cancer etiology from studies in farmers. *Scand J Work Environ Health* 18:209–215, 1992.

48. Pearce N, Bethwaite P. Increasing incidence of non-Hodgkin's lymphoma: occupational and environmental factors. *Cancer Res* 52(19 suppl):5496s–5500s, 1992.

49. Blair A, Linos A, Stewart PA, et al. Evaluation of risks for non-Hodgkin's lymphoma by occupation and industry exposures from a case-control study. *Am J Ind Med* 23:301–312, 1993.

50. Zahm SH, Blair A. Pesticides and non-Hodgkin's lymphoma. *Cancer Res* 52(suppl):5485s–5488s, 1992.

51. Zahm SH, Weisenburger DD, Babbitt PA, et al. Use of hair coloring products and the risk of lymphoma, multiple myeloma, and chronic lymphocytic leukemia. *Am J Public Health* 82:990–997, 1992.

52. Zahm SH, Hoffman-Goetz L, Dosemeci M, et al, Occupational physical activity and non-Hodgkin's lymphoma. *Med Sci Sports Exerc* 31:566–571, 1999.

53. Baris D, Zahm SH, Cantor KP, Blair A. Agricultural use of DDT and risk of non-Hodgkin's lymphoma: pooled analysis of three case-controlled studies in the United States. *Occup Environ Med* 55:522–527, 1998.

54. Adami J, Gridley G, Nyren O, et al. Sunlight and non-Hodgkin's lymphoma: a population-based cohort study in Sweden. *Int J Cancer* 80:641–645, 1999.

55. Hanada M, Delia D, Aiello A, et al. *bcl-2* gene hypomethylation and high-level expression in B-cell chronic lymphocytic leukemia. *Blood* 82:1820–1828, 1993.

56. Harris NL, Jaffe ES, Stein H, et al. A revised European-American classification of lymphoid neoplasms: a proposal from the International Lymphoma Study Group. *Blood* 84:1361–1392, 1994.

57. MacManus M, Hoppe RT. Is radiotherapy curative for stage I and II low-grade follicular lymphoma? Results of a long-term follow-up study of patients treated at Stanford University. *J Clin Oncol* 14:1282–1290, 1996.

58. Ezdinli EZ, Anderson JR, Melvin F, et al. Moderate versus aggressive chemotherapy of nodular lymphocytic poorly differentiated lymphoma. *J Clin Oncol* 3:769–775, 1985.

59. Johnson PWM, Rohatiner AZS, Whelan JS, et al. Patterns of survival in patients with recurrent follicular lymphoma: A 20-year study from a single center. *J Clin Oncol* 13:140–147, 1995.

60. Dana BW, Dahlberg S, Nathwani BN, et al. Long-term follow-up of patients with low-grade malignant lymphomas treated with doxorubicin-based chemotherapy or chemoimmunotherapy. *J Clin Oncol* 11:644–651, 1993.

61. Shipp MA, Harrington DP, Anderson JR, et al. Development of a predictive model for aggressive lymphoma: The International Non-Hodgkin's Lymphoma Prognostic Factors Project. *N Engl J Med* 329:987–994, 1993.

62. Hermans J, Krol ADG, van Groningen K, et al. International prognostic index for aggressive non-Hodgkin's lymphoma is valid for all malignancy grades. *Blood* 86:1460–1463, 1995.

63. Portlock CS, Rosenberg SA. No initial therapy for stages III and IV non-Hodgkin's lymphomas of favorable histologic types. *Ann Intern Med* 90:10–13, 1979.

64. Brice P, Bastion Y, Lepage E, et al. Comparison of low-tumor-burden follicular lymphomas between an initial no-treatment policy, prednimustine, or interferon alfa: a randomized study from the Group d'Etude des Lymphomes Folliculares. *J Clin Oncol* 15:1110–1117, 1997.

65. Portlock CS, Rosenberg SA, Glatstein E, Kaplan HS. Treatment of advanced non-Hodgkin's lymphomas with favorable histologies: preliminary results of a prospective trial. *Blood* 47:747–756, 1976.

66. Kimby E, Björkholm M, Gahrton G, et al. Chlorambucil/prednisone vs. CHOP in symptomatic low-grade non-

Hodgkin's lymphomas: A randomized trial from the Lymphoma Group of Central Sweden. *Ann Oncol* 5(suppl 2):567–571, 1994.

67. Weisdorf DJ, Andersen JW, Glick JH, Oken MM. Survival after relapse of low-grade non-Hodgkin's lymphomas: Implications for marrow transplantation. *J Clin Oncol* 10:942–947, 1992.

68. Cabanillas F, Velasquez WS, McLaughlin P, et al. Results of recent salvage chemotherapy regimens for lymphoma and Hodgkin's disease. *Semin Hematol* 25:47–50, 1998.

69. Wilson WH, Bryant G, Bates S, et al. EPOCH chemotherapy. Toxicity and efficacy in relapsed and refractory non-Hodgkin's lymphoma. *J Clin Oncol* 11:1573–1582, 1993.

70. Rodriguez MA, Cabanillas FC, Velasquez W, et al. Results of a salvage treatment program for relapsing lymphoma: MINE consolidated with ESHAP. *J Clin Oncol* 13:1734–1741, 1995.

71. Redman JR, Cabanillas F, Velasquez WS, et al. Phase II trial of fludarabine phosphate in lymphoma: An effective new agent in low-grade lymphoma. *J Clin Oncol* 10:790–794, 1992.

72. Hochster HS, Kim K, Green MD, et al. Activity of fludarabine in previously treated non-Hodgkin's low-grade lymphoma: Results of an Eastern Cooperative Oncology Group Study. *J Clin Oncol* 10:28–32, 1992.

73. Solal-Celigny P, Brice P, Brousse N, et al. Phase II trial of fludarabine monophosphate as first-line treatment in patients with advanced follicular lymphoma: a multicenter study by the Groupe d'Etude des Lymphomes de l'Adulte. *J Clin Oncol* 14:514–519, 1996.

74. Betticher DC, Fey MF, von Rohr A, et al. High incidence of infections after 2-chlorodeoxyadenosine (2-CDA) therapy in patients with malignant lymphomas and chronic and acute leukaemias. *Ann Oncol* 5:57–64, 1994.

75. Saven A, Emanuele S, Kosty M, et al, 2-Chlorodeoxyadenosine activity in patients with untreated, indolent non-Hodgkin's lymphoma. *Blood* 86:1710–1718, 1995.

76. Cummings FJ, Kim K, Neiman RS, et al. Phase II trial of pentostatin in refractory lymphomas and cutaneous T-cell disease. *J Clin Oncol* 9:565–571, 1991.

77. Hagenbeek A, Eghbali H, Monfardini S, et al. Fludarabine versus conventional CVP chemotherapy in newly diagnosed patients with stages III and IV low grade malignant non-Hodgkin's lymphoma. Preliminary results from a prospective randomized phase III clinical trial in 381 patients. *Blood* 92(suppl 1):315a (abstract 1294), 1998.

78. Klasa R, Meyer R, Shustik C, et al. Fludarabine versus CVP in previously treated patients with progressive low grade non-Hodgkin's lymphomas (lg-NHL). Proc ASCO 1999;18:9a (abstract 28).

79. Coiffier B, Neidhart-Berard EM, Tilly H, et al. Fludarabine alone compared to CHVP plus interferon in elderly patients with follicular lymphoma and adverse prognostic parameters: a GELA study. Groupe d'Etudes des Lymphomes de l'Adulte. *Ann Oncol* 10:1191–1197, 1999.

80. Foran JM, Oscier D, Orchard J, et al. Pharmacokinetic study of single doses of oral fludarabine phosphate in patients with "low-grade" non-Hodgkin's lymphoma and B-cell chronic lymphocytic leukemia. *J Clin Oncol* 17:1574–1579, 1999.

81. McLaughlin P, Hagemeister FB, Romaguera JE, et al. Fludarabine, mitoxantrone, and dexamethasone: An effective new regimen for indolent lymphoma. *J Clin Oncol* 14:1262–1268, 1996.

82. Velasquez W, Lew D, Miller T, Fisher R. SWOG 95–01: A phase II trial of a combination of fludarabine and mitoxantrone (FN) in untreated advanced low grade lymphoma. An effective, well tolerated therapy. Proc ASCO 1999.

83. Hochster H, Oken M, Winter J, et al. Prolonged time to progression (TTP) in patients with low grade lymphoma (LGL) treated with cyclophosphamide (C) and fludarabine (F)(ECOG 1481). Proc ASCO 1998;17:17a (abstract 66).

84. Dimopoulos MA, Kantarjian H, Estey E, et al. Treatment of Waldenstrom macroglobulinemia with 2-chlorodeoxyadenosine. *Ann Intern Med* 118:195–198, 1993.

85. Dimopoulos MA, O'Brien S, Kantarjian H, et al. Fludarabine therapy in Waldenström's macroglobulinemia. *Am J Med* 95:49–52, 1993.

86. Dimopoulos MA, Weber D, Delasalle KB, et al, Treatment of Waldenström's macroglobulinemia resistant to standard therapy with 2-chlorodeoxyadenosine: identification of prognostic factors. *Ann Oncol* 6:49–52, 1995.

87. Leblond V, Ben-Othman T, Deconinck E, et al. Activity of fludarabine in previously treated Waldenstrom's macroglobulinemia: a report of 71 cases. Groupe Cooperatif Macroglobulinemie. *J Clin Oncol* 16:2060–2064, 1998.

88. Cheson BD, Vena D, Foss F, Sorensen JM. Neurotoxicity of purine analogs: A review. *J Clin Oncol* 12:2216–2228, 1994.

89. Cheson BD. Immunologic and immunosuppressive complications of purine analogue therapy. *J Clin Oncol* 13:2431–2448, 1995.

90. Cheson BD, Frame J, Vena D, Sorensen JM. Tumor lysis syndrome as a rare complication of fludarabine therapy in chronic lymphocytic leukemia. *J Clin Oncol* 16:2305–2312, 1998.

91. Cheson BD, Vena D, Barrett J, Freidlin B. Second malignancies as a consequence of nucleoside analog therapy of chronic lymphoid leukemias. *J Clin Oncol* 17: 2454–2460, 1999.

92. McLaughlin P, Grillo-Lopez AJ, Link BK, et al. Rituximab chimeric anti-CD20 monoclonal antibody therapy of relapsed indolent lymphoma: half of patients respond to a four-dose treatment program. *J Clin Oncol* 16:2825–2833, 1998.

93. Solal-Celigny P, Salles G, Brousse N, et al. Rituximab as first-line treatment of patients with follicular lymphoma (FL) and a low-burden tumor: clinical and molecular evaluation. *Blood* 94(suppl 1):631a (abstract 2802), 1999.

94. Davis T, Levy R, White CA, et al. Retreatments with RITUXAN™ (Rituximab, IDEC C2B8) have significant efficacy, do not cause hama, and are a viable minimally toxic alternative in relapsed or refractory non-Hodgkin's lymphoma (NHL). *Blood* 90(suppl 1):509a (abstract 2269), 1999.

95. Czuczman MS, Grillo-Lopez AJ, White CA, et al. Treat-

ment of patients with low-grade B-cell lymphoma with the combination of chimeric anti-CD20 monoclonal antibody and CHOP chemotherapy. *J Clin Oncol* 17:268–276, 1999.

96. Lundin J, Osterborg A, Brittinger G, et al. CAMPATH-1H monoclonal antibody in therapy for previously treated low-grade non-Hodgkin's lymphomas: a phase II multicenter study. *J Clin Oncol* 16:3257–3263, 1998.

97. Kaminski MS, Zasadny KR, Francis IR, et al. Iodine-131-anti-B1 radioimmunotherapy for B-cell lymphoma. *J Clin Oncol* 14:1974–1981, 1996.

98. Vose J, Saleh M, Lister A, et al. Iodine-131 anti-B1 antibody for non-Hodgkin's lymphoma (NHL): overall clinical trial experience. Proc ASCO 1998;17:10a (abstract 38).

99. Liu SY, Eary JF, Petersdorf SH, et al. Follow-up of relapsed B-cell lymphoma patients treated with iodine-131-labeled anti-CD20 antibody and autologous stem-cell rescue. *J Clin Oncol* 16:3270–3278, 1998.

100. Witzig TE, White CA, Wiseman GA, et al. Phase I/II trial of IDEC-Y2B8 radioimmunotherapy for treatment of relapsed or refractory CD20(+) B-cell non-Hodgkin's lymphoma. *J Clin Oncol* 17:3793–3803, 1999.

101. Rohatiner AZS, Gregory W, Peterson B, et al. A meta-analysis (MA) of randomised trials evaluating the role of interferon (IFN) as treatment for follicular lymphoma (FL). Proc ASCO 1998;17:4a (abstract 11).

102. Fisher RI, Dana BW, Le Blanc M, et al. Alpha-interferon consolidation following intensive chemotherapy does not prolong the failure-free survival of patients with low-grade non-Hodgkin's lymphoma: results of a SWOG-8809, a randomized phase III study. *J Clin Oncol* 18:2010–2016, 2000.

103. Hsu FJ, Caspar C, Czerwinski D, et al. Tumor-specific idiotype vaccines in the treatment of patients with B-cell lymphoma: long term results of a clinical trial. *Blood* 89:3129–3135, 1997.

104. Bendandi M, Gocke CD, Kobrin CB, et al. Complete molecular remissions induced by patient-specific vaccination plus granulocyte-monocyte colony stimulating factor against lymphoma. *Nature Med* 10:1171–1177, 1999.

105. Waters JS, Webb A, Cunningham D, et al. Phase I clinical and pharmacokinetic study of bcl-2 antisense oligonucleotide therapy in patients with non-Hodgkin's lymphoma. *J Clin Oncol* 18:1812–1823, 2000.

106. van Besien K, Sobocinski KA, Rowlings PA, et al. Allogeneic bone marrow transplantation for low grade lymphoma. *Blood* 92:1832–1836, 1998.

107. Freedman AS, Gribben JG, Neuberg D, et al. High-dose therapy and autologous bone marrow transplantation in patients with follicular lymphoma. *Blood* 88:2780–2786, 1996.

108. Rohatiner AZS, Johnson PWM, Price CGA, et al. Myeloablative therapy with autologous bone marrow transplantation as consolidation therapy for recurrent follicular lymphoma. *J Clin Oncol* 12:1177–1184, 1994.

109. Freedman AS, Neuberg D, Mauch P, et al. Long-term follow-up of autologous bone marrow transplantation in patients with relapsed follicular lymphoma. *Blood* 94:3325–3333, 1999.

110. Friedberg JW, Neuberg D, Stone RM, et al. Outcome in patients with myelodysplastic syndrome after autologous bone marrow transplantation for non-Hodgkin's lymphoma. *J Clin Oncol* 17:3128–2135, 1999.

111. Offit K, Lo Coco F, Louie DC, et al. Rearrangements of the bcl-6 gene as a prognostic marker in diffuse large-cell lymphoma. *N Engl J Med* 331:74–80, 1994.

112. Miller TP, Dahlberg S, Cassady JR, et al. Chemotherapy alone compared with chemotherapy plus radiotherapy for localized intermediate-and high-grade non-Hodgkin's lymphoma. *N Engl J Med* 339:21–26, 1998.

113. Klimo P, Connors JM. MACOP-B chemotherapy for the treatment of diffuse large-cell lymphoma. *Ann Intern Med* 102:596–602, 1985.

114. Fisher RI, DeVita VT Jr, Hubbard SM, et al. Diffuse aggressive lymphomas: Increased survival after alternating flexible sequences of ProMACE and MOPP chemotherapy. *Ann Intern Med* 98:304–309, 1983.

115. Fisher RI, Longo DL, DeVita VT Jr, et al. Long-term follow-up of ProMACE-CytaBOM in non-Hodgkin's lymphomas. *Ann Oncol* 2(suppl 1):33–35, 1991.

116. Shipp MA, Yeap BY, Harrington DP, et al. The m-BACOD combination chemotherapy regimen in large-cell lymphoma: Analysis of the completed trial and comparison with the M-BACOD regimen. *J Clin Oncol* 8:84–93, 1990.

117. Armitage JO, Cheson BD. Interpretation of clinical trials in diffuse large-cell lymphoma. *J Clin Oncol* 6:1335–1347, 1988.

118. Fisher RI, Gaynor ER, Dahlberg S, et al. Comparison of a standard regimen (CHOP) with three intensive chemotherapy regimens for advanced non-Hodgkin's lymphoma. *N Engl J Med* 328:1002–1006, 1993.

119. Gascoyne RD, Aoun P, Wu D, et al. Prognostic significance of anaplastic lymphoma kinase (ALK) protein expression in adults with anaplastic large cell lymphoma. *Blood* 93:3913–3921, 1999.

120. Filippa DA, Ladanyi M, Wollner N, et al. CD30 (Ki-1)-positive malignant lymphomas: clinical, immunophenotypic, histologic, and genetic characteristics and differences with Hodgkin's disease. *Blood* 87:2905–2917, 1996.

121. Zinzani PL, Bendandi M, Martelli M, et al. Anaplastic large-cell lymphoma: Clinical and prognostic evaluation of 90 adult patients. *J Clin Oncol* 14:955–962, 1996.

122. Khouri IF, Romaguera J, Kantarjian H, et al. Hyper-CVAD and high-dose methotrexate/cytarabine followed by stem-cell transplantation: an active regimen for aggressive mantle-cell lymphoma. *J Clin Oncol* 16:3803–3809, 1998.

123. Hoskins PJ, Le N, Gascoyne RD, et al. Advanced diffuse large-cell lymphoma treated with 12-week combination chemotherapy: natural history of relapse after initial complete response and prognostic variables defining outcome after relapse. *Ann Oncol* 8:1125–1132, 1997.

124. Lee AYY, Connors JM, Klimo P, et al. Late relapse in patients with diffuse large-cell lymphoma treated with MACOP-B. *J Clin Oncol* 15:1745–1753, 1997.

125. Velasquez WS, McLaughlin P, Tucker S, et al. ESHAP—an effective chemotherapy regimen in refractory and relapsing lymphoma: a 4-year follow-up study. *J Clin Oncol* 12:1169–1176, 1994.

126. Philip T, Armitage JO, Spitzer G, et al. High-dose therapy and autologous bone marrow transplantation after fail-

ure of conventional chemotherapy in adults with intermediate-grade of high-grade non-Hodgkin's lymphoma. *N Engl J Med* 316:1493–1498, 1987.

127. Philip T, Guglielmi C, Hagenbeek A, et al. Autologous bone marrow transplantation as compared with salvage chemotherapy in relapses of chemotherapy-sensitive non-Hodgkin's lymphoma. *N Engl J Med* 333:1540–1545, 1995.

128. Haioun C, Lepage E, Gisselbrecht C, et al. Benefit of autologous bone marrow transplantation over sequential chemotherapy in poor-risk aggressive non-Hodgkin's lymphoma: updated results of the prospective study LNH87–2. Groupe d'Etude des Lymphomes de l'Adulte. *J Clin Oncol* 15:1131–1137, 1997.

129. Vose JM, Bierman PJ, Anderson JR, et al. Progressive disease after high-dose therapy and autologous transplantation for lymphoid malignancy: clinical course and patient follow-up. *Blood* 80:2142–2148, 1992.

130. Shipp MA, Abeloff MD, Antman KH, et al. International consensus conference on high-dose therapy with hematopoietic stem cell transplantation in aggressive non-Hodgkin's lymphomas: report of the jury. *J Clin Oncol* 17:423–429, 1999.

131. Collins RH Jr, Shpilberg O, Drobyski WR, et al. Donor leukocyte infusions in 140 patients with relapsed malignancy after allogeneic bone marrow transplantation. *J Clin Oncol* 15:433–444, 1997.

132. Coiffier B, Ketterer N, Haioun C, et al. A multicenter, randomized phase II study of rituximab (chimeric anti-CD20 mAb) at two dosages in patients with relapsed or refractory intermediate of high-grade NHL (IHG-NHL). *Blood* 90(suppl 1):510a (abstract 2271), 1997.

133. Coleman CN, Picozzi VJ Jr, Cox RS, et al. Treatment of lymphoblastic lymphoma in adults. *J Clin Oncol* 4:1628–1637, 1986.

134. Soussain C, Patte C, Ostronoff M, et al. Small noncleaved cell lymphoma and leukemia in adults. A retrospective study of 65 adults treated with the LMB pediatric protocol. *Blood* 85:664–674, 1995.

135. Lopez-Guillermo A, Cid J, Salar A, et al. Peripheral T-cell lymphomas: initial features, natural history, and prognostic factors in a series of 174 patients diagnosed according to the R.E.A.L. Classification. *Ann Oncol* 9:849–855, 1998.

21

Multiple Myeloma and Other Plasma Cell Dyscrasias

■ ■ ■

DAVID S. ROSENTHAL
LOWELL E. SCHNIPPER
RONALD P. MCCAFFREY
KENNETH C. ANDERSON

MALIGNANT PLASMA CELL DYSCRASIAS (e.g., multiple myeloma, plasmacytomas, and lymphoplasmacytic lymphoma, or Waldenström's disease) now are included in the Revised European-American Lymphoma (REAL) classification of lymphomas [1], as follows (see Chapter 20):

B-cell neoplasm
Peripheral B-cell neoplasm
 Plasma cell myeloma
 Lymphoplasmacytic lymphoma, immunocytoma.

Plasma cells represent the final stage in the maturation of B lymphocytes. Despite the reclassification, plasma cell malignancies often are discussed separately because of their unique clinical and laboratory presentation, in which uncontrolled proliferation of a neoplastic cell population leads to excessive secretion of monoclonal immunoglobulin or immunoglobulin subunits. Of several distinct clinical variants that have been recognized, the most common are multiple myeloma, which makes up approximately 75% of cases, and Waldenström's macroglobulinemia, which accounts for 20%; the remaining cases consist of such rare variants as the heavy-chain diseases characterized by the overproduction of immunoglobulin heavy-chain components [2].

Plasma cell dyscrasias can be understood best as clinical entities that result from the dysregulated proliferation of plasma cells or their precursors, with pathologic sequelae due to overproduction of their immunoglobulin products. These disorders are associated with a number of serious complications, the nature and treatment of which are discussed at the end of this chapter.

MULTIPLE MYELOMA

Multiple myeloma, the most common plasma cell dyscrasia, is a neoplasm characterized by massive hyperproliferation of malignant plasma cells. The main sites involved are the bones and bone marrow. The disease is characterized by the autonomous proliferation of marrow plasma cells and by the overproduction of a homogeneous population of normal immunoglobulin molecules (known variously as *monoclonal immunoglobulin, M spike,* or *M component*) or of the immunoglobulin light chains kappa or lambda.

Epidemiologic Features

Approximately 13,600 new cases of multiple myeloma will be diagnosed in the United States in 2000 [3]. Malignant plasma cell disorders are uncommon, accounting for only approximately 1% of all cancers in this country. Myeloma is rare among individuals younger than 40 years, but its incidence rises in subsequent decades and exhibits a slight male predominance. It is twice as high among blacks as among whites. Multiple myeloma does not appear to be caused by prior exposure to toxic substances (e.g., solvents that include benzene [4], paints, and pesticides), and no clusters of the disease have been observed. Evidence that this disease may develop after exposure to ionizing irradiation is equivocal and never was established firmly. Interestingly, an association with human herpesvirus 8 has been described [5], but the role of this virus in disease pathogenesis remains to be determined [6].

Pathogenesis

Experimental observations and a few case reports support the hypothesis that multiple myeloma may result from a sustained antigenic stimulus. Experimental myeloma can be produced in mice after repetitive intraperitoneal injection of mineral oil. The resulting disease is a monoclonal IgA plasma cell dyscrasia. Some individuals with chronic polyclonal hypergammaglobulinemia have developed multiple myeloma years later. Although in several of these cases the immunoglobulin produced in excessive amounts may have been related antigenically to a previous chronic disease, for the most part the proliferating plasma cells secreted an immunoglobulin directed against an antigen that could not be identified.

Multiple myeloma is characterized by excessive production of immunoglobulin molecules, by dysregulated proliferation of lymphoid or plasma cells in the marrow and, less often, in other tissues. Normal plasma cells represent the final stage in the maturation of B lympho-cytes. As B lymphocytes differentiate, they exhibit a sequence of immunologically recognizable phenotypic changes. These changes include the expression of surface antigens CD10 and, at a later stage, CD20, and the transient appearance of cytoplasmic mu chains followed by cytoplasmic immunoglobulin. However, after the final steps in maturation, the plasma cell exhibits only cytoplasmic, not surface, immunoglobulin and several plasma cell antigens (e.g., PCA-1, CD38, and CD9). The other B-cell antigens expressed earlier in differentiation normally are not detectable.

In multiple myeloma, the malignant clone extends from the pre-B-cell to plasma cell stage of differentiation. Often, myeloma cells display typical plasma cell surface antigens but, in addition, express B-cell-specific antigens in 20% to 30% of cases and, frequently, express antigens associated with such other hematopoietic lineages as CD2 and CD4 (T cells), glycophorin A (red blood cells), and CD41 (a megakaryocytic antigen). The importance of identifying antigens usually associated with other hematopoietic cell types is emphasized by a number of small studies that point to the prognostic importance of a specific immunophenotype [7].

Evidence suggests that some lymphocytes in patients with myeloma exhibit properties similar to those of the malignant plasma cells (e.g., the same M-protein idiotype, the immunophenotype), supporting the presence of cells derived from the same clonal lineage as that of the plasma cell [8]. Some investigators speculate that the early B cell is the target for the oncogenic change leading to full-blown myeloma.

Cytokines are important in the pathogenesis of multiple myeloma [9]. The plasma cell has a surface-membrane receptor for interleukin-6, which is known to be a growth and survival factor for myeloma cells. Interleukin-1 also is an important growth factor in this disorder, inasmuch as it has potent osteoclastic activity. Myeloma cells express a variety of adhesion molecules that mediate interaction with nonmalignant marrow stromal cells and extracellular matrix proteins and trigger the production of cytokines, which augment myeloma cell growth and survival [10].

B cells and plasma cells in normal individuals are polyclonal: The number of cells that express immunoglobulins containing kappa light chains is approximately equal to the number containing lambda light chains. In multiple myeloma, as in other malignant B-cell lymphoproliferative disorders, the neoplastic clone demonstrates light-chain restriction. The immunoglobulin produced by that clone is a single, light-chain type, and the heavy chain produced by the plasma cells also is identical in each cell of the tumor. The production of one specific immunoglobulin protein is characteristic of the malignant plasma cell population. Owing to a defect in the assembly of a mature immunoglobulin molecule, approximately 20% of the tumors produce only light chains, either kappa or lambda; the remainder produce intact immunoglobulin (approximately 55% producing IgG and approximately 20% producing IgA), with or without an overproduction of free light chains. Nearly 0.5% of patients secrete no immunoglobulin. For individual patients, each myeloma cell produces proteins that are identical in every part of the molecule, and high plasma concentrations of these homologous molecules contribute to the M spike.

Using fluorescence in situ hybridization (FISH), cytogeneticists have demonstrated aneuploidy in approximately 70% of patients, with the most frequent abnormalities involving chromosomes 13 (13q–) and 14 (14q+). Translocations involving the immunoglobulin switch region and multiple other partner chromosomes have been described [11]. These alterations may cause impaired apoptosis and subsequent resistance to therapy [12]. In patients with relapsed disease, *p53* mutations have been identified and may correlate with poor prognosis.

Clinical Staging

The diagnosis of multiple myeloma requires evidence of at least one of the following *major* findings [13]: (1) plasmacytoma; (2) marrow involved with at least 30% plasma cells or immature plasma cells; and (3) M protein of either IgG greater than 3.5 g/dl, IgA greater than 2.9 g/dl, or urine light-chain excretion greater than 1 g/24 hr. The presence of at least one of the following *minor* findings also is required: (1) marrow plasmacytosis greater than 10%; (2) M protein in serum and urine but less than levels described in (3) above; (3) lytic bone lesions; and (4) decreased normal immunoglobulins. The diagnosis is made if any two major findings are present; if plasmacytoma plus the first three minor findings are present; if the third major finding plus the first or third minor finding are present; or if no major findings but the first three minor *or* the first, second, and fourth minor findings are present.

LABORATORY ANALYSIS OF SERUM PROTEINS

Laboratory studies of the M component produced in plasma cell dyscrasias should include serum electrophoresis; quantitative immunoglobulin electrophoresis to define the absolute quantities of IgG, IgM, IgD, or IgE; and analytic immunoelectrophoresis or immunofixation to characterize the specific light- and heavy-chain types in the M component (Color Plate 21.1). Both serum and urine should be analyzed, and these tests may be used to follow the natural course of the illness or patient response to therapy.

Screening for multiple myeloma is not indicated in an asymptomatic population because no known advantage accrues to making a diagnosis before the disease becomes clinically evident. Furthermore, approximately 5% of otherwise normal adults older than age 70 will be found to have an M component, and most of them never will develop multiple myeloma.

DIFFERENTIAL DIAGNOSIS

Multiple myeloma must be distinguished from other disorders that may be associated with the production of an M protein detectable in the blood (e.g., chronic lymphocytic leukemia, non-Hodgkin's lymphoma, and amyloidosis). The presence of progressive, symptomatic disease (e.g., anemia, lytic bone lesions, hypercalcemia) distinguishes multiple myeloma from a far more common condition: monoclonal gammopathy of undetermined significance (MGUS) [14]. Patients with MGUS have no symptoms or bone lesions; have marrow plasma cell levels less than or equal to 10% and serum M components less than or equal to 3.5 g/dl for IgG and 2.0 g/dl for IgA; and rarely excrete light chains alone. In general, those affected are elderly, have minimal or no anemia, and have normal levels of other immunoglobulins. Although some patients (24%) ultimately develop multiple myeloma or a related disorder, most remain well. At present, discerning which patients with MGUS will develop myeloma is impossible.

SIGNS AND SYMPTOMS

A small percentage of patients will present with no symptoms attributable to multiple myeloma, but routine laboratory testing or laboratory work-up for a co-existing disorder reveal an abnormally high serum protein level or unexplained proteinuria. When multiple myeloma becomes symptomatic, several clinical clues can aid in the diagnosis.

Hematologic Features
Anemia is a common manifestation; myeloma always should be suspected in an elderly person with unexplained normochromic normocytic anemia and a high erythrocyte sedimentation rate due to high concentrations of immunoglobulin. In most affected patients,

suppression of some or all marrow cell lines may be far greater than would be expected solely on the basis of the apparent degree of bone marrow replacement by malignant cells. As the disease progresses, marrow displacement may become sufficiently extensive to explain the pancytopenia. The excessive production of immunoglobulin can lead to coagulation abnormalities by the formation of a nonspecific coating on platelets, which impairs their function by interfering with biochemical events that occur on their surfaces. Occasionally, a monoclonal immunoglobulin may interact specifically with a coagulation factor, producing a factor deficiency and hence a bleeding tendency.

Bone Abnormalities

Back pain is particularly common because of bone involvement and should suggest the diagnosis of multiple myeloma in patients with other incriminating signs or symptoms [15]. The bone lesions have both a cellular and a humoral aspect. Localized proliferation of malignant plasma cells in the marrow and bone may produce painful osteolytic lesions visible on plain films (Color Plate 21.2). Bone involvement may produce several important clinical problems (e.g., pathologic fractures) that increase pain and skeletal instability. Hypercalcemia manifested by weakness, nausea, or altered mental status may develop in patients with extensive bone disease.

Neurologic problems are an important cause of morbidity in multiple myeloma. Progressive vertebral osteolytic lesions with or without a paravertebral soft-tissue mass may produce spinal cord compression or radiculopathy. Plasma cell infiltration of the meninges is an infrequent complication. Sometimes, excess light chains may aggregate in tissue to form amyloid, resulting in neuropathy or nephropathy.

Effects of Excessive Monoclonal Protein

Although multiple myeloma is characterized by excessive production of monoclonal immunoglobulin, levels of normal immunoglobulins usually are depressed, because macrophages respond to the high total immunoglobulin level by producing a B-cell-inhibitory molecule. This action contributes to a general susceptibility to bacterial infections. Because patients with multiple myeloma are at risk for pneumococcal infection with sepsis, they should be vaccinated against these organisms. However, the immune defect that renders patients susceptible to infection also may diminish an appropriate response to this vaccine.

Occasionally, symptoms of multiple myeloma are related exclusively to the excessive protein production and not to the neoplastic cell mass. The hyperviscosity syndrome may develop when IgG levels exceed 7 g/dl or when IgA levels exceed 5 g/dl. This syndrome is characterized by fatigue, changes in mental status, focal or nonfocal neurologic changes, and visual changes along with a retinopathy characterized by sludging of blood in venules, hemorrhaging and, occasionally, papilledema (Color Plate 21.3). The increased viscosity also may precipitate angina pectoris or a bleeding disorder. In a few patients, the protein or protein aggregate may act as a cryoglobulin and can result in Raynaud's phenomenon or purpuric eruptions on exposure to the cold (or both).

Renal Abnormalities

Renal failure is a common problem in patients with multiple myeloma. Excessive production of light chains can cause a condition known as *myeloma kidney,* characterized by irreversible renal tubular damage (Color Plate 21.4). Hypercalcemic nephropathy and hyperuricemia secondary to degradation of a large tumor cell mass also may cause renal failure in multiple myeloma. In some cases, amyloid is deposited in the kidney and can cause renal failure. During the evaluation for possible multiple myeloma, the use of radiographic contrast dyes should be avoided whenever possible, as their presence in conjunction with the myeloma light chains may precipitate renal failure in dehydrated patients. If diagnostic dye studies are essential, hydration must be carefully maintained.

Plasmacytomas

Plasmacytomas may develop in both medullary and extramedullary locations. True solitary plasmacytomas are rare, and nearly all patients with solitary bone lesions later develop disseminated myeloma. In contrast, soft-tissue plasmacytomas often remain localized (the most common site being the gastrointestinal tract) and may be cured with local treatment [16]. The clinical presentation and age and gender distribution of localized plasma cell tumors differ substantially from those of multiple myeloma. When plasmacytomas present as osseous lesions, often they are associated with bone destruction and localized pain, and an associated neurologic syndrome of vertebral collapse occasionally occurs.

Pathologic Characteristics

Marrow examination, although essential, will not necessarily be diagnostic. Plasma cell reactions may occur in many clinical situations; although a clinician cannot diagnose multiple myeloma on the basis of bone marrow plasmacytosis alone, plasma cell levels greater than or equal to 30% usually are consistent with this disease (Color Plate 21.5). Immunohistochemical stains can distinguish polyclonal reactive plasma cell proliferation from neoplastic monoclonal proliferation.

Staging

Estimating the total-body tumor burden is possible in patients with multiple myeloma by determining the rate of cellular immunoglobulin synthesis, in vivo levels of immunoglobulin, and the in vivo rate of immunoglobulin catabolism. These measurements also have

Table 21.1 Staging of Multiple Myeloma

Stage[a]	Criteria	Tumor Burden[b]
I	Hemoglobin > 10 g/dl Normal Ca^{2+} Normal bones IgG < 5.0 g/dl IgA < 3.0 g/dl Urinary lambda *or* kappa chains < 4 g/24 hr	< 0.6 (low tumor burden)
II	Intermediate between stages I and III	> 0.6 to < 1.2 (intermediate tumor burden)

III	Hemoglobin < 8.5 g/dl
	
	or
	
	Ca^{2+} > 12.0 mg/dl
	
	or
	
	> 3 lytic bone lesions
	
	or
	
	IgG > 7.0 g/dl
	
	or
	
	IgA > 5.0 g/dl
	
	or
	
	Urinary lambda or
	  kappa chains > 12.0
	  g/24 hr
		> 1.2 (high tumor
		burden)

[a]Substages include A (renal function intact) and B (renal failure).
[b]Myeloma cell mass (cells $\times$ 10^{12}/m^2).

permitted the total-body tumor burden to be correlated with various clinical manifestations. As a result, a multiple myeloma staging system that has emerged categorizes patients as having a low, high, or intermediate tumor burden (Table 21.1) [17]. Patients who present with a low tumor burden (stage I) have no or mild anemia, no or minimal bone lesions, and protein concentrations lower than those in patients with a high tumor burden. Those with a high tumor burden (stage III) have more significant anemia, hypercalcemia, advanced osteolytic bone disease, and higher protein concentrations. Median survival for patients with stage I disease is longer than for those with stage III disease (four versus two years, respectively).

As it is an important prognostic factor and generally is associated with poor survival, the presence of renal failure is used to divide the main disease stages into substages: Patients with intact renal function are classified as being in substage A, whereas those with renal failure are in substage B. In addition to tumor burden, labeling index, and creatinine levels, other prognostic factors include age, elevated beta$_2$-microglobulin levels, and C-reactive protein, which has been shown to correlate directly with growth factor interleukin-6 [18].

Therapy

The staple of systemic therapy for multiple myeloma consists of chemotherapy with orally administered alkylating agents, often in conjunction with corticosteroids (Table 21.2) [19]. Chlorambucil, L-phenylalanine mustard (melphalan), and cyclophosphamide are equally effective. Melphalan combined with prednisone (MP) is the treatment used most commonly and results in a 50% objective response rate (almost always a partial re-

Table 21.2 Treatment of Multiple Myeloma

Chemotherapy
High-dose chemotherapy with stem-cell or autologous
  transplantation
Interferon
Irradiation
Supportive therapies
  Growth factors
  Bisphosphonates
  Antibiotics
New strategies
  Multidrug-resistant agents (cyclosporin, PSC-833)
  Interleukin-6 inhibitors
  Antiidiotype (vaccines)

sponse), with a mean duration of 1.5 to 2.0 years and median survival of 3 to 4 years [20]. The five-year survival of patients treated in this fashion is less than 20%. Researchers have attempted to improve on this unsatisfactory outcome by employing combinations of alkylating agents, vincristine, and prednisone. However, two large meta-analyses of nearly 6,000 aggregate patients treated in randomized trials comparing MP to various polychemotherapy programs have failed to show clearly that combination chemotherapy can improve outcome [21, 22].

As an alternative to MP, the protocol of continuous infusions of anthracycline, vincristine, and high-dose dexamethasone has proved effective in many patients [23]. Initially, this protocol was used in cases refractory to MP, but now it is recommended as a first-line therapy in potential high-dose chemotherapy–stem cell transplantation candidates because of the lesser chance of impairing normal marrow stem cells (a specific problem with alkylating agents). High-dose dexamethasone also is a simple alternative to MP [24].

The limited results attained with conventional chemotherapy have led to trials of more intensive treatments, such as high-dose melphalan therapy followed by infusion of autologous bone marrow or peripheral blood stem cells [25]. Marrow is harvested prior to chemotherapy in patients who have shown responsiveness to chemotherapy and, in some centers, is purged of myeloma cells either by selection of normal progenitor cells or by depletion of tumor cells [26, 27]. Overall complete response rates approach 40%, and most other patients develop partial response. The median progression-free survival is 24 to 36 months. A randomized trial has demonstrated superior response rates, in the form of overall and event-free survival, in patients treated with high-dose therapy and autografting, as compared with patients who received conventional therapy [28]. Attempts to improve outcome include more intensive ablative therapy [29], improved autograft purging [30], and immune therapies to treat minimal residual disease after transplantation [31]. Allografting in myeloma is associated with high toxicity and mortality [32, 33]. However, improved graft-versus-host disease prophylaxis, donor compatibility testing, and supportive therapy can reduce toxicity markedly [25]. This approach has further appeal, owing to the demonstrated graft-versus-myeloma effect of donor lymphocyte infusions to treat myeloma relapse after allografting [34, 35]. Ongoing studies are attempting to improve response rates and to reduce toxicity of high-dose therapy approaches and to use immune-based strategies (including adoptive immunotherapy and vaccination) to treat minimal re-

sidual disease after transplantation and thereby to improve outcome [31].

Studies evaluating the utility of interferon-α in myeloma demonstrate a slight increase in response rate and progression-free survival without altering overall survival [36]. This minimal benefit must be balanced against the side effects of interferon therapy [37].

Radiotherapy also can provide effective control in 80% to 90% of patients with solitary plasmacytomas, whether these tumors involve bone or soft tissue [16, 38]. In such cases, irradiation portals should encompass the lesion and should include adequate margins, although wide-field treatment of all regional lymph node groups is not indicated.

Because multiple myeloma may be accompanied by myriad complications, this possibility must be considered in the development of a comprehensive treatment plan. For example, a particular plan may necessitate treating the hyperviscosity syndrome or cryoglobulinemia with plasmapheresis until systemic chemotherapy begins to take effect. In patients with hypercalcemia, treatment with hydration, furosemide, bisphosphonates, dexamethasone, mithramycin, or calcitonin may be required to control the systemic disease. Intravenous bisphosphonates have been shown to abrogate the development of bony complications in myeloma and also may have antitumor activity [39, 40]. Physicians must be especially alert for signs of infection, which should be treated vigorously with antibiotics. The need for transfusions depends on affected patients' symptoms; in patients with persistent anemia and low erythropoietin levels, treatment with erythropoietin may be beneficial [41]. Granulocyte colony-stimulating factor or granulocyte-macrophage colony-stimulating factor may be helpful while affected patients are on chemotherapy.

Newer therapeutic techniques and strategies offer greater possibilities for the future [10]. Two primary promising areas are the enhancement of allogeneic and autologous immune responses as the basis for adoptive immunotherapy and vaccination approaches [31] and the use of novel drugs to target not only the tumor cell but its microenvironment. Already, thalidomide has been shown to induce responses in patients whose myeloma is refractory to all conventional therapies [42], and further elucidation of its mechanism of action on the tumor or the marrow microenvironment (or both) may derive novel, more potent, and better-tolerated therapies [43].

WALDENSTRÖM'S MACROGLOBULINEMIA

The central abnormality in Waldenström's macroglobulinemia is the uncontrolled proliferation of plasmacytoid lymphocytes, a cell type that occurs earlier than the plasma cell in the B-cell differentiation schema [44]. These cells secrete large amounts of a homogeneous immunoglobulin polymer, a pentamer containing five immunoglobulin molecules. Abnormal cells may be found in bone marrow, lymph nodes, and blood. The proliferation of abnormal cells and their product—monoclonal IgM molecules—is the pathophysiologic basis of the signs and symptoms in this disease.

Epidemiologic Factors

Two-thirds of patients with Waldenström's macroglobulinemia are men. The median age at the onset of symptomatic disease is 60 years.

Clinical Manifestations

Some patients will be asymptomatic and present only with an M spike, as in multiple myeloma. Many individuals present with the hyperviscosity syndrome and a history that includes insidious fatigue, oronasal bleeding, blurred vision, recurrent infections, weight loss, and manifestations of peripheral neuropathy. In contrast to multiple myeloma, no bone pain occurs in Waldenström's macroglobulinemia.

Physical examination reveals pallor, hepatosplenomegaly, and peripheral lymphadenopathy—findings similar to those of non-Hodgkin's lymphoma and distinctly different from those of multiple myeloma. Often, retinal hemorrhages, exudates, venous congestion, and vascular segmentation ("sausage formation") are seen on funduscopic examination. Sensory and motor peripheral neuropathy may be noted, as may auditory and vestibular dysfunction. Blood studies indicate mild anemia, with striking rouleaux formation on the smear. Bone marrow examination shows infiltration by many small lymphocytes, some of which have plasma cell characteristics. Infrequently, clearly identifiable plasma cells account for more than 10% of the marrow population. Serum protein electrophoresis reveals an M component, usually greater than 3 g/dl, which can be identified as IgM on immunoelectrophoresis with specific IgM antiserum. Bence Jones proteinuria is present in 20% of patients.

Waldenström's macroglobulinemia is characterized by progressive organ dysfunction, either as a direct result of local cellular infiltration or secondary to increased IgM. Median survival after diagnosis is three years. As the lymphoplasmacytoid cells proliferate in the hematopoietic space, bone marrow function becomes increasingly compromised. Rising plasma IgM levels increase viscosity, resulting in circulatory impairment, particularly in the central nervous system. The latter may produce transient neurologic signs (e.g., transient paresis, cranial neuropathies, and impaired cognition). Bleeding may occur as a result of protein interactions between the IgM and such physiologically important plasma proteins as fibrinogen or prothrombin. In approximately one-third of patients, the deposition of IgM in basement membranes leads to renal failure.

Therapy

Therapy is directed toward prompt recognition and treatment of the hyperviscosity syndrome and suppression of the abnormal proliferation of lymphoplasmacytoid cells. Historically, such alkylating agents as chlorambucil have been employed, producing remission in approximately 50% of patients, with corticosteroids added in treating patients with significant anemia. Several nucleoside analogs have been studied with gratifying results. Cladribine (2-chlorodeoxyadenosine) is an adenosine analog with substantial activity in this disease [44]. In one study of previously untreated patients, 80% had a durable response after only two cycles of treatment [45]. Another analog, fludarabine, also has been shown to be active in this disorder. Progressive disease has been treated with modest success using various combinations of cyclophosphamide, melphalan, vincristine, prednisone, and carmustine.

HEAVY-CHAIN DISEASES

The heavy-chain diseases are rare lymphoma-like disorders characterized by secretion of monoclonal immunoglobulin heavy-chain fragments by the neoplastic cells, which then show up in the plasma or urine [2]. To confirm the diagnosis, these molecules must be distinguished from other immunoglobulin fragments (e.g., light chains, Bence Jones proteins) found in several dysproteinemias, with or without intact immunoglobulin. Three variants of heavy-chain disease have been described in the literature.

IgA heavy-chain disease presents as a lymphoma-like proliferation of abnormal plasmacytoid cells in the lamina propria of the small intestine and mesenteric nodes and is associated with chronic diarrhea and malabsorption. Small-bowel biopsies reveal infiltration of the lamina propria by these cells, and similar cells may be found in bone marrow aspirates. Serum electrophoresis shows a distinctive increase in IgA heavy chains, or alpha chains. Although initially described as Mediterranean abdominal lymphoma, this condition has been identified in individuals of non-Mediterranean ancestry. Complete regression of symptoms and the disappearance of abnormal immunoglobulin fragments have been recorded in several patients treated with tetracycline for presumptive intestinal infections. These patients were believed to have been suffering from a polyclonal reactive process. However, IgA heavy-chain disease generally is fatal within five years. Cyclophosphamide, melphalan, and prednisone have been used to treat patients with advanced disease.

IgG heavy-chain disease presents insidiously as a non-Hodgkin's lymphoma-like illness characterized by lymphadenopathy, hepatosplenomegaly, and enlargement of Waldeyer's ring, with edema of the uvula and palate, weakness, weight loss, and anemia. The disease occurs in the fifth decade or later, with a male-female ratio of 2:1. Massive proteinuria and abnormal serum electrophoresis are characteristic clinical findings, and abnormal lymphoplasmacytoid cells are found on bone marrow or nodal biopsy. An analysis of abnormal urinary and plasma proteins shows that they are related to IgG heavy chains or other chains, usually the Fc fragments of IgG. Although melphalan, cyclophosphamide, and prednisone have been prescribed in an attempt to slow the abnormal cell proliferation, such treatment has not been successful.

IgM heavy-chain disease is the rarest heavy-chain disease. The few cases reported have been associated with chronic lymphocytic leukemia, which dominates the clinical course. Serum and immunoelectrophoretic analysis may reveal small amounts of monoclonal IgM heavy-chain (mu-chain) proteins in the plasma, which are thought to be produced by lymphoplasmacytoid cells within the bone marrow. Bence Jones proteinuria also has been noted in some cases.

SUMMARY

Multiple myeloma is a malignant neoplasm characterized by the unregulated proliferation of plasma cells in association with excess production of intact immunoglobulin molecules or their light-chain components. A definitive diagnosis depends on serum or urine protein electrophoresis in which an M component is detected in either of these body fluids, followed by immunoelectrophoresis or immunofixation to determine the specific proteins present and to measure their concentrations. The most common clinical sequelae of multiple myeloma are painful bone lesions, often accompanied by hypercalcemia related to the osteolysis that frequently accompanies this disease. Numerous organ systems can be affected either directly through plasma cell infiltration or indirectly through the destruction of bone and its attendant hypercalcemia, which ultimately may lead to renal failure; such bone destruction also may produce neurologic dysfunction.

Systemic chemotherapy is the primary treatment for the underlying disease, and bisphosphonates are used to abrogate progressive complications in bone. Radiotherapy is an important palliative treatment for painful bone lesions or solitary plasmacytomas, and hemodialysis may be required for patients who present with renal failure. Treatment offers substantial benefits in terms of both prolonging survival and improving quality of life. High-dose therapies, immune-based treatments, and novel therapeutic strategies targeting both the myeloma and other marrow cells offer potential for significant advances in the treatment of this presently incurable disease.

REFERENCES

1. Harris N, Jaffe E, Stein H, et al. A revised European-American classification of lymphoid neoplasms: a proposal from the International Lymphoma Study Group. *Blood* 84:1361–1392, 1994.
2. Anderson KC. Plasma cell tumors. In Holland JF, Frei III E, Bast RC, et al. (eds), *Cancer Medicine* (4th ed). Baltimore: Williams & Wilkins, 2000:2809–2828.
3. Greenlee RT, Murray T, Bolden S, et al. Cancer statistics, 2000. *CA Cancer J Clin* 50:7–33, 2000.
4. Bergsagel DE, Wong O, Bergsagel PL, et al. Benzene and multiple myeloma: appraisal of the scientific evidence. *Blood* 94:1174–1182, 1999.
5. Rettig MB, Ma HJ, Vescio RA, et al. Kaposi's sarcoma–associated herpesvirus infection of bone marrow dendritic cells from multiple myeloma patients. *Science* 276:1851–1854, 1997.
6. Berenson JR. Etiology of multiple myeloma: what's new? *Semin Oncol* 26:2–9, 1999.
7. Durie B, Grogan T. CALLA positive myeloma: an aggressive subtype with poor survival. *Blood* 66:229–232, 1985.
8. Pilarski LM, Jensen GS. Monoclonal circulating B cells in multiple myeloma. A continuously differentiating, possibly invasive, population as defined by expression of CD45

isoforms and adhesion molecules. *Hematol Oncol Clin North Am* 6:297–322, 1992.

9. Anderson KC, Lust JL. Role of cytokines in multiple myeloma. *Semin Hematol* 36:14–20, 1999.

10. Anderson K. Advances in the biology of multiple myeloma: therapeutic applications. *Semin Oncol* 26:10–22, 1999.

11. Bergsagel PL, Chesi M, Nardini E, et al. Promiscuous translocations into immunoglobulin heavy chains with regions in multiple myeloma. *Proc Natl Acad Sci USA* 93:13931–13936, 1996.

12. Tricot G, Sawyer JR, Jagannath S, et al. Unique role of cytogenetics in the prognosis of patients with myeloma receiving high-dose therapy and autotransplants. *J Clin Oncol* 15:2659–2666, 1997.

13. Malpas JS. Clinical presentation and diagnosis. In Malpas JS, Bergsagel DE, Kyle RA, Anderson KC (eds), *Myeloma: Biology and Management.* New York: Oxford University Press, 1998.

14. Kyle RA. "Benign" monoclonal gammopathy—after 20 to 35 years of follow-up. *Mayo Clin Proc* 68:26–36, 1993.

15. Kyle RA. Multiple myeloma: review of 869 cases. *Mayo Clin Proc* 50:29–40, 1975.

16. Dimopoulos MA, Goldstein J, Fuller L, et al. Curability of solitary bone plasmacytoma. *J Clin Oncol* 10:587–590, 1992.

17. Durie BGM, Salmon SE. A clinical staging system for multiple myeloma. Correlation of measured cell mass with presenting clinical features, response to treatment and survival. *Cancer* 36:842–854, 1975.

18. Bataille R, Boccadoro M, Klein B, et al. C-reactive protein and β_2-microglobulin produce a simple and powerful myeloma staging system. *Blood* 80:733–737, 1992.

19. Bataille R, Harousseau J-L. Multiple myeloma. *N Engl J Med* 336:1657–1664, 1997.

20. Bergsagel DE. Use a gentle approach for refractory myeloma patients. *J Clin Oncol* 6:757–758, 1988.

21. Gregory WM, Richards MA, Malpas JS. Combination chemotherapy versus melphalan and prednisolone in the treatment of multiple myeloma: an overview of published trials. *J Clin Oncol* 10:334–342, 1992.

22. Group MTsC. Combination chemotherapy versus melphalan plus prednisone as treatment for multiple myeloma: an overview of 6,633 patients from 27 randomized trials. *J Clin Oncol* 16:3832–3842, 1998.

23. Barlogie B, Smith L, Alexanian R. Effective treatment of advanced multiple myeloma refractory to alkylating agents. *N Engl J Med* 310:1353–1356, 1984.

24. Alexanian R, Barlogie B, Dixon D. High-dose glucocorticoid treatment of resistant myeloma. *Ann Intern Med* 105:8–11, 1986.

25. Schlossman SF, Anderson KC. Bone marrow transplantation in multiple myeloma. In Jones R (ed), *Current Opinions in Oncology,* 1999:102–108.

26. Seiden M, Schlossman R, Andersen J, et al. Monoclonal antibody–purged bone marrow transplantation therapy for multiple myeloma. *Leuk Lymphoma* 17:87–93, 1995.

27. Vescio R, Schiller G, Stewart K, et al. Multicenter phase III trial to evaluate CD34+ selected vs. unselected autologous peripheral blood progenitor cell transplantation in multiple myeloma. *Blood* 93:1–13, 1999.

28. Attal M, Harousseau JL, Stoppa AM, et al. Autologous bone marrow transplantation versus conventional chemotherapy in multiple myeloma: a prospective, randomized trial. *N Engl J Med* 335:91–97, 1996.

29. Barlogie B, Jagannath S, Desikan KR, et al. Total therapy with tandem transplants for newly diagnosed multiple myeloma. *Blood* 93:55–65, 1999.

30. Teoh G, Chen L, Urashima M, et al. Adenovirus vector-based purging of multiple myeloma cells. *Blood* 92:4591–4601, 1998.

31. Schlossman SF, Alyea E, Orsini E, et al. Immune based strategies to improve hematopoietic stem cell transplantation in multiple myeloma. In Dicke KA, Keating A (eds), *Autologous Marrow and Blood Transplantation.* Charlottesville, VA: Carden, Jennings, 1999:207–221.

32. Gahrton G, Tura S, Ljungman P, et al. Prognostic factors in allogeneic bone marrow transplantation for multiple myeloma. *J Clin Oncol* 13:1312–1322, 1995.

33. Bjorkstrand B, Ljungman P, Svensson H, et al. Allogeneic bone marrow transplantation versus autologous stem cell transplantation in multiple myeloma: a restrospective case-matched study from the European Group for Blood and Marrow Transplantation. *Blood* 88:4711–4718, 1996.

34. Lokhorst HM, Schattenberg JJ, Cornelissen JJ, et al. Donor lymphocyte infusions are effective in relapsed multiple myeloma after allogeneic bone marrow transplantation. *Blood* 90:4206–4211, 1997.

35. Alyea EP, Soiffer RJ, Canning C, et al. Toxicity and efficacy of defined doses of CD4+ donor lymphocytes for treatment of relapse after allogeneic bone marrow transplant. *Blood* 91:3671–3680, 1998.

36. Ludwig H, Cohen AM, Polliack A, et al. Interferon-alpha for induction and maintenance in multiple myeloma: results of two multicenter randomized trials and summary of other studies. *Ann Oncol* 6:467–476, 1995.

37. Ludwig H, Fritz E, Neuda J, et al. Patient preferences for interferon-alpha in multiple myeloma. *J Clin Oncol* 15:1672–1679, 1997.

38. Raje N, Anderson KC. Radiotherapy in the management of plasma cell tumors. *Med Oncol* 14:112–115, 2000.

39. Berenson JR, Lichtenstein A, Porter L, et al. Efficacy of pamidronate in reducing skeletal events in patients with advanced multiple myeloma. *N Engl J Med* 334:488–493, 1996.

40. Berenson JR, Lichtenstein A, Porter L, et al. Long-term pamidronate treatment of advanced multiple myeloma patients reduces skeletal events. *J Clin Oncol* 16:593–602, 1998.

41. Kyle RA. Maintenance therapy and supportive care for patients with multiple myeloma. *Semin Oncol* 26:35–42, 1999.

42. Singhal S, Mehta J, Desikan R, et al. Anti-tumor activity of thalidomide in refractory multiple myeloma. *N Engl J Med* 341:1565–1571, 1999.

43. Raje N, Anderson KC. Thalidomide: a revival story. *N Engl J Med* 341:1606–1609, 1999.

44. Dimopoulos MA, Alexanian R. Waldenström's macroglobulinemia. *Blood* 83:1452–1459, 1994.

45. Dimopoulos MA, Kantarjian H, Weber D, et al. Primary therapy of Waldenstrom's macroglobulinemia with 2-chlorodeoxyadenosine. *J Clin Oncol* 12:2694–2698, 1994.

22

Leukemia

∎ ∎ ∎

KENNETH B. MILLER
HOWARD M. GRODMAN

IN THE UNITED STATES, LEUKEMIAS CONSTITUTE approximately 3% of all cancers and account for 4.0% of all cancer deaths (annual death rate approximately 4.6 per 100,000) [1]. The leukemias are a heterogeneous group of disorders that are divided broadly into acute and chronic types. The acute leukemias are characterized by cells that demonstrate both proliferation and impaired differentiation. This imbalance between proliferation and maturation results in the rapid accumulation of immature blast cells in the bone marrow and blood. If untreated, acute leukemia usually is fatal in weeks to months. The chronic leukemias, in contrast, are characterized by an expanded population of cells that proliferate but retain their capacity to differentiate and mature. Generally, the chronic leukemias have an indolent course.

The leukemias are divided further into lymphoid, myeloid, and biphenotypic subtypes. The subtypes are defined by the predominant leukemic cell population, with the biphenotypic leukemias demonstrating characteristics of both lymphoid and myeloid lineages. Morphology, histochemical staining, immunophenotyping, cytogenetics, and molecular markers are used to define the leukemic subtype. Assigning the appropriate lineage and subtype to acute or to chronic leukemia is important in defining prognosis and selecting treatment. Advances in both the treatment of the leukemias and supportive therapy has led to an improvement in the prognosis and quality of life for patients with both acute and chronic leukemias.

The acute leukemias account for approximately 1.5% of all cancer deaths in the United States (annual death rate, 2.2 per 100,000) [1]. Approximately 12,900 new cases of acute leukemia occur annually. The incidence increases with age and has remained remarkably steady since the late 1960s. Acute myelocytic leukemia (AML) represents approximately 80% of all adult acute leukemias. Acute lymphocytic leukemia (ALL) is the most common leukemia in childhood, causing approximately 25% of all childhood cancer deaths (annual incidence, 4 per 100,000). It accounts for approximately 20% of adult acute leukemias. The incidence of acute leukemias gradually increases with age, with a peak incidence of 12.6 per 100,000 adults older than 65 years.

The chronic leukemias—chronic lymphocytic leukemia (CLL) and chronic myelocytic leukemia (CML)—are rare before the age of 20 but steadily increase in incidence thereafter. The incidence of CLL is one in 100,000 at age 40 and increases steadily to 100 in one million at age 70. CML tends to be a disease of middle age, with an incidence of 1.5 to 2.5 per 100,000 for persons aged 45 to 60 years and is rare before age 20.

CLINICAL PRESENTATION

Generally, the clinical manifestations of the leukemias are diverse and nonspecific, resulting from the leukemic cell infiltration of the bone marrow and other organs. In the chronic leukemias, the proliferation and accumulation of the leukemic cells in the bone marrow, lymph nodes, and spleen gradually replace the normal tissues, reflecting their indolent course. In the acute leukemias, the clinical signs and symptoms are related directly to the rapid infiltration of the leukemic cells in bone marrow, which results in suppression of normal hematopoiesis and causes anemia, neutropenia, and thrombocytopenia. Typically, patients with leukemia present with signs and symptoms of fatigue, malaise, and low-grade fevers, easy or spontaneous bruising due to decreases in red blood cells, neutrophils, and platelets, respectively. The clinical presentation of the leukemia depends, in part, on the subtype and the biological characteristics of the disease. Though lymphadenopathy and splenomegaly are common findings in the chronic leukemias at presentation, in many patients CLL and CML are diagnosed at the time of a complete blood count performed for an unrelated illness.

ETIOLOGIC CHARACTERISTICS

Leukemia results from the neoplastic proliferation of hematopoietic or lymphoid cells. A malignant cell is the result of a series of transformations that cause alterations in the chromosomes and the inappropriate expression of various oncogenes. These changes affect the growth and differentiation of the transformed cell.

Genetic factors, drugs, and environmental and occupational exposures variously have been implicated as possible leukemogenic agents in both children and adults (Table 22.1)[2]. Leukemogenesis is a multistep process that requires the susceptibility of a hematopoietic progenitor cell to inductive agents at multiple stages. No single factor has been shown to cause leukemia in all exposed individuals.

Evidence supporting a genetic predisposition for human leukemia comes from epidemiologic and family studies [3]. The highest incidence of leukemia in adults occurs in North America, western Europe, and Oceania, and the lowest is found in Asia and Latin America [4]. In contrast, the highest rate of childhood leukemia occurs in Asia and is lower in children in North America and India. Many reports cite multiple cases of both ALL and AML occurring within the same family [5]. As regards all types of leukemia, a threefold increase in the incidence of leukemia is seen among first-degree relatives of patients with acute leukemia.

Monozygotic twins exhibit an increased concordance for childhood leukemia. If one of affected twins develops leukemia before age 6, the first-year risk of leukemia occurrence in the second twin is as high as 25% [6]. The studies in twins are compatible with the occurrence of a genetic or a nongenetic intrauterine postzygotic event in utero, leading to involvement of both of such twins owing to the shared placental fetal circulation of monozygotic twins. The clinical presentation of leukemia in twins is atypical: The leukemia occurs before age 2; it occurs in both twins in close succession, typically in the same year; and it is the same morpho-

Table 22.1 Pathogenesis of Acute Leukemia

Toxins
Radiation
Chemicals (benzene)
Drugs
    Alkylating agents: cyclophosphamide, melphalan, chlorambucil
    Topoisomerase II inhibitors: anthracyclines, etoposide

Congenital disorders
Down's syndrome
Fanconi's anemia
Klinefelter's syndrome
Bloom's syndrome
Ataxia telangiectasia

Acquired disorders
Polycythemia vera
Agnogenic myeloid metaplasia
Myelodysplastic syndromes
Aplastic anemia
Paroxysmal nocturnal hemoglobinuria

logic and cytogenetic subtype. Nonidentical twin studies, however, do not demonstrate a similar concordance for acute leukemia [7].

The existence of a genetic predisposition to develop acute leukemia is suggested by the increased leukemia incidence associated with a number of congenital disorders, including Down's syndrome, von Recklinghausen's disease, congenital neurofibromatosis, Fanconi's anemia, ataxia telangiectasia, and Bloom's syndrome [8]. In Down's syndrome patients, the incidence of acute leukemia is 10 times that in the general population. The development of leukemia in persons with these disorders appears to be a multistep process rather than a single transforming event. Presumably, these genetic disorders result in a microenvironment permissive for chromosomal instability or in an increased sensitivity to DNA damage and a susceptibility to mutations.

Exposure to ionizing radiation and to a number of chemicals has been linked to the development of acute leukemia. The evidence linking radiation exposure and leukemia comes, in part, from the long-term follow-up of survivors of the atomic bomb explosions in Hiroshima and Nagasaki [9]. The latency time from exposure to the development of leukemia was between 5 and 21 years, and the risk was related to age at the time of exposure and to the radiation dose. In Hiroshima, a 30-fold increase was seen in the incidence of AML, ALL, and CML. The highest rates were observed in persons younger than 10 or older than 50 at the time of exposure. In Nagasaki, where victims were exposed to a higher amount of gamma radiation, the incidence of AML was even greater.

Exposure to even moderate doses of ionizing radiation appears to be associated with an increased risk for developing leukemia. Workers at radium plants and military personnel exposed to ionizing radiation during nuclear test explosions had a higher-than-expected incidence of AML [10]. Patients who received low doses of radiation for various benign disorders (e.g., ankylosing spondylitis, rheumatoid arthritis) developed AML at a greater-than-expected rate [11].

The chronic exposure to a number of chemicals has been associated with the development of acute leukemia [12]. Benzene is the chemical leukemogenic agent best studied and most widely used [13]. The chronic exposure to benzene and benzene derivatives is associated with a significant increase in the incidence of AML. Persons exposed to embalming fluid, ethylene oxides, and herbicides also appear to be at an increased risk for developing acute leukemia. Cigarette smokers and those chronically exposed to cigarette smoke appear to be at an increased risk of developing AML [14]. Heavy cigarette smoking is associated with the development of clonal, nonrandom, cytogenetic abnormalities. Metabolites of benzene, polonium 210, and various polycyclic aromatic hydrocarbons are found in cigarette smoke.

An increased incidence of acute leukemia occurs in patients who have received chemotherapy for a number of malignant and nonmalignant disorders. AMLs occurring after exposure to chemotherapy are called *secondary leukemias*. Alkylating agents, including cyclophosphamide, chlorambucil, busulfan, and mechlorethamine, have been associated with an increased risk for AML. Exposure to a combination of chemotherapy and radiotherapy further increases affected patients' risk of developing leukemia [15]. In patients with Hodgkin's disease, the cumulative risk of developing AML after treatment with alkylating agents increases steadily from 1 year after the start of treatment and reaches a peak of 13% at seven years [16]. The incidence of AML in patients treated with the regimen of mechlorethamine, vincristine (Oncovin), procarbazine, and prednisone is 3%, 4%, and 7% at three, five, and seven years, respectively. The actuarial risk is between 9% and 18% for these secondary AMLs after high-dose chemotherapy and radiotherapy administered as part of an autologous transplantation regimen for Hodgkin's disease and the non-Hodgkin's lymphomas.

Therapy-related secondary leukemias now represent 10% to 20% of all cases of AML [15]. These treatment-related leukemias are clinically and prognostically different from AML that occurs spontaneously. Usually, the secondary leukemias are preceded by a variable period of anemia, neutropenia, or thrombocytopenia. The bone marrow reveals dysplastic changes in one or more cell lines. In the blood, platelets may be large and exhibit abnormal granulation; neutrophils may be hypogranular or agranular, with pseudo-Pelger-Huët nuclei; and the red blood cells may be macrocytic, evincing coarse basophilic stippling and prominent anisocytosis. These morphologic abnormalities may be accompanied also by functional defects in platelet and neutrophils. The findings in the blood and bone marrow may precede the development of overt AML by many months. Clonal, nonrandom, cytogenetic abnormalities involving chromosomes 7, 5, and 8 occur in 50% to 90% of patients with therapy-related secondary leukemias [15].

A clinically and cytogenetically distinct group of secondary leukemias has been reported in individuals who have received one of the topoisomerase II inhibitors [17]. This group includes the epipodophyllotoxins eto-

poside and teniposide and the anthracyclines daunomy-
cin and doxorubicin. In contrast to alkylating agent–
related AML, the topoisomerase II therapy–related
leukemias are characterized by a shorter latency of onset, generally two to three years. Usually, these topoisomerase II–related secondary leukemias are associated
with chromosomal rearrangements involving chromosomes 11 and 21. The *MLL* gene (mixed lineage, or
myeloid-lymphoid leukemia), located on chromosome
11 at band q23, is the most frequent site of the leukemogenic translocation induced by topoisomerase II inhibitors. The treatment outcome for these patients is
much worse than that for patients who have de novo
AML and similar clinical and cytogenetic abnormalities.

Certain acquired diseases are associated with an
increased incidence of transformation to AML. The
myeloproliferative disorders (e.g., polycythemia vera,
primary thrombocythemia, and agnogenic myeloid
metaplasia) are associated with an increased incidence
of leukemic transformation that rises further with the
administration of chemotherapy and radiotherapy.

CHILDHOOD LEUKEMIAS

The annual incidence of cancer in children aged 0 to 14
years is approximately 13 cases per 100,000 population.
This represents perhaps 1% of all cancers in the Western industrialized world. Leukemia represents some
25% of all childhood cancers in the United States,
translating into an incidence of four per 100,000 children. Despite the relatively low incidence of the disease,
research and care of childhood cancer has had a dramatic impact on the therapy of cancer overall.

Acute leukemia in children is very different from the
adult version of the disease. ALL is the most common
malignancy in children and represents approximately
75% of all pediatric leukemias, most of the remainder
being AML. Chronic leukemias are rare in children. The
incidence of ALL in the United States is approximately
3.4 per 100,000 children aged 0 to 14 years [1]. The
incidence in white children is twice that of black children in the United States, and the ratio of boys to girls
is 1.2:1.

The incidence of ALL varies geographically, and the
disease is relatively rare in the Middle East and Africa.
White children experience a peak incidence of ALL at
approximately age 4, whereas black children exhibit no
such age peak. This peak has appeared in different
countries at different times. It occurred in Great Britain
in the 1920s, in the United States in the 1940s, and in
Japan in the 1960s. Some have suggested that these

times correspond to periods of major increases in industrialization in each of these countries. In contrast
to ALL, childhood AML shows no such peak. The ratio
of ALL to AML in childhood is approximately 4:1, although neonates are more likely to have AML than
ALL. Also in contrast to ALL, AML has exhibited little
change in the rate of its cure using conventional chemotherapy. Approximately 40% of these children experience prolonged disease-free survival.

ACUTE MYELOGENOUS LEUKEMIA

AML, also called *acute nonlymphocytic leukemia* or *acute
myeloblastic leukemia,* originally was described by the
German pathologist Virchow in 1847. It is not a single
disease but a group of neoplastic disorders characterized
by the proliferation and accumulation of immature hematopoietic cells in the bone marrow and blood. Gradually, these malignant cells replace and inhibit the
growth and maturation of normal erythroid, myeloid,
and megakaryocytic precursors. The clinical evaluation,
therapy, and prognosis of patients with AML has
changed dramatically over the last two decades from a
disease that was uniformly fatal to one that is potentially curable [18].

Clinical Manifestations

Usually, the presenting signs and symptoms of AML are
nonspecific and are related to the decreased production
of normal hematopoietic cells and the invasion of organs by the leukemic cells. Initially, patients usually
complain of a brief viruslike illness characterized by fatigue and malaise. Bleeding after mild trauma or easy
bruising are common presenting complaints and reflect
the low platelet count. Diffuse bone tenderness involving the long bones, ribs, and sternum is the initial clinical manifestation in 25% of patients. The bone pain,
which can be severe and migratory, is caused by the
expansion of the intramedullary space or direct involvement of the periosteum by the leukemic cells.

The findings on physical examination relate to leukemic cells' interference with normal hematopoiesis.
Typically, all three cell lines are affected. Anemia results
in pallor and the onset of cardiovascular symptoms,
such as tachycardia and shortness of breath. Thrombocytopenia results in petechiae and ecchymoses. Petechiae are most prominent in the lower extremities and
may appear suddenly after minor physical activity or
after standing for prolonged periods of time. Spleno-

megaly may occur in up to 50% of patients with AML, but the splenic enlargement usually is modest. A very large spleen at presentation suggests that the leukemia has evolved from an underlying prior myeloproliferative disorder. Lymphadenopathy is rare in AML, in contrast to ALL, in which peripheral lymphadenopathy may a be prominent presenting finding. Involvement of the thymus or hilar nodes is very uncommon in AML.

Skin involvement—leukemia cutis—occurs in approximately 10% of patients and usually presents as violaceous, raised, nontender plaques or nodules, which on biopsy are found to be infiltrated with blastlike cells. Skin involvement is more common with the monocytic and myelomonocytic subtypes. Chloromas (local collections of blasts) may present as isolated subcutaneous masses and may, therefore, be confused with a primary or metastatic carcinoma. The term *chloromas* reflects the greenish appearance of the masses seen on sectioning due to the presence of myeloperoxidase granules in the myeloblasts. Granulocytic sarcomas are more common in the M2 subtype of AML with the (8;21) translocation and leukocytosis. Gingival hyperplasia, due to leukemic cell infiltration, is more frequent in the monocytic leukemias (Color Plate 22.1) but may occur in all the leukemic subtypes. Initially, patients may present to their dentist complaining of painful gums, the new onset of progressive gingival disease, and gum bleeding after mild dental brushing.

Central nervous system (CNS) involvement is uncommon in AML. Patients who present with a high circulating blast count and the M4 subtype of AML with eosinophils (M4E) are at higher risk for developing CNS leukemia. Thirty-five percent of patients with the M4E variant associated with an inversion of chromosome 16 have evidence of CNS involvement.

Metabolic and electrolyte derangements are common in patients with AML. Hyperuricemia is frequent and is due to the increased turnover of the proliferating leukemic cells and subsequent purine catabolism. Hyperuricemia and hyperuricuria can develop before therapy is started. Typically, however, the uric acid level rises rapidly once therapy is initiated, owing to release of intracellular nucleic acids by the lysis of large numbers of cells. Therefore, maintaining adequate hydration is important, as is administering allopurinol prior to and during induction chemotherapy. Hypokalemia is common in the myelomonocytic and monocytic leukemias. These subtypes release large amounts of lysozyme (muramidase), which are toxic to renal tubular cells. Ineffective myelopoiesis or destruction of the leukemic cells after treatment results in the release of large amounts of this enzyme, thereby producing a proxi-

mal renal tubular dysfunction and leading to renal potassium wasting. Leukemic cells also can synthesize other factors with reninlike activity that may contribute to the development hypokalemia.

A spuriously low serum glucose level and arterial oxygen saturation can occur in the presence of high numbers of circulating blasts. A false elevation of blood potassium levels may occur with hyperleukocytosis due to the release of potassium from leukocytes undergoing lysis during clotting or due to prolonged storage of the sample prior to analysis. This phenomenon is more common in patients with a high blast count. If a spuriously elevated potassium level is suspected, the serum electrolyte studies should be repeated with an anticoagulated blood sample that is analyzed rapidly to prevent the in vitro lysis of leukemic blasts.

Patients who present with a high circulating blast count are at risk for a number of complications. The high number of circulating leukemic blasts increases the blood viscosity and is associated with small-vessel leukoblastic emboli that can result in leukostasis in the cerebral vessels. The leukemic blasts can infiltrate the arteriolar endothelial walls and cause a secondary hemorrhage. Suspected or developing CNS leukostasis requires emergency efforts to lower the blast count rapidly. Patients may complain of diffuse headaches and fatigue, which rapidly progress to confusion and coma.

The risk of CNS leukostasis rapidly increases when the blast count is greater than 50,000/mm^3. Pulmonary leukostasis is a serious potential problem for patients who present with high blast count. Leukocyte thrombi and plugging of pulmonary microvascular channels lead to vascular rupture and infiltration of the lung parenchyma, resulting in the sudden onset of shortness of breath and progressive dyspnea. Usually, chest radiography demonstrates a diffuse interstitial infiltrate. Hypercapnia, hypoxemia, and progressive respiratory acidosis are signs of pulmonary leukostasis. Pulmonary hemorrhage and leukostasis may mimic the signs and symptoms of a bacterial or fungal pneumonia. The prognosis for patients who develop symptomatic pulmonary leukostasis is very poor.

The perirectal and oral area are two important portals for infection in patients with leukemia. In such patients, the first signs of a perirectal infection may be induration and tenderness without other signs of inflammation or infection. Initially, patients may complain only of pain on defecation and diffuse anal tenderness. Early recognition and treatment of these potential sources of infection is important. Usually, perirectal abscesses are due to gram-negative bacteria and, in the setting of granulocytopenia, can progress rapidly to perirectal cellulitis and septicemia. Though digital rectal examinations generally are avoided in patients who are granulocytopenic, the perirectal area can be examined carefully and gently. Patients should be instructed about the importance of perirectal hygiene. Constipation should be avoided so as to prevent small mucosal tears.

Diagnosis

AML is classified according to the FAB classification, a system developed by a collaborating group of French, American, and British hematologists. The FAB classification was established in 1976 and has been modified and expanded over the last two decades to incorporate cytogenetics and immunophenotyping studies [18, 18a, 19]. Usually, the presumptive diagnosis of acute leukemia is apparent after examining affected patients and reviewing their blood smears. Most patients present with anemia, thrombocytopenia, and circulating blast forms, which are apparent on the peripheral blood smear. The total white blood cell count (WBC) may range from fewer than 1,000/mm³ to more than 200,000/mm³, with the majority of affected patients having a total WBC between 5,000 and 30,000/mm³. A bone marrow aspiration and biopsy is necessary to confirm the diagnosis and to define the leukemic subtype.

Many patients and physicians feel compelled to start treatment for AML immediately; in most instances, however, emergency therapy is not needed. Usually, treatment can be delayed until the necessary clinical and laboratory evaluations are available. Patients also may need time to accept the diagnosis and to address personal, financial, and family needs. As part of an initial evaluation, the psychological and emotional needs and concerns of affected patients and their families must be considered. Even in severely neutropenic and thrombocytopenic patients, a bone marrow biopsy and aspiration can be performed safely.

Local bleeding or infection at the site of the procedure is rare. The posterior iliac crest is the preferred site unless a patient has received prior radiotherapy to the pelvis or has evidence of an active infection at the site. The sternum is an alternate site for performing a bone marrow aspirate.

Cytogenetic studies are an important prognostic indicator and should be performed on all affected patients at the time of the initial bone marrow aspiration [20]. Cell-surface markers and molecular and enzyme studies are helpful for suspected lymphoid or biphenotypic leukemia. The bone marrow aspirate provides for quali-

tative assessment of bone marrow cellularity and morphology. The bone marrow biopsy allows for quantitative assessment of bone marrow cellularity, megakaryocyte number, and reticulin fibrosis.

The initial bone marrow sample in most patients with AML is hypercellular, with absent or decreased megakaryocytes. However, elderly patients or those with secondary or treatment-related AML may have a normal cellular or hypocellular bone marrow. Dysplastic myeloid and erythroid maturation may be noted. The prognostic significance of dysplasia in de novo AML is controversial. Frequently, trilineage dysplasia is associated with other poor prognostic features, including unfavorable chromosomal abnormalities. In addition, prominent dysplasia may suggest a prior exposure to hematotoxins or that the patient's leukemia evolved from a prior myelodysplastic syndrome or secondary to prior cytotoxic chemotherapy. Auer bodies or rods— reddish rodlike filaments of aggregated primary granules—may be present in the leukemic cells. These bodies (rods), first described by Dr. Joseph Auer, are primary azurophilic granules that have been incorporated into autophagic vacuoles. Auer rods are helpful in differentiating a myeloid from a lymphoid leukemia [21].

The number of blasts in the blood and bone marrow is the defining criterion to distinguish a myelodysplastic syndrome from acute leukemia and to subclassify the acute leukemias. The diagnosis of acute leukemia requires that at least 30% of either total nucleated cells or nonerythroid cells in the bone marrow are blast forms. Blasts must be distinguished from promyelocytes in the bone marrow count, because the latter are included with differentiated granulocytes. The determination of the number of *blasts* in the bone marrow is crucial, and the distinction between a blast and a promyelocyte can be difficult.

In patients with acute leukemia, the most important initial morphologic evaluation is to distinguish among AML, ALL, or one of the myelodysplastic syndromes. The prognosis and therapeutic strategies remain very different for adults with these disorders. In most cases, the morphologic evaluation and cytochemical stains will define the appropriate lineage. Cytogenetic studies define specific abnormalities associated with AML or myelodysplastic syndromes. In some cases, the morphologic distinction between an undifferentiated myeloblastic leukemia and a lymphoblastic leukemia can be difficult. Distinguishing AML with no or minimal differentiation, the monoblastic leukemias without differentiation, and some of the acute megakaryocytic leukemias from ALL can be difficult by morphologic studies or cytochemical stains alone. In such instances, the use

Table 22.2 Monoclonal Antibodies Commonly Used to Distinguish AML from ALL

AML	ALL
CD11	CD10 (CALLA)
CD13	CD2
CD14	CD3
CD15	CD4
CD33	CD5
CD41	CD19
CD61	CD20

AML = acute myelogenous leukemia; ALL = acute lymphoid leukemia; CD = cluster designation.

of monoclonal antibodies for lineage-associated markers is most important.

In the majority of cases of acute leukemia, morphologic features and cytochemistry are sufficient to assign the correct lineage. In approximately 15% of cases, however, the distinction between an immature AML variant and ALL cannot be made by morphologic analysis. The use of monoclonal antibodies that identify myeloid- and lymphoid-associated antigens is highly beneficial in such cases (Table 22.2). In ALL, the immunologic markers are important is assigning cell lineage, defining leukemia-specific subsets, and assessing prognosis. In AML, biochemical and immunologic markers have been applied less widely. The expression of these antibodies corresponds to the normal stages of myeloid and monocytic differentiation. None of the currently available myeloid monoclonal antibodies identifies leukemia-specific determinants. The monoclonal antibodies have been useful tools for defining the maturation and differentiation of normal myeloid and monocytic precursors. However, leukemic cells frequently express markers of multiple levels of maturation and different lineages. Therefore, unlike the morphologic classifications that attempt to place the predominant cell type within a specific defined group, immunophenotyping marker studies have demonstrated that AML cells are antigenically and morphologically heterogeneous.

Immunophenotyping has been most useful in distinguishing between AML and ALL and in defining hybrid or biphenotypic leukemias. In ALL, the immunophenotyping studies have defined functionally and prognostically relevant subgroups unrelated to both morphologic features and cytochemistry [22, 23]. Myeloid blasts also may express lymphoid-associated antigens. A meaningful proportion of myeloid blasts (20–45%) express lymphoid-associated antigens, most frequently CD2, CD7, and CD19. The prognostic significance of this phenotypic heterogeneity is unclear but, in most studies, it does not appear to be associated with a poorer response to treatment.

The use of immunophenotyping is particularly important in identifying AML with minimal differentiation (M0), erythroleukemia (M6), and megakaryoblastic leukemia (M7) (Color Plate 22.2). Immunophenotyping may help also in identifying subsets of patients who are at risk for shorter remission durations and resistant disease, such as CD34-positive AML, but the role of immunophenotyping as an independent prognostic indicator remains unclear. CD13 and CD33 are the most useful markers for identifying myeloid leukemias. Immunophenotyping has demonstrated the phenotypic heterogeneity and mixed-lineage differentiation of many myeloid leukemias.

The acute leukemias are classified according to the predominant neoplastic cell type. In the FAB classification, the myeloid leukemias are divided into eight categories on the basis of morphology, cytochemical staining, and immunologic phenotype of the predominant cell type (Table 22.3; see Color Plate 22.2). Initially, the classification system was proposed solely for morphologic definition of the subtypes of the acute leukemias. However, subsequently it has been expanded to include ultrastructural morphology, cytogenetics, immunophenotyping, and immunohistochemical markers. This classification system has been shown to be both clinically and prognostically useful. The FAB criteria are based on a Wright-Giemsa-stained blood smear and the bone marrow aspirate or biopsy. Four basic histochemical stains are described, including periodic acid–Schiff reagent, Sudan black, peroxidase, and esterase (specific and nonspecific). The FAB classification *does not* include hybrid or biphenotypic leukemias that cannot be classified on the basis of morphologic definition or cytochemistry alone. The classification system *does* try to take into account the heterogeneous nature of AML and recognizes that it is not a single disease but a group of disorders affecting the hematopoietic precursors in the bone marrow.

Subtypes of AML

M0 SUBTYPE (AML WITHOUT DIFFERENTIATION OR MATURATION)

The M0 subtype constitutes approximately 3% of all cases of AML [24]. On the basis of morphologic definition, differentiating the blasts from the L2 variant of

Table 22.3   Diagnostic Features of Acute Myelogenous Leukemia (AML)

FAB Type	Diagnostic Features

AML-M0
  AML with no evidence of
  myeloid maturation
	$\geq$ 30% blasts; < 3% blasts reactive to MPO, SBB, or NSE; immunophenotyping CD33- and CD13-positive

AML-M1 AML without maturation	$\geq$ 30% blasts; $\geq$ 3% blasts reactive to MPO or SBB; < 10% of marrow nucleated cells are promyelocytes or more mature neutrophils
AML-M2 AML with maturation	$\geq$ 30% blasts; $\geq$ 3% blasts reactive to MPO or SBB; 10% of marrow nucleated cells are promyelocytes or more mature neutrophils: t(8;21) cytogenetic abnormality

AML-M3
  Acute promyelocytic
  leukemia (APML)
	$\geq$ 30% blasts and abnormal promyelocytes; intense MPO and SBB reactivity; promyelocytes and blasts with multiple Auer rods: t(15;17) cytogenetic abnormality

AML-M4
  Acute meylomonocytic
  leukemia
	$\geq$ 30% myeloblasts, monoblasts, and promonocytes; $\geq$ 20% monocytic cells in marrow;$\geq$ 5 $\times$ 10^9/liter monocytic cells in blood; $\geq$ 20% neutrophils and precursors in marrow; monocytic cells reactive for NSE; abnormal eosinophils in M4e: Inv (16) chromosome abnormality

AML-M5a
  Acute monoblastic
  leukemia
	> 30% blasts; $\geq$ 80% monocytic cells; monoblasts $\geq$ 80% of monocytic cells; monoblasts and promonocytes NSE-positive; monoblasts usually MPO- and SBB-negative

AML-M5b
  Acute monocytic
  leukemia
	> 30% blasts; $\geq$ 80% monocytic cells; monoblasts < 80% of monocytic cells; promonocytes predominate; monoblasts and promonocytes NSE-postive; promonocytes may have scattered MPO- and SBB-positive granules

AML-M6 Acute erythroleukemia	> 30% blasts; $\geq$ 50% erythroblasts; $\geq$ 30% of nonerythroid precursors are myeloblasts; dysplastic erythroid precursors frequently PAS-positive

AML-M7
  Acute megakaryoblastic
  leukemia
	$\geq$ 30% blasts; $\geq$ 50% cells megakaryoblasts by electron microscopy; immunophenotyping CD41-positive (GP IIa/IIIb), CD61-positive (GP IIIa)

FAB = *F*rench, *A*merican, and *B*ritish collaborating hematologists; MPO = myeloperoxidase; SBB = Sudan black B; NSE = nonspecific esterase; CD = cluster designation; PAS = periodic acid–Schiff; GP = glycoprotein.

ALL is difficult. The blasts appear very immature, and fewer than 3% of the blast cells stain positive with myeloperoxidase or Sudan black B. Generally, lymphoid markers are negative except for the enzyme terminal deoxynucleotidyl transferase, which is expressed in more than 60% of the cases. Auer rods are absent. The use of immunophenotypic markers or ultrastructural myeloperoxidase is necessary to identify the myeloid lineage in this subtype. In approximately 30% of cases, the blasts mark with the T-cell markers CD4 and CD7. Myeloid-specific monoclonal antibodies (including CD13 and CD33) are positive. The stem cell antigen CD34 is associated strongly in the AML-M0 subtype. AML-M0 has a high incidence of complex karyotypes and frequent involvement of chromosomes 5, 7, 8, and 13. The M0 subtype is associated with a poor overall prognosis.

M1 SUBTYPE (AML WITHOUT MATURATION)

The M1 subtype accounts for 15% to 20% of AML cases. Auer rods are rare or absent. The bone marrow contains fewer than 3% promyelocytes and fewer than 10% maturing granulocytes. Some of the cells express CD7, an antigen present on early T cells.

M2 SUBTYPE (AML WITH MATURATION)

Myeloblastic leukemia with maturation (M2) is the most common subtype of AML and accounts for approximately 25% to 30% of all cases. The blasts demonstrate clear evidence of maturation to and beyond the promyelocyte. Usually, Auer rods are present, and the myeloblasts contain prominent azurophilic granules. Approximately half of affected patients with this subtype will have a translocation involving chromosomes 8 and 21 [t(8;21)]. However, other subtypes also express this cytogenetic finding. The (8;21)(q22;q22) translocation juxtaposes the *AML1* gene on chromosome 21 to the *ETO* (for "eight-twenty-one") gene on chromosome 8, which results in the production of the AML1-ETO fusion protein [25]. AML cells with the 8;21 translocation characteristically contain thin and elongated Auer rods, a basophilic cytoplasm, and indented

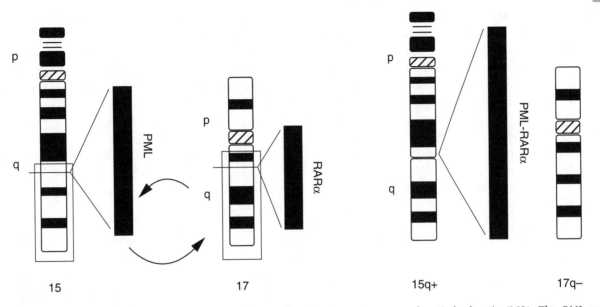

Figure 22.1 Representation of the t(15;17)(q22;q21) translocation in acute promyelocytic leukemia (M3). The *PML* gene at 15q22 is fused with part of the *RARα* (retinoic receptoralpha) gene from 17q21.

nuclei; abnormal granulocytic maturation with dysplastic granulocytes is common.

Generally, this subtype has a favorable prognosis, with a high remission induction rate after standard chemotherapy. The overall survival of patients with the 8;21 translocation generally is better than that associated with the other subtypes of AML.

M3 SUBTYPE (ACUTE PROMYELOCYTIC LEUKEMIA)

Acute promyelocytic leukemia (APL; M3) accounts for 5% to 10% of all cases of AML and is characterized by the presence of atypical promyelocytes in the bone marrow and peripheral blood [26]. APL is distinguished from other subtypes of AML by its distinctive morphologic features, younger patient age at presentation, specific chromosomal abnormality, associated coagulopathy, and unique response to treatment with retinoic acid. Auer rods may be so numerous as to form Auer bundles. Patients with this subtype present with a WBC lower than that of the other subtypes (usually fewer than 5,000/mm³). The M3 subtype has a characteristic cytogenetic finding: the 15;17 translocation, which is a balanced translocation from the long arm of chromosome 17 to the long arm of chromosome 15: t(15q+; 17q−; Fig. 22.1) This rearrangement fuses the promyelocytic leukemia gene on chromosome 15 with the retinoic acid receptor–alpha (*RARα*) gene on chromosome 17, resulting in a PML-RARα chimeric protein.

Cells that express the *PML-RARα* gene are uniquely sensitive to all-*trans*-retinoic acid, a vitamin A derivative [27]. The retinoic acid receptor is a member of a family of steroid hormone nuclear receptors important in the regulation and control of both normal and malignant cellular differentiation and proliferation. The translocation encodes for a novel DNA-binding protein that results in the expression of an abnormal messenger RNA transcript for *RARα* and confers a unique therapeutic sensitivity to one of its ligands: all-*trans*-retinoic acid. Myeloid differentiation appears to be blocked by the abnormal PML-RARα fusion protein. This abnormal receptor is the target of all-*trans*-retinoic acid treatment.

Treatment of APL with all-*trans*-retinoic acid results in differentiation of the leukemic cells; approximately 70% to 85% of patients attain a complete remission. Moreover, unlike standard induction therapy, treatment with oral all-*trans*-retinoic acid is not associated with bone marrow hypoplasia and the usual complications of cytotoxic chemotherapy. All-*trans*-retinoic acid induces leukemic cells to replicate and differentiate into cells capable of undergoing normal senescence and cell death. In patients in whom treatment fails or who relapse after treatment with all-*trans*-retinoic acid, low doses of arsenic trioxide can induce complete remission [28]. The clinical response to arsenic trioxide is associated with incomplete cytodifferentiation and may be related to the induction of apoptosis in leukemic cells.

Often, APL patients present with thrombocytopenia, prolongation of the thromboplastin and thrombin time, increased levels of fibrin degradation products, and hypofibrinogenemia. The coagulation disorder in APL results from at least three distinct mechanisms: disseminated intravascular coagulation, fibrinolysis, and proteolysis. The disseminated intravascular coagulation and fibrinolysis are attributed to the spontaneous or chemotherapy-associated release of a tissue factor with procoagulant activity present in the granules of the leukemic promyelocytes. APL cells overexpress annexin II, a cell-surface receptor for both plasminogen and its tissue activator, t-PA, which increases the production of the fibrinolytic protein plasmin [29]. The use of all-*trans*-retinoic acid with or without chemotherapy has changed the prognosis, course, and management of this leukemic subtype. Generally, the bleeding and clotting problems respond promptly to treatment with retinoic acid. The prognosis for patients with APL after treatment with all-*trans*-retinoic acid and chemotherapy is very favorable.

M4 SUBTYPE (ACUTE MYELOMONOCYTIC LEUKEMIA)

The M4 subtype accounts for 20% to 25% of all cases of AML. The cells have characteristics of both myelocytes and monocytes. Extramedullary disease, including gingival hypertrophy, leukemia cutis, and meningeal leukemia, is more common in this subtype than in the other myeloid leukemias. This subtype is morphologically similar to AML-M2; however, the blast count includes myeloblasts, monoblasts, and promonocytes that together must exceed 30%.

A variant of this subtype, called *acute myelomonocytic leukemia with abnormal eosinophils* (M4E) is characterized by the presence of myelomonocytic blasts and 5% to 30 % of morphologically and cytochemically abnormal eosinophils. Often, patients with the M4E subtype present with a high peripheral WBC (range = 30,000–100,000/mm³) and splenomegaly. CNS involvement is common in this variant. The M4E variant has a unique karyotypic abnormality of chromosome 16: an inversion of the long and short arm or a balanced translocation between two homologous chromosomes 16. The cytogenetic feature in both of these translocations is the break in the long arm of chromosome 16 at band q22. Patients with the M4E variant who undergo chemotherapy have a generally favorable prognosis [30].

M5 SUBTYPE (ACUTE MONOCYTIC LEUKEMIA)

The AML-M5 subtype represents 2% to 9% of all cases of AML. The monocytic leukemias are divided into two variants: a poorly differentiated monoblastic leukemia (M5a) and a differentiated monocytic leukemia (M5b).

The blasts in the M5a variant are poorly differentiated monoblasts, with rare granules and occasional cytoplasmic vacuoles. Usually, Auer rods are not seen. These cells morphologically resemble lymphoblasts of the L2 variant. The M5b variant consists of more differentiated monocytes, which have the typical lobulated monocytic nucleus. Auer rods also are rare.

The M5 subtype has an increased incidence of gingival hypertrophy and extramedullary disease involving the liver, spleen, and lymph nodes. The monocytic leukemias demonstrate a poorer overall response to treatment.

M6 SUBTYPE (ACUTE ERYTHROLEUKEMIA)

Acute erythroleukemia represents 3% to 5% of all cases of AML. The erythroblasts are morphologically abnormal, with multilobed nuclei, multiple nuclei, nuclear fragments, and giant pronormoblasts having megaloblastic features. Trilineage dysplasia is frequent, and differentiating this subtype from an evolving myelodysplastic syndrome is difficult. In such cases, the bone marrow has a high fraction of proerythroblasts without a myeloblastic component or dysplastic erythroid hyperplasia. Usually, Auer rods are not present.

Patients with erythroleukemia tend to be older at the time of diagnosis. Usually, the presenting complaints are associated with the development of anemia. The peripheral smear may exhibit only rare blast forms. Some patients present with peculiar rheumatic and immunologic findings, and up to one-third will complain of diffuse joint, abdominal, back, and chest pain. Frequently, the erythroleukemias are preceded by a myelodysplastic syndrome, and they generally respond poorly to treatment.

M7 SUBTYPE (ACUTE MEGAKARYOCYTIC LEUKEMIA)

Acute megakaryocytic leukemia (M7) represents 3% to 12% of all cases of AML. The incidence of acute megakaryocytic leukemia is higher in patients whose disease evolves from a prior myeloproliferative disorder, myelofibrosis, or chronic myelogenous leukemia. Megakaryoblasts are morphologically heterogeneous and vary from small round cells, resembling cells found in the L2 variant of ALL or in an undifferentiated M0 or M1 leukemia. Undifferentiated blasts may be surrounded by shed platelets and recognizable micromegakaryocytes. In the peripheral blood, megakaryocytic fragments are seen, along with large atypical cells with prominent cytoplasmic blebs representing megakaryoblasts. Typically, bone marrow aspirate yields a dry tap, and biopsy shows increased reticulin and fibrosis. The fibrosis is due to the local secretion of platelet-derived growth factors by the leukemic cells that stimulate the normal fibroblasts in the bone marrow. In many cases, megakaryocytic features may not be recognized, necessitating the use of monoclonal antibodies to specific platelet glycoproteins to define this subtype. Immunophenotyping with monoclonal antibodies to platelet glycoproteins IIb/IIIa, CD42b, CD61, or CD41 or to coagulation factor VIII–related antigen may be needed to identify the megakaryoblasts.

The clinical and hematologic features of the M7 subtype vary, reflecting evolution of the disease from a prior myeloproliferative disorder in many patients. Frequently, such patients present with hepatomegaly and splenomegaly and generally have a poor response to chemotherapy. A complete remission often is associated with reversal of the bone marrow fibrosis.

Predictors of Response

A number of defined clinical characteristics of leukemia are important prognostic factors (Table 22.4). Age is the most important prognostic variable for induction therapy. Patients older than 60 years tolerate intensive treatment poorly. In addition, such patients have an increased incidence of unfavorable prognostic variables, including FAB subtype and cytogenetic patterns (e.g., abnormalities of chromosomes 5, 7, and 8), the generally favorable cytogenetic and FAB types being less common in elderly patients. Cytotoxic chemotherapy in elderly patients is associated with a higher morbidity and mortality than in younger patients because of the presence of comorbid diseases, poor tolerance of prolonged pancytopenia and, perhaps, impaired drug metabolism and excretion.

Colony-stimulating factors have been shown to reduce the duration of neutropenia in elderly patients undergoing induction chemotherapy, but their overall effect on morbidity or mortality is unclear [31, 32]. The duration of disease remission in patients older than 60 years who attain complete remission is shorter than in young patients, and the role of postinduction chemotherapy in treating this group remains unclear.

Patients with secondary AML or a prior myelodysplastic syndrome or myeloproliferative disorder also respond poorly to standard chemotherapy regimens. Patients presenting with blast cell counts greater than 50,000/mm³ and signs of leukostasis also respond poorly to induction therapy. The pretreatment serum

Table 22.4 Prognostic Factors in Acute Myelogenous Leukemia

Clinical Factor	Favorable	Unfavorable
Age	< 50 yr	> 60 yr
Leukemia	De novo	Secondary
White blood cell count	< 10,000/mm³	> 50,000/mm³
FAB type	M3, M4Eo	M5a, M5b, M6, M7
Cytogenetics	t(15;17), inv16, normal cytogenetics	Abnormalities 5, 7, 11q
MDR expression	—	Expressed
Courses to complete remission	One	Multiple

FAB = *F*rench, *A*merican, and *B*ritish collaborating hematologists; MDR = multidrug resistance.

albumin level and performance status are important predictors of response: Patients with a low serum albumin level experience increased morbidity and mortality associated with induction chemotherapy.

The expression of multidrug resistance genes has been implicated in poor response to treatment [33]. Chemotherapy resistance in AML may be mediated by the multidrug resistance gene 1 (*MDR1*). *MDR1* encodes an adenosine triphosphate–binding transmembrane protein that extrudes a variety of antineoplastic compounds from the cells, including the anthracyclines. Twenty percent of de novo AML cases and 75% of secondary AML cases express *MDR1*. The *MDR1* phenotype is linked to other indicators of adverse outcome in AML, including expression of the CD34+ antigen on blast cells, advanced patient age, poor cytogenetic patterns, an immature phenotype, and unfavorable FAB subtypes. The *MDR1* phenotype identifies a group of high-risk, poor-prognosis leukemias.

A major determinant of the outcome of induction therapy is the capacity of affected patients to tolerate intensive therapy. Most patients who fail to attain a complete remission do so because of complications of induction chemotherapy. Resistant disease accounts for approximately 20% of all induction failures. The presence of prior medical problems and the pretreatment performance status are, therefore, important predictors of response.

In most trials, 60% to 80% of patients younger than 60 will attain a complete remission with induction therapy, and 40% to 70% will experience relapse in the first 18 to 24 months. The factors that determine remission duration are controversial and depend, in part, on the type of postinduction chemotherapy administered. Cytogenetic abnormalities, including t(8;21) and inv(l6), are associated with significantly longer remission duration and overall survival, whereas abnormalities of chromosomes 5, 7, and 11 are associated with a poorer response to treatment and shorter overall survival. FAB subtypes M0, M5, M6, and M7 are associated with a generally poorer prognosis, whereas the M2, M3, and M4E subtypes are associated with a better prognosis. Patients who require more than one course of induction chemotherapy to attain a complete remission also appear to have a shorter remission duration.

Treatment

The treatment of AML is divided into two phases: The first is remission induction, and the second is postinduction, consolidation, or maintenance therapy. The aim of remission induction therapy is to attain a complete remission, defined as the eradication of leukemic cells from the bone marrow and blood and establishment of normal hematopoiesis. Cytosine arabinoside and an anthracycline are the drugs used most frequently in induction chemotherapy. The complete remission rate depends on a number of variables, including the AML subtype and age of the patient. The remission rate in younger patients ($<$ 55 years) is 70% to 85%, whereas in older patients a remission rate of approximately 40% to 50% is exhibited.

Once remission has been achieved, postinduction therapy is required to prevent relapse. However, the optimal postinduction regimen has not yet been defined. In younger patients, three options are available: consolidation chemotherapy, autologous transplantation, and allogeneic transplantation from an HLA-matched sibling or other related or unrelated donor. Approximately 25% to 35% of patients who receive postinduction chemotherapy only will have a long-term remission, and 60% to 75% of patients will experience relapse within two years of attaining a complete remission. The use of high-dose cytarabine consolidation has improved the duration of the first remission for most younger AML patients [18].

The role of autologous transplantation remains controversial and is the subject of ongoing clinical investigations. Selected studies have shown an improvement in disease-free survival of an autologous bone marrow or stem cell transplantation performed in first remission [34–37]. However, the effect on overall survival remains unclear [38]. Differences in the outcome of these studies reflect patient selection, timing of the transplantation and, in randomized studies, the number of patients who actually complete their transplantation regimen.

Allogeneic bone marrow transplantation (BMT) from an HLA-matched donor has resulted in cure rates of 50% to 60% for recipients in first remission [39]. The relapse rate after an HLA-matched sibling donor transplantation is lower than 20%. The allogeneic effect mediated by the graft-versus-host disease is responsible, in part, for the improved long-term survival in recipients of an allogeneic transplant. However, the favorable effects of the transplantation are offset partially by the increased treatment-related toxicity associated with the prolonged period of immunosuppression and complications of graft-versus-host disease [35, 37]. Generally, allogeneic transplantations are reserved for patients younger than 55. The timing of the allogeneic transplantation for AML patients remains controversial and must be balanced against the risk of relapse and mortality and morbidity of the transplantation (Table 22.5).

The treatment of AML patients whose disease relapses remains controversial. A number of chemotherapeutic regimens have been used with varying success. The use of an allogeneic transplant in second remission or at the time of relapse improves survival as compared to the use of chemotherapy alone [40].

AML treatment is associated with a number of side effects. All patients who receive induction and consolidation chemotherapy will become pancytopenic and will require red cell and platelet support. All such patients also will become neutropenic and will, therefore, be at increased risk for serious infections.

Metabolic and electrolyte derangements are common in patients receiving antileukemic chemotherapy. Hyperuricemia occurs commonly, owing to the increased turnover of the proliferating leukemic cells and subsequent purine catabolism. In addition, antibiotic- and chemotherapy-induced nephropathy, diarrhea, and vomiting, and the development of hypomagnesemia variously contribute to the development of potentially life-threatening hypokalemia during treatment. The rapid lysis of leukemic cells—tumor lysis syndrome—can precipitate acutely a number of serious metabolic problems, owing to the release of intracellular phosphate, potassium, and urate and the rapid development of hyperuricemia, hyperkalemia, hyperphosphatemia, and hypocalcemia [41]. The consequences of the tumor lysis syndrome are related directly to the metabolic abnormalities: Hyperuricemia produces a urate nephropathy and acute renal failure; hyperkalemia is associated

Table 22.5   Comparison of Allogeneic and Autologous Transplantation

	Allogeneic Transplantation	Autologous Transplantation
Advantages	Graft-versus-leukemia effect Lower relapse rate	Patient < 65 yr No HLA match required No graft-versus-host disease Low transplant-related mortality and morbidity
Disadvantages	Patient < 55 yr HLA match required Graft-versus-host disease Prolonged immunosuppression Increased transplant-related morbidity and mortality	No graft-versus-leukemia effect Potential contamination of stem cells with leukemic cells Higher relapse rate

with potentially lethal cardiac arrhythmias; and hyperphosphatemia causes a reciprocal depression of the serum calcium level and progressive renal insufficiency and neurologic dysfunction.

Because patients with acute leukemia are at risk for the tumor lysis syndrome, metabolic and electrolyte abnormalities should be followed closely and should be corrected before and after treatment is initiated. Allopurinol and intravenous hydration should be started before the induction of chemotherapy. Serum electrolyte levels (including potassium, calcium, phosphate, and uric acid) and renal function should be monitored carefully during and after treatment.

ACUTE LYMPHOBLASTIC LEUKEMIA

ALL is the most common leukemia of childhood (see under "Childhood Leukemias") and accounts for 20% of all acute leukemias in adults [42]. It is a heterogeneous disorder, the classification of which rests on both morphologic and immunologic criteria. In the last two decades, a marked improvement has been made in the prognosis of both adult and childhood ALL. Remission rates of 60% to 80% and long-term survival of 25% to 40% in adults have been achieved through administration of prolonged, intensive, multidrug, chemotherapeutic regimens.

Clinical Characteristics

Like other acute leukemias, ALL generally presents with a two- to four-week history of malaise, fatigue, bone pain, bleeding, and bruising. The first symptoms may be a nonspecific upper respiratory infection that persists despite therapy. Patients may complain of constant pains in the back and limbs. The bone pain may be diffuse or localized to a single joint and can resemble acute arthritis. The joints may be swollen and tender and may mimic acute osteomyelitis. Headaches and lethargy reflect the anemia, and a purpuric rash or spontaneous or excessive bruising are manifestations of thrombocytopenia.

On examination, affected patients usually appear pale and exhibit generalized nontender lymphadenopathy and moderate splenomegaly. Patients with T-cell ALL may present with signs of mediastinal obstruction associated with a large anterior mediastinal mass and a pleural effusion. Presentation with acute renal failure can occur in patients with a high blast count and leukemic infiltration of the kidneys. Cranial nerve palsies, particularly involving the sixth and seventh nerves, may occur and are associated with CNS involvement. Abdominal pain may be due to bulky abdominal nodes typically found in the B-cell subtypes of ALL.

Classification

ALL is classified on the basis of both morphologic and immunologic studies [18a, 42]. The FAB system separates ALL into three groups: L1, L2, and L3 (Table 22.6; Color Plate 22.3). L1, seen most frequently in childhood, is characterized by small, homogenous lymphoblasts with scant cytoplasm, regular nuclei, and indistinct nucleoli. L2 lymphoblasts, typical of adult ALL, are larger and more variable. In L3 ALL (Burkitt's type), the lymphoblasts are large and display prominent vacuolated, deeply basophilic cytoplasm and prominent nucleoli.

Table 22.6 Classification of Acute Lymphoblastic Leukemia

Subtype	Frequency		Antigen Expression	FAB Classification
	Children	**Adults**		
Early pre–B cell	55–65%	50–60%	CD19+, CD22+, CD79a+, CD10+, CD7–, CD3–, cIg–, sIg–	L1, L2
Pre–B cell	20–25%	15–25%	CD19+, CD22+, CD79a+, CD10+, CD7–, CD3–, cIg+, sIg	L1, L2
B cell	2–3%	4–6%	CD19+, CD22+, CD79a+, CD10+, CD7–, CD3–, cIg+, sIg+	L3
T cell	10–15%	20–25%	CD19–, CD22–, CD79a–, CD10+, CD7+, CD3+, cIg–, sIg–	L1, L2

FAB = *F*rench, *A*merican, and *B*ritish collaborating hematologists; CD = cluster designation; cIg = cytoplasmic immunoglobulin; sIg = surface immunoglobulin; + indicates positive in > 50% of cases; – indicates positive in < 50% of cases.

The immunologic classification attempts to divide ALL into the predominant cell type and is more clinically relevant than is the morphologic classification (see Table 22.6). In children, approximately 20% of ALLs are of T-cell origin, 75% are precursor B cells, and 5% are more mature B cells, the so-called Burkitt-type ALL. In approximately 25% of cases of adult ALL, the lymphoblasts express both myeloid and lymphoid markers [43]. The correlation between morphologic and immunologic findings are presented in Table 22.6.

Diagnosis

Circulating lymphoblasts are commonly detected in patients with ALL. Distinguishing lymphoblasts from undifferentiated, immature myeloblasts may be difficult. Histochemistry and immunologic markers have proved invaluable in this regard. On histochemical staining, 75% of lymphoblasts stain positive with periodic acid–Schiff in a coarse staining pattern. Acid phosphatase staining may help in identifying lymphoblasts of T-cell origin. Cytogenetics are normal in one-third of ALL patients. The Philadelphia chromosome—t(9;22)—is the cytogenetic abnormality detected most frequently in adult ALL (20–30% of cases). The translocation in ALL is distinguished from that in CML by a unique *bcr-abl* fusion gene and a p190-kD protein product (not the p210 kD in typical CML). The t(8;14) translocation is associated with the L3 (Burkitt's) morphologic subtype and mature B-cell (smIg+) phenotype. The translocation t(4;11)(q21;q23) occurs in 3% to 6% of adult ALL patients. Usually, patients with t(4;11) show an early B-precursor phenotype. Generally, ALL with the t(4;11) translocation presents with a high total WBC count (> 100,000/mm³), coexpresses myeloid antigens, and has a poor prognosis.

Prognosis

Factors adversely affecting outcome have been defined for childhood and adult ALL (Table 22.7) [44]. Long-term, three-year survival varies from 50% to 60% to 10% to 25% for favorable and unfavorable subtypes, respectively. Low-risk, favorable criteria included B-cell precursor ALL, age between one and nine years, and a presenting leukocyte count of less than 50,000/mm³. Unfavorable prognostic factors include older age > 60), WBC counts greater than 50,000/mm³, a mediastinal mass, an L3 morphology, a Ph+ chromosome, t(4;11), rearrangement of the *MLL* gene, and a very elevated level of lactate dehydrogenase. Generally, adult patients present with one or more unfavorable prognostic factors.

Treatment

Treatment programs for adult ALL are based on regimens that have been used successfully in children and differ from therapy for AML in two important respects: Chemotherapy is prolonged (including the administration of maintenance therapy) for up to 18 months, and CNS prophylaxis is given routinely [45]. The most active drugs include anthracyclines, vincristine, prednisone, L-asparaginase, methotrexate, cyclophosphamide, cytosine arabinoside, 6-thioguanine, and 6-mercaptopurine. Combinations of these medications are administered routinely in various schedules over two years to most patients. Remission rates of 60% to 80%, similar to those of childhood ALL, now occur in most adults. However, unlike patients with childhood ALL, most adults with ALL will relapse within the first two years, and the overall survival is only 35% to 50%. CNS prophylaxis is part of the standard treatment of ALL and consists of intrathecal chemotherapy with methotrexate or cytosine arabinoside (or both). Adult patients with the L3 subtype [mature B-cell phenotype, t(8;14)] have a generally poorer prognosis. Generally, patients with the L3 subtype are older and present with an elevated WBC count, CNS disease, and extramedullary involvement. Patients with this subtype may require more intensive therapy than that of the standard ALL chemotherapy regimen.

Fewer than half of adult patients with ALL will be cured. Allogeneic BMT in first remission remains controversial but should be offered to those with high-risk disease (e.g., Ph chromosome–positive ALL). When BMT is performed in a second or subsequent remission, disease-free survival is approximately 20% to 30%. The results of allogeneic BMT in adult ALL are inferior to the results in AML.

Childhood ALL

The majority (85%) of children with ALL present with the favorable L1 subtype. The L2 and L3 subtypes are seen in 14% and 1%, respectively, of ALL children. The L2 and L3 subtypes have an intermediate and a poor prognosis, respectively, with standard ALL-type treatment [46]. The L3 phenotype represents patients with a mature B-cell leukemia that is morphologically and clinically similar to the high-grade, Burkitt's, and small, noncleaved-cell lymphomas [46]. The treatment of these children with lymphoma-type therapy has improved their overall survival [47].

The immunophenotyping classification of ALL is more clinically relevant than is morphology. Approximately 85% of childhood ALLs are of pre-B-cell origin, and 14% are of T-cell origin; the remaining 1% are malignancies arising from a mature B cell. The pre-B-cell ALLs share certain characteristics: They express the common ALL antigen CD10 (CALLA) on their cell surface and are HLA-negative, DR-positive, and CD19-positive and, possibly, CD20-positive. The earliest pre-B-cell lymphoblasts have no associated cytoplasmic immunoglobulin (so-called early pre-B-cell ALL). The more mature B cell has intracytoplasmic immunoglobulin. The most favorable prognosis is associated with early pre-B-cell and pre-B-cell ALL.

CLINICAL PRESENTATION

Children with ALL present with the signs and symptoms of the uncontrolled growth of leukemic cells in the bone marrow, lymphoid organs, and other sites of extramedullary spread. Children complain of a variable period of fatigue and easy bruising after minor trauma. Bone pain is a common presenting symptom and, in young children, the first sign may be a limp or refusal to walk. Symptoms may be present for days to several weeks before the diagnosis of ALL is made. On physical examination, hepatosplenomegaly is present in more than 60% of children, and more than 50% of those with ALL have generalized lymphadenopathy.

TREATMENT

Therapy stratification by risk factor has been a major advance in the treatment of childhood leukemia. This modality, along with prophylactic treatment of the CNS, has had a dramatic impact on the disease-free survival in pediatric leukemia. Therapy is targeted to affected patients' specific subtype and prognostic group [43].

Most pediatric treatment protocols for ALL divide patients into low-risk, standard- (average-) risk, and high-risk groups. The risk relates to the prognosis of subtype and determines the type and extent of treatment administered. The prognostic features include immunophenotype, age at diagnosis, cytogenetics, and presenting WBC count. Most children with ALL present with good risk features for age: They are between ages one and nine. Infants tend to do poorly. Structural abnormalities of chromosome 11q23 tend to confer a poorer prognosis. The t(4:1l)(q21;q23) translocation is the most frequent of these abnormalities and occurs in some 5% of pediatric ALL patients but is seen in more than 60% of infants with ALL [43, 48, 49].

The Philadelphia chromosome, the (Ph+)t(9;22)(q34;ql1) translocation, occurs in approximately 5% of childhood ALL. Children with the Ph+ chromosome tend to be older at diagnosis, have higher presenting WBC counts, and an increased incidence of CNS leukemia and the L2 morphology. The t(l;l9)(q23;pl3) and

Table 22.7 Adverse Prognostic Factors in Acute Lymphocytic Leukemia

Male gender
Age: children younger than 1 yr or older than 10 yr; adults older than 50 yr
White blood cell count > 15,000/mm³
Prolonged time to achieve remission (> 4 wk from start of treatment)
Philadelphia chromosome–positive: t(9;22)t(4;11)
MLL rearrangements
Very elevated lactate dehydrogenase
Hypodiploidy (< 45 chromosomes)

the t(8;14) cytogenetic abnormalities are associated with a higher relapse rate and shorter survival. In contrast, trisomy of chromosomes 4 and 10 is associated with a better response to treatment.

At diagnosis, a WBC count greater than 50,000/mm³ puts children at higher risk for other signs of increased tumor load, such as widened mediastinum and organomegaly and CNS disease, and is an important adverse prognostic factor. Ploidy, as determined by the DNA content of the leukemic cells by flow cytometry, is an important predictor of response. Children with a higher ploidy (> 50 chromosomes) have the best prognosis; a ploidy of 47 to 50 chromosomes and near-haploid chromosome number are associated with an intermediate and poor prognosis, respectively [44].

Children with CNS involvement that does not respond to intrathecal treatment have a prognosis poorer than do patients with no CNS disease or CNS disease that responds to treatment. The finding of CNS alone does not appear to correlate with an overall poorer prognosis. If the cerebrospinal fluid can be cleared of ALL blasts with intrathecal chemotherapy during induction therapy, the disease-free survival can approach that of patients without CNS disease.

The first goal of ALL therapy is to induce a complete remission with restoration of normal hematopoiesis. The induction regimen includes a glucocorticoid and vincristine plus asparaginase [42]. The complete remission rate in children ranges from 90% to 95%. After induction therapy, all children receive chemotherapy in the form of consolidation or intensification. These phases of treatment employ a variety of agents, including high-dose methotrexate, 6-mercaptopurine, epipodophyllotoxins, cytarabine, and asparaginase. The duration of treatment is determined in part by the risk factors but generally continues for 18 to 36 months. The optimal duration of treatment is the subject of ongoing clinical trials. Children with Ph+ ALL or leukemic cells that demonstrate the *MLL* rearrangement have a very poor prognosis and generally are considered for an allogeneic BMT during their first remission [48].

BIPHENOTYPIC LEUKEMIA

Refinement of histochemical, immunologic, and cytogenetic techniques has led to the frequent detection of leukemic blasts that share myeloid and lymphoid features [46]. These so-called biphenotypic leukemias coexpress cell-surface markers common to both forms of leukemia. The precise categorization of these leukemias is controversial (AML with lymphoid markers,

ALL with myeloid markers, or acute undifferentiated leukemia). The classification of all leukemias is based on the predominant cell type and does not attempt to address the biological makeup of the disease or the leukemogenic events. In many cases, defining a single lineage or cell type of a leukemic cell is impossible morphologically, cytochemically, or with the use of phenotypic markers. In an attempt to explain this phenomenon, a number of different terms have been used (e.g., *lineage infidelity; mixed-lineage leukemias; biphenotypic or bi-lineage leukemias; hybrid or biclonal leukemias; and lineage switches*). This terminology reflects the heterogeneous nature of these disorders and the lack of specificity of currently available markers. Though many of the reported cases reflect the lack of specificity of the phenotypic markers, there are clear examples of blasts that express markers of more than one lineage.

The monoclonal antibodies used to characterize lymphoid or myeloid leukemias recognize hematopoietic differentiation antigens. These antigens, which are expressed on a number of epithelial cells and overlapping subsets of hematopoietic cells, have important roles in the biological makeup of normal and malignant hematopoiesis. Leukemic cells can demonstrate cytochemical and phenotypic markers of both myeloid and lymphoid precursors. This phenomenon may reflect a fundamental abnormality of gene expression that is specific for the malignant clone.

The clinical significance of lymphoid antigen expression in myeloid leukemias is unclear. Lymphoid antigens may be positive in up to 48% of myeloid leukemias. The most common lymphoid antigens expressed in myeloid leukemias are CD2 and CD7, which are expressed in 34% and 42% of patients with AML, respectively. The presence of lymphoid-associated antigens does not appear to be associated with a uniformly poorer prognosis. A minority of acute leukemias have features of both myeloid and lymphoid lineages and are characterized as biphenotypic leukemias. The incidence of acute biphenotypic leukemia represents approximately 7% of all adult acute leukemias. In this setting, two distinct leukemic cell populations are noted on immunophenotyping.

The complete remission rates for the hybrid and biphenotypic leukemias are variable, as is their clinical course. The undifferentiated and minimally differentiated hybrid leukemias do poorly with standard induction chemotherapy. Monoclonal antibodies to cell-surface markers are necessary to define these morphologically atypical leukemias and should be part of the initial evaluation in patients who present with an atypical morphologic or clinical pattern.

Current models of hematopoietic differentiation are based on the evidence that normal pluripotential precursors give rise to committed precursors of a single cell lineage and then undergo a series of discrete developmental steps. The classification system used currently is based on the premise that leukemic cells adhere morphologically and immunologically to a single lineage. The cases of biphenotypic leukemias demonstrate the heterogeneity of these neoplastic disorders and support the concept that, in at least some acute leukemias, the transforming event occurs at the level of the pluripotential stem cell. Moreover, these data suggest that leukemic cells can differentiate, although aberrantly, and express differentiation markers.

CHRONIC MYELOGENOUS LEUKEMIA

CML is a clonal myeloproliferative disorder characterized by myeloid hyperplasia and progressive splenomegaly. The disorder results from the clonal expansion of a transformed hematopoietic progenitor cell. CML was the first human malignancy associated with a defined cytogenetic abnormality: the Philadelphia (Ph) chromosome.

Incidence and Epidemiologic Background

CML constitutes approximately 0.3% of all cancers in the United States and accounts for 15% to 20% of all leukemias in adults (annual incidence, 1.0–1.5 per 100,000 population). CML is rare in individuals younger than age 20 but occurs in all decades (median age = 40–50 years); 30% of patients with CML are age 60 or older. The incidence is slightly higher in male individuals than in female individuals (ratio = 1.3:1).

Etiologic Factors

The etiology of CML is unknown. The Ph chromosome—the hallmark of CML—originally was described by Nowel and Hungerford [50] in 1960 as shortened chromosome 22. Now, the Ph chromosome is known to represent a reciprocal translocation of genetic material between the long arms of chromosomes 9 and 22; t(9;22)(q34;q11). This transposes the large 3' segment of the c-abl gene from chromosome 9q34 to the 5' part of the bcr gene on chromosome 22q11, creating a hybrid bcr-abl gene (Fig. 22.2) The genomic breakpoint on chromosome 22 is clustered in a relatively small 5.8-kb

breakpoint cluster region (bcr). This bcr area is the central part of a large gene, the BCR gene, on chromosome 22. The translocation results in the juxtaposition of the 5' sequences from the BCR gene with the 3' ABL sequences derived from chromosome 9. The new chimeric gene, bcr-abl, is transcribed as an 8.45-kb mRNA and encodes a protein of molecular weight 210 kD that has tyrosine kinase activity. The p210 protein plays a pivotal role in the pathogenesis of CML. Virtually all cases of CML will show evidence of the bcr-abl rearrangement.

The translocation is seen also in 15% to 30% of adult patients with ALL. The c-abl gene is a protooncogene that encodes a tyrosine kinase with a molecular mass of 145 kD. The c-abl oncogene spans 230 kb and consists of 11 exons (a1–a11). In most cases of CML, the breakpoint in the abl oncogene occurs in the 5' part of the abl exon a2 [51]. Abl exons a2 to a11 are transposed into a region of the bcr gene between exons b1 and b5 on chromosome 22. The area is called the *major breakpoint cluster region* (M-bcr). This transposition creates a bcr-abl fusion mRNA of 8.5 kb, which translates into a 210-kD chimeric protein (p210). In Ph+ ALL, the breakpoint on chromosome 22 occurs near the 5' region of M-bcr within the minor breakpoint cluster region (m-bcr) and translates into a smaller bcr-abl transcript of 190 kD (p190). The p190 and the p210 chimeric proteins demonstrate higher tyrosine phosphokinase activity than does the normal c-abl protein. The mechanism by which the new chimeric bcr-abl gene alters stem cell kinetics remains unknown, but the expression of the fusion gene products appears to be, in part, responsible for the abnormal proliferation and malignant behavior of hematopoietic progenitor cells. In CML, the Ph chromosome is present in all cells derived from the transformed progenitor cells. The primary genetic translocation results in a genetic change that is permissive for additional cytogenetic translocations, accounting for progression of the disease.

Clinical Characteristics

Typically, CML follows a triphasic course: a chronic phase of variable length, followed by a short accelerated phase and a terminal blastic (blast crisis) phase (Color Plate 22.4). The chronic phase follows an indolent course. Approximately 50% of patients are asymptomatic at presentation, and diagnosis is obtained on a blood test usually done as part of the evaluation of an unrelated disorder. In patients with symptoms, the most frequent complaints are fatigue, abdominal fullness, left up-

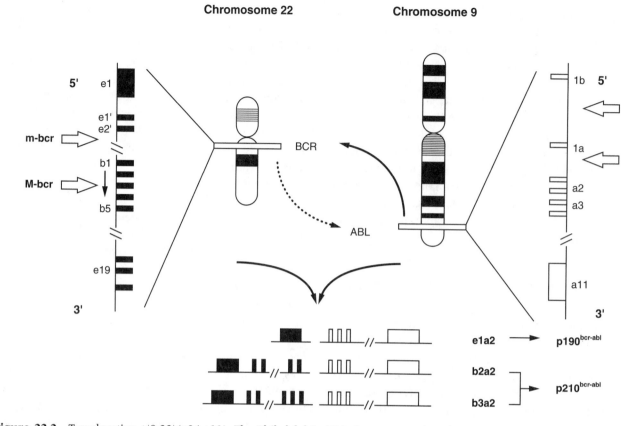

Figure 22.2 Translocation t(9;22)(q34;q11). The Philadelphia (Ph) chromosome is a shortened chromosome 22 that results from a translocation of 3'-*abl* segments of chromosome 9 to 5'-*bcr* segments on chromosome 22. Breakpoints in the *abl* gene are located 5' of exon a2 in most cases. Various breakpoint locations have been identified along the *bcr* gene on chromosome 22. Depending on where the breakpoint occurs, differently sized segments from *bcr* are fused together with the 3' sequences of the *abl* gene. This results in fusion messenger RNA molecules (e1a2, b2a2, b3a2, e19a2) of different lengths that are transcribed into different chimeric protein products (p190, p210).

per quadrant fullness, and decreased exercise tolerance. Early satiety and left upper quadrant fullness reflect the enlarged spleen, which is noted in approximately 80% of patients. Fever, night sweats, and weight loss are unusual features early in the chronic phase but are prominent findings in the accelerated and blast crisis.

Though patients in the chronic phase of CML generally are asymptomatic, without effective treatment all patients will enter the accelerated phase within three to five years from the time of diagnosis. The accelerated phase is characterized by enlargement of the spleen and progressive symptoms (Table 22.8). An increase in the basophil count (> 15%) and more immature cells in the blood or bone marrow confirm the transformation to the accelerated phase. Additional cytogenetic abnormalities are noted at this time, and affected patients may complain of intermittent fevers, night sweats, and unexplained weight loss. Generally, the accelerated phase is short (6–12 months) and is followed by a short

terminal blastic phase (blast crisis). Constitutional symptoms are pronounced during this period, and the spleen can enlarge rapidly. Patients complain of bone pain, weight loss, fevers, and night sweats. Progressive anemia and thrombocytopenia are common. The percentage of blast cells in the bone marrow and blood increases, and the appearance may resemble that of a patient with acute leukemia. Isolated foci of blasts—chloromas—can appear and present in soft tissues. Signs and symptoms of leukostasis can develop if the peripheral blast count is greater than 50,000/mm³.

The blast crisis represents the terminal phase of the disease for the majority of affected patients. Characterizing by standard morphologic methods the blast cells that appear in the terminal phase often is difficult. The majority (70%) of patients in the blast crisis have a myeloid transformation, with the remainder having lymphoid leukemias (20%) or mixed-lineage leukemias (10%).

Table 22.8   Clinical and Laboratory Features of Chronic Myelocytic Leukemia During Three Phases of the Disease

Feature	Phase		
	Chronic Phase	**Accelerated Phase**	**Blast Crisis**
Symptoms[a]	None or minimal	Moderate	Pronounced
Splenomegaly	Mild	May increase	May be marked
White blood cell count	Elevated	Erratic	High or low
Differential[b]	< 1–2% blasts on spectrum WBC	Increasing basophils and immaturity	Circulating blasts (often > 25%)
Hematocrit	Normal	May decrease	Low
Platelets	High or normal	Erratic	Low
LAP score	Low	May increase	Normal
Bone marrow	< 10% immature	Increased immaturity	> 30% blasts
Cytogenetics	Ph+	Ph+, additional abnormalities	Ph+, additional abnormalities
Median survival	3–4 yr	6–24 mo	2–4 mo

WBC = white blood cells; LAP = leukocyte alkaline phosphatase; Ph+ = Philadelphia chromosome.
[a]Fever, bone pain, night sweats, fatigue, weight loss.
[b]Promyelocytes and myeloblasts.

Laboratory Features and Initial Diagnostic Evaluation

Typically, patients in the chronic phase of CML have a leukocytosis with the full spectrum of myeloid maturation. Most of the myeloid cells are mature, but circulating myelocytes, promyelocytes, and blasts usually are noted. The hematocrit is normal, but approximately one-third of patients will present with thrombocytosis. An elevated serum lactate dehydrogenase and uric acid level may be noted, reflecting the increased turnover of myeloid precursors. The leukocyte alkaline phosphatase (LAP) score is low (< 10) in CML patients. This score is particularly helpful in differentiating CML from other causes of an elevated WBC count. The LAP score is elevated (> 100) in leukocytosis associated with an infection and a leukemoid reaction. However, in the accelerated and blastic phases, the LAP score increases to the normal range. Moreover, patients with CML and an intercurrent infection may have a normal LAP score, reflecting the response of residual normal marrow precursors.

The diagnosis of CML depends on demonstrating the Ph chromosome or its molecular equivalent, the *bcr-abl* rearrangement. In more than 90% of CML patients, the cytogenetic analysis demonstrates the Ph chromosome. In approximately 5% of such patients, the Ph chromosome is not detected, but the *bcr-abl* translocation is identified. These patients have CML that follows the usual clinical course.

Fluorescence in situ hybridization (FISH) allows for the analysis of both metaphase (dividing) and nondividing cells. FISH analysis can be performed on peripheral blood specimens and thus may avoid the need for bone marrow aspiration. FISH analysis is rapid and allows for the analysis of more cells than is possible with conventional cytogenetics.

The bone marrow aspirate and biopsy is hypercellular with myeloid hyperplasia. In the chronic phase, immature myeloid precursors constitute fewer than 10% of the marrow cells. In the accelerated and blastic phases, the proportion of blast forms gradually increases, and the bone marrow is similar to that found in acute leukemia.

Treatment

The natural history of CML has changed dramatically over the last decade. In the past, the median survival was less than three years, with less than 20% of patients surviving five years after diagnosis. Currently, the median survival is five to seven years, with 50% of patients alive at five years. The factors responsible for this change include earlier diagnosis, better supportive care, and more effective antileukemic therapies.

Hydroxyurea, a cell cycle–specific inhibitor of DNA synthesis, and busulfan, an alkylating agent, have been used to control the disease in patients with CML in the chronic phase. The majority of patients will respond to either of these oral chemotherapeutic agents. Cytogenetic and clinical remissions are rare and transient, and neither of the aforementioned agents affects progression of the disease. Treatment with either of these drugs will not prevent the inevitable transformation to the accelerated and blastic phases. Generally, hydroxyurea is tolerated better than is busulfan and may be associated with a longer duration of the chronic phase. In addition, busulfan has greater side effects, including delayed myelosuppression, increased marrow fibrosis, and idiosyncratic pulmonary reactions [52]. Splenic irradiation may be helpful to control a very large or painful splenomegaly.

Interferon-α induces clinical (hematologic) remissions in 70% to 80% of patients treated in the early chronic phase of CML. Interferon-α has been demonstrated to induce a cytogenetic response in 55% to 60%. The response to interferon is associated with a prolongation of the chronic phase and an increase in the median survival (89 months) [53]. Achieving a cytogenetic response after 12 months of therapy was associated with a significant survival benefit: five-year survivals of 90%, 88%, 76%, and 38%, respectively, for patients with complete, partial, minor, or no cytogenetic response. Interferon-α achieved rates of hematologic and cytogenetic responses higher than those from treatment with hydroxyurea or busulfan [54]. The combination of interferon-α and low doses of cytarabine may increase further the percentage of patients who have a cytogenetic response [55].

Treatment of patients in the accelerated phase and blast crisis is disappointing. Transient responses to antileukemic chemotherapy have resulted in the reestablishment of a brief second chronic phase. Interferon in not active in patients with CML in the accelerated phase or blast crisis. The lymphoid variant of the blast crisis is more responsive to treatment, with temporary remissions (second chronic phase) occurring in approximately 50% to 60% of patients and a median survival of 6 to 12 months.

Allogeneic BMT or stem cell transplantation achieves long-term overall survival in 50% to 80% of patients. It is most successful when performed early in the chronic phase within the first year of diagnosis, wherein long-term disease-free survival and cure rates are 40% to 70%. Application of allogeneic transplantation is limited by the availability of a matched donor and the toxicity of the transplant. Generally, transplantation is reserved for patients who are younger than 55 years and have no meaningful intercurrent medical problems. The mortality from transplantation within the first 100 days is approximately 20%. Toxicity relates to the preparative regimen and the development of graft-versus-host disease. Attempts to diminish the graft-versus-host disease have been associated with an increased relapse rate [56]. The allogeneic effect of the transplantation appears critical to controlling the CML. The timing and selection of patients for allogeneic transplantation remains controversial. However, patients who have a matched donor and are suitable for allogeneic transplantation should be offered this potentially curative option early in the course of their disease.

CHRONIC LYMPHOCYTIC LEUKEMIA

CLL is an indolent lymphoproliferative disorder characterized by lymphocytosis, lymphadenopathy, and splenomegaly. In the majority (95%) of cases, it is a neoplasm of B cells; T-cell CLL represents a rare subtype. CLL is an accumulative disease of long-lived B cells that express high levels of the antiapoptotic protein BCL2 and other genes that modulate apoptosis [56, 57]. The course of CLL depends on the stage of disease, with median survival ranging from more than 10 years (for early-stage disease) to less than 19 months (for advanced-stage illness). Immunologic abnormalities, including autoimmune hemolytic anemia and immune-mediated thrombocytopenia, reflect the abnormal immunoregulation inherent in this disease.

Incidence and Epidemiologic Background

CLL is the most common leukemia in adults and constitutes approximately 0.9% of all cancers (annual incidence, 2.9 per 100,000 population). CLL is a disease primarily of the elderly; 90% of all CLL cases occur in patients older than 50 years. Men are affected twice as frequently as are women.

Etiologic Factors

The cause of CLL remains unknown. Unlike the acute leukemias, CLL is not associated with prior exposure to irradiation or alkylating agents. No familial tendency is inherent in this disorder.

Clinical Characteristics

Often, patients with CLL present when an unexplained lymphocytosis is noted on a complete blood count obtained for another, unrelated disorder. Fatigue, shortness of breath, night sweats, and bleeding are rare at presentation and usually reflect a more advanced stage. Recurrent bacterial infections are a major cause of morbidity and mortality late in the disease. The incidence of viral infections, notably herpes zoster, approaches 20% in patients with advanced disease.

In the majority of patients, CLL is a chronic, indolent disorder that does not require immediate treatment. Most affected patients are asymptomatic at diagnosis, though they may demonstrate very elevated lymphocyte counts (> 200,000/mm³; Color Plate 22.5). Unlike those of the acute leukemias, signs and symptoms of leukostasis are rare, and emergency efforts to lower the lymphocyte count are not required. Generalized lymphadenopathy and splenomegaly are noted in up to two-thirds of patients at the time of diagnosis. Generally, the lymphadenopathy is small, diffuse, and nontender.

Transformation to a very aggressive form of lymphoma (Richter's syndrome) occurs in 3% to 10% of CLL cases. Unexplained fevers, rapid and disproportional growth of one or more lymph node groups, weight loss, night sweats, and abdominal pain serve as warning signs of this transformation. The transformation of CLL to an aggressive high-grade lymphoma is associated with a poor prognosis.

Laboratory Features

CLL is marked by the proliferation of small, mature-appearing lymphocytes, though variation in size is common. Typically, the peripheral smear reveals smudge cells reflecting disrupted lymphocytes. The diagnosis of CLL is suggested by a blood lymphocytosis (absolute lymphocyte count > 5,000/mm³) with mature-appearing lymphocytes and is confirmed by the characteristic immunophenotyping of monoclonal B cells [58]. The CLL cells express low-intensity surface immunoglobulin (IgM ± IgD) with monotypic light-chain expression; they also express other markers of B-cell lineage, including CD19, CD20, and CD23. Typically, the CLL B lymphocytes coexpress CD5, a normal T-cell antigen. The coexpression of CD5 distinguishes CLL from prolymphocytic leukemia, low-grade lymphomas, and hairy-cell leukemia. Mantle-cell lymphoma cells also mark with CD5 but do not express CD23. In CLL, a marrow aspirate or biopsy is not required to make the diagnosis.

Patients may present with anemia or thrombocytopenia resulting from bone marrow infiltration with CLL lymphocytes. Autoimmune anemia and thrombocytopenia also are common. Immunoregulatory abnormalities are common in CLL; more than 20% of patients develop a positive Coombs' (antiglobulin) test and tests for other autoantibodies. Hypogammaglobulinemia is common and may be profound. A monoclonal gammopathy is seen in 10% of affected patients.

Generally, cytogenetic studies are neither diagnostic nor clinically helpful in CLL. The most common finding is trisomy 12, which is noted in 20% of cases studied. Histologic analysis of lymph nodes reveals the same cells as are found in the peripheral blood, and the appearance is indistinguishable from that of a well-differentiated lymphocytic lymphoma.

Staging

Staging is based on physical findings and laboratory abnormalities. It is most helpful in classifying patients for study purposes and provides general guidelines of prognosis and indications for therapy. Two widely used classification schemes are those of Rai et al. [59] (Table 22.9) and Binet et al. [60] (Table 22.10).

Prognosis

The prognosis for CLL patients is determined mainly by clinical stage. However, for many patients, the course varies considerably, ranging from one to two years to more than 10 years. Assessing the activity of affected patients' disease is critical for evaluating the need for

Table 22.9 Rai Classification of Chronic Lymphocytic Leukemia

Stage	Clinical Features	Median Survival (mo.)
0	Lymphocytosis only (> 15,000/mm³)	150
I	Lymphocytosis and adenopathy	101
II	Lymphocytosis and hepatomegaly or splenomegaly	71
III	Lymphocytosis and anemia (hemoglobin < 11 g/dl)	19
IV	Lymphocytosis and thrombocytopenia (platelets < 100,000/mm³)	19

Note: The modified Rai classification further groups stages according to prognosis: stage 0, low-risk; stage I and stage II, intermediate-risk; stage III and stage IV, high-risk.
Source: Adapted from KR Rai, A Sawitsky, EP Cronkite, et al., Clinical staging of chronic lymphocytic leukemia. *Blood* 46:219–234, 1975. Used with permission of the American Society of Hematology (ASH) © 1975.

Table 22.10 Binet Classification of Chronic Lymphocytic Leukemia

Stage	Clinical Features	Median Survival (mo.)
A	Lymphocytosis and enlargement of three lymph node groups	108
B	Lymphocytosis and enlargement of > three lymph node groups	60
C	Lymphocytosis with anemia (hemoglobin < 10 g/dl) or thrombocytopenia (platelets < 100,000/mm³)	24

Source: Reprinted with permission of Wiley-Liss, Inc., a subsidiary of John Wiley & Sons, Inc., from JL Binet, A Auquier, G Dighiero, et al., A new prognostic classification of chronic lymphocytic leukemia: prognostic significance. *Cancer* 40:855–864, 1981.

treatment. Treating patients in the early stage of their disease does not prolong survival. Therefore, practitioners are advised to withhold treatment until evidence of progressive, symptomatic disease has been obtained. Though the staging systems are useful for defining prognosis, the course of individual elderly patients' illness may be complicated by other medical problems.

Treatment

CLL remains incurable with standard chemotherapy. Treatment early in the course of affected patients' disease has not been shown to prolong the indolent phase or to have an impact on survival [61]. Treatment is palliative and should be delayed until diseased patients are symptomatic. Patients with unexplained weight loss, night sweats, profound fatigue, symptomatic adenopathy, rapidly enlarging spleen, and progressive and symptomatic anemia and thrombocytopenia should be considered for treatment. Chlorambucil with or without prednisone is as effective as combination chemotherapy (cyclophosphamide, vincristine, and prednisone) for intermediate-stage patients (Rai stage I, II; Binet stage B). The role of more intensive, multiagent chemotherapy for patients with advanced CLL (Rai stage III, IV or Binet stage C) remains unclear.

Fludarabine, a purine analog, offers an alternative treatment for patients with symptomatic CLL. Fludara-

bine is associated with a better overall response rate and a longer duration of response, as compared to standard combination chemotherapy, in patients with symptomatic CLL [62]. However, fludarabine has not been shown to prolong the overall survival in patients with CLL. This and the other nucleoside analogs are potent immunosuppressive agents, and the risk for opportunistic infections after treatment is increased.

Radiotherapy to sites of bulk disease (lymph nodes and spleen) may provide palliative benefit. Allogeneic and autologous stem cell transplantation is being investigated as a potentially curative option for younger patients with CLL. The selection of patients and the timing of such transplantation in CLL remains unclear and must be weighed against the toxicity of the treatment.

Infections remain a major cause of morbidity and mortality in CLL. Prophylactic gamma globulin infusion for CLL patients and those with hypogammaglobulinemia is controversial, and its long-term benefit is unproved. Patients should receive pneumococcal, *Haemophilus influenzae,* and meningococcal vaccines; however, their response to these vaccines is blunted. All live vaccines should be avoided.

CLL VARIANTS

Prolymphocytic Leukemia

Prolymphocytic leukemia (PLL) is a rare, chronic B-lineage lymphoproliferative disorder that represents 1% to 10% of all lymphoid leukemias [63]. The majority of cases occur in men. The characteristic clinical features are prominent splenomegaly with minimal lymphadenopathy, lymphocytosis (100,000–500,000/mm³), and cutaneous involvement. A papular and nonpruritic rash is present in approximately one-third of patients and typically involves the face, torso, and arms.

Prolymphocytes are larger-than-usual, mature-appearing CLL lymphocytes. Typically, prolymphocytes contain generous amounts of cytoplasm and large prominent central nucleoli. The diagnosis of PLL requires that more than 50% of circulating lymphocytes be prolymphocytes (Color Plate 22.6). PLL is distinguished from CLL by intense surface immunoglobulin staining (as compared with the dim staining in CLL) and the absence of CD5 antigen expression. Most PLL cells stain with such B-cell markers as CD19, CD20, and CD24. Rare T-cell variants of PLL have been described. In T-PLL, the predominant phenotype is CD3-positive, CD4-positive, CD7-positive, and CD8-negative.

Generally, PLL follows an aggressive course (median survival > 3 years). PLL does not respond to treatment with chlorambucil, and remissions with anthracycline-based combination regimens have been short.

Hairy-Cell Leukemia

Hairy-cell leukemia (HCL) is a rare disorder representing 2% of all adult leukemias. The incidence of HCL is three cases per one million population; approximately 600 to 800 new cases are diagnosed each year [64]. The median age at onset is approximately 50 years (male-female ratio = 4:1). The disease is very rare in patients younger than 20 years and is characterized by infiltration of the bone marrow and spleen by lymphocytes with unusual hairlike projections. The etiology of HCL is unknown.

CLINICAL AND LABORATORY CHARACTERISTICS

HCL is an indolent disorder. The majority of affected patients present with anemia and splenomegaly, though lymphadenopathy is rare. Discomfort associated with the splenomegaly is unusual, and splenic infarction is rare. Fevers, night sweats, and weight loss are unusual early in the disease. Most patients (70%) present with pancytopenia with rare circulating hairy cells. A majority of the patients are leukopenic, with monocytopenia and thrombocytopenia. Untreated patients experience an increased incidence of infections, with an increased susceptibility to mycobacterial infection.

Hairy cells are larger than normal lymphocytes and exhibit reniform (kidney-shaped) nuclei. The irregular hairlike projections on these cells result in an ill-defined cell outline (Color Plate 22.7A). The cytoplasm may contain azurophilic granules or rod-shaped inclusions. Occasionally, parallel linear structures are present in the weakly basophilic cytoplasm, corresponding to the ribosomal lamellar complex on ultrastructural examination.

The vast majority of hairy cells mark with mature B-cell antigens, including surface immunoglobulin. Usually, these markers are CD25- (interleukin-2 receptor), CD11c-, and CD20-positive, and CD5-negative [65]. Acid phosphatase staining that is resistant to treatment with tartrate is a hallmark finding in HCL (in 95% of cases).

Infiltration of the spleen occurs in the red pulp, as distinct from the usual white-pulp involvement of other low-grade lymphoproliferative disorders. The bone marrow cannot be aspirated in more than 50% of patients (a condition termed *dry tap*) because of the increase in stromal reticulum fibers that characterize the disease. The bone marrow biopsy shows infiltration that may be either focal or diffuse. The bone marrow is infiltrated with cells that appear to be separated from one another by a clear zone (fried-egg pattern; Color Plate 22.7B).

TREATMENT

The course of HCL varies; up to 20% of patients may have prolonged survival without therapeutic intervention. Splenectomy was the traditional first-line approach for this disease, but the nucleoside analogs pentostatin and 2-chlorodeoxyadenosine now represent first-line treatment for the majority of patients [66]. In most patients with HCL, the response to treatment will be prolonged remissions and, perhaps, cure. Generally, the toxicities of the nucleoside analog are mild, though they include transient leukopenia and immunosuppression. Opportunistic infections may occur after treatment, reflecting the prolonged CD4 lymphopenia induced by the treatment.

SUMMARY

The leukemias are a heterogeneous group of disorders that affect individuals of all ages. The application of histochemical stains, cytogenetics, and immunologic, molecular, and biochemical markers have helped to define the lineage of the leukemic cell and to classify the leukemias. The application of new molecular studies and cell biology have aided in the classification and treatment of both acute and chronic leukemias. New therapies have changed the prognosis and treatment approaches for many patients with leukemia. Over the last decade, the prognosis of patients with leukemias has changed from uniformly fatal to potentially curable. Advances in cell biology have resulted in better diagnostic tools, have demonstrated the phenotypic heterogeneity of many leukemias, and have contributed to an understanding of leukemogenesis.

REFERENCES

1. Greenlee RT, Murray T, Bolden S, Wingo PA. Cancer statistics, 2000. *CA Cancer J Clin* 50:7–33, 2000.
2. Greaves MF. Aetiology of acute leukemia. *Lancet* 349:344–349, 1997.

3. Taylor GM, Birch JM. The hereditary basis of human leukemia. In Henderson ES, Lister TA, Greaves MF (eds), *Leukemia* (6th ed). Philadelphia: Saunders, 1996:210–245.

4. Linet MS. The leukemias: epidemiologic aspects. In Lilienfeld AM (ed), *Monographs in Epidemiology and Biostatistics*. New York: Oxford University Press, 1985:1.

5. Horwitz M, Goode EL, Jarvik GP. Anticipation in familial leukemia. *Am J Hum Genet* 59:990–998, 1996.

6. Fong C, Brodeur GM. Downs syndrome and leukemia: epidemiology, genetics, cytogenetics and mechanisms of leukemogenesis. *Cancer Genet Cytogenet* 28:55–76, 1987.

7. Keith L, Brown E. Epidemiologic study of leukemia in twins. *Acta Genet Med* 20:9–22, 1971.

8. Cartwright RA. Epidemiology of leukemia. In Whittaker JA, Holmes JA (eds), *Leukemia and Related Disorders*. Boston: Blackwell, 1998:1–30.

9. Ichimaru M, Tomognaga M, Amenomori T, Matsuo T. Atomic bomb and leukemia. *J Radiat Res (Tokyo)* 32 (suppl 2):14–19, 1991.

10. Stevens W, Thomas DC, Lyon J, et al. Leukemia in Utah and radioactive fallout from the Nevada test site. *JAMA* 264:585–591, 1990.

11. Adamson RH, Seiber SM. Chemically induced leukemia in humans. *Environ Health Perspect* 39:93–103, 1981.

12. Karp JE, Smith MA. The molecular pathogenesis of treatment-induced (secondary) leukemias: foundations for treatment and prevention. *Semin Oncol* 24:103–113, 1997.

13. Aksoy M, Erdern S. Follow-up study on the mortality and development of leukemia in 44 pancytopenic patients with chronic exposure to benzene. *Blood* 52:285–292, 1978.

14. McLaughlin JK, Hirubec Z, Linet MS, et al. Cigarette smoking and leukemia. *J Natl Cancer Inst* 81:1262–1263, 1989.

15. Smith MA, McCaffrey RP, Karp JE. The secondary leukemias: challenges and research directions. *J Natl Cancer Inst* 88:407–418, 1996.

16. Pedersen-Bjergaard J, Larsen SO. Incidence of acute nonlymphocytic leukemia, preleukemia, and acute myeloproliferative syndrome up to 10 years after treatment of Hodgkins disease. *N Engl J Med* 307:965–971, 1982.

17. Pedersen-Bjergaard J, Phillip P. Balanced translocations involving chromosome bands 11q23 and 21q22 are highly characteristic of myelodysplasia and leukemia following therapy with cytostatic agents targeting at DNA-topoisomerase II. *Blood* 78:1147–1148, 1991.

18. Lowenberg B, Downing JR, Burnett A. Acute myeloid leukemia. *N Engl J Med* 341:1051–1062, 1999.

18a. Harris NL, Jaffe ES, Diebold J, et al. World Health Organization classification of neoplastic diseases of the hematopoietic and lymphoid tissues: Report of the clinical advisory committee meeting—Airlie House, Virginia, November 1997. *J Clin Oncol* 17:3835–3849, 1999.

19. Bennett JM, Catovsky D, Daniel MT, et al. Proposed revised criteria for the classification of acute myeloid leukemia: a report of the French-American-British Cooperative Group. *Ann Intern Med* 105:620–625, 1985.

20. Grimwade D, Walker H, Oliver F, et al. The importance of diagnostic cytogenetics on outcome of AM: analysis of 1,612 patients entered into the MRC AML 10 Trial. *Blood* 92:1–13, 1998.

21. Jain NC, Cox C, Bennett JM. Auer rods in the acute myeloid leukemias: frequency and methods of demonstration. *Hematol Oncol* 5:197–202, 1987.

22. Catovsky D, Matutes E, Buccheri V, et al. A classification of acute leukemia for the 1990s. *Ann Hematol* 62:16–21, 1991.

23. Bradstock K, Matthews J, Benson E, et al. Prognostic value of immunophenotyping in acute myeloid leukemia. Australian Leukemia Study Group. *Blood* 84:1220–1225, 1994.

24. Amardori S, Venditti A, Del Poets G, et al. Minimally differentiated acute myeloid leukemia (AML-M0): a distinct clinico-biologic entity with poor prognosis. *Ann Hematol* 72:208–215, 1996.

25. Nucifora G, Birn DJ, Erickson P, et al. Detection of DNA rearrangements in the AML1 and ETO loci and the AML1/ETO fusion mRNA in patients with t(8;21) acute myeloid leukemia. *Blood* 81:883–888, 1993.

26. Fenaux P, Chomienne C, Degos L. Acute promyelocytic leukemia: biology and treatment. *Semin Oncol* 24:92–102, 1997.

27. Tallman MS, Andersen JW, Schiffer CA, et al. All-*trans*-retinoic acid in acute promyelocytic leukemia. *N Engl J Med* 337:1021–1027, 1997.

28. Soignet SL, Maslak P, Wang ZG, et al. Complete remission after treatment of acute promyelocytic leukemia with arsenic trioxide. *N Engl J Med* 339:1341–1348, 1998.

29. Menell JS, Cesarman GM, Jacovina AT, et al. Annexin II and bleeding in acute promyelocytic leukemia. *N Engl J Med* 340:994–1004, 1999.

30. Haferlach T, Gassman W, Loffler H, et al. Clinical aspects of acute myeloid leukemias of the FAB types M3 and M4Eo. The AML Cooperative Group. *Ann Hematol* 66:165–170, 1993.

31. Godwin JE, Kopecky KJ, Head D, et al. A double-blind placebo-controlled trial of granulocyte colony-stimulating factor in elderly patients with previously untreated acute myeloid leukemia: a Southwest Oncology Group Study (9031). *Blood* 91:3607–3615, 1998.

32. Stone RN, Berg DT, George SL, et al. Granulocyte-macrophage colony-stimulating factor after initial chemotherapy for elderly patients with primary acute myelogenous leukemia. *N Engl J Med* 332:1671–1677, 1995.

33. Advani R, Saba H, Tallman MS, et al. Treatment of refractory and relapsed acute myelogenous leukemia with combination chemotherapy plus the multidrug resistance modulator PSC 833. *Blood* 93:787–795, 1999.

34. Mitus A, Miller K, Schenkein D, et al. Improved survival for patients with acute myelogenous leukemia. *J Clin Oncol* 13:560–569, 1995.

35. Sierra J, Nrunet Maurr S, Granena A, et al. Feasibility and results of bone marrow transplantation after remission induction and intensification chemotherapy in de novo acute myeloid leukemia. Catalan group for bone marrow transplantation. *J Clin Oncol* 14:1353–1363, 1996.

36. Burnett AK, Goldstone AH, Stevens RMF, et al. Randomised comparison of autologous bone marrow transplantation to intensive chemotherapy for acute myeloid leuke-

mia in first remission: results of MRC-AML10 trial. UK Medical Research Council Adult and Children's Leukaemia Working Parties. *Lancet* 351:700–708, 1998.

37. Zittoun RA, Mandelli F, Willemze R, et al. Autologous or allogeneic bone marrow transplantation compared with intensive chemotherapy in acute myelogenous leukemia. European Organization for Research and Treatment of Cancer (EORTC) and the Gruppo Italiano Malattie Ematologiche Maligne dellAdulto (GIMEMA) Leukemia Cooperative Groups. *N Engl J Med* 322:17–23, 1995.

38. Cassileth PA, Harrington DP, Appelbaum FR, et al. Chemotherapy compared with autologous or allogeneic bone marrow transplantation in the management of acute myeloid leukemia in first remission. *N Engl J Med* 339:1649–1656, 1998.

39. Reiffers J, Stoppa AM, Attal M, et al. Allogeneic vs autologous stem cell transplantation vs chemotherapy in patients with acute myeloid leukemia in first remission: the BGMT 87 study. *Leukemia* 10:1874–1882, 1996.

40. Tomas F, Gomez Garcia de Soria V, Lopez L, et al. Autologous or allogeneic bone marrow transplantation for acute myeloblastic leukemia in second complete remission. Importance of duration of first complete remission in final outcome. *Bone Marrow Transplant* 17:979–984, 1996.

41. Harris KP, Hattersley JM, Feehally J, Walls J. Acute renal failure associated with haemotological malignancies: a review of 10 years experience. *Eur J Haematol* 47:119–122, 1991.

42. Pui CH, Evan WE. Acute lymphoblastic leukemia. *N Engl J Med* 339:605–615, 1998.

43. Pui CH. Acute lymphoblastic leukemia. *Pediatr Clin North Am* 48:831–846, 1997.

44. Smith M, Arthur D, Camitta B, et al. Uniform approach to risk classification and treatment assignment for children with acute lymphoblastic leukemia. *J Clin Oncol* 14:18–24, 1996.

45. Laport GF, Larson RA. Treatment of adult acute lymphoblastic leukemia. *Semin Oncol* 24:70–82, 1997.

46. Hanson CA, Abaza M, Sheldon S. Acute biphenotypic leukemia: immunophenotypic and cytogenetic analysis. *Br J Haematol* 84:49–60, 1993.

47. Bowman WP, Shuster JJ, Cook B, et al. Improved survival for children with B-cell acute lymphoblastic leukemia and stage IV small noncleaved-cell lymphoma; a Pediatric Oncology Group study. *J Clin Oncol* 14:1252–1261, 1996.

48. Behm FG, Raimondi SC, Frestedt JL, et al. Rearrangement of the MLL gene confers a poor prognosis in childhood acute lymphoblast leukemia regardless of presenting age. *Blood* 87:2870–2877, 1996.

49. Faderl S, Kantararjian HM, Talpaz M, et al. Clinical significance of cytogenetic abnormalities in adult lymphoblastic leukemia. *Blood* 91:3995–4019, 1998.

50. Nowel PC, Hungerford DA. A minute chromosome in human chronic granulocytic leukemia. *Science* 132:1497, 1960.

51. Cortes J, Talpaz M, Kantarajian H. Chronic myelogenous leukemia: a review. *Am J Med* 100:555–570, 1996.

52. Hehlmann R, Heimpel H, Hasford J, et al. Randomized comparison of busulfan and hydroxyurea in chronic myelogenous leukemia: prolongation of survival by hydroxyurea. *Blood* 82:691–703, 1993.

53. Kantarjian HM, Smith TL, O'Brien SM, et al. Prolonged survival in chronic myelogenous leukemia after cytogenetic response to interferon-alpha therapy. *Ann Intern Med* 122:254–261, 1995.

54. Chronic Myeloid Leukemia Trial Collaborative Group. Interferon alpha versus chemotherapy for chronic myeloid leukemia: a meta-analysis of seven randomized trials. *J Natl Cancer Inst* 89:1616–1620, 1997.

55. Kantarjian HM, O'Brien S, Smith TL, et al. Treatment of Philadelphia chromosome–positive early chronic-phase chronic myelogenous leukemia with daily doses of interferon alpha and low-dose cytosine arabinoside. *J Clin Oncol* 17:284–292, 1999.

56. Sehn LH, Alyea EP, Canning C, et al. Comparative outcome of T-cell depleted and non-T-cell-depleted allogeneic bone marrow transplantation for chronic myelogenous leukemia: impact of donor lymphocytes. *J Clin Oncol* 17:561–568, 1999.

57. Gottardi D, Alfarano A, DeLeo AM, et al. In leukemic CD5+ B cells the expression of BCL-2 gene family is shifted toward protection for apoptosis. *Br J Haematol* 94:612–618, 1996.

58. Cheson BD, Bennett JM, Grever M, et al. National Cancer Institute-sponsored Working Group guidelines for chronic lymphocytic leukemia: revised guidelines for diagnosis and treatment. *Blood* 87:4990–4997, 1996.

59. Rai KR, Sawitsky A, Cronkite EP, et al. Clinical staging of chronic lymphocytic leukemia. *Blood* 46:219–234, 1975.

60. Binet JL, Auquier A, Dighiero G, et al. A new prognostic classification of chronic lymphocytic leukemia: prognostic significance. *Cancer* 40:855–864, 1981.

61. Dighiero G, Maloum K, Desablens B, et al. Chlorambucil in indolent chronic lymphocytic leukemia. French Cooperative Group on Chronic Lymphocytic Leukemia. *N Engl J Med* 338:1506–1514, 1998.

62. Johnson S, Smith AG, et al. Multicenter prospective randomised trial of fludarabine versus cyclophosphamide, doxorubicin and prednisone (CAP) for treatment of advanced stage chronic lymphocytic leukemia. The French Cooperative Group on CLL. *Lancet* 347:1432–1438, 1996.

63. Stone RM. Prolymphocytic leukemia. *Hematol Oncol Clin North Am* 4:457–471, 1990.

64. Staines A, Cartwright RA. Hairy-cell leukemia: descriptive epidemiology and case control study. *Br J Haematol* 85:714–717, 1993.

65. Digiuseppe JA, Borowitz MJ. Clinical utility of flow cytometry in the chronic lymphoid leukemias. *Semin Oncol* 25:6–10, 1998.

66. Cheson BD, Sorensen JM, Vena DA, et al. Treatment of hairy cell leukemia with 2-chlorodeoxyadenosine via the Group C Protocol: a report of 979 patients. *J Clin Oncol* 16:3007–3015, 1998.

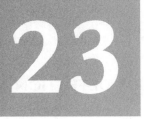

23

Malignant Melanoma

■ ■ ■

Marshall M. Urist
Martin J. Heslin
Donald M. Miller

Melanomas develop by malignant transformation of the melanocyte, a cell of neural crest origin that produces melanin pigment. Historically, the first published instance of a patient with melanoma was recorded by John Hunter (1728–1793) in 1787. The patient was a 35-year-old man with a secondary deposit in the neck. In an unpublished memoir presented to the faculty of medicine in 1806, René Laennec first described melanoma as a disease entity.

Most commonly, this cancer arises in the skin but is also found as a primary melanoma in the uveal tract (choroid, iris, ciliary body), upper aerodigestive tract, anal canal, rectum, and vagina. Melanoma accounts for nearly 4% of all cancers in the United States and is increasing in incidence. The worldwide incidence also is on the rise, a development that cannot be explained by any major change in diagnostic criteria. Recent research has advanced our understanding of cutaneous melanoma and its biological characteristics, natural history, and treatments. In the past, melanoma was notorious for its poor prognosis. The current 5-year survival rate of 88% represents a marked improvement over the last three decades.

BIOLOGICAL CHARACTERISTICS
Etiologic Features

The cause of melanoma is unknown. This tumor is believed to result from the combination of a susceptible phenotype (fair skin) and environmental factors (principally ultraviolet [UV] B light exposure). Although melanoma can occur in a familial pattern, the majority of cases appear to be sporadic. A personal or family history of nonmelanoma skin cancer also raises the risk of melanoma. This fact enhances the case for considering UV light a causative agent for both types of skin cancer. Intermittent intense sun exposure of untanned skin in younger individuals appears to be the most harmful combination.

Epidemiologic Factors

The estimated 2000 US incidence of new cases of melanoma of the skin is 47,700 (27,300 male and 20,400 female patients). The estimated number of deaths from melanoma in the same year is 7,700 (4,800 male and 2,900 female patients). This incidence represents 4% of cancers in male patients and 3% of cancers in female patients [1]. The trend in 5-year relative cancer survival rates has shown a significant improvement as follows: 80% in 1974 through 1976, 83% in 1980 through 1982, and 88% in 1989 through 1995.

The incidence of melanoma rose sharply for three decades and continues to increase. Nonetheless, the rate of rise has declined significantly for reasons that remain unclear. Although the rise is due partly to early recognition of pigmented lesions, it is not due to a change in the pathologic definition of the disease. Retrospective studies have shown that the pathologic criteria for the diagnosis of melanoma have not changed.

Pathogenesis

Risk factors for the development of melanoma in adults include multiple melanocytic nevi, fair skin, inability to tan, advancing age, and a history of melanoma. Additional factors include giant congenital melanocytic nevi, xeroderma pigmentosum, and chronic immunosuppression. Although the risk of development of melanoma is proportional to the number of benign nevi, whether these nevi are biological markers or actual precursors of risk is unclear. Ongoing prospective studies in large populations have been designed to help to clarify this issue. Certain types of moles, termed *atypical* or *dysplastic nevi,* are associated with a high incidence of melanoma (Color Plate 23.1). Usually, these nevi are larger than 6 mm in greatest diameter and exhibit uneven pigmentation and irregular borders. Most melanomas arise from preexisting nevi; however, they may appear also to arise de novo. Initially, the cell grows in a radial pattern that produces a flat, pigmented lesion on the skin. The appearance of a vertical growth component signals a rising risk of lymphovascular invasion. Regional lymph node enlargement is the most common first site of tumor spread. Although lymph nodes do act as filters for tumor cells, node involvement should be considered as a strong risk factor for further systemic metastases. The

most common sites of distant metastases are the brain, lung, and liver. As the tumor burden rises, metastases may appear in any tissue in the body.

PREVENTION AND EARLY DETECTION

Because UV irradiation is the risk factor associated most strongly with melanoma, efforts at prevention have focused on reduction of exposure to the sun and on the use of sunscreens. This emphasis is especially important in young persons because the damage from UV irradiation is thought to have lasting consequences. No strong evidence supports the use of sunscreens in the prevention of melanoma [2, 3]. Sunscreens actually may increase the risk by allowing susceptible individuals to remain in the sun longer without developing a burn. Equally unclear at present is the role of nonsolar UV irradiation (tanning beds) as a cause for melanoma. These lamps produce a level of UVB radiation lower than that in natural sunlight, and not all reports have shown a higher incidence among regular users. Still, the use of tanning beds is not advised, especially for individuals with fair skin or a history (personal or family) of any type of skin cancer.

Much of the improvement in prognosis for melanoma is attributed to early recognition. Public awareness programs sponsored by the American Cancer Society and other organizations have led to a rising cure rate for this potentially lethal disease. Physicians, nurses, patients, family members, and others should inquire into the nature of skin lesions. Changing or questionable nevi should be removed and analyzed.

DIAGNOSIS
Clinical Presentation

Classic melanoma arises in an asymptomatic, pigmented lesion having irregular borders and variable diameter and variably colored or black. A change in color, size (especially rapid growth), and shape and an extension of pigmentation outside the prior smooth margin of a mole should prompt suspicion of melanoma. A raised area within a previously flat mole with ulceration, bleeding, crusting, or pruritus should be considered a melanoma until proved otherwise.

Each of the four common histologic growth patterns of melanoma produces a characteristic physical appearance (Color Plates 23.2–23.5). Commonly, superficial spreading melanoma (70%) arises at the site of a preexisting nevus and is a flat lesion with irregular borders and colors (see Color Plate 23.2). Nodular melanomas make up 15% to 30% of melanoma cases and more commonly occur among older men (see Color Plate 23.3). These melanomas have vertical growth patterns, frequently without a recognizable antecedent mole. Often, their color is blue-black, but they also may be amelanotic. They may be polypoid, and their thickness portends a poor prognosis.

A lentigo maligna melanoma (1–5%) begins as a lentigo maligna (a type of in situ melanoma) that appears as a slowly expanding black to tan lesion with irregular borders larger than 3 cm (see Color Plate 23.4). Typically, such lesions are located on the face and neck of elderly, severely suntanned individuals. Approximately 5% of these melanomas are invasive, with vertical growth in a portion of the lesion that frequently becomes much darker and tends to ulcerate.

Acral lentiginous melanomas occur on the palms and soles or in nail beds (see Color Plate 23.5). Although this growth pattern constitutes only 2% to 8% of melanomas in white patients, it constitutes 35% to 60% of melanomas in dark-skinned patients, particularly blacks. Histologically, atypical melanocytes extend along the dermoepidermal junction as a manifestation of the lentiginous radial growth phase. Initially, the melanin can be seen through the epidermis as flat stains, and later a vertical growth phase may appear.

Subungual melanoma, considered to be a variant of acral lentiginous melanoma, occurs nearly equally among whites and blacks. This variant appears as brown or black discoloration under the nail bed, commonly in the great toe and thumb. The course is indolent; with ulceration, the lesion can be mistaken for a chronic paronychia. Most important is distinguishing subungual hematoma, a benign lesion, from subungual melanoma.

Melanomas may present also as enlarged regional lymph nodes or distant metastases. In such cases, the skin should be inspected carefully for evidence of a primary site. Because these melanomas can occur anywhere on the skin surface, clinical examinations should include the scalp, external auditory canal, nasal vestibule, nail beds, umbilicus, perianal skin, foreskin, labia, and web-space areas.

Diagnosis and Pathologic Determination

Any lesion suspected of being a melanoma should undergo biopsy. Most pigmented lesions are less than 1 cm in diameter and, therefore, are amenable to excisional biopsy. An incisional biopsy (shave biopsy, skin punch, or wedge excision) can be performed but may not provide all the information necessary for treatment decisions. This limitation occurs because the treatment is based on the tumor thickness and because the thickest area of the tumor may not be included in the incisional biopsy.

In some anatomic areas, total excision is not desirable because the wound cannot be closed or may cause a poor cosmetic result. In such instances, a full-thickness punch biopsy, carefully positioned in the most raised area of the tumor, is the procedure of choice.

When an excisional biopsy is performed, the margin should be minimal (1–2 mm), and the wound should not be enlarged for cosmetic purposes. In addition, the skin edges of the wound should not be elevated, because this may interfere with cutaneous lymphoscintigraphy.

Within the microscopical description of the tumor, the pathology report of an invasive melanoma should include the following: (1) tumor thickness in millimeters (Breslow's thickness), (2) level of invasion (Clark's level), (3) presence or absence of ulceration, regression, microsatellites, desmoplasia, neurotropism, (4) status of margins, and (5) histologic growth pattern. In cases in which a sentinel lymph node biopsy is performed, the tissue is examined by both standard hematoxylin-eosin staining and immunohistochemistry for S-100 antigen.

Staging System

Clinical staging of primary tumors is extremely inaccurate both in terms of estimating the thickness of the primary tumor and of judging the presence of regional lymph node metastases. Biopsy and pathologic interpretation are essential for proper diagnosis and staging. Pathologic staging of the primary melanoma is based on a microscopical assessment of thickness (in millimeters) and of level of invasion (Clark's levels I–V) [4]. Therefore, evaluation of the entire tumor—rather than a wedge or a punch biopsy—is advised. Regional nodes should be evaluated by physical examination. Enlarged regional nodes should be noted for staging. If the pathology report (or histology slides) of the primary melanoma is not available, the tumor is coded *TX*. If a primary tumor is not identified (i.e., an unknown primary), it is coded *T0*. The staging system adapted by the American Joint Committee on Cancer (AJCC) is based on tumor microstaging of the primary melanoma and the pattern of metastasis. This staging applies only to malignant melanoma of the skin (now including eyelids). The AJCC staging and grouping systems are sum-

Table 23.1   TNM Staging for Malignant Melanoma of the Skin

Classification	Definition
Primary tumor (pT)	
pTX	Primary tumor cannot be assessed
pT0	No evidence of primary tumor
pTis	Melanoma in situ (Clark's level I)
pT1	Tumor ≤ 0.75 mm thick and invades the papillary dermis (Clark's level II)
pT2	Tumor > 0.75 mm but < 1.5 mm thick and/or invades to papillary-reticular dermal interface (Clark's level III)
pT3	Tumor > 1.5 mm but < 4 mm thick and/or invades the reticular dermis (Clark's level IV)
pT3a	Tumor > 1.5 but < 3 mm thick
pT3b	Tumor > 3 but < 4 mm thick
pT4	Tumor > 4 mm thick and/or invades the subcutaneous tissue (Clark's level V) and/or satellite(s) within 2 cm of the primary tumor
pT4a	Tumor > 4 mm thick and/or invades the subcutaneous tissue
pT4b	Satellite(s) within 2 cm of the primary tumor
Regional lymph nodes (N)	
NX	Regional lymph nodes cannot be assessed
N0	Regional lymph node metastasis
N1	Metastasis ≤ 3 cm in greatest dimension in any regional lymph node(s)
N2	Metastasis > 3 cm in greatest dimension in any regional lymph node(s) and/or in-transit metastasis
N2a	Metastasis > 3 cm in greatest dimension in any regional lymph node(s)
N2b	In-transit metastasis
N2c	Both N2a and N2b
Distant metastasis (M)	
MX	Distant metastasis cannot be assessed
M0	No distant metastasis
M1	Distant metastasis
M1a	Metastasis in skin or subcutaneous tissue or lymph nodes(s) beyond regional nodes
M1b	Visceral metastasis

Source: Used with permission of the American Joint Committee on Cancer (AJCC), Chicago, Illinois. Reprinted from ID Fleming, JS Cooper, DE Henson, et al. (eds), *AJCC Cancer Staging Manual* (5th ed). Philadelphia: Lippincott-Raven, 1997: 163–167.

Table 23.2   AJCC/UICC Stage Grouping for Malignant Melanoma of the Skin

Stage 0	pTis	N0	M0
Stage I	pT1	N0	M0
	pT2	N0	M0
Stage II	pT3	N0	M0
Stage III	pT4	N0	M0
	Any pT	N1	M0
	Any pT	N2	M0
Stage IV	Any pT	Any N	M1

AJCC = American Joint Committee on Cancer; UICC = Union Internationale Contre le Cancer.
Source: Used with permission of the American Joint Committee on Cancer (AJCC), Chicago, Illinois. Reprinted from ID Fleming, JS Cooper, DE Henson, et al. (eds), *AJCC Cancer Staging Manual* (5th ed). Philadelphia: Lippincott-Raven, 1997: 163–167.

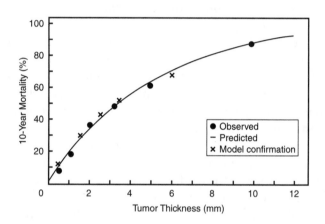

Figure 23.1   Observed and predicted 10-year mortality based on a mathematical model derived from tumor thickness.

marized in Tables 23.1 and 23.2. The 10-year mortality can be estimated using the graph in Figure 23.1.

Notably, two important weaknesses are seen in the current staging system. The first drawback is the absence of ulceration as a prognostic factor. Many studies have shown that ulceration is an independent risk factor for a poor outcome [5]. When ulceration is present (i.e., part of the tumor is missing), the high likelihood is that the measurement of thickness will be artificially low. The second drawback is the current classification of lymph node metastases by *size*, whereas the prognosis is well-known to be related to the *number* of lymph node metastases [6].

TREATMENT

Primary Tumors

The management of melanoma is based on a knowledge of tumor stage. Figure 23.2 summarizes the management of melanomas at stages 0, I, II, and III.

Treatment of the primary tumor is determined by the tumor thickness (Breslow's thickness) or by the level of invasion (Clark's level) [7]. The radius of excision

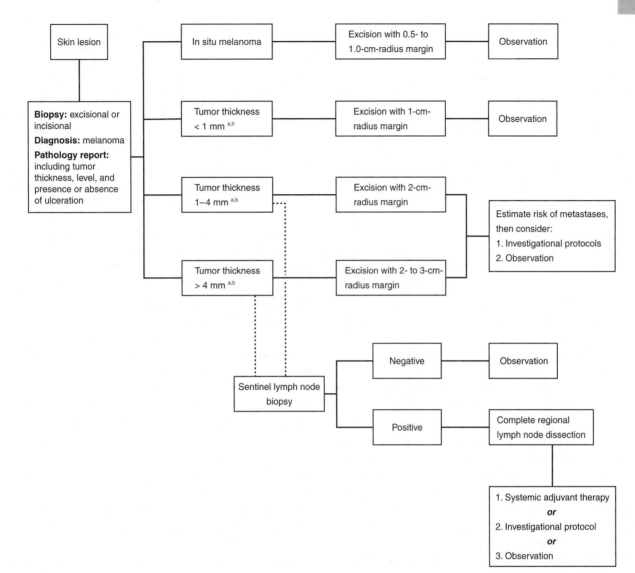

Figure 23.2 Algorithm for the management of melanoma. [a]Evaluation: When the diagnosis of invasive melanoma is made, all patients should have a complete history obtained and a physical examination. Symptoms and signs of metastatic disease should be investigated. Asymptomatic patients with normal physical examination results should undergo a metastatic evaluation appropriate to the risk of finding metastases. Tumor thickness < 1 mm requires no tests. Tumor thickness > 1 mm requires a minimum of a chest roentgenogram. Serum liver function tests, computed tomography, and magnetic resonance imaging scans are optional. [b]Patients with enlarged regional lymph nodes should undergo biopsy and, if the specimen is positive, complete dissection.

is measured from the edge of the lesion (if present) or the line of the biopsy scar. Recommended margins are based on prospective, randomized trials that have shown that larger margins of excision in the range of 3 to 5 cm are not associated with a higher survival as compared to smaller margins. The recommended margins are as follows: 3- to 5-mm radius for in situ melanoma; 1-cm radius for melanoma less than 1 mm thick; and 2-cm radius for melanoma 1 to 4 mm thick. Margins greater than 2 cm may be used for melanomas greater than 4 mm, but this group has not been studied

in controlled clinical trials. The risk of developing a local recurrence (tumor reappearing within 2 cm of the scar after wide local excision) increases with the thickness of the primary tumor [8]. For this reason, wider excisions of thick primary tumors may decrease the local recurrence rate. Most primary excision sites can be closed using skin-flap advancement techniques, thereby avoiding a skin graft. At one time, reduction in local recurrences and increase in survival rates were believed to result from prophylactic hyperthermic limb perfusion in patients with high-risk extremity primary tumors. In

1998, results from a randomized trial did not show a benefit for this form of adjuvant therapy [9].

A common site of first metastasis (after excision of the primary tumor) long has been observed to be the regional lymph node–bearing area. This finding led physicians to perform elective (also called *prophylactic*) lymph node dissection, which was thought to increase patient survival. Three prospective trials testing this hypothesis did not find a benefit to elective lymph node dissection; however, these studies did not control for all the factors known to affect the outcome in melanoma [10–12]. Recently, the results from a fourth randomized trial reported no overall benefit in survival for patients undergoing elective lymph node dissection. In contrast to the other three, this trial incorporated stratification for the important prognostic factors in melanoma. With this type of trial design, an analysis can detect subgroups of patients who might benefit from treatment. Patients with nonulcerated tumors 1 to 2 mm thick did show a significantly improved survival with elective lymph node dissection [13]. The question of elective lymph node dissection largely has become moot since the development of lymphatic mapping and sentinel lymph node biopsy.

A current capability is mapping the course of lymphatic drainage from sites on the skin to the regional lymph nodes that receive direct flow from the primary tumor. This node is called the *sentinel lymph node* (Color Plate 23.6) [14]. If tumor cells spread from the primary tumor to regional nodes, the sentinel node will be the first node in which the cells appear. Therefore, excision of this node can be used to test for the presence of melanoma cells and to identify those patients requiring lymph node dissection [15, 16]. When nodes are positive, consideration is given also to systemic adjuvant therapy. In general, a sentinel lymph node biopsy is recommended when the tumor thickness is greater than 1 mm. At this point, the chance of finding a positive node is greater than 3% to 5%. Important reminders are that sentinel lymph node biopsy is considered to be a staging (diagnostic) technique and that its therapeutic value is being evaluated in ongoing clinical trials. When sentinel lymph nodes are found to contain metastatic melanoma, a completion dissection of the node-bearing area should be performed.

Adjuvant Therapy

For several reasons, melanoma is an ideal disease for the development of an effective adjuvant treatment.

First, for a well-defined group of patients (those with nodal involvement or with thick primary lesions), the risk of recurrent disease is fairly high. Second, several current treatment modalities offer some likelihood of inducing response (immunotherapy, chemotherapy). Finally, no curative treatment exists for distant metastatic disease. Although many studies have investigated the possible activity of immunotherapy and chemotherapy in the adjuvant setting, none have shown a benefit until the recent adjuvant trials with high-dose interferon-α as a postsurgical adjuvant in AJCC stage III melanoma.

An Eastern Cooperative Oncology Group (ECOG) trial (EST 1684) tested the efficacy of interferon-α2b given intravenously at 20 MU/m²/day 5 days weekly for the first 4 weeks of therapy, followed by alternate-day therapy with 10 MU/m²/day, and 3 days weekly for the subsequent 11 months. At a median follow-up of 4.7 years, the ECOG trial showed almost a 1-year increase in median disease-free and overall survival for patients treated with interferon-α2b [17].

More recently, ECOG has conducted a three-arm adjuvant trial (EST 1690) for patients with deep primary melanoma (> 4 mm thick) or regional lymph node metastases. This study randomly assigned patients to high-dose therapy (as in EST 1684), low-dose therapy (interferon-α2b at a dose of 3 MU/day three times weekly for 2 years), or standard follow-up without treatment. The study accrued 642 patients and completed patient accrual in 1995. However, an interim analysis of the data from EST 1690 failed to demonstrate a statistically significant difference in overall survival between any arm, though showing an improvement in relapse-free survival on the high-dose interferon arm. The current standard adjuvant therapy for high-risk melanoma patients continues to be high-dose interferon-α2b.

Numerous clinical trials have not produced a current role for adjuvant chemotherapy in treating malignant melanoma outside a controlled clinical trial setting. Several pivotal clinical trials are seeking to determine the activity of chemoimmunotherapy or interleukin-2 (IL-2) in the treatment of patients with thick primary tumors or regional nodal metastases.

Surveillance

Follow-up of patients after initial treatment of melanoma is a combined effort on the part of patients and their physicians. In addition to looking for new or changing moles, patients should examine themselves on a monthly basis to detect recurrent melanoma in the skin, subcutaneous tissues, or lymph nodes. The most common sites of metastases are regional lymph nodes, lung, liver, and brain. In fact, most recurrences are diagnosed by patients rather than by their physicians. The frequency of periodic examinations by a physician is determined by the risk for recurrence. Patients with very early melanoma may not need to be examined more than once or twice yearly, whereas those with thicker tumors are followed up at closer intervals. The highest risk for recurrence is during the first 3 to 5 years after diagnosis; however, melanoma can recur many years later.

Routine laboratory tests and radiologic studies have very limited benefit in asymptomatic patients. Computed tomography and positron emission tomography scans and magnetic resonance imaging can be very helpful when the symptoms or signs of recurrence appear.

Metastases

Tumor spread away from the primary site is classified as a local, in-transit, regional, or distant metastasis. Local recurrences are defined as metastases appearing within 2 cm of the primary tumor excision scar. They are associated with a high risk of further recurrence, because 70% of patients die within 5 years of experiencing a local recurrence. Though often these sites can be excised surgically, prompt reappearance of the tumor is common.

In-transit metastases (dermal and subcutaneous tumor deposits) occur between the primary site and regional node-bearing areas. Often, they too are followed by other metastases. When in-transit metastases are limited to one extremity, isolated hyperthermic limb perfusion with melphalan can be the most effective form of therapy [18, 19].

Regional lymph node metastases are controlled best by a complete regional lymph node dissection. Affected patients' prognosis will be proportional to the number of involved nodes. Irradiation of the bed of the resection has been shown to reduce further the incidence of regional recurrence.

Treatment of distant metastatic disease has undergone considerable improvement in the last decade. For the first time, clinical studies are reporting that a significant proportion of patients undergo complete remission. A number of agents, including dacarbazine (DTIC), have single-agent response rates of 10% to 20% in the treatment of melanoma. Other active agents include cisplatin, nitrosoureas, thiotepa, and the taxanes. In the early 1990s, combinations of chemotherapeutic agents that were developed could induce response rates of 40% to 50%.

Legha et al. [20] reported a series of studies in which cisplatin-vinblastine-DTIC chemotherapy was combined with intravenous IL-2 and interferon-α [20, 21]. In these studies, the overall response rate was 60%, with a 21% to 23% complete remission rate. More important is that these investigators have shown that more than one-half of patients with complete remission are disease-free at 5 years [22]. This finding suggests that combinations of chemotherapy and immunotherapy may prolong life expectancy in a significant number of patients with metastatic melanoma. Though these results are extremely promising, these combinations have not yet been shown to be superior to single-agent chemotherapy in a prospective randomized trial. Several cooperative group trials are comparing combination chemoimmunotherapy to single-agent DTIC.

Despite melanoma's well-known tendency to disseminate widely, surgical resection of metastases can provide substantial palliation and, in some instances, long-term remissions. Patients with a long disease-free interval and with a small number of metastases appear to do better after resection than do those with short disease-free intervals or multiple metastatic lesions [23]. Generally, patients having involvement of multiple organs do not gain significant benefit from surgical treatment. Postoperative radiotherapy has been shown to be beneficial for patients with melanoma metastatic to the head and neck region [24].

The treatment of brain metastases in patients with malignant melanoma has been a very difficult problem. The development of stereotactic radiotherapy and the gamma-knife technology have allowed prolonged control of brain metastases in some patients [25, 26]. Previously, the median survival of melanoma patients with brain metastases was 4 to 6 weeks. With gamma-knife therapy, this survival has been improved substantially, with median survivals of up to 35 weeks.

Palliation

Patients with melanoma symptoms can be palliated with all three major treatment modalities. Surgical resection of metastases is the most reliable way to achieve a complete response if the risk of operation is low [27]. If unresectable disease is present, radiotherapy can be useful in the palliation of pain. Chemotherapy also can reduce the severity of symptoms; however, the average duration of response is relatively short.

INVESTIGATIONAL TREATMENT
Surgery

The unanswered questions about the treatment of primary melanoma center around the issue of smaller margins of excision for early melanoma. No results from prospective trials show that margins of less than 1 cm are adequate for tumors less than 1 mm thick. Some debate continues about the value of elective regional lymph node dissection; however, the introduction of sentinel lymph node biopsy largely has defused this issue. Unanswered questions about sentinel lymph node biopsy are being addressed in ongoing studies.

Chemotherapy and Immunotherapy
GENE THERAPY

Because the benefit of treating metastatic melanoma is limited, this tumor has been ideal for gene therapy trials [28, 29]. A large number of trials have tested various gene therapy approaches. The primary approach has been the development of recombinant vaccines or the development of cellular therapies using cytokine-transfected lymphocytes (or both modalities). Additionally, the use of retroviral vectors to deliver major histocompatibility antigens has been tested in clinical trials.

VACCINES

Although a randomized clinical trial has yet to show a statistically significant improvement in the survival of patients receiving vaccine therapy for melanoma, several studies have shown enhanced survival of patients who develop an immune response to a melanoma vaccine [30, 31]. These studies reported response rates as high as 40% for patients with metastatic disease treated with recombinant vaccines in conjunction with IL-2.

REHABILITATION
Sequelae of Therapy

Most resections of the primary tumor or biopsy of a regional lymph node do not lead to physical disabilities. A complete regional lymph node dissection is associated with a risk of swelling (lymphedema) and infection of the extremities (lymphangitis or cellulitis or both) but not in the head and neck. Precautions for patients who have undergone axillary or inguinal lymph node dissections include good personal hygiene, avoidance of injury to the skin of the extremity (trauma, chemicals, toxic plants, injections, and intravenous catheters), constricting garments, and repetitive motions of the extremity. Sustained physical therapy programs employing compression or massage techniques can prevent or reduce the development of lymphedema.

Genetic and Family Issues

Approximately 5% of all cases of cutaneous melanoma occur in persons with a familial predisposition. In these families, first-degree relatives of patients with melanoma have a twofold increase of their relative risk of melanoma. Familial melanoma is characterized by an increased risk of developing primary melanoma, a higher incidence of multiple primary lesions, and an earlier age of onset. Molecular characterization of kindreds of familial melanoma patients have suggested that the multiple tumor suppressor gene likely is involved in the development of this disease. This cell-cycle control gene appears to be inactivated by mutation in several of these kindreds. Interestingly, patients with an inherited mutation that predisposes them to melanoma have an even higher risk if they have extensive sun exposure.

Critically important is that family members of patients with a strong indication of inherited melanoma be followed closely for evidence of the development of new lesions. These individuals should be counseled carefully about the risk of sun exposure and the use of sunscreens.

REFERENCES

1. Greenlee RT, Murray T, Bolden S, Wingo PA. Cancer statistics, 2000. *CA Cancer J Clin* 50:7–33, 2000.
2. Naylor MF, Farmer KC. The case for sunscreens. A review of their use in preventing actinic damage and neoplasia. *Arch Dermatol* 133:1146–1154, 1997.
3. Wolf P, Quehenberger F, Mullegger R, et al. Phenotypic markers, sunlight-related factors and sunscreen use in patients with cutaneous melanoma: an Austrian case-control study. *Melanoma Res* 8:370–378, 1998.
4. American Joint Committee on Cancer. Malignant melanoma of the skin. In Fleming ID, Cooper JS, Henson DE, et al. (eds), *AJCC Cancer Staging Manual* (5th ed). Philadelphia: Lippincott-Raven, 1997:163–170.

5. Buzaid AC, Ross MI, Balch CM, et al. Critical analysis of the current American Joint Committee on Cancer staging system for cutaneous melanoma and proposal of a new staging system. *J Clin Oncol* 15:1039–1051, 1997.

6. Coit DG, Rogatko A, Brennan MF. Prognostic factors in patients with melanoma metastatic to axillary or inguinal lymph nodes. A multivariate analysis. *Ann Surg* 214: 627–636, 1991.

7. McDermott NC, Hayes, DP, al-Sader MH, et al. Identification of vertical growth phase in malignant melanoma. A study of interobserver agreement. *Am J Clin Pathol* 110: 753–757, 1998.

8. Soong SJ, Harrison RA, McCarthy WH, et al. Factors affecting survival following local, regional, or distant recurrence from localized melanoma. *J Surg Oncol* 67:228–233, 1998.

9. Koops HS, Vaglini M, Suciu S, et al. Prophylactic isolated limb perfusion for localized, high-risk limb melanoma: results of a multicenter randomized phase III trial. European Organization for Research and Treatment of Cancer Malignant Melanoma Cooperative Group Protocol 18832, the World Health Organization Melanoma Program Trial 15, and the North American Perfusion Group Southwest Oncology Group-8593. *J Clin Oncol* 16:2906–2912, 1998.

10. Veronesi U, Adamus J, Bandiera DC, Brennhovd IO, et al. Stage I melanoma of the limbs. Immediate versus delayed node dissection. *Tumori* 66:373–396, 1980.

11. Cascinelli N, Morabito A, Santinami M, et al. Immediate or delayed dissection of regional nodes in patients with melanoma of the trunk: a randomized trial. WHO Melanoma Programme. *Lancet* 351:793–796, 1998.

12. Sim FH, Taylor WF, Pritchard DJ, Soule EH. Lymphadenectomy in the management of stage I malignant melanoma: a prospective randomized study. *Mayo Clin Proc* 61:697–705, 1986.

13. Balch CM, Soong S, Ross MI, et al. Long-term results of a multi-institutional randomized trial comparing prognostic factors and surgical results for intermediate thickness melanomas (1.0 to 4.0 mm). Intergroup Melanoma Surgical Trial. *Ann Surg Oncol* 7:87–97, 2000.

14. Morton DL, Wen D-R, Wong JH, et al. Technical details of intraoperative lymphatic mapping for early stage melanoma. *Arch Surg* 127:392–399, 1992.

15. Ross MI, Reintgen DS. Role of lymphatic mapping and sentinel node biopsy in the detection of melanoma nodal metastases. *Eur J Cancer* 34(suppl 3):S7–S11, 1998.

16. Shivers SC, Wang X, Li W, et al. Molecular staging of malignant melanoma: correlation with clinical outcome. *JAMA* 280:1410–1415, 1998.

17. Kirkwood JM, Strawderman MH, Ernstoff MS, et al. Interferon alfa-2b adjuvant therapy of high risk resected cutaneous melanoma: the Eastern Cooperative Oncology Group Trial EST 1684. *J Clin Oncol* 14:7–17, 1996.

18. Vrouenraets BC, Hart GA, Eggermont AM, et al. Relation between limb toxicity and treatment outcomes after isolated limb perfusion for recurrent melanoma. *J Am Coll Surg* 188:522–530, 1999.

19. Brobeil A, Berman C, Cruse CW, et al. Efficacy of hyperthermic isolated limb perfusion for extremity-confined recurrent melanoma. *Ann Surg Oncol* 5:376–383, 1998.

20. Legha SS, Ring S, Eton O, et al. Development and results of biochemotherapy in metastatic melanoma. *Cancer J Sci Am* 3(suppl 1):S7–S8, 1997.

21. Legha SS, Ring S, Eton O, et al. Development of a biochemotherapy regimen with concurrent administration of cisplatin, vinblastine, dacarbazine, interferon alpha, and interleukin-2 for patients with metastatic melanoma. *J Clin Oncol* 16:1752–1759, 1998.

22. Legha SS. Durable complete responses in metastatic melanoma treated with interleukin-2 in combination with interferon alpha and chemotherapy. *Semin Oncol* 24:S39–S43, 1997.

23. Tafra L, Dale PS, Wanek LA, Ramming KP. Resection and adjuvant immunotherapy for melanoma metastatic to the lung and thorax. *J Thorac Cardiovasc Surg* 110:119–128, 1995.

24. Ang KK, Peters LJ, Weber RS, et al. Postoperative radiotherapy for cutaneous melanoma of the head and neck region. *Int J Otolaryngol* 30:795–798, 1994.

25. Seung SK, Sneed PK, McDermott MW, et al. Gamma knife radiosurgery for malignant melanoma breast metastases. *Cancer J Sci Am* 4:103–109, 1998.

26. Shiau CY, Sneed PK, Shu HK, et al. Radiosurgery for brain metastases: relationship of dose and pattern of enhancement to local control. *Int J Radiat Oncol Biol Phys* 37:375–383, 1997.

27. Ollila DW, Hsueh EC, Stern SL, Morton DL. Metastasectomy for recurrent stage IV melanoma. *J Surg Oncol* 71:209–213, 1999.

28. Gutzmer R, Guerry D. Gene therapy for melanoma in humans. *Hematol Oncol Clin North Am* 12:519–538, 1998.

29. Mastrangelo MJ, Sato T, Lattime EC, Maguire HC. Cellular vaccine therapies for cancer. *Cancer Treat Res* 94:35–50, 1998.

30. Morton DL, Ollila DW, Hsueh EC, et al. Cytoreductive surgery and adjuvant immunotherapy: a new management paradigm for metastatic melanoma. *CA Cancer J Clin* 49: 101–106, 1999.

31. Ollila DW, Kelley MC, Gammon G, Morton DL. Overview of melanoma vaccines: active specific immunotherapy for melanoma patients. *Semin Oncol* 14:328–336, 1998.

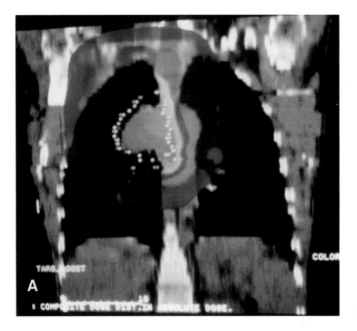

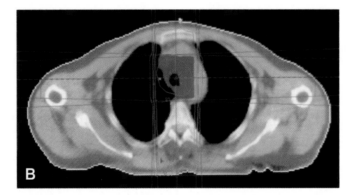

Color Plate 11.1 (A) Three-dimensional conformal radiation treatment plan for a right-sided T4 lung cancer. The color-wash display demonstrates that the high-dose region (*red*) conforms to the hatched target volume. *Blue* areas receive very low doses. Areas of underdosing and overdosing can be readily identified and appropriate action taken. These displays are invaluable (especially in conjunction with dose-volume histograms) and are available in axial, sagittal, and coronal planes. (B) Composite treatment plans for postoperative radiotherapy for a right lung T2N2 squamous cell carcinoma treated surgically by right upper lobectomy and mediastinal lymph node dissection. The computed tomographic scan is taken through the upper mediastinum, and the target volume is the *purple* oval shape. It is adequately covered by the 95% isodose line, which is the prescription isodose. The cord dose was 86%. Using 12-MV x-rays, 4,140 cGy was delivered with anterior and posterior ports, and then lateral fields received a further 900 cGy. The total dose to the cord was slightly more than 4,500 cGy (5,040 cGy × 0.86 ÷ 0.95).

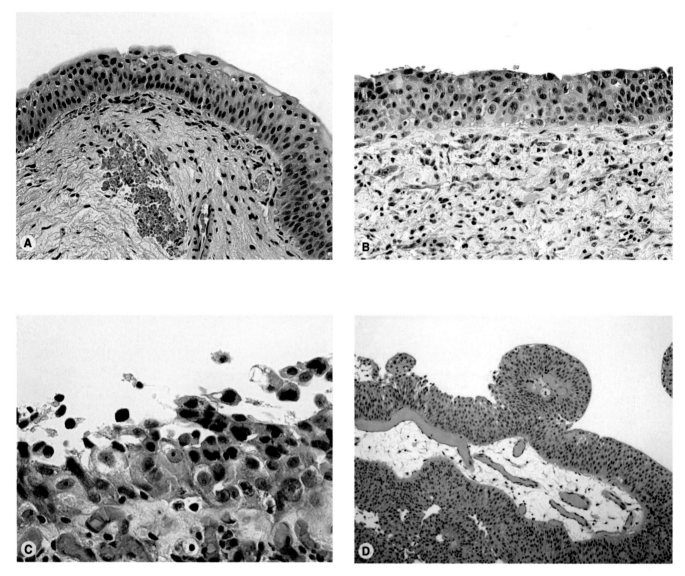

Color Plate 18.1 (A) Normal urothelium with umbrella cells covering the orderly epithelial layer of urothelial (transitional) cells. Nuclei are regular and bland and cytoplasm is abundant (magnification 200×). (B) Dysplastic urothelium. Note the disorder within the epithelial layer and the variation in cellular and nuclear detail (magnification 200×). (C) Carcinoma in situ (CIS). Note the increased disorder within the urothelial epithelium and pleomorphic nuclei and cells. Nucleoli are seen readily and mitoses, which often are aberrant, may appear throughout the urothelial layer. The urothelial epithelium is dyscohesive, with numerous cells partially or completely separated from the urothelium (magnification 400×). (D) Papillary neoplasm of low malignant potential. A thickened urothelial layer of orderly cells with minimal cytologic atypia is present in a papillary configuration (magnification 50×).

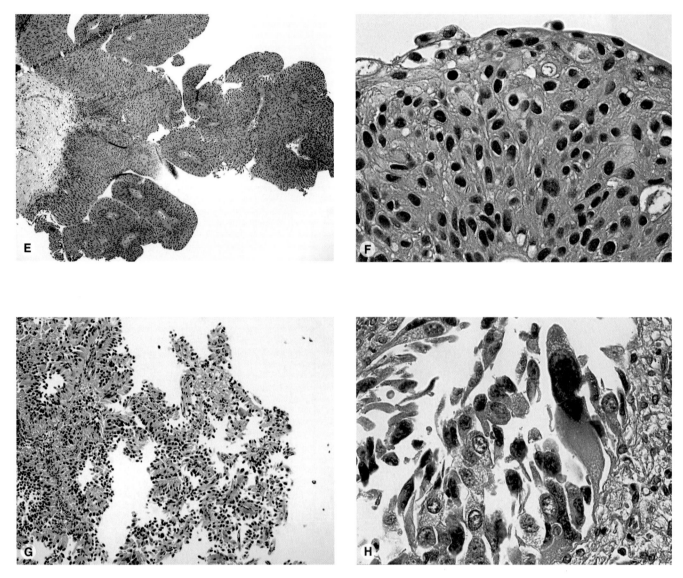

Color Plate 18.1 (continued) (E) Low-grade papillary urothelial carcinoma. A low-power view demonstrates the papillary configuration and architectural disorder. The urothelial layer often is thickened, and papillary fronds may be partially fused (magnification 25×). (F) Low-grade papillary urothelial carcinoma. A high-power view demonstrates the cytologic atypia present in low-grade urothelial carcinoma. Nuclear pleomorphism and hyperchromasia are demonstrated within a disordered urothelial layer (magnification 400×). (G) High-grade papillary urothelial carcinoma. Increased architectural and cytologic disorder is apparent even at low power. Marked variation is noted in cellular and nuclear details, and cellular dyscohesion is apparent (magnification 100×). (H) High-grade papillary urothelial carcinoma. A high-power view of the marked cytologic and nuclear atypia present. Numerous cells are separated from the urothelial component (magnification 400×).

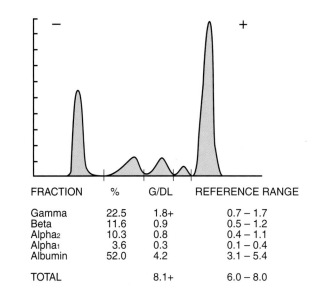

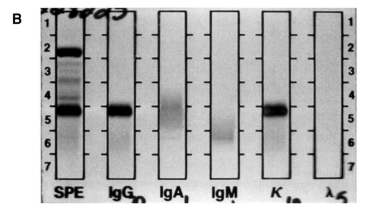

Color Plate 21.1 (A) Densitometric scan of serum protein electrophoresis run on cellulose acetate, showing a monoclonal gammopathy (spike) migrating in the gamma region. The area under the curve is expressed as a percentage for each region that, when multiplied by the total protein (expressed in grams per deciliter), results in the quantitative measurement of the amount of protein in each fraction. Because little or no normal protein remains in the gamma region, the amount of the "spike" or "M component" in this patient is equivalent to the amount in the gamma region (1.8 g/dl). In other examples, an attempt would be made to separate the area under the "spike" from the rest of the normal proteins present in that region. (B) Serum immunofixation electrophoresis revealing the presence of a band of restricted electrophoretic mobility in the IgG lane and a corresponding band in the kappa lane. Together, these bands establish the presence of an IgG kappa monoclonal gammopathy. *SPE* = serum protein electrophoresis.

The authors of Chapter 21 are deeply indebted to Dr. Richard L. Humphrey and Johns Hopkins University School of Medicine for graciously allowing us to use the color plates cited in this chapter.

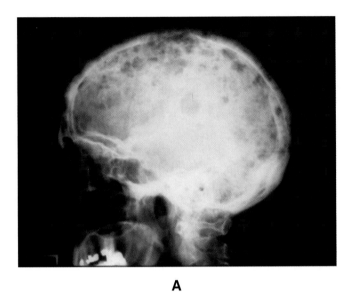

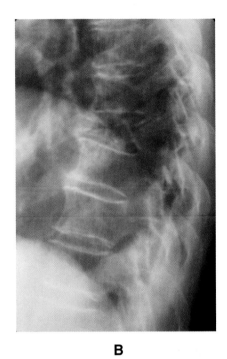

A

B

Color Plate 21.2 (A) Lateral skull radiograph from a patient with far advanced myeloma, showing multiple lytic ("punched-out") lesions throughout the calvarium. Despite the great number of these lesions, they usually are asymptomatic. (B) Lateral radiograph of the thoracic spine, showing generalized osteoporosis and collapse and anterior wedging of T10.

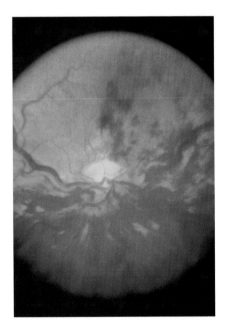

Color Plate 21.3 Fundus of a patient with severe hyperviscosity, revealing extensive retinal hemorrhages that can result in blindness when the macula is involved. The extent of the bleeding obscures the swollen veins with segmental constrictions described as "sausage links."

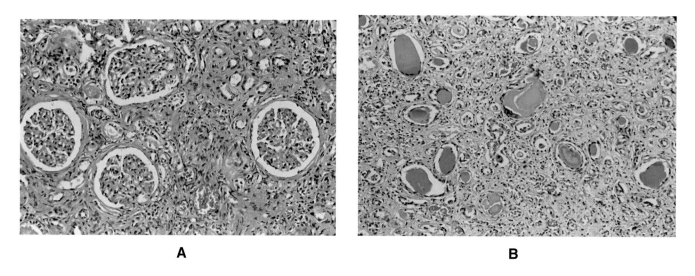

A   **B**

Color Plate 21.4   (A) Hematoxylin and eosin–stained renal biopsy from a patient with myeloma cast nephropathy. In the cortex, the glomeruli are largely intact but are spaced more closely because of the atrophy, scarring, and disappearance of the tubules. (B) Renal medulla of this patient, showing the same process of tubular destruction, with some of the tubular lumina occupied by amorphous, dense, eosinophilic casts that have resulted from the precipitation of a Bence Jones protein (free light chain).

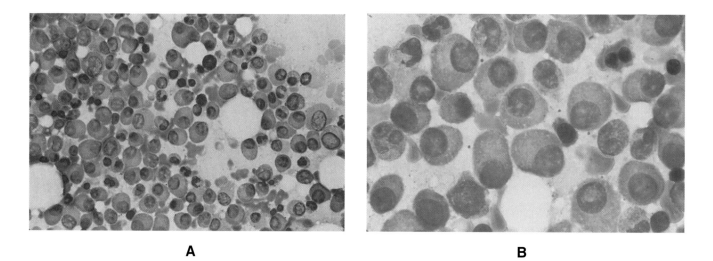

A   **B**

Color Plate 21.5   Wright-stained smears of bone marrow aspirate from a patient with multiple myeloma. (A) Even in this low-power view, the marrow clearly is shown to be replaced largely by plasma cells. (B) At high power, the cytologic features of the plasma cells include abundant blue cytoplasm, an eccentric purple nucleus, and a perinuclear clear zone. Some of the nuclei have a rather large nucleolus but, taken one at a time, the cells are not especially primitive. No binucleate or multinucleate forms or dividing cells are present, and the most significant abnormality is their markedly increased numbers.

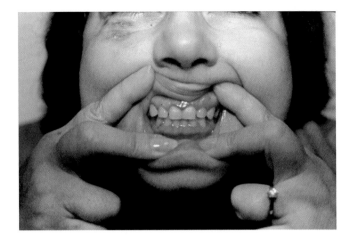

Color Plate 22.1 Gingival hypertrophy in a patient with acute myelogenous leukemia.

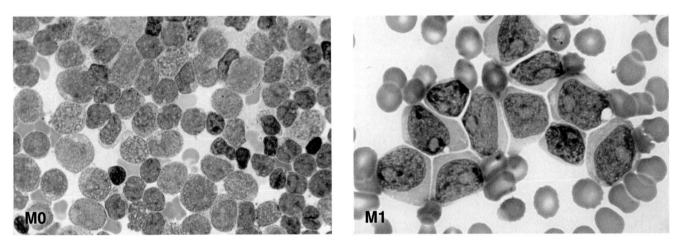

Color Plate 22.2 Morphologic appearance of acute myelogenous leukemia cells classified according to the FAB system: M0 and M1.

The editors are deeply indebted to Dr. Diane C. Farhi (Quest Diagnostics) for graciously allowing us to use Color Plates 22.2, 22.3 (L3), 22.4, and 22.7 and to Dr. C. Whitaker Sewell (Emory University School of Medicine) for graciously allowing us to use Color Plates 22.3 (L1 and L2) and 22.5 cited in this chapter.

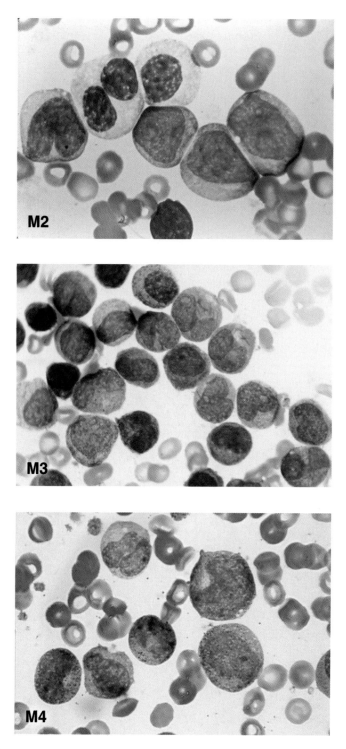

Color Plate 22.2 Morphologic appearance of acute myelogenous leukemia cells classified according to the FAB system: M2–M4.

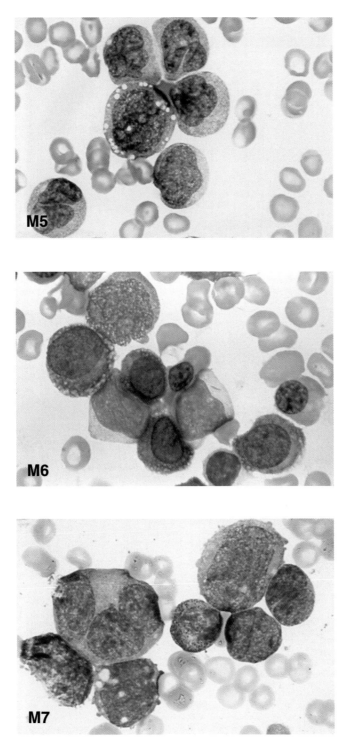

Color Plate 22.2 Morphologic appearance of acute myelogenous leukemia cells classified according to the FAB system: M5–M7.

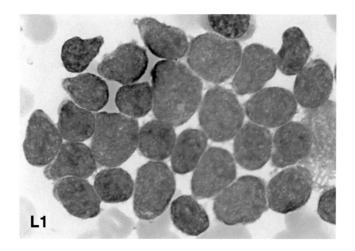

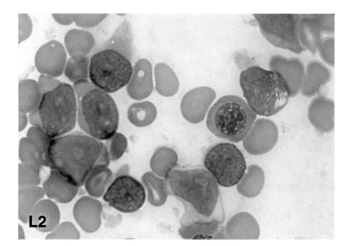

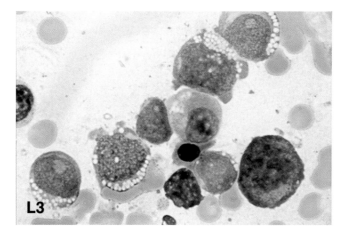

Color Plate 22.3 Morphologic appearance of acute lymphoblastic leukemia cells classified according to the FAB system: L1–L3.

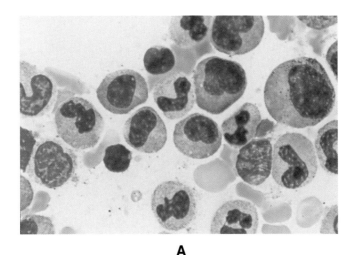

A

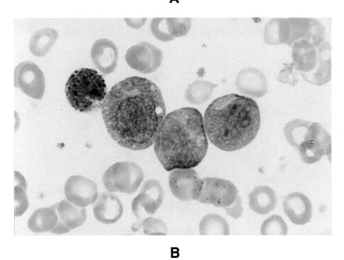

B

Color Plate 22.4 Chronic myelogenous leukemia (CML). (A) CML, stable phase (peripheral blood). Note leukocytosis with orderly maturation from immature to more mature white blood cells. (B) CML, accelerated phase (peripheral blood). Note the increased number of blasts (myeloblasts) and basophils.

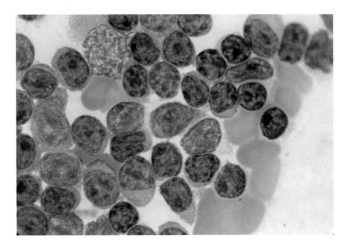

Color Plate 22.5 Chronic lymphocytic leukemia (peripheral blood). Lymphocytosis consisting of mature lymphocytes is noted, as is an occasional "smudge" cell.

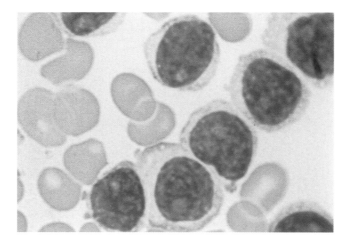

Color Plate 22.6 Prolymphocytic leukemia (peripheral blood). Prolymphocytes are larger than normal lymphocytes and have more generous cytoplasm. Nucleoli are prominent.

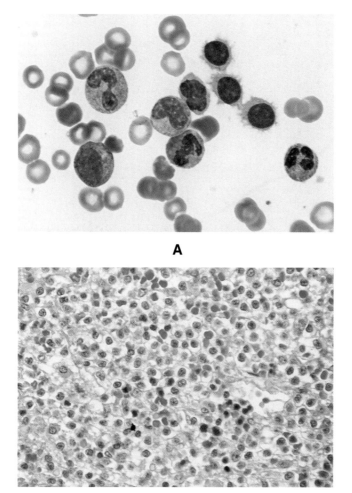

Color Plate 22.7 (A) Hairy cell leukemia (peripheral blood). Hairy cells have prominent cytoplasmic projections. Nuclei are round or folded. (B) Hairy cell leukemia (bone marrow biopsy). Histologic section demonstrates characteristic fried-egg appearance of hairy cells. Nuclei are separated by generous amounts of cytoplasm.

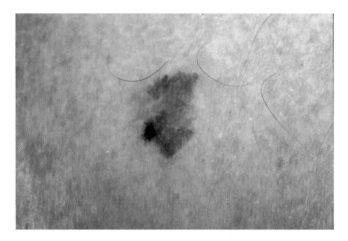

Color Plate 23.1   Melanoma arising from a dysplastic nevus (of the trunk).

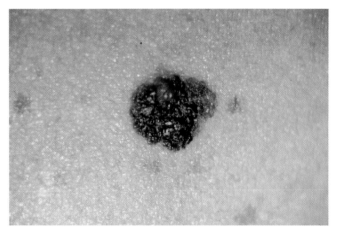

Color Plate 23.2   Superficial spreading melanoma.

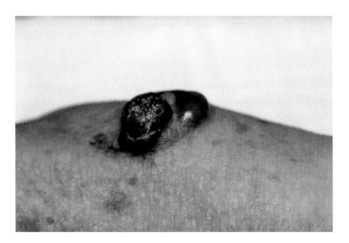

Color Plate 23.3   Nodular melanoma.

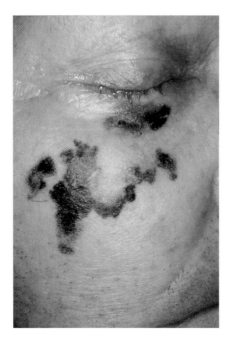

Color Plate 23.4 Lentigo maligna melanoma of the cheek.

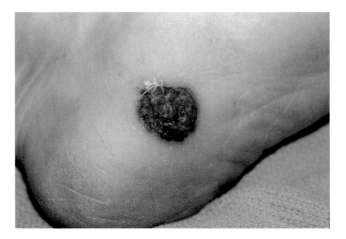

Color Plate 23.5 Acral lentiginous melanoma of the foot.

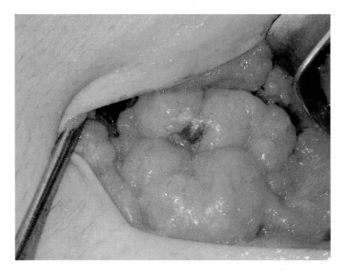

Color Plate 23.6 Sentinel lymph node.

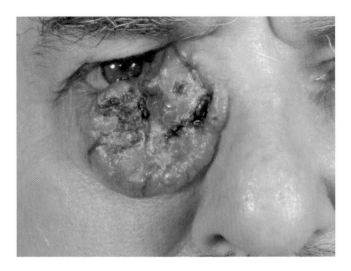

Color Plate 24.1 Ulcerated basal cell carcinoma characterized by a central ulceration and a rolled border.

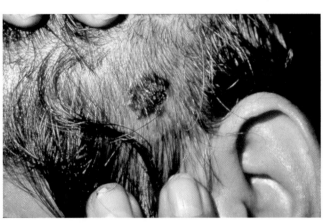

Color Plate 24.2 Pigmented basal cell carcinoma on the scalp. This pigmented lesion is difficult to distinguish from a melanocytic neoplasm.

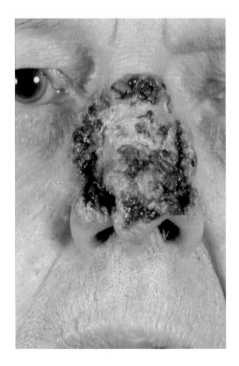

Color Plate 24.3 Large fungating, ulcerated basal cell carcinoma. This advanced neoplasm has been present for many years and has replaced a large portion of the nose.

The editors are deeply indebted to Dr. Carl Washington (Department of Dermatology, Emory University School of Medicine) for graciously allowing us to use the color plates cited in this chapter.

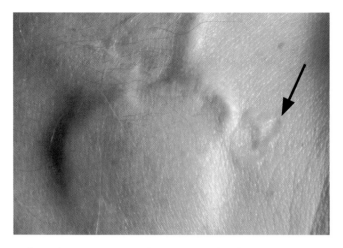

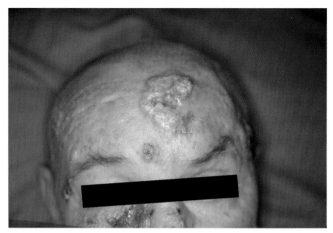

Color Plate 24.4   Morpheaform basal cell carcinoma. This depressed lesion (**arrow**) was present for many years on the chest of a middle-aged man. The elevation adjacent to the basal cell carcinoma is an implanted cardiac pacemaker.

Color Plate 24.5   Multiple squamous cell carcinomas on markedly sun-damaged skin in an elderly man.

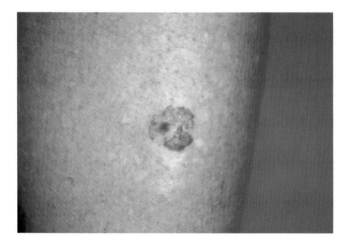

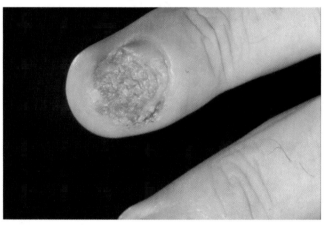

Color Plate 24.6   In situ squamous cell carcinoma. This scaly, slightly elevated plaque has been present for many years.

Color Plate 24.7   Squamous cell carcinoma of the periungual region.

24

Basal Cell and Squamous Cell Skin Cancer

■ ■ ■

John A. Carucci
Darrell S. Rigel
Robert J. Friedman

Nonmelanoma skin cancer (basal and squamous cell carcinoma) represents a major public health burden. Estimates predict that approximately 1.3 million new nonmelanoma skin cancers will be diagnosed this year in the United States, rendering the incidence of this type of neoplasm nearly equal in magnitude to the sum of all other cancers combined [1]. At current rates, one in five Americans will develop a skin cancer during their lifetime, with more than 97% of these being nonmelanoma skin cancer [2]. Some studies suggest a correlation between development of nonmelanoma skin cancer and risk for internal malignancy, although the precise nature of this relationship is yet to be defined [3, 4].

What should be noted is that nonmelanoma skin cancer is a preventable disease. Primary prevention behaviors include application of sunscreen, use of protective clothing, limit of sun exposure during peak hours, and avoidance of artificial sources of ultraviolet irradiation [5]. Secondary prevention behaviors include regular screening for skin cancer to promote early detection [6]. A recent study indicated that sun awareness education programs may inspire and support prevention behavior in children [7].

BASAL CELL CARCINOMA
Definition

Basal cell carcinoma (BCC) is a neoplasm of nonkeratinizing cells from the basal cell layer of the epidermis. Metastases are rare. However, BCC may result in extensive local damage if left untreated.

Epidemiologic Characteristics

BCC is the most common cancer in humans, accounting for 75% of all nonmelanoma skin cancers and almost

25% of all cancers diagnosed in the United States [8]. It occurs primarily on sun-exposed skin and rarely develops in dark-skinned persons [9, 10]. Currently, BCC affects men only slightly more often than women [8]. Once infrequent before the age of 40, BCC is becoming more common in younger individuals. Probably this is due to changes in fashion and lifestyle, leading to increased sun exposure and possibly coupled with depletion of the ozone layer [11].

Pathogenesis

Factors implicated in the development of BCC include exposure to ultraviolet light (UVL), mutations in tumor suppressor and regulatory genes, exposure to ionizing radiation, alterations in immunosurveillance, and selected inherited conditions. The factor implicated most frequently in the pathogenesis of BCC is exposure of the skin to UVL. The most damaging irradiation lies in the 290- to 320-nm (ultraviolet B [UVB]) range. Individuals at greatest risk of developing skin cancer are those living near the equator or in ozone-depleted areas [11,12]. Cumulative exposure to UVL over many years is necessary for the development of skin cancer. Therefore, individuals with outdoor professions or hobbies are at risk for developing BCC [13]. Light-skinned people who tend to burn easily are at increased risk for developing BCC. One study correlates heavy freckling or moles with a diameter of more than 5 cm in children with a tendency to develop BCC in adulthood [14]. The risk of BCC is decreased substantially in dark-skinned people and those who tan rather than burn [15].

Mutations in tumor suppressor genes and genes that regulate developmental pathways may be involved in the pathogenesis of BCC. Recent studies indicate that mutations in the tumor suppressor gene *p53* are present in 50% of BCC cases [16]. UVL may be involved in mutation of *p53;* Ananthaswamy et al. [17] demonstrated that application of sunscreen prevented development of mutations of tumor suppressor gene *p53* in mice exposed to UVL. This finding supports the potential protective role for sunscreens in skin cancer development.

Other studies indicate that the human patched gene is mutated in both sporadic and hereditary BCC. Inactivation of this gene may be a necessary step in the pathogenesis of BCC [18].

Ionizing radiation is an etiologic factor in BCC with a long latency period [19]. Davis et al. [19] stated that the latency period of skin cancer varies inversely with the dose of radiation. As with carcinomas caused by UVL, damage to DNA probably plays a critical role [20, 21]. Chemical factors associated with the development of BCC may include arsenic [22].

Immunosurveillance plays an unclear role in the pathogenesis of skin cancer. Marked increases in the incidence of squamous cell carcinoma (SCC) but only a slight variation in BCC development [23–25] are noted in immunosuppressed patients with lymphoma or leukemia and patients who have undergone transplantations. A potential link between UVL and immunosurveillance has been suggested by Gitierrez-Steil et al. [26], who demonstrated that UVL-induced BCC tumor cells express the Fas ligand (CD95L). These authors further showed that these cells were associated with CD95-bearing T cells undergoing apoptosis. In patients with depressed cellular immunity secondary to human immunodeficiency virus (HIV) infection, a higher frequency of more aggressive, infiltrative BCC has been demonstrated [27].

Inherited conditions associated with BCC include the basal cell nevus syndrome [28]. Alterations of the patched gene have been implicated in the basal cell nevus syndrome, which presents with frontal bossing, mental deficiency, odontogenic cysts, hyperkeratotic palmar pits, and numerous BCCs [29].

Biological Behavior

The behavior of BCC, including the potential to invade locally and metastasize, depends on stromal and angiogenic factors, growth characteristics, and propensity for the tumor to follow the anatomic path of least resistance. The stroma is critical for both initiating and maintaining the development of BCC. Usually, transplants of BCC devoid of stroma are unsuccessful [8]. In one study, Hernandez et al. [30] demonstrated that cultured BCC tumor cells stimulated collagenase production by fibroblasts. Many studies indicate that collagenase may contribute to the spread of BCC [31].

Tumor development also depends on a sufficient blood supply. BCC can elicit angiogenic factors, which may account also for the characteristic telangiectases. Often, large BCCs have necrotic centers, owing to an extreme radial distance from its blood supply [8, 32].

Generally, the growth rate of BCC is slow, the result of opposing forces of growth and tumor regression. The dominant phase dictates the rate at which the tumor enlarges [33]. BCCs are locally invasive and destructive. They follow the path of least resistance, a tendency that explains why invasion of bone, cartilage, and muscle is a late event. When an invasive BCC reaches these areas, it tends to migrate along the perichondrium, the periosteum, the fascia, or the tarsal plate [34–36]. This proclivity may contribute to high recurrence rates on the eyelid, nose, and scalp [34, 37–39].

Embryonic fusion planes offer little resistance and can lead to deep invasion and tumor spread, with extraordinarily high rates of recurrence after therapy. Susceptible areas include the inner canthus, the philtrum, the middle to lower chin, the nasolabial groove, the preauricular area, and the retroauricular sulcus [34–36, 40].

Usually, BCCs do not penetrate the subcutis because of an insufficient vascular supply. Perineural spread is uncommon and usually is seen with recurrent, aggressive lesions [41]. In one series, Niazi and Lamberty [42] noted perineural invasion in 0.178% of BCC cases. In all cases, perineural extension was associated with recurrent tumors that most often were located at the periauricular and malar areas. Perineural invasion may manifest with paresthesia, pain, weakness, or paralysis.

Metastatic BCC is rare, with incidence rates varying from 0.0028% to 0.1%, and rarely is noted in nonimmunosuppressed patients [8, 43]. Most commonly, this form of BCC occurs via lymphatic spread to regional nodes and hematogenous spread to long bones and lungs. When metastasis is present, usually the primary lesion is located on the head and neck area and has been long-standing. BCC may invade both the vasculature and the periosteum. Although the adenoid and basosquamous (metatypical) variants of BCC metastasize most often, all histologic subtypes may do so.

Clinical Manifestations

Variants of BCC include nodular, superficial, morpheaform, cystic, and basosquamous (BSCC), and fibroepithelioma of Pinkus [8–10]. Nodular (noduloulcerative) BCC is the most common type of primary lesion. Usually, it presents as a flesh-colored or pink translucent nodule with superimposed telangiectases. Ulceration may accompany growth of the tumor (Color Plate 24.1). The occasional presence of melanin accounts for the variable amount of visible pigment and may cause the lesion to appear black, resembling a melanocytic neoplasm (Color Plate 24.2) This melanin is produced by benign melanocytes and is taken up by macrophages found adjacent to nests of BCC. Over many years, these tumors can grow and invade deeply, destroying an eyelid, nose, or ear (Color Plate 24.3). The destruction may be so extensive that the ulcer's primary cause is not easily discernible. Close inspection of the ulcer's periphery, however, often reveals a pearly, telangiectatic rolled border.

Most often, the superficial multicentric variant of BCC is found on the trunk and extremities, although it may occur also in the head and neck region. Usually, the lesion is an erythematous, slightly scaly patch that typically has a rolled, translucent border. Atrophy and pigmentary alterations appear in areas in which regression has occurred. Lesions vary in size and may be single or multiple. Their appearance may resemble such benign inflammatory processes as nummular dermatitis and psoriasis. Early radial growth is responsible for the large size of these tumors; however, they also can penetrate vertically, forming nodules and ulceration. A high recurrence rate after surgical removal is caused by persistent subclinical centrifugal extension of the lesions.

The morpheaform BCC presents as an indurated sclerotic plaque of varying size, with occasional telangiectases, resembling a lesion of morphea (Color Plate 24.4). Clinically and histologically, this form also can mimic metastatic carcinoma. Morpheaform BCC infiltrates aggressively and subclinically, tending to recur after seemingly adequate treatment.

Cystic BCC is characterized by clear, blue cystic lesions containing a clear fluid that can be expressed with manipulation. When present on the face, the lesions resemble hidrocystomas. Occasionally, the cystic changes that can be seen histologically are fairly subtle clinically, thus giving the tumor the appearance of a common nodular BCC.

Basosquamous cell carcinoma (BSCC) is a histologic classification, although it is clinically more aggressive than are other BCCs. Some believe that its characteristics are more like those of SCC, with an increased incidence of metastasis and postoperative recurrences [44, 45]. The estimated incidence of metastasis for this type of BCC is 9.7% [44]. Histologic studies confirmed that BSCC shows staining patterns similar to those of both SCC and BCC. The presence of a transition zone supports the concept that BSCC represents a phenomenon of differentiation rather than of collision [46].

The fibroepithelioma of Pinkus is a rare variant of BCC usually found on the lower back. The lesion, a firm smooth nodule that is classically pedunculated, resembles a fibroma. It may represent spread of BCC via eccrine ducts [47].

Staging

The American Joint Committee on Cancer defines a TNM (*t*umor, *n*ode, *m*etastasis) staging system that applies to both BCC and SCC, with instructions for clinical and pathologic staging of the disease (Tables 24.1, 24.2)

Table 24.1 TNM Staging for Basal Cell and Squamous Cell Carcinoma of the Skin

Classification	Definition
Primary tumor (T)	
TX	Primary tumor cannot be assessed
T0	No evidence of primary tumor
Tis	Carcinoma in situ
T1	Tumor ≤ 2 cm in greatest dimension
T2	Tumor > 2 cm in greatest dimension but ≤ 5 cm in greatest dimension
T3	Tumor > 5 cm in greatest dimension
T4	Tumor invading deep extradermal structures (e.g., cartilage, skeletal muscle, or bone)
Regional lymph nodes (N)	
NX	Regional lymph nodes cannot be assessed
N0	No regional lymph node metastasis
N1	Regional lymph node metastasis
Distant metastasis (M)	
MX	Distant metastasis cannot be assessed
M0	No distant metastasis
M1	Distant metastasis
Histopathologic grade (G)	
GX	Grade cannot be assessed
G1	Well differentiated
G2	Moderately differentiated
G3	Poorly differentiated
G4	Undifferentiated

Notes: Staging excludes eyelid, vulva, and penis.
In the case of multiple simultaneous tumors, the tumor with the highest T category will be classified, and the number of separate tumors will be indicated in parentheses [e.g., T2(5)].
Source: Used with permission of the American Joint Committee on Cancer (AJCC), Chicago, Illinois. Reprinted from ID Fleming, JS Cooper, DE Henson, et al. (eds), *AJCC Cancer Staging Manual* (5th ed). Philadelphia: Lippincott-Raven, 1997:157–161.

Table 24.2 AJCC Stage Grouping for Basal Cell and Squamous Cell Carcinoma of the Skin

Stage	T	N	M
Stage 0	Tis	N0	M0
Stage I	T1	N0	M0
Stage II	T2	N0	M0
	T3	N0	M0
Stage III	T4	N0	M0
	Any T	N1	M0
Stage IV	Any T	Any N	M1

AJCC = American Joint Committee on Cancer.
Source: Used with permission of the American Joint Committee on Cancer (AJCC), Chicago, Illinois. Reprinted from ID Fleming, JS Cooper, DE Henson, et al. (eds), *AJCC Cancer Staging Manual* (5th ed). Philadelphia: Lippincott-Raven, 1997:157–61.

[48]. Clinical staging is based on physical examination of the lesion and lymph nodes. With fixed lesions, underlying bony structures should be imaged, especially if these lesions occur on the scalp. Pathologic staging requires resection of the entire site and confirmation of any lymph node involvement. For both clinical and pathologic staging, complete excision of the site and microscopical verification is necessary to determine the histologic type.

Treatment Overview

Common treatment options for BCC include destruction by electrodesiccation and curettage, cryosurgery, excision by either traditional or Mohs' technique, and

radiotherapy. Selection of the most appropriate therapy requires consideration of anatomic location, knowledge of histologic characteristics of the lesion, understanding of the potential for invasion and recurrence, and familiarity with the various treatment options. The primary goal in managing patients with BCC is complete removal of the lesion. Also important are the need for conservation of normal structure and function and for an optimal cosmetic result. Mohs' micrographic surgery provides superior cure rates while allowing for maximal conservation of normal tissue [49].

The anatomic location should be considered in selecting the appropriate treatment. Certain high-risk areas, including the inner canthus, philtrum, middle to lower chin, nasolabial groove, preauricular area, and the retroauricular sulcus, may be at increased risk for recurrence. Some anatomic structures, including the temporal branch of the facial nerve and the temporal artery, may be at increased risk for intraoperative injury.

Adequate treatment of BCC requires knowledge of the pathologic pattern of the neoplasm and of its varying modes of extension. Though some BCCs are small and superficial and behave in essentially a "biologically benign" manner as long as they are removed conservatively, others behave more aggressively and thus require more aggressive treatment. BCCs having infiltrative (morpheaform) features and those that invade deeper structures (e.g., cartilage or bone) require wider, deeper, and generally more extensive surgical extirpation.

Although BCCs enlarge slowly and seldom metastasize, their potential for aggressive local growth should not be underestimated in determining a treatment approach. The decision to perform repeated desiccation and curettage rather than surgical removal of a recurrent BCC eventually could result in extensive tissue destruction if the tumor depth is not appreciated sufficiently.

On diagnosis of BCC, optimal therapy may require

referral to an appropriately skilled expert. When multiple treatment options are suitable, clinicians should select the modality with which they have the most experience.

CURETTAGE AND ELECTRODESICCATION

Curettage and electrodesiccation is the method used most commonly by dermatologists in treating BCC [50, 51]. Less-than-optimal depth of curettage will lead to recurrence, and deeper treatment than is required to eradicate the tumor will merely contribute to poor cosmesis.

Cure rates using curettage and electrodesiccation have been reported to be as high as 95% [52], but only certain lesions are amenable to this form of therapy. Curettage and electrodesiccation should not be considered in most cases for BCC arising in areas characterized by a high rate of recurrence (e.g., eyelids, nose, lips, ears, scalp, temple, and embryonic fusion planes), because there is no confirmation of tumor destruction. Silverman et al. [53] stated that BCCs less than 6 mm in diameter, regardless of anatomic site, are treated effectively by curettage and electrodesiccation. Alternative forms of treatment should be considered for lesions greater than 1 cm in diameter, because curettage and electrodesiccation fail to remove tumor completely in the majority of primary BCCs greater than 1 cm and in recurrent BCC [34, 52].

Potential complications include hypertrophic scar, pigmentary alterations, and local recurrence. Some dermatologists have omitted electrodesiccation to optimize the cosmetic result and have achieved cure rates only slightly lower than those achieved by the combination of curettage and electrodesiccation [53]. Although the omission decreases the incidence of hypertrophic scarring, it does not prevent postinflammatory pigmentary alterations.

EXCISION

Surgical excision provides a specimen that can be histologically evaluated. If performed skillfully, excision can provide adequate cosmesis. Theoretically, excision is appropriate for most BCC, but it requires more time and experience than is involved in electrodesiccation and curettage. Normal tissue is sacrificed with traditional excisional surgery. The cure rates are inferior to those for Mohs' surgery in the treatment of recurrent BCC, morpheaform BCC, some large superficial multicentric BCCs, and BCC in high-risk areas [54–57]. Wolf and Zitelli [58] have shown that for nonmorpheaform BCC with a distinct border and a diameter of less than 2 cm, 4-mm clear margins were necessary to eliminate 98% of the lesions. These authors reported that the subclinical extension of the neoplasms was not uniform in all directions; in BCCs greater than 2 cm in diameter, subclinical spread was so irregular that the investigators could not offer advice regarding an appropriate margin.

The question as to the proper depth of the excision remains unanswered. For small primary BCCs, excision into fat generally is appropriate, because spread into the subcutis is rare. However, large recurrent or high-risk BCCs may infiltrate deeper into the subcutaneous tissue. Potential complications of traditional excisional surgery include postoperative infection, bleeding, and recurrence.

MOHS' MICROGRAPHIC SURGERY

Mohs' micrographic surgery permits superior histologic verification of complete removal, allows maximum conservation of tissue, and remains cost-effective as compared to traditional excisional surgery for nonmelanoma skin cancers [39, 59, 60]. It is the preferred treatment for large penetrating tumors; for morpheaform and recurrent, poorly delineated, high-risk, and incompletely removed BCC; and for those sites in which tissue conservation is imperative [59]. With the Mohs' technique, the tumor is removed in stages and is fully evaluated histologically, thus allowing maximal tissue conservation with superior margin control. Mohs' surgery is more time-consuming than is routine surgery and is not always as easily accessible. As this technique may be applied to the most aggressive BCC, other surgical specialists may be consulted for removal of a deeply invasive tumor or for repair of the resulting surgical defect [61]. Potential complications include postoperative infection and bleeding, as with any excisional surgery. High cure rates for high-risk and recurrent tumors are obtainable; one study showed an overall five-year cure rate of more than 96% [62].

RADIOTHERAPY

Radiotherapy is helpful in the treatment of some BCCs. Its major advantage is that normal tissue is spared, obviating the need for complicated surgical procedures. Often, it is preferred for BCC of the nose, ear, and periocular area, as reconstructive surgery is not required and functional integrity is not compromised [63]. Radiotherapy has been used also for palliation in inoperable BCC. However, it should not be used in young patients because of potential late irradiation sequelae.

Although one dose of radiation can treat a small BCC (< 1 cm) adequately, usually appropriate treatment consists of fractionated doses administered over several sessions to maximize cure and cosmesis. The skin of the head and neck endures the effects of radiotherapy better than does that of the trunk and extremities. The five-year cure rate for primary BCC treated with irradiation is 90% to 95%. Cure rates for recurrent BCC are poorer than those for primary lesions, an outcome probably owing to the subclinical spread of the neoplasm.

Potential complications of radiotherapy include scarring, cutaneous necrosis, and chronic irradiation dermatitis. Though surgical scars improve with time, cosmesis deteriorates after radiotherapy. At 9 to 12 years, only 50% of patients maintain satisfactory cosmetic results.

CRYOSURGERY

Cryosurgery may be used to treat BCC. A liquid nitrogen spray unit is required; cotton-tipped swabs in liquid nitrogen are not acceptable. A double freeze-thaw cycle to a tissue temperature of –50°C is required to destroy the tumor sufficiently. A margin of normal-appearing skin also should be frozen to ensure eradication of subclinical disease [64, 65].

Cryosurgery is recommended for BCC of the eyelid because the procedure preserves normal tissue and obviates the need for reconstructive surgery. In fractional cryosurgery, treatment is performed in stages until tumor size is reduced to less than 1 cm, at which point the final stage is performed. The advantage of this variation is that the final scar corresponds to the size of the final stage rather than to the size of the original tumor. In this anatomic area, cure rates as high as 97% have been reported for BCC less than 1 cm in diameter; the cure rate decreases with larger and recurrent lesions. Cure rates for cryosurgery of BCC in other areas are excellent (97–98%) for tumors less than 2 cm in diameter. Larger tumors and morpheaform, recurrent, and high-risk BCCs are more likely to recur after therapy.

Cryosurgery is not advised for BCC of the scalp. Lesions on the lower legs treated with cryosurgery heal slowly and often yield poor cosmetic results. Patients with blood dyscrasias, dysglobulinemia, cold intolerance, or autoimmune disease and those who are receiving immunosuppressive therapy may not be candidates for cryosurgery.

Potential complications include hypertrophic scarring and postinflammatory pigmentary changes. The occurrence of pain early during the thaw can be avoided by preoperative infiltration of the treatment area with a local anesthetic. Blistering, crusting, and swelling also can develop, but usually these effects resolve within a few weeks.

LASERS

The CO_2 laser has been used in the treatment of BCC and offers several advantages over conventional surgery. The sealing of small blood vessels and nerves provides a relatively bloodless surgical field and reduced postoperative pain. In a recent study, Humphreys et al. [66] reported ablation of primary superficial BCC with the high-energy pulsed CO_2 laser.

INTERFERON

Interferon has been used as an alternative therapy for noduloulcerative and superficial BCC. A study of 172 patients receiving intralesional injections of interferon-α_{2b} resulted in an 81% cure rate after a follow-up period of 1 year [67]. Single doses of 1.5 million IU were administered three times per week for 3 weeks, resulting in a total dose of 13.5 million IU. Attempts using lower doses were unsuccessful. Side effects from this therapy include fever, malaise, myalgias, chills, transient leukopenia, and injection site reactions.

RETINOIDS

Experience with the use of retinoids is limited; the process is used most often in patients with the basal cell nevus syndrome [68]. Partial regression of BCC has resulted from the use of 4.5 mg/kg/day of isotretinoin and 1 mg/kg/day of etretinate. Potential side effects limit the use of these agents for prolonged periods, and discontinuation of therapy can lead to relapse.

CHEMOTHERAPY

Chemotherapy is appropriate for locally aggressive or metastatic tumors. Otherwise, disseminated disease is associated with a poor prognosis, with an average survival of 10 to 20 months [45]. A complete systemic workup is required in evaluating affected patients for metastasis. Included are a thorough medical history, physical examination, complete blood counts, liver profile, chest roentgenography, bone and liver scans, and computed tomographic scans, when appropriate. Platinum-based cytotoxic therapy may be indicated when local therapy is inadequate or in cases of metastatic disease. Moeholt et al. [69] reviewed 53 cases of advanced BCC treated with platinum-based chemotherapy and showed an overall response rate of 83%, with complete remission observed in 37% of cases.

OTHER THERAPEUTIC MODALITIES

Other options for treating BCC include photodynamic therapy, intralesional 5-fluorouracil–epinephrine injectable gel, and electrochemotherapy with bleomycin [70–72].

Follow-Up

Regularly examining patients with BCC is imperative. Although most recurrences appear within 5 years, many can develop later. Subsequent new primary BCCs also can appear; 20% to 30% develop within 1 year of treatment of the original lesion [73]. Equally important is advising patients to avoid excessive sun exposure and to apply at regular intervals a sunscreen with a sun-protective factor of 15 whenever they are exposed to direct or reflected sunlight.

SQUAMOUS CELL CARCINOMA
Definition

SCC is a neoplasm of keratinizing cells that shows malignant characteristics including anaplasia, rapid growth, local invasion, and metastatic potential. If left untreated, SCC may metastasize to regional lymph nodes and distant sites.

Epidemiologic Characteristics

Nearly 200,000 cases of SCC are diagnosed in the United States each year, rendering it the second most common human cancer. The risk of occurrence increases with age and affected men tend to outnumber affected women [74]. In a large retrospective study, the mean ages at diagnosis of SCC were 68.1 and 72.7 years for men and women, respectively [75].

Many studies suggest that SCC depends on the total accumulated dose of solar irradiation (Color Plate 24.5) [76–79]. The relative risk of SCC for individuals with a history of excessive sun exposure is increased three to five and one-half times. Clearly, skin pigmentation protects against the induction of skin cancer. People of Celtic descent, with fair complexions, poor tanning abil-

ity, and a predisposition to sunburn, are at increased risk for developing SCC.

Some have suggested that psoriasis patients treated with oral psoralens and ultraviolet A (UVA) irradiation are at increased risk for development of SCC [76, 77]. The lamps in most commercial tanning booths emit light that is primarily in the UVA spectrum [78]. In a study by Van Weelden et al. [79], UVA was shown to be carcinogenic in mice. Whether the incidence of SCC in tanning booth patrons will increase remains to be seen. Another risk factor for development of SCC is exposure to arsenic [80].

Pathogenesis

The factors that initiate or promote the development of SCC are similar to those involved in BCC. They include exposure to ultraviolet radiation or chemicals, mutations in tumor suppressor genes, and alterations in immune response. In addition, chronic inflammation, viral transformation, and defective DNA repair are risk factors.

The evidence for an association with sunlight (i.e., UVL) is even stronger for SCC than for BCC. Actinic damage leads to actinic keratoses, which may undergo malignant transformation to invasive SCC [81]. The rate at which solar keratoses undergo invasive progression has been estimated to be as high as 20%. However, the risk of progression of a single actinic keratosis is likely to be much less [81].

The *p53* gene product acts as a tumor suppressor, and mutations in *p53* are associated with SCC. Recent studies have demonstrated that UVL may introduce mutations into tumor suppressor gene *p53*. Thus, UVL may be acting as both tumor initiator and tumor promoter [82].

Immunosuppression also may play a role in pathogenesis. Patients receiving immunosuppressive therapy and renal, cardiac, and bone marrow transplant recipients are prone to SCC [18, 19]. Skin cancers in such patients appear primarily on sun-exposed skin. This correlation suggests that immunosuppression and UVL act as cofactors in the development of SCC. HIV-infected patients tend to experience higher rates of SCC [83–88]. However, the exact correlation between HIV and the incidence of SCC has not yet been determined. UVL may be involved with immunosuppression. Exposure to UVB appears to interfere with the density and antigen-processing capability of Langerhans cells and may suppress production of T-helper 1 (Th1) cytokines interleukin-2 and interferon-γ through a mechanism involving the Th2 cytokine interleukin-4 [87]. It may be that UVB exposure contributes to a state of immune tolerance with regard to tumors, through alteration of these and other cellular and cytokine networks.

SCC has a tendency to develop in areas of chronic inflammation. It has been reported in lesions of discoid lupus erythematosus, chronic osteomyelitis, acne conglobata, lupus vulgaris, hidradenitis suppurativa, pilonidal sinus, thermal burns, and leg ulcers [88, 89].

The potential role of human papillomavirus (HPV) in the development of SCC has been studied. Eliezri et al. [90] demonstrated a correlation between the venereal spread of HPV-16 and the initiation of SCC. Epidermodysplasia verruciformis is a rare inherited disorder characterized by infection with multiple HPV types and development of SCC. It has been associated with HPV types 5 and 8 and, most recently, with types 20, 23, 38, DL40, and DL267 [91].

Xeroderma pigmentosum is a rare genetic disorder characterized by defective DNA excision repair and increased susceptibility to skin cancer [92]. Patients with xeroderma pigmentosum are unable to repair damage induced by UVL and show markedly increased incidence of both nonmelanoma skin cancer and melanoma.

Biological Behavior

The metastatic potential of SCC depends on a number of variables, including depth and degree of differentiation, presence of chronic inflammation at the site of the primary tumor, the anatomic location, and the presence of perineural invasion. SCC restricted to the epidermis is called *SCC in situ*, whereas invasive SCC is defined by dermal penetration. SCC in situ may arise also in association with preexisting actinic or arsenical keratosis. These lesions may be considered "biologically benign," without competence for metastasis if removed completely or otherwise destroyed.

Invasive SCCs that penetrate to the reticular dermis and subcutis tend to recur [93]. Immerman et al. [94] observed a 20% incidence of recurrence in 86 patients with invasive SCC. Patients with moderately or poorly differentiated neoplasms had a greater degree of recurrence. Invasive SCC can metastasize. The most common type arises on sun-damaged skin, often associated with actinic keratosis and solar elastosis. The incidence of metastasis of such lesions is low (3–5%). A higher incidence (10–30%) is associated with SCC arising on mucosal surfaces (lip, genitalia) and on sites of prior injury (scars, chronic ulcers) [95–97].

Approximately 10% to 40% of SCC cases develop at sites of preexisting inflammatory conditions. Tumors arising in areas of chronic inflammation are prone to metastasis. SCCs developing at burn scar sites reportedly have a metastatic rate of 18%, those developing in conjunction with chronic osteomyelitis a rate of 31%, and those arising in discoid lupus erythematosus a 30% metastatic rate [88, 98]. Although tumors are more likely to disseminate to regional lymph nodes than to organs, intravascular metastases to viscera have appeared in as many as 5% to 10% of all metastatic cases [89].

The incidence of metastasis from SCC arising in noninflamed, actinically damaged skin varies from 0.05% to 16.0% [98]. Although actinically induced tumors behave in a more biologically benign fashion than de novo SCC, all lesions have the potential to become invasive locally and to metastasize to draining lymph nodes.

Friedman et al. [99] demonstrated that all trunk and extremity primary SCCs that later developed local or nodal recurrence were at least 4 mm deep and penetrated into the reticular dermis or subcutis. Every fatal lesion was at least 10 mm deep and invaded the subcutis.

SCCs arising in nonglabrous mucocutaneous sites (lip, vulva, penis, perianal area) are more likely to metastasize than are those involving glabrous areas of the skin. The incidence of metastasis for SCC varies from 0.5% for patients with primary cutaneous SCC to 11% for patients with mucocutaneous labial lesions.

Distant metastases may occur also with perineural involvement. In one study [100], 14% of SCCs showed perineural spread, whereas rates as high as 36% have been found by other investigators [101]. Regional lymph node metastases and distant metastases were increased in patients with perineural involvement. SCC of the head and neck may metastasize to cervical lymph nodes and distantly to the central nervous system, the latter either hematogenously or via the perineural space, which directly connects to the subarachnoid space. High-risk areas include the midface, lip, and areas involving the mandibular branch of the trigeminal nerve. Although patients thus afflicted generally are asymptomatic, they show a lower 10-year survival (23% versus 88%) and a higher local recurrence rate (47% versus 7.3%) than do those without neural involvement. Despite poor prognosis, Mohs' micrographic surgery occasionally can achieve successful treatment in such patients [102].

Clinical Manifestations

SCC includes SCC in situ, invasive SCC, and verrucous carcinoma. SCC in situ may occur in a preexisting thermal, hydrocarbon, or arsenical keratosis. Invasive SCC is characterized by the potential to metastasize. Verrucous carcinoma is a low-grade lesion, and differentiating it from the common wart may be difficult.

Morphologic variants of SCC in situ include Bowen's disease, bowenoid papulosis, and erythroplasia of Queyrat. Usually, an intraepidermal carcinoma or a premalignant lesion precedes invasive SCC clinically. Most lesions consist of patches or plaques that may be covered with scale, crust, or ulceration (Color Plate 24.6). Usually, the lesions lack the pearly rolled border and superficial telangiectases found in BCC. Although most are red, hyperkeratotic SCCs or those that occur on mucocutaneous surfaces may be white. The clinical differential diagnosis includes other tumors (BCC, keratoacanthoma, adnexal neoplasm); precancerous lesions (actinic keratosis, Bowen's disease); and inflammatory disorders (psoriasis, eczema).

SCC may appear anywhere on the body. Though SCC on the trunk usually does not present a therapeutic challenge, SCC occurring on the nose, lip, nail bed, or penis may be troublesome. Small SCCs appearing on the trunk and extremities are treated easily, although advanced lesions may be aggressive. Factors associated with a poor prognosis included a low degree of histologic differentiation, location on the sacrum or perineum, and degree of lymphatic metastasis. SCC of the trunk and extremities may spread to the axillary and inguinal lymph nodes, whereas hand and foot tumors may metastasize to epitrochlear and popliteal nodes, respectively.

SCC of the nose was studied by Binder et al. [103], who found that 21 of 114 patients had involvement of underlying cartilage and bone. In 77% of these 21 individuals, lesions were more than 3 cm in diameter, and symptoms had been present for more than one year. The incidence of nodal metastasis in this study was 8%. In every patient who developed metastases, the cervical lymph nodes were involved (ipsilateral in six cases, bilateral in two, and contralateral in one), as was cartilage or bone, and all experienced symptoms for at least one year. Most had a primary lesion greater than 3 cm in diameter. Only one patient developed distant metastases.

The majority of SCCs on the lip arise from the lower lip in an area of chronic actinic cheilitis. The reported risk of metastasis from SCC of the lip has ranged from 5% to 37% [102].

SCC can occur also on the nail bed, nail folds, and matrix (Color Plate 24.7) [104]. If the nail matrix is affected, atrophy or loss of the nail plate can result. The differential diagnosis of these lesions includes paronychia, pyogenic granuloma, verrucae, nail dystrophies, and such tumors as glomus, keratoacanthoma, and melanoma.

SCC of the penis is rare in the Western hemisphere [105]. On the penis, it may develop within lesions of leukoplakia, erythroplasia of Queyrat, and balanitis xerotica obliterans. Verrucous carcinoma of the penis (Buschke-Lowenstein tumor) is histologically well differentiated, with features of a wart. However, it behaves clinically like an aggressive SCC; it may undergo malignant transformation and may metastasize [105–107].

Usually, penile SCC occurs between the ages of 40 and 60. It may present with a penile nodule, ulceration, discharge, edema, or inguinal adenopathy. The most common site of involvement is the glans. However, it can develop anywhere along the shaft. Metastasis to inguinal lymph nodes has been reported in 33% to 50% and is associated with poor prognosis [107].

Verrucous carcinoma, a subtype of low-grade SCC, can affect the cutaneous and mucosal surfaces [108]. Most often, this lesion occurs in middle-aged and elderly men. It is characterized by a warty exophytic neoplasm containing sinuses, with a greasy, malodorous discharge.

Staging

As previously noted, the American Joint Committee on Cancer includes a TNM staging system that applies to both SCC and BCC (see Table 24.1) [48]. Clinical staging is based on size of the primary lesion and on examination of lymph nodes. Pathologic staging requires resection and confirmation of lymph node involvement.

Treatment Overview

Many of the treatments for BCC are appropriate for SCC. The type of therapy should be selected on the basis of size of the lesion, anatomic location, depth of invasion, degree of cellular differentiation, and history of previous treatment. Essentially, treatment of SCC can follow any of three approaches: (1) destruction by curettage and electrodesiccation or cryosurgery; (2) removal by traditional excisional surgery or by Mohs' micrographic surgery; and (3) radiotherapy. Curettage and electrodesiccation can be used for small lesions arising in sun-damaged skin. Excisional surgery is indicated for larger, ill-defined lesions and for more extensive lesions that have invaded deeper structures. Rarely, regional lymph node dissection may be required in SCCs that have metastasized there. Radiotherapy is indicated for head and neck SCC in the absence of spread to bone or cartilage and of evidence of metastasis.

CURETTAGE AND ELECTRODESICCATION

SCCs greater than 2 cm in diameter are amenable to this form of therapy. Honeycutt and Jansen [109] reported a 99% cure rate for 281 SCCs after a four-year follow-up. Two recurrences were noted in lesions larger than 2 cm in diameter. Others have reported five-year cure rates of greater than 95% [110].

EXCISION

Surgical excision is another well-accepted treatment modality. Lesions larger than 3 cm in diameter on the scalp, forehead, and distal extremities are best treated by excision because of the poor healing qualities of the thin layers of subcutaneous tissue overlying bone. Usually, carcinomas of the eyelid and lip commissures are excised, because function and cosmesis can be better preserved. Carcinomas of the penis, vulva, and anus usually are treated by excision because of the frequent need for lymph node dissection and because of poor tolerance of these areas to irradiation. Surgical excision is the treatment of choice for verrucous carcinoma [111].

MOHS' MICROGRAPHIC SURGERY

Mohs' surgery is useful for SCCs that fall into one of the following groups: (1) recurrent SCC; (2) clinically ill-defined SCC; (3) SCC invading bone or cartilage; (4) carcinoma arising in late irradiation dermatitis; and (5) other SCC arising in areas at high risk for recurrence. This modality allows conservation of the maximum amount of tissue with preservation of function and enhanced cosmesis and is superior with regard to local recurrence [112].

RADIOTHERAPY

As with BCC, radiotherapy is excellent for elderly patients who have SCC and are unwilling to undergo surgery. It is especially suitable for lesions of the nose, lip, eyelid, and canthal region. Radiotherapy in a fractionated dose schedule is associated with a better cosmetic result and probably an enhanced therapeutic effect. The use of radiotherapy for verrucous carcinoma has been controversial because of the potential for anaplastic transformation or a high rate of metastasis (or both) [113].

CRYOTHERAPY

Cryotherapy for SCC is useful in selected patients. Lesions having a diameter between 0.5 and 2.0 cm and well-defined borders are amenable to this modality. This technique boasts exceptional cosmetic results and has achieved five-year cure rates as high as 96.1% [114].

OTHER THERAPEUTIC MODALITIES

Other treatment options have included the neodymium–yttrium aluminum garnet laser, photodynamic therapy, retinoids, 5-fluorouracil given either topically or systemically, and a combination of cisplatin and 5-fluorouracil [115–117]. Humphreys et al. [66] found that high-energy pulsed CO_2 was not sufficient to treat superficial SCC.

Follow-Up

Invasive SCC can be a potentially lethal neoplasm and warrants close follow-up with yearly total-body skin examinations. In one study, approximately 30% of patients with SCC developed a subsequent SCC; 54% of these recurrences were seen within the first year of follow-up [118]. The association between solar irradiation and the development of SCC is established firmly. Thus, an important step in follow-up is to advise patients to avoid excessive sun exposure and to apply sun block with a sun-protective factor of higher than 15.

REFERENCES

1. Greenlee RT, Murray T, Bolden S, Wingo PA. Cancer statistics, 2000. *CA Cancer J Clin* 50:7–33, 2000.
2. Rigel DS, Friedman RJ, Kopf AW. Lifetime risk for development of skin cancer in the U.S. population: current estimate now 1 in 5 (editorial). *J Am Acad Dermatol* 35:1012–1013, 1996.
3. Levi F, La Vecchia C, Te VC, et al. Incidence of invasive cancers following basal cell skin cancer. *Am J Epidemiol* 147:722–726, 1998.
4. Levi F, Randimbison L, La Vecchia C, et al. Incidence of invasive cancers following squamous cell skin cancer. *Am J Epidemiol* 146:734–739, 1997.
5. Cummings SR, Tripp MK, Herman NB. Approaches to

the prevention and control of skin cancer. *Cancer Metastasis Rev* 16:309–327, 1997.

6. Wolfe JT. The role of screening in the management of skin cancer. *J Cutan Med Surg* 3:230–235, 1999.

7. Gooderham MJ, Guenther L. Sun and the skin: evaluation of a sun awareness program for elementary school students. *J Cutan Med Surg* 3:230–235, 1999.

8. Miller SJ. Biology of basal cell carcinoma. *J Am Acad Dermatol* 24:1–13, 161–175, 1991.

9. Goldberg LH. Basal cell carcinoma. *Lancet* 347:663–667, 1996.

10. Lear JT, Smith AG. Basal cell carcinoma. *Postgrad Med J* 73:538–542, 1997.

11. Jankowski J, Cader AB. The effect of depletion of the earth ozone layer on the human health condition. *Int J Occup Med Environ Health* 10:349–364, 1997.

12. Martens WJ. Health impacts of climate change and ozone depletion: an ecoepidemiologic modeling approach. *Environ Health Perspect* 106(suppl 1):241–251, 1998.

13. Marks R, Jolley D, Dorevitch AP, Selwood TS. The incidence of non-melanocytic skin cancers in an Australian population: results of a five-year prospective study. *Med J Aust* 150:475–478, 1989.

14. Kricker A, Armstrong BK, English DR, Heenan PJ. Pigmentary and cutaneous risk factors for non-melanocytic skin cancer: a case-control study. *Int J Cancer* 48:650–662, 1991.

15. Thissen MRTM, Neumann MHA, Schouten LJ. A systemic review of treatment modalities for primary basal cell carcinomas. *Arch Dermatol* 135:1177–1183, 1999.

16. Barrett TL, Smith KJ, Hodge JJ, et al. Immunohistochemical nuclear staining for p53, PCNA, and Ki-67 in different histologic variants of basal cell carcinoma. *J Am Acad Dermatol* 37:430–437, 1997.

17. Ananthaswamy HN, Loughlin SM, Ullrich SE, Kripke ML. Inhibition of UV-induced p53 mutations by sunscreens: implications for skin cancer prevention. *J Invest Dermatol Symp Proc* 3:52–56, 1998.

18. Gailani MR, Bale AE. Developmental genes and cancer: role of patched gene in basal cell carcinoma of the skin. *J Natl Cancer Inst* 89:1103–1109, 1998.

19. Davis MM, Hanke W, Zollinger TW, et al. Skin cancer in patients with chronic radiation dermatitis. *J Am Acad Dermatol* 20:608–616, 1989.

20. Cadet J, Berger M, Douki T, et al. Effects of UV and visible radiation on DNA-final base damage. *Biol Chem* 378:1275–1286, 1997.

21. Garssen J, Vandebriel RJ, van Loveren H. Molecular aspects of UVB-induced immunosuppression. *Arch Toxicol Suppl* 19:97–109, 1997.

22. Hsu CH, Yang SA, Wang JY, et al. Mutational spectrum of p53 gene in arsenic related skin cancers from the blackfoot disease endemic area of Taiwan. *Br J Cancer* 80:1080–1086, 1999.

23. Ramsay HM, Fryer A, Strange SC, Smith AG. Multiple basal cell carcinomas in a patient with acute myeloid leukemia and chronic lymphocytic leukemia. *Clin Exp Dermatol* 24:281–282, 1999.

24. DiGiovanna JJ. Posttransplantation skin cancer: scope of the problem, management, and role for systemic retinoid chemoprevention. *Transplant Proc* 30:2771–2778, 1998.

25. Dreno B, Mansat E, Legoux B, Litoux P. Skin cancers in transplant patients. *Nephrol Dial Transplant* 13:1374–1379, 1998.

26. Gutierrez-Steil C, Wrone-Smith T, Sun X, et al. Sunlight-induced basal cell carcinoma tumor cells and ultraviolet-B-irradiated psoriatic plaques express Fas ligand (CD95L). *J Clin Invest* 101:33–39, 1998.

27. Oram Y, Orengo I, Griego RD, et al. Histologic patterns of basal cell carcinoma based upon patient immunostatus. *Dermatol Surg* 21:611–614, 1995.

28. Hall J, Johnson KA, McPhillips JP, et al. Nevoid basal cell carcinoma syndrome in a black child. *J Am Acad Dermatol* 38:363–365, 1998.

29. Negano T, Bito T, Kallassy M, et al. Over expression of the human homologue of *Drosophila* patch (PTCH) in skin tumors: specificity for basal cell carcinoma. *Br J Dermatol* 140:287–290, 1999.

30. Hernandez AD, Hibbs MS, Postlethwaite AE. Establishment of basal cell carcinoma in culture: evidence for a basal cell carcinoma derived factor(s) which stimulates fibroblasts to proliferate and release collagenase. *J Invest Dermatol* 85:470–475, 1985.

31. Barsky SH, Grossman DA, Bhuta S. Desmoplastic basal cell carcinomas possess unique basement membrane–degrading properties. *J Invest Dermatol* 88:324–329, 1987.

32. Arbiser JL. Angiogenesis and the skin: a primer. *J Am Acad Dermatol* 34:486–497, 1996.

33. Franchimont C, Pierard GE, van Cauwenberge D, et al. Episodic progression and regression of basal cell carcinomas. *Br J Dermatol* 106:305–310, 1982.

34. Mora RG, Robins P. Basal cell carcinoma in the center of the face: special diagnostic, prognostic, and therapeutic considerations. *J Dermatol Surg Oncol* 4:315–321, 1978.

35. Bailin PL, Levine HL, Wood BF, Tucker HM. Cutaneous carcinoma of the auricular and periauricular region. *Arch Otolaryngol Head Neck Surg* 106:692–696, 1980.

36. Levine HL, Bailin PL. Basal cell carcinoma of the head and neck: identification of the high risk patient. *Laryngoscope* 90:955–961, 1980.

37. Binstock JH, Stegman SJ, Tromovitch TA. Large, aggressive basal cell carcinomas of the scalp. *J Dermatol Surg Oncol* 7:565–569, 1981.

38. Roenigk RK, Ratz JL, Bailin PL, Wheeland RG. Trends in the presentation and treatment of basal cell carcinomas. *J Dermatol Surg Oncol* 12:860–886, 1986.

39. Rosen HM. Periorbital basal cell carcinomas requiring ablative craniofacial surgery. *Arch Dermatol* 123:376–378, 1987.

40. Gullane PJ. Extensive facial malignancies: concepts and management. *J Otolaryngol* 15:44–48, 1986.

41. Terashi H, Kurata S, Tadokoro T, et al. Perineural and neural involvement in skin cancers. *Dermatol Surg* 23:259–265, 1997.

42. Niazi ZB, Lamberty BG. Perineural infiltration in basal cell carcinoma. *Br J Plast Surg* 46:156–157, 1993.

43. Christian MM, Murphy CM, Wagner RF Jr. Metastatic basal cell carcinoma presenting as unilateral lymphedema. *Dermatol Surg* 24:1151–1153, 1998.

44. Borel DM. Cutaneous basosquamous carcinoma: review of the literature and report of 35 cases. *Arch Pathol* 95:293–297, 1973.

45. Farmer ER, Helwig EB. Metastatic basal cell carcinoma: a clinicopathologic study of 17 cases. *Cancer* 46:748–757, 1980.

46. Jones MS, Helm, KF, Maloney ME. The immunohistochemical characteristics of the basosquamous cell carcinoma. *Dermatol Surg* 23:181–184, 1997.

47. Stern JB, Haupt HM, Smith RR. Fibroepithelioma of Pinkus. Eccrine duct spread of basal cell carcinoma. *Am J Dermatopathol* 16:585–587, 1994.

48. Fleming ID, Cooper JS, Henson DE, et al. (eds). *AJCC Cancer Staging Manual* (5th ed). Philadelphia: Lippincott-Raven, 1997.

49. Shriner DL, McCoy DK, Goldberg, DJ, Wagner RF. Mohs' micrographic surgery. *J Am Acad Dermatol* 39:79–97, 1998.

50. Spencer JM, Tannenbaum A, Sloan L, Amonette RA. Does inflammation contribute to the eradication of basal cell carcinoma following curettage and electrodesiccation? *Dermatol Surg* 23:625–630, 1997.

51. Jensen P. Use of curettage in the treatment of skin tumors. *Tidsskr Nor Laegeforen* 117:3245–3246, 1997.

52. Salasche SJ. Status of curettage and desiccation in the treatment of primary basal cell carcinoma. *J Am Acad Dermatol* 10:285–287, 1984.

53. Silverman MK, Kopf AW, Grin CM, et al. Recurrence rates of treated basal cell carcinomas: II. Curettage and electrodesiccation. *J Dermatol Surg Oncol* 17:720–726, 1991.

54. Rowe DE, Carroll RJ, Day CL. Mohs' surgery is the treatment of choice for recurrent (previously treated) basal cell carcinoma. *J Dermatol Surg Oncol* 15:424–431, 1989.

55. Salasche SJ, Amonette RA. Morpheaform basal cell epitheliomas: a study of subclinical extensions in a series of 51 cases. *J Dermatol Surg Oncol* 7:387–394, 1981.

56. Sloane JP. The value of typing basal cell carcinomas in predicting recurrence after surgical excision. *Br J Dermatol* 96:127–132, 1977.

57. Dublin N, Kopf AW. Multivariate risk score for recurrence of cutaneous basal cell carcinomas. *Arch Dermatol* 119:373–377, 1983.

58. Wolf JE, Zitelli JA. Surgical margins for basal cell carcinoma. *Arch Dermatol* 123:340–344, 1987.

59. Nelson BR, Railan D, Cohen S. Mohs' micrographic surgery for nonmelanoma skin cancers. *Clin Plast Surg* 24:705–718, 1997.

60. Cook J, Zitelli JA. Mohs' micrographic surgery: a cost analysis. *J Am Acad Dermatol* 39:698–703, 1998.

61. Baker SR, Swanson NA, Grekin RC. An interdisciplinary approach to the management of basal cell carcinomas of the head and neck. *J Dermatol Surg Oncol* 13:1095–1106, 1987.

62. Julian CG, Bowers PW. A prospective study of Mohs' micrographic surgery in 2 English centers. *Br J Dermatol* 136:515–518, 1997.

63. Halpern JN. Radiation therapy in skin cancer. A historical perspective and current applications. *Dermatol Surg* 23:975–978, 1997.

64. Zacarian SA. *Cryosurgery for Skin Cancer and Cutaneous Disorders.* St Louis: Mosby, 1985.

65. Goncalves JC. Fractional cryosurgery. A new technique for basal cell carcinoma of the eyelids and periorbital area. *Dermatol Surg* 23:475–481, 1997.

66. Humphreys TR, Malhorta R, Scharf MJ, et al. Treatment of superficial basal cell carcinoma and squamous cell carcinoma in situ with a high-energy pulsed carbon dioxide laser. *Arch Dermatol* 134:1247–1252, 1998.

67. Cornell RC, Greenway HT, Tucker SB, et al. Intralesional interferon therapy for basal cell carcinoma. *J Am Acad Dermatol* 23:694–700, 1990.

68. Levine N. Role of retinoids in skin cancer treatment and prevention. *J Am Acad Dermatol* 39:S62–S66, 1998.

69. Moeholt K, Aagaard H, Pfeiffer P, Hansen O. Platinum based cytotoxic therapy in basal cell carcinoma—a review of the literature. *Acta Oncol* 35:677–682, 1996.

70. Bissonette R, Lui H. Current status of photodynamic therapy in dermatology. *Dermatol Clin* 15:507–519, 1997.

71. Nonsurgical treatment of basal cell carcinomas with intralesional 5-fluorouracil/epinephrine injectable gel. *J Am Acad Dermatol* 36:72–77, 1997.

72. Glass LF, Jaroszeski M, Gilbert R, et al. Intralesional bleomycin-mediated electrochemotherapy in 20 patients with basal cell carcinoma. *J Am Acad Dermatol* 37:596–599, 1997.

73. Robinson JK. Risk of developing another basal cell carcinoma: a 5-year prospective study. *Cancer* 60:118–120, 1987.

74. Levi F, LaVechia CL, Te VC, Mezzanote G. Descriptive epidemiology of skin cancer in the Swiss canton of Vaud. *Int J Cancer* 42:811–816, 1988.

75. Aubry F, MacGibbon B. Risk factors of squamous cell carcinoma of the skin. *Cancer* 55:907–911, 1985.

76. Lear JT, Tan BB, Smith AG, et al. A comparison of risk factors for malignant melanoma, squamous cell carcinoma, and basal cell carcinoma in the UK. *Int J Clin Pract* 52:145–149, 1998.

77. Stern RS, Lunder EJ. Risk of squamous cell carcinoma and methoxsalen (psoralens) and UV-A radiation (PUVA). A meta-analysis. *Arch Dermatol* 134:1582–1585, 1998.

78. Rivers JK, Norris PG, Murphy GM, et al. UVA sunbeds: tanning, photoprotection, immunological changes and acute adverse effects. *Br J Dermatol* 120:767–777, 1989.

79. Van Weelden H, Van der Putte SC, Toonstra J, Van der Leun JC. UVA-induced tumors in pigmented hairless mice and the carcinogenic risks of tanning with UVA. *Arch Dermatol* 282:289–294, 1990.

80. Col M, Col C, Soran A, et al. Arsenic related Bowen's disease, palmar keratosis and skin cancer. *Environ Health Perspect* 107:687–689, 1999.

81. Schwartz RA. The actinic keratosis. A perspective and update. *Dermatol Surg* 23:1009–1019, 1997.

82. Brash DE, Ziegler A, Jonason AS, et al. Sunlight and sunburn in human skin cancer: p53, apoptosis, and tumor promotion. *J Invest Dermatol Symp Proc* 1:136–142, 1996.

83. Gmeinhart B, Hinterberger W, Greinix HT, et al. Anaplastic squamous cell carcinoma (SCC) in a patient with

chronic cutaneous graft-versus-host disease (GVHD). *Bone Marrow Transplant* 23:1197–1199, 1999.

84. Veness MJ, Quinn DI, Ong CS, et al. Aggressive cutaneous malignancies following cardiothoracic transplantation: the Australian experience. *Cancer* 85:1758–1764, 1999.

85. Jensen P, Hansen S, Moller B, et al. Skin cancer in kidney and heart transplant recipient and different long-term immunosuppressive therapy regimens. *J Am Acad Dermatol* 40:177–186, 1999.

86. Dover JS, Johnson RA. Cutaneous manifestations of human immunodeficiency virus infections. *Arch Dermatol* 127:1383–1391, 1991.

87. El-Ghorr AA, Norval M. The role of interleukin-4 in ultraviolet B light–induced immunosuppresssion. *Immunology* 92:26–32, 1997.

88. Phillips TJ, Salman SM, Bhawan J, Rogers GS. Burn scar carcinoma. Diagnosis and management. *Dermatol Surg* 24:561–565, 1998.

89. Goldman GD. Squamous cell cancer: a practical approach. *Semin Cutan Med Surg* 17:80–95, 1998.

90. Eliezri YD, Silverstein SJ, Nuovo GJ. Occurrence of human papillomavirus type 16 DNA in cutaneous squamous and basal cell neoplasms. *J Am Acad Dermatol* 23:836–842, 1990.

91. De Villiers EM. Human papilloma viruses in skin cancer. *Biomed Pharmacother* 52:26–33, 1998.

92. Woods CG. DNA repair disorders. *Arch Dis Child* 78:178–184, 1998.

93. Dzubow LM, Rigel DS, Robins P. Risk factors for local recurrence of primary cutaneous squamous cell carcinomas. *Arch Dermatol* 118:900–902, 1982.

94. Immerman SC, Scanlon EF, Christ M, Knox KL. Recurrent squamous cell carcinoma of the skin. *Cancer* 51:1537–1540, 1983.

95. Yerushalmi J, Grunwald MH, Halevy DH, et al. Lupus vulgaris complicated by metastatic squamous cell carcinoma. *Int J Dermatol* 37:934–935, 1998.

96. Bowman PH, Hogan DJ. Leg ulcers: a common problem with sometimes uncommon etiologies. *Geriatrics* 54:43–50, 1999.

97. Eroglu A, Camilbel S. Risk factors for locoregional recurrence of scar carcinoma. *Br J Surg* 84:1744–1746, 1997.

98. Dinehart SM, Pollack SV. Metastases from squamous cell carcinomas of the skin and lip. *J Am Acad Dermatol* 21:241–248, 1989.

99. Friedman HI, Cooper PH, Wanebo HJ. Prognostic and therapeutic use of microstaging of cutaneous squamous cell carcinoma of the trunk and extremities. *Cancer* 56:1099–1105, 1985.

100. Goepfert H, Dichtel WJ, Medina JE, et al. Perineural invasion in squamous cell skin carcinoma of the head and neck. *Am J Surg* 148:542–547, 1984.

101. Carter RL, Foster CS, Dinsdale EA, Pittam MR. Perineural spread by squamous cell carcinomas of the head and neck: a morphological study using antiaxonal and anti-myelin monoclonal antibodies. *J Clin Pathol* 36:269–275, 1983.

102. Breuninger H, Holzschuh J, Schaumburg Lever G, et al. Desmoplastic squamous epithelial carcinoma of the skin and lower lip. A morphologic entity with great risk of metastasis and recurrence. *Hautarzt* 49:104–108, 1998.

103. Binder SC, Cady B, Catlin D. Epidermoid carcinoma of the skin of the nose. *Am J Surg* 116:506–512, 1968.

104. Mikhail GR. Subungual epidermoid carcinoma. *J Am Acad Dermatol* 11:291–298, 1984.

105. Soria JC, Fizazi K, Piron D, et al. Squamous cell carcinoma of the penis: multivariate analysis of prognostic factors and natural history in monocentric study with a conservative policy. *Ann Oncol* 8:1089–1098, 1997.

106. Fernandez Gomez JM, Rebade Rey CJ, Perez Garcia FJ, et al. Epidermoid carcinoma of the penis. Review of 30 cases. *Arch Esp Urol* 50:243–252, 1997.

107. Chiu TY, Huang HS, Lai MK, et al. Penile cancer in Taiwan—20 years experience at National Taiwan University Hospital. *J Formos Med Assoc* 97:673–678, 1998.

108. Kao GF, Graham JH, Helwig EB. Carcinoma cuniculatum (verrucous carcinoma of the skin): a clinicopathologic study of 46 cases with ultrastructural observations. *Cancer* 49:2395–2403, 1982.

109. Honeycutt WM, Jansen GT. Treatment of squamous cell carcinoma of the skin. *Arch Dermatol* 108:670–672, 1973.

110. Kibarian MA, Hruza GJ. Nonmelanoma skin cancer. Risks, treatment options, and tips on prevention. *Postgrad Med* 98:39–56, 1995.

111. Spiro RH. Verrucous carcinoma then and now. *Am J Surg* 176:3939–3997, 1998.

112. Rowe DE, Carroll RJ, Day CL. Prognostic factors for local recurrence, metastasis, and survival rates in squamous cell carcinoma of the skin, ear, and lip. Implications for treatment modality selection. *J Am Acad Dermatol* 26:976–990, 1992.

113. Smith RRL, Kuhajda FP, Harris AE. Anaplasttherapy. *Am J Otolaryngol* 6:448–452, 1985.

114. Kuflik EG, Gage AA. The five year cure rate achieved by cryosurgery for skin cancer. *J Am Acad Dermatol* 24:1002–1004, 1991.

115. Meyskens FL Jr, Gilmartin E, Alberts DS, et al. Activity of isotretinoin against squamous cell cancers and preneoplastic lesions. *Cancer Treat Rep* 66:1315–1319, 1982.

116. Brunner R, Landthaler M, Haina D, et al. Treatment of benign, semimalignant, and malignant skin tumors with the Nd:YAG laser. *Lasers Surg Med* 5:105–110, 1985.

117. Odom RB. Fluorouracil. In Epstein E, Epstein NE Jr (eds), *Skin Surgery* (6th ed). Philadelphia: Saunders, 1987:396–400.

118. Frankel DH, Hanusa BH, Zitelli JA. New primary nonmelanoma skin cancer in patients with a history of squamous cell carcinoma of the skin. Implications and recommendations for treatment and follow up. *J Am Acad Dermatol* 26:720–726, 1992.

25

Pediatric Solid Tumors

■ ■ ■

Karen C. Marcus

Cancer is diagnosed annually in approximately 8,400 US children younger than age 15. Cancer is the second major cause of mortality in this population (see Chapter 1). Childhood cancers differ from adult cancers as regards their origins and histologic subtypes, their etiologic characteristics, their response to treatment, and the outcomes. In the adult population, epithelial cancers are most common, and many are related to environmental carcinogens. More commonly, pediatric malignancies are of hematopoietic origin or are primary central nervous system (CNS) tumors. This chapter reviews the epidemiologic factors, pathologic features, clinical presentation, and treatment of pediatric solid tumors. Despite the small number of cases of childhood cancers (in contrast with the numbers in the adult population), great strides have been made in the treatment of pediatric malignancies. In addition, major advances in cancer genetics and the molecular biological characteristics of cancer have been gained through research on these tumors. The improvements in the treatment of childhood cancers have come about largely through cooperative groups that have been established. They include the National Wilms' Tumor Study Group (NWTSG), the Children's Cancer Group (CCG), the Pediatric Oncology Group (POG), the Intergroup Rhabdomyosarcoma Study Group, and the Intergroup Ewing's Sarcoma Study Group. These organizations have performed multiinstitutional, prospective randomized trials to define treatment standards and to advance understanding of pediatric solid tumors. The recently established Children's Oncology Group, a merger of the CCG, the POG, the Intergroup Rhabdomyosarcoma Study Group, and the NWTSG, will continue to improve methods of cancer treatment in children.

Because of the rarity of childhood cancers, children with this diagnosis should be referred to cancer centers with expertise in pediatric cancer treatment. Such centers provide the multidisciplinary team approach to the care of pediatric cancer patients. This team of pediatric specialists includes oncologists, surgeons, irradiation oncologists, anesthesiologists, radiologists, nurses, psychologists, and child life specialists. Successful treatment of childhood cancer also demands knowledge of the potential for late treatment toxicities that can have devastating consequences as affected children mature. Among these late effects are growth abnormalities, cardiac sequelae, neurocognitive effects, sterility, and the development of second, treatment-induced cancers. Many of these toxicities are unavoidable, depending on the treatment required to eradicate disease; however, every attempt to minimize such late effects must be made in parallel with the improvements in cancer treatments.

The most common pediatric malignancies are acute leukemia, non-Hodgkin's lymphoma (NHL); Hodgkin's disease (HD); and primary CNS tumors. Neuroblastoma, Wilms' tumor, rhabdomyosarcoma, and retinoblastomas are the solid tumors occurring most commonly in children.

- Acute lymphoblastic leukemia   23%
- CNS tumors   21%
- Neuroblastoma   7%
- NHL   6%
- Wilms' tumor   6%
- Hodgkin's disease   5%
- Acute myelogenous leukemia   4%
- Rhabdomyosarcoma   4%
- Retinoblastoma   3%
- Osteosarcoma   3%
- Ewing's sarcoma   2%
- Other   16%

The etiology of most childhood malignancies is unknown, although some solid tumors do occur in association with recognized genetic defects. Bilateral retinoblastoma occurs with mutations of the retinoblastoma tumor suppressor gene *RB1* [1]. Wilms' tumor occurs in association with mutations in the *WT1* gene in the Denys-Drash syndrome (consisting of intergender disorders, mesangial sclerosis, and Wilms' tumor) and in the WAGR syndrome (consisting of Wilms' tumor, aniridia, genitourinary abnormalities, and mental retardation) [2, 3]. Rhabdomyosarcomas, soft-tissue and bone sarcomas, brain tumors, adrenocortical cell carcinomas, premenopausal breast cancers, and acute leukemias are seen in patients with the Li-Fraumeni syndrome with *p53* gene mutations [4, 5].

The mechanism of tumor development proposed by Knudson—the two-hit hypothesis—provides an explanation for hereditary retinoblastoma and, by extension,

for other tumors wherein the loss of function of a remaining normal allele results in tumor development [6]. A mutation occurring as a new germinal mutation is transmitted from a carrier or affected parent. A tumor would develop only if a second event occurs, resulting in the loss of function of the remaining normal allele. This loss of heterozygosity can occur by several mechanisms, including a nondisjunction loss, nondisjunction reduplication, mitotic recombination, gene conversion, deletion, or point mutation [7]. The end result is the lack of a normal gene product. How this lack leads ultimately to the development of a malignant tumor is not known directly. The genetic explanation of most childhood solid tumors is likely to be more complex than that of the mechanisms described here.

NON-HODGKIN'S LYMPHOMA

Epidemiologic Factors and Genetic Background

NHL represents approximately 10% of pediatric cancers. The incidence of NHL increases steadily throughout life and occurs in boys two to three times more often than in girls. For unknown reasons, the average annual incidence increased in the United States by almost 30% during the last two decades [8]. Numerous factors have been linked to an increased risk of NHL. Immunodeficiency syndromes, such as severe combined immunodeficiency syndrome, Wiskott-Aldrich syndrome, common variable immunodeficiency, ataxia telangiectasia, and the X-linked lymphoproliferative syndrome, are associated with an increased risk of developing a lymphoma [9, 10]. Children with an acquired immunodeficiency, such as that secondary to human immunodeficiency virus infection or immunosuppressive therapy after solid-organ or bone marrow transplantation, greatly increases the risk of developing a malignant lymphoma or a lymphoproliferative disorder [11, 12]. Most of the lymphomas that occur in patients with abnormalities of the immune system (either constitutional or acquired) are large B-cell or Burkitt tumors in subtype. Monoclonal Epstein-Barr virus (EBV) DNA has been identified in tumor tissue from many such patients, implicating an early role for the virus in tumor development [13]. One explanation for this effect is the inability of the immunodeficient host to generate an adequate T-lymphocyte response (EBV-specific cytotoxic T cells) against B cells that are infected latently with EBV. Most often, the EBV is found in African (endemic) cases of Burkitt's lymphoma. Until re-

Table 25.1 Non-Hodgkin's Lymphomas of Childhood

Histologic Subtype	Frequency (%)	Immunophenotype	Associated Nonrandom Chromosomal Translocations
Undifferentiated Burkitt's lymphoma, non-Burkitt's lymphoma	30–40	B	t(8;14)(q24.1;q32.3) t(8;22)(q24.1;q11) t(2;8)(p11–13;q24.1)
Lymphoblastic lymphoma	30–40	T or pre-B	t(11;14)(p13;q11) t(11;14)(p15;q11) t(7;19)(q35;p13) t(10;14)(q24;q11) t(1;14)(p32–34;q11) t(8;14)(q24;q11) t(1;7)(p34;q34)
Large-cell lymphoma	30	B, T, mixed, null cell	t(2;5)(p23;q35)

cently, EBV was thought to be absent in sporadic cases. More recently, aberrant expression of the viral genome has been identified in cases of sporadic Burkitt's lymphoma that were considered negative by standard screening techniques [14]. Thus, the pathogenic role of EBV in Burkitt's lymphoma is becoming clearer.

Pathologic Classification

The NHLs that occur in children almost always are diffuse. Using the Revised European-American Lymphoma Classification, pediatric NHLs generally fall into the following categories: precursor-B and precursor-T lymphoblastic lymphoma; small, noncleaved-cell lymphomas (Burkitt's and non-Burkitt's lymphoma); diffuse large B-cell lymphoma; or anaplastic large-cell lymphoma (T- and null-cell types) [15]. The frequency, immunophenotype, and associated chromosomal translocations are shown in Table 25.1.

Presentation and Diagnosis

The clinical presentation of NHL in children depends on the histologic background, the extent of disease, and the primary site of disease. More often, NHLs in children are extranodal. They involve abdominal structures in approximately one-third of cases, the mediastinum in one-third of cases, and the head and neck in one-third of cases. The majority of patients will have advanced disease at diagnosis, with disease spreading by hematogenous dissemination. Cytopenias suggest bone marrow infiltration. Patients who have lymphoblastic lymphoma or Burkitt's lymphoma with greater than 25% marrow involvement are considered to have acute lymphoblastic leukemia. Cranial nerve palsies or cerebrospinal fluid pleocytosis are indicative of CNS involvement.

The most common sites are related to the histologic subtypes. Burkitt's lymphoma involves the abdomen or the head and neck. Generally, endemic Burkitt's lymphoma presents as a jaw mass, although abdominal tumors also occur. These tumors grow rapidly, and patients are at risk of developing tumor lysis syndrome when therapy is begun. Alkalinization, vigorous hydration, and the administration of allopurinol are indicated to decrease the risk of development of this syndrome [16]. The small, noncleaved-cell lymphomas are of B-cell immunophenotype and represent 30% to 40% of childhood NHLs. The chromosomal translocations seen most frequently are t(8;14)(q24;q32), t(2;8)(p11;q24), and t(8;22)(q24;q11) [17].

Often, lymphoblastic lymphoma presents with a mediastinal mass, frequently with an associated pleural effusion. The mediastinal mass can grow rapidly, causing airway compromise or compression of the superior vena cava. Prompt initiation of chemotherapy is indicated after diagnostic material has been obtained. Although the occurrence of a primary abdominal tumor in patients with lymphoblastic lymphoma is rare, involvement of such abdominal organs as the liver and spleen can occur. These lymphomas, representing 30% of childhood NHL, most often are of the T-cell immunophenotype. Some patients with a non-T-cell immunophenotype present with peripheral adenopathy or isolated bone involvement [17].

Large-cell lymphomas in children can present with an anterior mediastinal mass, an abdominal mass, skin involvement, or bone involvement. Less frequently,

Table 25.2 Recommended Studies for Evaluation of Non-Hodgkin's Lymphoma Patients

Physical examination
Complete blood count
Serum chemistries
  Electrolytes
  Calcium, phosphorus
  Liver function
  Lactate dehydrogenase
  Uric acid
  Renal function
Human immunodeficiency virus test
Bilateral bone marrow biopsies and aspirates
Cerebrospinal fluid cytology
Imaging studies
  Chest radiogram
  Chest-abdomen-pelvis computer tomogram
  ^{67}Ga
  Thallium scan (optional)
  Positron emission tomogram (optional)

Table 25.3 Murphy Staging System for Childhood Non-Hodgkin's Lymphoma

Stage	Definition
I	Single tumor (extranodal) or single nodal site, excluding mediastinum or abdomen
II	Single tumor (extranodal) with regional nodal involvement on same side of diaphragm: (a) two or more nodal areas; (b) two single extranodal tumors with or without regional nodal involvement; primary gastrointestinal tract tumor (usually ileocecal) with or without mesenteric nodal involvement, completely resected
III	Tumor on both sides of the diaphragm: (a) two single extranodal tumors; (b) two or more nodal areas; all primary intrathoracic tumors (mediastinal, thymic, pleural); all extensive primary intraabdominal disease; all primary epidural or paraspinal tumors
IV	Any of the preceding with bone marrow involvement ($< 25\%$) or initial central nervous system involvement

Source: Reprinted with permission from SE Murphy, Classification, staging and end results of treatment of childhood non-Hodgkin's lymphomas: dissimilarities from lymphomas in adults. *Semin Oncol* 7:332–339, 1980. Copyright © 1980, W. B. Saunders Co., Philadelphia.

large-cell lymphomas occur in other extranodal or nodal sites. Spread to the bone marrow or to the CNS is less frequent than that in small, noncleaved-cell lymphomas or lymphoblastic lymphomas. Large-cell lymphomas in children can be of T-cell, B-cell, or indeterminate phenotype. Thirty percent of childhood large-cell lymphomas have anaplastic features, including abundant cytoplasm, atypical lobulated nuclei, and prominent nucleoli [18]. Generally, anaplastic large-cell lymphomas in children are CD30-positive, have a chromosomal translocation t(2;5), and are of T-cell lineage. Often, these lymphomas involve extranodal sites, including bone and skin, and are considered a separate clinicopathologic classification with a favorable prognosis [18].

Evaluation and Staging

The evaluation of patients with NHL includes complete blood counts with differential counts; analysis of serum electrolyte levels, calcium, phosphorus, uric acid, and lactate dehydrogenase; a test for human immunodeficiency virus; cerebrospinal fluid analysis; bilateral bone marrow biopsies and aspirates; and renal and liver function tests. Radiographic imaging should include computed tomography (CT) of the chest, abdomen, and pelvis. Gallium scans and thallium scans are performed as part of the staging in many institutions, as are bone scans. The use of positron emission tomography scans is increasing in diagnosis and after response to treat-

ment at some centers. A recommended list for evaluation is found in Table 25.2.

The staging system used for pediatric NHL is the Murphy Staging System shown in Table 25.3 [19]. This system differs from that used in staging adult NHL and reflects such patterns of presentation and involvement as frequent extranodal disease, CNS disease, bone marrow disease, and noncontiguous spread of disease. Accurate staging and pathologic classification are critical in determining the appropriate therapy, including the duration, intensity, and expected outcome.

Treatment and Outcome

Owing to the systemic nature of NHL, chemotherapy is the mainstay of treatment for all patients. Surgery plays a limited role except for obtaining diagnostic material and for biopsy of areas suspicious for residual disease. Radiotherapy is used for such emergency situations as intracranial involvement, spinal cord compression, airway compromise, or compression of the superior vena cava. In addition, patients who have advanced disease, do not enter a complete remission after induction therapy, and have pathologically proved residual disease are given consolidative radiotherapy. The treatment regimens differ on the basis of histology and the stage of disease. CNS prophylaxis is given with intrathecal chemotherapy.

BURKITT'S AND LARGE-CELL NHL

Patients with stage I or stage II Burkitt's lymphoma or large-cell lymphoma receive cyclophosphamide, vincristine, prednisone, doxorubicin (Adriamycin), and methotrexate. Protocols may vary, with some differences in which agents are used and in the length of therapy. The 5-year event-free survival for patients with early-stage, large-cell NHL or with early-stage Burkitt's lymphoma is 85% to 95% [20]. Randomized trials in children with early-stage NHL have shown the absence of benefit of involved-field irradiation [20]. Patients with stage III and stage IV Burkitt's lymphoma receive similar agents with the addition of high-dose methotrexate and other chemotherapeutic drugs, including ifosfamide, cytarabine, and cisplatin. The expected event-free survival at 3 years is 75% to 85%. The agents used to treat children with advanced-stage large-cell lymphoma include vincristine, prednisone, doxorubicin, cyclophosphamide, methotrexate, thioguanine, and mercaptopurine. The 3-year event free survival for these patients is 50% to 70%.

LYMPHOBLASTIC LYMPHOMA

Children with early-stage lymphoblastic lymphoma receive Adriamycin, vincristine, prednisone, and cyclophosphamide, as well as oral mercaptopurine and oral methotrexate for maintenance therapy. CNS prophylaxis is given with intrathecal therapy for children with low-stage NHL and head and neck primary lesions. Patients with advanced stage lymphoblastic lymphoma are treated with regimens similar to therapy for acute lymphoblastic leukemia (see Chapter 22).

HODGKIN'S DISEASE
Epidemiologic Factors

HD represents approximately 5% of childhood cancers, with a US annual incidence of 7 per 1 million in children younger than age 15. There is a bimodal age distribution that peaks between 15 and 34 and is followed by a plateau until age 40, after which it increases steadily

with age [21]. The male-female ratio of HD in children is 3 : 1 a ratio much higher than that in adults [22]. The age-specific incidence rates in developing countries is the inverse of that seen in the United States, with rates higher in younger children than in adults in Third World countries. Additionally, the risk that a close relative of a patient with HD will develop the disease is increased slightly; most such cases involve two siblings or a parent and child [23]. The etiology of HD remains unknown. Some interest is generated in the possible association of HD with a history of EBV-related infectious mononucleosis. Patients with a history of such infection are at increased risk of developing HD [24]. The actual role of EBV in the pathogenesis of HD is not established.

Pathologic Classification

The pathologic classification of HD is the Rye modification of the Lukes-Butler classification. HD is classified in four categories: lymphocyte-predominant (LP), nodular sclerosis, mixed-cellularity, and lymphocyte-depleted [25]. The frequency of subtypes in children differs from that in adults. A higher percentage of children than adults have LP histologic characteristics. The majority of patients with LP HD have localized, very early-stage disease. The mixed-cellularity subtype occurs most commonly in children younger than 10 years. Most often, nodular sclerosing HD occurs in adolescents. Lymphocyte-depleted HD is rare in children, and affected patients frequently present with advanced disease.

The cell of origin in HD is unknown. Reed-Sternberg cells characteristic of HD have been postulated as activated lymphoid cells of B- and T-cell lineage; they elaborate cytokines responsible for the various histologic subtypes. No specific monoclonal antibody is directed against the Reed-Sternberg cell, although CD15 (Leu M1) and CD30 (Ki-1) are expressed by Reed-Sternberg cells in most cases of HD. The notable exception is the LP subtype, in which the neoplastic cells often express leukocyte common antigen or CD45 but do not express CD15 or CD30.

Presentation and Evaluation

Most cases of HD arise in lymph nodes. Often, patients present with enlarged lymph nodes, which in children is a frequent physical finding secondary to benign causes. Usually, the lymph nodes involved with HD are nontender and are described as firm and rubbery. Nodes may be enlarged for weeks or months. Suspicious lymph nodes must be subjected to biopsy. A thorough history is recorded. Special attention is given to the presence of "B" symptoms: unexplained weight loss of 10% over 6 months, drenching night sweats, and unexplained fevers of 101°F or higher on three occasions. A careful physical examination is performed. A biopsy of the suspicious node or mass is required to establish the diagnosis. All patients undergo laboratory studies, including complete blood counts, renal function tests, liver function tests, and erythrocyte sedimentation rate analysis. Patients with HD have altered cellular immunity but relatively normal humoral immunity. Radiographic imaging with plain-film chest radiography and CT of the chest, abdomen, and pelvis are recommended. CT of the neck is performed for patients with any neck adenopathy. Gallium scanning now is being used by most institutions, and bone scanning is performed for patients with bony pain or elevated alkaline phosphatase levels.

Staging

The staging system used for HD is the Ann Arbor Staging System (Table 25.4) [26]. This system does not include an assessment of bulk or disease, which is known to have prognostic significance. A clinical stage is assigned on the basis of the history and on results of physical examination, laboratory studies, radiographic studies, and biopsy. Surgical staging, including splenectomy in children with HD, is controversial. Unless the results of the staging laparotomy will be used to determine the treatment—particularly unless radiotherapy alone is being considered—surgical staging is not indicated. Most often, treatment of HD in children (see discussion later) includes chemotherapy, either in combination with radiotherapy or alone. Therefore, little justification exists for surgical staging.

Treatment

The appropriate therapy for pediatric patients with HD is determined by the age of affected children and the stage and extent of their disease. The use of six cycles of chemotherapy with involved-field radiotherapy was introduced at Stanford and has served as a model to improve outcome and to minimize late effects [27]. That pioneering study used nitrogen mustard, vincristine, procarbazine, and prednisone and a sliding scale of irra-

Table 25.4 Ann Arbor Staging Classification for Hodgkin's Disease

Stage	Definition
I	Involvement of a single lymph node region (I) or of a single extralymphatic organ or site (I_E)
II	Involvement of two or more lymph node regions on the same side of the diaphragm (II) or localized involvement of an extralymphatic organ or site and one or more lymph node regions on the same side of the diaphragm (II_E)
III	Involvement of lymph node regions on both sides of the diaphragm (III), may be accompanied by involvement of the spleen (III_S) or by localized involvement of an extralymphatic organ or site (III_E) or both (III_{SE})
IV	Diffuse or disseminated involvement of one or more extralymphatic organs or tissues, with or without associated lymph node involvement

Note: The absence or presence of fever exceeding 38°C (100.4°F) for 3 consecutive days, night sweats, or unexplained loss of 10% or more of body weight in the 6 months preceding diagnosis is designated by the suffix A or B, respectively.

Source: Reprinted with permission of the American Association for Cancer Research from PP Carbone, HS Kaplan, K Musshoff, et al., Report of the committee on Hodgkin's disease staging. *Cancer Res* 31:1860–1861, 1971.

diation doses based on patient age. Many other institutions and cooperative group studies have subsequently adopted and modified this approach.

Children with early-stage, nonbulky disease can be treated successfully with combination chemotherapy, such as doxorubicin, bleomycin, vinblastine, and dacarbazine, and low-dose involved-field radiotherapy. Survival rates of more than 90% are expected for such children. Children with more advanced disease also are treated with combined-modality therapy. Often, more intensive chemotherapy is used in addition to involved-field radiotherapy, resulting in long-term survivals of more than 80%. Radiotherapy alone is considered only for patients who are fully grown and who have limited disease, as proved by surgical staging. The treatment of children with relapsed HD depends on the initial therapy and the duration of complete response. Salvage therapy is very successful for patients who had been treated with radiotherapy alone, although fewer and fewer children are being treated in this way. Patients can be treated with non-cross-resistant chemotherapy for salvage. The concept of non-cross-resistant chemotherapy incorporates several factors: Each agent is individually active; the agents differ in their mechanisms of action; and toxicities do not overlap. Patients who do not respond to nitrogen mustard, vincristine, procarbazine, and prednisone combined with doxorubicin, bleomycin, vinblastine, and dacarbazine have a poor prognosis. In some cases, high-dose chemotherapy with bone marrow or peripheral blood stem-cell rescue or allogeneic bone marrow transplantation have been successful [28, 29].

Follow-Up and Late Effects

The recommended follow-up of children treated for HD includes recording a history and performing a physical examination, chest radiography, and complete blood counts every 3 months for the first year, quarterly for the second 2 years, and semiannually thereafter. Chest-neck and abdominal-pelvic CT scans and ^{67}Ga scans are performed annually, as are thyroid function and pulmonary function tests in those children who received neck or thoracic irradiation, respectively. Any clinical suspicion of recurrence should prompt an appropriate immediate investigation. Any female patient who received thoracic irradiation should undergo mammography 8 to 10 years after treatment and annually thereafter.

The current goals of treating HD are to improve the outcome for poor-risk patients and to minimize late toxicities in patients whose outcome is favorable. The acute toxicities of HD treatment in children include nausea and vomiting, myelosuppression, mucositis, and hair loss and are similar to those in adults. The late effects of therapy include thyroid dysfunction, musculoskeletal abnormalities, reproductive difficulties, cardiac toxicity, pulmonary toxicity, and second tumors. Second cancers after pediatric HD include solid tumors and secondary leukemias and lymphomas. The median time to the development of leukemias is shorter than that to the development of solid tumors. The incidence of leukemia is related to the administration of chemotherapy, and that of solid tumors is associated with irradiation. Most commonly, the solid tumors are breast tumors (in girls) and sarcomas, melanomas, and thyroid cancers [30]. The actuarial risk at 20 years (reported from Stanford) is 9.7% for boys, 16.8% for girls, and 9.2% for breast cancer [30]. Relapse of HD increased the risk of a second cancer [30], further emphasizing the important goal of initial cure of disease (see Chapter 20).

RHABDOMYOSARCOMA
Epidemiologic Factors

The most common malignant tumor of soft tissues in children is rhabdomyosarcoma (RMS). In the United States, 4.5 cases occur per 1 million infants and children younger than age 15 (approximately 250 new cases per year). The incidence is slightly higher in boys and is lower in Oriental children. The median age at diagnosis is 4 years. Families with Li-Fraumeni syndrome and children with neurofibromatosis type 1 disease are at increased risk of developing RMS [31, 32]. The RMS cell of origin is a mesenchymal cell, which normally matures into skeletal muscle, smooth muscle, fat, fibrous tissue, bone, or cartilage. RMSs are believed to come from those mesenchymal cells that were committed to the skeletal muscle lineage, although these tumors can display evidence of multilineage.

Genetic Background and Pathologic Classification

RMSs are identified on the basis of characteristic light-microscopical, immunohistochemical, electron-microscopical, and molecular genetic features. These tumors are composed of small, round, blue cells that often exhibit cross-striations under the light microscope. The immunohistochemical features include positive staining for the muscle proteins actin and myosin and for desmin, myoglobin, MyoD, and Z-band protein. The two major variants of RMS are the embryonal and alveolar subtypes, which have characteristic appearances under the light microscope and distinguishing molecular markers. The chromosomal translocation characteristic of the alveolar subtype is t(2;13)(q35;q14), which can be identified using reverse transcriptase–polymerase chain reaction. This tool provides confirmatory evidence of the alveolar subtype. The loss of heterozygosity of chromosome 11p15 can be used to identify the embryonal subtype [33].

Presentation

RMS can originate from many sites. The most frequent site of origin is the head and neck (35%); the most common site within the head and neck is the orbit. Other head and neck sites are the parameninges, which include the nasopharynx, paranasal sinuses, middle ear, mastoid, and pterygoid-infratemporal fossa; the scalp; the buccal mucosa; the oropharynx; the larynx; and the neck [34]. Tumors in the orbit present with proptosis and, occasionally, with ophthalmoplegia or periorbital edema. Tumors in nonorbital parameningeal sites produce nasal or sinus obstruction, sinusitis, epistaxis, and aural obstruction. Cranial nerve palsies can occur with invasion of the base of the skull and meningeal extension. Most often, RMS of the head and neck is embryonal. Regional nodal involvement from RMS arising in the head and neck is infrequent.

The second most frequent site for RMS is the genitourinary tract, accounting for more than 20% of all cases of RMS. Tumors can arise in the bladder and prostate, the paratesticular area, the vagina, and the uterus [35]. Bladder tumors grow intraluminally and can produce urinary obstruction and hematuria. Often, children with genitourinary RMS present with a pelvic mass, a mass in the scrotum in patients with paratesticular tumors, or grapelike masses in the vagina (botryoid tumors), which can break off and appear in the diaper. Abdominal masses may be present in patients with retroperitoneal primary lesions or owing to the involvement of paraaortic nodes. Nodal involvement is present in 26% of cases arising in the paratesticular area and in 20% to 40% of cases in such other genitourinary sites as the bladder and prostate. The majority of RMSs in the genitourinary tract are of the embryonal subtype.

Most often, RMS of the extremity leads to a mass or swelling of the affected limb. The mass may be painful, but the presence of pain varies. Tumors arising in the extremity represent 20% of RMS. Regional nodal involvement is common (approximately 12%), particularly if the histologic characteristic of the tumor is alveolar, which is the more likely subtype in extremity tumors. RMS can occur in the trunk, perineal-perianal region, biliary tract, heart, breast, and ovary. In some cases, a primary site cannot be determined.

Diagnosis and Evaluation

The most common metastatic sites of RMS are the lung, bone marrow, bones, liver, and brain. In addition, the regional nodes can be targets of tumor spread, the frequency of which varies by site and histology. Evaluation of children with RMS requires participation by pathologists, radiologists, surgeons, pediatric oncologists, and irradiation oncologists. The diagnostic studies include complete blood count; liver function tests; CT scanning and magnetic resonance imaging (MRI) of the primary tumor; CT scanning of the lungs and of the abdomen and pelvis for primaries arising in these sites; bone scan; and bone marrow aspirates and biopsies. Biopsy (most often an incisional biopsy) is required for all patients for whom future resection is planned. Immediate surgical excision no longer is necessary unless the resection will not cause significant functional morbidity. Lymph node biopsy is performed for clinically enlarged or suspicious

nodes. The site of the primary tumor influences the likelihood of nodal disease and will be a determining factor also in surgical management.

The staging of RMS is critical in determining appropriate treatment and of the prognosis. Patients with localized tumors that can be resected completely have a better prognosis than do those with regional or distant disease. The clinical grouping system (Table 25.5) was developed by the Intergroup Rhabdomyosarcoma Study (IRS) group in 1972 and is based on the results of initial surgical resection. A revised staging system has

Table 25.5   Clinical Grouping of Rhabdomyosarcoma

Group	Definition
Group I	Localized disease, completely resected. Regional nodes not involved: A. Confined to muscle or organ of origin. B. Contiguous involvement; infiltration outside muscle or organ of origin through fascial planes; includes gross and microscopic confirmation of complete resection. Any lymph nodes inadvertently removed must be negative or patient is considered group IIB or IIC.
Group II	Gross total resection with evidence of regional spread: A. Grossly resected tumor with microscopic residual disease. Surgeon believes all tumor removed (grossly), but pathologist finds tumor at the margin, and additional resection to achieve negative margin not feasible. No gross residual tumor. No evidence of regional lymph node involvement. B. Regional disease with involved lymph nodes, completely resected with no microscopic residual disease. C. Regional disease with involved nodes, grossly resected but with evidence of microscopic residual disease and histologic involvement of most distal regional lymph node (from the primary site) in the dissection.
Group III	Incomplete resection with gross residual disease: A. After biopsy only. B. After gross or major resection of the primary tumor.
Group IV	Metastatic disease present at onset (lung, liver, bone, bone marrow, brain, distant muscle or nodes). The presence of positive cytology in the cerebrospinal, pleural, and peritoneal fluids as well as implants on the pleural or peritoneal surface are considered group IV.

Source: Reprinted with permission of Wiley-Liss, Inc., a subsidiary of John Wiley & Sons, Inc., from HM Mauer, EA Gehan, M Beltangady, The Intergroup Rhabdomyosarcoma Study II. *Cancer* 71:1904–1922, 1993.

Table 25.6 TNM Staging of Rhabdomyosarcoma

Stage	Site	Tumor Invasiveness	Tumor Size	Nodal Involvement	Metastases
1	Orbit; H/N (nonparameningeal); genitourinary (nonbladder or prostate);	T1 or T2	a or b	N0, N1, Nx	M0
2	Bladder, prostate; extremity; parameningeal; retroperitoneal; trunk	T1 or T2	a	N0 or Nx	M0
3	Bladder, prostate	T1 or T2	a	N1	M0
	Extremity; parameningeal; retroperitoneal, trunk	T1 or T2	b	N0, N1, Nx	M0
4	All	T1 or T2	a or b	N0 or N1	M1

T1 = confined to anatomic site of origin; T2 = extension; a = < 5 cm in diameter; b = > 5 cm in diameter; N0 = nodes not clinically involved; N1 = nodes clinically involved; NX = clinical status of nodes unknown; M1 = distant metastases present.
Source: Used with permission from ID Fleming, JS Cooper, DE Henson, et al. (eds), *AJCC Cancer Staging Manual* (5th ed). Philadelphia: Lippincott-Raven, 1997:149–156.

been developed on the basis of the TNM (tumor-node-metastasis) system (Table 25.6). This system is less dependent on such factors as surgical excision at diagnosis, which can be affected by the aggressiveness of a local surgeon. It also takes into consideration the site of the primary tumor and its size, and nodal involvement. The clinical grouping system is used in conjunction with the TNM system to determine the role of radiotherapy (discussed later).

Treatment

The treatment of RMS involves surgery for possible removal of the primary tumor, chemotherapy for cytoreduction of the primary tumor and treatment of microscopic and gross metastases, and radiotherapy for control of local or regional residual disease. The randomized clinical trials carried out by the IRS have helped to determine the current therapeutic recommendations. Combination chemotherapy is a component of treatment for all patients. The IRS-I was initiated in 1972 and was followed by subsequent IRS trials [36]. These trials and many other studies of more limited numbers of patients have helped to establish the treatment for all stages of RMS, with current and future trials designed to improve the outcome. These trials have found vincristine, dactinomycin, and cyclophosphamide to be among the most active agents against RMS, and they would be considered standard therapy outside of a protocol [37]. The IRS-IV piloted the use of etoposide and ifosfamide along with hyperfractionated radiotherapy for children with group III disease [38]. The final results of IRS-IV have not been published, and

the next IRS trial (now open) seeks to define further the appropriate therapy for RMS.

Radiotherapy is indicated for all patients with microscopic or macroscopic residual disease. Patients with completely resected tumors with negative margins do not require adjuvant radiotherapy [39]. Patients with microscopic residual disease receive 4,140 cGy in standard fractions (180 cGy per fraction), whereas patients with gross residual or unresectable disease receive 5,040 cGy with standard fractionation. The IRS-IV trial was designed to test hyperfractionated radiotherapy for children with gross residual disease using twice-daily fractions of 110 to 5,940 cGy.

Patients receive initial chemotherapy with radiotherapy started at week 9 unless they present with a primary tumor in the parameningeal region and demonstrate bony erosion of the base of the skull with intracranial extension. Such patients begin radiotherapy on day 0 [40]. The pilot study ran from 1988 to 1991; the IRS-IV trial opened in 1991 and closed in 1997. The goal of the hyperfractionated radiotherapy was to increase the biologically effective dose by 10% without increasing the late effects [40]. Until the results of this trial are reported to confirm the benefit of this approach, hyperfractionated radiotherapy is not considered as standard treatment. To minimize late effects while improving local control, conformal radiotherapy techniques generally are used at most centers (Fig. 25.1).

Outcome

The progression-free survival of patients based on the IRS-II and IRS-III trials reported by clinical grouping

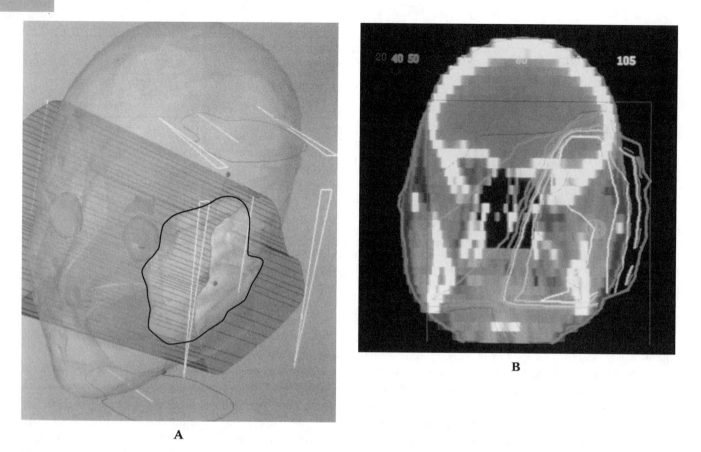

A

B

Figure 25.1 (A) Conformal radiotherapy reconstructed image for treatment of a rhabdomyosarcoma of the infratemporal fossa. The tumor is outlined in black. Multiple noncoplanar beams are used to treat the tumor volume and to limit the dose delivered to critical normal structures. (B) Coronal images of a radiation therapy planning computed tomography with isodose curves superimposed displaying dose distribution.

was more than 80% for patients in clinical group I, approximately 70% for those in clinical group II, 60% for those in group III, and 30% for those in group IV [41]. The current strategies for improving outcome and decreasing late effects of the survivors include the development of risk-based therapies. Children with low-risk disease would be those with embryonal histology and stage I, group I or II disease; stage I, group III disease (orbit only); and stage II, group I disease (Dr. Holcombe Grier, personal communication, 1999). Children with alveolar histologic features at all sites, groups I through III, and those children who are younger than age 10 and have group IV disease and embryonal histologic features are considered to have intermediate-risk disease. Those who are older than 10 years and have group IV disease or all children with group IV alveolar disease are considered to have high-risk disease. With this approach, therapy can be tailored to maximize tumor control and to minimize late effects in patients with favorable characteristics, while identifying patients with

unfavorable characteristics, those for whom more intensive therapy is indicated.

RETINOBLASTOMA

Epidemiologic Factors and Genetic Background

Retinoblastoma is the most common malignant ocular tumor afflicting children, with an annual incidence of 3.9 cases per 1 million US children younger than 15 years. Two-thirds of these cases are unilateral, and the remainder are bilateral. The median age at diagnosis of unilateral retinoblastoma is 2 years for boys and 1 year for girls; the median age at diagnosis of bilateral disease is less than 1 year for both genders. Retinoblastoma occurs as either a sporadic mutation (60% of cases) or an inherited form. All patients with bilateral disease are believed to have the autosomal dominant form, even if no other family members have the disease. Such children carry the germline mutation.

Approximately 10% of patients with unilateral disease also have the heritable form with a germline mutation and are capable of transmitting the disease to offspring [42]. The genetic defect is the loss of heterozygosity at the retinoblastoma gene (RB) locus that predisposes the child to the development of retinoblastoma. Alteration of both copies of the retinoblastoma gene leads to malignant tumor development. Patients with the inherited form of the disease possess a germline mutation at the RB locus. The second mutation ("hit") at the RB site leads to malignant tumor growth [43]. Patients with sporadic (nonheritable) disease have two somatic mutations. The putative location for the RB gene was confirmed by linkage studies in heredity retinoblastoma families [44].

The RB1 gene, localized to the 13q14.1 region, has been cloned and sequenced [45]. The RB1 gene now is considered to be a tumor suppressor gene. The loss of function of the protein, which normally suppresses cell growth, contributes to oncogenic transformation by removing the restraints on cell proliferation [46]. Mutations in the RB1 gene disrupt this regulation, allowing cells to enter a proliferative state, unchecked by the usual mechanisms [46]. Patients with the heritable form of retinoblastoma are also at increased risk of developing other second tumors, primarily osteogenic sarcomas [47].

Pathologic Classification

A retinoblastoma is composed of small round cells with scant cytoplasm and a deeply staining nucleus, resembling embryonal retinal cells. It appears grossly as a white, friable tumor with dense calcifications. Tumors that arise from the internal nuclear layer, the nerve fiber layer, the ganglion cell layer, or the external nuclear layer grow toward the subretinal space, pushing the retina inward and leading to retinal detachment [48]. This type of retinoblastoma is known as the exophytic type. Tumors that arise from the inner layers of the retina and grow toward the vitreous are known as the endophytic type.

Presentation and Evaluation

Frequently, children present with leukokoria (white-eye reflex), strabismus, conjunctival erythema, and de-

creased visual acuity; conversely, the disorder may be detected on routine eye examination. Leukokoria can result also from nonneoplastic conditions, such as Toxocara canis infection and retrolental fibroplasia secondary to prolonged oxygen administration at birth [49].

The physical examination of children with retinoblastoma can reveal a white pupillary reflex, esotropia, exotropia, decreased acuity, or pain due to glaucoma or uveitis after tumor necrosis. Tumors near the macula can be seen with direct ophthalmoscopy; tumors at the periphery of the retina may not be apparent with direct visualization. All children with suspected retinoblastoma must undergo examination of both eyes under general anesthesia. In addition to the examination under anesthesia, a complete blood count, urinalysis, and renal and liver function tests should be performed. CT is useful in defining the extent of the intraocular tumor and in assessing extraocular spread.

Retinoblastoma can metastasize to the CNS and bone marrow in patients with advanced intraocular disease. A lumbar puncture and bone marrow aspiration and biopsy can be performed under anesthesia at the time of the examination. Radionuclide bone scanning is indicated for patients with extensive ocular disease, positive bone marrow, or bony symptoms that could suggest bone metastases.

Staging and Treatment

All patients undergo examination of both eyes under anesthesia; each eye is staged separately. The staging system used most often is that of Reese and Ellsworth (Table 25.7) [50]. The staging correlates with the likelihood of preserving useful vision. Patients with group IV or group V disease have a low likelihood of vision in the affected eye.

Indications for enucleation include extensive retinal damage and disruption, with no possibility of restoring useful vision; tumor in the anterior chamber; neurovascular glaucoma; and bilateral cases with extensive disease and no possibility of restoring vision. At the time of enucleation, 10 to 15 mm of optic nerve should be removed. Children with limited unilateral or bilateral tumors can be treated with photocoagulation or cryotherapy [51]. Photocoagulation successfully controlled retinoblastoma in 80% of cases [50]. Megavoltage radiotherapy can irradiate the retinal tumor with relative sparing of the posterior lens surface. Meticulous daily field placement is required. The dose of irradiation needed is 40 to 45 Gy [52]. Focal techniques of episcleral radio-

Table 25.7   Staging System of Reese and Ellsworth

Stage	Description
IA	Solitary tumor < 4 disc diameters at or behind the equator
IB	Multiple tumors < 4 disc diameters all at or behind the equator
IIA	Solitary tumor 4–10 disc diameters at or behind the equator
IIB	Multiple tumors 4–10 disc diameters behind the equator
IIIA	Any tumor anterior to the equator
IIIB	Solitary tumors > 10 disc diameters behind the equator
IVA	Multiple tumors, some > 10 disc diameters
IVB	Any tumor extending anterior to the ora serrata
VA	Massive tumors involving more than one-half the retina
VB	Vitreous seeding

Source: Reprinted with permission of Elsevier Science from AB Reese, RM Ellsworth, The evaluation and current concept of retinoblastoma therapy. *Trans Am Acad Ophthalmol Otolaryngol* 67:164–172, 1963.

active plaques also have been used to treat small tumors in early-stage disease [53].

Although the survival from retinoblastoma is more than 90%, patients with bilateral disease are at increased risk for the development of second malignancies [47]. Most (but not all) these recurrences are within the irradiation field. Several researchers are investigating the role of chemotherapy in the management of retinoblastoma patients as front-line therapy to eliminate the need for external-beam radiotherapy [54]. The goals of this approach are to improve eye salvage and to decrease the risk of irradiation-induced second tumors. Although no randomized trials exist, protocols using such agents as vincristine, carboplatin, and etoposide have shown promise and are in progress [55].

WILMS' TUMOR
Epidemiologic Factors and Genetic Background

Wilms' tumor is a primary malignant tumor of the kidney. Median age at diagnosis is 41.5 months for unilateral cases in boys and 46.9 months in girls. Bilateral cases present earlier, at a median age of 29.5 months and 32.6 months for boys and girls, respectively [56]. Children with Wilms' tumor may have other anomalies that include aniridia, hemihypertrophy, cryptorchidism, and hypospadias.

Some syndromes include Wilms' tumor. These syndromes are the Beckwith-Wiedemann syndrome of aniridia, hemihypertrophy, and Wilms' tumor; the Denys-Drash syndrome of hermaphroditism, renal disease (glomerulonephritis or nephrotic syndrome), and Wilms' tumor; and the WAGR syndrome of Wilms' tumor, aniridia, genitourinary anomalies, and mental retardation [57–59].

The study of Wilms' tumor has revealed much information about the mechanisms of tumor development. Several chromosomal abnormalities have been associated with Wilms' tumor, including the interstitial deletion of chromosome 11 at band p13, trisomy 8, and trisomy 18. In patients with the WAGR syndrome, the deletion encompasses a number of contiguous genes, including the aniridia gene *PAX6* and the Wilms' tumor suppressor gene *WT1* [60]. The germline absence of the *PAX6* allele leads to aniridia, and the germline mutation or deletion of the *WT1* gene results in genitourinary defects [61]. In contrast to effects of such other tumor suppressor genes as *RB1*, the consequences of *WT1* gene deletion are restricted to those organs that normally express the gene. *WT1* expression may be required for differentiation of renal blastemic cells, glomerular epithelium, and renal vesicles, as these cells in the kidney normally express the *WT1* gene [62].

Pathologic Classification

Wilms' tumor is thought to be derived from primitive metanephric blastemic cells. Although most Wilms' tumors are single tumors, 5% are bilateral, and 7% are multifocal in one kidney [63]. Classically, Wilms' tumor is composed of three cell types: blastemic, stromal, and epithelial. Anaplastic Wilms' tumors contain cells with giant polypoid nuclei. Tumors are considered focally anaplastic if the anaplastic features are confined strictly to a single focus within the tumor; tumors with more extensive anaplasia are considered to be diffusely anaplastic.

Two other variants of renal tumors still are grouped with Wilms' tumor but have higher rates of relapse and death and have patterns of metastasis different from those of classic Wilms' tumor. These variants are clear-cell sarcoma of the kidney and rhabdoid tumor. Clear-cell sarcoma is associated with a higher rate of bony metastases. The cell of origin of rhabdoid tumors remains elusive and is associated with separate neuroectodermal tumors of the brain [64]. Precursor lesions to Wilms' tumor—nephrogenic rests—are found in the normal kidney of 30% of patients with Wilms' tumor

[65]. Congenital mesoblastic nephroma is a tumor of infancy separate from Wilms' tumor and curable by nephrectomy [66].

Presentation and Evaluation

Most often, Wilms' tumor presents as an abdominal mass. Abdominal pain, hematuria, fever, and hypertension also can occur. The initial evaluation of children with an abdominal mass includes a recorded history and a physical examination. The presence of other genitourinary anomalies or other associated characteristics, such as aniridia, macroglossia, or hemihypertrophy, should be noted. Often, obtaining abdominal ultrasonography is the first and easiest step, and this radiographic study will differentiate a solid from a cystic mass and often can identify the origin of any mass present. Abdominal ultrasonography also can demonstrate the patency of the inferior vena cava. A complete blood count, tests of liver and renal functions, determination of serum calcium levels, and urinalysis should be performed.

An MRI or CT scan of the abdomen is obtained to evaluate the mass further and to assess the presence of lymph nodes and extension of the tumor into other structures, including the liver or spleen. A chest radiograph is obtained to look for pulmonary metastases. CT of the chest is a more sensitive test for identifying pulmonary metastases, but it will also identify lesions that may not be tumors; for equivocal lesions, a biopsy is prudent.

A bone scan should be obtained for patients with clear-cell sarcoma and for all patients who have Wilms' tumor and pulmonary or hepatic metastases or bony symptoms. An MRI of the brain is indicated for children with clear-cell sarcoma and the rhabdoid variant, as both have a propensity to develop metastases to the brain.

Staging

The staging system used for Wilms' tumor is that developed by the NWTSG. The system is presented in Table 25.8.

Treatment

The NWTSG has performed a series of prospective randomized trials with multifactorial design [67]. These trials have included almost 2,000 children with Wilms' tumor and have been able to arrive at treatment recom-

Table 25.8 National Wilms' Tumor Study Group Staging System for Wilms' Tumor

Stage	Definition
I	Tumor limited to the kidney, completely excised; renal capsule with an intact outer surface; tumor not ruptured or sampled for biopsy prior to removal (fine-needle aspiration excluded); vessels of renal sinus not involved; no evidence of tumor at or beyond the margins of resection
II	Tumor extended beyond kidney but completely excised; regional extension (e.g., penetration of renal capsule or extensive invasion of renal sinus); blood vessels outside renal parenchyma, including vessels of renal sinus, with possible tumor; biopsy performed prior to resection, excluding fine-needle aspiration; spillage before or during surgery confined to the flank and not involving the peritoneal surface; no evidence of tumor at or beyond the margins of resection
III	Residual nonhematogenous tumor present, confined to the abdomen; any of the following: lymph nodes within the abdomen or pelvis involved by tumor; intrathoracic or other extraabdominal lymph nodes considered stage IV; tumor penetrating peritoneal surface tumor; implants found on peritoneal surface; gross or microscopic tumor remaining postoperatively; tumor not completely resectable because of local infiltration into vital structures; or tumor spillage not confined to the flank before or during surgery
IV	Hematogenous metastases (lung, liver, bone, brain, etc.) or lymph node metastases outside the abdominopelvic region
V	Bilateral renal involvement present at diagnosis; each side staged individually

Source: Reprinted with permission of Wiley-Liss, Inc., a subsidiary of John Wiley & Sons, Inc., from GJ D'Angio, N Breslow, JB Beckwith, et al., Treatment of Wilms' tumor: results of the Third National Wilms' Tumor Study. *Cancer* 64:349–360, 1989.

mendations by stage. The recommendations include initial surgery for most patients, with postoperative therapy as outlined below:

- *Stage I favorable or anaplastic histology:* vincristine and dactinomycin; no abdominal irradiation
- *Stage II favorable histology:* vincristine and dactinomycin; no abdominal irradiation
- *Stage III favorable histology:* vincristine, dactinomycin, and doxorubicin; abdominal irradiation
- *Stage IV favorable histology:* vincristine, dactinomycin, and doxorubicin; abdominal irradiation for abdominal tumor at stage III; whole-lung irradiation for patients with pulmonary metastases visible on chest radiograph; lung irradiation for those

with pulmonary metastases evident by CT (only if elected by treating institution)

- *Stage II to stage IV anaplastic histology:* vincristine, doxorubicin, cyclophosphamide, and etoposide; abdominal irradiation; pulmonary irradiation for pulmonary metastases
- *Stage I to stage IV clear-cell sarcoma:* vincristine, doxorubicin, cyclophosphamide, and etoposide; abdominal irradiation; pulmonary irradiation for pulmonary metastases
- *Stage I to stage IV rhabdoid:* carboplatin, cyclophosphamide, and etoposide

Children with Wilms' tumor of all stages displaying favorable histology have an expected long-term survival of more than 80%. Children with advanced-stage anaplastic disease or one of the other variants have not faired as well, but the current NWTSG trial V is exploring the use of such agents as platinum-containing regimens and etoposide to improve the outlook for such patients [68].

EWING'S SARCOMA/PRIMITIVE NEUROECTODERMAL TUMORS
Background and Epidemiologic Factors

Ewing's sarcoma is a member of the family of primitive neuroectodermal tumors (PNET) that occur as either osseous or soft-tissue tumors. (These tumors are distinct from the PNET arising in the CNS, despite the common name.) Ewing's sarcoma is the second most common bone tumor occurring in children. The most frequent site for Ewing's sarcoma is the femur, usually in the diaphysis. The pelvis represents the second most common site; other sites include the pubis, sacrum, ileum, ischium, humerus, vertebrae, ribs, skull, and other flat bones. Extraosseous Ewing's sarcoma without bony involvement also can occur. The annual incidence of Ewing's sarcoma is approximately 2.7 cases per 1 million white US children younger than age 15 [69]. This tumor rarely presents in black or Asian children.

Pathologic Features

The characteristic pathologic findings of Ewing's sarcoma include densely packed, regularly shaped, small, glycogen-containing cells with round to oval nuclei. The majority of Ewing's sarcomas have a characteristic chromosomal translocation: t(11;22)(q24;q12) [70]. In addition to this chromosomal translocation, other nonrandom translocations also are seen in the PNET family of tumors; the majority of the translocations include t(11;22). Molecular cloning of the breakpoints of the t(11;22) translocation has localized further the rearrangement sites to the *EWS* gene on chromosome 22 and the *FLI1* gene on chromosome 11. The t(11;22)(q24;q12) translocation results in a rearrangement of the *FLI1* gene and fusion of the *FLI1* and *EWS* genes. Other rearrangements have been seen less frequently in Ewing's tumors, involving the *EWS* and such other genes as *ERG*, closely related to the *FLI1* gene and a transcription factor of the Ets family [71, 72]. In all the *EWS* rearrangements identified thus far, a hybrid RNA that is produced fuses a portion of the *EWS* gene to an Ets transcription factor.

Diagnosis

Children with Ewing's sarcoma can present with pain, a palpable mass, tenderness, or redness. Fever is noted in 28% of patients. Some patients present with a limp, back pain, neurologic symptoms, or pain with respiration depending on the sites of involvement. Approximately 25% of patients will have metastatic disease at diagnosis. The most common sites of metastases are the lungs, the bone marrow, and other bones. The evaluation of children suspected of having a Ewing's sarcoma includes recording a general history, performing a physical examination, and evaluating the primary and potential sites of distant disease. In addition, laboratory studies are performed: complete blood count, liver and renal function tests, and analysis of lactate dehydrogenase levels. The primary tumor should be evaluated with MRI and, in some cases, with CT as well; the lungs should be scanned for evidence of metastases (Fig. 25.2). Patients with primary tumors of the rib can have an associated pleural effusion. A bone scan and bilateral bone marrow aspirates and biopsies are also indicated to look for other hematogenous metastases.

Treatment

Not long after Ewing's sarcoma first was described in 1921 by James Ewing, the ability of radiotherapy to control this tumor locally was recognized. At the same time, more than 90% of patients with Ewing's sarcoma ultimately would succumb to pulmonary metastases, demonstrating the systemic nature of this tumor. Chemotherapy to control micrometastatic disease and treat-

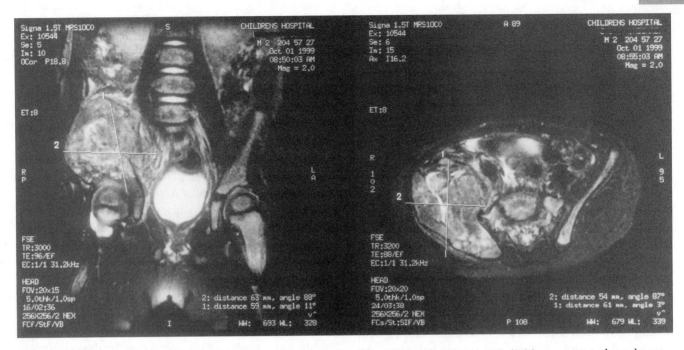

Figure 25.2 T_2-weighted magnetic resonance image of a child with a pelvic Ewing's sarcoma/primitive neuroectodermal tumor involving the right iliac bone with a large soft-tissue mass.

ment directed at the primary tumor are the mainstays of therapy for Ewing's sarcoma. Local control of the primary tumor can be achieved with surgery, radiotherapy, or a combination of both. Larger tumors (> 8 cm or > 100 cm³ by volume) have correlated with a decrease in local control [73, 74]. No randomized trials have shown an improvement in survival with resection rather than radiotherapy, although nonrandomized trials have shown some such improvement in survival [75]. This improvement has been attributed to inclusion of larger, unresectable tumors in the radiotherapy-alone groups. Long-term morbidity of both treatment and resectability are considered in determining the optimal local control of the primary lesion. In addition to impairment of growth of irradiated bones is the 10% to 20% risk of an irradiation-induced tumor at 10 or more years after treatment [76]. Radiotherapy can control Ewing's sarcoma in more than 80% of patients in the modern chemotherapy era [77, 78]. The current standards for radiotherapy of Ewing's sarcoma include the use of tailored radiotherapy fields with adequate margins of 2 to 5 cm and doses of 55 Gy for gross disease and 45 to 50 Gy for microscopic disease.

The efficacy of chemotherapy in eradicating micrometastatic disease in Ewing's sarcoma has been demonstrated in multiinstitutional prospective trials. In 1973, the Intergroup Ewing's Sarcoma Study I was undertaken to compare three treatment regimens for patients with nonmetastatic disease. Those three regimens were vincristine, dactinomycin, and cyclophosphamide (VAC) plus local radiotherapy to local tumor; VAC with doxorubicin plus local radiotherapy to local tumor; and VAC with prophylactic bilateral pulmonary irradiation plus local radiotherapy to local tumor. This trial demonstrated that doxorubicin resulted in an improvement in disease-free survival and overall survival [79]. Subsequent trials demonstrated that more intensive therapy and, most recently, the addition of ifosfamide and etoposide to vincristine, Cytoxan, and doxorubicin improve the disease-free survival significantly from 50% to 69% ($p = .0005$) [80]. Children with metastatic disease treated aggressively with chemotherapy, local therapy to the primary tumor, and either whole-lung irradiation or total-body irradiation have achieved 3-year relapse-free survivals of 34% to 43%, indicating that some of these patients can be treated successfully [81, 82].

Late Effects

The late effects of therapy for children treated for Ewing's sarcoma include those related to chemotherapy, surgery, and radiotherapy. Late effects of chemotherapy are chiefly those related to anthracyclines, alkylating agents, and epipodophyllotoxins. These toxicities are cardiac dysfunction, infertility, and secondary leuke-mias, respectively [76, 83]. Functional late effects secondary to surgery vary greatly, depending on the nature and extent of surgery. The late effects of radiotherapy include abnormalities of bone growth, fibrosis, risk of bone fracture, and secondary malignancy [76].

Relapse and Palliation

Current trials are investigating dose intensification for patients with localized disease and the addition of new agents and high-dose (myeloablative therapy) for patients with metastatic disease. Treatment of a relapse is guided by the prior therapy. Patients treated previously with radiotherapy might benefit from surgery. Similarly, patients who had been treated with surgery could benefit from radiotherapy. Additional chemotherapy would be indicated also to assess response and to treat subclinical systemic disease. Reasonable palliation can also be achieved in patients by using radiotherapy, chemotherapy or, in some cases, surgery.

OSTEOSARCOMA
Epidemiologic Factors

Osteosarcoma (OS) is the most common malignant tumor of bone in children. The tumor is of mesenchymal origin, typically occurring in the metaphysis of long bones. The median age at diagnosis is 15 years, as appearance of the tumor is associated with the adolescent growth spurt. Annually, 5.6 cases per 1 million children occur in the United States, with a slight male predominance after age 13. Children with heritable retinoblastoma have a markedly increased risk of developing OS: approximately 1% per year in irradiated sites and 0.5% per year in nonirradiated sites [84].

Tumor suppressor genes (see "Retinoblastoma") play a role in the development of OS. Two genes implicated in OS are the retinoblastoma or *RB* gene and the *p53* tumor suppressor gene associated with the Li-Fraumeni syndrome. Despite the association of the *RB* gene with OS, not all tumors have *RB* mutations. Another tumor suppressor gene, *p53*, is now believed to be a causative factor in some cases of OS [85]. Although the exact mechanisms involved are under continued evaluation, *p53* is believed to regulate the transition from the G_1 to the S phase of the cell cycle [86].

The molecular mechanisms underlying the development of OS are not fully elucidated. Multiple genes are likely to be involved, with specific alterations of combinations of genes ultimately leading to tumorigenesis.

Pathologic Features

Most OSs arise in the medullary canal, spread centrifugally along the medullary canal, break through the cortex and the periosteum, and develop a soft-tissue mass. The notable exceptions, parosteal and periosteal OS, both arise in the cortex. A pseudocapsule may form from compressed tumor cells, with a fibrovascular zone of reactive tissue and an inflammatory component. The malignant cells break through the capsule to form satellite lesions. Skip metastases occur in 20% of cases. The majority of OSs are classic, further categorized as osteoblastic, fibroblastic, or chondroblastic. The other, less frequently occurring types of OS include telangiectatic, periosteal, and parosteal tumors. The latter form is more common in adults, often presenting in the femur and associated with a more indolent biology. The periosteal type may occur at any age and progresses at a rate intermediate between that of the parosteal and that of the remaining types of OS (see Chapter 26).

Presentation and Evaluation

Most children with OS present with pain, a swelling secondary to a soft-tissue mass or, occasionally, a fracture. Because these tumors tend to occur in adolescents, the pain or swelling may be attributed erroneously to sports-related trauma. More than 60% of OSs occur around the knee, including the distal femur, proximal tibia, or fibula; 10% occur in the proximal humerus; 10% occur in the trunk; and the remainder occur in such other bones as the skull and mandible.

The initial evaluation includes plain-film radiographs of the primary site, often revealing the sunburst sign, characteristic of horizontal bony spicules of new bone surrounding the tumor as it has broken through the cortex. Also typical on plain-film radiographs is the Codman's triangle resulting from the periosteal new bone at the margin of the tumor. CT scans demonstrate the cortical destruction, and MRI scans can best delineate the soft-tissue component and can search for skip metastases and intramedullary spread.

Surgeons also may require an arteriogram to determine the potential for limb-sparing surgery. The initial biopsy should be performed by a surgeon experienced in bone tumors. An open biopsy is preferable to a fine-needle aspiration. If a soft-tissue mass is present, that tissue is subjected to biopsy, as it most likely contains viable tumor.

The most common site of OS metastases is the lung, with other bones being the second most common site. Metastatic disease will be found in 10% to 20% of patients at the time of initial diagnosis. Hence, a CT scan to seek pulmonary metastases and a nuclear bone scan to seek other bony metastases are indicated in the initial evaluation of patients with OS.

Management

The management of OS includes complete surgical resection of the tumor and the administration of systemic chemotherapy. Historically, amputations were used for primary tumors in the extremities. More recently, particularly in the modern chemotherapeutic era, use of limb-sparing procedures has become more widespread. Although the primary tumor could be controlled with surgery, historical studies indicated that 80% of patients ultimately would succumb to metastatic disease [87].

Two prospective, randomized controlled trials in the 1980s demonstrated the improvement in survival with the use of adjuvant systemic chemotherapy in OS [88, 89]. The most active agents used in treating OS are doxorubicin, cisplatin, high-dose methotrexate, ifosfamide, and Cytoxan. Presurgical chemotherapy is being used more widely, and the histologic tumor response to chemotherapy provides prognostic information [90]. Patients with a poor response to presurgical chemotherapy are at high risk for the development of recurrence and can be identified. The relapse-free survivals of children with nonmetastatic OS in the modern chemotherapeutic era are 50% to 77% [91, 92].

Radiotherapy in the management of the primary tumor in OS is reserved for unresectable lesions or, in some selected cases, for preoperative or postoperative treatment or for palliation of symptoms. The vast majority of OS patients will undergo surgical resection; however, for those patients who refuse aggressive surgery or have unresectable disease, Albrecht et al. [93] reported the use of 50 to 70 Gy of photon irradiation in conjunction with chemotherapy to control primary OS.

Patients with close surgical margins and a poor response to presurgical chemotherapy may be at higher risk for local recurrence. Such patients sometimes are given postoperative radiotherapy to decrease local recurrence. The control of microscopic disease with radiotherapy in this setting is more likely to be successful than is primary radiotherapy to treat the gross tumor.

However, patients with poor response to chemotherapy and inadequate resections have a poorer outcome regardless of the addition of local radiotherapy [94]. Patients who develop pulmonary metastases can have long-term survival if all overt metastatic occurrences can be resected surgically. With aggressive treatment, including resection and systemic chemotherapy, a 30% to 40% 5-year survival after relapse has been reported [95].

Late Effects

Survivors of OS treated with multiagent chemotherapy and surgery are at risk for late complications of therapy [88]. These sequelae include cardiotoxicity related to doxorubicin, ototoxicity from cisplatin, and renal tubular and glomerular damage from ifosfamide and cisplatin. Fertility also may be affected after the use of such alkylating agents as cyclophosphamide and ifosfamide.

Musculoskeletal complications of limb-sparing surgery, such as fracture of a prosthesis or leg-length discrepancy, also can occur. Patients who have OS and a genetic predisposition may be at risk also for other malignancies, such as germline mutations of *p53*, as in the Li-Fraumeni syndrome.

Though much progress has been made in the treatment of OS and in the understanding of this tumor's cancer biology, still more work lies ahead to improve the outcome and to diminish the late sequelae of this tumor. Ongoing investigations of specific molecular targets seek to add to or enhance the agents already in use [88].

GERM-CELL TUMORS

Germ-cell tumors are neoplasms that derive from the totipotential primordial germ cells. These tumors can be germinomatous or embryonal. Pure germ-cell tumors are called *germinomatous* and are either seminomas (if presenting in boys) or dysgerminomas (if presenting in girls). The tumors with embryonal differentiation can be embryonal carcinomas, teratomas, endodermal sinus tumors, or choriocarcinomas. Germ-cell tumors containing a mixture of germ cells and embryonal cells are classified by their most malignant component.

The location of these tumors along the midline is a manifestation of the migration of the germ cells during embryonal development. Tumors can present in the sacrococcygeal area, the retroperitoneum, the mediastinum, the neck, and the pineal gland (see "Pineal Tumors").

Epidemiologic Factors

The presacral and sacrococcygeal teratomas that occur in newborns and young infants almost always are benign, whereas 65% of those occurring after age 6 months are malignant. Frequently, children with presacral or sacrococcygeal teratomas have congenital anomalies of the vertebrae, the genitourinary system, or the anorectum. The incidence of malignant germ-cell tumors in all ages in the United States is 2 to 3 per 1 million live births [96]. Children with germ-cell tumors can present with an external midline mass, a pelvic mass, a buttock mass, paralysis, or signs of urinary or fecal obstruction. Tumors arising in the testes can cause unilateral painless testicular enlargement. In prepubertal boys, the most common malignant tumor of the testes is the yolk sac tumor. Testicular tumors in adolescents have histologic features similar to those in affected adults. Ovarian tumors in girls can be dysgerminoma, teratoma (mature or immature), yolk sac tumors, embryonal carcinoma, or choriocarcinoma. Tumors presenting in the chest can cause respiratory signs and symptoms.

Diagnosis

Radiographic evaluation after thorough history and physical examination includes CT scanning of the chest, abdomen, and pelvis and a bone scan. Serum markers of the beta subunit of human chorionic gonadotropin and alpha-fetoprotein are indicated prior to surgery. If a malignant tumor is suspected or for tumors arising in older children, a biopsy should be performed, and preoperative chemotherapy should be used to allow maximum preservation of normal structures. The evaluation of children with a painless testicular mass includes ultrasonography of the testes, serum markers, and plain-film chest radiography. All scrotal masses are explored through an inguinal incision. A transscrotal biopsy should not be performed. Radiographic evaluation with CT scanning of the chest, abdomen, and pelvis is performed.

Staging

Pediatric cooperative groups have developed staging systems for ovarian and testicular tumors. Special note should be made that the presence of mature glial tissue does not step up the staging of stage I disease in a patient [97].

Treatment

Surgical resection of presacral and sacrococcygeal teratomas is the treatment of choice for benign tumors. In treating testicular germ-cell tumors, the effectiveness of chemotherapy has decreased the need for retroperitoneal lymph node dissections for nongerminomatous germ-cell tumors. Patients with stage I disease (i.e., those with disease limited to the testicle after complete resection via high inguinal orchiectomy; without clinical radiographic or histologic evidence of disease beyond the testes; and no elevation of tumor markers after surgery) should be observed closely. Boys with stage II or stage III disease; microscopic, residual, transscrotal orchiectomy with spill of tumor; or retroperitoneal nodal disease or elevated serum markers should receive chemotherapy, possibly followed by debulking surgery. The chemotherapeutic regimen currently includes cisplatin, etoposide, and bleomycin, based on a regimen developed in 1974 by Einhorn [98] using these three agents to treat disseminated testicular cancers.

For ovarian tumors, surgical exploration allows removal of the primary tumor and permits adequate staging. The ipsilateral pelvic lymph nodes and paraaortic and pericaval nodes at the level of the renal vessels should be examined and subjected to biopsy. The contralateral ovary should be examined carefully. Chemotherapy is highly effective for malignant ovarian germ-cell tumors.

The prognosis for germ-cell tumors depends on disease stage, with disease-free survivals of more than 90% for localized disease and 50% to 70% for more advanced disease. Children and adolescents with ovarian immature teratoma without foci of embryonal carcinoma, choriocarcinoma, or germinoma and stage I or stage II disease can be treated with surgical resection alone and can be observed [99]. Usually, those girls who developed recurrence can be salvaged with conventional-dose cisplatin, etoposide, and bleomycin chemotherapy.

NEUROBLASTOMA

Epidemiologic Factors

Neuroblastoma (NBL) is the fourth most common pediatric malignancy, representing 8% to 10% of cancers in children younger than age 15. The median age at diagnosis is 2 years; however, one-half of all malignancies diagnosed in the first month of life and one-third of all malignancies diagnosed in the first year of life are NBL

[100]. Despite great strides in the understanding of the tumor's biological makeup, the disease often takes a progressive clinical course. NBL is unique among human cancers in its ability to undergo spontaneous differentiation and regression. Disseminated NBL can regress spontaneously in a subset of infants with metastatic disease involving the liver, skin, and limited infiltration of the bone marrow. Residual microscopic disease after a resected localized NBL rarely results in recurrence of disease.

The tumor's unique clinical behavior has been known for several years; however, recent research in the molecular biological features of NBL led to advances in the treatment of the disease [101–104].

Presentation

NBL is a tumor of the autonomic nervous system and can occur anywhere this tissue is found. The most common sites are the abdomen (with an adrenal primary), in the spinal ganglia, in the thoracic ganglia, or in the pelvis (primarily in the organ of Zuckerkandl). Presentation of patients varies, depending on the site and extent of disease. Patients can present with an abdominal or flank mass, with respiratory symptoms from a thoracic primary tumor, with Horner's syndrome from a cervicothoracic primary lesion, or with bladder symptoms resulting from a pelvic primary tumor. Children with advanced disease that involves the bone marrow might appear pale or bruise easily or can experience bone pain, fever, or general failure to thrive. A syndrome combining opsoclonus (rapid multidirectional eye movements) and polymyoclonus (truncal ataxia) occurs in approximately 5% of patients, generally with early-stage NBL [105].

Diagnosis and Evaluation

The diagnostic evaluation of patients in whom NBL is suspected includes an investigation of the primary tumor. Often, abdominal ultrasonography will demonstrate a mass, or plain-film radiography will show calcifications. The diagnosis of NBL is established if an unequivocal pathologic diagnosis is made from tumor tissue or if the bone marrow contains unequivocal tumor cells and the urine contains increased catecholamine metabolites (vanillylmandelic acid or homovanillic acid levels greater than 3 standard deviations above the mean per milligram of creatinine for age) [106]. Imaging of the primary tumor either by CT scan or MRI is

performed, as is a search for metastases. The metastatic evaluation includes bone marrow aspiration and biopsy, nuclear bone scan, and an abdominal CT or ultrasonography to evaluate the liver. The ^{131}I or ^{123}I metaiodobenzylguanidine (MIBG) scan is becoming a standard part of the evaluation of NBL [107].

Staging

The staging system now recommended for NBL is known as the *International Neuroblastoma Staging System* (INSS; Table 25.9). Prior to the development of this staging system, three major staging systems had been used worldwide. Although these various systems provided similar results in distinguishing low-stage patients from high-stage patients, they embodied substantial dif-

Table 25.9 International Neuroblastoma Staging System

Stage	Definition
1	Localized tumor with complete gross excision, with or without microscopic residual disease; representative ipsilateral lymph nodes negative for tumor microscopically (lymph nodes adherent to and removed with primary possibly positive)
2A	Localized tumor with incomplete gross excision; representative ipsilateral nonadherent lymph nodes negative for tumor microscopically
2B	Localized tumor with or without complete gross excision, with ipsilateral nonadherent lymph nodes positive for tumor; enlarged contralateral lymph nodes negative microscopically
3	Unresectable unilateral tumor infiltrating across the midline, with or without regional lymph node involvement; or localized unilateral tumor with contralateral regional lymph node involvement; or midline tumor with bilateral extension by infiltration (unresectable) or by lymph node involvement
4	Any primary tumor with dissemination to distant lymph nodes, bone, bone marrow, liver, skin, other organs (except as defined for stage 4S)
4S	Limited to infants younger than 1 yr and localized primary tumor (as defined for stage 1, 2A, or 2B) with dissemination limited to skin, liver, or bone marrow (or all). Bone marrow involvement must be < 10% of total nucleated cells identified as malignant on bone marrow biopsy or aspirate; more extensive bone marrow involvement stage 4

Source: Reprinted with permission from GM Brodeur, RC Seeger, A Barrett, et al., International criteria for diagnosis, staging, and response to treatment in patients with neuroblastoma. *J Clin Oncol* 6:1874–1881, 1988.

ferences that precluded comparisons regarding individual patients and a variety of clinical situations. The INSS was developed by an international conference and was presented for discussion at the Fourth International Research Symposium on Advances in Neuroblastoma Research in Philadelphia in May 1987. In addition to a new, mutually accepted staging system, criteria for the diagnosis of NBL and strict definitions of response were established [106].

Evaluation of the tumor tissue by pediatric pathologists is critical for assessment of the Shimada histologic classification. Shimada et al. [108] developed a histologic classification of NBL on the basis of the stroma (stroma-rich versus stroma-poor, according to the presence or absence of schwannian spindle-cell stroma), the extent of differentiation, and the mitotic-karyorrhectic index. Patients' ages were incorporated into the prognostic scheme of these researchers (Table 25.10).

Tumor Biology

In addition to clinical staging, the assessment of biological markers has become an important component of the workup and actually may be the most critical determinant in guiding therapy. Several chromosomal abnormalities of NBL cells have been identified. One is the partial monosomy of the short arm of chromosome 1. These deletions are found in 70% to 80% of patients with near-diploid tumors. The deletions vary in their proximal breakpoints, but the region of consistent deletion is mapped to sub-bands of 1p36, and loss of heterozygosity occurs for the deleted alleles. Further abnormalities include that of chromosome 17; double-minutes or extrachromosomal chromatin bodies; homogeneously staining regions that are a cytogenetic

manifestation of gene amplification in which the amplified sequences are integrated chromosomally; and variability in modal karyotypes.

The majority of tumors studied cytogenetically have modal karyotypes in the diploid range; however, many tumors that have been studied are hyperdiploid or near-triploid. Often, the hyperdiploid and near-triploid tumors in infants have increased chromosomal numbers without any identifiable structural rearrangements. Such patients have a relatively favorable prognosis. Frequently, patients with near-diploid tumors and older patients with hyperdiploid tumors do have structural rearrangements that predict a more aggressive course. Flow-cytometric analysis of human NBL cells also can demonstrate changes in DNA content [101, 109–112].

Some of the foregoing biological properties have been shown to demonstrate clinical significance in NBL patients. Amplification of N-myc was found in approximately 25% of primary tumors and was correlated strongly with advanced disease [102, 103]. Independent of age and stage of the patients, however, N-myc amplification was associated in several studies with rapid tumor progression and poor clinical outcome [102–104, 113–115]. These studies suggest that N-myc amplification is a marker of aggressive biological tumor properties in some patients. Loss of heterozygosity of 1p is associated strongly with N-myc amplification, and both of these markers are associated with poor patient outcomes [116]. Deletion of the short arm of chromosome 1 (1p) has been established as an indicator of tumor aggressivity [117]. The unbalanced gain of genetic material in chromosome 17 (gain of segment 17q21-qter) now has been shown to be a powerful prognostic indicator of adverse outcome in NBL patients [118].

Although the pathogenesis of NBL is unknown, the tumor is believed to derive from the sympathoadrenal cells of the neural crest. Studies of neurotrophic factors and their tyrosine kinase receptors in NBL have shown a correlation between the expression of the nerve growth factor receptor TRKA and clinical outcome [119]. Brodeur et al. [115] studied the expression of TRKA in tumors from 77 NBL patients and 5 ganglioglioma patients. They found a high level of expression in 82% of the NBL samples. All patients who had stages I, II, and IVS tumors (by the CCG staging system) without N-myc amplification showed high TRKA expression. This outcome was contrasted to 10 of 11 tumors with N-myc amplification that demonstrated low TRKA expression [119]. TRKA expression was strongly correlated with survival; the 5-year survival of patients with high expression was 86%, as compared to 14% survival in the patients with low TRKA expression ($p < .001$).

Table 25.10 Clinical, Histologic, and Biological Markers and Risk Group Assignment

Factor	Low Risk	Intermediate Risk	High Risk
Age (yr)	< 1	> 1	> 1
Stage	1, 2, 4S	3, 4	3, 4
N-myc status	Nonamplified	Nonamplified	Amplified
DNA ploidy	Hyperdiploid	Near-diploid	Near-diploid
Shimada classification	Favorable	Favorable or unfavorable	Unfavorable

Note: Patients can have some markers that fall into different risk strata. Treatments are based on all factors considered together for a given patient.

Although the biological role of nerve growth factor and TRKA in NBL is unknown, some theorize that the expression of these factors reflects the propensity of NBL to regress or differentiate.

Treatment

NBL can be divided into genetically distinct groups on the basis of biological properties. When these biological characteristics are combined with clinical properties, patients can be stratified into risk groups, and therapy can be tailored for patients on the basis of these clinical and biological groupings. The modalities employed in the management of NBL include surgery, chemotherapy, and radiotherapy. Surgery plays a role in the establishment of the diagnosis, in obtaining sufficient tissue for biological studies and for molecular characterization of a tumor, and in excising a primary tumor when feasible. Often, complete or even partial resection of a primary tumor is sufficient therapy and is the treatment of choice in favorable patients. Second-look surgery or postinduction chemotherapy is used in situations in which an initial tumor is unresectable but can be rendered resectable with chemotherapy. These modalities are used also to assess response to chemotherapy and to follow induction chemotherapy with removal of residual disease.

NBLs respond to several chemotherapeutic agents, including doxorubicin, cisplatin, melphalan, cyclophosphamide, etoposide (VP-16), and teniposide (VM-26). Combination chemotherapy has been used to exploit differences in mechanism of action and differences in toxicities and to avoid development of drug resistance. The effectiveness of chemotherapy in treating NBL has been evaluated in several clinical trials [100]. NBL is also sensitive to ionizing irradiation [120]. Low doses of fractionated radiotherapy with total doses in the range of 15 to 30 Gy are effective [121]. Very low-dose radiotherapy (3–6 Gy in three to four fractions) has been given to neonates with respiratory compromise secondary to massive hepatomegaly (stage 4S). Radiotherapy doses of 18 to 30 Gy have been used to treat regional disease, including lymph node drainage areas. The role of local radiotherapy in the treatment of children with localized NBL depends on the risk group and is controversial. Some studies demonstrate a survival advantage with the use of radiotherapy, and other studies show no such advantage [122]. Localized NBL compromises a spectrum of patients whose prognosis depends on several factors both clinical and biological.

Patients with NBL are assigned to risk groups on the basis of clinical and biological features. The clinical factors include the age and stage of affected patients, and the biological features are N-myc status, Shimada histology, and DNA ploidy. Table 25.10 shows the risk assignment using these criteria. Evans et al. [123] described the successful management of children with stage 1, stage 2A, stage 2B, and stage 4S disease without adjuvant therapy. The results were an event-free survival of 86% for patients given no adjuvant therapy after initial surgery, as compared to 52% event-free survival for those who were given adjuvant therapy. That study emphasized the importance of recognizing clinical and biological factors in determining treatment.

The Children's Cancer Study Group reported the treatment of children with stage 3 NBL on the basis of risk grouping. Children with unfavorable characteristics received intensive multimodality therapy, with autologous bone marrow transplantation in some cases. Children with INSS stage 3 disease and favorable characteristics underwent chemotherapy followed by delayed surgery and radiotherapy to gross residual disease after surgery [124]. Children of any age and with favorable biological characteristics had a 4-year event-free survival of 100%. Children who were older than 1 year and had unfavorable biological characteristics had a 4-year event-free survival of 54%; those who were younger than 1 year and had at least one unfavorable biological marker had an event-free survival of 90%.

These studies demonstrate both the current approach to the treatment of NBL using risk grouping and the success of this approach. Although the best treatment of advanced disease remains to be determined, disease in such children generally is treated aggressively, often with myeloablative regimens with or without total-body irradiation, and treatment is followed by bone-marrow or stem-cell rescue. The goals of risk-related treatment are to improve the outcome in patients with unfavorable markers and at the same time to spare the patients with more favorable markers both the short- and the long-term toxicities of unnecessary treatment.

A recently published randomized trial compared continuation chemotherapy to a high-dose chemotherapy with total-body irradiation intensification for patients with high-risk NBL [125]. Subsequently, patients were randomly assigned to the addition of 13-cis-retinoic acid for 6 months after completion of cytotoxic therapy. This trial showed that treatment with myeloablative therapy and autologous transplantation improved the event-free survival in these high-risk patients and that the addition of cis-retinoic acid was beneficial for both groups of patients. Cis-retinoic acid appears to be most effective in patients with minimal residual disease. This agent seems to act by decreasing proliferation and inducing differentiation of NBL cells and may be a promising additional therapy in patients who have high-risk disease and have achieved a minimal disease state [125].

MEDULLOBLASTOMA

Epidemiologic Factors

Brain tumors in children account for approximately 20% of childhood cancers. Of them, medulloblastoma is the most common CNS tumor [126]. Medulloblastoma is a primitive tumor thought to be derived from multipotential cells in the external granular layer of the cerebellum. The World Health Organization classification of brain tumors (see Chapter 28) defines medulloblastoma as an embryonal tumor. PNETs that arise in the posterior fossa are called *medulloblastomas*. The median age at diagnosis is 5 to 6 years, although 30% present before age 3.

Diagnosis and Staging

The most common presenting symptoms of medulloblastoma are headache, vomiting, and nausea. Most frequently, the observed signs are papilledema, ataxia or other gait disturbance, and cranial nerve deficits. Patients with suspected brain tumors should undergo MRI (Fig. 25.3). Medulloblastomas are seeding tumors with a propensity to disseminate throughout the neuraxis. A spinal MRI and cerebrospinal fluid evaluation should be performed on all patients. The staging of medulloblastoma is based on the surgical assessment of the tumor's extent and on radiographic imaging (Table 25.11). In the Langston modification of the Chang staging system, children with total or near-total resection (< 1.5 cm²) and M0 disease are considered to be at standard risk. Patients with more advanced disease are considered to be at high risk.

Treatment

The approach to management involves an attempt to resect all gross tumor completely. Operative mortality is rare (< 2%), but surgical morbidity occurs in up to 40% of cases and can include the posterior fossa syndrome of mutism, pharyngeal dysfunction, respiratory dys-

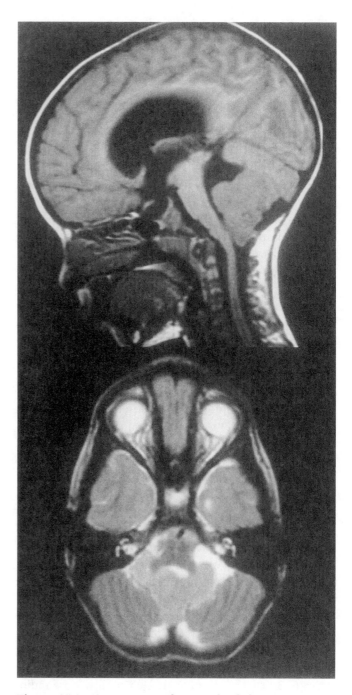

Figure 25.3   T₁- (upper) and T₂-weighted (lower) magnetic resonance images of a child with a medulloblastoma filling the inferior fourth ventricle and causing marked hydrocephalus.

function, and ataxia [127]. Generally, these operative sequelae are reversible over the months after surgery. Resection of all or nearly all gross tumor is associated with an improved outcome [128].

Craniospinal axis irradiation (CSI) postoperatively is essential in the management of medulloblastoma. Within a decade after Cushing's first description of this tumor, CSI was reported as effective therapy [129, 130].

Table 25.11 Langston Modification of Chang Staging for Medulloblastoma

T1	Tumor < 3 cm in diameter
T2	Tumor ≥ 3 cm in diameter
T3a	Tumor > 3 cm with extension into aqueduct of Sylvius or foramen of Luschka (or both)
T3b	Tumor > 3 cm with extension into brainstem
T4	Tumor > 3 cm with extension past aqueduct of Sylvius or foramen magnum
M0	No gross subarachnoid or hematogenous metastasis
M1	Microscopic tumor cells in cerebrospinal fluid
M2	Gross nodular seeding beyond primary site in the cerebellar or cerebral subarachnoid space
M3	Gross nodular spinal seeding
M4	Metastases outside the cerebrospinal axis

Source: Modified by J Langston from CH Chang, EM Housepian, C Herbert Jr, An operative staging system and a megavoltage radiotherapeutic technic for cerebellar medulloblastomas. *Radiology* 93:1351–1359, 1969.

After CSI, a boost dose of radiotherapy is given to the posterior fossa or to the area of original disease in those with supratentorial presentations. Medulloblastoma is a relatively radiosensitive tumor. The standard dose to the craniospinal axis has been 35 to 36 Gy, with the final dose to the tumor bed being 54 to 55 Gy. Medulloblastoma is also a chemosensitive tumor, with high response rates to such alkylating agents as cyclophosphamide and platinum [131, 132].

The combination of chemotherapy and reduced-dose CSI in patients has been studied; for patients who are between ages 3 and 10 and have nondisseminated medulloblastoma, the 5-year progression-free survival was 79% [133]. The reduced doses used were 23.4 Gy of CSI, with the full dose of 55 Gy being delivered to the tumor bed. The goal of the combined chemotherapy and lower-dose irradiation is to minimize the late effects on neurocognitive development and growth while maintaining disease control.

Several studies have sought to evaluate the effectiveness of chemotherapy in high-risk medulloblastoma patients who have either residual disease greater than 1.5 cm³ or CNS dissemination. In a randomized trial performed by the CCG, patients with T3b, T4, or metastasis-positive disease had a statistically improved 5-year disease-free and overall survival when receiving chemotherapy in addition to radiotherapy and a 46% disease-free and 57% overall survival as compared to 0%, and 19% for those not receiving chemotherapy [134]. Packer et al. [135] reported the use of adjuvant lomustine (CCNU), vincristine, and cisplatin in children with high-risk medulloblastoma. These children received vincristine during radiotherapy, followed by eight cycles of chemotherapy after radiotherapy. The 5-year disease-free survival was 85%, although some patients included in this trial would no longer be considered at high risk.

The current approach to treating children with medulloblastoma is to assign patients to risk groups on the basis of the extent of disease, which includes the intraoperative surgical and postoperative radiographic assessments. Children with T1 to T3 disease, no metastases, and a gross resection are considered standard-risk; those with T4 or M1 through M4 disease or residual tumor are considered high-risk. In the current Intergroup POG/CCG study, children with less than 1.5 cm³ of residual tumor are eligible for standard-risk treatment. The expected 5-year disease-free survival for children with medulloblastoma is approximately 60%, although reports of disease-free survivals of 80 to 90% have been made by single institutions with the use of chemotherapy [126]. The current goals of the treatment of medulloblastoma are to increase the survival of children with high-risk disease, to decrease the toxicity in children with standard-risk disease, and to identify new prognostic factors to tailor treatments and to improve outcomes.

Most recurrences in patients with nondisseminated disease (M0) at diagnosis are in the posterior fossa, although almost one-half of these relapses are associated also with concurrent dissemination elsewhere in the CNS. Treatment of recurrences with high-dose chemotherapy and autologous stem-cell rescue has shown some promise [136].

BRAINSTEM GLIOMAS
Epidemiologic Factors

Brainstem gliomas are glial tumors arising in the midbrain, pons, or medulla, though the majority of brainstem gliomas occur in the pons. They can be either diffusely infiltrative or focally discrete lesions. Usually, the pontine lesions are diffusely infiltrative and expand into the midbrain or the medulla and the cerebellopontine peduncles (Fig. 25.4). Owing to their location, brainstem gliomas are not subjected routinely to biopsy. Studies in which histologic workup has been performed reveal that approximately one-half are fibrillary astrocytomas and one-half are anaplastic astrocytomas or glioblastomas [137]. Most commonly, brainstem gliomas present in children between the ages of 3 and 9.

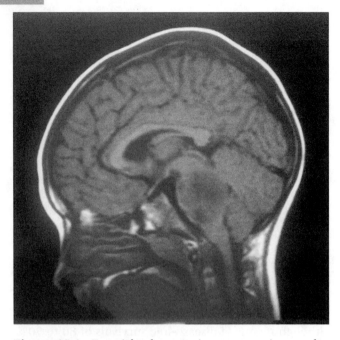

Figure 25.4 T$_1$-weighted magnetic resonance image of a child with a pontine glioma, demonstrating the infiltrative tumor with pontine expansion.

Diagnosis

Brainstem gliomas produce symptoms of ataxia and such cranial nerve palsies as diplopia, facial asymmetry, and swallowing and speech difficulties. The morbidity of biopsy coupled with the lack of therapeutic options based on histologic characteristics argue against the need for biopsy unless the radiologic imaging is unusual. In such situations, a stereotactic biopsy is performed to confirm the diagnosis.

The dorsally exophytic tumors of the brainstem may require a ventriculoperitoneal shunt to relieve hydrocephalus, and these tumors can be considered for subtotal resection. This subgroup can be associated with a 5-year survival rate of 75% after subtotal resection. Pathologically, such tumors tend to be juvenile pilocytic astrocytomas (JPAs) [137].

Treatment

The primary treatment for most brainstem gliomas is radiotherapy. The pontine tumors are uniformly fatal, but patients do experience a temporary improvement in relief from symptoms. The use of hyperfractionated radiotherapy has been studied by several institutions and by cooperative groups. Initial reports showed modest im-

provements in survival as compared to conventional once-a-day fractionation [138, 139]. The majority of children treated with hyperfractionated radiotherapy are steroid-dependent. Other late toxicities (e.g., hearing loss and leukoencephalopathy) have been reported [140]. With further follow-up, conventional once-a-day fractionation appears to be as efficacious as hyperfractionated irradiation for diffuse brainstem gliomas. The median survival for children with diffusely infiltrative pontine gliomas is 9 to 12 months. Chemotherapy has shown little efficacy, although ongoing trials are exploring new agents and new classes of agents.

HIGH-GRADE MALIGNANT GLIOMAS
Epidemiologic Factors and Pathologic Classification

Malignant gliomas represent approximately 8% to 12% of pediatric brain tumors and 15% of glial tumors [141]. Half to two-thirds of these gliomas are anaplastic astrocytomas, 30% to 40% are glioblastomas, and the remainder are anaplastic oligodendrogliomas and mixed gliomas. The histologic grading system used most commonly is the three-tiered system consisting of astrocytoma, anaplastic astrocytoma, and glioblastoma multiforme [142]. Most often, high-grade malignant gliomas occur in the cerebral hemispheres and thalamus. Up to one-third of these tumors present in children younger than 5 years.

Treatment

The treatment of high-grade malignant gliomas involves aggressive surgical resection for tumors in the cerebral hemispheres, although tumors in some regions, such as the thalamic region, rarely can be resected fully [143]. After resection, radiotherapy is indicated except in children younger than age 3; these youngsters often are placed on chemotherapeutic protocols to delay radiotherapy so as to avoid the significant neurocognitive effects of the latter treatment mode in this age group [126]. Generally, radiotherapy is administered to the tumor with a 2-cm margin (judged from MRI scans) with doses of 54 to 60 Gy in conventional fractionation. Radiosurgical boosts can be given to small areas of residual disease after conventional fractionated radiotherapy, as in adults [144].

Chemotherapy in pediatric high-grade gliomas has been studied by the CCG. Combination postoperative irradiation and chemotherapy with vincristine, CCNU, and prednisone produced an improvement in progression-free survival superior to postoperative irradiation alone [145]. The outcome of children with high-grade gliomas is better than that of adults, although long-term survival remains only 15% to 30% for those with anaplastic astrocytomas and 10% to 15% for those with glioblastomas. Children who are able to undergo complete resections do have a superior prognosis (as high as 40% to 60% in some series) [143].

LOW-GRADE GLIOMAS
Epidemiologic Factors

Low-grade gliomas comprise 40% of pediatric brain tumors and include several histologic subtypes. The tumors can be astrocytomas, oligodendrogliomas, mixed gliomas, and mixed neuroepithelial tumors. Most often, astrocytomas are supratentorial and frequently occur in the optic system pathways and in the thalamus. Tumors of the optic pathway almost always are low-grade astrocytomas, obviating biopsy confirmation in most cases. Children with neurofibromatosis type 1 have an increased risk of developing optic pathway gliomas. In one series of 42 children, 41% with these tumors had neurofibromatosis type 1 [146]. Infratentorial astrocytomas involve the cerebellum or the brainstem (Fig. 25.5). JPA is one of the more common pediatric astrocytomas. This tumor has an indolent course and, on MRI, has a characteristic appearance of a well-circumscribed, uniformly enhancing lesion.

Pathologic Features

Low-grade astrocytomas in children include JPA, fibrillary astrocytomas, gemistocytic astrocytomas, protoplasmic astrocytomas, and giant-cell and pleomorphic xanthoastrocytomas. Microscopically, JPAs show parallel arrays of glial fibers. Oligodendrogliomas occur less frequently in children and sometimes are diagnosed in patients with a history of seizures.

Mixed oligodendrogliomas and astrocytomas also can occur in children. Low-grade gliomas can be multifocal and ultimately can result in disseminated disease. Tumor dissemination occurs either at diagnosis or at progression in 20% of children with JPA [147, 148]. Malignant transformation occurs in 10% to 15% of children with low-grade astrocytomas [149].

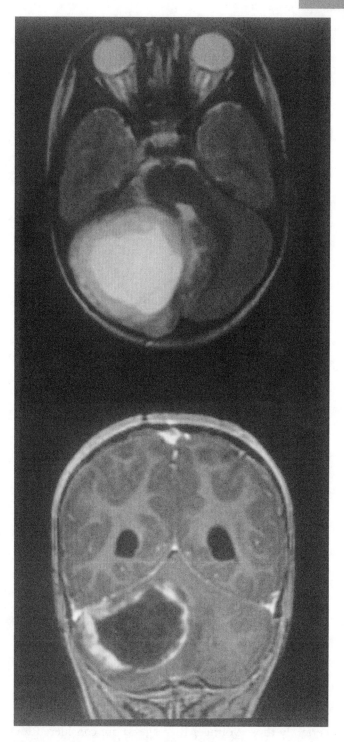

Figure 25.5 T_2- (upper) and T_1-weighted (lower) magnetic resonance images of a child with a right cerebellar astrocytoma, showing a large, peripherally enhancing cyst with mass effect on the fourth ventricle.

Presentation and Diagnosis

Children with low-grade astrocytomas present with a long history of rather nonspecific symptoms. Signs and symptoms of increased intracranial pressure can be present, particularly in midline tumors and tumors of the cerebellum wherein cerebrospinal fluid obstruction can occur. Neck stiffness and head tilt can result from increased intracranial pressure brought on by cerebellar tumors. Seizures occur in almost 75% of children with tumors of the cerebral hemispheres. Tumors of the optic pathways can cause loss of vision. Tumors of the hypothalamic region can result in neuroendocrine deficits.

Treatment

The most important aspect of managing low-grade astrocytomas of the cerebral hemispheres in children is resection. In modern series, complete resection is possible in 70% to 90% of cases. Gross total resection confirmed by postoperative MRI is associated with nearly 100% long-term disease control [150]. After subtotal resection, pediatric patients can be observed if they are neurologically stable. At the time of disease progression, reoperation is considered.

Radiotherapy is reserved for patients with inoperable progressive disease. No overall survival benefit accrues to the addition of radiotherapy immediately after subtotal resection [150]. Fractionated radiotherapy using conformal techniques (e.g., stereotactic radiotherapy delivering doses of 54 Gy) is recommended when radiotherapy is used [151]. The overall survival rates for children with low-grade astrocytomas treated with subtotal resection and radiotherapy are reported variously as 67% to 100% at 5 years and 63% to 89% at 10 years [152, 153].

Chemotherapy for low-grade astrocytomas has been used in recent years to delay or avoid radiotherapy in very young patients. Children younger than age 5 (and certainly those younger than age 3) are considered for chemotherapy using such agents as vincristine and carboplatin. Overall response rates to chemotherapy are 70% to 100%, although complete responses are unusual [154, 155]. Chemotherapy seems to delay (or, in some cases, avoid) the need for radiotherapy for childhood low-grade astrocytomas, although generally these tumors have an indolent course, calling into question the efficacy of any cytotoxic treatment [156].

EPENDYMOMA

Epidemiologic Factors

Ependymoma is the third most common brain tumor of childhood. These tumors arise from the ependymal lining cells of the ventricular system and can arise throughout the CNS. The majority of ependymomas occur intracranially; approximately 10% arise along the spinal cord. Two-thirds occur in the posterior fossa. Ependymomas can occur in children of all ages, with a median age at diagnosis of between 3 and 5 years, although infants also can develop this tumor.

Pathologic Features

Pathologically, ependymomas are classified as ependymoma (cellular, papillary, epithelial, clear-cell, or mixed), anaplastic ependymoma, myxopapillary ependymoma (generally arising within the conus medullaris and filum terminale), or subependymoma [157]. The tumor known as an *ependymoblastoma* is classified as a primitive neuroectodermal tumor, with an incidence, behavior, and outcome different from those of ependymoma.

Presentation and Diagnosis

Children with ependymoma can present with nausea and vomiting, headache, head tilt, hearing loss, or other cranial nerve dysfunction. Fewer than 15% of children will present with CNS dissemination [158]. The evaluation of children with a suspected ependymoma includes recording a complete history, conducting a physical examination, obtaining MRI scans of the brain and the spine, and examining the lumbar cerebrospinal fluid (Fig. 25.6).

Treatment

Initial surgical resection is critical in the management of ependymoma. After surgical resection, a postoperative MRI is performed to aid in the assessment of postoperative residual disease. Gross total resection is possible in approximately 50% of cases and appears to correlate with outcome [159]. The incidence of postoperative neurologic complications, including the posterior fossa syndrome, is approximately 40% [160].

Although surgical resection plays an important role in the management of ependymoma, surgery alone re-

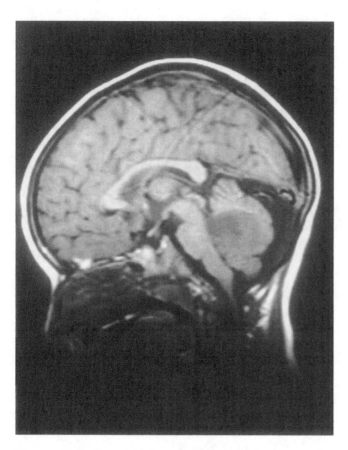

Figure 25.6 T_1-weighted magnetic resonance image of a child with an anaplastic ependymoma demonstrating a hypointense mass filling the fourth ventricle.

sults in poor survival. Radiotherapy is indicated for the treatment of ependymoma. The 5-year progression-free survival of patients with intracranial ependymoma from several institutions treated with resection and radiotherapy is 40% to 60% [161, 162]. The current standard radiotherapeutic protocol for a posterior fossa ependymoma is to treat the posterior fossa but not to treat the entire craniospinal axis in patients with no evidence of dissemination. Recent series with modern imaging fail to show a benefit to CSI [163]. The dose of irradiation recommended in most protocols is 50 to 55 Gy. The use of three-dimensional conformal radiotherapy techniques may decrease the late neurologic toxicity and, at the same time, permit increased dose and, possibly, increased local tumor control.

Ependymomas do respond to chemotherapy; however, no proved benefit to chemotherapy has been demonstrated in ependymoma for children older than 3 years [126]. Various chemotherapeutic regimens have been studied in protocols designed to delay or even eliminate radiotherapy in very young children [164]. The drugs that have been used include cisplatin, etopo-

side, carboplatin, vincristine, cyclophosphamide, and CCNU. Such other agents as topotecan, a topoisomerase I inhibitor, are being studied in patients with unresectable disease [165].

Treatment of Relapse

The majority of relapses of ependymoma occur in the primary site, although 10% of patients will develop metastases elsewhere in the neuraxis. Treatment of recurrence can include reoperation, chemotherapy, and reirradiation using stereotactic radiosurgery [126]. This technique delivers a single large fraction of radiotherapy to a focal site without giving an additional dose to the remainder of the prior irradiation field. Stereotactic radiosurgery also can play a role in boosting sites of residual gross tumor after initial resection [126].

PINEAL TUMORS
Epidemiologic Factors

Tumors arising in the pineal region of the brain account for 0.5% to 2.0% of pediatric brain tumors. Three major types of tumors occur in this area: germ-cell tumors, pineal parenchymal tumors, and astrocytomas. Approximately 50% to 66% of pineal tumors are germ-cell tumors, pineal parenchymal tumors make up 17% of tumors, and astrocytomas comprise 15%. Germ-cell tumors have a peak age incidence of 10 to 14 years, pineal parenchymal tumors occur in the first decade of life, and astrocytomas occur in two age peaks: 2 to 6 years and 12 to 18 years [166, 167].

Presentation and Evaluation

Most commonly, children with tumors in the pineal area present with nonspecific signs of increased intracranial pressure. If such tumors extend anteriorly and caudally and involve the tectal area and compress the midbrain, Parinaud's syndrome can occur. This syndrome is manifested by the paralysis of upward gaze, slight dilatation of the pupils that react to accommodation but not to light, conversion nystagmus, and eyelid retraction. The preoperative evaluation should include a high-resolution MRI of the brain and the spine. Measurement of serum alpha-fetoprotein and the beta subunit of human chorionic gonadotrophin and the cerebrospinal fluid levels of these germ-cell tumor markers also should be obtained. A biopsy of a pineal region tumor should be performed, if possible, because the appropriate therapy and the patient's prognosis are determined by a tumor's histologic makeup. Almost 90% of patients with pineal tumors will have hydrocephalus and increased intracranial pressure. Third ventriculostomy has become the procedure of choice to control obstructive hydrocephalus. Aggressive surgical resections can be associated with significant morbidity in this location and generally are not performed.

Treatment

Once a diagnosis has been made, the appropriate therapy can be determined. Germinomas are radiosensitive tumors; thus, the recommended dose to the primary tumor is approximately 50 Gy. The appropriate volume for nonmultiple midline cases of germinoma without cerebrospinal fluid dissemination is controversial. Some centers recommend whole-brain radiotherapy to 25 Gy, with a boost to the primary tumor. Others recommend low-dose full CSI, as these tumors do have the propensity to seed the neuraxis. The control rates are 90% with local and whole-brain irradiation or with CSI [168, 169]. Germinomas also are chemosensitive, and the use of chemotherapy to reduce the dose or volume of irradiation (or both) have been advocated by some to reduce the toxicities of irradiation.

REFERENCES

1. Yandell DW, Campbell TA, Dayton SH, et al. Oncogenic point mutations in the human retinoblastoma gene: their application to genetic counseling. *N Engl J Med* 321:1689–1695, 1989.
2. Coppes MJ, Higuchi M, Liefers GJ, et al. Inherited *WT1* mutation in Denys-Drash syndrome. *Cancer Res* 52:6125–6128, 1992.
3. Call KM, Glaser T, Ito CY. Isolation and characterization of a zinc finger polypeptide gene at the human chromosome 11 Wilms' tumor locus. *Cell* 60:509–520, 1990.
4. Li FP, Fraumeni JF, Mulvihill JJ, et al. A cancer family syndrome in twenty-four kindreds. *Cancer Res* 48:5358–5362, 1988.
5. Santibanez-Koref MF, Birch JM, Hartley AL, et al. p53 germline mutations in Li-Fraumeni syndrome. *Lancet* 338:1490–1491, 1991.
6. Knudson AG. Mutation and cancer: statistical study of retinoblastoma. *Proc Natl Acad Sci USA* 68:820–823, 1971.
7. Cavenee WK, Dryja TP, Phillips RA, et al. Expression of recessive alleles by chromosomal mechanisms in retinoblastoma. *Nature* 305:779–784, 1989.

8. Ries LAG, Miller BA, Hankey BF (eds). *SEER Cancer Statistics Review, 1973–1991.* [NIH Pub. No. 94–2789.] Bethesda: National Cancer Institute, 1994.
9. Filipovich AH, Mathur A, Kamat D, Shapiro RS. Primary immunodeficiencies: genetic risk factors for lymphoma. *Cancer Res* 52(suppl):s5465–s5467, 1992.
10. Taylor A, Metcalfe J, Thick J, Mak Y. Leukemia and lymphoma in ataxia telangiectasia. *Blood* 87:423–436, 1996.
11. Reynolds R, Saunders LD, Layefsky ME, Lemp GF. The spectrum of acquired immunodeficiency syndrome (AIDS) associated malignancies in San Francisco, 1980–1987. *Am J Epidemiol* 137:19–30, 1993.
12. Fischer A, Blanche S, LeBidois J, et al. Anti-B cell monoclonal antibodies in the treatment of severe B-cell lymphoproliferative syndrome following bone marrow and organ transplantation. *N Engl J Med* 324:1451–1456, 1991.
13. Anagnostopoulos I, Herbst H, Niedobiteck G, Stein H. Demonstration of monoclonal EBV genomes in Hodgkin's disease and k-1 positive anaplastic large cell lymphoma by combined southern blot and in situ hybridization. *Blood* 74:810–816, 1989.
14. Razzouk BI, Srinivas S, Sample CE, et al. Epstein-Barr virus DNA recombination and loss in sporadic Burkitt's lymphoma. *J Infect Dis* 173:529–535, 1996.
15. Harris N, Jaffe E, Stein H, et al. A revised European American classification of lymphoid neoplasms: a proposal from the International Lymphoma Study Group. *Blood* 84:1361–1392, 1994.
16. Sandlund, JT, Hutchison RE, Crist WM. Non-Hodgkin's lymphoma. In Fernbach DJ, Vietti TJ (eds), *Clinical Pediatric Oncology* (4th ed). St Louis: Mosby–Year Book, 1991:337–353.
17. Sandlund JT, Downing JR, Crist WM. Non-Hodgkin's lymphoma in childhood. *N Engl J Med* 334:1238–1248, 1996.
18. Sandlund JT, Pui CH, Santana VM, et al. Clinical features and treatment outcome for children with CD30+ large-cell non-Hodgkin's lymphoma. *J Clin Oncol* 12:895–898, 1994.
19. Murphy SE. Classification, staging and end results of treatment of childhood non-Hodgkin's lymphomas: dissimilarities from lymphomas in adults. *Semin Oncol* 7:332–339, 1980.
20. Link MP, Shuster JJ, Donaldson SS, et al. Treatment of children and young adults with early-stage non-Hodgkin's lymphoma. *N Engl J Med* 337:1259–1266, 1997.
21. MacMahon B. Epidemiology of Hodgkin's disease. *Cancer Res* 26:1189–1201, 1966.
22. Fraumeni J, Li F. Hodgkin's disease in childhood: an epidemiologic study. *J Natl Cancer Inst* 42:681–691, 1969.
23. Fraumeni J. Family studies in Hodgkin's disease. *Cancer Res* 34:1164–1165, 1974.
24. Muñoz N, Davidson R. Infectious mononucleosis and Hodgkin's disease. *Int J Cancer* 22:10–13, 1978.
25. Lukes RJ, Butler JJ. Report of the nomenclature committee. *Cancer Res* 26:1063–1081, 1966.
26. Carbone PP, Kaplan HS, Musshoff K, et al. Report of the

committee on Hodgkin's disease staging. *Cancer Res* 31:1860–1861, 1971.

27. Donaldson S, Link MP. Combined modality treatment with low-dose radiation and MOPP chemotherapy for children with Hodgkin's disease. *J Clin Oncol* 5:742–749, 1987.

28. Applebaum FR, Sullivan KM, Buckner CD. Allogeneic marrow transplantation in the treatment of MOPP-resistant Hodgkin's disease. *J Clin Oncol* 3:1490–1497, 1985.

29. Horning SJ, Negrin RS, Chao JC, et al. Fractionated total-body irradiation, etoposide, and cyclophosphamide plus autografting in Hodgkin's disease and non-Hodgkin's lymphoma. *J Clin Oncol* 12:2552–2558, 1994.

30. Wolden SL, Lamborn KR, Cleary SF, et al. Second cancers following pediatric Hodgkin's disease. *J Clin Oncol* 16:536–544, 1998.

Rhabdomyosarcoma

31. Li FP, Fraumeni JF, Mulvihill JJ, et al. A cancer family syndrome in twenty-four kindreds. *Cancer Res* 48:5358–5362, 1988.

32. Matsui I, Tanimura M, Kobayashi N, et al. Neurofibromatosis type 1 and childhood cancer. *Cancer* 72:2746–2754, 1993.

33. Mao L, Lee DJ, Tockman MS, et al. Microsatellite alterations in clonal marking for the detection of human cancer. *Proc Natl Acad Sci USA* 91:9871–9875, 1994.

34. Rodary C, Gehan EA, Flamant F, et al. Prognostic factors in 951 non-metastatic rhabdomyosarcomas in children: a report from the International Rhabdomyosarcoma Workshop. *Med Pediatr Oncol* 19:89–95, 1991.

35. Shapiro E, Strother D. Pediatric genitourinary rhabdomyosarcoma. *J Urol* 148:1761–1768, 1992.

36. Mauer HM, Gehan EA, Beltangady M. The Intergroup Rhabdomyosarcoma Study II. *Cancer* 71:1904–1922, 1993.

37. Pappo AS, Shapiro DN, Crist WM, Mauer HM. Biology and therapy of pediatric rhabdomyosarcoma. *J Clin Oncol* 13:2123–2139, 1995.

38. Arndt C, Tefft M, Gehan EA, et al. A feasibility, toxicity, and early response study of etoposide, ifosfamide, and vincristine for the treatment of children with rhabdomyosarcoma: a report from the Intergroup Rhabdomyosarcoma Study (IRS) IV pilot study. *J Pediatr Hematol Oncol* 19:124–129, 1997.

39. Teft M, Lindberg RD, Gehan EA. Radiation therapy combined with systemic chemotherapy of rhabdomyosarcoma in children: local control in patients enrolled in the Intergroup Rhabdomyosarcoma Study. *Monogr Natl Cancer Inst* 56:75–81, 1981.

40. Donaldson SS, Asmar L, Breneman J, et al. Hyperfractionated radiation in children with rhabdomyosarcoma-results of an Intergroup Rhabdomyosarcoma Pilot Study. *Int J Radiat Oncol Biol Phys* 32:903–911, 1995.

41. Crist W, Gehan EA, Ragab AH, et al. The Third Intergroup Rhabdomyosarcoma Study. *J Clin Oncol* 13:610–630, 1995.

Retinoblastoma

42. Vogel F. Genetics of retinoblastoma. *Hum Genet* 52:1–54, 1979.

43. Knudson A. Mutation and cancer: statistical study of retinoblastoma. *Proc Natl Acad Sci USA* 68:820–823, 1971.

44. Sparkes RS, Murphree AL, Lingua RW, et al. Gene for hereditary retinoblastoma assigned to chromosome 13 by linkage esterase D. *Science* 219:971–983, 1983.

45. Ward P, Packman S, Loughman W, et al. Location of the retinoblastoma susceptibility genes and the human esterase D locus. *J Med Genet* 21:92–95, 1984.

46. Weinberg RA. The retinoblastoma protein and cell cycle control. *Cell* 81:323–330, 1995.

47. Eng C, Li FP, Abramson DH, et al. Mortality from second tumors among long-term survivors of retinoblastoma. *J Natl Cancer Inst* 85:1121–1128, 1993.

48. Zimmerman LE. Retinoblastoma and retinocytoma. In Spencer WH (ed), *Ophthalmic Pathology: An Atlas and Textbook* (3rd ed). Philadelphia: Saunders, 1983:1292.

49. Nelson LB. Abnormalities of the pupil and iris. In Behrman RE, Kliegman RM, Arvin AM (eds), *Behrman: Nelson's Textbook of Pediatrics* (15th ed). Philadelphia: Saunders, 1996:1770–1772.

50. Reese AB, Ellsworth RM. The evaluation and current concept of retinoblastoma therapy. *Trans Am Acad Ophthalmol Otolaryngol* 67:164–172, 1963.

51. Shields CL. Recent developments in the management of retinoblastoma. *J Pediatr Ophthalmol Strabismus* 36:8–18, 1999.

52. Hernandez JC, Brady LW, Shields JA, et al. External beam radiation for retinoblastoma: results, patterns of failure, and a proposal for treatment guidelines. *Int J Radiat Oncol Biol Phys* 35:125–132, 1996.

53. Amendola BE. Radiotherapy of retinoblastoma. A review of 63 children treated with different irradiation techniques. *Cancer* 66:21–26, 1990.

54. Shields CL, De Potter P, Himelstein BP, et al. Chemoreduction in the initial management of intraocular retinoblastoma. *Arch Ophthalmol* 114:1330–1338, 1996.

55. Gallie BL. Chemotherapy with focal therapy can cure intraocular retinoblastoma without radiotherapy. *Arch Ophthalmol* 114:1321–1328, 1996.

Wilms' Tumor

56. Breslow N, Olshan A, Beckwith JB, Green DM. Epidemiology of Wilms' tumor. *Med Pediatr Oncol* 21:172–181, 1993.

57. Miller RW, Fraumeni JF, Manning MD. Association of Wilms' tumor with aniridia, hemihypertrophy and other congenital malformations. *N Engl J Med* 270:922–927, 1964.

58. Drash A, Sherman F, Hartmann WH, Blizzard RM. A syndrome pseudohemaphroditism, Wilms' tumor, hypertension and degenerative renal disease. *J Pediatr* 76:585–593, 1970.

59. Coppes MJ, Huff V, Pelletier J. Denys-Drash syndrome: relating a clinical disorder to genetic alteration in the tumor suppressor gene *WT1*. *J Pediatr* 123:673–678, 1993.

60. Ton CCT, Hirvonen H, Miwa H. Positional cloning and characterization of a paired box- and homeobox-containing gene from the aniridia region. *Cell* 67:1059–1074, 1991.

61. Huang A, Campbell CE, Bonetta L, et al. Tissue, developmental, and tumor-specific expression of divergent transcripts in Wilms' tumor. *Science* 250:991–994, 1990.

62. Pritchard-Jones K, Fleming S, Davidson D, et al. The candidate Wilms' tumour gene is involved in genitourinary development. *Nature* 346:194–197, 1990.

63. Breslow NE, Beckwith JB, Ciol M, Sharpies K. Age distribution of Wilms' tumor: report from the National Wilms' Tumor Study. *Cancer Res* 48:1653–1657, 1988.

64. Weeks, DA, Beckwith JB, Mierrrau GW, et al. Rhabdoid tumor of the kidney: a report of 111 cases from the National Wilms' Tumor Study Pathology Center. *Am J Surg Pathol* 13:439–458, 1989.

65. Beckwith JB, Kiviat NE, Bonadio J. Nephrogenic rests, nephroblastomatosis and the pathogenesis of Wilms' tumor. *Pediatr Pathol* 10:1–36, 1990.

66. Howell CG, Othersen HE, Kiviat NE, et al. Therapy and outcome in 51 children with mesoblastic nephroma: a report of the National Wilms' Tumor Study. *J Pediatr Surg* 17:826–831, 1982.

67. D'Angio GJ, Breslow N, Beckwith JB, et al. Treatment of Wilms' tumor: results of the Third National Wilms' Tumor Study. *Cancer* 64:349–360, 1989.

68. National Wilms' Tumor Study Committee. Wilms' tumor: status report, 1990. *J Clin Oncol* 9:877–887, 1991.

Ewing's Sarcoma

69. Gurney JG, Davis S, Severson RK, et al. Trends in cancer incidence among children in the US. *Cancer* 78:532–541, 1996.

70. Whang-Peng J, Triche TJ, Knutsen T, et al. Cytogenetic characterization of selected small round cell tumors of childhood. *Cancer Genet Cytogenet* 21:185–208, 1986.

71. Zucman J, Melot T, Desmaze C, et al. Combination generation of variable fusion proteins in the Ewing's family of tumors. *EMBO J* 12:4481–4487, 1993.

72. Delattre O, Zuchman J, Melot T, et al. The Ewing's family of tumors: a subgroup of small, round-cell tumors defined by specific chimeric transcripts. *N Engl J Med* 331:294–299, 1994.

73. Evans R, Nesbit M, Askin F, et al. Local recurrence, rate and sites of metastases, and time to relapse as a function of treatment regimen, size of primary and surgical history in 62 patients presenting with non-metastatic Ewing's sarcoma of the pelvic bones. *Int J Radiat Oncol Biol Phys* 11:129–136, 1985.

74. Arai Y, Kun LE, Brooks MT, et al. Ewing's sarcoma: local control and patterns of failure following limited-volume radiation therapy. *Int J Radiat Oncol Biol Phys* 21:1501–1508, 1991.

75. Sailer SI, Harmon DC, Mankin HJ, et al. Ewing's sarcoma: surgical resection as a prognostic factor. *Int J Radiat Oncol Biol Phys* 15:43–52, 1988.

76. Kuttesch Jr JF , Wexler LE, Marcus RE, et al. Second malignancies after Ewing's sarcoma: radiation dose dependency of secondary sarcomas. *J Clin Oncol* 14:2818–2825, 1996.

77. Dunst J, Jurgens H, Sauer R, et al. Radiation therapy in Ewing's sarcoma: an update of the CESS 86 trial. *Int J Radiat Oncol Biol Phys* 32:919–930, 1995.

78. Donaldson SS, Torrey M, Link MP, et al. A multidisciplinary study investigating radiotherapy in Ewing's sarcoma: end results of POG #8346. *Int J Radiat Oncol Biol Phys* 42:125–135, 1998.

79. Nesbit Jr ME , Gehan EA, Burgert EO, et al. Multimodal therapy for the management of primary nonmetastatic Ewing's sarcoma of bone: a long-term follow-up of the first intergroup study. *J Clin Oncol* 8:1664–1674, 1990.

80. Grier H, Krailo M, Link M, et al. Improved outcome in non-metastatic Ewing's sarcoma (EWS) and PNET of bone with the addition of ifosfamide (I) and etoposide (E) to vincristine (V), adriamycin (Ad), cyclophosphamide (C) and actinomycin (A): a Children's Cancer Group (CCG) and Pediatric Oncology Group (POG) report (abstract). *Proc Am Soc Clin Oncol* 1994;13:421.

81. Burdach S, Jurgens H, Peters C, et al. Myeloablative radiochemotherapy and hematopoietic stem-cell rescue in poor-prognosis Ewing's sarcoma. *J Clin Oncol* 11:1482–1488, 1993.

82. Horowitz ME, Kinsella TJ, Wexler LH. Total-body irradiation and autologous bone marrow transplant in the treatment of high-risk Ewing's sarcoma and rhabdomyosarcoma. *J Clin Oncol* 11:1911–1918, 1993.

83. Nicholson SH, Mulvihill JJ, Bynre J. Late effects of therapy in adult survivors of osteosarcoma and Ewing's sarcoma. *Med Pediatr Oncol* 20:6–12, 1992.

Osteosarcoma

84. Wong FL, Boice JD, Abramson DH, et al. Cancer incidence after retinoblastoma: radiation dose and sarcoma risk. *JAMA* 278:1262–1267, 1997.

85. Lavigueer A, Maltby V, Mock D, et al. A high incidence of lung, bone, and lymphoid tumors in transgenic mice overexpressing mutant alleles of the p53 oncogene. *Mol Cell Biol* 9:3982–3991, 1989.

86. Chang F, Syrjnan S, Syrjnan K. Implications of the p53 tumor-suppressor gene in clinical oncology. *J Clin Oncol* 13:1009–1022, 1995.

87. Dome JS, Schwartz CL. Osteosarcoma. In Walterhouse DO, Cohn SL (eds), *Diagnostic and Therapeutic Advances in Pediatric Oncology*. Boston: Kluwer, 1997:215–251.

88. Link MP, Goorin AM, Miser AW, et al. The effect of adjuvant chemotherapy on relapse-free survival in patients with osteosarcoma of the extremity. *N Engl J Med* 314:1600–1606, 1986.

89. Eilber F, Giuliano A, Eckardt J, et al. Adjuvant chemotherapy for osteosarcoma: a randomized prospective trial. *J Clin Oncol* 5:21–26, 1987.

90. Davis AM, Bell RS, Goodwin PJ. Prognostic factors in os-

teosarcoma: a critical review. *J Clin Oncol* 12:423–431, 1994.

91. Bacci G, Picci P, Ferrari S, et al. Primacy chemotherapy and delayed surgery for nonmetastatic osteosarcoma of the extremities: results in 164 patients preoperatively treated with high doses of methotrexate followed by cisplatin and doxorubicin. *Cancer* 72:3227–3238, 1993.

92. Miser J, Arndt C, Smithson W, et al. Treatment of high-grade osteosarcoma with ifosfamide, mesna, adriamycin, high-dose methotrexate with or without cisplatin. Results of two pilot trials. *Proc Am Soc Clin Oncol* 13:421, 1994.

93. Albrecht MR, Henze G, Habermalz JH, Ruhl U. *Osteosarcoma—a radioresistant tumor? Long-term evaluation after multidrug chemotherapy and definitive irradiation of the primary instead of radical surgery.* Paper presented at the Radiation Therapy for Children and Cancer Meeting, Philadelphia, PA, July 24, 1994.

94. Davis A, Bell R, Goodwin P. Prognostic factors in osteosarcoma: a critical review. *J Clin Oncol* 12:423–431, 1994.

95. Pastorino U, Gasparini M, Tavecchio L, et al. The contribution of salvage surgery to the management of childhood osteosarcoma. *J Clin Oncol* 9:1357–1362, 1991.

Germ-Cell Tumors

96. Malogolowkin M, Mahour G, Krailo M, Ortega J. Germ cell tumors in infants and children: a 45-year experience. *Pediatr Pathol* 10:231–241, 1990.

97. Calder CJ, Light AM, Rollason TP. Immature ovarian teratoma with mature peritoneal metastatic deposits showing glial, epithelial, and endometrioid differentiation: a case report and review of the literature. *Int J Gynecol Pathol* 13:279–282, 1994.

98. Einhorn LH. Clinical trials in testicular cancer. *Cancer* 71:3182–3184, 1993.

99. Cushing B, Giller R, Ablin A, et al. Surgical resection alone is effective treatment for ovarian immature teratoma in children and adolescents: a report of the Pediatric Oncology Group and the Children's Cancer Group. *Am J Obstet Gynecol* 181:353–358, 1999.

Neuroblastoma

100. Cohn SL, Meitar D, Kletzel M. Neuroblastoma: solving a biologic puzzle. In Walterhouse DO, Cohn SL (eds), *Diagnostic and Therapeutic Advances in Pediatric Oncology.* Boston: Kluwer, 1997:125–162.

101. Look AT, Hayes FA, Shuster JJ, et al. Clinical relevance of tumor cell ploidy and *N-myc* gene amplification in childhood neuroblastoma. *J Clin Oncol* 9:581–591, 1991.

102. Brodeur GM, Seeger RC, Schwab M, et al. Amplification of *N-myc* in untreated human neuroblastomas correlates with advanced disease stage. *Science* 224:1121–1124, 1984.

103. Seeger RC, Brodeur GM, Sather H, et al. Association of multiple copies of the *N-myc* oncogene with rapid progression of neuroblastomas. *N Engl J Med* 313:1111–1116, 1985.

104. Brodeur GM, Seeger RC, Sather H, et al. Clinical implications of oncogene activation in human neuroblastomas. *Cancer* 58:541–545, 1986.

105. Altman AJ, Baehner RL. Favorable prognosis for survival in children with coincident opsomyoclonus and neuroblastoma. *Cancer* 37:846–852, 1976.

106. Brodeur GM, Seeger RC, Barrett A, et al. International criteria for diagnosis, staging, and response to treatment in patients with neuroblastoma. *J Clin Oncol* 6:1874–1881, 1988.

107. Geatti O, Shapiro B, Sisson JC, et al. Iodine-131 metaiodobenzylguanidine scintigraphy for the location of neuroblastoma: preliminary experience in ten cases. *J Nuclear Med* 26:736–742, 1985.

108. Shimada H, Chatten J, Newton Jr WA, et al. Histopathologic prognostic factor in neuroblastic tumors. Definition of subtypes of ganglioneuroblastoma and an age-linked classification of neuroblastomas. *J Natl Cancer Inst* 73:405–416, 1984.

109. Christiansen H, Lampert F. Tumour karyotype discriminates between good and bad prognostic outcome in neuroblastoma. *Br J Cancer* 57:121–126, 1988.

110. Look AT, Hayes FA, Nitsche R, et al. Cellular DNA content as predictor of response to chemotherapy in infants with unresectable neuroblastomas. *N Engl J Med* 311:231–235, 1984.

111. Gansler T, Chatten J, Varello M, et al. Flow cytometric DNA analysis of neuroblastoma. Correlation with histology and outcome. *Cancer* 58:2453–2458, 1986.

112. Oppedal BR, Storm-Mathisen I, Lie SO, Brandtzaeg P. Prognostic factors in neuroblastoma. Clinical, histologic, immunohistochemical features and DNA ploidy in relation to prognosis. *Cancer* 62:772–780, 1988.

113. Seeger RC, Wada R, Brodeur GM, et al. Expression of *N-myc* by neuroblastomas with one or multiple copies of the oncogene. *Prog Clin Biol Res* 271:41–49, 1988.

114. Brodeur GM. Patterns and significance of genetic changes in neuroblastomas. In Pretlow TP, Pretlow TG (eds), *Biochemical and Molecular Aspects of Selected Tumors.* Orlando, FL: Academic Press, 1991:251–276.

115. Brodeur GM, Hayes FA, Green AA, et al. Consistent *N-myc* copy number in simultaneous or consecutive neuroblastoma samples from sixty individual patients. *Cancer Res* 47:4248–4253, 1987.

116. Fong CT, Dracopoli NC, White PS, et al. Loss of heterozygosity for chromosome 1p in human neuroblastomas: correlation with *N-myc* amplification. *Proc Natl Acad Sci USA* 86:3753–3757, 1989.

117. Ambros IM, Zellner A, Roald B, et al. Role of ploidy, chromosome 1p, and Schwann cells in the maturation of neuroblastoma. *N Engl J Med* 334:1501–1511, 1996.

118. Bown N, Cotterill S, Lastowska M, et al. Gain of chromosome arm 17q and adverse outcome in patients with neuroblastoma. *N Engl J Med* 340:1954–1961, 1999.

119. Nakagawara A, Arima M, Atar CG, et al. Inverse relationship between *trk* expression and *N-myc* amplification in human neuroblastomas. *Cancer Res* 52:1364–1368, 1992.

120. Deacon JM, Wilson PA, Peckham MJ. The radiobiology of human neuroblastoma. *Radiat Oncol* 3:201–209, 1985.
121. Rosen EM, Cassady JR, Frantz CN, et al. Neuroblastoma: the Joint Center for Radiation Therapy/Dana Farber Cancer Institute/Children's Hospital Experience. *J Clin Oncol* 2:719–732, 1984.
122. Matthay KK, Sather HN, Seeger RC, et al. Excellent outcome of stage II neuroblastoma is independent of residual disease and radiation therapy. *J Clin Oncol* 7:236–244, 1989.
123. Evans, AE, Silber JH, Arkady S, D'Angio GJ. Successful management of low-stage neuroblastoma without adjuvant therapies: a comparison of two decades, 1972 through 1981 and 1982 through 1992, in a single institution. *J Clin Oncol* 14:2405–2410, 1996.
124. Matthay KK, Perez C, Seeger RC, et al. Successful treatment of Stage III neuroblastoma–based prospective biologic staging: a Children's Cancer Group Study. *J Clin Oncol* 16:1256–1264, 1998.
125. Matthay KK, Villablanca JG, Seeger RC, et al. Treatment of high-risk neuroblastoma with intensive chemotherapy, radiotherapy, autologous bone marrow transplantation, and 13-*cis*-retinoic acid. *N Engl J Med* 341:1165–1173, 1999.

Medulloblastoma

126. Kun LE. Brain tumors: challenges and directions. *Pediatr Clin North Am* 44:907–917, 1997.
127. Cochrane DD, Gustavsson B, Poskitt KP, et al. The surgical and natural morbidity of aggressive resection for posterior fossa tumors in childhood. *Pediatr Neurosurg* 20:19–29, 1994.
128. Jenkin D, Goddard K, Armstrong D, et al. Posterior fossa medulloblastoma in childhood: treatment results and a proposal for a new staging system. *Int J Radiat Oncol Biol Phys* 19:265–274, 1990.
129. Gushing H. Experiences with the cerebellar medulloblastoma: a critical review. *Acta Pathol Microbiol Scand* 7:1–86, 1930.
130. Cutler EG, Sosman MC, Vaughan WW. Place of radiation in the treatment of cerebellar medulloblastoma: report of 20 cases. *AJR Am J Roentgenol* 35:429–453, 1936.
131. Friedman HS, Cakes WJ. The chemotherapy of posterior fossa tumors in childhood. *J Neurooncol* 5:217–219, 1987.
132. Heideman RL, Kovnar EH, Kellie SJ, et al. Preirradiation chemotherapy with carboplatin and etoposide in newly diagnosed embryonal pediatric GNS tumors. *J Clin Oncol* 13:2247–2254, 1995.
133. Packer RJ, Goldwein J, Nicholson HS, et al. Treatment of children with medulloblastoma with reduced-dose craniospinal radiation therapy and adjuvant chemotherapy: a Children's Cancer Group Study. *J Clin Oncol* 17:2127–2136, 1999.
134. Evans A, Jenkin D, Sposto R, et al. The treatment of medulloblastoma: results of a prospective randomized trial of radiation with and without CCNU, vincristine and prednisone. *J Neurosurg* 72:575–582, 1990.
135. Packer R, Sutton L, Elterman R, et al. Outcome for children with medulloblastoma treated with radiation and cisplatin, CCNU and vincristine chemotherapy. *J Neurosurg* 81:690–698, 1994.
136. Mahoney DH, Strother D, Camitta B, et al. High-dose melphalan and cyclophosphamide with autologous bone marrow rescue for recurrent/progressive malignant brain tumors in children: a pilot Pediatric Oncology Group study. *J Clin Oncol* 14:382–388, 1996.

Brainstem Gliomas

137. Barkovich AJ, Krischer J, Kun LE, et al. Brainstem gliomas: a classification system based on magnetic resonance imaging. *Pediatr Neurosurg* 16:73–83, 1991.
138. Freeman CR. Hyperfractionated radiotherapy for diffuse intrinsic brain stem tumors in children. *Pediatr Neurosurg* 24:103–110, 1996.
139. Packer RJ, Boycott JM, Zimmerman RA, et al. Outcome of children after treatment with 7800 cGY of hyperfractionated radiotherapy. *Cancer* 74:1827–1834, 1994.
140. Freeman CR, Bourgouin PM, Sanford RA, et al. Long-term survivors of childhood brainstem gliomas treated with hyperfractionated radiotherapy: clinical characteristics and treatment-related toxicities. *Cancer* 77:555–562, 1996.

High-Grade Malignant Gliomas

141. Duffner PK, Cohen ME, Myers MH, et al. Survival of children with brain tumors: SEER program 1973–1980. *Neurology* 36:597–601, 1986.
142. Burger PC, Vogel FS, Green SE, et al. Glioblastoma multiforme and anaplastic astrocytoma: pathologic criteria and prognostic implications. *Cancer* 56:1106–1111, 1985.
143. Campbell JW, Pollack IF, Martinet AJ, et at. High-grade astrocytomas in children: radiologically complete resection is associated with an excellent long-term prognosis. *Neurosurgery* 38:258–264, 1996.
144. Dunbar SF, Tarbell NJ, Kooy HM, et al. Stereotactic radiotherapy for pediatric and adult brain tumors: preliminary report. *Int J Radiat Oncol Biol Phys* 30:531–539, 1994.
145. Sposto R, Ertel IJ, Jenkin RD, et al. The effectiveness of chemotherapy for treatment of high-grade astrocytoma in children: results of a randomized trial. A report from the Children's Cancer Study Group. *J Neurooncol* 7:165–177, 1989.

Low-Grade Gliomas

146. Tao ML, Barnes PD, Billett AC, et al. Childhood optic chiasm gliomas: radiographic response following radiotherapy and long-term clinical outcome. *Int J Radiat Oncol Biol Phys* 39:579–587, 1997.

147. Gajjar A, Bhargava R, Jenkins JJ, et al. Low-grade astrocytoma with neuraxis dissemination at diagnosis. *J Neurosurg* 83:67–71,1995.

148. Pollack IF, Hurtt M, Pang D, et al. Dissemination of low grade intracranial astrocytomas in children. *Cancer* 73:2869–2878, 1994.

149. Dirks PB, Jay V, Becher LE, et al. Development of anaplastic changes in low-grade astrocytomas of childhood. *Neurosurgery* 34:68–78, 1994.

150. Pollack IF, Claassen D, Al-Shboul Q, et al. Low-grade gliomas of the cerebral hemispheres in children: an analysis of 71 cases. *J Neurosurg* 82:536–547, 1995.

151. Shaw EG, Scheithauer BW, O'Fallon JR. Management of supratentorial low-grade gliomas. *Oncology* 7:97–107, 1993.

152. Leibel SA, Sheline GE, Wara WM, et al. The role of radiation therapy in the treatment of astrocytomas. *Cancer* 35:1551–1557, 1975.

153. Bloom HJ, Glees J, Bell J. The treatment and long-term prognosis of children with intracranial tumors: a study of 610 cases, 1950–1981. *Int J Radiat Oncol Biol Phys* 18:723–745, 1990.

154. Packer RJ, Sutton LN, Bilaniuk LT, et al. Treatment of chiasmatic/hypothalamic gliomas of childhood with chemotherapy: an update. *Ann Neurol* 23:79–85, 1988.

155. Friedman HS, Krisher JP, Burger P, et al. Treatment of children with progressive or recurrent brain tumors with carboplatin or iproplatin: a Pediatric Oncology Group randomized phase II study. *J Clin Oncol* 10:249–256, 1992.

156. Freeman CR, Farmer JP, Montes J. Low-grade astrocytomas in children: evolving management strategies. *Int J Radiat Oncol Biol Phys* 41:979–987, 1998.

Ependymomas

157. Rorke LB, Gilles FH, Davis RL, Becker LE. Revision of the World Health Organization classification of brain tumors for childhood brain tumors. *Cancer* 56:1869–1886, 1985.

158. Kovnar E, Kun L, Burger P, Krischer J, and the Pediatric Oncology Group. Patterns of dissemination and recurrence in childhood ependymoma: preliminary results of the Pediatric Oncology Group 8532. *Ann Neurol* 30:457, 1991.

159. Pollack I, Gerszten PC, Martinet AJ, et al. Intracranial ependymomas of childhood: long-term outcome and prognostic factors. *Neurosurgery* 37:655–667, 1995.

160. Cochrane DD, Gustavsson B, Poskitt KP, et al. The surgical and natural morbidity of aggressive resection for posterior fossa tumors in childhood. *Pediatr Neurosurg* 20:19–29, 1994.

161. Rousseau P, Habrand JL, Sarrazin D, et al. Treatment of intracranial ependymomas of children: review of a 15-year experience. *Int J Radiat Oncol Biol Phys* 28:381–386, 1993.

162. Goldwein JW, Laehy JM, Packer RJ, et al. Intracranial ependymomas in children. *Int J Radiat Oncol Biol Phys* 19:1497–1502, 1990.

163. Goldwein JW, Corn BW, Finaly JL, et al. Is craniospinal irradiation required to cure children with malignant (anaplastic) intracranial ependymomas? *Cancer* 67:2766–2771, 1991.

164. Duffner PK, Horowitz ME, Krischer JP, et al. Postoperative chemotherapy and delayed radiation in children less than three years of age with malignant brain tumors. *N Engl J Med* 328:1725–1731, 1993.

165. Needle MN, Goldwein JW, Grass J, et al. Adjuvant chemotherapy for the treatment of intracranial ependymoma of childhood. *Cancer* 80:341–347, 1997.

Pineal Tumors

166. Packer RJ, Sutton LN, Rosenstock JG, et al. Pineal region tumors of childhood. *Pediatrics* 78:97–101, 1984.

167. Edwards MSB, Hudgins RJ, Wilson CB, et al. Pineal region tumors in children. *J Neurosurg* 66:689–697, 1988.

168. Dattoli MJ, Newall J. Radiation therapy for intracranial germinoma: the case for limited volume treatment. *Int J Radiat Oncol Biol Phys* 19:429–433, 1990.

169. Lindstadt D, Wara WM, Edwards MSB, et al. Radiotherapy of primary intracranial germinomas: the case against routine craniospinal irradiation. *Int J Radiat Oncol Biol Phys* 15:291–297, 1988.

26

Sarcomas of Soft Tissue and Bone

■ ■ ■

Alan W. Yasko
Shreyaskumar R. Patel
Alan Pollack
Raphael E. Pollock

INCIDENCE

Soft-tissue sarcomas are a group of extremely rare, anatomically and histologically diverse malignant neoplasms of mesodermal tissue origin. These tumors constitute approximately 1% of adult malignancies and 7% of pediatric malignancies. Soft-tissue sarcomas can develop in patients of all ages, with approximately 20% arising in patients younger than age 40, 30% in patients between ages 40 and 60, and 50% in patients older than 60. In the United States, approximately 8,100 new cases of soft-tissue sarcoma are diagnosed annually, and approximately 4,600 patients die from this disease per year. The age-adjusted incidence is approximately 2 cases per 100,000 persons.

Bone sarcomas also are extremely rare and represent only 0.2% of all new cancer diagnoses; approximately 2,500 new cases occur in the United States annually. Osteosarcoma is the most common primary bone sarcoma, accounting for approximately 20% of all malignancies of bone. The annual incidence is approximately three cases per million persons. An observed biphasic pattern of osteosarcoma incidence shows a peak in adolescence as a primary sarcoma and in the elderly as a secondary sarcoma associated with Paget's disease and irradiated bone. Chondrosarcoma is one-half as common as is osteosarcoma and is observed mostly in adults. Ewing's sarcoma is the second most common bone malignancy in children, representing an annual incidence of one case per million persons. All other bone sarcomas are rare, each accounting for fewer than 1% of primary bone sarcomas.

EPIDEMIOLOGIC FACTORS AND ETIOLOGIC FEATURES

Most soft-tissue sarcomas are sporadic, with no specific identifiable etiologic agent. Infrequently, a predisposing factor is identified. Almost all sarcomas due to antecedent etiologic factors are high-grade tumors, a classic example of which is an irradiation-induced sarcoma. By definition, an irradiation-induced sarcoma arising in soft tissue or bone can develop no sooner than 3 years after completion of a course of therapeutic radiotherapy; frequently, these lesions will develop decades later. Typically, such lesions are osteosarcoma or malignant fibrous histiocytoma.

Phenoxy herbicide exposure in forestry workers has been linked with subsequent sarcoma development. Other agents implicated in the etiology of soft-tissue sarcoma include exposure to dioxin, vinyl chloride, arsenic, and Thorotrast, a thorium-based suspension formerly used as a contrast agent in radiologic studies.

Chronic lymphedema is a factor predisposing to the subsequent development of lymphangiosarcoma. Typically, these extremely aggressive sarcomas arise in a chronically lymphedematous extremity. Originally, this clinical entity was described as the *Stewart-Treves syndrome* in reference to the rise of lymphangiosarcoma in the chronically edematous upper extremity of breast carcinoma patients treated with radical mastectomy.

Exposure to alkylating chemotherapeutic agents, such as cyclophosphamide used in the treatment of acute lymphocytic leukemia, has been associated with subsequent development of osteosarcoma in a small percentage of acute lymphocytic leukemia patients. Melphalan, procarbazine, nitrosoureas, and chlorambucil have been associated with the subsequent development of bone sarcomas. Bone sarcomas can develop in association with benign neoplastic and nonneoplastic conditions. Osteosarcoma can develop in the abnormal bone associated with Paget's disease and with other benign processes (e.g., fibrous dysplasia). Chondrosarcoma can develop from a benign osteochondroma. Malignant fibrous histiocytoma can be observed to arise in areas of bone infarction.

Though at the time of presentation patients frequently report a recent history of trauma, no scientific evidence directly connects such injury to the inception of soft-tissue or bone sarcomas. Instead, such traumatic episodes are thought to call attention to a specific body part or location, thereby increasing the likelihood of detecting an otherwise painless and frequently innocuous soft-tissue mass or bone lesion.

Several genetic conditions are related to the development of soft-tissue sarcoma. They include neurofibromatosis, tuberous sclerosis, basal-cell nevus syndrome, Gardner's syndrome, and Li-Fraumeni syndrome. Genetic factors implicated in sarcomagenesis include mutations in the *RB1* and *p53* tumor suppressor genes, the genes mutated most commonly in soft-tissue sarcoma. The importance of *RB1* and *p53* mutations is suggested by their high incidence of mutation in hereditary retinoblastoma and Li-Fraumeni syndrome families. Ultimately, as many as 10% of patients with neurofibromatosis will develop neurofibrosarcoma. In Gardner's syndrome, familial adenomatous polyps are associated with the subsequent development of intraabdominal desmoid tumors, particularly in the root of the mesentery. The overall incidence of desmoid tumors in Gardner's syndrome patients is approximately 8% to 12%.

CLINICAL IMPLICATIONS
Sites of Disease

Soft-tissue sarcomas arise predominantly in the extremities, although they may develop from any site in the body. Approximately 45% of soft-tissue sarcomas develop in the lower extremities, most commonly in the thigh; 15% are located in the upper extremity, 15% in the trunk, 15% in the retroperitoneum, and 10% in the head and neck.

Bone sarcomas can arise in any bone and within any region of a given bone. Osteosarcoma is the most common bone sarcoma and arises most frequently in the long bones of the lower extremity. In general, osteosarcomas arise near the ends of the bone in the metaphyseal region. Approximately 45% of these sarcomas arise in the femur, 18% in the tibia, 11% in the humerus, 8% in the pelvis, 6% in the jaw, 3% in the fibula, and 9% in other sites. Chondrosarcomas also occur most frequently in the extremities (45%), with a predominance in the femur. The pelvic bones collectively represent the most frequent site of development of chondrosarcomas (25%). Other common sites of chondrosarcoma are the ribs and the scapula. Ewing's sarcomas (including primitive neuroectodermal tumors) have a predilection for the long tubular bones, followed in frequency by the flat bones of the pelvis and ribs. In affected patients, the primary bone sites of Ewing's sarcoma are the lower extremity (approximately 37%), the pelvis (23%), the ribs (18%), the upper extremities (12%), the spine (7%), and craniofacial areas (3%). Malignant fibrous histiocytoma of bone occurs most often in the region of the knee, in the distal femur–proximal tibia. Chordomas are located most commonly in the sacrococcygeal region and in the base of the skull (90%); occasionally, presentation in the cervical and lumbar vertebrae also is observed.

Natural History

Soft-tissue sarcomas grow centrifugally, causing compression of surrounding normal structures. A zone of compressed reactive tissue forms a pseudocapsule that often is mistaken by inexperienced clinicians as the boundary of a benign lesion. Fingerlike tentacles of tumor extend through and beyond the pseudocapsule for some distance, and secondary satellite tumors may form independent of the primary mass. Soft-tissue sarcomas tend to spread longitudinally along muscle compartments, nerve and fascial sheaths, and other such anatomic tissue planes. This potential for local extension must be taken into account in the planning of surgery and radiotherapy. Frequently, bone, fascia, peritoneum, and pleura act as natural tissue barriers. However, aggressive tumors may invade across such boundaries, and such spread commonly occurs in large tumors. Usually, soft-tissue sarcomas metastasize by hematogenous spread. Lymphatic involvement is observed much less frequently. Approximately 10% of soft-tissue sarcoma patients present with detectable distant disease. The lung is the most common site of metastasis for soft-tissue sarcomas.

Bone sarcomas exhibit varied patterns of bone destruction but characteristically are associated with a mixed pattern of bone lysis and new bone formation with indistinct margins. As do soft-tissue sarcomas, malignant bone tumors characteristically expand centrifugally, infiltrate adjacent bone, penetrate the periosteum, and extend into the soft tissues. Frequently, local extension of tumor along the capsule and ligaments of adjacent joints is observed. In skeletally immature patients, tumor extension across the growth plates at the ends of the bone commonly is seen, although direct intraarticular involvement is less common. Pathologic fracture secondary to structural weakening of the involved bone is not uncommon.

Bone sarcomas metastasize by hematogenous spread. The lung is the most common site of distant disease. Other bony sites and lymph nodes are much less common and usually reflect advanced disseminated disease. The rate of detectable metastasis at presentation for high-grade bone sarcomas is approximately 10% to 20%.

Patterns of Failure

Surgical extirpation of the soft-tissue sarcoma with negative margins is the most important factor in reducing local failure. Surgery in conjunction with radiotherapy as an adjuvant local therapy significantly reduces the risk of local tumor recurrence. Local failure rates of 5% to 20% for soft-tissue sarcomas of the extremity and trunk are typical when modern conservative surgical and radiotherapy techniques are used. The propensity for distant metastasis depends greatly on histologic grade and size of a tumor.

The incidence of metastasis in high-grade soft-tissue sarcomas is 20% overall and 50% when the primary tumor diameter is greater than 5 cm. The incidence of metastasis in intermediate-grade soft-tissue sarcomas with a diameter of less than 5 cm is 3% overall and 20% when the tumor diameter is greater than 5 cm. Low-grade tumors rarely metastasize.

The most common site of first distant failure is the lung (approximately 50%), followed in frequency by liver, bone and, to a lesser degree, skin. Liver metastases and peritoneal sarcomatosis are frequent features of retroperitoneal sarcomas. Myxoid liposarcomas tend to metastasize to fat-bearing intraabdominal sites, rather than to the lung, as the first site of failure. Lymph node metastasis is uncommon and typically is observed in fewer than 4% of soft-tissue sarcomas. However, some histologic subtypes metastasize more frequently to lymph nodes, including clear-cell sarcoma (28%), epithelioid sarcoma (23%), angiosarcoma (12%), synovial sarcoma (12%), and rhabdomyosarcoma (11%).

Local control of bone sarcomas depends primarily on the adequacy of the surgical procedure to achieve wide oncologic margins. For low-grade bone sarcomas, the sole predictor of outcome is the adequacy of the surgical margin achieved at the time of tumor extirpation. Low-grade malignancies metastasize in fewer than 10% of patients for whom a primary tumor has been treated by appropriate surgery. For high-grade sarcomas, the response of the tumor to induction chemotherapy is the most significant predictor of patient outcome. For high-grade chemotherapy-sensitive sarcomas (osteosarcoma, Ewing's sarcoma, malignant fibrous histiocytoma), local control is predicated on both response to chemotherapy and adequacy of surgical margins. Local recurrence rates are reported to be between 5% and 10% for patients with extremity high-grade osteosarcoma. High-grade osteosarcomas, Ewing's sarcomas, and high-grade chondrosarcomas are highly metastatic; more than 80% spread distantly when only definitive local therapy is used.

The lung is the most frequent site of distant failure for bone sarcomas. Distant osseous sites, bone marrow, and lymph nodes are infrequent sites of distant failure and usually are detected in patients with progressive disease after the development of pulmonary metastases.

Survival Statistics

Survival for patients with soft-tissue sarcomas is related closely to the stage of the disease. The 5-year survival rate is approximately 75% for patients with early-stage disease and less than 20% for patients with advanced disease. For patients with bone sarcomas, survival also is related closely to the stage of disease. Patients with localized, low-grade bone sarcomas have survival rates of more than 90%. An exception may be patients with chordomas that typically exhibit a protracted clinical course. Most patients with chordoma succumb to relentless local disease progression at 10 to 15 years after initial treatment. Patients with localized high-grade sarcomas treated with contemporary multiagent chemotherapy and appropriate surgery experience a 60% to 75% long-term survival. Patient survival is poor for those who present with metastatic disease (< 15%).

WORKUP AND STAGING
Diagnosis

The clinical presentation of patients with soft-tissue sarcomas depends in large part on the primary tumor site. Because the majority (60%) of soft-tissue sarcomas arise in the extremities, patients present most commonly with an asymptomatic mass. Less frequently observed is localized painful swelling. Rarely does a patient present with pain without a palpable mass. Usually, retroperitoneal sarcomas (15%) and visceral sarcomas (15%) are discovered once they have achieved a considerable size, and usually retroperitoneal sarcomas present with an abdominal mass often associated with vague abdominal pain. Visceral sarcomas present with nonspecific symptoms related to the site of origin (e.g., abdominal symptoms for gastrointestinal sarcomas or pelvic symptoms for uterine sarcomas).

In contrast, most patients with bone sarcomas will seek medical attention because of localized pain. The character of the pain varies, depending on the pathologic process, the site and extent of tumor involvement, and the presence of impending or established pathologic fracture. Usually, pain is localized, dull, continuous, deep-seated, and present at rest and at night and usually is exacerbated by motion or weight bearing on an affected limb. Typically, recent trauma and exacerbation of low-grade discomfort prompt medical attention, at which time the underlying neoplasm is detected. Usually, any localized soft-tissue swelling is associated with tenderness and a palpable firm, deep, fixed mass.

Perilesional inflammation induced by the tumor may result in soft-tissue edema, synovitis, and joint effusion that may compromise the range of motion of the affected extremity.

In general, blood studies are unremarkable in patients with soft-tissue and bone sarcomas. Anemia and leukocytosis can be observed in patients with Ewing's sarcoma and elevated levels of alkaline phosphatase, and lactate dehydrogenase can be detected in patients with osteosarcoma and Ewing's sarcoma. An abnormal glucose tolerance test has been observed in some patients with chondrosarcoma.

Radiologic Considerations

Although optimal imaging of primary tumor depends on the anatomic site of involvement, the evaluations used for soft-tissue and bone sarcomas are different. For extremity and pelvic soft-tissue sarcomas, magnetic resonance imaging (MRI) is regarded as the imaging modality of choice. MRI provides multiplanar delineation of the tumor and enhanced contrast between the tumor and adjacent neurovascular structures, muscle, and bone (Fig. 26.1). In the retroperitoneum and abdomen, usually computed tomography (CT) provides anatomic definition of the tumor. Other imaging studies, including plain radiographs of the extremity and angiography, rarely (if ever) are indicated for accurate soft-tissue sarcoma staging and treatment planning.

In contrast, the initial evaluation of a suspected bone sarcoma should include conventional radiography. Biplanar views reveal the anatomic location of a tumor within the affected bone and its relationship to the adja-

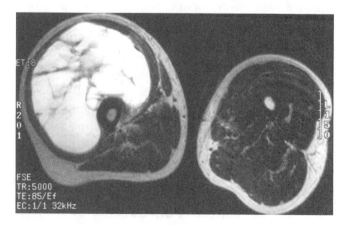

Figure 26.1 Magnetic resonance image of the thigh in a 37-year-old man, demonstrating a large, deep-seated, malignant fibrous histiocytoma abutting the femur and displacing the femoral vessels.

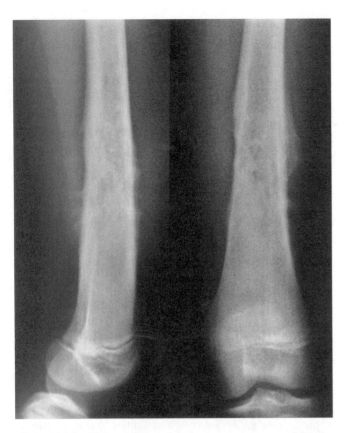

Figure 26.2 Plain radiographs of an osteosarcoma arising in the distal femur of a 14-year-old boy. Note mixed osteoblastic and osteolytic changes within the bone. Periosteal reaction and tumor extension into the soft tissues are common findings in primary malignant tumors of bone.

cent joints and growth plates. The pattern of bone destruction, characteristics of a periosteal reaction, matrix production within the lesion, and presence of a soft-tissue mass are important in the formulation of the differential diagnosis and staging evaluation (Fig. 26.2). Commonly, the diagnosis of the primary neoplasm can be made presumptively on the basis of this initial radiographic evaluation; however, usually other studies are indicated to define more clearly the local extent of disease. Usually, local staging studies include CT and MRI of the affected bone.

A CT scan provides valuable information regarding the reactive response of bone to a tumor and provides excellent detail of changes in cortical and cancellous bones, including mineralization within the lesion and surrounding soft tissues. MRI complements the CT scan by demonstrating the relational anatomy between normal and diseased tissues. The extent of bone-marrow and soft-tissue involvement is visualized optimally using this technique. The relation of the tumor to vital adjacent neural, vascular, and joint structures is deline-

ated best by MRI. Cross-sectional images afforded by CT and MRI are critical for delineating the local extent of the disease for tumors arising in the spine and pelvis. Technetium 99m bone scans are performed primarily to screen the skeleton for polyostotic involvement and to obtain early detection of skeletal metastases for bone sarcomas. Periosteal involvement by soft-tissue sarcoma also can be detected using this technique.

Imaging of the chest is a critical part of the staging of both soft-tissue sarcomas and bone sarcomas, in view of the propensity of these lesions to metastasize to the lung. Biplanar chest radiography is sufficient for patients at a low risk of developing pulmonary metastases, such as low-grade sarcomas, and may be sufficient for patients with small (< 5-cm-diameter) primary, intermediate, or high-grade soft-tissue sarcomas. For accurate staging, a chest CT should be performed in all patients with high-grade bone sarcomas and for all large (> 5-cm-diameter), intermediate, or high-grade soft-tissue sarcomas.

Biopsy Considerations

Biopsy is a critical step in the diagnosis of soft-tissue and bone sarcomas. Successful execution of a biopsy requires a working knowledge of sarcomas and their treatment. Expertise in procuring adequate tissue and analyzing limited samples of these rare tumors reduces errors in diagnosis. A biopsy may be performed as a surgical (open) or percutaneous (closed) procedure. Currently, most tumors are subjected to surgical biopsy. The biopsy incision must be placed appropriately, and the biopsy should be performed properly to optimize the yield of diagnostic tissue, yet it should not compromise the definitive surgical procedure. The use of longitudinal skin incisions parallel to the long axis of an extremity, limited tissue flaps, meticulous hemostasis, and avoidance of the joint and the plane of adjacent neurovascular structures all are critical. Relatively small, superficial soft-tissue masses (< 3 cm in diameter) can be removed by excisional biopsy with clear margins. Biopsies of larger lesions should be incisional or should be performed using needle-biopsy techniques.

Experience with percutaneous biopsy at large referral centers has resulted in a growing application of fine-needle aspiration and cutting-core biopsy for the diagnosis of bone lesions. These minimally invasive procedures have been shown to be safe, highly accurate, and economic diagnostic methods when performed by experts in percutaneous musculoskeletal biopsy techniques. Usually, percutaneous biopsies are performed under local anesthesia for adult patients and under conscious sedation or general anesthesia for children. The accuracy of percutaneous biopsy has reached 90% in some centers but remains highly variable overall, reflecting the differing levels of clinical experience and cytopathologic expertise available to diagnose these rare neoplasms on limited tissue samples.

Biopsy-obtained tissue may be processed for standard histologic and cytologic preparations, immunohistochemical studies, electron microscopy, flow cytometry, and molecular studies, as indicated. The histopathologic diagnosis always should be interpreted in the context of the clinical presentation and radiographic features of the primary lesion. The primary concern with needle-biopsy techniques is the limited amount of tissue that can be obtained to establish the diagnosis and to use for research investigations.

Regardless of the technique used, the biopsy procedure should be performed by personnel expert in the management of extremity sarcomas. A recent multiinstitutional study found that when a biopsy is performed at a referring institution, biopsy-related problems occur three to five times more frequently than when the procedure is performed at a center in which the definitive surgical resection is to be performed [1]. Problems associated with poorly performed surgical biopsies, such as misoriented biopsy incisions, postoperative hematoma formation, or infection, may necessitate more radical resections or can necessitate amputation rather than limb salvage while increasing the incidence of local tumor recurrence. Therefore, the recommended approach is that open biopsies be planned carefully and be performed at the center in which the definitive surgery is to be undertaken. Even when a well-executed surgical biopsy is performed, excising the surgically created biopsy site in continuity with the resected tumor specimen is necessary to minimize the incidence of local recurrence. Resection of overlying skin, fat, fascia, and muscle to incorporate the biopsy site may necessitate a more complex wound closure requiring soft-tissue transfer if the initial biopsy is created without consideration of the ultimate tumor resection.

Histopathologic Classification

The most common classification scheme for both soft-tissue sarcoma and bone sarcoma is based historically on putative histogenesis. In this schema, a pathologist identifies certain architectural, cytoplasmic, and nuclear characteristics that suggest that a neoplastic cell resembles, and therefore might derive from, a specific tissue. Accordingly, this histogenic concept proposes that liposarcoma has a putative cell of origin in adipose tissue, rhabdomyosarcoma in skeletal muscle, leiomyosarcoma in smooth muscle, chondrosarcoma in cartilage, osteosarcoma in bone, and so on. A more modern concept based on experimental and clinical observations is that all sarcomas develop from primitive multipotential mesenchymal cells. Fortunately, this newer concept has little impact on sarcoma classification. Malignancies exhibiting morphologic and histochemical evidence of lipoblastic or rhabdomyoblastic differential are still classified as liposarcoma and rhabdomyosarcoma, for example, even though they are now believed to have developed from multipotential mesenchymal cells rather than dedifferentiating from mature adipose tissue or striated muscle. Most large studies suggest that the most common extremity soft-tissue sarcoma histologic subtype is malignant fibrous histiocytoma (40%) followed by liposarcoma (25%) [2]. In the retroperitoneum, liposarcoma is the most common histopathologic determination, followed in frequency by leiomyosarcoma and malignant fibrous histiocytoma. At least 25 distinct histopathologic subtypes are enumerated in the soft-tissue sarcoma family (Fig. 26.3), and a similar number of distinct bone sarcomas are listed (Table 26.1). Bone sarcomas may arise from any cellular constituent of bone, including osteogenic, chondrogenic, fibrogenic, hematopoietic, and other elements.

Classification systems are most reproducible for the better-differentiated tumors and make use of standard light microscopy, electron microscopy and, increasingly, immunohistochemistry. However, as the degree of histologic differentiation moves from well differentiated to undifferentiated, the determination of cellular type becomes increasingly more difficult. Despite immunohistochemical techniques and electron microscopy, determining the cell of origin for many spindle-cell and round-cell soft-tissue tumors is particularly difficult and sometimes impossible. Because of these difficulties, disparities are observed in up to 40% of histopathologic diagnoses, even among expert sarcoma pathologists. Cytogenetic analysis may be useful for sarcoma classification. Specific clonal abnormalities of chromosome number or arrangement for certain sarcomas, such as the translocations $t(11;22)(q24;q12)$ in Ewing's sarcomas/primitive neuroectodermal tumors and $t(12;16)$ $(q13–14;p11)$ in myxoid liposarcomas, may be useful in sarcoma classification and, possibly, prognosis.

Clearly, light microscopy alone lacks the necessary precision to form a basis for prediction of ultimate bio-

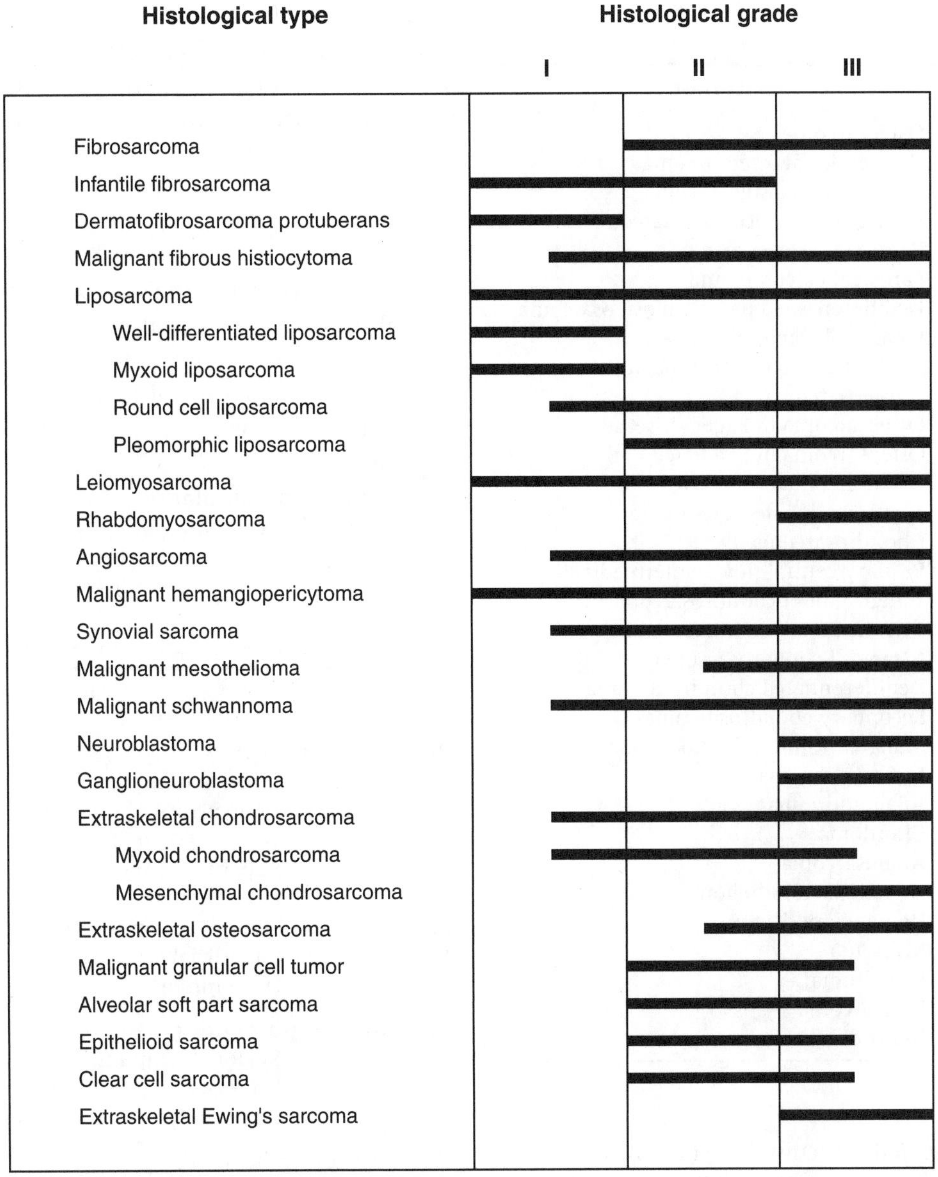

Figure 26.3 Estimated range of degree of malignancy of soft-tissue sarcomas, based on histologic type and grade. Grade within the overall range depends on specific histologic features such as cellularity, cellular pleomorphism, mitotic activity, amount of stroma, infiltrative or expansive growth, and necrosis. (Reprinted with permission from FM Enzinger, SW Weiss, *Soft Tissue Tumors* [3rd ed]. St Louis: Mosby, 1995.)

logical behavior. In fact, such complicated issues as local tumor recurrence and tumor dissemination may be driven by such underlying molecular characteristics as the acquisition of critical mutations in various tumor suppressor genes or oncogene activation and amplification. Ultimately, these latter factors may prove to be more important than the information that can be derived by light-microscopical examination. Molecular characteristics have not been incorporated yet into current staging systems. Increased understanding of molecular genetics may yield a coupling of histopathologic classification and molecular determinations of the factors that drive sarcomagenesis, proliferation, and metastasis.

Staging

The relative rarity of soft-tissue sarcomas, their anatomic heterogeneity, and a multiplicity of histologic

Table 26.1　Classification of Common Malignant Bone Tumors

Histologic Type	Tumor
Osteogenic	Osteosarcoma
	Conventional osteosarcoma
	Telangiectatic osteosarcoma
	High-grade surface osteosarcoma
	Periosteal osteosarcoma
	Parosteal osteosarcoma
	Dedifferentiated parosteal osteosarcoma
	Small-cell osteosarcoma
	Well-differentiated intramedullary osteosarcoma
	Osteosarcoma in Paget's disease
	Osteosarcoma in irradiated bones
	Osteosarcoma of the jaw
	Multicentric osteosarcoma
Chondrogenic	Chondrosarcoma
	Primary central (low-, intermediate-, high-grade) chondrosarcoma
	Mesenchymal chondrosarcoma
	Clear-cell chondrosarcoma
	Dedifferentiated chondrosarcoma
	Secondary chondrosarcomas
Histiocytes	Malignant fibrous histiocytoma
Unknown	Ewing's sarcoma
	Adamantinoma
Notochordal	Chordoma
Vascular	Angiosarcoma
	Hemangioendothelioma
	Hemangiopericytoma
Hematopoietic	Myeloma
	Lymphoma
Lipogenic	Liposarcoma
Neurogenic	Neurofibrosarcoma

subtypes have created difficulty in establishing a functional system that accurately stages all presenting forms of this disease. The recently revised TNM (tumor-node-metastasis) staging system of the American Joint Committee on Cancer (AJCC) and the Union Internationale Contre le Cancer (UICC) is the system now employed most widely for staging soft-tissue sarcoma [3]. This system is a revision of the initial AJCC system published in 1977, is based on the conventional TNM staging criteria, but incorporates histologic grade as a staging parameter. All soft-tissue sarcoma subtypes are included except dermatofibrosarcoma protuberans, a condition that has minimal malignant potential.

The AJCC/UICC staging system recognizes four distinct histologic grades of tumors, ranging from well differentiated to undifferentiated. The features that define grade include cellularity, differentiation, pleomorphism, necrosis, and number of mitoses. However, the criteria for grading are neither specific nor standardized. Many

pathologists consider that mitotic activity, nuclear atypia, and degree of necrosis are the most important pathologic features suggestive of grade. Histologic grade and tumor size are the most important factors in determining clinical stage (Tables 26.2, 26.3). Tumor size is substaged further as *a* (superficial tumor arising outside the investing muscle bundle fascia) or *b* (deep tumor that arises beneath the fascia or invades the fascia). Nodal status is part of the staging system; however, the overall incidence of nodal metastasis is only approximately 3% to 5%. In light of the rarity of nodal disease, some advocate that nodal metastases be grouped with other distant disease sites rather than as a separate staging entity.

An additional limitation of the current staging system is that the dependence on grading criteria remains

Table 26.2　TNM Staging System for Soft-Tissue Sarcomas

Classification	Definition
Primary tumor (T)	
TX	Primary tumor cannot be assessed
T0	No evidence of primary tumor
T1	Tumor $\leq$ 5 cm in greatest dimension
T1a	Superficial tumor[a]
T1b	Deep tumor[a]
T2	Tumor > 5 cm in greatest dimension
T2a	Superficial tumor[a]
T2b	Deep tumor[a]
Regional lymph nodes (N)	
NX	Regional lymph nodes cannot be assessed[b]
N0	No regional lymph node metastasis
N1	Regional lymph node metastasis
Distant metastasis (M)	
MX	Distant metastasis cannot be assessed
M0	No distant metastasis
M1	Distant metastasis
Histopathologic grade (G)	
GX	Grade cannot be assessed
G1	Well differentiated
G2	Moderately differentiated
G3	Poorly differentiated
G4	Undifferentiated

[a]Superficial tumor is located above the superficial fascia without invasion of the fascia; deep tumor is located either exclusively beneath the superficial fascia, or superficial to the fascia with invasion of or through the fascia, or superficial and beneath the fascia. Retroperitoneal, mediastinal, and pelvic sarcomas are classified as deep tumors.
[b]Because of the rarity of lymph node involvement in sarcomas, the designation *NX* may not be appropriate and could be considered *N0* if no clinical involvement is evident.
Source: Used with permission of the American Joint Committee on Cancer (AJCC), Chicago, Illinois. Reprinted from ID Fleming, JS Cooper, DE Henson, et al. (eds), *AJCC Cancer Staging Manual* (5th ed). Philadelphia: Lippincott-Raven, 1997:149–156.

Table 26.3   AJCC Stage Grouping for Soft-Tissue Sarcoma

Stage IA (low-grade, small, superficial and deep)	G1–2	T1a–1b	N0	M0
Stage IB (low-grade, large, superficial)	G1–2	T2a	N0	M0
Stage IIA (low-grade, large, deep)	G1–2	T2b	N0	M0
Stage IIB (high-grade, small, superficial, deep)	G3–4	T1a–1b	N0	M0
Stage IIC (high-grade, large, superficial)	G3–4	T2a	N0	M0
Stage III (high-grade, large, deep)	G3–4	T2b	N0	M0
Stage IV (any metastasis)	Any G	Any T	N1	M0
	Any G	Any T	N0	M1

AJCC = American Joint Committee on Cancer.
Source: Used with permission of the American Joint Committee on Cancer (AJCC), Chicago, Illinois. Reprinted from ID Fleming, JS Cooper, DE Henson, et al. (eds), *AJCC Cancer Staging Manual* (5th ed). Philadelphia: Lippincott-Raven, 1997:149–156.

subjective and is prone to discord among expert sarcoma pathologists. Yet another limitation of the present staging system is that it does not take into account the anatomic heterogeneity of these lesions. The current staging system is very effective for extremity sarcomas but is applied also to lesions in the trunk, retroperitoneum, and head and neck. In these latter locations, the staging factors may not be as pertinent, given both the anatomic constraints to resection and the variability in the predominant histologic subtypes in each of these anatomic locations. Stage for stage, the prognosis for patients with retroperitoneal and visceral sarcomas is poorer overall than that for patients with extremity lesions. Although site is not incorporated as a specific component of the current AJCC/UICC staging system, outcome data must be interpreted on a site-specific basis because of the impact of location on survival.

The surgical staging system for bone sarcomas adopted by the Musculoskeletal Tumor Society is based on the observation that bone sarcomas behave similarly regardless of histologic type. The staging system is based on tumor grade (I, low-grade; II, high-grade), tumor extent (A, intraosseous involvement only; B, extraosseous extension), and presence of metastasis regardless of the extent of local tumor (III). As regards similar tumor types, patients with axial skeletal sarcomas have a poorer prognosis than that for patients with extremity sarcomas.

Prognostic Factors

Establishing the clinical profile of patients with extremity soft-tissue sarcoma who are at high risk for recurrence clearly is possible. Such patients present with a large (at least 5-cm-diameter), high-grade, deep-seated tumor. The adverse prognostic significance of these specific factors has been demonstrated in prospective data from the Memorial Sloan-Kettering Cancer Center [2]

and from a recent report of the French Federation of Cancer Centers [4]. In addition to the foregoing factors, outcome is affected by specific histopathologic subtypes: microscopically positive surgical margin, locally recurrent disease, or nonextremity location.

The adverse prognostic factors for local recurrence in soft-tissue sarcomas differ from those predictive of either distant metastasis or tumor-related mortality. Factors predictive of local recurrence include patient age of 50 or older, local recurrence presentation, microscopically positive margin, and fibrosarcoma or malignant peripheral nerve sheath tumor histology (Table 26.4). Factors predictive of distant recurrence include size ($\geq$ 5-cm diameter), high grade, deep location, local recurrence at presentation, leiomyosarcoma histology, or nonliposarcoma histology. Finally, disease-specific survival is predicated on size ($\geq$ 10-cm diameter), deep location, local recurrence at presentation, leiomyosarcoma or peripheral nerve sheath tumor histology, microscopically positive margin, or lower-extremity site. As can be discerned readily, several of these factors do not appear in the current soft-tissue sarcoma-staging system. Until such time as these factors are incorporated into staging systems, astute clinicians will bear these considerations in mind in designing follow-up and treatment strategies.

Though bone tumors are a diverse disease cluster, several factors are relevant to prognosis in this group. Most studies have demonstrated that tumor response to preoperative chemotherapy, as measured histologically from a resected specimen, is the most powerful predictor of survival. Patient outcome is affected adversely by metastasis at presentation, long duration of symptoms (> 6 months), high grade or unfavorable histologic subtype, size and tumor volume, and axial skeleton primary tumor. Transarticular skip metastases also portend an increase in the incidence of distant metastasis and reduced survival. For low-grade malignant bone

Table 26.4   Multivariate Analysis of Prognostic Factors in Patients with Soft-Tissue Sarcoma of an Extremity

End Point	Adverse Prognostic Factor	Relative Risk
Local recurrence	Age > 50 yr	1.6
	Local recurrence at presentation	2.0
	Microscopically positive margin	1.8
	Fibrosarcoma	2.5
	Malignant peripheral nerve tumor	1.8
Distant recurrence	Size 5.0–9.9 cm	1.9
	Size > 10.0 cm	1.5
	High grade	4.3
	Deep location	2.5
	Local recurrence at presentation	1.5
	Leiomyosarcoma	1.7
	Nonliposarcoma histology	1.6
Disease-specific survival	Size > 10.0 cm	2.1
	Deep location	2.8
	Local recurrence at presentation	1.5
	Leiomyosarcoma	1.9
	Malignant peripheral nerve tumor	1.9
	Microscopically positive margin	1.7
	Lower-extremity site	1.6

Note: Adverse prognostic factors identified are independent by Cox regression analysis.
Source: Adapted with permission from PWT Pisters, DHY Leung, J Woodruff, et al., Analysis of prognostic factors in 1,041 patients with localized soft tissue sarcomas of the extremities. *J Clin Oncol* 14:1679–1689, 1996.

tumors, adequacy of surgery for the local tumor is the most significant predictor of patient outcome.

PRIMARY MULTIMODALITY TREATMENT

Surgery

Contemporary management of soft-tissue sarcomas includes a multidisciplinary approach using some combination of surgery, radiotherapy, and chemotherapy specific for tumor type and stage of disease. Most patients with bone sarcomas are treated with systemic chemotherapy and surgery with selective use of radiotherapy (i.e., Ewing's sarcoma/primitive neuroectodermal tumor). The surgical management of soft-tissue sarcomas and bone sarcomas has evolved along with the emergence of effective adjuvant therapies and advances in diagnostic imaging modalities. Although complete extirpation of the tumor has remained the primary objective of surgery, the nature and scope of the approach taken to accomplish this goal has resulted in more conservative yet technically challenging operative strategies.

Tumor extirpation with wide negative margins is recognized as the surgical approach to optimize local tumor control; this strategy is applicable to all soft-tissue sarcomas and bone sarcomas. A wide excision removes the primary tumor en bloc, along with its reactive zone and a cuff of normal tissue in all planes, and can be accomplished by limb-sparing surgery or by amputation.

Surgical oncologists are obligated to determine the feasibility of performing a limb-sparing procedure on the basis of the clinical presentation, stage of disease, local extent of tumor, involvement of adjacent vital structures, and tumor response to preoperative chemotherapy or irradiation (or both). The principal goal of limb conservation is to maintain a sensate and functional extremity. The extent of a resection for an extremity sarcoma determines the functional deficit and the type of soft-tissue or bone reconstruction needed to achieve the desired goal. If a clinical situation is not suitable to achieve satisfactory surgical margins with a limb-sparing surgery, amputation is required.

For extremity sarcomas, limb-salvage procedures have supplanted amputation as the principal method to eradicate primary sarcomas, regardless of histology or grade, as long as this procedure can be accomplished without compromising local tumor control or patient survival. In optimizing patient outcome, the emergence of limb-salvage approaches have necessitated close cooperation of surgical, medical, and radiation oncologists to coordinate patient treatment. Refinements in surgical techniques and advances in bioengineering have increased to 95% or greater the percentage of patients eligible for limb-salvage surgery in most major sarcoma treatment centers. Experience with this approach has resulted also in improved function and cosmesis.

Frequently, soft-tissue sarcomas are large and deep-seated at presentation and subsequently often lie adjacent to or involve major blood vessels, nerves, and bone. Frequently, these anatomic constraints to resection create difficulty in achieving a wide surgical margin while preserving limb viability and function. Frequently, sharp dissection in a perineural, periadventitial, or subperiosteal plane is necessary to achieve resection of all gross disease while preserving function. Therefore, the size of the negative margin obtained may be small by necessity. A general recommendation cannot be made regarding the specific quantitative soft-tissue margin needed for all possible sarcoma presentations. The surgical approach is an attempt to maximize preservation of function, but tumor control is the higher priority.

Frequently, soft-tissue reconstruction is necessary to provide reliable wound coverage after tumor extirpation. This procedure is particularly important when preoperative irradiation is a component of the multimodality treatment. Irradiation creates a suboptimal tissue bed susceptible to wound breakdown, seroma and hematoma formation, and infection [5]. Consequently, adequate soft-tissue reconstruction has been critical in the contemporary success of limb-preservation surgery in extremity sarcoma. Local or free transfers of nonirradiated autologous tissues can obliterate dead space after tumor extirpation and can provide a reliable and expedient scaffold for uncomplicated wound closure. Moreover, healthy, well-vascularized, nonirradiated soft tissue can protect underlying blood vessels, nerves, and bones and can withstand the mechanical forces of tension, compression, and shear that occur across joints and in the hands and feet. An immediate one-stage extirpation-reconstruction procedure results in predictable wound coverage, has a low associated failure rate, can reduce perioperative morbidity and duration of hospitalization, and can facilitate the restoration of function [6].

Involvement of major neurovascular structures of affected limbs, which often prompts a recommendation of amputation, is not always an absolute contraindication to limb salvage. If sacrifice of these structures is necessary to achieve negative surgical margins, a complex reconstruction of the deficient tissue (soft tissue, bone, major blood vessels, and nerves) may be performed at the time of tumor resection in an attempt to optimize patient functional outcome (Fig. 26.4). Major arterial and venous reconstruction has been performed successfully to maintain limb viability without compromising oncologic margins. Multiple cable nerve grafts and vascularized nerve grafts in compromised tissue beds have been used to maximize motor function and to restore protective sensation in critical areas that will be needed for long-term preservation of a viable and functional extremity.

Most frequently, bone sarcomas involve the long bones and extend into the adjacent soft tissues. Very often, satisfactory oncologic resection requires sacrifice of the tumor-bearing bone segment in continuity with the adjacent soft-tissue component.
Skeletal reconstruction alternatives have expanded in parallel with advances in biomechanical engineering, prosthesis design, metallurgy, allograft biology, and microvascular techniques. Preoperative planning is essential, and surgeons must coordinate chemotherapy schedules and anticipated post–chemotherapy cycle bone marrow recovery with the time needed to procure a customized prosthesis or other reconstructive materials. Options for skeletal and joint reconstruction include biological, mechanical, or composite biological-mechanical implants. Current methods of skeletal and joint defect reconstruction after sarcoma excision include prosthetic arthroplasty, osteoarticular allografts, allograft-prosthesis composites, and vascularized and nonvascularized large-segment autogenous bone grafts and large-segment allografts.

Because most bone sarcomas arise in the metaphysis of the long bone near the joint, the majority of the procedures performed for these tumors involve resection of both the segment of tumor-bearing bone and the adjacent joint (osteoarticular resection). Usually, reconstruction is achieved by a prosthetic arthroplasty or osteoarticular allograft to maintain a mobile joint or by an arthrodesis of the joint for durable but nonmobile joint function (Fig. 26.5).

Less frequently encountered is the situation wherein a sarcoma arises within the diaphysis or shaft region of the long bone. Ewing's sarcoma, adamantinoma, and a small percentage of osteosarcomas may arise in the shaft of a bone sufficiently distant from the adjacent joint for successful local control without joint sacrifice. In such an approach, the tumor-bearing segment of bone alone is resected (intercalary resection). Most commonly, large-segment bone allografts are used to reconstruct the resultant bony defect (Fig. 26.6). Rarely, involvement along the length of the bone may be so extensive that adequate resection and reconstruction require a resection both of whole-bone resection and of the proximal and distal joints. Whole-bone and adjacent prosthetic arthroplasty is used to reconstruct this massive defect.

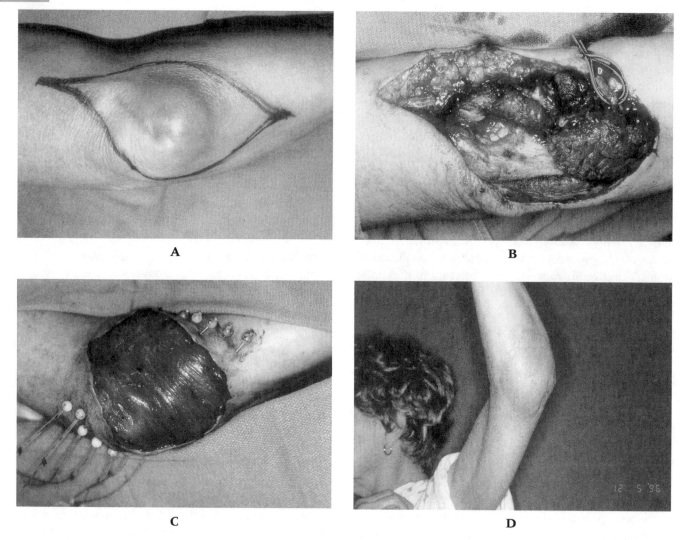

Figure 26.4 Soft-tissue malignant fibrous histiocytoma arising about the elbow in a 68-year-old woman. (A) Planned extent of resection outlined intraoperatively. (B) Surgical wound after wide local excision of the malignant mass, resulting in a large soft-tissue defect and exposed adjacent bone. (C) Free latissimus dorsi muscle flap placed over interstitial catheters inserted for adjuvant radiotherapy. (D) Clinical result after healing of the skin graft and muscle flap.

Pelvic resections present a unique clinical challenge. A tumor arising in the pelvis can involve a segment of nonarticular bone, the acetabulum, or both these structures. The extent of the skeletal resection determines the functional deficit and drives the decision about the type of reconstruction (if any) needed to optimize function. If wide margins can be achieved without compromising the viability of the limb, an internal hemipelvectomy (with preservation of the limb) can be considered as a viable alternative to hindquarter amputation. Sarcomas arising within the sacrum and vertebral column are rare. Because of the unique anatomic challenges of these locations, such tumors rarely are amenable to wide local excision.

The pelvis can be left unreconstructed when a tumor does not involve the acetabulum and hip joint. Such a pelvis is without significant functional deficit. In contrast, resection of the hip joint without reconstruction results in suboptimal function because the extremity is unstable and weak about the hip region and is associated with shortening relative to the contralateral extremity (Fig. 26.7). Restoration of a disrupted pelvic ring or reconstruction of the hip joint may yield better function, but too few cases of any type of reconstruction have been performed to demonstrate superiority of one method over another.

Periacetabular resections can be reconstructed with a large-segment allograft pelvis-hip prosthesis composite implant (Fig. 26.8), pelvifemoral arthrodesis, or prosthetic spacer reconstruction (saddle prosthesis). In all

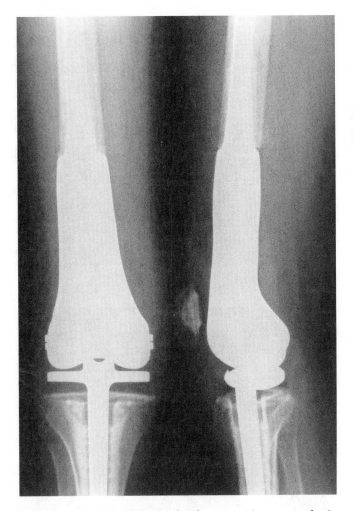

Figure 26.5 Plain radiographs demonstrating a prosthetic arthroplasty of the knee after resection of a primary malignant tumor arising in the distal femur. This reconstruction provides immediate stability and allows early weight bearing and range of motion of the joint.

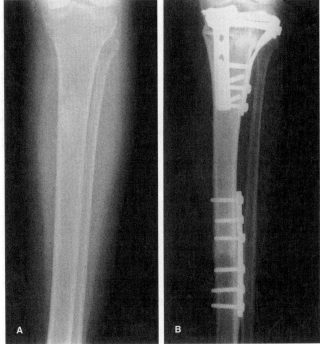

Figure 26.6 (A) Plain radiograph of an osteosarcoma of the shaft of the tibia in a 41-year-old woman. The tumor is amenable to resection without sacrificing the adjacent joint to achieve a satisfactory wide surgical margin. (B) Reconstruction of the bone defect was performed with a large-segment, intercalary bone allograft.

series, a high complication rate has been reported in association with the various available reconstructive methods. Deep infection is the most serious complication of pelvic surgery that can compromise the survival of the reconstruction and limb. In the absence of complications, lower-extremity function and ambulation may be facilitated, at least over the short-term interval.

Tumors arising in an immature skeleton pose a reconstructive challenge, particularly in patients with substantial projected growth of the involved extremity. When the surgical resection includes sacrifice of the principal growth plate of a long bone, standard limb-salvage techniques can result in an appreciable limb-length discrepancy, leading to a functional deficit and a cosmetically undesirable result regardless of the mode of reconstruction. Therefore, the surgical management

of bone sarcomas in skeletally immature patients, with few exceptions, has been standard amputation or Van Nes rotationplasty (intercalary amputation).

For skeletally immature patients with extremity bone sarcomas, the advent of the expandable prosthesis offers an alternative to amputation or rotationplasty. The goals of surgical reconstruction in patients in this group are maintaining a mobile joint and providing a mechanism to accommodate for the loss of the bone growth center. The prosthesis is designed to be lengthened surgically to achieve periodic limb expansion. The need for multiple surgical procedures during the period of affected patients' skeletal growth must be anticipated with this reconstructive approach. At skeletal maturity, the expandable prosthesis can be exchanged for a non-expandable prosthetic arthroplasty, or an arthrodesis can be performed if a more durable reconstruction is desired. Even if wide surgical margins can be achieved without amputation, anatomic limitations, prosthetic design, and mechanical constraints restrict universal application, particularly in very young patients.

The reconstruction method chosen should have the lowest possible associated rate of early postoperative

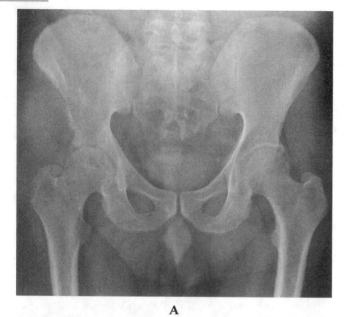

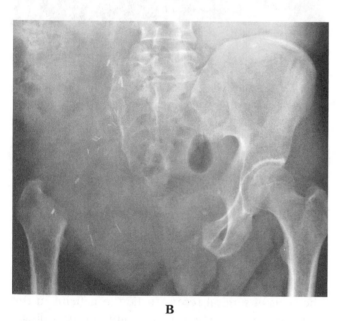

Figure 26.7 (A) Plain radiograph of the pelvis demonstrating a destructive process in the ilium and acetabulum, which proved to be an osteosarcoma. (B) After preoperative chemotherapy, a wide excision of the tumor was performed by internal hemipelvectomy.

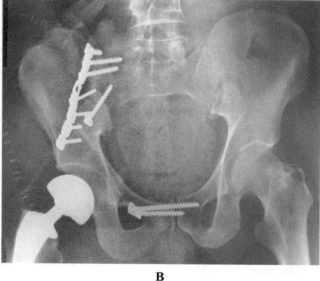

Figure 26.8 (A) Radiographic evidence of destruction of the periacetabular bone. Needle biopsy revealed a high-grade chondrosarcoma. A wide excision of the tumor-bearing portion of the pelvis was performed. (B) Reconstruction of the pelvis and hip joint was accomplished using a large-segment bone allograft and arthroplasty of the hip, in an attempt to optimize lower-extremity function.

complications to avoid a delay in the resumption of adjuvant chemotherapy. Wound-healing problems and infection are the most common complications observed early in the postoperative period.

Late functional outcome and complications depend on site and reconstruction method. However, no reconstruction currently being performed to preserve mobile joint function will last the lifetime of long-term cancer survivors. Variously, loss of fixation, mechanical fail-

ures, polyethylene component debris due to wear, and late infection have compromised the long-term durability of prosthetic reconstructions. Survival of prosthetic reconstructions after segmental bone resections are approximately 70% to 80% at 5 years and 60% to 70% at 10 years [7]. Allogeneic segmental bone graft fracture, infection, and nonunion secondary to resorption limit the usefulness of currently available biological reconstruction alternatives.

Adequate soft-tissue coverage is critical to the success of any limb-salvage procedure. Multiple intraoperative factors contributing to compromised wound healing include surgical elevation of extensive soft-tissue flaps, resection of large segments of bone and surrounding soft tissues, insertion of a massive prosthesis or allograft, and long duration of the surgical procedure. These considerations, coupled with the deleterious effects of chemotherapy or irradiation (or both) on soft-tissue and bone healing, leave affected patients extremely vulnerable to wound-associated complications and to deep infection. This risk is compounded during the period of early postoperative adjuvant chemotherapy, when drug-induced bone marrow suppression leads to loss of neutrophil-granulocyte function. The development of the aforementioned complications during this period can place both limb and patient at risk and often prompts amputation. However, local transposition muscle flaps and free tissue transfers have proved extremely useful in providing a healthy, well-vascularized soft-tissue envelope to cover the reconstruction. The liberal use of these methods has reduced significantly the incidence of wound-healing problems and deep infections associated with limb salvage procedures, especially those complications occurring after resection and reconstruction of the proximal tibia.

Radiotherapy

The standard practice for the treatment of soft-tissue sarcomas is radiotherapy in combination with surgical resection. Several randomized studies support the use of radiotherapy in contemporary management of soft-tissue sarcomas of the extremities and trunk. These studies demonstrated a significant improvement in local disease-free survival when radiotherapy is combined with limb-sparing surgical excision of the tumor [8, 9]. Improved local control is most significant for patients with high-grade sarcomas.

Radiotherapy may be administered preoperatively, postoperatively, or in both periods. Most often, radiotherapy is given via external beam; however, interstitial implants (brachytherapy) also may be used to deliver irradiation locally (Fig. 26.9). Considerable debate has sought to determine which method results in the best local control rate, but no randomized trials have offered a definitive conclusion. Overall, control rates are similar for these approaches and are approximately 10% to 20%. Advocates of preoperative radiotherapy argue that smaller fields and lower doses are necessary (typically, 50 Gy in 25 fractions over 5 weeks), reduc-

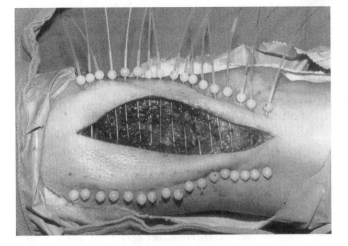

Figure 26.9 Interstitial catheters inserted in the surgical bed for adjuvant radiotherapy (brachytherapy) after resection of a large, high-grade, soft-tissue sarcoma in the thigh. A high dose of radiation can be delivered to the tumor bed in the perioperative period, with maximal sparing of adjacent normal tissues.

ing acute morbidity and cost. However, preoperative external-beam radiotherapy is associated also with a four- to fivefold increase in delayed wound healing and in complications requiring intervention (e.g., infection, débridement, grafting) as compared to surgery in a non-irradiated field. Preoperative radiotherapy is contraindicated when vascular reconstruction within the irradiated field is anticipated. Typically, postoperative external-beam radiotherapy is administered at doses of 60 to 66 Gy, with the higher doses used for positive or uncertain margins. The radiotherapy field is larger because the entire surgical field with a margin of undisturbed tissue must be irradiated.

In contrast to its use in soft-tissue sarcomas, the use of radiotherapy in the primary treatment of bone sarcomas is rare. The role for radiotherapy in the treatment of bone sarcomas is restricted to the management of Ewing's sarcoma/primitive neuroectodermal tumor [10]. These small-cell tumors are radiosensitive, and doses of irradiation of 45 to 55 Gy have been effective as primary local therapy. Although in most centers contemporary management of these tumors includes surgery as the primary local treatment, often radiotherapy is used as a local adjuvant to surgery to produce cytoreduction preoperatively, to facilitate surgical excision of large tumors, and to consolidate local treatment after surgical resection, particularly if tissue margins after surgical resection are inadequate or are positive for microscopic disease. In some instances, radiotherapy may be the preferred modality for local treatment (e.g., for certain pelvic or extremity tumors wherein the functional outcome may be unacceptable to an affected patient, or for unresectable tumors). No prospective randomized studies have defined the relative role of radiotherapy and surgery for the local treatment of these tumors.

Long-term complications of radiotherapy may include bone necrosis, pathologic fracture (30%), growth-plate arrest with limb shortening in skeletally immature patients, soft-tissue fibrosis, joint contracture, and secondary malignancies (< 10%).

Chemotherapy

A clearly defined role for systemic therapy in patients with soft-tissue sarcomas is limited to the subset of patients with small-cell sarcomas (e.g., extraskeletal Ewing's sarcoma/primitive neuroectodermal tumor, rhabdomyosarcoma), to patients with overt metastatic disease, and to those patients at high risk for distant micrometastases. Patients in this latter category include patients with large (> 5-cm-diameter), high-grade, primary soft-tissue sarcomas.

The issue of adjuvant chemotherapy in all other soft-tissue sarcomas remains controversial. Several prospective randomized trials have evaluated the role of adjuvant chemotherapy in localized soft-tissue sarcomas. Only two of these studies demonstrated a significant overall patient survival advantage with the addition of chemotherapy. Doxorubicin and ifosfamide are the two agents most active in soft-tissue sarcoma. Both these drugs have a positive dose-response curve [11]. Several other chemotherapeutic agents, including dacarbazine (DTIC), cisplatin, and methotrexate, have minimal activity in soft-tissue sarcomas. Dactinomycin, vincristine, and etoposide are active only in small-cell sarcomas, including extraskeletal Ewing's sarcoma/primitive neuroectodermal tumor, and rhabdomyosarcoma.

A formal meta-analysis of the 14 adjuvant chemotherapy trials conducted between 1973 and 1990 and involving 1,555 patients with soft-tissue sarcoma revealed a significant improvement in local recurrence-free interval ($p = .016$); distant recurrence-free interval ($p = .0003$); overall recurrence-free survival ($p = .0001$); and a trend toward improved overall survival ($p = .12$) at a median follow-up of 9.4 years [12]. Nonetheless, most studies have been flawed, and so adjuvant chemotherapy for soft-tissue sarcomas still must be considered as investigational.

Chemotherapy has been applied also in the treatment of low- and intermediate-grade soft-tissue sarcomas. Desmoid tumors are locally aggressive neoplasms with no metastatic potential. Patients with desmoid tumors are cured routinely by surgery with or without radiotherapy. In select situations wherein desmoids present as large primary tumors requiring amputation, for a local recurrence within a previously operated and irradiated field, or when the desmoid is part of Gardner's syndrome with mesenteric fibromatosis encasing the mesenteric vasculature, chemotherapy has been effective in cytoreduction, enabling less radical surgical procedures. Systemic chemotherapy with doxorubicin and dacarbazine results in response rates in excess of 60%, and similar results have been published using weekly administration of methotrexate and vinblastine [13]. Tamoxifen, toremifene (a triphenylethylene derivative chemically related to tamoxifen), and progesterone also have activity in patients with desmoid tumors. However, their response rates range between 15% and 25%. Intermediate-grade tumors, such as myxoid liposarcoma, myxoid malignant fibrous histiocytoma, and extraskeletal myxoid chondrosarcoma, can metastasize but tend to have an indolent natural history as compared to high-grade sarcomas. Myxoid variants of liposarcoma and malignant fibrous histiocytoma respond to standard doxorubicin-based chemotherapy in a manner comparable to that of other soft-tissue sarcomas [14, 15].

One of the major deterrents to adjuvant chemotherapy has been the difficulty in justifying exposure to the significant toxicities of these drugs for potentially nonresponding patients. Even in the best of circumstances, only 30% to 50% of the patients with soft-tissue sarcomas will respond to standard chemotherapeutic regimens. Therefore, a better approach to this problem might be to administer chemotherapy before surgical resection, thereby enabling identification of patients with responsive disease while facilitating limb-sparing surgery with better functional results in patients whose sarcoma had be cytoreduced. In addition, with continually improving supportive care due to the availability of bone marrow–stimulating growth factors, better antiemetics, and antibiotics, the morbidity of chemotherapy has been diminished significantly, rendering reasonable and justifiable the treatment of a high-risk population in a controlled neoadjuvant clinical trial research setting.

The role of chemotherapy for patients with bone sarcomas is established more clearly. Prospective, randomized trials conducted in the 1980s and evaluating chemotherapy for patients with osteosarcoma have shown significant improvement in patient survival when chemotherapy is administered. Contemporary management of high-grade bone sarcomas includes preoperative chemotherapy, followed by limb-salvage surgery (or amputation if indicated), followed by postoperative chemotherapy. Active drugs include doxorubicin, ifosfamide, cisplatin, and high-dose methotrexate with leucovorin rescue. These agents have been used with comparable success in various permutations and combinations. Through use of these approaches, long-term survival and cure rates in extremity osteosarcoma in the range of 60% to 80% can be anticipated [16, 17].

Malignant fibrous histiocytoma of bone is considered by many as part of the osteosarcoma spectrum and is, therefore, comparably managed. Multiagent chemotherapeutic regimens for Ewing's sarcoma have increased the survival for this disease from 5% to 10% to up to 75% [18]. Several chemotherapeutic agents, including doxorubicin, cyclophosphamide, ifosfamide, etoposide, vincristine, and dactinomycin, have significant activity in treating this tumor.

Conventional chondrosarcomas are resistant to standard sarcoma chemotherapy, and surgical resection of primary or recurrent tumors, including pulmonary metastases, is the mainstay of therapy. Two specific histologic chondrosarcoma subtypes must be considered as exceptions to this general rule. Dedifferentiated chondrosarcoma is a tumor in which a low-grade chondrosarcoma dedifferentiates with recurrence into a high-grade component consistent with osteosarcoma or a malignant fibrous histiocytoma. The high-grade component of these tumors can demonstrate a response to chemotherapy. Mesenchymal chondrosarcoma is another extremely rare subtype composed of a small-cell element that is responsive to systemic chemotherapy. This latter lesion is treated as is Ewing's sarcoma.

SURVEILLANCE

Rational cost-effective follow-up for patients who have been treated successfully for soft-tissue or bone sarcoma requires an understanding of the relationship between the risk of recurrence and the amount of time elapsed after treatment. Long-term follow-up studies demonstrate that approximately 80% of patients who develop recurrent disease will do so within the first 3 years after therapy. In addition, patients who are alive without recurrence at 5 and 10 years after therapy apparently still carry a risk for a subsequent late recurrence. Consequently, a follow-up strategy should be most intense during the first several posttreatment years and, while less frequent thereafter, still must be continued for at least 10 years after the completion of therapy. All sur-

veillance strategies incorporate follow-up physical examinations and appropriate imaging of the site of the primary tumor (MRI, CT, or ultrasonography for soft-tissue sarcomas and biplanar radiography for bone sarcomas) and chest posteroanterior and lateral views regularly. Such precautionary assessments are more frequent immediately after completion of treatment (every 2–4 months) for 2 years; are less frequent thereafter (every 4–6 months) for 3 years; and ultimately occur annually for an affected patient's lifetime.

TREATMENT OF RELAPSE
Local Recurrence

Contemporary multimodality treatment of soft-tissue and bone sarcomas has allowed more conservative approaches to primary tumor extirpation without sacrificing local tumor control or compromising patient survival. Anatomic constraints on both the extent of the surgical resection and the dose of irradiation have resulted in a higher incidence of local recurrence for patients with retroperitoneal (40%) and head and neck soft-tissue sarcomas (50%) and for pelvic bone sarcomas (35 %). In contrast, local recurrence rates consistently have been in the range of 5% to 10% for high-grade extremity soft-tissue and bone sarcomas (median time to local recurrence, < 24 months after the index surgical procedure).

For soft-tissue sarcoma recurrences, the local treatment depends on the clinical presentation and on prior treatment of the primary tumor. Usually, patients for whom only surgery has been performed are addressed with irradiation (50–65 Gy) and surgical excision. Patients for whom irradiation was part of the initial treatment of the primary tumor may be addressed with re-excision and additional irradiation using external-beam radiation or brachytherapy.

Local tumor recurrence is an adverse prognostic factor for patient survival in both soft-tissue and bone sarcomas. A strong association appears to exist between local recurrence and the development of subsequent metastasis, leading to tumor-specific mortality. Although the role of chemotherapy for locally recurrent high-grade soft-tissue sarcoma remains uncertain, doxorubicin-based chemotherapy regimens may provide a local control advantage and may be of value for patients at high risk for the development of systemic disease. To maximize knowledge gain, chemotherapy should be given only under the aegis of a clinical trial.

For low-grade bone sarcomas, usually excision of the

local recurrence is sufficient to achieve local tumor control. Recurrence of high-grade bone sarcomas is associated with an extremely poor prognosis. Restaging followed by reinduction chemotherapy is indicated in affected patients. Commonly, local tumor control is achieved by limb amputation, owing to the inability to achieve adequate surgical margins about the recurrence. If recurrent tumor is amenable to a wide excision, a limb-sparing procedure could be considered.

Metastasis

Lungs constitute the most common initial site of metastases for the vast majority of soft-tissue and bone sarcomas. Resection of pulmonary metastases is a valid option for a select group of patients with few nodules and a long disease-free interval, which implies a more a favorable prognosis. This approach has been reported to result in a 5-year disease-free and overall survival of 10% to 35% [19]. For the remaining majority of patients, combination chemotherapy continues to be the only available treatment modality, with complete response rates of less than 10% and a very limited potential for cure. With varying degrees of success, several investigators have attempted to improve these results by combining doxorubicin and ifosfamide (with mesna) with or without dacarbazine (MAID regimen). Severe myelosuppression seems to be the dose-limiting toxicity of these combinations and mandates dose reductions and further erosion of the already compromised dose intensity of the individually active drugs, which in turn may be responsible for the lack of improvement in complete responses or overall survival.

Approximately 30% to 40% of patients who have osteosarcoma and develop pulmonary metastasis can be salvaged with reinduction chemotherapy and metastasectomy. Patients with extrapulmonary metastases or unresectable pulmonary metastases have a uniformly poor prognosis. Ewing's sarcoma is a curable tumor even in the presence of clinically detectable metastatic disease if treated with appropriate chemotherapy.

EXPERIMENTAL THERAPEUTIC APPROACHES
Isolated Limb Perfusion

Hyperthermic isolated limb perfusion (HILP) is an investigational technique that is being evaluated in the treatment of soft-tissue sarcoma. In this experimental approach, the circulation to an extremity is isolated from that of the remainder of the body. Then chemotherapeutic agents are perfused directly into that extremity at supranormal temperatures. In this manner, the effective drug administration gradient created is 5 to 50 times greater than that which might be attained via systemic routes. Historically, other agents that have been used in regional perfusion include nitrogen mustard, dactinomycin, and doxorubicin. Hyperthermia to 41°C has been shown to potentiate the effect of chemotherapeutic agents in preclinical laboratory studies, which is the rationale underlying the use of supranormal temperature perfusates. Complications of isolated limb perfusion include infection, chronic damage to skin, muscle, and nerve, extremity edema, and both arterial and venous thrombosis.

HILP has been evaluated for the treatment of extremity sarcomas in the context of locally advanced tumors amenable only to amputation at presentation. It may be indicated to control the primary tumor in patients who have locally advanced and synchronous distant disease and for whom survival is anticipated to be short (6–9 months). Contemporary treatment algorithms for HILP have included high-dose tumor necrosis factor–α, interferon–γ, and melphalan [20]. Despite some reports of extremely high response rates in patients with localized extremity soft-tissue sarcomas, this approach does not address the systemic micrometastases, the major deterrent to survival in most high-risk patients. This approach remains investigational and is being evaluated further in the United States in a multicenter trial conducted by the National Cancer Institute.

Dose-Intensive Chemotherapy

The major thrust of clinical research over the last few years has been dose intensification of the commercially available agents by using myelostimulatory growth factors. The basic rationale for trials evaluating higher-dose intensity lies in the linear dose-response relationship that has been established for doxorubicin and ifosfamide [21]. The ultimate goal is to increase the quality of response sufficiently to bring about a favorable impact on survival. The advent and availability of such growth factors as granulocyte colony-stimulating factor and granulocyte-macrophage colony-stimulating factor have helped to minimize the morbidity related to neutropenia; however, the use of thrombopoietin, a platelet-specific growth factor, to ameliorate dose-limiting thrombocytopenia remains under study. Though the strategy of dose intensification with growth factor support appears promising, confirmation of a positive impact on survival remains unknown.

Reinfusion of growth factor–stimulated and harvested autologous peripheral blood progenitor cells may hold promise for allowing a greater dose intensification for chemotherapy. This approach has the advantage of negating the need for general anesthesia for marrow harvest and exploits the fact that platelet recovery generally is more rapid than that after autologous marrow transplantation.

New Drugs and Approaches

Though current dose intensification with growth factor support seems promising, newer and more effective drugs offer the best hope for future progress. Paclitaxel, topotecan (a topoisomerase I inhibitor), and taxotere have been studied in recent trials, with mixed response rates. Gemcitabine is being used in clinical trials with some encouraging early results. Immunotherapy trials in sarcomas have been limited. Response rates to interferon-α alone or in combination with 5-fluorouracil have been reported to be less than 10%.

Molecular Therapy Regimens

Because of the relative rarity of soft-tissue and bone sarcomas, establishing the development of concerted research programs involving multicenter trials and basic research efforts has been difficult. It is probably unrealistic to anticipate that further refinements in current surgical, radiotherapeutic, and chemotherapeutic approaches will have a marked impact on the 5-year 50% overall survival rate that has been essentially static for the last 20 years. For new gains to be made, increased understanding of the underlying molecular determinants of sarcomagenesis, proliferation, and metastasis will be needed. Through this understanding, specific molecularly targeted therapeutic programs can be created. Future treatment strategies might include modulating genetic mutation in tumor suppressor genes, such as *p53* and *RB1*, or repressing amplification of oncogenes, such as growth and angiogenesis factors, and other promoters of proliferation.

Preclinical studies have demonstrated that restoration of normal wild-type *p53* into soft-tissue sarcomas bearing mutated *p53* markedly decreases tumorigenicity of human sarcoma xenografts implanted into SCID mice [22]. The mechanisms underlying this sarcoma growth suppression include induction of cell-cycle regulatory proteins, such as p21, and inhibition in the production of vascular endothelial growth factor, which is produced at extremely high levels in tumors with mutated *p53*. In the future, such molecularly based strategies might be delivered topically to sarcomas via isolated limb or regional perfusion, as demonstrated recently in the preclinical context [23].

SUPPORTIVE CARE

Rehabilitation

Currently, an achievable goal for the majority of patients with soft-tissue and bone sarcomas is freedom from disease with long-term resumption of nearly normal function. Successful functional outcomes are predicated on the efforts of physiatrists, physical and occupational therapists, and nursing personnel to establish congruent expectations, to implement therapies tailored to individual patients, and to encourage efforts to achieve targeted goals.

The primary focus of inpatient rehabilitation therapy is to facilitate mobilization, thereby preventing such complications as decubitus ulcers, deep venous thrombosis, pneumonia, muscle wasting, and generalized weakness associated with prolonged bed rest. Transfers, gait training, stair climbing, muscle strengthening, and range-of-motion exercises are initiated in the immediate postoperative period. Evaluation of equipment needs for home and workplace is performed prior to hospital discharge. Preoperative instruction and practice in the safe performance of daily living activities also are provided, because postoperative range-of-motion restrictions or bracing may complicate self-care. Prior to discharge, assessment and implementation of outpatient-supervised or self-guided therapy programs are completed to minimize chronic conditions, such as lymphedema, soft-tissue and joint contractures, and myofascial pain syndromes. Because pain control is a critical component in successful acute rehabilitation, the adequacy of analgesia is evaluated and adjusted according to need.

A rehabilitation regimen is dynamic, and adjustments in the therapeutic intervention are matched to the rate of progress toward achieving optimal function. Physiatric management strategies include the use of orthoses to support involved extremities, modifiable ambulation devices, and adaptive equipment (e.g., bathtub benches, elevated commode seats, hospital beds, special chairs). Such environmental adaptations as access ramps, bathroom grab bars, and widened doorways can increase safety and accessibility while reducing effort and fatigue.

Subacute physiatric interventions may include flexibility or endurance exercises, scar-massage instruction to reduce the risk of contractures and skin breakdown, and ongoing assessment of patient protection of insensate skin. Vocational assessments that are made include recommendations regarding work-site modifications, disability services, or referral to local or state vocational rehabilitation and retraining programs. Sexual function may be affected by pain, restricted mobility, or role changes. Discussion of such issues with patients and partners may help in creating solutions to resolve problems or to identify appropriate medical interventions.

Quality-of-Life Considerations

Although advances in technology and refinements in surgical techniques have resulted in more tissue-conserving tumor resections, the impact these advances have had on patient quality of life is unclear. The general belief is that a favorable impact of treatment on patient quality of life would be predicated on (1) preserving those structures necessary for function, (2) harmonizing patient expectations with necessary treatments to control the tumor, and (3) implementing a rehabilitation program that can be followed over the long term to optimize these considerations.

Although most quality-of-life studies include measures of physical, psychosocial, economic, and global well-being, the majority of studies analyzing the non-oncologic outcome for patients treated for sarcomas focus on the functional outcome of treatment for patients with extremity tumors specific for the site and extent of surgery [24]. Usually, those studies that have examined broader indices have been designed to compare patients who have undergone limb-sparing tumor resections with those who have undergone amputation. Recent studies suggest that no measurable global benefit in quality of life is provided by either limb-sparing surgery or amputation [25].

Any measure of quality of life is a dynamic rather than a static process and mandates periodic reassessment. Local tumor recurrence, wound-related complications, or failure of mechanical and biological reconstructions can have a significant impact on a sarcoma patient's quality of life over time. These developments can result in repeated hospitalizations, time lost from work or school, loss of social interaction during acute recuperative periods, increased stress on family and other interpersonal relationships, and financial burdens. Few data address the impact of late complications on limb function and quality of life. Long-term follow-up studies are necessary to elucidate patients' true experience. Improved methodologies are needed to document better the impact that multimodality therapy has on quality of life for patients with a limb malignancy.

The improved ability to identify individuals at risk and to intervene proactively early in the clinical course of disease will increase the number of long-term sarcoma survivors. Measures that can be anticipated to maximize quality of life while improving sarcoma control include introduction of less debilitating surgical procedures coupled with increasingly sophisticated reconstructions, genetic strategies that destroy tumors more selectively, less toxic radiotherapy (such as conformational approaches), and more selective use of systemic chemotherapy in better defined contexts with enhanced supportive care. Though much progress has been made, the success of future treatment approaches in dealing with sarcoma patients will depend on the ongoing cooperative efforts of multidisciplinary sarcoma teams of medical, surgical (general and orthopedic), and irradiation oncologists; plastic surgeons; pathologists; radiologists (interventional and diagnostic); psychiatrists; physiatrists; physical and occupational therapists; nurses; and researchers.

REFERENCES

1. Mankin HJ, Mankin CJ, Simon MA. The hazards of the biopsy, revisited. Members of the Musculoskeletal Tumor Society. *J Bone Joint Surg Am* 78:656–663, 1996.
2. Pisters PWT, Leung DHY, Woodruff J, et al. Analysis of prognostic factors in 1,041 patients with localized soft tissue sarcomas of the extremities. *J Clin Oncol* 14:1679–1689, 1996.
3. American Joint Committee on Cancer. Soft tissue sarcoma. In Fleming ID, Cooper JS, Henson DE, et al. (eds), *AJCC Cancer Staging Manual* (5th ed). Philadelphia: Lippincott-Raven, 1997:149–156.
4. Coindre JM, Terrier P, Bui NB, et al. Prognostic factors in adult patients with locally controlled soft tissue sarcoma: a study of 546 patients from the French Federation of Cancer Centers Sarcoma Group. *J Clin Oncol* 14:869–877, 1996.
5. Bell RS, Mahoney J, O'Sullivan B, et al. Wound healing complications in soft tissue sarcoma management: comparison of three treatment protocols. *J Surg Oncol* 46:190–197, 1991.
6. Reece GP, Gillis T, Pollock RE. Lower extremity salvage after radical resection of malignant tumor in the groin and lower abdominal wall. *J Am Coll Surg* 185:260–267, 1997.
7. Malawer MM, Chou LB. Prosthetic survival and clinical results with use of large-segment replacements in the

treatment of high-grade bone sarcomas. *J Bone Joint Surg Am* 77:1154–1165, 1995.

8. Pisters PWT, Harrison LB, Leung DHY, et al. Long-term results of a prospective randomized trial of adjuvant brachytherapy in soft tissue sarcoma. *J Clin Oncol* 14:859–868, 1996.

9. Yang JC, Chang AE, Baker AR, et al. Randomized prospective study of the benefit of adjuvant radiation therapy in the treatment of soft tissue sarcomas of the extremity. *J Clin Oncol* 16:197–203, 1998.

10. Donaldson SS, Torrey M, Link MP, et al. A multidisciplinary study investigating radiotherapy in Ewing's sarcoma: end results of POG:8346. Pediatric Oncology Group. *Int J Radiat Oncol Biol Phys* 42:125–135, 1998.

11. Patel SR, Vadhan-Raj S, Burgess MA, et al. High-dose ifosfamide in bone and soft-tissue sarcomas—results of phase 2 and pilot studies. Dose-response and schedule dependence. *J Clin Oncol* 15:2378–2384,1997.

12. Sarcoma Meta-Analysis Collaboration. Adjuvant chemotherapy for localised resectable soft-tissue sarcoma of adults: meta-analysis of individual data. *Lancet* 350:1647–1654, 1997.

13. Patel SR, Evans HL, Benjamin RS. Combination chemotherapy in adult desmoid tumors. *Cancer* 72:3244–3247, 1993.

14. Patel SR, Burgess MA, Plager C, et al. Myxoid liposarcoma—experience with chemotherapy. *Cancer* 74:1265–1269, 1994.

15. Patel SR, Plager C, Papadopoulos N, et al. Myxoid malignant fibrous histiocytoma—experience with chemotherapy. *Am J Clin Oncol* 18:528–531, 1995.

16. Proviser AJ, Ettinger LJ, Nachman JB, et al. Treatment of nonmetastatic osteosarcoma of the extremity with preoperative and postoperative chemotherapy: a report from the Children's Cancer Group. *J Clin Oncol* 15:76–84, 1997.

17. Meyers PA, Gorlick R, Heller G, et al. Intensification of preoperative chemotherapy for osteogenic sarcoma: results of the Memorial Sloan-Kettering (T12) protocol. *J Clin Oncol* 16:2452–2458, 1998.

18. Picci P, Bohling T, Bacci G, et al. Chemotherapy-induced tumor necrosis as a prognostic factor in localized Ewing's sarcoma of the extremities. *J Clin Oncol* 15:1553–1559, 1997.

19. Roth JA, Putnam JB, Wesley MN. Deferring determinants of prognosis following resection of pulmonary metastasis from osteogenetic and soft tissue sarcoma patients. *Cancer* 55:1361–1366, 1985.

20. Eggermont ANM, Koops HS, Klausner JM, et al. Isolated limb perfusion with tumor necrosis factor and melphalan for limb salvage in 186 patients with locally advanced soft tissue extremity sarcomas: the cumulative multicenter European experience. *Ann Surg* 224:756–765, 1996.

21. Patel SR, Vadhan-Raj S, Burgess MA, et al. Dose-intensive therapy does improve response rates—updated results of studies of Adriamycin and ifosfamide with growth factors in patients with untreated soft-tissue sarcomas. *Am J Clin Oncol* 21:317–321, 1998.

22. Pollock RE, Lang A, Ge T, et al. Wild-type *p53* and a *p53* temperature-sensitive mutant suppress human soft tissue sarcoma by enhancing cell cycle control. *Clin Cancer Res* 4:1985–1994, 1998.

23. Milas M, Feig B, Yu D, et al. Isolated limb perfusion in the sarcoma bearing rat: a novel preclinical gene delivery system. *Clin Cancer Res* 3:2197–2204, 1997.

24. Davis AM, Bell RS, Badley EM, et al. Evaluating functional outcome in patients with lower extremity sarcoma. *Clin Orthop* 358:90–100, 1999.

25. Rougraff BT, Simon MA, Kneisl JS, et al. Limb salvage compared with amputation for osteosarcoma of the distal end of the femur. A long-term oncological, functional and quality-of-life study. *J Bone Joint Surg Am* 76:649–656, 1994.

27

Cancer of the Thyroid and Parathyroid Glands

■ ■ ■

Scott A. Hundahl
Orlo H. Clark

THYROID CANCER

Although busy primary-care physicians encounter thyroid disease relatively frequently, the scarcity of malignant neoplasms of the thyroid renders their study problematic. Few prospective randomized trials have been performed, and most of what is known about the behavior of these neoplasms derives from retrospective series, epidemiologic studies, and registry data. Additionally, the prolonged survival of patients with papillary and follicular thyroid cancer—the most common types—renders prospective cohort studies difficult. Despite these problems and continued controversy regarding management, recent clinical studies have enhanced our understanding of thyroid cancer behavior significantly.

Table 27.1 summarizes current world-standard incidence and mortality rates for thyroid cancer based on global surveillance data collected by the International Agency for Research on Cancer [1]. In the United States, the American Cancer Society estimates that thyroid cancer will account for approximately 1.5% of incident cancers and 0.2% of cancer deaths in 2000 [2].

Table 27.2 summarizes the proportional incidence (for the United States) of each type of thyroid cancer on the basis of National Cancer Data Base (NCDB) accessions between 1985 and 1995 (53,856 thyroid cancers of the 5,561,125 total cancer cases; approximately 1% of total NCDB cases during this period) [3].

Descriptive epidemiologic characteristics for both papillary and follicular thyroid cancer may be summarized as follows: Incidence for women exceeds that for men by a factor of approximately 2.5; whites and Asians appear to be overrepresented in most studies; and the median age at diagnosis is a bit earlier for papillary car-

We offer special thanks to Dr. Michael Bornemann, MD, FACP, and to Ms. Kate Poole for assistance in preparing this manuscript.

Table 27.1 Incidence and Mortality Rates for Thyroid Cancer

	Incidence	Mortality
Men	1.0	0.3
Women	2.6	0.6

Note: World standard rates per 100,000 population.
Source: Data derived from MD Parkin, P Pisani, J Ferlay, Global cancer statistics. *CA Cancer J Clin* 49:33–64, 1999.

Table 27.2 Proportional Incidence of Various Types of Thyroid Cancer

Histology	No. of Cases	Percentage
Papillary	42,686	79.2
Follicular	6,764	12.6
Medullary	1,928	3.6
Oncocytic (Hürthle)	1,585	2.9
Undifferentiated or anaplastic	893	1.7
Total	53,856	100.0

Source: Data derived from SA Hundahl, ID Fleming, AM Fremgen, HR Menck, A National Cancer Data Base report on 53,856 cases of thyroid carcinoma treated in the US, '85–'95. *Cancer* 83:2638–2648, 1998.

cinoma (40–45 yr) than for follicular carcinoma (48–53 yr). Oncocytic carcinomas (also called *Hürthle cell carcinomas*) behave as a slightly more aggressive form of follicular cancer but present similarly. Medullary thyroid carcinomas (MTCs) tend to present in the initial decades for familial disease and later for sporadic disease. Anaplastic or undifferentiated thyroid carcinoma, which is rare, afflicts those in the later decades of life [3, 4].

Detection, Diagnosis, and Staging

The vast majority of thyroid cancers present as a palpable nodule in the neck. Key aspects of history for thyroid cancers patients include presence of voice change, upper aerodigestive symptoms, growth of the nodule, and family history. Special attention should be devoted to examination of the neck. Examination of the thyroid and neck by standing behind affected patients and gently compressing the soft tissues of the anterior neck with the fingers, one side at a time, is recommended. Having such patients minimally nod forward enhances the examination. As such patients swallow, the thyroid gland will move cephalad, whereas lymph nodes will tend to remain in place. The lower neck should be examined carefully for adenopathy. In all patients with voice change and all who have undergone previous head and neck surgery, direct or indirect laryngoscopy should be performed to assess vocal cord function and to rule out aerodigestive pathologic processes.

Although some autopsy studies have documented a very high incidence of undetected thyroid nodules in elderly patients, particularly women [5], approximately 1% to 6% of adults in the general population have nodules detectable on routine examination [6]. Most such nodules prove benign, the incidence of malignancy in such nodules being only 5% to 10% [7]. However, patients with a history of head and neck irradiation, particularly if such treatment occurred in childhood, have a much higher incidence of malignancy (later in this chapter) [8, 9].

Usually, papillary thyroid cancers and MTCs are firm to palpation. Follicular neoplasms tend to be softer and can mimic benign colloid nodules. Anaplastic thyroid cancers feel poorly marginated and "woody." Most patients with anaplastic cancer present with a history of very rapid tumor growth. Cervical adenopathy, if due to thyroid cancer, usually is found in the middle and lower jugular nodes, the central neck, and the lateral triangle. Sometimes, metastatic lymphadenopathy is the first sign of a thyroid malignancy. Almost always, the primary tumor is situated within the ipsilateral lobe of the thyroid gland and may be occult. Neck ultrasonography is very helpful in evaluating any patient with an equivocal finding or with a subtle abnormality.

Although the appearance of a central neck nodule remains the most common mode of presentation, afflicted relatives of patients with familial-type MTC (including those with multiple endocrine neoplasia type 2 syndromes [MEN2]) are being identified increasingly through genetic testing for point mutations of the *ret* protooncogene on chromosome 10 [10–12]. This method of detection, usually before the onset of clinical disease, represents a diagnostic revolution in progress. At this point, however, genetic diagnosis plays a significant role only in familial MTC and the related familial MEN2A and MEN2B syndromes. Because 3% to 7% of patients with papillary thyroid cancer give a history of familial disease, genetic diagnosis someday may play a role in this disease as well.

In addition to assessing for hyperthyroidism with a serum thyroid-stimulating hormone (TSH), fine-needle aspiration (FNA) with or without ultrasonographic guidance has supplanted other modalities for the initial evaluation of thyroid nodules [11, 13–17]. FNA using a 10-ml syringe and a 22- or 23-gauge needle mounted on a one-handed aspiration device is relatively straightforward. With a patient positioned supine and having a

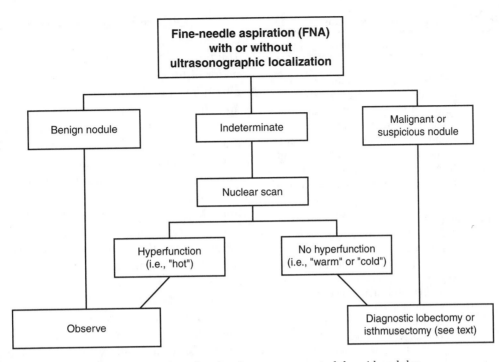

Figure 27.1 Algorithm for the management of thyroid nodules.

rolled towel beneath the shoulders and the neck extended, the nodule is fixed in place between thumb and forefinger, the skin is swabbed with alcohol or iodine solution, and the tip of the needle is placed within the mass. Then aspiration proceeds while the needle is rotated slightly and is moved in and out within the mass. With suction fully released, the needle then is withdrawn. After the specimen-containing needle has been disconnected from the syringe, the syringe's plunger can be repositioned, the needle can be remounted, and the specimen can be blown onto a glass slide. Smears are prepared, and then the slides are sprayed with high-alcohol hair spray or are allowed to air-dry (or both), according to the cytologist's preference. Unless a cytologist is available to stain and read the slides immediately, at least two or three passes (i.e., four to six slides) are recommended. When palpating thyroid nodules is difficult, ultrasonographic guidance should be used [15, 17]. When the specimen is inadequate, repeat aspiration should be arranged. When the aspirate is bloody, the patient should have a repeat biopsy while sitting up (to decrease venous congestion). Using a 25- or 30-gauge needle in this situation also helps.

Malignant aspirates should prompt surgical intervention. Aspirates suggesting follicular cells should be judged equivocal, as FNA cannot distinguish reliably between benign and malignant disease. In the face of such a result, however, evidence of a suppressed TSH level

and a nuclear thyroid scan that clearly reveals the nodule to be hyperfunctional ("hot") can spare the patient an unnecessary surgical procedure, because such hyperfunctional, hot nodules rarely are malignant [18]. Equivocal or suspicious aspirates from nodules that are not clearly hyperfunctional (i.e., "warm" or "cold") should prompt a diagnostic lobectomy and isthmusectomy (Fig. 27.1).

Sometimes, benign nodules can be managed with hormonal suppression (i.e., enough thyroid hormone to suppress TSH to subnormal levels), which generally suppresses the formation of new nodules. Two prospective randomized trials have shown that this practice does not appear to alter the behavior of the index nodule significantly [19, 20], although other prospective studies do support its usefulness. Surgery is recommended for those nodules that grow despite suppression, regardless of initial cytologic results. Repeat FNA, or even diagnostic surgical lobectomy or isthmusectomy, should be considered for nodules that fail to regress after six months of hormonal suppression. Additionally, in any patient with a history of neck irradiation or a family history of thyroid carcinoma, the threshold for surgical treatment should be low, particularly because FNA may be less sensitive in such patients [17].

Cysts constitute a special situation. After aspiration of cyst contents, most practitioners recommend ultrasonography to rule out a residual solid component.

Table 27.3 TNM Staging for Thyroid Neoplasms

Classification	Definition
Primary tumor (T)[a]	
TX	Primary tumor cannot be assessed
T0	No evidence of primary tumor
T1	Tumor ≤ 1 cm in greatest dimension, limited to the thyroid
T2	Tumor > 1 cm but < 4 cm in greatest dimension, limited to the thyroid
T3	Tumor > 4 cm, limited to the thyroid
T4	Tumor of any size extending beyond the thyroid capsule
Regional lymph nodes (N)[b]	
NX	Regional lymph nodes cannot be assessed
N0	No regional lymph node metastasis
N1	Regional lymph node metastasis
N1a	Metastasis in ipsilateral cervical lymph node(s)
N1b	Metastasis in bilateral, midline, or contralateral cervical or mediastinal lymph node(s)
Distant metastasis (M)	
MX	Distant metastasis cannot he assessed
M0	No distant metastasis
M1	Distant metastasis

[a]All categories may be subdivided: (a) solitary tumor; (b) multifocal tumor.
[b]Regional nodes are the cervical and upper mediastinal lymph nodes.
Source: Used with permission of the American Joint Committee on Cancer (AJCC), Chicago, Illinois. Reprinted from ID Fleming, JS Cooper, DE Henson, et al. (eds), *AJCC Cancer Staging Manual* (5th ed). Philadelphia: Lippincott-Raven, 1997:59–61.

Should such a solid component be seen, an ultrasonographically guided FNA of this area is performed, with treatment as outlined earlier [21, 22]. Alternatively, some clinicians simply collapse the cyst by repeat aspiration and then liberally aspirate the area of the lesion with additional passes.

Tables 27.3 and 27.4 describe the American Joint Committee on Cancer's TNM (*tumor, node, metastasis*) staging for thyroid malignancies [23]. The staging system for this site has remained unchanged since 1987. Review of registry data reveals a number of common staging errors for this site: (1) failing to appreciate that staging for papillary or follicular neoplasms changes according to age of the patient, (2) failing to appreciate that all anaplastic or undifferentiated carcinomas are classified as stage IV by definition, and (3) continuing to classify the tumor (T) designation according to size when the tumor extends beyond the capsule of the thyroid gland.

Differentiated Thyroid Cancer

The term *differentiated thyroid cancer* encompasses three major histologic subtypes: papillary carcinoma (80% of all thyroid neoplasms), follicular carcinoma (12.5%), and oncocytic (or Hürthle cell) carcinoma (3%). Microscopically, papillary carcinomas are characterized by areas of papillary fronds and enlarged, elliptical nuclei with thickened membranes, small nucleoli, intranuclear grooves, and intranuclear inclusions. The majority of papillary carcinomas contain varying degrees of follicular growth. The term *mixed papillary and follicular carcinoma* is no longer used, having been superseded simply by *papillary carcinoma* [24, 25]. Such tumors readily invade lymphatic spaces, leading to both a high incidence of multifocality and a high incidence of nodal metastases.

A tumor with purely follicular or trabecular growth and without the characteristic papillations or nuclear features seen in papillary carcinoma is termed a *follicular carcinoma*. Such tumors tend to be surrounded by a fibrous capsule, and invasion of this capsule, or invasion of blood vessels within the tumor, distinguishes a follic-

Table 27.4 AJCC Stage Grouping for Thyroid Neoplasms

Papillary or follicular (age < 45 yr)			
Stage I	Any T	Any N	M0
Stage II	Any T	Any N	M1
Stage III		Undefined	
Stage IV		Undefined	
Papillary or follicular (age ≥ 45 yr)			
Stage I	T1	N0	M0
Stage II	T2	N0	M0
	T3	N0	M0
Stage III	T4	N0	M0
	Any T	N1	M0
Stage IV	Any T	Any N	M1
Medullary			
Stage I	TI	N0	M0
Stage II	T2	N0	M0
	T3	N0	M0
	T4	N0	M0
Stage III	Any T	N1	M0
Stage IV	Any T	Any N	M1
Undifferentiated (anaplastic)*			
Stage IV	Any T	Any N	Any M

AJCC = American Joint Committee on Cancer.
*All cases are stage IV.
Source: Used with permission of the American Joint Committee on Cancer, Chicago, Illinois. Reprinted from ID Fleming, JS Cooper, DE Henson, et al. (eds), *AJCC Cancer Staging Manual* (5th ed). Philadelphia: Lippincott-Raven, 1997:59–61.

ular carcinoma from a follicular adenoma (hence the difficulty in distinguishing between these two entities on the basis of FNA cytology). Lymphatic spread is less common with follicular carcinomas, but they have a higher incidence of distant metastases [26, 27].

Oncocytic carcinoma (also known as *Hürthle cell carcinoma*) represents a variant of follicular carcinoma with a slightly worse prognosis. Given the confusion accompanying the fact that the cell originally described by Hürthle in 1894 subsequently proved to be a parafollicular C cell (the cell of origin for medullary carcinoma), *oncocytic carcinoma* is the term currently favored for this relatively rare variant [22, 28].

Autopsy studies from some geographic areas have revealed a very high incidence of occult thyroid cancer (14–24%) when glands from those dying of nonthyroid causes are analyzed using fine step-sectioning techniques [29, 30]. This finding contrasts markedly with the aforementioned incidence of clinically apparent thyroid cancer, a relatively rare disease (see Table 27.1). On this basis, one might question the significance of the so-called occult or minimal papillary carcinomas that predominate in these autopsy studies, particularly when they represent merely microscopic foci. Nodal metastases from such entities have been described, however [31].

Risk Factors

External-beam irradiation to the head and neck region, particularly during childhood, appears to be associated with a markedly increased risk of papillary carcinoma of the thyroid [8, 32]. The effect of exposure to ingested radioactive isotopes used in diagnostic and therapeutic scans appears negligible, probably owing to differing radiobiological effects, but exposure due to other ingested isotopes or due to radioactive fallout (e.g., that associated with the Chernobyl disaster) does appear to increase the risk of developing thyroid cancer [28, 33–36].

Other factors identified in epidemiologic studies over the years warrant mention, although they appear to be associated with a small relative risk. Dietary iodine deficiency may increase the incidence of follicular carcinomas, as does the ingestion of cruciferous, goitrogenic vegetables. Ingestion of seafood, shellfish, and diets high in iodine appear to be associated with papillary carcinomas, particularly where active volcanoes are close to fishing grounds, as in Hawaii and Iceland. Chronic elevation of TSH levels also may increase the incidence of differentiated thyroid carcinoma [28, 35].

Genetic Factors

Although the hereditary nature of MTC long has been appreciated, evidence for genetic predisposition to differentiated carcinoma has not been as clear. Evidence of familial aggregation in papillary carcinoma has been reported [37, 38]. Also, recent work has documented a number of oncogenes involved in papillary carcinoma, principally the *ret* protooncogene (which is involved also in MTC but through a different mechanism). The *ret* protooncogene, not normally expressed in follicular cells, codes for a tyrosine kinase receptor. In papillary carcinoma, as a result of chromosome 10 rearrangement, the *ret* protooncogene is "turned on" inappropriately as a result of relocation downstream of normally expressed promoters. The result is overproduction of tyrosine kinase activity. As many as 25% of sporadic papillary carcinomas demonstrate translocations involving *ret* [39–42], but the prevalence varies considerably from country to country. Translocations of *ret* tend to be seen more frequently in pediatric thyroid cancer patients and in patients with a history of radiation exposure.

Primary Treatment

For patients with equivocal FNA results (e.g., atypical follicular cells) and no evidence of hyperthyroidism or hyperfunctional characteristics on nuclear scan, a diagnostic ipsilateral complete thyroid lobectomy and isthmusectomy should be performed. Frozen section of the resected lobe fails to identify reliably the fine nuclear changes seen in follicular variants of papillary carcinoma and the microscopic capsular or vascular invasion seen in follicular carcinomas. Therefore, many practitioners now question its utility if an FNA has been performed previously [28, 43]. Permanent sections revealing differentiated carcinoma unappreciated at the time of surgery raise the inevitable question of whether to reoperate to perform completion thyroidectomy (see later). Sublobar resection or nodulectomy should be avoided, as these procedures can seriously compromise subsequent treatment for cancer.

CONTROVERSY

The optimal extent of surgical treatment for differentiated carcinoma of the thyroid remains somewhat controversial, but less so than previously. A brief overview of pertinent information is warranted.

Pathologists have identified a very high incidence of

contralateral disease in patients in whom differentiated thyroid cancer has been diagnosed and who are undergoing total thyroidectomy. In one study of 39 primary cases and 11 secondary cases, contralateral disease was identified in 88%, usually in the thyroid isthmus or nodes [44]. On the basis of this finding and because it facilitates adjuvant therapy with ^{131}I, total thyroidectomy with limited node dissection became established as the most common surgical treatment for this disease. The pathologic diagnosis of contralateral disease in such studies was based on 50-μm sectioning of the whole gland and inclusion of even the smallest foci. As noted, autopsy studies from some geographic areas using the same methods have revealed an implausibly high incidence of thyroid carcinoma (as high as 14–24%) in asymptomatic individuals dying of other causes [29, 30]. Thus, the significance of occult microcarcinomas has been questioned. Rare nodal metastases from such foci have been described, however [31].

Complications associated with thyroid surgery figure prominently in the treatment controversy. Notable are permanent hypoparathyroidism (which, if treated inadequately, can lead to life-threatening hypocalcemic tetany) and injury to the recurrent or superior laryngeal nerves (causing vocal impairment if unilateral and warranting permanent tracheostomy if bilateral). With unilobar operations, hypoparathyroidism does not occur, and recurrent nerve injury in recent series is less than 0.7%. With total thyroidectomy, the incidence of hypoparathyroidism increases to 1% to 9%, and the incidence of recurrent laryngeal nerve injury also increases [28, 44–47].

The majority of patients with differentiated carcinoma of the thyroid gland are considered to be low-risk (i.e., to have a favorable prognosis) and enjoy superb long-term survival even when treated with ipsilateral lobectomy and isthmusectomy. A number of different prognostic scoring systems have been proposed: the AMES (age, metastasis, extent, size) system [48]; the AGES (age, grade, extent, size) system [49, 50]; the DAMES (DNA aneuploidy, age, metastasis, extent, size) system [51]; the MACIS system (metastasis, age, completeness of resection, invasiveness, and size) [52]; the Clinical Class system [47]; the Mazzaferri system [53]; the GAMES (grade, age, metastases, extent, size) system [54]; and of course, the TNM system [23]. These systems capitalize on the adverse effect of the following factors: age beyond 40 to 50 years, presence of distant metastases, large tumor size, extension outside the capsule of the thyroid gland, and adverse histologic factors (e.g., high tumor grade, aneuploidy, extensive capsular

invasion by follicular carcinomas). For patients with low-risk disease as defined by AMES, AGES, MACIS, or GAMES criteria, 20-year determinate survival is approximately 99% [50, 52, 55]. Interestingly, even for patients with distant metastases or advanced, incurable neck disease, these prognostic factors (especially age) hold true [56].

Total or near-total thyroidectomy facilitates adjuvant radioactive iodine (^{131}I) treatment that is difficult in the face of a remaining, intact lobe [44]. Although oncocytic (Hürthle cell) carcinomas do not concentrate ^{131}I well, the modality has proved its benefit as an adjuvant treatment for patients with papillary and follicular carcinomas. Three studies have documented decreased local and regional failure rates with ^{131}I ablation of remnant thyroid elements or subsequent adjuvant treatment with [131]I (or both) [47, 53, 57]. In a Cox regression model of 1,355 cases followed up by questionnaire to determine outcomes, cancer death (8% overall) appeared to be reduced by ^{131}I administration [53]. Other studies also document survival benefit for some subgroups [47, 57].

For low-risk patients—because of their excellent prognosis, the lower morbidity associated with complete ipsilateral lobectomy and isthmusectomy (versus total thyroidectomy), the opportunity for effective salvage treatment for recurrences in the remaining lobe (< 8% at 1020 years in most series), and other factorsparticipants in a Canadian consensus conference in 1993 specified that routine total thyroidectomy should no longer be the treatment of choice [58].

RECOMMENDATIONS

For patients who are undergoing diagnostic lobectomy or isthmusectomy and whose cancer is not identified by frozen section, the entire specimen should be step-sectioned and examined microscopically. If cancer is discovered, the majority of such patients will fall into the low-risk subgroup (Table 27.5), and reoperation to address the contralateral lobe will not be required. For those at higher risk, reoperation and the subsequent use of ^{131}I should be considered (Fig. 27.2).

For patients in the low-risk subgroup, complete ipsilateral lobectomy and isthmusectomy with resection of adjacent neck nodes is adequate, provided the contralateral lobe appears normal. Many surgical experts with (documented) negligible complication rates proceed to total or near-total thyroidectomy even for this subgroup, but this approach no longer is routine. Should involved nodes be detected intraoperatively, functional

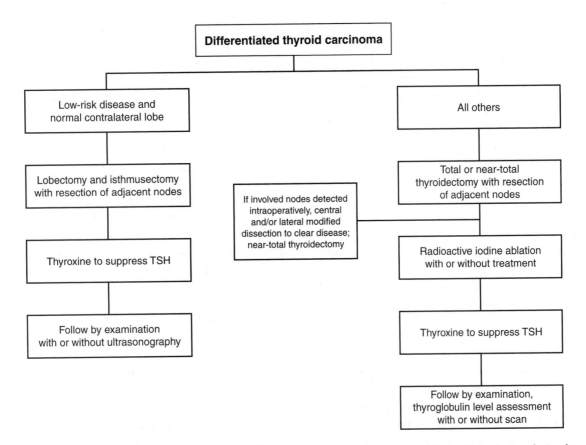

Figure 27.2 Algorithm for the management of primary differentiated thyroid cancer. *TSH* = thyroid-stimulating hormone.

dissection of the central and lateral neck—whatever is necessary to clear apparent disease—should be performed, and a total or near-total thyroidectomy should be considered. Most practitioners advocate the use of postoperative adjuvant ^{131}I for patients with involved nodes (see Fig. 27.2).

Higher-risk patients should be treated by total or near-total thyroidectomy with resection of adjacent central neck nodes. If detected intraoperatively, positive nodes are treated as noted earlier. Postoperatively, thyroid hormone therapy is withheld, and TSH levels are allowed to rise. At a minimum of six weeks postoperatively and at least six weeks after discontinuing all levothyroxine use, or two weeks after discontinuing liothyronine (Cytomel) use, residual thyroid remnants are ablated with [131]I. Affected patients should undergo serum TSH, thyroglobulin, and pregnancy tests (when appropriate) prior to treatment. Also, such patients should be on a low-iodine diet at least two weeks prior to treatment.

Management of the parathyroids deserves mention. Even in patients undergoing a unilateral resection, every parathyroid gland should be preserved meticu-

Table 27.5 Low-Risk Subgroup of Patients with Differentiated Carcinoma, GAMES Criteria

Grade	Low-grade histology[a]
Age	< 45 yr
Metastases	No distant metastases
Extent	No extrathyroidal extension
Size	≤ 4 cm[b]

[a]In this system, histologic grade is defined simply as follows: low-grade neoplasm, typical papillary; high-grade neoplasm, pure follicular or oncocytic (Hürthle cell). High-grade neoplasms also include aggressive papillary variants such as "tall cell."
[b]Some experts modify the GAMES cutoff for size, preferring a lower figure of ≤ 1.5–2.0 cm.
Note: The GAMES criteria derive from a combination of the AGES system (*a*ge, *g*rade, *e*xtent, *s*ize) and AMES system (*a*ge, *m*etastasis, *e*xtent, *s*ize).

lously, because some such patients may someday undergo a contralateral procedure. If devascularized during dissection, parathyroid glands should be preserved in isotonic saline and, after their identity has been confirmed by frozen section, should be implanted as 1-mm slivers of tissue into the base of the sternocleidomastoid muscle. Usually, the site is marked with a nonabsorbable suture. Such implanted tissue usually becomes active after six to eight weeks and helps to avoid the dire complication of permanent hypoparathyroidism. (For technical details concerning the surgical treatment of thyroid cancer, the reader is referred to recent chapters in surgical atlases [59, 60].)

Outside of periods of preparation for ^{131}I procedures, all patients should take daily levothyroxine in a dose sufficient to suppress their TSH to subnormal levels (i.e., TSH < 0.1 µU/ml).

Follow-up for low-risk patients treated by ipsilateral lobectomy or isthmusectomy consists of periodic neck examination (with or without neck ultrasonography), an annual chest roentgenogram, and an annual TSH evaluation to confirm appropriate suppression. Generally, ^{131}I scanning is not performed in such patients, as radioiodine will move preferentially to the functioning residual gland.

For those who have been treated by total or near-total thyroidectomy and have undergone successful ablation with ^{131}I, the thyroglobulin level can be used as a sensitive marker for recurrence. In this group of patients, ^{131}I scans are helpful in detecting and localizing recurrence. Some clinicians also recommend ultrasonography for such patients, as recurrences cannot always be visualized on radioiodine scanning.

Adjuvant Treatment

Outside of periods of preparation for ^{131}I procedures, all patients should take daily levothyroxine in a dose sufficient to suppress their TSH to subnormal levels but not to the extent that produces symptoms of hyperthyroidism or excessive elevation of free thyroxine (T_4). High T_4 levels are associated with increased risk of osteoporosis and cardiac arrhythmias.

Patients who are in the higher-risk categories and should have undergone total or near-total thyroidectomy as their surgical treatment also are given adjuvant ^{131}I therapy. This therapy starts with ablation of remnants of normal thyroid tissue in the neck (when present) and along the embryonic tract of the thyroglossal duct. TSH levels should be higher than 30 µU/ml for optimal ablation; in a patient who has undergone total thyroidectomy, six weeks without levothyroxine or two weeks without liothyronine (assuming administration of no other thyroid hormones during the six-week postoperative period) usually is sufficient to elevate TSH to this level. Human recombinant TSH (Thyrogen) has

been used to enhance diagnostic thyroid scanning, but its use to facilitate radioiodine treatment remains experimental. For two weeks prior to radioiodine treatment, affected patients should be on a low-iodine diet (i.e., no seafood or iodized salt). On the basis of a prospective, randomized trial by Bal et al. [61], a dose of approximately 50 mCi successfully ablates remnant thyroid tissue in 80% of patients, and larger doses up to 150 mCi do not appear more successful. Nuclear Regulatory Commission regulations specify that beyond a certain threshold of radioiodine (30–50 mCi, depending on restrictions of a given hospital's license), isolation and hospitalization is required. To avoid hospitalization, many attempt ablation doses below the threshold requiring mandatory isolation, but this alternative often is unsuccessful. Recalling that on nuclear scans thyroid carcinomas usually are cold relative to normal thyroid tissue, one should appreciate that the presence of normal thyroid tissue can competitively inhibit the uptake of ^{131}I by a tumor.

Sublethal irradiation "stunning" as a result of previous scans can thwart uptake of ^{131}I by otherwise sensitive cancer cells. The likelihood of this appears to increase with prolonged delay between scanning and therapeutic doses and may occur after inadequate ablation of normal thyroid tissue [28, 62, 63].

Treatment of Subsequent Nodal or Distant Metastases

Prior to initiation of treatment with ^{131}I, bulk disease should be excised surgically whenever feasible, depending on site and anticipated morbidity. This "reserves" the ^{131}I for microscopic residual disease. In unusual situations, when localized recurrence is not surgically treatable and the disease no longer is susceptible to ^{131}I, systemic doxorubicin combined with hyperfractionated radiotherapy can be helpful [28, 64, 65].

Prognosis

Figure 27.3 depicts 10-year overall relative survival for 53,856 patients with cases of thyroid carcinoma accessioned to the NCDB between 1985 and 1995. In the United States during this period, the vast majority of papillary and follicular thyroid carcinoma patients presented with low-stage disease (papillary, 57% stage I, 14% stage II; follicular, 41% stage I, 27% stage II)—hence the superb overall survival [3].

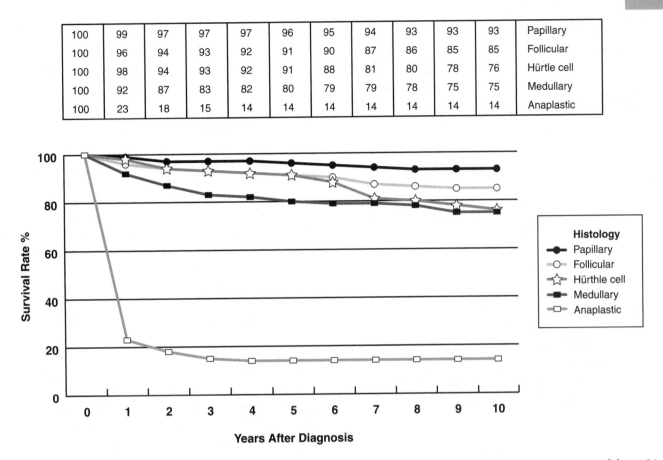

100	99	97	97	97	96	95	94	93	93	93	Papillary
100	96	94	93	92	91	90	87	86	85	85	Follicular
100	98	94	93	92	91	88	81	80	78	76	Hürtle cell
100	92	87	83	82	80	79	79	78	75	75	Medullary
100	23	18	15	14	14	14	14	14	14	14	Anaplastic

Figure 27.3   Overall 10-year relative survival of 53,856 patients with thyroid carcinoma, by histology. (Reprinted from SA Hundahl, ID Fleming, AM Fremgen, HR Menck, A National Cancer Data Base report on 53,856 cases of thyroid carcinoma treated in the US, '85–'95. *Cancer* 83:2638–2648, 1998. Copyright ©1998 American Cancer Society. Used with permission of Wiley-Liss, Inc., a subsidiary of John Wiley & Sons, Inc.)

Table 27.6 depicts five-year relative survival by TNM stage for the same cohort [3]. However, such five-year survival rates do not translate into cure. The natural history of differentiated thyroid cancer is long, and attributable deaths can occur 20 or more years after diagnosis.

MEDULLARY CARCINOMA

Only 3.5% to 7.0% of all thyroid cancers are MTCs, yet these tumors account for approximately 17% of all thyroid cancer deaths [3, 12]. Approximately 75% of patients with MTC have sporadic (i.e., nonfamilial) tumors and present with a solitary thyroid nodule, although some patients present with only palpable cervical lymph nodes or, less commonly, with distant (usually liver or bone) metastases. Approximately 35% of patients with MTC have palpable nodes at presentation, and some

50% are found to have lymphadenopathy at thyroidectomy [66]. Although most patients with MTC are asymptomatic, some have a mild aching sensation or pain in the neck, and the tumor may be tender to palpation.

Diagnosis

Evaluation begins with FNA. Usually, experienced cytologists can diagnose MTC by cytologic examination but, occasionally, they can state only that affected patients have cancer of unknown etiology. In such patients, the slides should be stained for calcitonin, thyroglobulin, carcinoembryonic antigen (CEA), and amyloid. A blood sample also should be obtained for calcitonin and CEA. Obtaining the results of a blood calcitonin level from the clinical laboratory often takes longer than do stains. Because poorly differentiated MTCs may stain poorly on immunochemical testing,

Table 27.6 TNM Stage-Stratified Five-Year Relative Survival Rates (By Histology)

Histology	Relative Survival Rate (%)			
	Stage I	Stage II	Stage III	Stage IV
Papillary	100	100	94	48
Follicular	99	99	82	47
Oncocytic	96	94	76	49
Medullary	98	98	73	40
Anaplastic (undifferentiated)	—	—	—	14

Source: Data derived from SA Hundahl, ID Fleming, AM Fremgen, HR Menck, A National Cancer Data Base report on 53,856 cases of thyroid carcinoma treated in the US, '85–'95. *Cancer* 83:2638–2648, 1998.

however, documenting an increased blood CEA and calcitonin level is still useful as this finding strongly suggests MTC. Additionally, all patients with MTC must be tested to determine whether they have MEN2A or MEN2B and a possible coexistent pheochromocytoma before a definitive thyroid operation is performed.

Genetics

All patients with MTC, whether familial or sporadic, should be tested for the presence of an *ret* point mutation on chromosome 10 that codes for a transmembrane receptor tyrosine kinase protein, the ligand of which is a neurotrophine called *glial-derived nerve growth factor* [10, 67]. Detection of such *ret* point mutations can facilitate screening of offspring. Perhaps 25% of patients with MTC have familial disease, and a number of associated point mutations in *ret* have been described (Fig. 27.4) [10, 12]. Testing for an *ret* mutation should be carried out even in patients with no family history of MTC, because such patients may have a de novo mutation [68]. Such mutations occur in approximately 10% of patients with MEN2A and in up to 50% of patients with MEN2B.

Familial MTC and Early Detection

Familial MTC occurs in three forms: (1) familial MTC alone, (2) familial MEN2A with MTC, pheochromocytomas, and hyperparathyroidism; and (3) familial MEN2B with MTC, pheochromocytomas, a marfanoid habitus, mucosal neuromas, and ganglioneuromatosis. Some patients with familial MTC and MEN2A (and,

rarely, MEN2B) also have Hirschsprung's disease and lichen planus amyloidosis [69, 70].

All first-degree relatives of patients with familial MTC and a known *ret* mutation should be screened for the same *ret* mutation. Patients who test positive should be tested a second time and, if again they test positive and are older than six years, should be treated by a prophylactic total thyroidectomy. Prior to thyroidectomy, such individuals also should have ultrasonography to evaluate the thyroid gland for abnormalities; a basal and stimulated calcitonin test; a blood calcium test to diagnose possible coexisting hyperparathyroidism; and urinary epinephrine, norepinephrine, and metanephrine analyses to diagnose coexistent pheochromocytomas.

Primary Treatment and Extent of Operation

In all patients in whom MTC has been diagnosed preoperatively, concomitant pheochromocytoma should be ruled out with the aforementioned urinary tests. In unprepared patients with pheochromocytoma, general anesthesia can induce life-threatening hypertension and tachyarrhythmias.

Medullary carcinoma of the thyroid gland should be regarded as a surgical disease. The extent of surgical treatment varies somewhat according to the specific situation, however. For patients with familial MTC, total thyroidectomy and a meticulous central neck dissection (and full bilateral modified neck dissection if nodes are involved) constitutes standard therapy [71, 72]. Patients with sporadic MTC and tumors smaller than 2 cm should undergo total thyroidectomy and central neck dissection. For patients with sporadic MTC and tumors larger than 2 cm, modified radical neck dissection should be added, because the incidence of nodal metastases in such patients approximates 60%. For MEN2B patients who have more aggressive disease, total thyroidectomy, central neck dissection, and bilateral modified radical neck dissection on the side on which primary tumor is detected is recommended. Also, in patients with MTC and MEN2A, any abnormal parathyroid glands should selectively removed.

In patients who are younger than age 6, are identified by genetic testing, and are *ret* oncogene–positive but who have no thyroid abnormalities on ultrasonography and have a normal basal and stimulated calcitonin level, simple total thyroidectomy is recommended. For patients whose disease is detected by screening for *ret* mutations, in whom any thyroid abnormality ap-

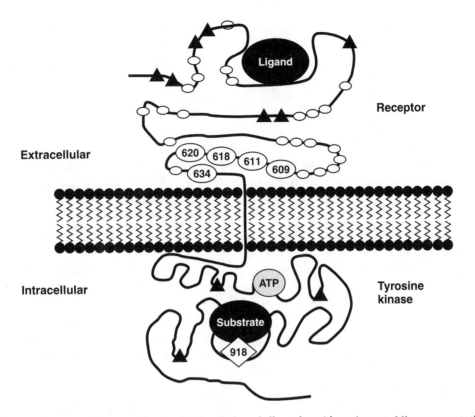

Figure 27.4 The *ret* point mutations associated with familial medullary thyroid carcinoma. Missense mutations associated with multiple endocrine neoplasia type 2A (MEN2A) and familial non-MEN medullary thyroid cancer have been found in codons encoding extracellular cysteine residues (codons 609, 611, 618, 620, and 634). A missense mutation associated with MEN2B has been found in the tyrosine kinase domain (codon 918). *ATP* = adenosine triphosphate.

pears on ultrasonographic examination of the thyroid or an increased basal or pentagastrin-or calcium-stimulated calcitonin level is determined, or who are more than 9 years old, total thyroidectomy and a central neck dissection is recommended.

During the total thyroidectomy, it is preferable to preserve the parathyroid glands in situ unless they cannot be dissected free from the thyroid gland on a vascular pedicle. In the latter case, the parathyroid gland should undergo biopsy to confirm its identity and should be autotransplanted. When necessary, in MEN2A patients, autotransplantion of the parathyroid glands to the nondominant forearm is preferred, whereas in familial MTC and MEN2B patients, transplantation to the ipsilateral or contralateral sternocleidomastoid muscle is preferred. This difference in approach is used because only MEN2A patients are at higher risk of subsequently developing hyperparathyroidism. All parathyroid glands, whether left in position or autotransplanted, should be marked carefully with a clip or stitch to help to identify them if affected patients subsequently develop recurrent MTC or primary hyperparathyroidism.

A few patients who are *ret*-positive with familial MTC may have normal thyroid glands without C-cell hyperplasia or detectable MTC [73, 74]. Some 11% of patients having prophylactic thyroid operations have positive nodes. This situation is more common in older children (> 9 years) and in patients with more than microscopic primary thyroid cancers. A controversial issue is whether prophylactic central neck dissection is necessary in children who are younger than age 6 and have MEN2A and in those who are younger than age 9 and have familial MTC with normal stimulated calcitonin levels and a normal ultrasonographic examination. Prophylactic central neck dissection at the time of total thyroidectomy in children younger than age 6 is no longer recommended, provided such patients have a normal basal and stimulated calcitonin level and a normal ultrasonographic examination. Central neck dissection does subject patients to a small but increased risk of hypoparathyroidism; in that situation, the risk of microscopic nodal disease is scant [73].

Also controversial is whether a prophylactic, unilateral, modified lateral radical neck dissection is indicated in patients with sporadic or familial MTC and thyroid cancers smaller than 2 cm. Studies document that more than 60% of patients with primary MTC greater than 2 cm have lymph node metastases in the ipsilateral neck [75, 76]. Therefore, both prophylactic and therapeutic ipsilateral modified radical neck dissection is recommended for such patients. Prophylactic neck dissection is also recommended for virtually all patients with MEN2B because such patients have the worst prognosis, with only approximately 35% being alive at five years. Finally, this procedure is recommended for all adults who have MTC and lymph node metastasis in the central neck.

Contralateral prophylactic modified radical neck dissection for patients with sporadic ipsilateral MTC does not seem warranted, but it is recommended for patients with familial MTC because the latter have bilateral disease. A Swedish cooperative study by Bergholm et al. [77] of 247 patients with MTC documented that the overall survival rate of patients with MTC was 69% at 10 years and 65% at 15 years. When patients who had familial MTC and were diagnosed by screening methods were removed from the study group, the mortality was 61% at 10 and 54% at 15 years. Similarly, Girelli et al. [78] recently reported that survival was 95% at 10 and 20 years, respectively, for patients with MTC confined to the thyroid gland but fell to 55% and 29% for stage III and stage IV patients, respectively, at 10 years. However, in the study of Bergholm et al. [77], only 10% of patients with sporadic MTC were calcitonin-negative; thus, most such patients have residual MTC. With increasing serum calcitonin levels, recurrence of tumor increases [78].

The initial operation constitutes the best opportunity to cure MTC. Studies confirm that cure correlates not only with less extensive disease but with more extensive initial treatment [71, 76, 79]. In particular, removal of lymph nodes in patients with MTC should be especially meticulous; in contrast to the experience in patients with papillary or follicular thyroid cancer, nodal metastases cannot be ablated with ^{131}I, and the presence of nodes is associated with a measurably worse outcome. Technical details concerning the actual conduct of surgery are well described in current surgical atlases [59, 60].

Six weeks postoperatively, all patients should have repeat calcitonin and CEA level tests. In patients with a low calcitonin level, provocative testing with pentagastrin or calcium can be carried out to determine whether calcitonin increases. In patients with a persistently elevated calcitonin or CEA level (or both), magnetic resonance imaging (MRI) or computed tomography (CT) scanning of the neck and superior mediastinum should be performed. If an ipsilateral modified radical (functional) neck dissection has not been performed already, it should be, regardless of the scanning results [71, 80]. In patients with markedly elevated calcitonin levels after definitive surgery for MTC and with no evidence of cancer, the cause almost invariably is the small, multiple hepatic metastases seen so frequently with such tumors. Occasionally, these lesions can be identified by CT scan or laparoscopy or by documenting increased calcitonin levels in the hepatic veins after pentagastrin stimulation [81].

Adjuvant Therapy and Therapy for Residual Disease

In the absence of residual disease, no additional therapy other than thyroid hormone administration is recommended. For patients with residual MTC that could not be eliminated surgically, the use of external-beam radiotherapy, ^{131}I ablation therapy, and chemotherapy is controversial. Although MTCs neither trap iodine nor have TSH receptors, benefit from a single ablative dose of ^{131}I has been reported [82, 83]. Small deposits of MTC situated immediately adjacent to some residual normal thyroid tissue may be ablated by such treatment. Frequently, external-beam radiotherapy is administered when residual tumor is present; some studies show benefit [84], whereas others do not [85]. In addition, although the combination of cyclophosphamide, dacarbazine, and vincristine, or dacarbazine and fluorouracil, or bleomycin, doxorubicin, and cisplatin has achieved some partial responses, chemotherapy has not proved to be very effective [86]. Recently, treatment with radioiodinated CEA was recommended [87]. Patients with liver metastases may benefit from radiofrequency ablation [88].

What should be emphasized, however, is that patients with persistent or recurrent MTC can live for many years with few or no adverse effects from their tumors. For most patients with high calcitonin levels after definitive surgery and no identifiable disease, treatment is not recommended until a tumor has been documented and localized. Selective venous catheterization for calcitonin levels has been reported to be helpful in some patients [89], as has sestamibi, thallium, and metaiodobenzyl guanidine (MIBG) scanning [12, 90, 91], but these by no means are reliable. Positron emission tomography scanning also can detect small tumor deposits of MTC. Unfortunately, however, calcitonin levels usually remain elevated after such metastases are destroyed, suggesting additional unrecognized metastatic deposits.

Prognosis

Figure 27.3 and Table 27.6 summarize overall survival rates for patients with MTC. Tumors larger than 2 cm, positive nodes, and distant metastases constitute major adverse prognostic factors. Male gender and advancing age also adversely influence prognosis, but their effects are not as pronounced as in differentiated thyroid cancer [3]. Also, patients with MEN2B and medullary carcinoma experience the worst outcomes, with only perhaps 35% of patients being alive at five years.

ANAPLASTIC THYROID CANCER

Background

Anaplastic and undifferentiated thyroid cancers—neoplasms with a notoriously dire prognosis—account for only 1% to 1.5% of thyroid malignancies [3, 92]. Often, papillary or follicular thyroid carcinoma coexists with anaplastic thyroid cancer, suggesting that differentiated thyroid cancers can dedifferentiate to become anaplastic cancers [93]. Several histologic variants of anaplastic thyroid cancer include large- or giant-cell, spindle-cell, and small-cell types. When patients are considered to have small-cell anaplastic thyroid cancer, excluding thyroid lymphoma or MTC is important, as these tumors may appear histologically to be similar to small-cell undifferentiated tumors. The prognosis associated with thyroid lymphoma and MTC is considerably better than that associated with anaplastic thyroid cancer [3, 24].

Usually, anaplastic thyroid cancer afflicts the elderly. Typically, affected patients reveal a history of rapid enlargement of a preexisting nodule or goiter. At the time of diagnosis, the mass often is fixed because of its large size or because of invasion into the adjacent soft tissues. In contrast to patients with differentiated thyroid cancer, patients with anaplastic thyroid cancer often have localized symptoms because of rapid tumor growth and because of the invasive nature of these tumors. Hoarseness due to invasion of the recurrent laryngeal nerve is relatively common. Hypothyroidism due to extensive destruction of the gland by tumor can occur.

Differential diagnosis includes thyroid lymphoma, squamous cell cancers, carcinosarcomas, teratomas, plasmacytomas, subacute thyroiditis, and hemorrhage within the thyroid. Usually, the diagnosis can be made by FNA. However, often these tumors are associated with hemorrhagic necrosis that can dilute the sample so that malignant cells are missed.

In contrast to the experience in patients with differentiated carcinoma or medullary carcinoma, CT or MRI scanning is helpful in patients with anaplastic thyroid cancer because the tumors usually are fixed, and precise delineation is difficult. Chest roentgenography or even chest CT should be performed, but bone scan and spot radiographs are used selectively, depending on presence of bone pain, elevated alkaline phosphatase, and the like. Airway evaluation and management are particularly important in such patients.

Treatment and Prognosis

Once the diagnosis of anaplastic thyroid cancer has been confirmed by FNA, cytologic examination, or core needle biopsy, uncommon patients with a mobile, potentially curable tumor should be treated initially by total thyroidectomy and all detectable disease should be removed. In addition, treatment with external-beam radiotherapy and chemotherapy is recommended.

However, most patients present with fixed thyroid masses that are not resectable to tumor-free margins. For such patients, a modification of the treatment plan used at the Karolinska Hospital in Sweden may be used. Briefly, this program includes (1) intravenous bleomycin, 5 mg, 1 to 2 hours before radiotherapy, and 5-fluorouracil, 500 mg intravenously, before every second treatment; (2) 30 Gy of irradiation in three weeks using megavoltage irradiation; (3) thyroidectomy removing as much tumor and thyroid as is safe approximately two to three weeks after completion of the initial chemotherapeutic and radiotherapeutic regimens; and (4) approximately two weeks postthyroidectomy, an additional 15 Gy of irradiation along with chemotherapy similar to that used preoperatively [94]. Using this therapeutic strategy, three of the 19 patients in the Swedish study were alive 31, 61, and 80 months after treatment, respectively, and no one died of suffocation from recurrent central neck disease, although the remaining 16 died from their thyroid cancers. Though these results are far superior to historic results with combination radiotherapy and chemotherapy [92, 95] they mirror recent NCDB results [3]. Recently, taxol has shown some promise both in vitro and in vivo [96].

PARATHYROID CANCER
Background

Parathyroid cancer ranks among the rarest of neoplasms. Among NCDB cases (1985–1995) in the United States, it constitutes only 0.01% of cases [97]. Among patients with primary hyperparathyroidism, it occurs in 0.5% of cases [98–100]. In contrast to benign parathyroid tumors, which are more common in women, parathyroid cancer afflicts men and women equally. Apparently, no racial, socioeconomic, or geographic predisposition is evidenced by parathyroid cancer. However, it does occur more frequently in patients with familial hyperparathyroidism and in individuals exposed to low-dose therapeutic radiation [99, 101]. Approximately 94% of patients with parathyroid cancer exhibit marked hypercalcemia, but 6% of patients have nonfunctioning parathyroid cancers and are normocalcemic [99, 100].

Dealing with patients with parathyroid cancer—a once-in-a-lifetime experience for most clinicians—presents challenges on three levels: (1) recognizing a parathyroid cancer (versus the far more common parathyroid adenoma) early enough to treat properly; (2) identifying the precise clinical and pathologic criteria used to diagnose parathyroid cancer; and (3) managing the disease and associated hypercalcemia, particularly in patients with metastases.

Recognition and Diagnosis

In marked contrast to the majority of patients who present with parathyroid adenomas or hyperplastic parathyroid glands, most patients with primary hyperparathyroidism due to parathyroid cancer present with profound hypercalcemia (i.e., serum calcium > 13.5 mg/dl). The symptoms in patients with parathyroid cancer are similar to those of primary hyperparathyroidism due to benign tumors but often are more profound [98, 99]. Thus, many patients have painful bones, kidney stones, abdominal groans, psychic moans, and fatigue overtones." Perhaps separating symptoms into categories of *neuropsychiatric* and *somatic* is best. The former, for example, would include fatigue, change in mood, depression, weakness, loss of memory, lack of motivation, or lack of energy, whereas the latter would include musculoskeletal aches, dyspepsia, constipation, pruritus, polydipsia, polyuria, and nocturia. Associated conditions or complications of primary hyperparathyroidism include hypertension, osteoporosis, nephrolithiasis, nephrocalcinosis, gout or pseudogout, peptic ulcer disease, and pancreatitis.

Numerous studies have documented that patients with even mild primary hyperparathyroidism have more symptoms and associated conditions than do age- and gender-matched patients without hyperparathyroidism [100–103]. Some patients who feel relatively well (asymptomatic) preoperatively note an improved state of well-being after successful parathyroidectomy [101–104]. Patients with parathyroid cancer are more likely to experience symptoms and are more likely to have associated conditions (including nephrolithiasis and osteitis fibrosa cystica) than are patients with parathyroid adenomas or hyperplastic parathyroid glands [98]. They also are more likely to present with coma or profound stupor and with pancreatitis, because these clinical manifestations occur more frequently in patients with profound hypercalcemia. However, when patients with parathyroid cancer are matched with patients who have large benign parathyroid tumors and comparable hypercalcemia, clinical manifestations are similar [100].

Approximately 50% of patients with parathyroid cancer have palpable neck mass versus perhaps 4% of patients with parathyroid adenomas. The size of the parathyroid tumor correlates directly with the degree of hypercalcemia and the serum parathyroid hormone (PTH) level [105]. Despite this correlation, Fuller Albright's dictum—"[W]hen one feels a mass in the neck of a patient with primary hyperparathyroidism it is usually a thyroid nodule not a parathyroid tumor"—still is usually true. From a clinical point of view, however, the neck should be examined carefully in any patient with profound hypercalcemia because, if the patient has a palpable mass, the risk of parathyroid cancer increases dramatically from some 1% of all patients with primary hyperparathyroidism to approximately 50%.

Laboratory data in patients with primary hyperparathyroidism and parathyroid cancer are similar to those relating to other patients with primary hyperparathyroidism (hypercalcemia, hypophosphatemia, hyperchloremia) and an elevated chloride-phosphorus ratio (> 33). Patients with parathyroid cancer are more likely to have an elevated alkaline phosphatase level (approximately 75%), abnormal renal function study results, and hypomagnesemia.

Localization studies for patients with primary hyperparathyroidism include sestamibi scanning, ultrasonography, MRI, and CT scanning. Sestamibi is used the most frequently and certainly is valuable for surgeons doing unilateral explorations or focal explorations. Because some 80% to 85% of patients with primary hyperparathyroidism have solitary parathyroid adenoma as the cause, most patients who have a positive sestamibi scan result will be treated successfully by excision of the identified lesion. However, in the 15% to 20% of patients who have more than one abnormal parathyroid gland, localization studies are only approximately 30% accurate [104]; for this reason, preoperative localization tests generally are not cost-effective. What should be emphasized is that diagnosis of primary hyperparathyroidism is a function of metabolic testing, not of localization studies.

In the setting of parathyroid cancer, however, both primary and metastatic parathyroid cancers frequently can be identified by sestamibi scanning. Also, in patients with persistent or recurrent primary hyperparathyroidism, selective venous catheterization for PTH is helpful and can lateralize the tumor or can localize metastatic parathyroid cancer outside the neck [105]. This study is especially useful when noninvasive localization study results are negative or equivocal.

Usually, patients with parathyroid cancer have locally invasive tumors, and approximately 15% have adjacent lymph node metastases. In addition, lung, bone, and liver metastases may be present [98, 100]. The presence of a gray-brown or gray-white parathyroid gland with gross evidence of fibrosis (particularly if associated with calcium levels greater than 13.5) or an unusually firm or large gland should alert involved surgeons to the presence of a possible parathyroid cancer [97, 98, 100].

Pathologists have a difficult time in diagnosing parathyroid carcinoma on cytologic or histologic grounds alone [98, 100]. Gross evidence of invasiveness at the time of surgery, combined with the aforementioned clinical characteristics, probably is more reliable. Microscopical evidence of capsular or vascular invasion is helpful but not pathognomonic. Microscopical evidence also includes thick fibrous bands, pleomorphic cells growing in a trabecular pattern, and high mitotic activity [98, 100]. DNA aneuploidy has been regarded as useful by some researchers [98] but not by others [100].

Primary Surgical Treatment

In addition to the usual preoperative evaluation, including detailed neck examination and laryngoscopy, correction of metabolic abnormalities (particularly of hypercalcemia) is essential. Often, forced hydration, saline replacement, and brisk diuresis with Lasix suffice to correct hypercalcemia but, in some patients presenting with hypercalcemic crisis, administration of a diphos-

phonate or mithramycin may be required. In rare cases, hemodialysis is performed.

Because these tumors implant so notoriously, early recognition and complete en bloc resection are particularly important [97, 98, 100, 106, 107]. The initial operation constitutes the best opportunity for cure. It is recommended that an en bloc resection be performed, which includes at least the ipsilateral thyroid gland, adjacent nodes, and any adherent strap muscles or other structures. In instances in which the recurrent laryngeal nerve is invaded and a paralyzed cord has been documented preoperatively, the nerve should be resected to accomplish an en bloc resection. In the face of doubt as to the nature of a parathyroid mass, particularly if it has the foregoing characteristics, performing a complete en bloc procedure (such as this) is preferable to a piecemeal approach.

Although identification of all parathyroid glands (usually four) as a matter of routine is preferred, we recognize that in the setting of a parathyroid cancer, some do not. Because patients with parathyroid cancer are, in fact, more likely to have abnormalities of the other parathyroid glands and because leaving such glands behind risks persistent hypercalcemia—creating the mistaken impression of unresected or metastatic disease—we see value in identifying all parathyroid glands. When nodes are involved (approximately 20% of primary cases), a central and lateral node dissection sufficient to clear all disease is recommended.

An important step immediately after surgery is to check serum calcium and phosphate levels. The PTH level should be checked on the morning after the operation. Affected patients are more prone to postoperative hypocalcemia because of "bone hunger." PTH is a primary phosphaturic, and elevations of serum phosphate suggest inadequate PTH. If serum phosphate rises above 5.5 mg/dl postoperatively, the cause more likely is hypoparathyroidism.

Postoperative follow-up should include neck examination and checking the serum calcium and PTH levels every three months for two years and then every six months. Most patients who experience recurrent disease do so within three years, and the PTH level often increases before hypercalcemia redevelops.

Treatment of Persistent, Recurrent, and Metastatic Disease

Regional disease, and even metastatic disease amenable to surgical treatment, should be treated surgically, as often this modality palliates hypercalcemia [98, 100].

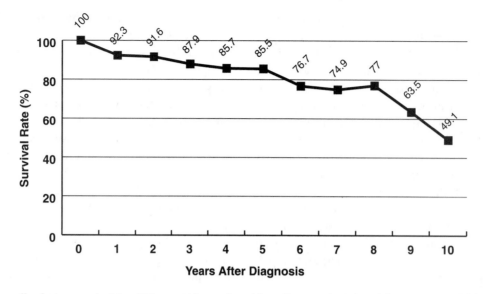

Figure 27.5   Overall relative survival for 286 cases of parathyroid carcinoma. (Reprinted from SA Hundahl, ID Fleming, AM Fremgen A, HR Menck, Two hundred eight-six cases of parathyroid carcinoma treated in the United States 19851995: a National Cancer Data Base Report. The American College of Surgeons Commission on Cancer and the American Cancer Society. *Cancer* 86:538–544, 1999. Copyright ©1999 American Cancer Society. Used with permission of Wiley-Liss, Inc., a subsidiary of John Wiley & Sons, Inc.)

However, this rarely results in cure [108], though long-term survivors have been reported [100]. Because more patients die from hypercalcemia than from the growth or spread of the tumor [100] and because tumor progression usually is slow, repeat resection has particular value in this disease.

When surgery fails to be effective, external irradiation or chemotherapy may be tried, although usually they are not helpful [100, 109]. A treatment regimen combining fluorouracil, cyclophosphamide, and dacarbazine or combining methotrexate, doxorubicin, cyclophosphamide, and lomustine has been reported to be effective in some patients [99, 100].

For medical palliation of hypercalcemia in patients with otherwise uncontrollable disease, etidronate and pamidronate are helpful. The problem with these and other agents (e.g., calcitonin, mithramycin, gallium nitrate) is that patients with high tumor burden usually become quickly refractory to treatment [109].

Prognosis

Figure 27.5 depicts 10-year relative survival for 286 patients with parathyroid carcinoma accessioned to the NCDB between 1985 and 1995 [97]. The depicted curve is steeper than that derived from the 95-case series reported by Sandelin et al [98], and the 10-year relative survival rate of 49.1% is lower. This difference may

stem from the inclusion of "histologically equivocal" cases by Sandelin et al [98], for which superior survival was demonstrated. Studies so far fail to offer compelling evidence supporting the value of tumor size or nodal status as significant prognostic factors [97], but a staging system based on these has been proposed [110].

REFERENCES

1. Parkin MD, Pisani P, Ferlay J. Global cancer statistics. *CA Cancer J Clin* 49:33–64, 1999.
2. Greenlee RT, Murray T, Bolden S, Wingo PA. Cancer statistics, 2000. *CA Cancer J Clin* 50:7–33, 2000.
3. Hundahl SA, Fleming ID, Fremgen AM, Menck HR. A National Cancer Data Base Report on 53,856 cases of thyroid carcinoma treated in the US, '85–'95. *Cancer* 83: 2638–2648, 1998.
4. Correa P, Chen VW. Endocrine gland cancer. *Cancer* 75: 338–352, 1995.
5. Denham MJ, Willis EJ. A clinico-pathological survey of thyroid glands in old age. *Gerontology* 26:160–166, 1980.
6. Vander JB, Gaston EA, Dawber TR. The significance of non-toxic nodules: final report of a 15 year study of the incidence of thyroid malignancy. *Ann Intern Med* 69:537–540, 1968.
7. Mazzaferri EL. Thyroid cancer in thyroid nodules: finding a needle in the haystack. *Am J Med* 93:359–362, 1992.
8. Schneider AB, Ron E, Lubin J, et al. Dose-response relationships for radiation-induced thyroid cancer and thyroid nodules: evidence for the prolonged effects of radia-

tion on the thyroid. *J Clin Endocrinol Metab* 77: 362–369,1993.

9. Shore RE. Issues and epidemiological evidence regarding radiation-induced thyroid cancer. *Radiat Res* 131:98–111, 1992.

10. Doris-Keller H, Dou S, Chi D, et al. Mutations in the *RET* proto-oncogene are associated with MEN 2A and FMTC. *Hum Mol Genet* 2:851–856, 1993.

11. Gagel RF, Goepfert H, Callender DL. Changing concepts in the pathogenesis and management of thyroid carcinoma. *CA Cancer J Clin* 46:261–283, 1996.

12. Marsh DJ, Learoyd DL, Robinson, BG. Medullary thyroid carcinoma: recent advances and management update. *Thyroid* 5:407–424, 1995.

13. Piromallii D, Martclli G, Del Prato I, et at. The role of fine needle aspiration in the diagnosis of thyroid nodules: analysis of 795 consecutive cases. *J Surg Oncol* 50:247–250, 1992.

14. Hamburger JI, Husain M. Semiquantitative criteria for fine-needle biopsy diagnosis: reduced false-negative diagnosis. *Diagn Cytopathol* 14:14–17, 1988.

15. Walfish PG, Hazani E, Strawbridge HT, et at. Combined ultrasound and needle aspiration cytology in the assessment and management of hypofunctioning thyroid nodule. *Ann Intern Med* 87:270–274, 1977.

16. Jones AJ, Aitman TJ, Edmonds CJ, et al. Comparison of fine needle aspiration cytology, radioisotopic and ultrasound scanning in the management of thyroid nodules. *Postgrad Med J* 66:914–917, 1990.

17. Rosen IB, Azadian A, Walfish PG, et al. Ultrasound-guided fine needle aspiration biopsy in the management of thyroid disease. *Am J Surg* 166:346–349, 1993.

18. Kenady DE, Schwartz RW. Thyroid: diagnostic techniques. *Curr Opin Oncol* 2:87–94, 1990.

19. Gharib H, James EH, Charboneau JW, et al. Suppressive therapy with levothyroxine for solitary thyroid nodules: a double-blind controlled clinical study. *N Engl J Med* 317:70–75, 1987.

20. Cheung PSY, Lee JMH, Boey JH. Thyroxine suppression of benign thyroid nodules: a prospective randomized study. *World J Surg* 13:818–821, 1989.

21. Clark OH, Okerlund MD, Cavalieri RR, Greenspan FS. Diagnosis and treatment of thyroid, parathyroid, and thyroglossal duct cysts. *J Clin Endocrinol Metab* 48:983–988, 1979.

22. McLeod MK, Thompson NW. Hürthle cell neoplasms of the thyroid. *Otolaryngol Clin North Am* 23:441–452, 1990.

23. Fleming ID, Cooper JS, Henson DE, et al. *AJCC Cancer Staging Manual* (5th ed). Philadelphia: Lippincott-Raven, 1997.

24. LiVolsi VA. *Surgical Pathology of the Thyroid*. Philadelphia: Saunders, 1990.

25. Tielens ET, Sherman SI, Hruban RH, Ladenson PQ. Follicular variant of papillary thyroid carcinoma: a clinico-pathologic study. *Cancer* 73:424–431, 1994.

26. LiVolsi VA, Asa SL. The demise of follicular carcinoma of the thyroid gland. *Thyroid* 4:233–236, 1994.

27. Cooper DS, Schneyer CR. Follicular and Hürthle cell carcinoma of the thyroid. *Endocrinol Metab Clin North Am* 19:577–591, 1990.

28. Fraker DL, Skarulis M, Livolsi V. Thyroid tumors. In De-

Vita VT, Hellman S, Rosenberg SA (eds), *Cancer—Principles and Practice of Oncology* (5th ed). Philadelphia: Lippincott-Raven, 1997:1629–1651.

29. Franssila KO, Harach HR. Occult papillary carcinoma of the thyroid in children and young adults. A systemic autopsy study in Finland. *Cancer* 58:715–719, 1985.

30. Fukunaga FH, Lockett LJ. Thyroid carcinoma in the Japanese in Hawaii. *Arch Pathol* 92:6–13, 1971.

31. Allo MD, Christianson W, Koivunen D. Not all "occult" papillary carcinomas are "minimal." *Surgery* 104:971–976, 1988.

32. Ron E, Kleinerman RA, Boice JD Jr, et al. A population-based case-control study of thyroid cancer. *J Natl Cancer Inst* 79:1–12, 1987.

33. Hundahl SA. Perspective: National Cancer Institute summary about estimated exposures and thyroid doses received from iodine-131 in fallout after Nevada atmospheric nuclear bomb tests. *CA Cancer J Clin* 48:285–298, 1998.

34. Hamilton TE, van Belle G, LoGerfo JP. Thyroid neoplasia in Marshall islanders exposed to nuclear fallout. *JAMA* 258:629–636, 1987.

35. Nikiforov Y, Gnepp DR. Pediatric thyroid cancer after the Chernobyl disaster. *Cancer* 74:748–766, 1994.

36. Ron E. Thyroid cancer. In Schottenfeld D, Fraumeni JF (eds), *Cancer Epidemiology and Prevention*. New York: Oxford University Press, 1996:1000–1021.

37. Ron E, Kleinerman RA, LiVolsi VA, et al. Familial non-medullary thyroid cancer. *Oncology* 48:309–311, 1991.

38. Stoffer SS, Van Dyke DL, Bach JV, et al. Familial papillary carcinoma of the thyroid. *Am J Med Genet* 25:775–782, 1986.

39. Santoro M, Carlomagno F, Hay ID, et al. *RET* oncogene activation in human thyroid neoplasms is restricted to the papillary cancer subtype. *J Clin Invest* 89:1517–1522, 1992.

40. Gagel RF, Goepfert H, Callender D. Changing concepts in the pathogenesis and management of thyroid carcinoma. *CA Cancer J Clin* 46:261–283, 1996.

41. Grieco M, Santoro M, Berlingieri MT, et al. PTC is a novel rearranged form of the *RET* proto-oncogene and is frequently detected in vivo in human thyroid papillary carcinomas. *Cell* 60:557–563, 1990.

42. Bongarzone I, Butti MG, Coronelli S, et al. Frequent activation of RET proto-oncogene by fusion with a new activating gene in papillary thyroid carcinomas. *Cancer Res* 54:2979–2985, 1994.

43. Hamburger JI, Husain M. Contribution of intraoperative pathology evaluation to surgical management of thyroid nodules. *Endocrinol Metab Clin North Am* 19:509–522, 1990.

44. Clark RL, White EC, Russell WO. Total thyroidectomy for cancer of the thyroid: significance of intraglandular dissemination. *Ann Surg* 149:858–866, 1959.

45. Brooks JR, Starnes HF, Brooks DC, Pelkey JN. Surgical therapy for thyroid carcinoma: a review of 1249 solitary thyroid nodules. *Surgery* 104:940–946, 1988.

46. Flynn MB, Lyons KJ, Tarter JW, Ragsdale TL. Local complications after surgical resection for thyroid carcinoma. *Am J Surg* 168:404–407, 1994.

47. DeGroot LJ, Kaplan EL, McCorinick M, Straus FH. Natu-

ral history, treatment, and course of papillary thyroid carcinoma. *J Clin Endocrinol Metab* 71:414–424, 1990.

48. Cady B, Rossi R. An expanded view of risk-group definition in differentiated thyroid carcinoma. *Surgery* 104:947–953, 1988.

49. Hay ID. Papillary thyroid carcinoma. *Endocrinol Metab Clin North Am* 19:545–576, 1990.

50. Hay JD, Grant CS, Taylor WF, McConahey WM. Ipsilateral lobectomy versus bilateral lobar resection in papillary thyroid carcinoma: a retrospective analysis of surgical outcome using a novel prognostic scoring system. *Surgery* 102:1088–1095, 1987.

51. Pasieka JL, Zedenius J, Auer G, et al. Addition of nuclear DNA content to the AMES risk-group classification for papillary thyroid cancer. *Surgery* 112:1154–1160, 1992.

52. Hay ID, Bergstralh EJ, Goellner JR, et al. Predicting outcome in papillary thyroid carcinoma: development of a reliable prognostic scoring system in a cohort of 1779 patients surgically treated at one institution during 1940 through 1989. *Surgery* 114:1050–1058, 1993.

53. Mazzaferri El, Jhiang SM. Long-term impact of initial surgical and medical therapy on papillary and follicular thyroid cancer. *Am J Med* 97:418–428, 1994.

54. Shaha AR, Loree TR, Shah JP. Intermediate risk group for differentiated carcinoma of the thyroid. *Surgery* 116:1036–1041, 1994.

55. Shaha AR, Shah JP, Loree TR. Low-risk differentiated thyroid cancer: the need for selective treatment. *Ann Surg Oncol* 4:328–333, 1997.

56. Rossi RL, Cady B, Silverman ML, et al. Surgically incurable well-differentiated thyroid carcinoma. *Arch Surg* 123:569–574, 1988.

57. Samaan N, Schultz PN, Hickey RC, et al. The results of various modalities of treatment of well differentiated thyroid carcinoma: a retrospective review of 1,599 patients. *J Clin Endocrinol Metab* 75:714–720, 1992.

58. Pasieka JL, Rotstein LE. Consensus conference on well-differentiated thyroid cancer: a summary. *Can J Surg* 36:298–310, 1993.

59. Clark OH. Total thyroidectomy and lymph node dissection for cancer of the thyroid. In Nyhus LM, Baker RJ (eds), *Masters of Surgery* (2nd ed). Boston: Little, Brown, 1992:204–215.

60. Wells SA. Total thyroidectomy and lymph node dissection for cancer. In Nyhus LM, Baker RJ, Fischer JE (eds), *Masters of Surgery* (3rd ed). Boston: Little, Brown, 1997:496–507.

61. Bal C, Padhy AK, Jana S, et al. Prospective randomized clinical trial to evaluate the optimal dose of ^{131}I for remnant ablation in patients with differentiated thyroid carcinoma. *Cancer* 77:2574–2580, 1996.

62. Park HM. Stunned thyroid after high-dose I-131 imaging. *Clin Nucl Med* 17:501–502, 1992.

63. Park HM, Perkins OW, Edmondson JW, et al. Influence of diagnostic radioiodines in the uptake of ablative doses of iodine-131. *Thyroid* 4:49–54, 1994.

64. Ekman ET, Lundell G, Tennvall J, et al. Chemotherapy and multimodality treatment in thyroid carcinoma. *Otolaryngol Clin North Am* 23:523–527, 1990.

65. Robbins J, Merino MJ, Boice JD, et al. Thyroid cancer: a lethal endocrine neoplasm. *Ann Intern Med* 115:133–147, 1991.

66. Gharib H, McConahey WM, Tiegs RD, et al. Medullary thyroid carcinoma: clinicopathological features and long-term follow-up of 65 patients treated during 1946 through 1970. *Mayo Clin Proc* 67:934–940, 1992.

67. Jing S, Wen D, Yu Y, et al. GDNF-induced activation of the ret protein tyrosine kinase is mediated by GDNFR-alpha, a novel receptor for GDNF. *Cell* 85:1113–1124, 1996.

68. Schuffenecker I, Ginet N, Goldgar D, et al. Prevalence and parental origin of de novo *RET* mutations in multiple endocrine neoplasia type 2A and familial medullary thyroid carcinoma. Le Groupe d'Etude des Tumeurs a Calcitonine (letter). *Am J Hum Genet* 60:233–237, 1997.

69. Mulligan LM, Eng C, Attie T, et al. Diverse phenotypes associated with exon 10 mutations of the *ret* proto-oncogene. *Hum Mol Genet* 3:2163–2167, 1994.

70. Romeo G, Ronchetto P, Luo Y, et al. Point mutations affecting the tyrosine kinase domain of the *RET* proto-oncogene in Hirschsprung's disease. *Nature* 367:377–378, 1994.

71. Tisell LE, Hansson G, Jansson S, Salander H. Reoperation in the treatment of asymptomatic metastasizing medullary thyroid carcinoma. *Surgery* 99:60–66, 1986.

72. Fushshuber PR, Loree TR, Hicks WL, et al. Medullary carcinoma of the thyroid: prognostic factors and treatment recommendations. *Ann Surg Oncol* 5:81–86, 1998.

73. Kebebew E, Treseler P, Siperstein AE, et al. Normal thyroid pathology in patients underoing thyroidectomy for *RET* germline mutation: a report of three cases and review of the literature. *Thyroid* 9:127–131, 1999.

74. Decker RA, Peacock ML. Occurrence of MEN 2A in familial Hirschsprungs disease: a new indication for genetic testing of the *RET* proto-oncogene. *J Pediatr Surg* 33:207–214, 1998.

75. Chung GC, Beahrs OH, Sizemore GW, Woolner LH. Medullary carcinoma of the thyroid gland. *Cancer* 35:695–704, 1975.

76. Duh QY, Sanebo JJ, Greenspan FS, et al. Medullary thyroid carcinoma. *Arch Surg* 124:1206–1210, 1989.

77. Bergholm U, Adami HO, Bergstrom R, et al. Long-term survival in sporadic and familial medullary thyroid carcinoma with special reference to clinical characteristics as prognostic factors. The Swedish MTC Study Group. *Acta Chir Scand* 156:37–46, 1990.

78. Girelli ME, Nacamulli D, Pelizzo MR, et al. Medullary thyroid carcinoma: clinical features and long-term follow-up of seventy-eight patients treated between 1969 and 1986. *Thyroid* 8:517–523, 1998.

79. Moley JF. Medullary thyroid cancer. In Clark OH, Duh QY (eds), *Textbook of Endocrine Surgery*. Philadelphia: Saunders, 1997:108–118.

80. Moley JF, Dilley WG, DeBenedetti RN. Improved results of cervical reoperation for medullary thyroid carcinoma. *Ann Surg* 225:734–743, 1997.

81. Gautvik KM, Talle K, Hager B, et al. Early liver metastases in patients with medullary carcinoma of the thyroid gland. *Cancer* 63:175–180, 1989.

82. Deftos LJ, Stein MF. Radioiodine as an adjunct to surgical

treatment of medullary thyroid carcinoma. *J Clin Endocrinol Metab* 50:967–968, 1980.

83. Riccabona G, Dielthelm L, Schmid K. When is medullary thyroid carcinoma medullary thyroid carcinoma? *World J Surg* 10:745–752, 1986.

84. Briefly J, Tsang R, Simpson WJ, et al. Medullary thyroid cancer: analyses of survival and prognostic factors and the role of radiation therapy in local control. *Thyroid* 6:305–310, 1996.

85. Samaan NA, Schultz PN, Hickey RC. Medullary thyroid carcinoma: prognosis of familial versus sporadic disease and the role of radiotherapy. *J Clin Endocrinol Metab* 67:801–805, 1988.

86. O'Doherty MJ, Coakley AJ. Drug therapy alternatives in the treatment of thyroid cancer. *Drugs* 55:801–812, 1998.

87. Juweid M, Sharkey RM, Swayne LC, et al. Improved selection of patients for operation for medullary thyroid cancer by imaging with radiolabeled anticarcinoembryonic antigen antibodies. *Surgery* 122:1156–1165, 1997.

88. Siperstein AE, Rogers SJ, Hansen PD, et al. Laparoscopic thermal ablation of hepatic neuroendocrine tumor metastases. *Surgery* 122:1147–1155, 1997.

89. Abdelmoumene N, Schlumberg M, Gardet P, et al. Selective venous sampling catheterization for localization of persisting medullary thyroid carcinoma. *Br J Cancer* 69:1141–1144, 1994.

90. Hoefnagel CA, Delprat CC, Zanin D, et al. New radionuclide tracers for the diagnosis and therapy of medullary thyroid carcinoma. *Clin Nucl Med* 13:159–165, 1988.

91. Hoefnagel CA, Delprat CC, Valdes Olmos RA. Role of 131-I metaiodobenzylguanidine therapy in medullary thyroid carcinoma. *J Nucl Biol Med* 35:334–336, 1991.

92. Rosen IB, Asa SL, Brierley JD. Anaplastic carcinoma of the thyroid gland. In Clark OH, Duh QY (eds), *Textbook of Endocrine Surgery*. Philadelphia: Saunders, 1997: 127–132.

93. Nishiyama RH, Dunn EL, Thompson NW. Anaplastic spindle-cell and giant-cell tumors of the thyroid gland. *Cancer* 30:113–127, 1972.

94. Wemer B, Abele J, Alveryd A, et al. Multinodal therapy in anaplastic giant cell thyroid cancer. *World J Surg* 8:64–70, 1984.

95. Nel CJC, van Heerden JA, Goellner JR, et al. Anaplastic carcinoma of the thyroid: a clinicopathologic study of 82 cases. *Mayo Clin Proc* 60:51–58, 1985.

96. Ain KB, Tofiq S, Taylor KD. Antineoplastic activity of taxol against human anaplastic thyroid carcinoma cells

lines in vitro and in vivo. *J Clin Endocrinol Metab* 81:3650–3653, 1996.

97. Hundahl SA, Fleming ID, Fremgen AM, et al. Two hundred eight-six cases of parathyroid carcinoma treated in the United States 1985–1995: a National Cancer Data Base Report. The American College of Surgeons Commission on Cancer and the American Cancer Society. *Cancer* 86:538–544, 1999.

98. Sandelin K, Auer G, Bondeson L, et al. Prognostic factors in parathyroid cancer: a review of 95 cases. *World J Surg* 16:724–731, 1992.

99. Sandelin K. Parathyroid carcinoma. In Clark OH, Duh QY (eds), *Textbook of Endocrine Surgery*. Philadelphia: Saunders, 1997:439–443.

100. Obare T, Fujimoro Y. Diagnosis and treatment of patients with parathyroid carcinoma: an update and review. *World J Surg* 15:738–746, 1991.

101. Mallette LE, Bilezikian JP, Ketcham AS, et al. Parathyroid carcinoma in familial hyperparathyroidism. *Am J Med* 57:642–646, 1974.

102. Levin K, Galante M, Clark OH. Parathyroid carcinoma versus parathyroid adenoma in patients with profound hypercalcemia. *Surgery* 101:649–660, 1987.

103. Chan A, Duh QY, Katz MH, et al. Clinical manifestations of primary hyperparathyroidism before and parathyroidectomy. A case control study. *Ann Surg* 222:402–414, 1995.

104. Pasieka JL, Parsons LL. Prospective surgical outcome study of relief of symptoms following surgery in patients with primary hyperparathyroidism. *World J Surg* 22:513–518, 1998.

105. Burney RE, Jones KR, Coon JW, et al. Assessment of patient outcomes after operation for primary hyperparathyroidism. *Surgery* 120:1013–1018, 1996.

106. Hakaimm AG, Esselstyn CB. Parathyroid carcinoma: 50-year experience at the Cleveland Clinic Foundation. *Cleve Clin J Med* 60:331–335, 1993.

107. Wang C, Gaz R. Natural history of parathyroid carcinoma. Diagnosis, treatment, and results. *Am J Surg* 149:522–527, 1985.

108. Van Heerden JA, Weiland LH, ReMine WH, et al. Cancer of the parathyroid glands. *Arch Surg* 114:475–480, 1979.

109. Fraker DL. Parathyroid tumors. In DeVita VT, Hellman S, Rosenberg SA (eds), *Cancer—Principles and Practice of Oncology* (5th ed). Philadelphia: Lippincott-Raven, 1997:1652–1659.

110. Shaha AR, Shah JP. Parathyroid carcinoma—a diagnostic and therapeutic challenge. *Cancer* 86:378–380, 1999.

28

Cancer of the Central Nervous System and Pituitary Gland

■ ■ ■

LISA M. DEANGELIS
JEROME B. POSNER

THE INCIDENCE OF SEVERAL TYPES OF BRAIN tumors is increasing. Brain tumors have surpassed acute lymphocytic leukemia as the most common childhood cancer [1]. Malignant brain tumors also appear to be increasing substantially in adults, particularly in the elderly. The apparent increase in adults may be due in part to better detection with powerful imaging techniques, such as magnetic resonance imaging (MRI), or to the fact that most brain tumors occur in old age, a cohort whose numbers are increasing [2]. However, the data may represent a true increase in brain tumors [3].

Despite the fear and pessimism regarding central nervous system (CNS) tumors, progress in diagnosis and treatment is being made: Better diagnostic techniques, such as MRI and stereotactic needle biopsy, have led to earlier diagnosis, which in some instances improves therapy. Such new imaging techniques as functional MRI [4] allow surgeons to excise tumors more radically, because brain structures vital for CNS function (i.e., eloquent areas) can be identified accurately both prior to and during surgery, allowing for more extensive resection. These techniques are particularly important because for most CNS tumors, surgery is the most effective treatment. New techniques of radiotherapy (e.g., conformal field irradiation, stereotactic radiotherapy, and stereotactic radiosurgery) allow more potent attack on tumors while sparing normal CNS tissue. New chemotherapeutic agents and novel combinations of established agents have demonstrated efficacy in treating certain brain tumors. Much excitement has been generated by preliminary studies of gene therapy and of antiangiogenesis factors. Thus, though CNS tumors remain largely intractable, in recent years survival has improved [5], particularly in children [1] but in adults as well.

This chapter is divided into two major sections. The first section discusses the general principles of diagnosis and treatment of CNS tumors. The second section discusses the management of specific intracranial tumors.

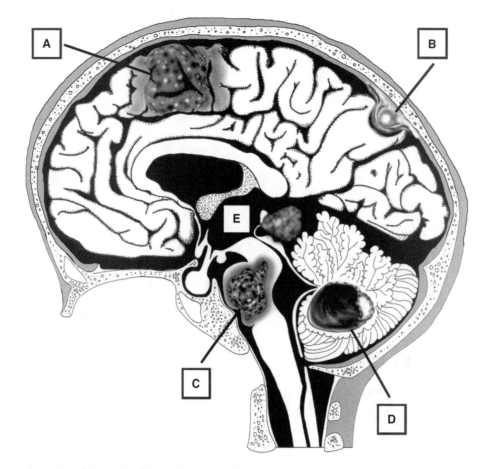

Figure 28.1   Sagittal section of the brain illustrating some of the tumors discussed: diffuse astrocytoma *(A)*, meningioma compressing but not invading the brain *(B)*, brainstem glioma *(C)*, hemangioblastoma of the cerebellum *(D)*, and pineal region tumor compressing the superior colliculus *(E)*.

Though this division inevitably may lead to some redundancy, many of the principles of diagnosis and treatment and many fundamental biological characteristics of CNS tumors apply to all CNS tumors. Shorter sections are devoted to spinal tumors and metastases. Several recently published book-length comprehensive reviews provide more details [6–10].

ANATOMIC CONTEXT

Several factors render CNS tumors unique (Fig. 28.1). The CNS is encased in unyielding bone: the brain in the skull and the spinal cord in the vertebral column. As a tumor grows within the bony cavity of the skull or spine, it first displaces blood and cerebrospinal fluid (CSF) and then compresses and shifts neural structures, causing neural dysfunction. Also, the CNS is composed of multiple structures, each with a different function.

Thus, even a small brain tumor in a critical area (e.g., brainstem, internal capsule, or parietal cortex) may cause severe symptoms.

Under normal circumstances, CNS structures are protected from toxins and other deleterious substances in the blood by blood-CNS barriers. As CNS tumors grow, they create "neovessels" that lack a normal blood-CNS barrier, allowing proteins and other potentially noxious substances to enter the tumor and diffuse into the surrounding normal tissue, causing edema and further compressing normal neural tissue.

Additionally, clearance of edema from the CNS is slow because the brain lacks lymphatics. However, lymphatics do drain CSF, particularly when intracranial pressure (ICP) is increased [11].

The terms *benign* and *malignant* do not apply strictly to most CNS tumors in the same way that they apply to tumors outside the CNS. Tumors within the parenchyma of the brain or spinal cord are rarely truly benign, because surgery rarely cures. Most histologically benign tumors infiltrate normal tissue extensively, preventing total resection and allowing tumor recurrence. Furthermore, tumors not resected may dedifferentiate into biologically more aggressive tumors. Brain tumors rarely are truly biologically malignant because they seldom metastasize, except occasionally within the CNS itself. The difficulty of pathologic discrimination and the absence of systemic or nodal metastases render standard staging systems used for systemic cancers inapplicable for CNS tumors. Thus, the terms *low-grade* and *high-grade* in classifying CNS tumors are more appropriate than are the terms *benign* and *malignant*.

The factors that are important in determining the prognosis of CNS tumors include histopathologic characteristics and location of the lesion; age, extent of surgery, and performance status of the patient; and irradiation or chemotherapeutic sensitivity of the lesion. Mitoses, vascular proliferation, and necrosis indicate an aggressive tumor with a poor prognosis. The location of the tumor determines symptomatology, surgical resectability, and (as a result of both) prognosis. Patients' age is an important prognostic factor. For certain tumors, such as malignant gliomas, children fare better than do adults, and young adults fare better than do older adults. In adults with malignant gliomas, age is the single most important prognostic factor. In contrast, adults with brainstem gliomas usually fare better than children. Although controversial, most evidence suggests that the extent of surgery is also an important prognostic factor [12]. In meningiomas, total surgical resection is curative, as it is for ependymomas of the spinal cord. Malignant gliomas never are cured by surgery, but the less tumor that remains after resection, the better the prognosis.

Patients' performance status is another important prognostic factor. Relatively asymptomatic patients have a better prognosis than do those who are paralyzed or suffer other crippling neurologic symptoms. The sensitivity of a tumor to irradiation and chemotherapy are additional important prognostic factors. Histopathologically malignant pineal region germinomas are cured by irradiation, and an increasing number of CNS lymphomas appear to be cured by chemotherapy. Poor sensitivity to irradiation and chemotherapy render the malignant glioma a highly intractable tumor. Physicians must consider all these prognostic factors in prescribing treatment and discussing prognosis with patients and their families.

EPIDEMIOLOGIC FACTORS

For 2000, the American Cancer Society predicted the occurrence of 16,500 new cases of primary brain and other CNS cancers (9,500 in male patients and 7,000 in female patients) [13]. This incidence is more than twice that of Hodgkin's disease and more than one-half that of melanoma. These data do not include metastases to brain and spinal cord or such so-called benign tumors as meningiomas and pituitary tumors. CNS cancers will kill approximately 13,000 persons in 2000. Brain tumors are the third leading cause of cancer death in men ages 20 to 39 and the fifth in women of that age [13].

As a cause of disability and death, metastases to the CNS are far more common than are primary CNS tumors. Although exact data are not available, one estimate suggests that in excess of 100,000 individuals a year will die having suffered from symptomatic intracranial metastases and that as many as 80,000 patients a year will suffer spinal cord compression as a result of metastatic tumor [9]. Although most CNS metastases appear late in the course of a patient's cancer, a significant number of patients with cancer present with CNS symptoms. Physicians always must consider metastatic disease as a possible cause of neurologic symptoms and signs in any patient with cancer.

CNS tumors can occur at any age. Some tumors, such as medulloblastoma and brainstem glioma, are more common in children than in adults, whereas others, such as glioblastoma multiforme and meningioma, are more common in adults. Overall, primary brain tumors have a bimodal incidence, with a small peak in infancy and childhood and then a consistent rise with age. At one time, brain tumors were believed to be less common in the very old, but that notion probably resulted from less aggressive evaluation of elderly patients with neurologic disability.

Epidemiologic data from the Mayo Clinic indicate an annual 19.1 per 100,000 age-adjusted incidence rate for primary brain tumors from 1950 to 1989. The annual rates were 11.8 per 100,000 for symptomatic tumors and 7.3 per 100,000 for asymptomatic tumors [14]. Moreover, current evidence suggests that the incidence of primary CNS tumors is increasing. This increase is especially marked for CNS lymphoma in both immunocompromised (predominantly those infected with human immunodeficiency virus [HIV]) and immunocompetent hosts. Once a rare CNS tumor usually identified only at autopsy, CNS lymphoma has become an important consideration in the diagnosis and treatment of undiagnosed brain tumors. Evidence also suggests that

Table 28.1   Histologic Classification of Central Nervous System Tumors

Tumors of neuroepithelial tissue
  Astrocytic tumors
    Astrocytoma
    Anaplastic (malignant) astrocytoma
    Glioblastoma multiforme
    Pilocytic astrocytoma
    Pleomorphic xanthoastrocytoma
    Subependymal giant-cell astrocytoma
  Oligodendroglial tumors
    Oligodendroglioma
    Anaplastic (malignant) oligodendroglioma
  Ependymal tumors
    Ependymoma
    Anaplastic (malignant) ependymoma
    Myxopapillary ependymoma
    Subependymoma
  Mixed gliomas
    Oligoastrocytoma
    Anaplastic (malignant) oligoastrocytoma
  Choroid plexus tumors
    Choroid plexus papilloma
    Choroid plexus carcinoma
  Neuronal and mixed neuronal-glial tumors
    Gangliocytoma
    Dysembryoplastic neuroepithelial tumor
    Ganglioglioma
    Anaplastic (malignant) ganglioglioma
    Central neurocytoma
  Pineal parenchymal tumors
    Pineocytoma
    Pineoblastoma
  Embryonal tumors
    Medulloblastoma
    Primitive neuroectodermal tumor

Tumors of cranial and spinal nerves
  Schwannoma
  Neurofibroma

Tumors of the meninges
  Meningioma
  Hemangiopericytoma
  Melanocytic tumor
  Hemangioblastoma

Primary central nervous system lymphomas

Germ-cell tumors
  Germinoma
  Embryonal carcinoma
  Yolk sac tumor (endodermal sinus tumor)
  Choriocarcinoma
  Teratoma
  Mixed germ-cell tumors

Cysts and tumor-like lesions
  Rathke cleft cyst
  Epidermoid cyst
  Dermoid cyst
  Colloid cyst of the third ventricle

Table 28.1   Histologic Classification of Central Nervous System Tumors (*continued*)

Tumors of the sellar region
  Pituitary adenoma
  Pituitary carcinoma
  Craniopharyngioma

Metastatic tumors

Source: Abridged and modified from P Kleihues, WK Cavenee (eds), *World Health Organization Classification of Tumors: Pathology and Genetics of Tumors of the Central Nervous System.* Lyon: IARC Press, 2000.

the incidence of glial tumors is increasing. For example, a recent study using data from the Florida Cancer Registry [15] comparing the incidence of brain tumors from 1981 to 1984 and from 1986 to 1989 showed a consistently significant increase in the incidence of all primary brain tumors in patients older than 65 years, with the largest increase among those older than 85. Because noninvasive neuroimaging has improved ascertainment substantially, the exact increase in incidence, if any, is unknown.

CLASSIFICATION

The World Health Organization (WHO) classifies CNS tumors by their patterns of differentiation and presumed cell of origin [16]. Table 28.1 lists the tumors discussed in this chapter; Figure 28.1 depicts some of these. Approximately 70% of symptomatic primary CNS tumors arise within the parenchyma of the brain and spinal cord; they are mostly of neuroepithelial origin, primarily from glial cells (usually astrocytes) or their precursors. The remainder arise from meninges or pituitary or pineal glands. Recent evidence suggests that oligodendrogliomas may be more common than previously believed, an important observation because these tumors are chemosensitive. That neuroepithelial tumors are among the most common brain tumors is not surprising, because 90% of the cells within the brain and spinal cord are glia. They include astrocytes, oligodendrocytes, and ependymal cells. The 100 billion neurons in the adult CNS, mostly postmitotic, or their precursors, are a rare source of CNS neoplasm.

Occasionally, CNS tumors arise from cells not normally found in the nervous system. These include germ-cell tumors with histologic features identical to those of the testis and ovary that grow in or around the pineal gland and the suprasellar area; primary lymphomas of the nervous system; and metastases from cancers arising elsewhere in the body (systemic cancer). Tumors arising from malmigration of the germ-cell layers include craniopharyngioma and dermoid and epidermoid tumors.

ETIOLOGIC FEATURES

Environmental Risk Factors

Although a large number of studies have examined the relationship between the environment and occurrence of brain tumors (Table 28.2), only two unequivocal risk factors have been identified: ionizing radiation and immunosuppression [17–29]. Low-dose irradiation to the scalp for the treatment of tinea capitis increases the incidence of meningiomas 10-fold over the incidence in nonirradiated individuals [30]; many are anaplastic or frankly malignant. Under similar conditions, glial tumors are increased threefold. Higher-dose irradiation given to treat intracranial or extracranial cancers, including prophylactic irradiation for leukemia, increases the incidence of both gliomas and sarcomas. Dental radiography and cosmic rays are not risk factors.

Immunosuppression, either acquired (e.g., immunosuppressive agents, such as those given after organ transplantation; HIV infection) or genetic (e.g., Wiskott-Aldrich syndrome), increases the incidence of primary CNS lymphomas (PCNSLs) and, in the case of HIV infection, also gliomas. Often, PCNSLs in patients immunosuppressed by HIV infection or after T-cell-depleted allogeneic transplant are driven by preexisting Epstein-Barr virus infection of B lymphocytes. When a lymphoma occurs in an immunosuppressed patient, it is twice as likely to be a PCNSL as a lymphoma outside the CNS.

Other studies of environmental risk factors are substantially less convincing than those already noted [19, 20]. Some investigators report that industrial exposure to polyvinyl chloride or dietary exposure to N-nitroso compounds could be a risk factor [20, 23], but others have failed to substantiate these findings. Head trauma has been reported as a risk factor for the development of glial tumors and meningiomas [26], but the evidence in support of that risk is unconvincing. A recent concern is that exposure to electromagnetic fields from high-tension power lines, computer terminals, or cellular telephones may cause brain tumors. A few epidemiologic studies support exposure to electromagnetic irradiation as a cause of brain tumors, but others fail to find an association [see ref. 19 for a review of this topic].

Table 28.2 Risk Factors Related to Central Nervous System Tumors

Risk Factor	Reference
Definitive	
Ionizing irradiation	[17]
Immunosuppression	[18]
Acquired (AIDS)	
Genetic	
Possible	
Electromagnetic fields	[19]
Diet	[20, 21]
N-nitroso compounds	[20]
Aspartame	[22]
Occupation (petroleum industry)	[23]
Chemicals	
Hair dyes and sprays	
Pesticides	[24, 25]
Head injury	[26]
Medications	
Infections	
Cysticercosis	[27]
Varicella-zoster	[28]
SV40	[29]

AIDS = acquired immunodeficiency syndrome; SV = simian virus.

The WHO and the American Health Foundation are investigating the risk factor of cellular telephones.

Olney et al. [22] have proposed that the recent increase in malignant brain tumors may be due to ingestion of aspartame, a dipeptide sugar substitute consisting of aspartic acid and phenylalanine. These amino acids are known to be active in the CNS, but the evidence that they are a risk factor for brain tumors remains weak for several reasons: (1) Brain tumors appear to be increasing predominantly in the elderly, the group least likely to use sugar substitutes; (2) these products have been on the market for only a few years, and it appears reasonable to presume that decades would be required for such a risk factor to exert its effect; and (3) women use aspartame-containing products more frequently than do men, but gliomas are more common in men. The same sort of reasoning applies to the connection between cellular telephones and brain tumors.

According to other studies, hair dyes, pesticides, formaldehyde, and industrial or occupational substances may cause brain tumors [21–25], but in none has the hypothesis been confirmed. If any of these substances turn out to be true risk factors, each can be responsible for only a small proportion of brain tumors.

Table 28.3   Hereditary Syndromes Associated with Brain Tumors

Syndrome	Mode of Inheritance	Tumor Type	Involved Chromosomes	Gene	Reference
Li-Fraumeni syndrome	AD	Glioma, medulloblastoma	17p13	*TP53*	[31]
Tuberous sclerosis	AD	Subependymal giant-cell astrocytoma, cortical tubers, glioma	9q34, 16p13	*TSC1*, *TSC2*	[32]
Neurofibromatosis type 1 (von Recklinghausen's disease; NF1)	AD	Glioma (optic nerve) astrocytoma, glioblastoma	17q11	*NF1*	[33, 34]
Neurofibromatosis type 2 (NF2)	AD	Meningioma, schwannoma (bilateral acoustic neuroma), ependymomas	22q12	*NF2*	[35]
Multiple endocrine neoplasia type 1 (MEN1)	AD	Pituitary	11q13	*Menin*	[36]
Retinoblastoma	AD	Retinoblastoma	13q14	*RB1*	[37]
Basal cell nevus syndrome (Gorlin's syndrome)	AD	Medulloblastoma	9q22	*PTCH*	[38]
Turcot's syndrome (hereditary nonpolyposis colorectal cancer syndrome [HNPCC])	AR or AD	Brain tumors of diverse histology, including glioblastoma and medulloblastoma	5q21 2p16 3p21 7p22	*APC* *hMLH2* *hMLH1* *hPMS2*	[39]
von Hippel-Lindau disease	AD	Hemangioblastoma	3p25–20	*VHL*	[40]
Cowden's syndrome	AD	Dysplastic cerebellar gangliocytoma, meningioma, astrocytoma	10p23	*PTEN (MMAC1)*	[41]
Rhabdoid predisposition syndrome	AD	Choroid plexus carcinoma, medulloblastoma, primitive neuroectodermal tumors	22q11	*hSNFS/ INI1*	[42]

AD = autosomal dominant; AR = autosomal recessive.

Genetic Risk

A few inherited diseases predispose to the development of primary CNS tumors (Table 28.3) [31–42]; many are associated with specific systemic cancers or other disorders as well. Neurofibromatosis is associated with a glioma in as many as 15% of patients with neurofibromatosis type 1 (NF1, von Recklinghausen's disease) and with schwannoma, meningioma and, less commonly, ependymoma in patients with NF2. Both NF1 and NF2 tumor suppressor genes have been cloned and sequenced. The gene coding for the von Hippel-Lindau (VHL) tumor suppressor protein has been cloned and sequenced; absence of the protein is responsible for hemangioblastomas of the cerebellum, retina, and other areas of the nervous system in VHL disease [40]. Together, these familial syndromes account for fewer than 5% of CNS tumors. However, one study reported that 7% of patients with newly diagnosed glial tumors and without a known genetic disorder had at least one blood relative with a glial tumor, suggesting that other familial factors remain to be discovered [43].

SYMPTOMS AND SIGNS

CNS tumors cause neurologic symptoms by one or more of four mechanisms:

- The tumor invades, irritates, and replaces normal tissue. This mechanism is particularly characteristic of infiltrating gliomas but rarely occurs with meningiomas, pineal region tumors, or metastases.
- The tumor and surrounding edema compress normal tissue and its blood vessels, causing distortion and ischemia.
- The tumors obstruct CSF pathways, causing hydrocephalus.
- Large brain tumors, peritumoral edema, and hydrocephalus can herniate normal cerebral structures under the falx cerebri, through the tentorium cerebelli, or through the foramen magnum, often causing acute neurologic decompensation.

As a result of these mechanisms, patients may have generalized symptoms caused by raised ICP, focal symptoms caused by ischemia and compression, or false localizing symptoms caused by shifts of cerebral or spinal structures. Generalized or false localizing symptoms are particularly likely to be caused by slow-growing tumors that reach a large size in the relatively silent frontal lobe, whereas focal symptoms occur with even small tumors in more functionally important areas of the brain (e.g., the motor strip and brainstem) or in the spinal cord.

Generalized Symptoms and Signs

Headache, the most common symptom of increased ICP, is the first symptom in approximately 40% of patients with a brain tumor [44]. Interestingly, headache is more frequent in those with a history of nontumoral headache. Most brain tumor headaches are nonspecific; however, a brain tumor should be suspected when headache is present on the patient's awakening from sleep but disappears within 1 hour (severe headaches that awaken one from sleep are more likely due to nontumoral causes), when headaches begin in a middle-aged or an older person who has not previously experienced them, or when the character or severity of headache in a chronic headache sufferer suddenly changes. Localized headache is a reliable indicator of laterality but does not mark the precise location of the tumor. For example, a right frontal headache indicates that the tumor is on the right but does not indicate that the tumor is frontal; it could be occipital or even cerebellar.

Vomiting with or without preceding nausea, particularly on awakening, is a common symptom of brain tumor in children but is less common in adults. Acute headache followed immediately by vomiting is characteristic of a brain tumor and indicates increased ICP; by contrast, a more prolonged headache that is followed by vomiting several hours later is characteristic of a migraine.

Papilledema occurs frequently in children and young adults but is less common in older patients. Usually, papilledema is asymptomatic but may cause transient episodes of visual blurring or blindness.

Mental changes begin with irritability and progress to apathy. Patients sleep longer, seem preoccupied when awake, and often fail to initiate activity, including conversation; however, if they are spoken to, usually they respond appropriately. In adults, psychiatric consultation for the treatment of what is thought to be depression frequently is obtained before a brain tumor is suspected.

Often, episodic symptoms that include headache, visual loss, altered consciousness, and sometimes tran-

sient weakness of the extremities are precipitated by rising from a recumbent position or by coughing or sneezing. They are caused by plateau waves (abrupt increases that occur in an already elevated ICP and last for 5–20 minutes). Plateau waves are not seizures; they respond to a decrease in the ICP but do not respond to anticonvulsant therapy.

Neck or back pain is the most common symptom of spinal tumor. As with brain tumors, spinal tumors often present with nocturnal or early morning neck or backache that often improves in the first few hours after arising. The pain is not worsened by activity. Unlike the pain of a herniated intervertebral disc, spinal tumor pain tends to be worse in recumbency and better when an affected patient is upright. Usually, the pain begins as a local pain at the site of the tumor, but it may radiate in a radicular or funicular pattern to other areas of the body.

Focal Symptoms and Signs

Seizures are the most common focal sign of a brain tumor. Focal seizures are particularly common in patients who have tumors (e.g., meningiomas) that compress the cortex or arise in or near the motor strip or the temporal lobe. Often, focal seizures caused by frontal or temporal foci produce behavioral or emotional symptoms that sometimes are confused with panic attacks or psychological disorders. Such episodic symptoms as a hemiparesis or aphasia without clear seizure activity can last for hours to days and then resolve. These episodes may respond to anticonvulsants. Generalized convulsions caused by brain tumors are also focal in onset, arising from an asymptomatic focal discharge. Depending on the growth rate of the tumor, seizures may be present for months to years before other symptoms develop. Any patient with focal or generalized seizures that begin in adulthood should undergo diagnostic evaluation for a brain tumor (see "Diagnosis").

The characteristics of other focal symptoms and signs of a brain tumor depend on the site of the lesion. These focal symptoms and signs are the same as those of CNS infection, stroke, or other structural diseases of the brain or spinal cord.

False Localizing Symptoms

False localizing symptoms are caused by shifts of cerebral structures. Diplopia may result from displacement or compression of the abducens nerve at the base of the brain. Hemianopsia may be caused by tentorial herniation that compresses the posterior cerebral artery. A number of other cranial nerve palsies associated with shifts of brainstem structures also may occur. Spinal cord tumors may cause funicular symptoms as false localizing signs. For example, a cervical spinal cord tumor may present as sciatica or the sensation of a tight band around the chest or abdomen.

DIAGNOSIS

All adults with new-onset seizures and all patients with papilledema or new focal motor or sensory signs require MRI [45] with the injection of contrast material (gadolinium DPTA). Patients with behavioral or personality changes should be evaluated with MRI if drowsiness, apathy, or memory loss accompanies the psychiatric symptoms or if the psychiatric symptoms are atypical. Patients with headache alone require MRI only if the headache has begun recently, has changed in character, or fails to respond to headache therapy. A negative MRI scan almost always rules out a tumor as the cause of the patient's symptoms or signs.

MRI identifies tumors that computed tomography (CT) misses and distinguishes tumors from arteriovenous malformations. Except for biopsy, other laboratory tests are unnecessary. The increased water content of tumors and their surrounding edema yield a hypointense (darker than normal brain) T_1-weighted image and a hyperintense (lighter than normal brain) T_2-weighted image. (T_1 and T_2 refer to the proton relaxation time for the acquisition of MRI data.) When the blood-brain barrier is disrupted, gadolinium leaks across and enters the brain tumor's extracellular space, causing hyperintensity (enhancement) on T_1-weighted images. Usually, hemorrhage appears hyperintense on T_1-weighted images and hypointense on T_2-weighted images but varies depending on the age of the hemorrhage. Identifying calcifications on MRI is difficult, but they are seen easily on CT scan. Although brain edema gives the same unenhanced MR signal as that of infiltrating tumor, the two can be distinguished: Edema spares the cortex, producing fingerlike projections of T_2-weighted hyperintensity between normal-appearing cortical gyri, whereas infiltrating tumor involves the cortex, changing the cortical signal.

Furthermore, in low-grade gliomas, edema often is absent, and infiltrating tumor may have the appearance of a well-defined border on T_2-weighted MRI scans, whereas edema typically has blurred, indistinct radiographic borders. Usually, high-grade gliomas exhibit contrast enhancement, with the T_1-weighted image showing an enhanced rim of irregular shape and thickness that surrounds a hypointense center; the T_2-weighted image shows only hyperintensity. Although the enhancement does not encompass the entire infiltrating margin, it represents a clinically useful approximation of tumor volume. A metastasis has a regular and spherical rim. Metastases are much more likely than are gliomas to be multiple; 50% of patients with metastases have multiple lesions, whereas only 5% of patients with gliomas have multifocal disease. Of patients with PCNSL, 20% to 40% have multiple tumors that are located periventricularly and usually exhibit diffuse contrast enhancement, have poorly circumscribed margins as compared with gliomas and metastases, and usually are surrounded by less edema than are these other tumors. On T_2-weighted images, PCNSL has relatively low signal intensity as compared with the high signal intensity of the surrounding edema. The MRI scan of immunocompromised patients with PCNSL may not demonstrate enhancement or may show ring enhancement. Basal ganglia involvement is more common in these patients.

Although MRI may suggest the histologic diagnosis (i.e., most low-grade tumor do not contrast enhance, whereas most high-grade tumors do), only biopsy is definitive [46]. An exception to this rule occurs in PCNSL, in which lumbar puncture or, if the eyes are involved, vitrectomy may yield malignant cells, obviating the necessity of brain biopsy. In other tumors, lumbar puncture poses a risk of cerebral herniation and rarely contributes to diagnosis. Positron emission tomography (PET) with positron-emitting radionuclides and magnetic resonance spectroscopy may prove to be useful noninvasive methods for determining the histologic type and degree of malignancy of a brain tumor.

TREATMENT

The histologic nature and location of a neoplasm and the general condition of a patient determine therapy. However, certain general principles apply to all CNS neoplasms.

Corticosteroids

Corticosteroids dramatically relieve the symptoms of brain and spinal cord tumors, reducing edema and, thus, decreasing ICP. Symptomatic improvement may begin within minutes, and patients often become asymptomatic within 24 to 48 hours. The mechanisms by which corticosteroids exert these effects are not understood well. One mechanism may be the decrease by corticosteroids of the flux of water-soluble agents across the disrupted blood-brain barrier. Unintended effects are inhibition of the entry of chemotherapeutic agents into the tumor and reduction of the apparent contrast enhancement on MRI (and CT).

Corticosteroids are indicated in all symptomatic patients with brain and spinal cord tumors, with the exception of those suspected of having PCNSL. In such patients, because of their lympholytic effects, corticosteroids may cause tumor necrosis, precluding definitive diagnosis. When PCNSL is suspected, corticosteroids should be withheld until a biopsy has established the diagnosis. Usually, the corticosteroid administered is dexamethasone, 16 mg/day. Once begun, the administration of a corticosteroid is continued until the patients' symptoms are relieved and ICP is diminished. Then the drug is tapered to the lowest dose commensurate with good neurologic function; often, it can be discontinued completely after surgery or irradiation.

Anticonvulsants

Patients who have focal or generalized seizures should be treated with antiepileptic drugs (AEDs). No evidence provides information about which drug is best, though phenytoin, carbamazepine, and valproate are the drugs prescribed most often. No evidence supports the use of AEDs prophylactically in brain tumor patients who have not had seizures [47]. Furthermore, side effects, drug interactions, and complications of AEDs are more common in patients with CNS tumors [48]. One exception is that prophylactic AEDs probably reduce the incidence of perioperative seizures and should be given immediately before and for several weeks after tumor resection [49].

Surgery

Although surgery for patients with brain or spinal cord tumors rarely is curative, it is the most important treatment for patients with accessible tumors other than PCNSL. Surgery establishes the diagnosis, relieves ICP, and improves symptoms and seizure control. In addition, the use of modern surgical techniques by a skilled neurosurgeon and the administration of corticosteroids to prevent postoperative swelling reduce the risk of worsening of neurologic function. Although some controversy surrounds the role of surgery in patients with gliomas, the preponderance of evidence indicates that more complete surgical removal of a tumor improves both the duration of survival and quality of life. If a tumor exhibits contrast enhancement before surgery, a postoperative contrast-enhanced MRI scan obtained within 3 days of resection accurately predicts the extent of residual tumor and thereby helps to establish the prognosis; surgeons' clinical estimates of the extent of resection are not reliable [12].

Radiotherapy

Postoperative radiotherapy prolongs the duration of survival and improves the quality of life in patients with high-grade tumors (e.g., anaplastic astrocytoma or glioblastoma multiforme), but its role in patients with low-grade (particularly asymptomatic) tumors is uncertain. After total resection of pilocytic astrocytomas, radiotherapy is not required. In asymptomatic patients with low-grade astrocytomas or oligodendrogliomas, radiotherapy may be deferred safely until symptoms develop. Brain and spinal cord gliomas should be treated with high doses of irradiation (5,500–6,000 cGy in fractions of 180–200 cGy for brain tumors and 4,500–5,000 cGy for spinal tumors) delivered to a limited field that encompasses the tumor and its immediate surroundings. Stereotactic radiosurgery (in which a single high dose of ionizing irradiation in multiple narrow beams is directed to a precise intracranial location by stereotaxy) is used in some centers to treat metastasis and to "boost" conventional irradiation for glioma. However, its efficacy has not been established [50]. Stereotactic radiosurgery given in several fractions is called *fractionated stereotactic radiotherapy.* Heavy-particle irradiation (e.g., protons, neutrons) may have a role to play, especially in tumors of the skull base [51]. Radiotherapy at doses required to treat most brain tumors can be neurotoxic, especially to children and the elderly [52].

Chemotherapy

The response of most gliomas to chemotherapy is limited, but the addition of nitrosoureas or procarbazine to radiotherapy increases the survival of some patients with high-grade gliomas [53]. Predicting which patients will respond to chemotherapy is impossible; therefore, all patients who have high-grade gliomas and are not entered into experimental protocols should be treated with a combination of radiotherapy and a nitrosourea or other lipid-soluble chemotherapeutic agent. This approach is justified in part because the toxicity profile of these agents is acceptable. A number of other chemotherapeutic agents are undergoing clinical trials, but none has proved superior to carmustine (BCNU) or procarbazine.

Other Therapeutic Modalities

Several therapeutic techniques, including immunotherapy, gene therapy, and antiangiogenesis agents, are under investigation; one or more ultimately may prove useful.

SPECIFIC INTRACRANIAL TUMORS

Diffuse Astrocytic Tumors

Astrocytic tumors are the most common clinically symptomatic brain tumor. Tumors of astrocytic origin can be divided into those that diffusely infiltrate local and distant brain structures and those that are more focal (Table 28.4).

Diffuse astrocytomas range from low-grade (astrocytoma) to extremely high-grade (glioblastoma multiforme). They are more common in adults than in children and generally arise in the cerebral hemispheres, although they may affect the brainstem, cerebellum, or spinal cord. Diffuse astrocytic tumors of the brainstem (pontine or brainstem gliomas) are more common in children. Low-grade tumors have a tendency to progress to a higher-grade phenotype. High-grade tumors may arise either by progression from a lower grade or as de novo tumors.

Diffuse astrocytic tumors can be divided by histologic characteristics into astrocytoma, anaplastic astrocytoma, and glioblastoma multiforme. Also included in

Table 28.4 Tumors of Astrocytic Origin

Diffuse astrocytic tumors (fibrillary astrocytomas)
  Astrocytoma
  Anaplastic astrocytoma
  Glioblastoma multiforme
  Gliomatosis cerebri
  Brainstem glioma

Focal astrocytic tumors
  Pilocytic astrocytoma
  Pleomorphic xanthoastrocytoma
  Subependymal giant-cell astrocytoma
  Diffuse astrocytic tumor

this group are some tumors that diffusely infiltrate the entire brain: gliomatosis cerebri, which may be of any grade or of mixed grade. Almost by definition, diffuse astrocytomas are not amenable to surgical cure.

Usually, focal astrocytomas are tumors of the young and often are found in specific portions of the neuraxis, such as the cerebellum or temporal lobe. They may have a "malignant" histologic appearance but usually are indolent in biological behavior and often are amenable to surgical cure. Such tumors include pilocytic astrocytomas, pleomorphic xanthoastrocytomas, and subependymal giant-cell astrocytomas. Diffuse astrocytic tumors are considered first as a whole because the biological characteristics of, symptomatologic traits of, diagnostic approach to, and treatment of such tumors are similar. Differences in the management of specific diffuse astrocytomas are considered later in this section.

INCIDENCE

Diffuse astrocytic tumors represent approximately 30% of primary intracranial tumors but more than 60% of clinically symptomatic tumors. The incidence varies, depending on ascertainment, but generally ranges between five and seven new patients per 100,000 population per year. A recent study by Polednak and Flannery [54] gave incidence rates of 2.1 for glioblastoma and 2.2 for astrocytoma using data for American whites in a recent Surveillance, Epidemiology, and End Results (SEER) survey between 1983 and 1987. Radhakrishnan et al. [14] found the age-specific incidence rate for malignant astrocytomas (anaplastic astrocytomas and glioblastomas) was highest in those persons in the 75- to 84-year-old group. In that study, the age and population distribution of primary intracranial neoplasms in Rochester, MN (1950–1989), was 3.6 per 100,000 per year for malignant astrocytomas, 90% of which were symptomatic. The incidence of low-grade astrocytomas was 1.3 per 100,000 per year, of which 0.9 were symptomatic. These figures can be contrasted with meningiomas, which had a rate of 7.8 per 100,000 per year, of which only 2.0 were symptomatic (Table 28.5).

Several studies addressed the question of whether the incidence of astrocytic tumors is increasing [14]; the studies arrived at somewhat different conclusions. In the Mayo Clinic series, the average annual age- and gender-adjusted incidence rates of primary intracranial neoplasms per 100,000 per year rose from 17.0 in the period 1950 through 1969 to 19.7 during the interval 1970 through 1989. Symptomatic tumors with corre-

Table 28.5 Neoplasms by Histologic Type at the Mayo Clinic, 1950 to 1989

Tumor Type	All Patients		Symptomatic Patients	
	Percentage of Total	Rate	Percentage of Total	Rate
Malignant astrocytoma	18	3.6	26	3.3
Low-grade astrocytoma	7	1.3	8	0.9
Meningiomas	40	7.8	16	2.0

Note: Average age- and gender-adjusted incidence rate per100,000 per year.
Source: Modified from K Radhakrishnan, B Mokri, JE Parisi, et al., The trends in incidence of primary brain tumors in the population of Rochester, Minnesota. *Ann Neurol* 37:67–73, 1995.

sponding rates were 9.5 and 12.5 in those same periods. These changes were not statistically significant. For malignant astrocytomas, the tumor type that many investigators claim is increasing dramatically in frequency, the symptomatic average annual incidence rates were 2.94 in 1950 through 1969 and 3.27 in 1970 through 1989. These figures also are not statistically significant: The incidence of malignant astrocytomas actually dropped from 0.53 to 0.18 during these two periods.

Other studies report a dramatic increase in astrocytomas, particularly high-grade astrocytomas, in the elderly [15, 22]. The most dramatic data are those of Olney et al [22]. The incidence of astrocytomas, anaplastic astrocytomas, and glioblastomas rose from 45 tumors per million population per year in 1975 to 53 in 1992, a significant figure. Anaplastic astrocytomas and glioblastomas increased, and astrocytomas decreased. The decrease in astrocytomas with an increase in anaplastic tumors may, of course, be attributed to neuropathologists' changes in interpretation of microscopical slides. A similar study from the French Cancer Registry between 1983 and 1989 indicates that malignant astrocytomas increased 5% per year in persons older than age 65 [55]. A study from the Florida Cancer Center found a risk increase of 1.32 for glioblastoma patients older than 65, comparing the years 1981 to 1984 to the years 1986 to 1989 [15].

Thus, most data support an increase in astrocytic tumor incidence, particularly higher-grade tumors in the elderly. The meaning of the increase is controversial: Some investigators have suggested that 20% or more of the apparent increase is due to better ascertainment by improved imaging. More accurate and less invasive modern diagnostic techniques lead physicians to perform such diagnostic tests as MRI on neurologically ill elderly patients for whom they would not order angiography. In addition, elderly patients generally are more vigorous now than in the past, leading them to

demand—and physicians to consider—more extensive workup when neurologic symptoms appear. Others have suggested that with an aging population, an increase in tumors of the elderly is statistically inevitable [2]. Because vascular disease and cancer are the two leading causes of death in the elderly (stroke being the leading neurologic cause of death), decreases in cerebrovascular disease incidence through better lifestyle and medical treatment very well may introduce an apparent increase in brain tumors.

ETIOLOGIC FEATURES

With the exception of ionizing irradiation and immunosuppression, no risk factor has been established unequivocally as a cause of sporadic diffuse astrocytomas. Diffuse astrocytomas occurring in an irradiation portal are reported with both high- and low-dose radiotherapy. Ron et al. [30] found that the relative risk of glioma after low-dose irradiation for tinea capitis was 2.6. With the higher radiotherapy doses required to treat childhood malignancies, the increase was sevenfold in those who survive more than three years after initial treatment. Although other environmental risk factors have been proposed as causes of astrocytic tumors, none has been proved. The risk factors implicated most frequently include the ingestion of nitrosamines, work in the petroleum industry, exposure to electromagnetic irradiation, and ingestion of aspartame (see Table 28.2).

Familial Tumors

A few familial disorders are associated with astrocytomas. Occasionally, astrocytomas complicate NF1 and NF2, the Li-Fraumeni syndrome, and Turcot's syndrome (see Table 28.3). A specific astrocytoma—the subependymal giant-cell astrocytoma—complicates tuberous sclerosis. The Li-Fraumeni syndrome is an autosomal dominant disorder characterized by multiple primary neoplasms in children and young adults, predominantly soft-tissue sarcomas, osteosarcomas, and breast cancer.

The syndrome results from a *p53* germline mutation. Approximately 12% of families with this germ line mutation have brain tumors. Approximately 75% of such tumors are of astrocytic origin and include both low-grade and high-grade tumors. Alteration of the *p53* gene occurs in approximately 50% of sporadically arising astrocytic tumors.

Turcot's syndrome consists of a group of autosomal dominant (and possibly autosomal recessive) disorders characterized by multiple colorectal neoplasms, neuroblastomas, and malignant neuroepithelial tumors, including glioblastomas. Glioblastomas in Turcot's syndrome result from an alteration in the genes *MLH1* and *PSM2*, which are found on chromosomes 3 and 7, respectively.

Genetic Alterations

Two major genetic mutations mark the change from a differentiated astrocyte or neuroepithelial precursor cell to an astrocytoma: *p53* mutations or overexpression of platelet-derived growth factor A (PDGF-A) or platelet-derived growth factor receptor–alpha (PDGF-α) [56]. Genetic changes in low-grade astrocytomas, which includes the loss of heterozygosity on chromosome 19q or alteration in the retinoblastoma tumor suppressor gene, mark the transition of low-grade tumors to anaplastic tumors. Several other genetic changes, including mutations in the *PTEN* gene, loss of expression of *DCC,* or amplification of PDGF, lead to glioblastoma multiforme. Some glioblastomas arise by progressive increase in grade from low-grade to high-grade (secondary glioblastoma). Others apparently arise de novo (primary glioblastoma). Differentiating between primary and secondary glioblastomas may be difficult and cannot be achieved on a molecular basis alone. If histologic evidence of both low-grade and high-grade astrocytoma is found in the same tumor at surgery, the glioblastoma is secondary. An MRI scan that shows both nonenhancing and enhancing tumor, or progression from nonenhancing to enhancing tumor, suggests a secondary tumor. Sudden growth of an intensely enhancing tumor on the background of a previously normal scan suggests a primary glioblastoma. Usually, primary glioblastomas occur in people older than 60 years, and the prognosis is worse than for secondary glioblastomas, which are more likely to occur in people younger than 50.

In approximately 40% of glioblastomas multiforme, the epidermal growth factor receptor is truncated with a frame deletion of approximately 30 amino acids. The truncated form is constitutively active (i.e., active without need for binding by its ligand). The truncated receptor is not found in normal glial cells and thus forms a potential target for therapy directed at a specific tumor protein.

PATHOLOGIC DETERMINATION

Most astrocytomas have a gray or yellow appearance. They may contain cysts, granular areas, and zones of firmness or gelatinous softening. Sometimes, a single large cyst filled with clear fluid is present. In some tumors, focal calcification gives the tumor a gritty feeling. Distinguishing low-grade from high-grade diffuse astrocytomas grossly is impossible. Owing to their infiltrative nature, diffuse astrocytomas usually show blurring of the gross anatomic boundaries, and the point at which tumor stops and edema begins cannot be identified grossly. High-grade astrocytomas are more likely than low-grade tumors to appear well-demarcated from surrounding normal brain tissues, but even when the boundaries appear distinct macroscopically, usually the microscope shows tumor infiltration of normal tissue. Microscopic cysts are less characteristic of high-grade tumors, but areas of granularity, opacity, and soft consistency are common. In glioblastoma multiforme, hemorrhage and necrosis may be grossly visible. Generally, hemorrhage and necrosis are not found in anaplastic astrocytomas or low-grade astrocytomas.

Microscopically, tumor cells may infiltrate far beyond the gross bulk of the tumor. The histologic criteria used to grade astrocytic tumors include nuclear atypia, mitotic activity, necrosis, and endothelial proliferation. Although cell proliferation indices, as measured by MIB-1 reaction, predict a poor prognosis, evidence of apoptosis is a good prognostic sign.

WHO uses a four-tiered system, reserving grade I for pilocytic astrocytomas and the other three grades for astrocytoma, anaplastic astrocytoma, and glioblastoma multiforme, respectively (Table 28.6). The St. Anne–Mayo Clinic system uses four grades, with their grades 1 and 2 corresponding to WHO grade II. Often, distinguishing astrocytomas from anaplastic astrocytomas is difficult, leading to some disagreement between pathologists over interpreting individual tumors. The difficulty is compounded by the recent increase in use of stereotactic needle biopsy to establish the diagnosis, a method that gives neuropathologists a very small sample to examine. Because of the well-known heterogeneity of brain tumors, the smaller the sample, the less likely the

Table 28.6 Comparison of World Health Organization (WHO) and St. Anne–Mayo Clinic Classification of Astrocytomas

WHO Grade	WHO Designation	St. Anne–Mayo Designation	Histologic Criteria
I	Pilocytic astrocytoma		Rosenthal fibers, piloid cells
II	Astrocytoma (low-grade diffuse)	Astrocytoma grade 1	Zero criteria
		Astrocytoma grade 2	One criterion, usually nuclear atypia
III	Anaplastic astrocytoma	Astrocytoma grade 3	Two criteria, usually nuclear atypia and mitosis
IV	Glioblastoma	Astrocytoma grade 4	Three of previous four criteria plus endothelial proliferation or necrosis (or both)

tumor will be graded accurately. In controlled trials of the treatment of diffuse astrocytomas, an important step is to have one pathologist examining all the tumors, thereby ensuring consistency if not absolute accuracy.

Two important characteristics of diffuse astrocytic tumors are invasion of normal brain and angiogenesis. Unlike cancers elsewhere in the body, which usually have the capacity not only to invade surrounding tissue but to metastasize distantly, astrocytomas usually invade and may spread widely within the CNS but rarely metastasize outside it. Normal glial cells are motile in vitro and probably in vivo as well; this property is enhanced in glioma cells. The degree of motility appears to be related directly to the histologic grade of the cell line [57]. Migration follows white-matter pathways. The corpus callosum is among the major pathways for spread of astrocytomas. The anterior commissure is another route of migration. These two routes allow tumors to spread from one hemisphere to the other. Stereotactic needle biopsy of both tumor and surrounding normal brain indicate a variable degree of invasion into normal brain by brain tumors.

Some tumors exhibit little or no invasion, and the tumor is apparently grossly (as well as microscopically) well circumscribed. In other tumors, cells can be found several centimeters from the apparent border of the tumor into normal brain. A series of steps is necessary to allow astrocytoma cells to invade surrounding normal brain: cell-cell interaction, proteases, integrins, motility, and growth factors.

Cell-cell interactions must be loosened. Adhesion molecules, such as neural cell adhesion molecule (NCAM), promote cell-cell interaction. Lack of NCAM in glioma cells may loosen that interaction. Proteases must be exuded to degrade the extracellular matrix. Proteases are expressed by glioma cells and some, particularly metalloproteases, probably are important for invasion. Integrins (transmembrane glycoproteins that

integrate extracellular matrix components with the cytoskeleton and the transcriptional machinery) are overexpressed in glioma cells. Interaction between integrins and extracellular matrix components, including tenascin, fibronectin, and osteopontin, are necessary for invasion to occur. CD44, a glycoprotein receptor for several extracellular matrix components, including hyaluronic acid, is expressed weakly in astrocytomas but more strongly in anaplastic astrocytomas and glioblastomas. This receptor mediates invasion by glioma cells. Growth factors, including transforming growth factor–beta$_1$, contribute to the spread of tumor cells within the CNS.

Invasion not only renders complete removal of diffuse astrocytic tumors impossible; it allows the tumors to appear at multiple places in the brain. Some 5% of diffuse astrocytomas are said to be multicentric. A multicentric glioma is a clinical challenge because the imaging may resemble that of brain metastases. So-called multicentric gliomas may represent spread from a single focus, with the areas of grossly apparent tumor being connected by bridges of microscopic glioma cells. In its most florid form, gliomas can invade the entire brain (gliomatosis cerebri).

The second major factor in growth of gliomas is angiogenesis [58, 59]. Both the tumor and the clinician depend on angiogenesis. The tumor needs new blood vessels to grow beyond a size that can be nourished by diffusion from normal brain, a few millimeters in diameter at best. The clinician relies on the fact that the neovasculature induced by the tumor is fenestrated, lacking a normal blood-brain barrier and leading to contrast enhancement on the MRI scan. The major vasoactive factor involved in angiogenesis in glial tumors is the vascular endothelial growth factor and its receptors FLK-1 and FLT-1. The growth factors elaborated by tumor cells have their effect not on the tumor but on the normal brain vasculature, promoting the growth of capillaries. These neovessels lack a blood-brain barrier, which leads not only to contrast enhancement but to passage of serum components into the brain tumor, in turn leading to brain edema. Normal brain immediately surrounding the tumor also may have a partially disrupted barrier, additionally promoting brain edema. However, because tumor cells may infiltrate so widely, many tumor cells at the edge receive their blood supply from normal capillaries and would continue to be nourished even in the absence of angiogenesis. Thus, the role of antiangiogenesis therapy in the treatment of gliomas may be limited.

Blood vessels affected by the vasoactive growth factors do not themselves appear to become neoplastic, although the exuberant growth of endothelial cells often seen in glioblastoma multiforme (endothelial proliferation), and the fact that they have an elevated labeling index, have led some to believe that these vessels may themselves become neoplastic. Experimental evidence in a non-CNS animal tumor indicates that angiogenesis can be inhibited repetitively without development of resistance to the antiangiogenesis agent. This phenomenon differs from the effect in neoplasms that, because of their genetic instability, usually become resistant to an agent after repetitive treatment.

DIAGNOSIS

Signs and Symptoms

Table 28.7 lists the presenting symptoms and signs in patients with diffuse astrocytoma. Low-grade astrocytomas are more likely than their higher-grade counterpart to present with seizures, either focal or generalized. Even grand mal seizures caused by brain tumors are focal at onset, though the focal origin may be silent or unrecognized. Occasional seizures over many months or years without the development of other neurologic symptoms is a characteristic of astrocytomas. Generally, with anaplastic astrocytomas, seizures (if they are the presenting symptom) are joined rapidly by other neuro-

Table 28.7 Symptoms and Signs of Glioma

Generalized
  Headache
  Mental status alterations
  Personality change
  Decreased consciousness

Focal
  Focal seizures
  Weakness or sensory changes (or both)
  Visual-field defect
  Aphasia

logic symptoms. Higher-grade lesions are more likely to present with such focal neurologic symptoms as memory loss, personality change, contralateral motor or sensory symptoms, and visual-field deficits.

When patients present with seizures, the neurologic examination may be entirely normal. On the other hand, on examination patients may have focal deficits of which they are unaware. Examples include difficulty with recent memory and mild contralateral motor signs. Sometimes, when they are questioned directly, members of a patient's family are aware of a personality change of which the patient is unaware. The most frequent personality change is that of apathy, often leading patients (particularly those with frontal lobe tumors) to consult a psychiatrist for depression.

Imaging

The first step in evaluating patients suspected of harboring an astrocytoma is MRI [60]. This examination should be performed in any adult who presents with an unprovoked seizure for which no immediate explanation is available. A normal MRI scan essentially rules out a diffuse astrocytoma as a cause of such patients' symptoms, and no further workup is required. Difficulty in interpreting the MRI scan of a tumor may occur in older patients who have multiple areas of white-matter hyperintensity related to vascular disease but not differentiated from a focal area of nonenhancing hyperintensity that eventually is revealed to be the tumor. The tumor hyperintensity is immediately subcortical and somewhat diffuse, different from the more focal periventricular hyperintense images of vascular disease. Usually, malignant gliomas, glioblastoma multiforme, and anaplastic tumors contrast enhance (Fig. 28.2), whereas lower-grade tumors do not (Fig. 28.3). However, many exceptions occur.

Histologic Identification

In most instances, if a suspected diffuse astrocytoma is encountered on an MRI scan, craniotomy and removal of as much tumor as is technically feasible is the best diagnostic *and* therapeutic approach. Because most evidence indicates that the more complete the resection of either low- or high-grade tumors, the better the prognosis, brain tumor surgery should be performed by experienced tumor neurosurgeons using the most modern techniques of localization and stereotaxy. The best series indicate an operative mortality of approximately 1% and worsening of neurologic symptoms and signs (usually transient) in 5% to 10%. In some instances—usually because of the location of the tumor in eloquent or vital areas—surgical extirpation is not feasible. In such cases, a stereotactic needle biopsy should be performed to establish the diagnosis before definitive treatment is begun. Important precautions are to establish that the abnormality on the MRI scan is indeed a diffuse astrocytoma and to grade the tumor, because grading affects treatment.

Stereotactic needle biopsy is not without problems. Although the procedure is performed easily, the small sample retrieved may render establishment of a diagnosis difficult for the neuropathologist. Even when pathologists can establish a diagnosis of diffuse astrocytoma, they may be unable to grade the tumor accurately because of sampling error. Neurosurgeons performing a stereotactic needle biopsy of a suspected diffuse astrocytoma should aim for what appears to be the highest-grade area. This site can be established either by areas of contrast enhancement on the MRI scan or by areas of hypermetabolism on the PET scan (see next section). The second major problem with stereotactic needle biopsy consists of two possible complications. The first is bleeding. Although the overall rate of symptomatic bleeding in patients who undergo stereotactic needle biopsy is approximately 1%, the rate is substantially higher in patients with diffuse astrocytoma, particularly those with high-grade lesions. In one study, as many as 6% of patients with glioblastoma multiforme bled after stereotactic needle biopsy. Complications are fewer in lower-grade tumors but still are greater than 1%.

The second complication is neurologic worsening without bleeding. Little in the literature addresses this complication, but we have found a significant number of patients (particularly those with widespread and diffuse tumors) whose neurologic condition worsens substantially after stereotactic needle biopsy. Most recover over several days to a few weeks, but some do not. Two types of neurologic worsening are possible: One is an increase in focal signs (e.g., hemiparesis); the second is an alteration of mental status without focal signs. Some of our patients who demonstrate memory loss or personality change may, after a stereotactic needle biopsy, become and remain lethargic or confused without making a substantial recovery.

Positron Emission Tomography

We perform PET scans in some patients with putative low-grade diffuse astrocytomas prior to biopsy [61]. The PET scan is performed with fluorodeoxyglucose to measure glucose metabolism. If the PET scan is hypometabolic (i.e., glucose metabolism less than normal white matter) in patients who have a nonenhancing lesion,

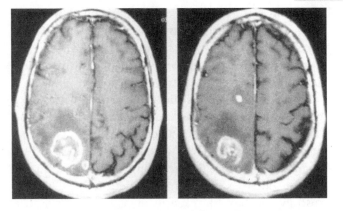

Figure 28.2 Glioblastoma multiforme. T_1-weighted, gadolinium-enhanced axial image at two levels in a patient with a glioblastoma multiforme. Patient shows three apparently discrete contrast-enhancing lesions surrounded by edema. Resection revealed a glioblastoma multiforme. Note the thick, irregular contrast-enhancing rim of the larger tumor and the hypointensity (edema) surrounding the area of contrast enhancement.

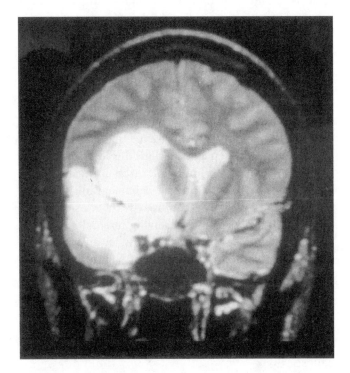

Figure 28.3 Astrocytoma. Coronal T_2-weighted image of a patient with many years of temporal lobe seizures and gradually developing memory loss. The tumor is hyperintense on the T_2-weighted image, does not contrast enhance, and is not surrounded by a significant amount of edema, although the tumor mass causes a shift of the ventricles. The patient's condition improved after a debulking operation.

suffer only seizures controllable by anticonvulsants, and have no other neurologic symptoms or signs, we may elect to follow them clinically rather than with biopsy or treatment (see "Treatment"). If a generally hypometabolic PET scan shows an area of hypermetabolism, a neurosurgeon can direct the stereotactic needle biopsy to that area because treatment is determined by the highest grade in a heterogeneous tumor.

Magnetic Resonance Spectroscopy

Recent evidence suggests that magnetic resonance spectroscopy may have the capacity of distinguishing diffuse astrocytomas from other intrinsic tumors of the brain and may play a role in noninvasively establishing the grade of astrocytoma [62]. The data are preliminary, and the technique should still be considered experimental.

Differential Diagnosis

Some lesions must be considered in the differential diagnosis of diffuse astrocytomas: oligodendroglioma, focal astrocytic tumors, cerebral infarct, metastasis, multiple sclerosis, and brain abscess. In addition to such other glial tumors as oligodendrogliomas and ependymomas, two main nonneoplastic lesions should be considered in the differential diagnosis. The first is ischemic infarction. Often, older patients with diffuse astrocytomas present with transient symptoms presumably due to seizures. Unlike the short-lived focal seizures occurring with other epileptic lesions, these episodes may last many minutes to hours, often are associated with abnormalities of cognition and behavior, and (because of their length) may be confused with transient ischemic attacks or even small resolving cerebral infarcts. A CT scan without contrast may show an area of hypodensity that is interpreted as cerebral infarction. However, CT hypodensity associated with diffuse astrocytomas is restricted to white matter and usually does not involve cortex. On the contrary, cerebral infarction generally is triangular, with the base at the cortical surface. Often, a contrast-enhanced MRI scan establishes the diagnosis.

The second important distinction occurs in patients with large contrast-enhancing lesions that are caused by demyelinating disease and have the appearance of a high-grade diffuse astrocytoma. One distinction between demyelinating lesions and glioblastoma is that the contrast-enhancing ring usually is incomplete in demyelinating disease but is complete in glioblastoma. However, usually these lesions cannot be distinguished easily on MRI scan, and biopsy may be necessary. Neurologists and neurosurgeons are obligated to call the neuropathologist's attention to the possibility of demyelinating disease, because the macrophages in a demyelinating lesion may be misinterpreted as tumor cells and patients might be subjected to major resection and radiotherapy. Radiotherapy appears particularly damaging in patients with demyelinating disease, and the distinction, therefore, is vital.

Functional Magnetic Resonance Imaging

Functional MRI prior to surgery and cortical mapping during surgery play important roles in the treatment of diffuse astrocytomas. Functional MRI can identify not only sensory and motor areas but language areas that cannot be identified at neurosurgery unless an affected patient is operated on under local anesthesia [4]. Mapping during the course of the procedure can identify motor areas. These tests are particularly important in patients with diffuse astrocytomas. The bulk of the tumor may be distant from eloquent areas, but a portion may impinge on an eloquent area (i.e., motor, language, or visual cortex). By knowing the exact location of these areas, surgeons can plan the approach appropriately. Many patients with diffuse astrocytomas who are suffering from focal neurologic symptoms improve after decompression of a tumor from an eloquent area.

TREATMENT

The treatment of diffuse astrocytomas depends on their grade: The optimum treatment of low-grade tumors (i.e., astrocytoma) is not established. In particular, current evidence indicates that radiotherapy delivered when affected patients first present with the disorder does not improve survival over radiotherapy delivered when such patients demonstrate tumor progression. The treatment plan must be individualized, but certain general rules and recommendations can be made.

If the tumor is in a relatively silent area of the brain (e.g., right frontal lobe), an attempt should be made to remove the tumor, regardless of whether it is causing neurologic symptoms and signs other than controllable seizures. Patients who undergo a gross total resection of a low-grade tumor are not cured but survive longer and better than do those who are not operated on.

Patients whose tumors involve eloquent areas and who are asymptomatic save for focal seizures, particularly if a PET scan is hypometabolic, can be followed without treatment. Some patients may be followed for many years without substantial growth of the lesion. In the absence of biopsy, however, whether these tumors are astrocytomas, oligodendrogliomas, or something else cannot be ascertained.

Symptomatic patients should undergo tumor removal to the extent feasible or should undergo at least a stereotactic needle biopsy when resection cannot be done. After a diagnosis is established, radiotherapy should be delivered to a limited field encompassing the visible tumor on MRI scan and a 2-cm margin. The treatment should be delivered in fractions no larger than 180 cGy, to a total dose of 50 to 54 Gy. No evidence at present indicates that radiosurgery, brachytherapy, or irradiation sensitizers have any role to play in the initial treatment of astrocytoma, but they may help when the tumor recurs.

Anaplastic Astrocytomas and Glioblastoma Multiforme

The conventional treatment of anaplastic astrocytoma and glioblastoma multiforme is to remove as much of the tumor as is surgically feasible, to deliver radiotherapy to a limited field encompassing the tumor and a 2.5- to 3-cm margin to a dose of 60 Gy at 180 cGy fractions, and to follow that treatment with chemotherapy. Two conventional chemotherapeutic regimens—BCNU alone and procarbazine, lomustine (CCNU), and vincristine (PCV)—are outlined in Table 28.8.

One study indicates that PCV chemotherapy is superior to BCNU for anaplastic astrocytomas but not for glioblastoma multiforme; however, this finding was identified in a post hoc subgroup analysis within an overall negative study. Although a number of phase II trials have shown that other chemotherapeutic agents are effective (Table 28.9), none have been shown to be superior to BCNU or PCV; only temozolamide has been shown to be superior to procarbazine in relapsed patients. No evidence indicates that chemotherapy given prior to radiotherapy or concomitant with radiotherapy promotes either quality or duration of survival.

With respect to anaplastic astrocytoma and glioblastoma, little question remains that radiotherapy improves quality and duration of life. In the original Brain Tumor Study Group controlled trial, median survival increased from 14 to 45 weeks with radiotherapy. The study demonstrated a direct correlation between the amount of irradiation and the duration of survival. However, the maximally feasible dose is approximately 5,940 cGy given in 180 cGy fractions to a limited field. At present, no evidence substantiates that hyperfractionated radiotherapy, radiosurgery, or brachytherapy are better than standard radiotherapy as indicated earlier, even when a maximum of 12,000 cGy has been delivered to the tumor.

Likewise, no evidence demonstrates that any other chemotherapy approach increases survival, although

Table 28.8 Conventional Chemotherapy of Malignant Glioma

Drug	Standard Dose and Route
BCNU (carmustine)	200–240 mg/m² IV every 6–8 wks
PCV, standard	
Procarbazine	60 mg/m² PO on days 8–21 repeated every 6 weeks
CCNU	110 mg/m² PO day 1 repeated every 6 weeks
Vincristine	1.4 mg/m² (maximum, 2 mg) IV on days 8 and 29 repeated every 6 weeks
PCV, intensive	
Procarbazine	75 mg/m²
CCNU	130 mg/m²
Vincristine	1.4 mg/m² (no cap)

IV = intravenous; PO = per os; CCNU = 1-(2-chloroethyl)-3-cyclohexyl-1-nitrosourea [lomustine].

Table 28.9 Some Chemotherapeutic Agents Used in Glioma Patients

Abbreviation	Drug Name
AraC	Cytosine arabinoside
AZQ	Arazidinylbenzoquinone
BCNU	1,3-bis(2-chloroethyl)-1-nitrosourea [carmustine]
CCNU	1-(2-chloroethyl)-3-cyclohexyl-1-nitrosourea [lomustine]
CDDP	Cisplatin
DAG	Dianhydrogalactitol
DBD	Dibromodulcitol
DTIC	Imadazole carboxamide [dacarbazine]
5-FU	5-Fluorouracil
HU	Hydroxyurea
MeCCNU	Methyl-1-(2-chloroethyl)-3-cyclohexyl-1-nitrosourea [semustine]
Miso	Misonidazole
MTX	Methotrexate
PCB	Procarbazine
PCNU	1-(2-chloroethyl)-3-(2,6-dioxo-3-piper-idyl)-1-nitrosourea
TEM	Temozolamide
VCR	Vincristine
VM-26	Teniposide
VP-16	Terazanate, etoposide

one study indicates that a biodegradable polymer containing carmustine implanted into the tumor bed for recurrent malignant glioma increases survival over a placebo implantation. Some studies of the use of adjuvant chemotherapy indicate modest effects; others do not. However, adjuvant treatment, regardless of chemotherapeutic agent, probably benefits approximately only 15% to 20% of patients.

Presently, newer forms of treatment, including immunotherapy, gene therapy, antiangiogenesis therapy, antisense therapy, and the like, have not been shown to be efficacious.

Inevitably, patients with anaplastic astrocytoma or glioblastoma multiforme relapse after treatment. In many circumstances, a second surgical procedure will improve symptoms and increase survival. Irradiation beyond the 60 cGy given originally is not feasible, but interstitial therapy, other chemotherapeutic agents, and experimental therapeutic techniques can be considered at that point.

Gliomatosis Cerebri

Sometimes, diffuse astrocytomas infiltrate the brain so widely as to involve the entire brain with or without the presence of an identifiable focal lesion. Such diffuse infiltration is called *gliomatosis cerebri*. The pathologic identity of the disorder is astrocytoma that may vary from low to high grade and may differ in grade from area to area. Rarely, an oligodendroglioma may present with the syndrome of gliomatosis cerebri. The symptoms may be either diffuse (i.e., headaches, papilledema, cognitive changes) or focal, including corticospinal tract abnormalities and seizures. Some patients present with brainstem or even spinal cord signs, as occasionally the entire neuraxis may be infiltrated. Usually, the MRI scan is characterized by hyperintensity on a T_2-weighted image, either diffusely or multifocally. On some occasions, areas of contrast enhancement are seen, with diffuse or multifocal nonenhancing areas. On rare occasions, the scan reveals no abnormality of signal intensity but simply diffuse enlargement of the brain leading to ventricles and sulci that are smaller than would be expected for affected patients' age. When gliomatosis cerebri is suspected, a stereotactic needle biopsy will establish the diagnosis. The needle biopsy should be directed toward the most abnormal area of the brain. The prognosis is poor; more than one-half the patients die within a year of symptom onset, and less than one-fourth survive more than 3 years.

Gliomatosis cerebri is treated with radiotherapy. Unlike focal anaplastic astrocytomas or glioblastoma, the irradiation is delivered to the entire brain to a total dose of 60 Gy. In patients in whom biopsy or scan evidence of anaplasia is present, chemotherapy with carmustine or PCV can be applied after the irradiation, although its efficacy is not known.

Brainstem Glioma

The most common brainstem gliomas are diffuse astrocytomas of varying grade; they are centered in the pons and usually occur in childhood (see Chapter 25). Tumors that occur in adulthood differ little in signs and symptoms from those in children, usually beginning with cranial nerve palsies (especially diplopia) and subsequently evolving to cause long-tract signs. Hydrocephalus is uncommon. The diagnosis is verified by MRI scan. The tumors appear histologically identical to astrocytomas in other areas of the brain. If the tumor is dorsally exophytic, likely it is a pilocytic astrocytoma or ganglioglioma, and biopsy is safe. Some neurosurgeons recommend stereotactic needle biopsy even when the tumor remains within the confines of the brainstem, but others believe the complication rate is too high and that MRI scan suffices to make the diagnosis. Some neurosurgeons recommend partial excision if tumors are exophytic. Most of the lesions are relatively diffuse in the brainstem and cannot be approached surgically. Focal radiotherapy is the treatment of choice. Our own experience is that the prognosis is better in adults than it is for children, with 50% of adults living longer than 5 years. Adjuvant chemotherapy has not been shown to be effective. Tumors that arise in the midbrain or medulla have a prognosis better than tumors that arise within the pons. The reason for this variance is unknown.

Sometimes, a peculiarly low-grade tumor affects the midbrain. These tumors have variously been called *tectal gliomas* or *pencil gliomas of the aqueduct*, depending on their appearance on MRI scan. They present in adolescence or early adulthood with hydrocephalus, the symptoms of which can be relieved by shunting of the cerebral ventricles. Many such tumors appear to require no additional treatment, as they do not grow; as long as the hydrocephalus is relieved, affected patients remain asymptomatic, often for many years. On evidence of tumor growth on scan or if symptoms of brainstem dysfunction develop, radiotherapy is the treatment.

PROGNOSIS

Table 28.10 lists the prognosis for diffuse astrocytoma. The median survival for glioblastoma multiforme (grade IV) is approximately 1 year, with 15% to 20% of patients surviving more than 2 years but fewer than 5% surviving for more than 3 years [63]. Occasionally, patients survive for a long term, particularly the very young. In anaplastic astrocytomas (grade III), the median survival is approximately 3 years, with 10% to

Table 28.10   Prognosis for Diffuse Astrocytoma with Conventional Therapy

Tumor Type	Median Survival	1-Yr Percentage*	2-Yr Percentage*	5-Yr Percentage*
Astrocytoma	4 yr	90	80	45
Anaplastic astrocytoma	2 yr	75	70	15
Glioblastoma	10 mo	45	20	2

*Percentage of total number of patients surviving.

15% surviving beyond 5 years. Clearly, new therapeutic regimens must be developed.

Focal Astrocytic Tumors

Focal astrocytic tumors affect predominantly children and young adults and differ from diffuse astrocytomas in that they tend to be well circumscribed and, if accessible, may be cured surgically. Even though low-grade, contrast enhancement tends to be the rule rather than the exception, these tumors may have a pleomorphic histologic appearance that, when combined with the contrast enhancement, often leads physicians to believe that they are dealing with a highly malignant neoplasm. Such patients should not be treated by immediate radiotherapy or chemotherapy but should be followed up clinically after surgery alone. A careful review by an expert neuropathologist is essential in making the diagnosis. Uncommonly, these generally low-grade tumors may recur aggressively and even seed the leptomeninges (see Chapter 25).

PILOCYTIC ASTROCYTOMA

Pilocytic astrocytoma is the most common glioma in childhood and corresponds to the WHO grade I astrocytoma (Fig. 28.4). The tumor can occur anywhere in the neuraxis but characteristically arises in certain areas, including the optic nerve or chiasm (optic glioma), hypothalamus (hypothalamic glioma), or cerebellum (cerebellar astrocytoma) [64]. Pilocytic astrocytoma may arise also within the basal ganglia, the brainstem, or the spinal cord. Symptoms depend on the location of the tumor. The tumors are identified on MRI scan as hypointense on a T_1-weighted image, hyperintense on a T_2-weighted image, sometimes cystic, and either uniformly and intensely contrast-enhancing or having focal areas of contrast enhancement. The presence, absence, or degree of enhancement has no prognostic significance. The treatment is surgery. Some lesions located in the

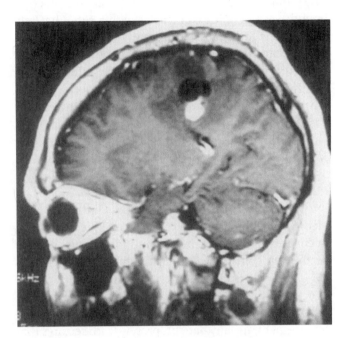

Figure 28.4   Pilocytic astrocytoma in a middle-aged man. This sagittal contrast-enhanced magnetic resonance image shows a solidly enhancing mass below a cyst and surrounded by edema. Originally, the tumor was thought to be a malignant glioma, but careful neuropathologic review revealed it to be a low-grade pilocytic astrocytoma. Surgery was the only treatment.

basal ganglia or brainstem may not be surgically approachable except for draining of a symptomatic cyst, in which case radiotherapy may be necessary after the cyst is drained. In those lesions that are surgically approachable, even partial removal may result in long-term remission without radiotherapy. Late recurrence may be seen even 20 to 30 years after the initial treatment, but that eventuality is rare.

Pilocytic astrocytomas arising in the optic nerve are a common complication of NF1. Some 15% of optic gliomas are associated with NF1. The percentage is even higher in those with bilateral tumors. The tumors grow slowly and may remain static through many years, even without treatment.

Regarding their pathologic features, most pilocytic astrocytomas are grossly well-circumscribed, although they show some microscopic infiltration. The exception is the optic nerve glioma and some diffuse variants of the cerebellar astrocytoma that tend to infiltrate normal structures. The tumor is characterized by pilocytes or hair cells with long projections that extend in bipolar fashion from the cell body and give the tumor a fibrillar background. The tumor contains Rosenthal fibers—brightly eosinophilic intracytoplasmic masses—that help to establish the diagnosis. The tumors are highly vascular, giving them the contrast enhancement on MRI scan. With the exception of those patients suffering from NF1, pilocytic astrocytomas do not have specific molecular genetic abnormalities. Some show an increase in p53 protein, and occasional tumors may show a loss of chromosome 17q, including the region encoding the *NF1* gene.

PLEOMORPHIC XANTHOASTROCYTOMA

Pleomorphic xanthoastrocytoma, usually encountered in children and young adults, tends to arise superficially in the temporal lobe, often involving the meninges [65]. Its name is derived from its pleomorphic appearance and the lipidized glial fibrillary acidic protein (GFAP)—expressing tumor cells. Because of cortical involvement, usually patients present with seizures that may be present for many years before the diagnosis is established. On MRI scan, the tumor mass appears as an inhomogeneous mixed-signal-intensity mass that is well circumscribed, often contrast enhances, and may be cystic (Fig. 28.5). Usually, surrounding edema is modest, as would befit a very slow-growing tumor.

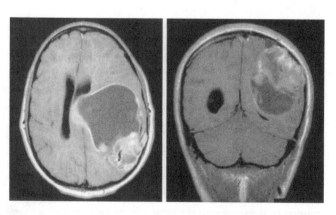

Figure 28.5 Axial and coronal contrast-enhanced images of an 18-year-old boy with progressive headache. The tumor, which originally appeared malignant pathologically, was a pleomorphic xanthoastrocytoma. The patient has made a complete recovery, with surgery as the only treatment.

No specific cytogenetic or molecular genetic abnormalities characterize this tumor, but *p53* missense mutations have been described in some patients and epidermal growth factor receptor (EGFR) amplification also has been described.

Treatment for the disorder is surgery. The pleomorphic appearance of the tumor and its invasion of the leptomeninges often suggest to physicians that they are dealing with a malignant tumor. Usually, expert neurologic examination establishes the diagnosis, and no treatment after surgery (beyond careful follow-up) is indicated. Occasionally, the tumors recur and sometimes seed the leptomeninges, but these occurrences are the exception.

SUBEPENDYMAL GIANT-CELL ASTROCYTOMA

Subependymal giant-cell astrocytoma is a low-grade tumor and typically arises as a single lesion or multiple lesions, lining the walls of the lateral ventricles [66]. Usually, the tumor occurs in patients suffering from tuberous sclerosis and generally affects children, although the disorder in infants and adults also has been reported. The tumors show a mixed glial-neuronal phenotype. Their characteristic site within the walls of the ventricle and the other stigmata of tuberous sclerosis (see Chapter 25) help to establish the diagnosis. Surgical treatment is necessary only when the tumor obstructs the ventricular system, causing hydrocephalus, but this development is uncommon.

Oligodendrogliomas

Oligodendroglial tumors have assumed increasing importance because some are highly chemosensitive, leading to experimental protocols using high-dose chemotherapy with stem-cell support and without radiotherapy in selected patients [67]. Usually, oligodendrogliomas are tumors of young and middle-aged adults, and usually they are found within the cerebral hemispheres, particularly the frontal lobe. Posterior fossa or spinal cord oligodendrogliomas are uncommon. The tumors grow slowly and often present with seizures that, before modern imaging techniques, often were the only recognizable symptom for many years before a diagnosis was established. In some patients, neurologic signs begin suddenly with a hemorrhage into the tumor.

The MRI result is similar to that of an astrocytic tumor except that oligodendrogliomas often contain calcium. Calcifications are visualized poorly on MRI but are seen clearly on CT scan. Cysts are present in some

20%, and hemorrhage occurs in perhaps 10%, giving the tumor mixed signal intensity on both T_1- and T_2-weighted images. Usually, oligodendrogliomas do not contrast enhance, whereas anaplastic oligodendrogliomas do.

Oligodendrogliomas are composed of a uniform cell population. An artifact of fixation imparts a perinuclear halo or fried-egg appearance to the oligodendroglial cells. GFAP staining may be positive or negative. Pathologic grading of oligodendroglial tumors is in a fashion similar to that of astrocytic tumors, although nuclear atypia and mitotic figures may have less ominous implications in oligodendroglial tumors. The close correlation between histopathologic changes and survival found in astrocytomas is not as clear in oligodendrogliomas. Some oligodendrogliomas develop all the aggressive histologic characteristics of glioblastoma multiforme and then must be treated as such.

No histochemical marker permits distinguishing oligodendrogliomas unequivocally from astrocytomas. As a result, the diagnosis of oligodendroglioma may vary from 5% to 25% in glial tumors in various surgical series. In recent years, an increase in the number of oligodendroglial tumors has been identified, probably resulting from greater concern on the part of neuropathologists to identify these chemosensitive tumors. At least one-third of oligodendrogliomas contain astrocytic components. When those components are sufficiently prominent, the tumor is called a *mixed glioma* (i.e., oligoastrocytoma). Some controversy concerns whether these tumors should be treated in a fashion different from that used for pure oligodendroglial tumors.

The most common molecular genetic changes in oligodendrogliomas is the loss of chromosomes 19q and 1p. In addition, approximately one-half of oligodendroglial tumors overexpress EGFR without *EGFR* gene amplification. More malignant tumors may lose 9p and 10p and also overexpress CDK4. Current evidence suggests that those oligodendroglial tumors with deletions of 19q and 1p are highly sensitive to treatment with chemotherapeutic agents (usually PCV), whereas tumors not possessing these deletions are less sensitive.

The treatment of oligodendrogliomas is surgery when the tumors are accessible. If resection is not feasible, a stereotactic biopsy may be performed for a tissue diagnosis. A gross total resection of an oligodendroglioma may lead to a prolonged remission. If the tumor is low-grade and a gross total resection has been achieved, many physicians recommend no further treatment, delaying radiotherapy until such time as the tumor recurs. For substantial residual tumor, conventional treatment is irradiation. However, patients who are asymptomatic except for well-controlled seizures may be followed until progression. Chemotherapy has been effective in some patients who have low-grade oligodendrogliomas and symptoms that require treatment. Further studies on the molecular genetics of these tumors may well alter current approaches.

All anaplastic oligodendrogliomas should be treated in the postoperative period despite the degree of resection. The conventional treatment is radiotherapy followed by chemotherapy, but many investigators are reversing this approach and beginning with chemotherapy (usually with PCV). If residual tumor appears to respond to the chemotherapy, PCV can be continued, radiotherapy can be administered, or experimental treatment with high-dose thiotepa and stem cell rescue can be considered.

The prognosis for low-grade oligodendrogliomas is good, with a 5-year survival rate of approximately 80% and a 10-year survival rate of near 50%. Anaplastic oligodendrogliomas and glioblastomas multiforme arising from oligodendrogliomas have a much worse prognosis.

Ependymomas

Ependymomas are tumors that arise from the ependymal cells that line the ventricular system and the central canal of the spinal cord [68]. They account for some 10% of childhood intracranial tumors (30% of those arising in children younger than 3 years old) and for 5% of adult intracranial tumors. They are the most frequent neuroepithelial tumor of the spinal cord, accounting for more than 50% of spinal gliomas (see "Specific Spinal Tumors"). The tumor exhibits a slight preponderance of males. The age-related incidence is bimodal, with the major peak at 5 years and a smaller peak at approximately 35 years.

Ependymomas can arise anywhere ependymal cells are present. A particular site of predilection is the fourth ventricle, where they grow within the ventricular system (Fig. 28.6). Unlike in brainstem gliomas, hydrocephalus is an early finding. Supratentorial ependymomas arise also from ependymal structures but grow into the parenchyma of the hemisphere and may have no clearly obvious intraventricular component. The histologic features of ependymomas are perivascular pseudorosettes (tumor cells arranged radially around blood vessels) and ependymal rosettes (columnar cells arranged around a central lumen). The diagnosis can be established unequivocally in problematic cases by electron microscopy, wherein tumor cells show the elaborate cilia and microvilli of normal ependyma. Generally,

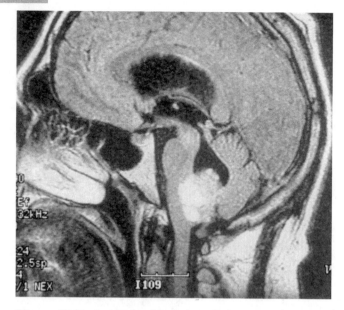

Figure 28.6 Contrast-enhanced sagittal image of an ependymoma obstructing the fourth ventricle and causing hydrocephalus. This tumor occurred in a middle-aged man; only a partial resection was possible.

the tumors are low-grade but may be aggressive and spread via the CSF to seed the meninges and even rarely metastasize to extraneural structures, primarily the lungs. Many, but not all, studies have found histologic features to be of no import as a prognostic factor independent of tumor location, extent of resection, and age at diagnosis.

MRI scan demonstrates a mass lesion that is heterogeneously hypointense and isointense on a T_1-weighted image and hyperintense on a T_2-weighted image, which may or may not contrast enhance; edema may be prominent. Hemorrhage may be present. Calcification, seen best on CT scan, is present in approximately 15% of ependymomas.

A number of different mutations have been described in ependymomas, none characteristic. One report describes a 50% incidence of allelic loss on the short arm of chromosome 17 in pediatric ependymomas; *p53* mutations are rare. Unlike most glial tumors, the prognosis is worse in children than in adults, probably because posterior fossa ependymomas are more common in children. Their fourth ventricular location renders resecting them difficult, and often they cause severe neurologic disability leading to premature death.

The treatment of ependymomas is surgery. A gross total resection is highly desirable, but the location of the tumor, particularly when it involves structures at the floor of the fourth ventricle, frequently renders that impossible. Surgical removal should be followed by radiotherapy. Despite the fact that some 10% of posterior fossa tumors eventually seed the leptomeninges, usually they do so in the setting of local recurrence, so that radiotherapy is delivered to the site of the tumor and not to the entire neuraxis. If symptomatic leptomeningeal seeding develops later, additional radiotherapy can be prescribed. No role is found for adjuvant chemotherapy at this time.

Isolated reports describe recurrent ependymomas responding to chemotherapy, particularly carboplatin and several other chemotherapeutic agents [68]. These reports render chemotherapy worth trying in patients in whom surgery and radiotherapy have failed.

The overall prognosis of brain ependymomas is better than that for most other glial tumors. Five-year survival rates are approximately 80%, and 10-year survival rates are nearly 50%. Anaplastic ependymomas are more invasive and more likely to spread by CSF pathways than are their lower-grade counterpart. Thus, the prognosis is worse. Eventually, most patients succumb to local recurrence rather than to metastatic disease.

Choroid Plexus Tumors

Choroid plexus papillomas and choroid plexus carcinomas are rare, accounting for fewer than 1% of all intracranial tumors [69]. The tumors originate from the epithelium of the choroid plexus of the cerebral ventricles and typically occur in children. Choroid plexus tumors are the most common intracranial tumor in the first year of life. However, these tumors also occur in adults. The most common site in children is the lateral ventricle. In adults, fourth ventricular tumors are more common. Most choroid plexus tumors cause symptoms by hydrocephalus. Usually, the hydrocephalus results from obstruction of CSF pathways by the tumor mass, but in a few children, a possible excess production of CSF may overwhelm spinal fluid absorptive pathways, leading to enlargement of the ventricular system. Occasionally, choroid plexus tumors present with an intraventricular hemorrhage.

MRI or CT scans show an intensely contrast-enhancing lobulated intraventricular mass that may be calcified. The histologic makeup of the majority of such tumors shows them to be benign, although even benign tumors occasionally may seed the subarachnoid space. Some 20% of tumors are malignant (choroid plexus carcinoma) and always seed the leptomeninges along CSF pathways. Some evidence suggests a possible role for simian virus 40 or a related DNA virus in pathogenesis.

The treatment of choroid plexus tumors is surgical removal. The 5-year survival after gross total removal is approximately 80%. Choroid plexus carcinomas should receive radiotherapy in the postoperative period even after a gross total removal. If cytologic or clinical evidence points to subarachnoid seeding, whole neuraxial irradiation may be required. No specific chemotherapeutic agent has been found to be active when tumors recur.

Neuronal and Mixed Neuronal-Glial Tumors

The WHO classification of tumors of neuronal origin includes the central neurocytoma and the gangliocytoma. Mixed neuronal-glial tumors include dysembryoplastic neuroepithelial tumors, ganglioglioma, and paraganglioma of the cauda equina (see "Specific Spinal Tumors"). Some evidence suggests that medulloblastoma, neuroblastoma, and primitive neuroectodermal tumors of the brain also may be of neuronal origin (see "Embryonal Tumors").

CENTRAL NEUROCYTOMAS

A central neurocytoma may arise from subependymal matrix cells, close to the lateral ventricles, and presents as an intraventricular mass usually within the frontal horn of one or both lateral ventricles. Their appearance of uniform, round cells originally had led pathologists to mistake them for oligodendrogliomas. Neuronal markers, including synaptophysin (a marker of neuronal synaptic vesicles) and, more recently, two nuclear neuronal antibodies (anti-Hu and Neu N) identify the cells of these and other such tumors as gangliocytomas to be of neuronal origin [70]. Generally, these tumors develop in patients between the ages of 20 and 40 and occur with equal frequency in both genders. Usually, affected patients present with signs of increased ICP due to ventricular obstruction. The MRI scan shows normal to high signal intensity on both T_1- and T_2-weighted images and uniform enhancement after gadolinium injection. Some tumors have a honeycomb appearance on unenhanced T_1-weighted images (Fig. 28.7). Gain of chromosome 7 has been reported in some tumors, but *p53* mutations are not detectable. Central neurocytomas are benign and are treated surgically. Even with incomplete surgical removal, radiotherapy may be withheld until evidence of tumor regrowth. Those neurocytomas

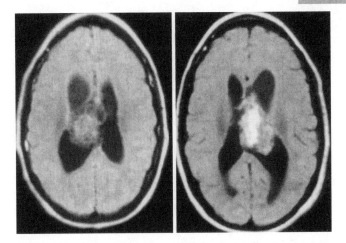

Figure 28.7 Unenhanced (left) and contrast-enhanced (right) magnetic resonance images of a central neurocytoma.

with a labeling index greater than 2%, so-called atypical neurocytomas, are more likely to recur and show aggressive behavior.

DYSEMBRYOPLASTIC NEUROEPITHELIAL TUMORS

Dysembryoplastic neuroepithelial tumors of mixed glial and neuronal origin, unlike most neuroepithelial tumors, involve predominantly the cerebral cortex rather than white matter and present with a long history of focal or generalized seizures [69]. Usually, they occur in infants and children but have been reported in young and, occasionally, elderly adults. The MRI scan identifies a largely cortical tumor, usually in the temporal lobe. Sometimes, the overlying calvarium is deformed, attesting to the slow growth of such tumors. Most do not contrast enhance, but some do. The mass effect is minimal, with no surrounding edema. Usually, cyst formation is not identified on MRI scan, although microcysts usually are present in the tumor. Before the development of sophisticated imaging techniques, these tumors often were discovered at epilepsy surgery. The treatment of dysembryoplastic neuroepithelial tumors is surgery. The patient should be followed by serial MRI without further intervention unless the tumor recurs.

GANGLIOGLIOMAS AND GANGLIOCYTOMAS

Gangliogliomas and gangliocytomas, which usually occur in children or young adults, occasionally are encountered in the elderly [69]. Usually, the tumors are composed of ganglion cells (neurons) or a combination of neurons and glial cells. When such tumors are composed of ganglion cells alone, they are called *gangliocytomas* and, when part of a mixture, they are called *gangliogliomas*. The majority are supratentorial and often involve the temporal lobe or other peripheral portions of the brain, where they may scallop the calvarium by their long-standing pressure. Seizures are the common presenting complaint. Usually, the MRI scan shows a well-circumscribed solid tumor or a cyst (50%) with a mural nodule. Most tumors contrast enhance, although the enhancement may be modest in 30% to 40%. Some are calcified. In addition to the neoplastic neurons and glial cells, perivascular lymphocytic infiltration is common. The astrocytic component may appear pilocytic. Sometimes, mitotic figures can be identified. Usually, the tumors are benign, although in some instances they may be anaplastic, or the glial component may dedifferentiate into a malignant lesion [71]. The treatment is surgery, with clinical follow-up; many patients require no additional therapy.

PINEAL PARENCHYMAL TUMORS

Several tumors arise in or near the pineal gland [72]. Altogether, the tumors of the pineal region represent only 1% of intracranial tumors in adults and approximately 8% in children. They include germ-cell tumors (25%), pineal parenchymal tumors (25%) [72], glial tumors (20%), meningiomas (20%), and other lesions, among them cysts and vascular anomalies. Approximately one-third of pineal region masses (see Chapter 25) are benign, including meningiomas, teratomas, and epidermoids. Germ-cell tumors, including germinoma, choriocarcinoma, and yolk sac tumors, presumably arise from embryonal rests in the midline of the brain, mostly near the pineal but also in the suprasellar area and rarely within the basal ganglia. These tumors affect predominantly children but also may affect some adults. The diagnosis and treatment in adults is similar to that in children.

Two types of pineal parenchymal tumors are identified: the relatively low-grade pineocytoma and the high-grade pineoblastoma. The higher-grade tumors are found in children and young adults; the lower-grade tumors are found in older adults. Both tumors can seed the leptomeninges, and both are rarely cured.

Usually, tumors of the pineal region present with hydrocephalus from the enlarging mass compressing the Sylvian aqueduct (see Fig. 28.1E). Because the superior and inferior colliculi immediately underlie the pineal gland, the compressing mass also may cause eye movement abnormalities, specifically Parinaud's syndrome (paralysis of upward gaze, light-near pupillary dissociation, and convergence nystagmus) and some hearing loss. Other signs result from brainstem or cerebellar compression, including gait ataxia. The pineal gland produces melatonin, a hormone involved in sleep regulation; thus, sleep disorder may be a symptom of a pineal tumor.

MRI scans show an enhancing mass. Often, leptomeningeal dissemination can be identified by enhancement of the cerebral or spinal meninges. Usually, pineal region masses cannot be distinguished by clinical symptoms or imaging alone, but the exceptions are teratomas that contain fat (which is hyperintense on a T_1-weighted image) or bone (which is hypointense on a T_2-weighted image). Sometimes, examination of the spinal fluid will reveal tumor markers, such as the beta subunit of human chorionic gonadotropin (β-HCG) or alpha-fetoprotein, identifying a nongerminomatous germ-cell tumor. Occasionally, cytologic examination reveals primitive neuroectodermal cells suggesting that a pineal parenchymal tumor has seeded the leptomeninges. Because lumbar puncture may be dangerous in a patient with severe noncommunicating hydrocephalus, an alternate approach is to perform a shunting procedure and to sample CSF from the lateral ventricle. In the majority of cases, a definitive diagnosis can be established only by biopsy of the tumor mass.

Because of the potential danger of surgery in and around the pineal gland (though much lessened by modern neurosurgical techniques), some investigators have recommended radiotherapy without biopsy. Germinomas are cured by radiotherapy [73]. The other tumors arising in that area are not curable (meningiomas being an exception). Accordingly, if affected patients respond rapidly to radiotherapy, the diagnosis of germinoma is ensured, and such patients are cured. Other tumors initially may respond but generally relapse. However, modern neurosurgical techniques usually permit a safe approach to the pineal gland and, sometimes, gross total removal of tumors in that area. This capability affords the establishment of a definitive diagnosis and substantially permits debulking of the tumor if further therapy is necessary. This approach seems the most straightforward and, for the patient, beneficial for both diagnosis and treatment.

Pineoblastomas are highly malignant tumors that infiltrate surrounding structures and also seed the leptomeninges. Sometimes, these tumors occur in children with retinoblastoma of both eyes (trilateral retinoblastoma). Radiotherapy is the treatment of choice. A variety of chemotherapeutic agents have been tried. Only approximately one-half of patients survive for 5 years

[74]. Pineocytomas grow more slowly. A recent study suggested that pineocytomas do not metastasize and yield 1-, 3-, and 5-year survival rates of 100%, 100%, and 67%, respectively. Radiotherapy to the site of the tumor is the treatment of choice after diagnosis by biopsy or surgical removal.

Embryonal Tumors

Several tumors of uncertain cell of origin, including so-called medulloepitheliomas, central neuroblastoma, medulloblastoma, and supratentorial primitive neuroectodermal tumors, are classified by the WHO as embryonal tumors. The most important is the medulloblastoma [75], a primitive neuroectodermal tumor that arises in the cerebellum, usually the vermis. These tumors are the most common malignant CNS tumor of childhood, accounting for 20% of childhood brain tumors (see Chapter 25); at least 20% of such tumors occur in young adults. Although the peak incidence is between 5 and 8 years, a smaller peak occurs between 20 and 30 years. Male persons are affected twice as often as are female persons. Usually, the tumor arises in the vermis of the cerebellum and compresses the fourth ventricle. Symptoms are related to hydrocephalus and to direct cerebellar involvement. In addition to exhibiting signs of generalized increase in ICP (hydrocephalus), patients develop gait ataxia, usually with relative sparing of the extremities. Dizziness, vertigo, and nystagmus also may be present. Nausea and vomiting are common in children but less so in adults.

Medulloblastomas have a strong tendency to spread by subarachnoid pathways and to seed the leptomeninges. Extraneural metastases occur in some 5% of patients, usually to bone and sometimes in lymph nodes or liver. Patients who have undergone ventriculoperitoneal shunting may develop deposits in the peritoneal cavity. The diagnosis is suggested strongly by the location and prominent enhancement of the tumor on MRI scan.

Often, the histopathologic appearance of the tumor is that of a poorly differentiated neuroectodermal neoplasm, sometimes having Homer-Wright rosettes or palisading tumor cells. The cells can express either neuronal or glial markers (or both). Most medulloblastomas are anti-Hu-positive. A number of chromosomal abnormalities, including isochromosome 17q in 50% of patients and various abnormalities of chromosome 1, have been described. Both *p53* mutations and 17p deletions also are common.

The tumors are treated in both adults and children by maximally feasible surgical resection. Regardless of whether a gross total resection has been performed, radiotherapy is delivered to the entire neuraxis, with a boost given to the posterior fossa. Chemotherapy, usually including a nitrosourea and vincristine, prolongs survival in high-risk patients and may be beneficial in standard-risk patients.

Good prognostic factors in adults include age (older), gender (female), extent of disease (localized), and complete surgical resection. Generally, such patients have a 5-year survival of greater than 60% [76]. Higher-risk patients and those without gross surgical removal or with some evidence of leptomeningeal seeding may live as long when chemotherapy is added. In one small series, women with localized disease had a 5-year survival rate of 90% [76].

Tumors of Cranial and Peripheral Nerves

Schwannomas and neurofibromas arise from the coverings of peripheral and cranial nerves. Schwannomas, as the name indicates, arise from Schwann cells. Neurofibromas contain cells with features of Schwann cells, fibroblasts, and perineural cells. Usually, tumors of both types are benign and can be cured surgically. A significant number of patients with schwannomas and neurofibromas suffer from neurofibromatosis. (Only acoustic neuromas are considered in this section; spinal tumors are considered later.)

Schwannomas of the auditory nerve, so-called acoustic neurinomas, actually arise from Schwann cells covering the vestibular portion of nerve VIII, either in the cerebellopontine angle or in the internal acoustic canal. Usually, they are tumors of middle age and affect men and women equally. Bilateral acoustic neuromas, present in approximately 5% of patients, are pathognomonic of NF2. The tumors are benign and grow slowly, compressing the eighth cranial nerve and causing hearing loss and tinnitus. Because vestibular function is lost slowly and is compensated, vertigo is an uncommon symptom of acoustic neuroma, although it may be present in a few patients. If the tumors grow to be large, they may compress the cerebellum and brainstem, causing gait ataxia and hydrocephalus. Numbness in the face from involvement of the trigeminal nerve and facial paralysis from involvement of the facial nerve also can be features.

All patients with unilateral hearing loss that is not clearly cochlear in origin should undergo MRI, with special emphasis on the acoustic nerves. Acoustic neuromas will be revealed as well-delineated, solidly (or sometimes cystically) contrast-enhancing masses somewhere along the eighth cranial nerve. Often, they are located in and expand the internal auditory meatus, a location in which meningiomas are not found. When located in the cerebellopontine angle rather than in the internal auditory meatus, distinguishing acoustic neuromas from meningiomas may be difficult. When these tumors are very small, surgery may not only cure the tumor but conserve hearing in up to 75% of patients. However, once the tumor grows beyond 2.5 cm, the likelihood of preserving hearing is less, and other neurologic deficits such as facial weakness may occur as a result of surgery. Total surgical removal of the tumor is curative, and no further therapy is necessary.

Recently, some investigators have recommended radiosurgery [77] or fractionated stereotactic radiotherapy [50] as treatment for small acoustic neuromas [77], particularly in the elderly or infirm. Local control is achieved in the vast majority of patients, and hearing and facial power often are preserved. Delayed effects of radiotherapy on the acoustic and facial nerve, however, can occur, and how stereotactic radiosurgery will compare with surgical therapy over decades is unclear.

Meningeal Tumors

Several different kinds of tumor arise in the meninges covering the brain and spinal cord. Meningiomas (benign, atypical, or frankly malignant) are the most common of such tumors. Hemangiopericytomas once were considered a subtype of meningioma but now are recognized as a separate tumor type. Hemangioblastoma, a tumor of uncertain cell origin usually found in the cerebellum, often connects with the meninges and is classified with meningeal tumors. Sarcomas of mesenchymal, nonmeningothelial origin rarely can arise in the meninges. The meninges also contain melanocytes that may give rise to either relatively indolent melanocytomas or frankly malignant melanomas. These primary tumors of the CNS must be distinguished from melanomas metastatic to the leptomeninges (see "Leptomeningeal Tumors"). Only meningiomas and hemangiopericytomas are considered here.

MENINGIOMA

Meningiomas arise from cells of the arachnoid membrane. Most are benign and are treated successfully by surgical removal. Atypical or frankly malignant meningiomas have a high likelihood of local recurrence, but metastases are rare. Meningiomas account for approximately 20% of all primary brain tumors. Because they are slow-growing, meningiomas may reach gigantic size before becoming symptomatic. Alternately, many meningiomas remain small and are discovered only as incidental findings at autopsy or, fortuitously, during imaging of the brain for unrelated symptoms. As many as 1% to 2% of patients may have an incidental meningioma found at autopsy. Typically, patients with NF2 and other families with hereditary predisposition to meningiomas have multiple meningiomas. Perhaps 5% of meningiomas are atypical, and approximately 1% are frankly malignant.

Meningiomas are tumors of adults occurring with a peak incidence at roughly age 45. Women are affected more commonly than are men, and the presence or history of breast cancer is a risk factor [78]. Other risk factors include prior irradiation and, in some series, prior head injury. Frequently, meningiomas express progesterone receptors, but they rarely express estrogen receptors. Some grow when women are pregnant and become symptomatic. These tumors can occur anywhere in the intracranial or intraspinal cavity. Characteristic areas are the optic nerve sheath, the cavernous sinus, and the parasagittal area of the hemispheres. The thoracic spinal cord is a characteristic location for meningiomas of women. Because so many meningiomas occur at the base of the brain and because parasagittal meningiomas often invade the sagittal sinus, approaching them surgically may be difficult. If gross total surgical removal (including the involved dura) is possible, most patients are cured, although approximately 20% relapse at some future time.

Meningiomas are slow-growing tumors that compress the brain but rarely invade it. They do not cause much edema, so-called secretory meningiomas that secrete vascular endothelial growth factor being exceptions. When they compress brain substance, usually they cause seizures initially, followed by focal neurologic signs. When they compress cranial nerves in the cavernous sinus or the optic nerve, they cause diplopia or visual loss, respectively. Frequently, they also invoke an osteoblastic response in the surrounding bone, called *hyperostosis,* which can be identified on plain skull films. Hyperostosis may cause symptoms by compressing cranial nerves at the skull base. Meningiomas may spread along the dura (en plaque meningioma), impairing several cranial nerves.

The tumor's diagnosis is suggested by neuroimaging. A typical meningioma is hypointense or isointense with brain on a T_1-weighted image, usually is hypointense on a T_2-weighted image, and intensely and uniformly contrast enhances. Heavily calcified meningiomas may not contrast enhance, but a CT scan will reveal the calcification and also may show surrounding hyperostosis. Typically, meningiomas have an enhancing dural tail that spreads out from the body of the tumor, an uncommon finding in other tumors of the dura, including metastasis. A large tumor compressing brain but not causing edema probably is a meningioma.

Meningiomas are subclassified into a number of histologic types, most of which have no clinical significance. Even the most benign meningioma may have pleomorphic nuclei and occasional mitoses; however, frequent mitoses, regions of hypercellularity, small cells with a high nucleus-to-cytoplasm ratio, necrosis, and brain invasion indicate a more aggressive tumor. Mutations in the *NF2* gene are detected in perhaps 60% of sporadic meningiomas. Some other meningiomas contain deletion of chromosome 22 outside the *NF2* region. Single meningiomas are monoclonal tumors. Current evidence from NF2 meningiomas indicates that in patients with multiple meningiomas, the multiple tumors are genetically identical.

If a meningioma is to be treated, it should be approached surgically. Surgery will establish the diagnosis, cure most meningiomas, and debulk those that cannot be excised completely. Increasing evidence substantiates that a number of meningiomas do not grow. Such tumors either are found incidentally or may cause seizures without other focal signs. If affected patients have only seizures that can be controlled easily by anticonvulsant medication, the tumor can be followed up with serial MRI. If the tumor does not grow, no further treatment may be necessary. This finding may be especially important when the tumors are at the base of the brain and approaching them surgically is difficult without causing neurologic damage.

In those patients in whom only partial resection or no resection is possible, radiotherapy either may prevent further growth of the tumor or may cause some shrinkage but rarely, if ever, eradicates the tumor. Radiosurgery is being advocated increasingly for tumors smaller than 3 cm in surgically difficult areas, such as near a patent sagittal sinus [79] or at the base of the brain [50]. No established chemotherapy is used to treat meningiomas, although some investigators have advocated hydroxyurea or mifepristone (RU-486).

HEMANGIOPERICYTOMAS

Originally believed to be a variant of meningioma called *angioblastic meningioma* (as were hemangioblastomas), the hemangiopericytoma now is recognized as being a distinct tumor of uncertain cellular origin and having a much worse prognosis than that of meningioma. CNS hemangioblastomas are meningeal and are approximately 2% as common as meningiomas. Unlike meningiomas, they are more frequent in men than in women, often appearing in early middle age. The signs and symptoms are indistinguishable from those of meningioma and, with certain exceptions, they also are indistinguishable on imaging. Hyperostosis of bone, so common in meningiomas, does not occur in hemangiopericytomas; instead the nearby bone is lytic. Calcification also does not occur in hemangiopericytomas. Nevertheless, the tumor usually is believed preoperatively to be a meningioma.

The tumor's histologic appearance differs from that of meningioma in possessing a dense reticulin network surrounding the tumor cells. The presence of wide and branching vascular spaces, so-called staghorn sinusoids, and the absence of epithelial membrane antigen also distinguish these tumors from meningiomas. Calcification and psammoma bodies are absent. Also unlike meningiomas, hemangiopericytomas demonstrate no changes in chromosome 22. Instead, they possess rearrangements of chromosome 12 and q13, and alterations of chromosome 19, 6, and 7 have been reported [80].

The treatment of hemangiopericytomas is surgery. Unlike the outcome in meningiomas, recurrence is inevitable, although often after many years. Irradiation delays recurrence and should follow surgical resection. Unlike meningiomas, these tumors frequently metastasize distantly to bones, lungs, and liver.

HEMANGIOBLASTOMA

Hemangioblastomas are benign tumors of uncertain origin that usually occur in the cerebellum but may appear anywhere in the nervous system, including the cerebral hemispheres and spinal cord [81]. In some 25% of patients, hemangioblastomas occur as part of the VHL syndrome, a disorder characterized by hemangioblastomas in the CNS and retina; renal cell carcinoma; pheochromocytoma; and cysts in various visceral organs. In patients with VHL disease, the tumors are associated with deletion of the *VHL* tumor suppressor gene. Hemangioblastomas are the most common primary tumor of the cerebellum in adults; however, they are much less common than is metastasis to the cerebellum. The tumors tend to occur in middle age, with a slight female preponderance.

The clinical symptoms of hemangioblastoma are those of the slow-growing tumor within the parenchyma of the CNS or the retina. Because most of the tumors occur in the cerebellum, ataxia and vertigo are the tumor's most common clinical symptoms. Some patients develop hydrocephalus from obstruction of the fourth ventricle. Like renal cell carcinoma, hemangioblastomas have the capacity to secrete erythropoietin. Significant secretion of that agent produces erythrocytosis, a finding that can help with the diagnosis in approximately 20% of patients with cerebellar hemangioblastomas.

Usually, hemangioblastomas can be identified on MRI scan as largely cystic with an intensely enhancing mural nodule. The cyst fluid is hyperintense on a T_2-weighted image. Often, the tumor contains hypointense flow voids, a result of its vascularity. The treatment is surgery, with complete excision resulting in cure. Often, even tumors in the brainstem and spinal cord can be excised completely. For tumors that cannot be excised completely, radiotherapy should follow subtotal resection. Radiosurgery may provide results better than those obtained from standard radiotherapy [82]. Those patients with VHL disease should undergo imaging of the entire nervous system because often the tumors are multiple, and small asymptomatic tumors might warrant treatment before symptoms develop. An abdominal CT scan also should be performed to assess a patient for renal carcinomas.

Hematopoietic Tumors

Both lymphomas (usually B-cell, but occasionally T-cell) and "histiocytic" tumors (i.e., Langerhans cell histiocytosis, Erdheim-Chester disease, hemophagocytic lymphohistiocytosis) can arise within the nervous system. (Lymphomas only are discussed here.)

Most CNS lymphomas are metastatic. Usually, metastatic lymphomas spread to the leptomeninges rather than to the brain parenchyma. Lymphomas that arise within the CNS (PCNSLs) also may affect the leptomeninges but usually grow in the parenchyma of the brain as well. PCNSLs may arise also within the eye (strictly speaking, an ocular lymphoma, but with a strong predilection for subsequent involvement of the CNS). At one time a very rare tumor, the incidence of PCNSLs has increased, both in immunocompromised hosts (usually persons with the acquired immunodeficiency syndrome [AIDS]) and in immunocompetent hosts [83].

PCNSLs affect all ages and both genders. Those patients with inherited immunodeficiency (i.e., Wiskott-Aldrich syndrome) develop such lymphomas in childhood, those with AIDS develop them in their thirties, and immunocompetent hosts generally develop them when they are older than 60.

The tumor can arise anywhere in the nervous system but prefers periventricular areas of the brain and brainstem (Fig. 28.8). Approximately 40% of PCNSL tumors are multiple, multiplicity being the rule in immunocompromised patients. Some 15% of patients have ocular involvement at presentation. Most patients with PCNSL develop leptomeningeal involvement either at onset or later in the course of the disease. In addition to immunocompromise, the history of a previous cancer appears to be a risk factor for PCNSL. A previous or concomitant malignant neoplasm has been found in up to 17% of immunocompetent patients with PCNSL.

Histopathologic types and molecular genetics of PCNSLs are similar to those arising outside the nervous system. The source of the B (or occasionally T) lymphocytes that cause lymphoma in the nervous system is unknown. Possibly the cells are transformed elsewhere in the body and then traffic into the nervous system, where they find sanctuary against the body's immune mechanisms. A second possibility is that normal cells traffic into the CNS as part of an inflammatory response and become transformed there. However, no evidence suggests that PCNSL is more common in patients with previous inflammatory diseases such as multiple sclerosis or encephalitis.

The tumor's signs and symptoms depend on its site. Because the tumors often are deep, seizures are less common and behavioral changes and focal signs are more common than those in gliomas. Usually, ocular

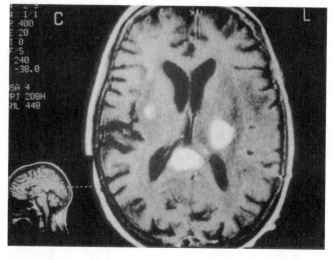

Figure 28.8 Contrast-enhanced T_1-weighted image of a patient with a primary lymphoma of the central nervous system. Note that two of the three tumors are deep near the ventricular system. They uniformly contrast enhance. They are not surrounded by a significant amount of edema, and the edges are not sharp. The patient had a complete response to chemotherapy.

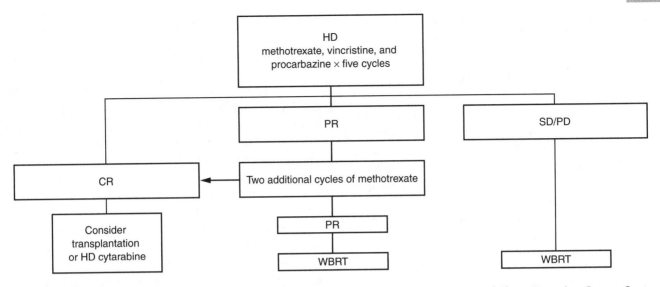

Figure 28.9 Treatment algorithm for primary central nervous system lymphomas at Memorial Sloan-Kettering Cancer Center. Methotrexate, 3.5 g/m²; vincristine, 1.4 mg/m²; and procarbazine, 100 mg/m² for 1 week at alternate cycles. *PR* = partial response; *SD/PD* = stable disease/progressive disease; *CR* = complete response; *HD* = high-dose; *WBRT* = whole-brain radiotherapy.

involvement presents with visual blurring or "floaters;" the symptoms may mimic uveitis.

Several diagnostic tests contribute to identifying PCNSL. In patients with ocular involvement, slit-lamp ophthalmoscopy identifies cells in the vitreous, and vitrectomy can identify those cells as malignant. In patients with leptomeningeal symptoms, examination of the CSF may reveal a monoclonal population of B cells, establishing lymphoma as the cause of the meningeal syndrome. In patients with brain lesions, MRI scan reveals one or more deeply situated, intensely, and uniformly contrast-enhancing masses with poorly demarcated edges and little or no surrounding edema. In occasional patients, particularly those with Epstein-Barr virus–driven lymphomas associated with bone marrow transplantation, contrast enhancement may be absent. The tumor is highly invasive, and autopsy usually reveals tumor well beyond the areas of abnormality seen on the MRI scan.

If PCNSL is suspected, corticosteroids should be withheld until just before a stereotactic needle biopsy has been performed. Steroids may cause rapid necrosis in PCNSL, rendering the biopsy specimen uninterpretable and preventing a clinician from differentiating lymphoma from an inflammatory CNS disease, such as multiple sclerosis or sarcoidosis.

The treatment of PCNSL is evolving. Many patients are responsive to corticosteroids that sometimes can obliterate PCNSL for months or years. However, corticosteroids are not curative, and usually the PCNSL re-curs after several months. Often, radiotherapy leads to complete disappearance of a PCNSL, but recurrence is inevitable, and median survival is only approximately one year. More recently, a number of investigators have treated PCNSL with chemotherapy using high-dose methotrexate with leucovorin rescue as the primary drug, combined with other drugs that cross the blood-brain barrier. Figure 28.9 outlines the Memorial Sloan-Kettering Cancer Center current protocol.

Age is an important risk factor. Patients older than 60 years not only have a poorer prognosis but are more likely to suffer severe neurotoxicity (usually dementia) from radiotherapy if they survive more than a year. Accordingly, several protocols call for treatment with chemotherapy alone in patients older than age 60, reserving radiotherapy for relapse.

Chemotherapy alone appears to result in prolonged remission (5 years, as compared with 1 year after irradiation). Some investigators have used intraarterial mannitol to open the blood-brain barrier prior to intravenous injection of chemotherapy, but no evidence supports this technique as a significant advantage over conventional routes of administration.

Cysts and Tumor-like Lesions

Occasionally, rests of embryonal tissue remaining in the nervous system after neural tube closure can develop into tumor-like cysts. They include Rathke's pouch tumors, dermoid and epidermoid tumors, lipomas, and colloid cysts of the third ventricle.

DERMOIDS AND EPIDERMOIDS

Representing perhaps 2% of intracranial tumors, epidermoid tumors contain cellular debris, keratin, and cholesterol confined within a squamous epithelial capsule. They occur in the cerebellopontine angle, in the suprasellar region, fourth ventricle, and spinal canal [84]. Usually, symptoms are caused by local mass effect, but occasionally recurrent aseptic meningitis results from leakage of irritating cyst contents, including cholesterol and fatty acids, into the CSF.

Dermoid tumors are less common and contain, in addition to the squamous epithelial cells, mature dermal elements, including hair follicles, sweat glands, and sebaceous glands. Usually, they occur in the midline posterior fossa, suprasellar region, or spinal canal. Some dermoids are associated with a dermal sinus tract to the skin surface, occasionally a source of repeated episodes of bacterial meningitis.

The diagnosis is suggested by MRI scan. Usually, epidermoids are hyperintense relative to CSF on a T_1-weighted image and either isointense or hyperintense on a T_2-weighted image [85]. They do not contrast enhance. In dermoids, lipomatous elements are hyperintense on both T_1- and T_2-weighted images [86].

Both epidermoids and dermoids are benign and are treated by surgical excision. The excision may not be complete because tumors adhere to surrounding neural and vascular structures. However, after partial removal of lesions, affected patients may experience a prolonged remission and may not require further therapy.

COLLOID CYSTS

Colloid cysts occur within the third ventricle at the foramen of Monro [87]. They contain a liquid center with a high protein content and cause symptoms by obstructing the ventricular system. Pressure waves in a patient with severe hydrocephalus can lead to herniation and sometimes death [88].

The treatment for colloid cysts is surgery. Occasionally, drainage of the cyst content through a stereotactically placed needle may relieve symptoms permanently but, in most instances, the cyst wall must be removed surgically to effect cure. Because the tumors are benign and create symptoms only by causing hydrocephalus, shunting of the lateral ventricles may suffice as treatment, especially on elderly and frail patients.

Miscellaneous Tumors

CRANIOPHARYNGIOMAS

Believed to arise from remnants of Rathke's pouch, the craniopharyngiomas (benign tumors) account for 1% to 4% of intracranial tumors, the maximum reported incidence being 2.5 patients per million per year [89]. The tumors are more common in children but can occur at any age. Their histopathologic characteristics divide them into two types: the adamantinomatous type and the papillary type. The former occurs in childhood and contains cholesterol-rich cysts that can elicit a chronic inflammatory reaction; usually, it is calcified. The latter occurs in middle age, has less tendency to calcify, is less often cystic, and often is confined to the third ventricle.

Usually, craniopharyngiomas originate above the sella. A minority originate within the sella, causing sellar enlargement and mimicking a pituitary adenoma. Ectopic craniopharyngiomas may involve the optic nerve, the sphenoid bone, and even the cerebellopontine angle. The tumors may grow into the third ventricle to cause hydrocephalus. Because they contain irritating substances, craniopharyngiomas may cause an intense glial reaction, with adherence to surrounding blood vessels and neural structures.

The clinical symptoms are similar to those of large pituitary adenomas (see "Tumors of the Pituitary Gland") and include endocrine dysfunction, cognitive changes, and visual complaints, bitemporal hemianopia in particular. Hydrocephalus is a late symptom.

Usually, an MRI scan reveals the craniopharyngioma as a suprasellar mass containing both solid and cystic components. The cysts are hypointense on a T_2-weighted image and variable on a T_1-weighted image. Usually, the solid tumor enhances, as does the wall of the cyst. Calcifications may or may not be present. Identifying calcium on an MRI scan is difficult; it gives a low signal on a T_2-weighted image within the solid tumor but is seen easily as hyperdense on a CT scan, where it is virtually diagnostic.

The management of craniopharyngiomas is controversial. Surgery is difficult because of the tendency of the tumor to adhere to the optic chiasm and the hypothalamus. If the tumor can be removed completely without unacceptable risk, it should be. After total resection, no further treatment is required, although a recurrence rate of up to 25% has been reported. If the tumor cannot be removed completely, subtotal resection followed by radiotherapy is the standard treatment. The best reports of such treatment indicate a remission rate of 90% after four years and a 10-year survival of 78%. Recurrence can be treated with a second surgery.

Experimental treatment has included intracavitary irradiation with ^{32}P or ^{90}Y colloidal suspension and stereotactic radiosurgery. Most tumors amenable to treatment by stereotactic radiosurgery probably are amenable also to a surgical approach.

CHORDOMAS

Chordomas are bone tumors that probably arise from remnants of the embryonic notochord and affect the CNS by compression. The majority of the tumors are located in either the clivus (35%) [69] or the sacrum (50%) [90]; others are located elsewhere in the spine. Men are affected twice as frequently as women, and usually the tumors present in middle or old age. The tumors grow slowly but, although histologically benign, cannot be completely removed surgically and tend to recur. Distant metastasis, usually to the lung or bone (and occasionally skin), occurs late in the course of the disease in approximately 10% of patients.

The symptoms depend on site (see "Specific Spinal Tumors" for spinal chordomas). Cranial chordomas grow within the skull base, causing cranial nerve palsies and sometimes brainstem compression. Either CT or MRI defines the lesion, which causes destruction of the skull base in association with a calcified soft-tissue mass that does not enhance.

Surgical approach to the tumors at the base of the skull is difficult, but modern surgical techniques have allowed more radical excision, which probably delays recurrence. Radiotherapy in the postoperative period also delays recurrence; radiosurgery and heavy-particle therapy (i.e., protons) appear more effective than doses of conventional irradiation with photons. Local recurrence, however, is still a common complication of this tumor and usually occurs within approximately three years of the original resection. Further resection, stereotactic radiosurgery, and proton-beam radiation have been advocated for the treatment of recurrent chordomas at the skull base.

Tumors of the Pituitary Gland

ANATOMY

The pituitary sits in the sella turcica, surrounded anteriorly, posteriorly, and inferiorly by bone. Its superior surface is covered by dura called the *diaphragma sella*, through which passes the pituitary stalk connecting the pituitary gland with the hypothalamus (Fig. 28.10). In approximately 20% of individuals, the diaphragma sella is incompetent, potentially allowing CSF from the suprasellar cistern to enter the sella turcica. Lateral to the pituitary gland are the paired cavernous sinuses that contain the carotid artery, the nerves to the external ocular muscles (oculomotor [cranial nerve III], trochlear [cranial nerve IV], and abducens [cranial nerve VI]), and the first division of the trigeminal nerve (cranial nerve V). Below the bone that encases the inferior aspect of the pituitary gland is the sphenoid sinus. Above the diaphragma sella within the suprasellar cistern is the optic chiasm that contains crossing fibers of the optic nerve from each of the paired retinas. Above the optic chiasm is the hypothalamus, which secretes the releasing factors that regulate pituitary function and transmits them to the pituitary gland via the stalk.

Actually, the pituitary gland is two structures: an anterior portion (adenohypophysis) that is true endocrine tissue and a posterior portion (neurohypophysis) that is an extension of the hypothalamus (i.e., neural tissue). Both portions secrete hormones. The anterior pituitary secretes growth hormone (GH), prolactin (PRL), adrenocorticotropic hormone (ACTH), thyroid-stimulating hormone (TSH), and the gonadotropins luteinizing hor-

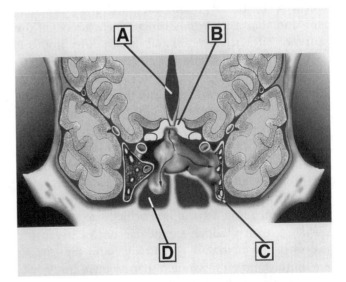

Figure 28.10 How pituitary adenomas cause nonendocrine symptomatology. A pituitary adenoma can grow superiorly above the diaphragma sella to compress the optic chiasm *(B)* or even the third ventricle *(A)*. It can grow laterally to compress the cavernous sinus *(C)* that contains the carotid artery, the oculomotor nerves, and the first division of the trigeminal nerve. It can grow inferiorly to invade the sphenoid sinus *(D)*, sometimes leading to cerebrospinal fluid leak.

Table 28.11 Classification of Pituitary Adenomas

Cell Type	Percentage of Clinical Prevalence	Hormone Secreted	Endocrine Syndrome
Lactotroph	27	Prolactin	Galactorrhea, amenorrhea
Somatotroph	21	Growth hormone ± prolactin	Acromegaly
Corticotroph	8	Adrenocorticotropic hormone	Cushing's syndrome ± Nelson's syndrome
Thyrotroph	1	Thyroid-stimulating hormone	None or hyperthyroidism
Gonadotroph	6	Follicle-stimulating hormone, luteinizing hormone	None or hypogonadism
Null cell	35	None	Hypopituitarism

Source: Data adapted from K Thapar, K Kovacs, ER Laws, Pituitary tumors. In PM Black, JS Loeffler (eds), *Cancer of the Nervous System.* Cambridge, MA: Blackwell, 1997:363–403.

mone and follicle-stimulating hormone. The posterior pituitary secretes arginine vasopressin, an antidiuretic hormone, and oxytocin, a regulator of smooth-muscle contraction important for lactation and uterine contraction.

EPIDEMIOLOGIC FACTORS

Pituitary tumors are the third most common primary intracranial neoplasm, exceeded only by gliomas and meningiomas and accounting for 10% to 15% of all primary intracranial neoplasms encountered in clinical practice [91]. Tumors of the anterior pituitary are common and almost uniformly benign [91]. Tumors of the posterior pituitary are rare and do not differ from tumors that arise elsewhere in the brain. The incidence of pituitary tumors ranges from 1 to 14 per 100,000 annually in various clinical series, and the prevalence of tumors at autopsy varies from 5% to 25%. In one autopsy series, incidental pituitary adenomas larger than 2 mm (and thus identifiable on MRI scan) were found in 1.7% of the population [92]. An additional 4.4% of pituitary glands had other lesions greater than 2 mm (i.e., focal hyperplasia, Rathke cysts). Another series reported a 9% incidence of lesions of unspecified size [93]. Thus, not all pituitary lesions identifiable on MRI scan are necessarily symptomatic. Clinically, pituitary tumors are more common in women than in men, but in autopsy series, they appear to be equally common in both genders.

CLASSIFICATION

Pituitary tumors can be classified in several ways. As regards size, microadenomas are tumors less than 1 cm in diameter, and macroadenomas are all those larger

than 1 cm. Microadenomas cause symptoms by secreting excessive amounts of hormones not under normal feedback control from the hypothalamus. Macroadenomas can cause their symptoms either by excessive hormone secretion or by compressing normal glandular or neural structures.

According to endocrine function, pituitary adenomas are divided into two types: those that secrete hormones and those that are chemically inactive. Chemically inactive adenomas can cause symptoms only when they grow large enough to compress other structures (i.e., become macroadenomas). Table 28.11 contains a classification of such tumors by clinical syndrome.

Almost all pituitary adenomas are histologically benign [94]. They are identified microscopically by uniformity of cells with disruption of the normal acinar patterns. Usually, the tumors are well demarcated by a pseudocapsule consisting of reticulin and compressed normal gland. Usually, mitoses and proliferative indices obtained are low, but invasiveness is common. Dural invasion, cellular pleomorphism, cellularity, necrosis, and aneuploidy do not necessarily imply an aggressive biological activity [95]. Mitotic activity and *p53* immunoreactivity may imply decreased likelihood of cure. Immunohistochemistry and electron microscopy are very useful techniques because they can define the hormones secreted by the tumor and thus allow for a functional classification [96].

Pituitary tumors arise clonally from a single cell type within the pituitary gland (see Table 28.11). Some pituitary adenomas secrete the hormones for which their cell of origin was designed, whereas others lose the capacity to secrete hormone. Virtually all pituitary adenomas escape feedback control and, thus, if they secrete hormones, they do so excessively, leading to endocrine abnormalities.

ETIOLOGIC FEATURES

The etiology of pituitary adenomas is unknown. The only known genetic defect causing pituitary tumors is that of the multiple endocrine neoplasia syndrome type I (MEN1) [97, 98]. This autosomal dominant condition is characterized by spontaneous development of tumors of the anterior pituitary, pancreatic islets, and parathyroid glands. Pituitary adenomas, usually associated with GH, ACTH, or PRL hypersecretion, occur in approximately 25% of such patients. MEN1 is associated with both microadenomas and macroadenomas, mostly PRL-secreting. The genetic abnormality is allelic loss of a tumor suppressor gene called *menin* at 11q13 (see Table 28.3) [98]. MEN1 patients account for no more than a few percent of pituitary tumors. Rarely, deletion of both menin alleles can occur sporadically.

Other genetic abnormalities have been found in some pituitary tumors [94]. The expression of *c-myc* expression correlates with clinical aggressiveness, and *ras* oncogene mutations, although rare in pituitary adenomas, mark an invasive tumor. G-protein oncogene mutations have been found in 30% to 40% of patients with acromegaly. This mutation in the alpha chain of the G-protein results in constitutive activity of adenylate cyclase. Adenomas with these G-protein mutations are significantly smaller than are those without mutations and may be more sensitive to such inhibitory factors as somatostatin or dopamine. Amplification of *v-fos* and point mutations in *H-ras* oncogenes has been shown in isolated prolactinoma cases. A number of growth factors have been identified in the pituitary, and growth factor–mediated autocrine and paracrine stimulation are believed to be important in pituitary tumor development.

CLINICAL FINDINGS

Pituitary adenomas cause their symptoms by abnormal hormone secretion (found in approximately 70% of pituitary adenomas) or by compression of normal glandular and neural structures [99]. As macroadenomas outgrow the sella turcica, they compress neural structures, including ocular motor nerves laterally and the optic chiasm and hypothalamus superiorly. An occasional pituitary adenoma erodes the floor of the sella turcica and presents as a mass in the sphenoid sinus or nasopharynx.

Endocrine Abnormalities

Table 28.11 lists the various syndromes caused by hypersecretion of particular hormones. The clinical symptoms are detailed in the paragraphs on specific tumor

Table 28.12 Some Symptoms and Signs of Pituitary Failure

Gonadotroph failure
Loss of libido
Impotence
Osteoporosis

Thyrotroph failure
Fatigue, malaise
Apathy, slow cognition
Myalgias
Carpal tunnel syndrome
Constipation
Delayed reflexes

Somatotroph failure
Reduced strength (muscle mass)
Central obesity
Premature atherosclerosis
Depression, anxiety, emotional lability

Corticotroph failure
Fatigue
Weight gain
Hypoglycemia

Vasopressin (posterior pituitary)
Polydipsia
Frequent urination (especially nocturia)
Thirst

types (see later). By compressing surrounding normal glandular elements, macroadenomas can lead to hyposecretion of one or more pituitary hormones.

Gonadotrophs are most vulnerable. Often, loss of libido, amenorrhea, and impotence are the presenting symptoms in patients with large pituitary adenomas (Table 28.12). TSH and GH are the next most vulnerable hormones. GH deficiency has subtle but important effects in adults [100]. Hypothyroidism, with its vague and protean symptoms of fatigue and malaise, may be a confusing presenting complaint. Hypoadrenalism is rare.

PRL levels may be elevated in patients with nonsecreting pituitary adenomas, because the hypothalamus inhibits normal release of this hormone. Dopamine is the most important PRL inhibitory factor. Thus, compression by a macroadenoma of the pituitary stalk decreases the output of most anterior pituitary hormones but may increase output of PRL. The increased level of this hormone caused by stalk compression rarely exceeds 200 ng/ml. Although diabetes insipidus is a common finding in pituitary metastases and transiently after pituitary surgery, it almost never is a presenting complaint of pituitary adenoma. Sudden pituitary failure may be caused by pituitary apoplexy (see next section).

Nonendocrine Findings

Frequently, headache is an early tumor symptom probably due to stretching of the diaphragma sella. The headache is nonspecific, usually felt as a dull bifrontal or vertex ache and, like the pain from other brain tumors, often is more intense in the morning. In some patients, as the tumor grows and the diaphragma sella is ruptured, the headache disappears. As the tumor grows superiorly, above the diaphragma sella, it first encounters the optic chiasm. Compression of that structure may lead to bitemporal hemianopia of which affected patients often are unaware. Thus, the first sign of a pituitary tumor may be manifested as an automobile accident attributable to a patient's lack of peripheral vision. Depending on the exact location of the optic structures and on the site of suprasellar tumor growth, one optic nerve anterior to the chiasm may be compressed, causing unilateral visual loss with optic atrophy. If the tumor grows laterally rather than anteriorly, it compresses the cavernous sinus, causing ptosis (oculomotor nerve), diplopia (oculomotor, trochlear, or abducens nerve), or facial numbness (trigeminal nerve). Very large pituitary adenomas can compress the hypothalamus, causing dementia, drowsiness, hypophagia or hyperphagia, emotional disturbances, and obstructive hydrocephalus from compression of the third ventricle.

For reasons not entirely understood, both large and small pituitary adenomas have a tendency to either bleed or infarct spontaneously, causing pituitary apoplexy [101]. Usually, the vascular insult occurs spontaneously, but it may result from cerebral angiography or during provocative endocrine testing; it also occurs with greater frequency in pregnant women. The result is sudden enlargement of the pituitary tumor and spillage of hemorrhagic or necrotic material into the suprasellar cistern and the subarachnoid space. The clinical symptoms include sudden onset of visual loss, ocular palsies, acute hypopituitarism, and alteration in consciousness, varying from confusion to coma. Fever and nuchal rigidity may suggest the diagnosis of bacterial or viral meningitis. The CSF may contain blood or white cells, the latter in response to spilled necrotic material. Most patients respond to conservative treatment, replacing absent hormones and using corticosteroids to suppress inflammation. In some patients, emergency decompression of the enlarged pituitary is necessary to relieve symptoms. Untreated pituitary apoplexy can be fatal.

DIAGNOSIS

If a pituitary abnormality is suspected, high-resolution MRI with gadolinium enhancement and 1-mm sections through the pituitary fossa will establish the diagnosis in most instances, even when microadenomas are as small as 2 to 3 mm. Physicians suspecting a pituitary adenoma should indicate to involved radiologists that they require "fine sections" and rapid imaging during bolus contrast administration, particularly for a suspected microadenoma. With macroadenomas, the MRI also establishes the spatial relationships between the tumor and important surrounding neural structures. Characteristically, the tumor is isointense on a T_1-weighted image and variably isointense to hypointense on a T_2-weighted image. Immediately after injection of contrast, the tumor is hypointense on a T_1-weighted image as compared to normal gland, which has no blood-brain barrier. Later, it becomes isointense. Approximately 10% of prolactinomas calcify and are seen best on CT scan. Contrast may not be necessary to evaluate patients postoperatively [102]. Occasionally, a CT scan of the pituitary fossa is indicated. It is particularly valuable in identifying acute hemorrhages in patients with pituitary apoplexy and may help with the differential diagnosis of pituitary tumors versus meningiomas by identifying the hyperostosis of bone characteristic of meningioma.

A second approach to diagnosis is measurement of hormones in the blood. Both hypersecretion and hyposecretion of pituitary hormones can be identified by blood measurement. Hormone measurement not only helps to establish the diagnosis of the tumor cell type but is useful to follow tumor response to treatment and to identify posttreatment hypopituitarism. Careful neuroophthalmologic examination with special attention to visual fields and ocular movements will determine whether macroadenomas have interfered substantially with neurologic function. Occasional patients whose tumor has eroded the floor of the sella may develop a CSF leak. All patients with macroadenomas should be questioned concerning the presence of rhinorrhea. If rhinorrhea is present, measurement of the nasal fluid for transferrin will determine whether the fluid is CSF.

In most instances, MRI scans will distinguish pituitary neoplasms from other masses of the sella turcica. MRI cannot, of course, distinguish pituitary adenomas from the much rarer pituitary carcinomas [95]; that can be accomplished only by biopsy. Distinguishing tumors of neurohypophyseal origin, which are fairly rare, from those of adenohypophyseal origin may be difficult. Generally, tumors of nonpituitary origin, such as craniopharyngiomas, germ-cell tumors, meningiomas, and hypothalamic gliomas, are easily distinguishable because they either spare the pituitary fossa or invade it only after filling the suprasellar area. Dermoids and epidermoids, Rathke's cleft cysts, and the empty sella syndrome have an MRI signal intensity that differs from that of pituitary tumors.

One problem in diagnosis involves metastasis to the pituitary gland [103]. Carcinomas of the breast have a predilection to metastasize to the pituitary, but other cancers also may metastasize. Unlike pituitary adenomas, usually the first symptom of metastatic pituitary disease is diabetes insipidus from invasion of either the pituitary stalk or the neurohypophysis. Sometimes, the tumor also invades the subarachnoid space, allowing establishment of a diagnosis of metastatic tumor by examination of the CSF. Occasionally, a diagnosis is not possible on the basis of imaging or CSF examination, and biopsy is the only option. Carotid aneurysms rarely mimic pituitary adenoma, and MRI scan characteristics easily distinguish these.

The most difficult differential diagnosis is between certain inflammatory conditions and pituitary adenoma: Often, lymphocytic hypophysitis and giant-cell granulomas of the pituitary present with hypopituitarism, particularly hypothyroidism; diabetes insipidus is common [104, 105]. Such lesions enlarge the sella and mimic pituitary adenomas on MRI scan. Because the treatment of these tumors is nonsurgical (i.e., corticosteroid therapy), physicians should consider that all patients (particularly pregnant or postpartum young women) with rapidly developing hypothyroidism and an enlarging sella turcica might be suffering from an inflammatory condition and should consider initiating a trial of steroids.

TREATMENT

Surgery

The treatment for most pituitary adenomas is surgery. Neurosurgeons with extensive experience in pituitary surgery have substantially better results than will those less experienced. In most patients, the tumor can be reached by a transsphenoidal approach. A few tumors that are very large or that have grown laterally into the cavernous sinus may require a transfrontal approach. Microadenomas not causing symptomatic hormonal dysfunction may just be followed, and some prolactinomas [106] and GH-secreting adenomas [107] may be treated successfully with pharmacologic therapy (see later).

Surgery is both safe and efficacious. Generally, operative mortality and morbidity rates from several series are 0.5% and 2.2%, respectively [91]. The most common complication is CSF rhinorrhea predisposing to meningitis. Rare complications include traumatic injury to the hypothalamus resulting in coma or death, laceration of the carotid artery, and damage to the optic chiasm. Diabetes insipidus also may be a complication of surgery (usually transient) but is controlled easily by appropriate hormonal therapy. Postoperative hypopituitarism is uncommon and also can be controlled by hormonal therapy.

Radiotherapy

Radiotherapy using doses of 45 to 50 Gy in 180-cGy fractions also is effective at reducing tumor growth in some patients but generally is inferior to surgery and, in the long run, may be accompanied by more late complications, including hypopituitarism, optic nerve, hypothalamic, or temporal lobe damage and, as a late delayed effect, secondary tumors [108]. Even when radiotherapy is effective, elevated hormone levels may take years to normalize. Irradiation probably should be reserved for persistent or recurrent medically refractory hypersecreting adenomas or should be administered postoperatively to patients with invasive or large, incompletely removed tumors [109]. Radiosurgery may produce more rapid hormonal and clinical responses with toxicity similar to or less than that of conventional radiotherapy [110], but it cannot be used for large tumors or those near (< 3 mm) the optic nerve or chiasm.

Pharmacologic Therapy

Some pituitary adenomas have proved sensitive to pharmacologic treatment. Secreting tumors that require therapy can be treated with dopamine agonists to inhibit the output of PRL. These drugs substantially reduce the size of prolactinomas and control their growth. Bromocriptine and pergolide are the agents used most frequently, but cabergoline is more effective, is tolerated better, and probably is currently the drug of choice [111, 112]. Somatostatin and its analogs, such as octreotide, have been used in the management of tumors associated with acromegaly [107]. However, the degree of tumor shrinkage obtained is not as dramatic as with dopamine agonist therapy for prolactinomas. In selected patients, somatostatin analogs may be primary therapy, but usually they are reserved to control symptoms if surgery and irradiation fail.

SPECIFIC TUMORS

Prolactinomas

PRL-secreting pituitary adenomas are the most common clinically recognized tumor of the pituitary gland, accounting for approximately one-third of symptomatic tumors. These adenomas occur in both genders but are most common in young women and in older men. Usually, women present with amenorrhea and galactorrhea as a consequence of PRL excess. Men present either with headache and visual loss from the enlarging mass or (sometimes) with impotence. The lack of early endocrine symptoms in men may explain why tumors in men generally are larger than those in women when recognized. Fewer than 10% of PRL-secreting microadenomas evolve into macroadenomas; the others seem not to grow after they are identified, or they even may regress spontaneously [91]. The diagnosis is made on the basis of MRI and PRL levels. A PRL level in excess of 200 ng/ml is diagnostic of a prolactinoma, whereas levels in excess of 1,000 ng/ml suggest that the prolactinoma is invasive.

The treatment of choice is pharmacologic [112]. In women with the amenorrhea-galactorrhea syndrome, dopamine agonist therapy can restore appropriate hormonal levels and allow for pregnancy. PRL levels are controlled in almost all microadenomas [111]; some 60% of patients with macroadenomas respond with more than 80% tumor shrinkage [112]. The drugs are discontinued during pregnancy and are resumed after pregnancy. A risk remains, however, of accelerated tumor growth during pregnancy in patients with macroadenoma. In men with asymptomatic microadenomas, treatment is unnecessary. Macroadenomas can be treated successfully by dopamine agonist therapy. The treatment must be maintained for life, and the lesion tends to scar. Some neurosurgeons believe that the scarring renders subsequent surgery more difficult [113], although the final outcome usually is the same. If drugs fail or cannot be tolerated by affected patients, surgery is effective. The surgical cure rate for microadenomas is as high as 75%, higher if PRL levels are less than 100 ng/ml and lower if levels are more than 200 ng/ml; the cure rate is approximately 30% for macroadenomas and even lower for invasive tumors. Symptomatic recurrence occurs in perhaps 25% of patients. Risk factors for recurrence include basal PRL levels of more than 400 ng/ml, macroadenoma, male gender, and prolonged preoperative dopamine agonist therapy [113]. PRL levels can be followed to determine the effectiveness of therapy. Radiotherapy should be reserved for patients in whom both pharmacologic therapy and surgery fail. Radiosurgery may be superior to conventional irradiation.

GH-Secreting Adenomas

GH excess from pituitary adenomas results in pituitary gigantism in children and acromegaly in adults. Coarsening of facial features, separation of teeth, and en-

largement of the hands and feet characterized by an increase in shoe and glove size are signs of acromegaly. Patients may develop diabetes mellitus. With further tumor growth, hypopituitarism and visual complaints develop. Headache, carpal tunnel syndrome, and arthritic pain are common complications of acromegaly. The diagnosis can be made by inspection of affected patients and is supported by elevation of GH observed after a glucose load and by elevation of insulinlike growth factor 1 in the serum. Sometimes, the tumors are too small to be identified by MRI, in which case ectopic acromegaly caused by carcinoids or small-cell lung cancer must be considered.

The treatment of choice for most GH-secreting adenomas is surgery, although recent evidence warrants a trial of octreotide as primary therapy for some patients, giving response rates of more than 60% [107]. Dopamine agonists are effective in some patients, usually at high doses [111]. Biochemical cure, as defined by normalization of insulinlike growth factor 1 levels or basal or glucose-suppressed GH levels of 2 ng/ml or less, can be achieved in almost 90% of patients with microadenomas and in 55% of patients with macroadenomas [114]. Tumor recurrence is uncommon. Risk factors for recurrence include basal GH levels of more than 40 ng/ml, macroadenoma, invasive adenoma, and an abnormal postoperative glucose tolerance test [114]. Radiotherapy can be delivered to invasive tumors or to those that fail to yield to biochemical cure, but it rarely is curative. Often, long-term treatment with a somatostatin analog is required.

ACTH-Secreting Adenomas

Approximately 15% of pituitary adenomas secrete ACTH. This secretion leads to two distinct clinical syndromes: Cushing's disease and Nelson's syndrome. Seventy-five percent of patients with Cushing's disease are women, usually in their third and fourth decades. Patients characteristically develop deposition of fat in the face (moon facies), supraclavicular fossae, abdomen (central obesity), and back of the neck (buffalo hump). Muscle atrophy leads to thin extremities, accentuating the central obesity. Hirsutism, thinness, and hyperpigmentation of the skin and vascular fragility lead to diffuse ecchymoses and purple abdominal striae. Proximal weakness is manifested first by difficulty in getting off the toilet seat and subsequently in climbing stairs. Patients may develop hypertension, glucose intolerance, and osteoporosis. The disorder, untreated, is life-threatening, with a 5-year mortality of approximately 50%. The diagnosis is made by (1) elevated levels of 24-hour urinary free cortisol, (2) loss of ACTH suppression by glucocorticoids, and (3) elevated ACTH levels. Some cancers (especially small-cell lung cancer) secrete ACTH-like substances and cause Cushing's syndrome (see Chapter 11), and ACTH-secreting pituitary adenomas often are too small to identify on MRI scan, conditions sometimes necessitating measurement of ACTH in blood from the inferior petrosal sinus of both cavernous sinuses, the venous drainage of the pituitary gland, to verify a pituitary origin of excessive ACTH secretion.

Transsphenoidal exploration of the pituitary gland can lead to curative resection of more than 70% of microadenomas and 30% of macroadenomas. Persistence or recurrence of tumor is not uncommon. Pharmacologic blocking agents, such as mitotane, ketoconazole, and metyrapone, have some effect but probably should be used only after failure of surgical intervention. The same caution applies to radiotherapy that, however, controls more than 80% of tumors in cases of failed transsphenoidal surgery [115]. In some instances, bilateral adrenalectomy is necessary to ameliorate the potentially fatal hyperadrenocorticalism.

Nelson's syndrome occurs in approximately 10% to 15% of patients who have Cushing's disease and undergo bilateral adrenalectomy. The high levels of ACTH stimulate melanocyte-stimulating hormone. Affected patients develop diffuse hyperpigmentation and expansion of the sella turcica. Surgery cures only 25%. Radiotherapy may help to control tumor growth.

TSH-Secreting Adenomas

TSH-secreting adenomas account for some 1% of all pituitary tumors. Most patients present with hyperthyroidism with unrepressed TSH levels. By the time the diagnosis is established—often after thyroid ablation has been carried out—usually the tumor is macroscopic in size and has invaded parasellar structures. Most tumors also secrete GH or PRL, helping to establish the diagnosis of a pituitary lesion rather than a thyroid lesion. The treatment is surgery, with adjunctive radiotherapy in cases of invasion. Surgery cures approximately 25% of tumors. In some instances, use of a somatostatin analog has reduced TSH levels but generally does not reduce the tumor mass.

Gonadotropin-Secreting Pituitary Adenomas

Gonadotropic adenomas secrete follicle-stimulating hormone and luteinizing hormone. They account for 5% to 15% of pituitary adenomas. Usually, they are macroadenomas [116] and present with visual loss and hypopituitarism. These lesions can cause hypogonadism with diminished libido in men and amenorrhea in premenopausal women, but usually they are asymptom-

atic until they compress normal tissue. Microadenomas do not require treatment unless they are symptomatic. Macroadenomas should be treated surgically. Persistence or recurrence of tumors occurs in perhaps 40% of patients [116]. Residual tumor may respond to radiotherapy.

Nonsecreting Pituitary Adenomas

Nonfunctioning pituitary adenomas account for approximately one-third of clinically recognized pituitary adenomas and most incidental tumors encountered at autopsy. The tumors present as macroadenomas with headache, visual disturbances, and symptoms of pituitary failure. PRL may be elevated because of pituitary stalk compression. Generally, these tumors occur in individuals older than 50 years, are diagnosed by MRI, and are treated surgically. Visual abnormalities are reversed in most patients and, if normal preoperatively, endocrine function is preserved.

Symptomatic recurrence develops in fewer than 10% of patients after gross total resection [109]. Radiotherapy reduces the rate of tumor regrowth after surgery [117, 118]. Risk factors for recurrence include macroadenoma, invasive adenoma, plurihormonal adenoma, silent ACTH adenoma, and oncocytoma [119].

Pituitary Carcinoma

Pituitary carcinoma is rare; fewer than 100 cases have been reported [95]. The diagnosis is established when tumors of anterior pituitary origin, previously believed to be adenomas, cause distant metastases or disseminate into the subarachnoid space. Often, the tumors declare themselves with clinical evidence of invasion of the intracranial or spinal leptomeninges. Extraneural metastases to the mediastinum and lymph nodes also occur. The tumors may be hormonally active or hormonally silent. Once distant metastases develop, radiotherapy and standard anticancer chemotherapy may be tried but usually are ineffective. Usually, the metastatic disease is responsible for death.

Posterior Pituitary Tumors

Posterior pituitary tumors are rare. The most common of these tumors is the granular cell tumor, usually an incidental finding at autopsy. If the tumor causes symptoms, usually diabetes insipidus is the first symptom, a rare finding with pituitary adenomas.

Astrocytomas, usually low-grade, also occur in the posterior pituitary. The most common tumor of the neurohypophysis is a metastasis. The most common primary tumor is breast cancer, with lung and prostate cancer being less common. In most cases, diabetes insipidus is the first symptom. At least 20% of patients presenting with diabetes insipidus to a general hospital are discovered to have metastatic breast cancer as the cause.

PRIMARY INTRASPINAL TUMORS
General Considerations

Tumors affecting the spine are common, but most are metastatic. Primary tumors of the spinal column or spinal cord are only perhaps 10% to 20% as frequent as are primary intracranial tumors (Fig. 28.11). However, fully one-third of patients with systemic cancer, particularly those suffering from breast, lung, and prostate cancer, develop vertebral metastasis during life, many of which are symptomatic (see "CNS Metastases"). The exact incidence and relative frequency of different types of spinal tumors are not known; data in the literature vary, depending on patterns of referral to the center reporting the data. In one population-based survey, the annual incidence of primary intraspinal neoplasms was five per million for women and five per million for men.

Spinal tumors are classified by their location in relation to the spinal cord and its coverings (i.e., extradural and intradural but extramedullary and intramedullary; Table 28.13) and, within each of these groups, by histologic features. Unlike intracranial tumors, intraspinal tumors (except those involving the vertebral bodies themselves) are more likely to be benign than malignant. Thus, meningiomas and schwannomas within the spinal canal outnumber gliomas.

Clinical Findings

Often, the symptoms of extradural, intradural, or intramedullary tumors are indistinguishable [120]. By far, pain is the most common first symptom and may be the *only* symptom for many weeks or months before the appearance of other neurologic signs. The pain of spinal tumors, whatever their location, often is exacerbated by coughing or straining, maneuvers that increase intraspinal pressure. The pain may be classified into four types: local, radicular, referred, or funicular.

Local pain is the most common presenting complaint in extradural tumors. Usually, local pain is steady and aching, not sharp or shooting. It is present at the site of the lesion and often is accompanied by local tenderness to percussion, especially when the tumor involves the

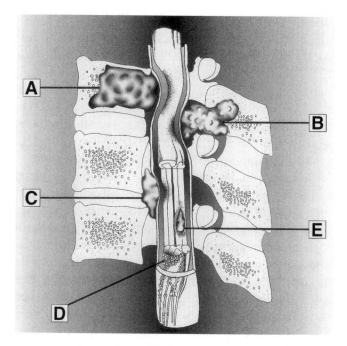

Figure 28.11 Sagittal section of the spinal column illustrating some of the tumors discussed. Tumors can arise in and collapse the vertebral body *(A)* or bones of the posterior spinal elements *(B)*. Extramedullary, intradural tumors can compress the spinal cord and cause edema, as do extradural tumors *(C)*. Tumors may also arise in or metastasize to the leptomeninges *(D)*. Tumors can arise within the spinal cord itself *(E)*.

posterior elements of the vertebral body. Characteristically, the pain is worse in the lying position and often is relieved by sitting or standing. As the disease progresses, many patients find they can sleep only in the sitting position. If the tumor causes spinal instability, pain may be present only on movement and may be relieved when the patient is still. When nerve roots are involved, many patients with or without local pain develop pain in the distribution of that nerve root (i.e., radicular pain).

Characteristically, radicular pain is sharp and radiates down an arm or leg or encompasses the chest or abdomen in a bandlike distribution. Referred pain is pain at a distance from the site of the tumor but not in a radicular distribution. For example, involvement of the L1 vertebral body can cause pain over the sacroiliac joint, sometimes leading physicians to undertake a fruitless search for a lesion at the site of the referred pain. Funicular pain is caused when spinal cord sensory fibers are compressed or invaded by tumor. The pain mimics radicular or referred pain but is defined less sharply, rendering patient description of it more difficult. Often, it is exacerbated when the spinal cord is stretched by neck flexion or straight-leg raising.

Table 28.13   Classification of Primary Spinal Tumors

Extradural (primary bone tumors)
Myeloma
Chordoma
Osteogenic sarcoma
Chondrosarcoma
Hemangioma
Aneurysmal bone cyst

Intradural-extramedullary
Schwannoma
Meningioma
Neurofibroma
Ependymoma
Arachnoid cyst
Lipoma
Dermoid-epidermoid

Intramedullary
Ependymoma
Astrocytoma
Hemangioblastoma
Dermoid-epidermoid
Hemangioma
Paraganglioma
Lipoma
Schwannoma
Endodermal cyst

Motor symptoms include upper motor neuron weakness beginning in the legs and characterized by spasticity, hyperactive reflexes, and extensor plantar responses. Lower motor neuron weakness due to involvement of anterior horn cells at the site of the lesion is characterized by atrophy, fasciculations, and hyporeflexia. The combination of lower motor neuron weakness of the arms and upper motor neuron weakness of the legs from a cervical cord tumor may mimic amyotrophic lateral sclerosis.

Generally, sensory changes are characterized by paresthesias and sensory loss that begin distally and ascends proximally. Dissociated sensory loss (i.e., loss of pain and temperature sensation with preservation of vibration and position sense or preservation of sensation in sacral segments) has been attributed to intramedullary lesions, but it does not reliably distinguish intramedullary from extramedullary tumors. Often, patients who complain of paresthesias in the lower extremities and have vibratory and position loss are misdiagnosed as suffering from a peripheral neuropathy. The preservation of Achilles reflexes in such patients should lead physicians to suspect a spinal lesion instead and consequently to perform appropriate investigations.

Autonomic dysfunction, consisting of disturbances of bladder, bowel, and sexual function, usually occurs late in the course of most spinal tumors, although often it is a presenting symptom (after pain) of tumors of the conus medullaris or cauda equina. Occasionally, patients with intramedullary cervical cord tumors present with autonomic dysfunction. Vascular or sudomotor changes in one or both legs (warm, dry foot) may result from compression of sympathetic fibers in the spinal cord.

Ataxia in the absence of other neurologic abnormalities may be a presenting complaint of an upper thoracic spinal cord tumor. Headache resulting from increased ICP caused by hydrocephalus is an unusual presenting complaint of spinal cord tumors. Otherwise silent spinal cord tumors may exude protein into the subarachnoid space, interfering with normal absorption of CSF and leading to hydrocephalus. The resulting headache and other symptoms of hydrocephalus may be present in the total absence of symptoms of spinal cord dysfunction.

Diagnosis

An MRI of the entire spine in the sagittal plane should be performed in any patient in whom a spinal cord tumor is suspected clinically. Additional axial images are obtained from areas of clinical or radiologic abnormality. The axial images allow visualization both of paravertebral structures and of vertebral bodies and spinal cord. The imaging should be performed first without contrast, then should be repeated after gadolinium injection if intradural or intramedullary disease is suspected. The MRI scan will identify both primary and metastatic vertebral tumors and will distinguish them from intradural and intramedullary lesions. Usually, no other diagnostic test is necessary. In occasional patients with leptomeningeal tumors, CSF evaluation for malignant cells and biochemical tumor markers may be necessary, but this assessment should follow rather than precede MRI. Proceeding directly to MRI is a better care practice and is more cost-effective in any patient suspected of harboring a spinal cord tumor. Roentgenography, radionuclide bone scans, and CT scans are both less sensitive and less specific and usually lead to an MRI scan in patients if symptoms persist.

Usually, MRI scans distinguish tumors from inflammatory and hemorrhagic spinal lesions by size, location, and signal characteristics. Almost always, tumors spare the avascular intervertebral disc, whereas infections often cross the disc space, causing contrast enhancement of the disc cartilage. The location and signal characteristics also help to distinguish benign from malignant lesions. Most extradural tumors are malignant; intradural but extramedullary lesions usually are benign even though they enhance intensely with contrast, and intramedullary lesions are either benign or malignant.

The major problem in diagnosis is deciding which patients with back or neck pain require imaging. Back and neck pain are common, and spinal tumors are rare. Many patients with spinal tumors suffer prolonged back or neck pain and eventually develop neurologic disability before their physicians decide that the back pain is serious. A few clues help physicians to decide which patients to select for imaging. Most spinal tumors occur in the thoracic region, a site of benign back pain that is less common than lumbar or cervical areas. Characteristically, pain from spinal tumors is worse in the recumbent position and usually is exacerbated by coughing, sneezing, or straining at stool. Usually, benign back pain is lessened in the recumbent position and is not affected substantially by raising intraspinal pressure. Back pain from spinal tumors gradually worsens in both duration and severity, whereas benign back pain generally remains static or decreases after onset.

Treatment

Often, corticosteroids ameliorate the pain associated with spinal tumors and sometimes relieve other neurologic symptoms. Short-term treatment with high doses of corticosteroids (i.e., dexamethasone, 100 mg/day) may allow an otherwise incapacitated patient to lie flat for diagnostic MRI or other necessary procedures. The corticosteroids should be tapered as rapidly as possible after more definitive therapy is begun. As with PCNSL, steroids should be withheld until biopsy if lymphoma is suspected.

Surgery is the principal form of treatment for all primary intraspinal tumors and for some metastatic tumors. Because most intraspinal tumors are benign, the goal of surgery is cure. In those tumors that cannot be removed totally, such as astrocytomas of the spinal cord, the goal is to establish the diagnosis and to relieve symptoms by debulking the tumor (when possible). Technical improvements in neuroanesthesia, microsurgery, spinal stabilization, intraoperative neurophysiologic monitoring, and ultrasonography have allowed surgeons to operate on the spinal cord successfully and with little morbidity. For those tumors that are malignant or cannot be resected completely, radiotherapy should be delivered in the postoperative period. Although the value of radiotherapy in the treatment of spinal cord tumors, such as astrocytomas or incompletely removed ependymomas, still is disputed, most investigators believe that radiotherapy is beneficial.

Little evidence supports the role of chemotherapy in the treatment of malignant spinal tumors. However, because these tumors have histologic traits similar to those of other CNS tumors, if surgery and radiotherapy fail, chemotherapy should be considered.

Specific Spinal Tumors

Primary tumors of the spinal cord, spinal nerves, and spinal meninges are identical to their intracranial counterparts. As the details of those tumors have been discussed in previous sections, only factors relevant to the spinal location are discussed here.

CHORDOMA

Spinal chordomas are tumors that grow slowly over several years and usually occur in the sacral region [121]. They are believed to arise from notochord remnants and are locally invasive. Although benign in histologic appearance, spinal chordomas may metastasize hematogenously. Typically, affected patients present with local pain that may be present for years before bladder and bowel dysfunction develop from compression of the cauda equina. Sometimes, the tumor can be felt over the sacrum posteriorly or by digital rectal examination anteriorly. Bone destruction and compression of neural elements are identified on MRI scan. The histologic diagnosis can be established by CT-guided needle biopsy. Radical surgical resection is the treatment of choice but is not always possible. The tumor cannot be cured by surgical resection, but after debulking, its slow growth often allows many years of remission before recurrence or metastasis. Radical resection should be followed by radiotherapy. Stereotactic radiosurgery [122] and heavy-particle radiotherapy [123] may be more effective than is standard radiotherapy. No chemotherapy is known to be effective.

Chordomas may present in vertebral bodies other than the sacrum. In the cervical spine, chordomas often cause a mass anterior to the vertebral body that compresses the esophagus and causes dysphagia as an early symptom.

SCHWANNOMA

Schwannoma is the most common intradural extramedullary tumor. These tumors may occur in patients with neurofibromatosis, where multiple schwannomas are the rule, or as isolated lesions in patients with no known genetic defect. In many instances, schwannomas form "dumbbell tumors" extending through the intervertebral foramen into the abdominal or thoracic cavity. Usually, patients present with local or radicular pain and later with symptoms of spinal cord compression (i.e., motor weakness, sensory and autonomic changes). The diagnosis is established by MRI scan, and the treatment is surgical removal. Schwannomas almost always are benign and curable if resected totally.

MENINGIOMAS

Spinal meningiomas can be a symptom of neurofibromatosis or can occur sporadically [124]; they are more frequent in middle-aged women. Usually, they are located in the thoracic spine and may be painless, presenting with symptoms of gradually progressive spinal cord compression. In many instances, the first symptoms are paresthesias in the lower extremities, leading physicians to a mistaken diagnosis of peripheral neuropathy. Spinal meningiomas virtually always are benign and can be cured by surgical resection. Unlike those afflicted with spinal cord compression from metastatic tumors, patients who are substantially paralyzed from meningiomas may make a complete recovery after successful surgical resection.

EPENDYMOMAS

Spinal ependymomas can arise either within the spinal cord itself or at the filum terminale, just caudal to the spinal cord [68]. Usually, ependymomas of the filum terminale are of the myxopapillary subtype, whereas intramedullary and cerebral ependymomas usually are of the cellular variety. Intramedullary ependymomas present with pain and other spinal cord symptoms (as described). On MRI scan, characteristically they contain cysts, and they contrast enhance. The tumor may be hemorrhagic. The tumors are well circumscribed and usually amenable to complete surgical resection leading to cure (Fig. 28.12). Usually, resection is followed by radiotherapy. Tumors of the filum terminale are identified as contrast-enhancing masses involving the cauda equina. These tumors, although reasonably well circumscribed, often cannot be removed completely un-

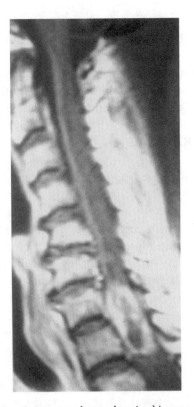

Figure 28.12   Contrast-enhanced sagittal image of the cervical spinal cord showing an ependymoma. The patient has had 2 years of progressive neurologic symptoms. A complete resection was possible.

less multiple roots of the cauda equina are sacrificed, leading to considerable neurologic disability. If the tumors are removed only partially, radiotherapy should follow.

ASTROCYTOMAS

Generally, spinal astrocytomas are low-grade but infiltrative tumors and frequently are associated with cysts or syrinx formation. The tumor may be localized over several segments or occasionally may involve the entire length of the spinal cord. The diagnosis is established by MRI scan, which shows a hyperintense abnormality on the T_2-weighted image that runs several segments and may or may not contrast enhance. A cyst within the tumor or syrinx can be identified also by the MRI scan. A syrinx expands the cord, is isointense or slightly hypointense on a T_1-weighted image, and is hyperintense on a T_2-weighted image. Unlike ependymomas, astrocytomas are not cured by surgery. Surgery can establish the diagnosis, can debulk the tumor partially, and may relieve the symptoms of the syrinx by drainage. Although the benefits of radiotherapy are not established, most investigators believe that after surgery, astrocytomas of the spinal cord should be treated with radiotherapy. The role of chemotherapy in tumors that recur or have a malignant appearance is not established.

PARAGANGLIOMAS

Paragangliomas are benign tumors of neural crest origin and usually are associated with peripheral structures, such as the carotid body (chemodectoma) or jugular ganglia (glomus jugulare tumor). Rarely, they occur in the CNS, in the filum terminale of the cauda equina. They are more common in men than in women and occur in both young and older adults [125]. Patients present with low back pain and subsequently may go on to develop cauda equina symptoms (i.e., urinary retention, leg weakness and sensory loss, loss of lower-extremity deep tendon reflexes). On a T_1-weighted image, the MRI scan shows a mass that is isointense with the spinal cord and is uniformly enhancing. The tumor's treatment is surgical. Most tumors do not recur, but some recur locally or seed the meninges or metastasize to bone. In such instances, radiotherapy may be helpful. Rarely, intracranial tumors have been reported.

OTHER SPINAL CORD TUMORS

Other less common intramedullary tumors, including hemangioblastomas, epidermoid and dermoid tumors, and teratomas, are treated surgically and often are cured. Extramedullary intradural tumors, in addition to the neurofibroma, schwannoma, and meningioma, include extramedullary hemangioblastoma and drop metastasis from malignant brain tumors. Occasional patients suffering medulloblastoma of the cerebellum or a pineal region tumor may present with spinal symptoms due to drop metastasis. Generally, these tumors intensely contrast enhance on MRI scan and often are multiple rather than single. Extradural bone tumors, such as osteogenic sarcomas and chondrosarcomas, are treated as they are when they occur elsewhere in the body.

CNS METASTASES

Metastatic tumors to the brain and spinal column are far more common than are primary tumors. Because their symptoms of cognitive dysfunction, seizures, and paralysis are the same as those of primary tumors, they substantially diminish the quality of life of otherwise stable patients suffering from cancer elsewhere in the body. Furthermore, because the blood-brain barrier offers sanctuary for tumor cells that otherwise might be exposed to effective chemotherapy, the incidence of CNS metastases appears to be increasing as more effective therapy is developed for the systemic cancer. The brain is increasingly the sole site of relapse in such relatively chemosensitive disorders as breast cancer.

Usually, although CNS metastases develop late in the course of the cancer, exceptions occur. Brain metastasis may be the presenting symptom in as many as 10% of lung cancer patients who are otherwise asymptomatic and in whom the tumor has not been discovered. Conversely, routine brain scans in 5% to 10% of patients with newly diagnosed lung cancer show asymptomatic metastatic brain lesions. Epidural spinal cord compression is the presenting sign of cancer in approximately 20% of patients who present with spinal cord symptoms at a general hospital. Often, careful attention to the development of neurologic symptoms in patients being treated for cancer can establish the diagnosis of CNS metastasis early and allow for effective treatment of the neurologic disorder, thereby improving the quality of such patients' lives. In most patients with CNS metastasis, if the diagnosis is made when the neurologic symptoms are mild, the patients' nervous system continues to function well after treatment. Conversely, patients with severe neurologic disability generally respond poorly to treatment. (A comprehensive review of CNS metastases has been published [9].)

Intracranial Metastases

Metastatic tumors can affect any portion of the intracranial cavity, including the skull, epidural or subdural spaces, cranial leptomeninges, cranial nerves within the subarachnoid space, the brain itself, and the pituitary and pineal glands. Although metastases to the calvarium are fairly common, particularly in patients with widespread bony metastases, usually they are asymptomatic. The most common symptomatic intracranial metastatic lesion occurs in the parenchyma of the brain. Approximately 20% of patients who die of cancer suffer from at least one intracranial metastasis. Roughly three-fourths of such patients have experienced symptoms from the intracranial metastasis during life. Tumors that commonly metastasize to the brain include lung (particularly small-cell lung) and breast cancer and malignant melanoma. Ovarian and prostate cancer are examples of tumors that rarely metastasize to the brain but appear to be increasing in frequency as better systemic therapy becomes available.

Most metastases reach the brain by hematogenous spread through the arterial system, implying that the tumor also has the opportunity to metastasize to other organs. Because they spread via the arterial system, tumor emboli tend to lodge at the gray matter–white matter junction in the terminal ends of the arterial supply, the so-called watershed areas. Most tumors are distributed between the supratentorial and infratentorial compartments in proportion to the weight and blood supply of these structures (i.e., 85% to cerebral hemispheres, particularly frontal and parietal lobes in the distribution of the middle cerebral artery, and 15% to the posterior fossa, particularly the cerebellum). Certain tumors, however, particularly those arising from the pelvis (prostate, uterus, or gastrointestinal tract), have a predilection to metastasize to the cerebellum. Unlike those in children, primary cerebellar tumors are uncommon in adults so that metastasis must be among the leading diagnostic considerations in any patient suffering from a cerebellar tumor.

Most metastases in the brain grow as spherical masses, displacing rather than destroying brain tissue and creating edema in the surrounding white matter. Although edema of the white matter surrounds virtually all metastatic tumors, its amount varies. Some small tumors are surrounded by massive amounts of edema, and some large tumors are surrounded by lesser amounts. Approximately 50% of brain metastases are multiple. However, more than 70% of patients exhibit three or fewer lesions on MRI scan; such patients should be considered for focal therapy (see "Treatment"). Because multicentric primary brain tumors other than PCNSL are uncommon, patients with multiple brain tumors must be suspected of harboring metastases until proved otherwise.

Dural metastases are somewhat less common than are metastases to the parenchyma of the brain. They are particularly likely to occur in patients with breast and prostate cancer. They may be single or multiple and, because their MRI scan appearance mimics that of meningioma, the differential diagnosis may be difficult. This effect is particularly true in women with breast cancer, because the incidence of meningiomas is greater in that population as compared to the general female population.

CLINICAL FEATURES

Because metastatic intracranial tumors grow more rapidly than do their primary counterparts, the evolution of neurologic signs and symptoms usually is faster. The specific neurologic signs and symptoms are, however, identical to those of primary intracranial tumors. Usually, symptoms evolve over weeks, although sometimes they develop gradually or have an apoplectic onset. On rare occasions, a tumor embolus temporarily occludes a vessel large enough to cause a transient ischemic attack. Affected patients may recover from the acute vascular compromise only to relapse several months later when the tumor embolus has grown. Acute symptoms may be caused by seizures or by hemorrhage into the tumor. All metastatic tumors can bleed, but melanomas and germ-cell tumors have the greatest propensity for this characteristic.

DIAGNOSIS

Characteristically, MRI scan identifies within the white matter one or more spherical lesions that exhibit contrast enhancement and are surrounded by edema. Usually, the tumor itself is relatively low in signal intensity on a T_2-weighted image and usually is hypointense on a T_1-weighted image. Melanomas, because melanin is paramagnetic, and such other tumors as germ-cell and renal tumors, because of hemorrhage, may produce a hyperintense T_1-weighted image signal. With smaller lesions, the contrast enhancement may be uniform; with larger lesions, a symmetric rim of contrast enhancement surrounds a central unenhanced area. In some instances, increasing the dose of contrast (i.e., double- or triple-dose gadolinium) will reveal small metastases not seen otherwise. The MRI appearance of metastases differs from that of primary gliomas in that the former are rounder and have a more regular contrast-enhancing rim. Metastases differ from primary lymphomas in that the latter uniformly contrast enhance, tend to be surrounded by somewhat less edema, and have an irregular rather than a smooth margin. Dura-based metastases differ from meningiomas in that generally they cause more edema in the underlying brain (a finding unusual with meningiomas) and may lack the enhancing dural tail characteristic of meningioma (Fig. 28.13).

In certain clinical settings (e.g., multiple cerebral lesions in patients known to have active cancer), MRI is diagnostic. If the MRI scan is atypical or if such patients are not known to have cancer, biopsy may be required. In one series of presumed single brain metastasis in patients known to have cancer, biopsy revealed an 11% error rate [126]; several of the lesions were benign (i.e., inflammatory) and others revealed a second malignancy. The differential diagnosis includes primary brain tumors, inflammatory lesions (including brain ab-

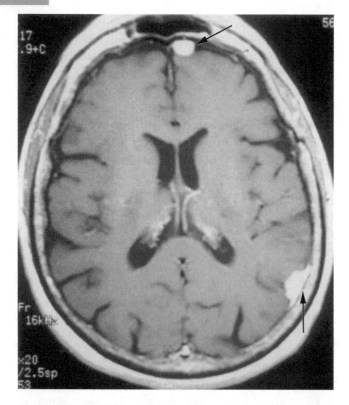

Figure 28.13 Two meningiomas (arrows) in a patient with known breast cancer. The patient was asymptomatic. Magnetic resonance imaging of the brain was done as part of an evaluation looking for metastatic disease. Note the dural tail on the posterior tumor. No treatment was administered.

scesses and demyelinating disease [multiple sclerosis]), and a rare, enhancing demyelinating disorder that complicates 5-fluorouracil-levamisole therapy in patients with colon cancer.

Any patients who have known cancer and develop symptoms of brain dysfunction should receive MRI before and after injection of gadolinium contrast. This precaution includes patients who experience confusion and are thought to be suffering from metabolic encephalopathy. At least 15% of such patients are found to have brain metastases as the cause of their confusion, even in the absence of other more focal signs of brain disease. Patients who have lung cancer or malignant melanoma and are about to undergo major surgical procedures probably should also undergo an MRI.

TREATMENT

The choice of treatment for brain metastasis is determined in part by the number and location of the meta-

static lesions and in part by the state of affected patients' systemic cancer. Patients with one to three metastases in the brain—particularly if located in noneloquent brain areas—are candidates for focal therapy (i.e., surgery or radiosurgery). Patients with widespread or terminal systemic cancer, even when the brain metastasis is single and surgically accessible, are less likely to be candidates for surgery than are patients whose only site of cancer is the brain. Nevertheless, symptomatic treatment should be delivered to all patients with brain metastases, because treatment can improve the quality of life at least temporarily.

Corticosteroids

Corticosteroids are used to treat brain metastases in the same manner as they are used to treat primary brain tumors. The response of neurologic symptoms in patients with brain metastases is even more dramatic than that in patients with primary brain tumors. Such diffuse symptoms as headache and lethargy respond dramatically, and even such focal symptoms as hemiparesis may resolve completely. The usual dose is 16 mg of dexamethasone (or its equivalent) per day, except in patients who are deteriorating rapidly, in which case higher doses can be used. If such patients do not respond within 24 hours, the dose should be doubled and increased either until a response is achieved or until a dose of approximately 100 mg/day is reached. After more definitive therapy has been administered, the steroids can be tapered to tolerance. Many patients, particularly those with multiple brain metastases, remain steroid-dependent for life.

Anticonvulsants

Anticonvulsants are used in brain metastases in the same manner as they are used in primary brain tumors.

Radiotherapy

For patients with multiple metastases or for those whose systemic cancer is terminal, the treatment of choice is whole-brain radiotherapy (WBRT). The standard treatment consists of 10 fractions of 300 cGy each. Most patients will have a temporary clinical response to irradiation, but such treatment rarely sterilizes the brain metastasis, and usually patients relapse after several months. Moreover, the 300-cGy fractionation schedule that allows the treatment to be completed within 2 weeks may cause late-delayed irradiation encephalopathy in patients who live more than a year. Accordingly, if the prognosis of the systemic tumor is greater than a year, the fractionation schedule should be changed.

One schedule is 200 cGy in 20 fractions, a dose biologically equivalent to the 10 fractions of 300 cGy but theoretically less toxic to normal brain. At the end of radiotherapy, corticosteroids should be tapered to tolerance. Some patients will be able to discontinue the corticosteroids, but others remain corticosteroid-dependent.

WBRT may be indicated also in patients who have undergone surgery or radiosurgery for treatment of single or a few brain metastases. Current evidence suggests that patients who undergo surgical resection of a single brain metastasis suffer fewer CNS relapses if they receive WBRT in the postoperative period [127]. Similar considerations may apply also to patients who are treated focally with radiosurgery (see next section).

Radiosurgery

Radiosurgery is becoming an increasingly popular modality for the treatment of one or a few brain metastases. In one series, as many as seven lesions were treated radiosurgically [128]. Most series report local control of brain metastases in 80% to 90% of patients so treated [129]. Generally, tumors resistant to WBRT (e.g., melanoma and renal cell carcinoma) appear to be particularly amenable to radiosurgery, perhaps because of the large dose of irradiation delivered as a single fraction. Usually, toxicity to surrounding tissue is modest, although necrosis of the tumor may lead to edema and exacerbation of neurologic symptoms. These necrotic lesions may require surgical resection. Radiosurgery has been applied successfully to such surgically inaccessible areas as the basal ganglia and brainstem. Because it has not yet been compared to surgical removal of a single brain metastasis in a controlled trial, its exact role in the treatment of such metastases is not established.

Surgery

Controlled trials demonstrate that surgery is superior to WBRT in patients with a single brain metastasis in a surgically accessible site. The surgery probably should be followed by WBRT to sterilize remaining tumor cells at the surgical site and microscopic tumor deposits elsewhere in the brain. Patients treated with surgery live longer and are less likely to die a neurologic death than are those treated with WBRT alone, their quality of life is improved, and their dependence on potentially toxic corticosteroids is decreased. Surgical mortality is low (approximately 1%), and surgical morbidity, usually transient, occurs in only perhaps 5% to 10% of patients. Most patients recover from the surgery rapidly and are ready for discharge in a few days. At least one comparative but uncontrolled trial suggested that surgical removal is superior to radiosurgery both in terms of survival and toxicity [130].

Chemotherapy

Many oncologists believe that brain metastases are not amenable to chemotherapy because of the blood-brain barrier. However, many chemotherapeutic agents are lipid-soluble and easily cross the blood-brain barrier, distributing with the brain blood flow. Water-soluble drugs enter a brain metastasis because of disruption of the blood-brain barrier caused by neovascularization of the tumor. Current evidence suggests that if effective chemotherapeutic agents are available for the primary cancer, they will be roughly as effective in treating brain metastases from that primary site. Often, choriocarcinomas, breast cancer, and small-cell lung cancer respond as well in the brain as they do elsewhere in the body. Accordingly, for patients who have asymptomatic brain metastases and active systemic tumor and are about to undergo systemic chemotherapy, other treatment of the brain metastases might be deferred until their response to chemotherapy has been assessed. If the tumor is causing significant neurologic symptoms, surgery or irradiation or both should be administered.

Spinal Metastases

Whereas the majority of intracranial metastases are within the parenchyma of the brain itself, usually the spinal cord is compressed by tumors that metastasize to the bones of the spinal column, particularly the vertebral bodies. Intramedullary spinal cord metastases are uncommon. In contrast to brain tumors, tumors within the substance of the spinal cord are more likely to be primary than metastatic.

Tumors metastasize to the vertebral body hematogenously. The spread may be either arterial or venous by Batson's plexus (a valveless collection of epidural veins). Other modes include spread along lymphatics and direct extension from retroperitoneal or posterior mediastinal tumors. Individual tumors drain differently into Batson's plexus and thus reach different portions of the vertebral column. The breast drains principally by the azygos vein into the thoracic level of the plexus. Cervical cancers metastasize to lumbar spine and sacrum, usually to the left side, probably representing direct drainage from tumor-bearing lymph nodes. Prostate tumors drain through the pelvic venous plexus, reaching Batson's plexus in the pelvis and lower spine. Some tumors, by contrast, drain principally via the pulmonary vein into the left atrium and reach the vertebral body via the arterial circulation. Once a vertebral body is infiltrated by metastatic tumor, spinal cord compression occurs either by direct tumoral expansion into the epidural space or by destruction of the vertebral body, leading to spinal instability and bony compression of the spinal cord.

CLINICAL FINDINGS

The clinical symptoms of metastatic spinal tumors do not differ from those of primary tumors except that usually the more rapid growth of metastatic tumors causes symptoms to develop more rapidly. Also, because most metastatic spinal tumors involve bone, back pain almost always is the earliest symptom. Usually, the back pain is present for weeks to months before other neurologic symptoms appear. Typically, the pain is worse at night in the recumbent position. Many patients are unable to lie down to sleep, and some have so much pain they are unable to lie on the MRI table for imaging. Often, corticosteroids ameliorate the pain and allow adequate imaging studies. Because most metastatic spinal tumors are in the thoracic area (approximately 70%), the lumbosacral area (20%), and the cervical area (10%), the back pain is most likely to be thoracic, an area not usually affected by the more common degenerative causes of low back and neck pain. Nevertheless, any neck or back pain in patients known to have cancer should prompt an immediate search for spinal metastases. This step is particularly important because patients treated for spinal metastases before they develop significant neurologic disability are likely to remain functional, whereas those treated after significant disability develops are likely to remain disabled [9]. Thus, once such neurologic symptoms as weakness, sensory changes, or autonomic dysfunction develop, a spinal metastasis becomes a neurologic emergency.

DIAGNOSIS

The diagnosis is made on MRI scan. Noncontrast MRI identifies bony metastases in virtually every instance and is more sensitive than plain roentgenography or radionuclide scanning. MRI also reveals accompanying changes, such as vertebral body collapse and epidural mass lesions. Contrast-enhanced scans identify both the uncommon intramedullary metastasis and the leptomeningeal metastases. MRI scan also allows examination of the paravertebral space for those tumors that invade the spinal canal through the intervertebral foramen but do not involve bone directly. Myelograms are performed rarely except in patients who are ineligible for MRI (i.e., those having a cardiac pacemaker).

Although MRI scans identify tumors involving the spine, they cannot identify the nature of such tumors. Most metastases develop in patients known to have cancer, and imaging alone provides an adequate diagnosis. Epidural hemorrhage and abscesses can be distinguished by MRI characteristics, but these are rare. Occasionally, needle biopsy under CT control is necessary to establish a definitive diagnosis before therapy is prescribed.

TREATMENT

Corticosteroids
As does the brain, the compressed spinal cord swells, so edema probably is responsible for some of the symptoms arising from tumor. Corticosteroids are extremely effective in relieving pain related to spinal cord compression, but their role in relieving other neurologic symptoms is less clear. Because spinal cord compression is a neurologic emergency, such definitive treatment as radiotherapy or surgery is undertaken immediately, allowing no time adequately to assess the effects of corticosteroids alone. However, some patients who receive corticosteroids clearly respond with improvement of their neurologic signs. The definitive dose of corticosteroids is not established. For patients with severe pain or for patients with rapidly progressing neurologic symptoms, some investigators have recommended a bolus of 100 mg of dexamethasone followed by a rapidly tapering dose [9]. For patients with less pain or those who are neurologically stable, standard doses (e.g., 16 mg/day) often will suffice. Usually, pain is relieved within a matter of hours after an intravenous bolus of dexamethasone. Physicians should be aware that when intravenous dexamethasone is given rapidly, patients may complain of severe genital burning. Patients should be warned of that possibility; if it occurs, the infusion should be slowed. Once affected patients are neurologically stable and other treatment has been instituted, the steroids can be tapered rapidly.

Radiotherapy
Radiotherapy is delivered to areas involved by tumor with a margin of two vertebral bodies on either side. The usual dose is 10 fractions of 300 cGy each. More than 90% of patients who are ambulatory when treatment begins will remain ambulatory. Approximately one-half of the patients who have some weakness will regain ambulation. Rarely, a paraplegic patient will recover. Recovery may take many weeks after completion

of radiotherapy, so absence of immediate response does not indicate treatment failure.

Surgery

The role of surgical decompression in the treatment of spinal cord compression is not established. By general agreement, surgical treatment should be offered to patients who have spinal cord compression and already have received maximum radiotherapy or to patients whose spinal cord compression results from spinal instability. Often, spinal instability can be recognized by the fact that affected patients have pain only on movement and are free of pain when still. Some investigators recommend surgery for patients whose tumors are known to be radioresistant and for those without a cancer diagnosis when spinal cord compression develops.

Surgical decompression can be accomplished either by laminectomy or by vertebral body resection. Regardless of the approach taken, surgeons should attempt not only to decompress the spinal cord but to remove as much tumor as possible so that affected patients may respond better to subsequent treatment with radiotherapy or chemotherapy. When epidural tumors are decompressed, often a stabilization procedure is required as well. At present, no definitive evidence indicates that surgical treatment is superior to radiotherapy in most cases.

For patients who have received prior irradiation either for treatment of abdominal or mediastinal tumor or for prior spinal cord compression, reirradiation after development of cord compression may be effective in relieving symptoms and in allowing such patients to remain ambulatory [131]. Although reirradiation increases the risk of irradiation damage to the spinal cord, the risk is less than that of paraplegia from the tumor.

Leptomeningeal Tumors

Some tumors, particularly lymphomas, leukemias, and breast cancer, have a predilection to seed the leptomeninges, often sparing brain and spinal cord parenchyma. The tumor may be microscopic or can cause mass lesions within the subarachnoid space. The leptomeninges may be the only site of relapse in patients with treated leukemia and breast cancer. Malignant cells can reach the leptomeninges (1) by direct extension from a brain or spinal cord tumor (surgically treated posterior fossa metastases being particularly likely to lead to subsequent leptomeningeal dissemination); (2) by the arterial circulation; (3) by veins from bone marrow of the skull or vertebral bodies; or (4) by growth along cranial or peripheral nerves into the subarachnoid space. Once cells have reached the subarachnoid space, they can be disseminated by CSF flow. Approximately 8% of cancer patients have leptomeningeal metastases at autopsy, and the incidence appears to be increasing.

CLINICAL FINDINGS

Leptomeningeal metastases cause their clinical symptoms in one of several ways. They may obstruct CSF pathways, leading to hydrocephalus with increased ICP and symptoms of headache and cognitive decline. Also, they may invade the Virchow-Robin spaces (the spaces through which penetrating pial arteries enter the brain) and interfere with the blood supply of the brain, causing symptoms of brain ischemia. Additionally, they may invade cranial or peripheral nerves within the subarachnoid space, causing neuropathy with the attendant symptoms of pain, paralysis, and sensory loss. Finally, they may irritate the leptomeninges, causing symptoms reminiscent of a chronic meningitis with headache, nuchal rigidity, and pain on straight-leg raising (thus, the term *carcinomatous meningitis*). Because of widespread involvement within the CNS, symptoms may involve virtually any portion of the neuraxis, either alone or in combination.

The diagnosis is established in one of two ways. MRI scans may demonstrate enhancement of the leptomeninges, ventricular surface, cranial nerves, or spinal roots. The enhancement may be linear, resembling blood vessels, or ventricular or subarachnoid masses may be seen. In the appropriate setting, such findings are diagnostic of leptomeningeal metastases. Examination of CSF may yield either malignant cells on cytologic examination (diagnostic of leptomeningeal metastases) or positive biochemical tumor markers (which may be diagnostic in the appropriate setting). Distinguishing leptomeningeal leukemia or lymphoma from inflammatory disorders of the nervous system may be difficult; both false-positive and false-negative results may complicate cytologic diagnosis of these tumors. However, the presence of clonal lymphoid cells within the CSF is diagnostic. Inflammatory cells are virtually all T cells. B cells are present only when the meninges are invaded by B-cell tumors.

With regard to solid tumors invading the leptomeninges, the initial cytologic evaluation is positive in only some 50% of patients. Though false-negative findings are common, false-positive results almost never occur. When cytologic examination is negative, such tumor markers as carcinoembryonic antigen and prostate-specific antigen help to establish the diagnosis of leptomeningeal invasion. Other markers, such as β-glucuronidase, lactic acid (or lactate) dehydrogenase, and β_2-microglobulin, are found in patients with both leptomeningeal tumors and inflammatory lesions and thus are less diagnostically helpful.

TREATMENT

Corticosteroids sometimes relieve symptoms transiently, but they play a minor role in the treatment of leptomeningeal tumor except for tumors that are intrinsically responsive to corticosteroids (e.g., breast cancer, leukemia, and lymphoma). Whole neuraxial irradiation compromises the bone marrow and decreases affected patients' ability to tolerate further chemotherapy. Intrathecal drugs, particularly methotrexate and cytarabine, are effective in treating meningeal leukemia and lymphoma and have some effect on such solid tumors as breast cancer. However, for most other tumors, response to therapy is minimal. Some evidence suggests that a slow-release preparation of cytarabine is more effective and less toxic than is methotrexate. Because leptomeningeal tumors disrupt the blood-brain barrier, parenteral treatment with high-dose chemotherapy (i.e., high-dose methotrexate with leucovorin rescue) may ameliorate the symptoms of leptomeningeal metastases in some instances. Newer techniques, including monoclonal antibodies conjugated with radionuclides, are being tested, but the response to treatment of leptomeningeal tumors, particularly from solid tumors, usually is poor.

REFERENCES

1. Bleyer WA, Sposto R, Sather H. In the United States, pediatric brain tumors and other nervous system tumors (NST) are now more common than childhood acute lymphoblastic leukemia (ALL) and have a 3-fold greater national mortality rate (abstract). *Proc Am Soc Clin Oncol* 17:1498, 1998.
2. Riggs JE. Rising primary malignant brain tumor mortality in the elderly. A manifestation of differential survival. *Arch Neurol* 52:571–575, 1995.
3. Smith MA, Freidlin B, Ries LAG, et al. Trends in reported incidence of primary malignant brain tumors in children in the United States. *J Natl Cancer Inst* 90:1269–1277, 1998.
4. Schulder M, Maldjian JA, Liu WC, et al. Functional image-guided surgery of intracranial tumors located in or near the sensorimotor cortex. *J Neurosurg* 89:412–418, 1998.
5. Davis FG, Freels S, Grutsch J, et al. Survival rates in patients with primary malignant brain tumors stratified by patient age and tumor histological type: an analysis based on Surveillance, Epidemiology, and End Results (SEER) data, 1973–1991. *J Neurosurg* 88:1–10, 1998.
6. Levin VA. *Cancer in the Nervous System.* New York: Churchill Livingstone, 1996:474.
7. Black PM, Loeffler JS. *Cancer of the Nervous System.* Cambridge, MA: Blackwell, 1997:935.
8. Kaye AH, Laws JER. *Brain Tumors.* New York: Churchill Livingstone, 1995:990.
9. Posner JB. *Neurologic Complications of Cancer.* Philadelphia: Davis, 1995:482.
10. Vecht CJ. *Handbook of Clinical Neurology.* New York: Elsevier, 1997.
11. Boulton M, Armstrong D, Flessner M, et al. Raised intracranial pressure increases CSF drainage through arachnoid villi and extracranial lymphatics. *Am J Physiol* 275:R889–R896, 1998.
12. Albert FK, Forsting M, Sartor K, et al. Early postoperative magnetic resonance imaging after resection of malignant glioma: objective evaluation of residual tumor and its influence on regrowth and prognosis. *Neurosurgery* 34:45–61, 1994.
13. Greenlee RT, Murray T, Bolden S, Wingo PA. Cancer statistics, 2000. *CA Cancer J Clin* 50:7–33, 2000.
14. Radhakrishnan K, Mokri B, Parisi JE, et al. The trends in incidence of primary brain tumors in the population of Rochester, Minnesota. *Ann Neurol* 37:67–73, 1995.
15. Werner MH, Phuphanich S, Lyman GH. The increasing incidence of malignant gliomas and primary central nervous system lymphoma in the elderly. *Cancer* 76:1634–1642, 1995.
16. Kleihues P, Burger PC, Scheithauer BW. *Histological Typing of Tumours of the Central Nervous System* (2nd ed). Berlin: Springer, 1993:112.
17. Pollak L, Walach N, Gur R, et al. Meningiomas after radiotherapy for tinea capitis—still no history. *Tumori* 84:65–68, 1998.
18. Goedert JJ, Cote TR, Virgo P, et al. Spectrum of AIDS-associated malignant disorders. *Lancet* 351:1833–1839, 1998.
19. Salvatore JR, Weitberg AB, Mehta S. Nonionizing electromagnetic fields and cancer: a review. *Oncology* 10:563–574, 1996.
20. Kaplan S, Novikov I, Modan B. Nutritional factors in the etiology of brain tumors—potential role of nitrosamines, fat, and cholesterol. *Am J Epidemiol* 146:832–841, 1997.
21. Lee M, Wrensch M, Mike R. Dietary and tobacco risk factors for adult onset glioma in the San Francisco Bay Area (California, USA). *Cancer Causes Control* 8:13–24, 1997.
22. Olney JW, Farber NB, Spitznagel E, et al. Increasing brain tumor rates: is there a link to aspartame? *J Neuropathol Exp Neurol* 55:1115–1123, 1996.
23. Rodvall Y, Ahlbom A, Spannare B, et al. Glioma and occupational exposure in Sweden, a case-control study. *Occup Environ Med* 53:526–537, 1996.
24. Bohnen NI, Kurland LT. Brain tumor and exposure to pesticides in humans: a review of the epidemiologic data. *J Neurol Sci* 132:110–121, 1995.
25. Pogoda JM, Preston-Martin S. Household pesticides and

risk of pediatric brain tumors. *Environ Health Perspect* 105:1214–1220, 1997.

26. Inskip PD, Mellemkjaer L, Gridley G, et al. Incidence of intracranial tumors following hospitalization for head injuries (Denmark). *Cancer Causes Control* 9:109–116, 1998.

27. Del Brutto OH, Castillo PR, Mena IX, et al. Neurocysticercosis among patients with cerebral gliomas. *Arch Neurol* 54:1125–1128, 1997.

28. Wrensch M, Weinberg A, Wiencke J, et al. Does prior infection with varicella-zoster virus influence risk of adult glioma? *Am J Epidemiol* 145:594–597, 1997.

29. Huang HT, Reis R, Yonekawa Y, et al. Identification in human brain tumors of DNA sequences specific for SV40 large T antigen. *Brain Pathol* 9:33–42, 1999.

30. Ron E, Modan B, Boice JD Jr, et al. Tumors of the brain and nervous system after radiotherapy in childhood. *N Engl J Med* 319:1033–1039, 1988.

31. Tomlinson GE. Familial cancer syndromes and genetic counseling. *Cancer Treat Res* 92:63–97, 1997.

32. Young J, Povey S. The genetic basis of tuberous sclerosis. *Mol Med Today* 4:313–319, 1998.

33. Gutmann DH, Aylsworth A, Carey JC, et al. The diagnostic evaluation and multidisciplinary management of neurofibromatosis 1 and neurofibromatosis 2. *JAMA* 278:51–57, 1997.

34. Feldkamp MM, Gutmann DH, Guha A. Neurofibromatosis type 1: piecing the puzzle together. *Can J Neurol Sci* 25:181–191, 1998.

35. Pollack IF, Mulvihill JJ. Neurofibromatosis 1 and 2. *Brain Pathol* 7:823–836, 1997.

36. Asa SL, Somers K, Ezzat S. The MEN-1 gene is rarely down-regulated in pituitary adenomas. *J Clin Endocrinol Metab* 83:3210–3212, 1998.

37. Mulligan G, Jacks T. The retinoblastoma gene family: cousins with overlapping interests. *Trends Genet* 14:223–229, 1998.

38. Wicking C, Bale AE. Molecular basis of the nevoid basal cell carcinoma syndrome. *Curr Opin Pediatr* 9:630–635, 1997.

39. Foulkes WD. A tale of four syndromes: familial adenomatous polyposis, Gardner syndrome, attenuated APC and Turcot syndrome. *Q J Med* 88:853–863, 1995.

40. Decker HJ, Weidt EJ, Brieger J. The von Hippel-Lindau tumor suppressor gene. A rare and intriguing disease opening new insight into basic mechanisms of carcinogenesis. *Cancer Genet Cytogenet* 93:74–83, 1997.

41. Eng C. Genetics of Cowden syndrome: through the looking glass of oncology. *Int J Oncol* 12:701–710, 1998.

42. Sevenet N, Sheridan E, Amram D, et al. Constitutional mutations of the *hSNF5/INI1* gene predispose to a variety of cancers. *Am J Hum Genet* 65:1342–1348, 1999.

43. Ikizler Y, Van Meyel DJ, Ramsay DA, et al. Gliomas in families. *Can J Neurol Sci* 19:492–497, 1992.

44. Forsyth PA, Posner JB. Headaches in patients with brain tumors: a study of 111 patients. *Neurology* 43:1678–1683, 1993.

45. Gilman S. Imaging the brain. Second of two parts. *N Engl J Med* 338:889–896, 1998.

46. Hall WA. The safety and efficacy of stereotactic biopsy for intracranial lesions. *Cancer* 82:1749–1755, 1998.

47. Glantz MJ, Cole BF, Friedberg MH, et al. A randomized, blinded, placebo-controlled trial of divalproex sodium prophylaxis in adults with newly diagnosed brain tumors. *Neurology* 46:985–991, 1996.

48. Grossman SA, Hochberg F, Fisher J, et al. Increased 9-aminocamptothecin dose requirements in patients on anticonvulsants. *Cancer Chemother Pharmacol* 42:118–126, 1998.

49. De Santis A, Baratta P, Bello L, et al. Early postoperative seizures and endovenous phenytoin. Preliminary clinical data. *J Neurosurg Sci* 40:207–212, 1996.

50. Chang SD, Adler JR Jr, Hancock SL. Clinical uses of radiosurgery. *Oncology* 12:1181–1191, 1998.

51. Krengli M, Liebsch NJ, Hug EB, et al. Review of current protocols for proton therapy in USA. *Tumori* 84:209–216, 1998.

52. Reddick WE, Mulhern RK, Elkin TD, et al. A hybrid neural network analysis of subtle brain volume differences in children surviving brain tumors. *Magn Reson Imaging* 16:413–421, 1998.

53. Huncharek M, Muscat J. Treatment of recurrent high-grade astrocytoma: results of a systematic review of 1,415 patients. *Anticancer Res* 18:1303–1311, 1998.

54. Polednak AP, Flannery JT. Brain, other central nervous system, and eye cancer. *Cancer* 75:330–337, 1995.

55. Fleury A, Menegoz F, Grosclaude P, et al. Descriptive epidemiology of cerebral gliomas in France. *Cancer* 79:1195–1202, 1997.

56. Merzak A, Pilkington GJ. Molecular and cellular pathology of intrinsic brain tumours. *Cancer Metastasis Rev* 16:155–177, 1997.

57. Chicoine MR, Silbergeld DL. The in vitro motility of human gliomas increases with increasing grade of malignancy. *Cancer* 75:2904–2909, 1995.

58. Wesseling P, Ruiter DJ, Burger PC. Angiogenesis in brain tumors; pathobiological and clinical aspects. *J Neurooncol* 32:253–265, 1997.

59. Roberts WG, Palade GE. Neovasculature induced by vascular endothelial growth factor is fenestrated. *Cancer Res* 57:765–772, 1997.

60. Leeds NE, Jackson EF. Current imaging techniques for the evaluation of brain neoplasms. *Curr Opin Oncol* 6:254–261, 1994.

61. Roelcke U. PET: brain tumor biochemistry. *J Neurooncol* 22:275–279, 1994.

62. Preul MC, Caramanos Z, Collins DL, et al. Accurate noninvasive diagnosis of human brain tumors by using magnetic resonance spectroscopy. *Nature Med* 2:323–325, 1996.

63. Scott JN, Rewcastle NB, Brasher PMA, et al. Long-term glioblastoma multiforme survivors: a population–based study. *Can J Neurol Sci* 25:197–201, 1998.

64. Morreale VM, Ebersold MJ, Quast LM, et al. Cerebellar astrocytoma: experience with 54 cases surgically treated at the Mayo Clinic, Rochester, Minnesota, from 1978 to 1990. *J Neurosurg* 87:257–261, 1997.

65. Tonn JC, Paulus W, Warmuth-Metz M, et al. Pleomorphic xanthoastrocytoma: report of six cases with special consideration of diagnostic and therapeutic pitfalls. *Surg Neurol* 47:162–169, 1997.

66. Shepherd CW, Scheithauer BW, Gomez MR, et al. Subependymal giant cell astrocytoma: a clinical, pathological, and flow cytometric study. *Neurosurgery* 28:864–868, 1991.

67. Brandes AA, Fiorentino MV. Clinical, pathological and therapeutic aspects of oligodendroglioma. *Cancer Treat Rev* 24:101–111, 1998.

68. McLaughlin MP, Marcus RB Jr, Buatti JM, et al. Ependymoma: results, prognostic factors and treatment recommendations. *Int J Radiat Oncol Biol Phys* 40:845–850, 1998.

69. Schiff D, Wen PY. Uncommon brain tumors. *Neurol Clin* 13:953–974, 1995.

70. Gultekin SH, Dalmau J, Graus Y, et al. Anti-Hu immunolabeling as an index of neuronal differentiation in human brain tumors—a study of 112 central neuroepithelial neoplasms. *Am J Surg Pathol* 22(2):195–200, 1998.

71. Rumana CS, Valadka AB. Radiation therapy and malignant degeneration of benign supratentorial gangliogliomas. *Neurosurgery* 42:1038–1043, 1998.

72. Schild SE, Scheithauer BW, Haddock MG, et al. Histologically confirmed pineal tumors and other germ cell tumors of the brain. *Cancer* 78:2564–2571, 1996.

73. Aoyama H, Shirato H, Kakuto Y, et al. Pathologically proven intracranial germinoma treated with radiation therapy. *Radiother Oncol* 47:201–205, 1998.

74. Chang SM, Lillis-Hearne PK, Larson DA, et al. Pineoblastoma in adults. *Neurosurgery* 37(3):383–390, 1995.

75. Provias JP, Becker LE. Cellular and molecular pathology of medulloblastoma. *J Neurooncol* 29:35–43, 1996.

76. Le QT, Weil MD, Wara WM, et al. Adult medulloblastoma: an analysis of survival and prognostic factors. *Cancer J Sci Am* 3:238–245, 1997.

77. Pollock BE, Lunsford LD, Norén G. Vestibular schwannoma management in the next century: a radiosurgical perspective. *Neurosurgery* 43:475–481, 1998.

78. Markopoulos C, Sampalis F, Givalos N, et al. Association of breast cancer with meningioma. *Eur J Surg Oncol* 24:332–334, 1998.

79. Kondziolka D, Flickinger JC, Perez B, et al. Judicious resection and/or radiosurgery for parasagittal meningiomas: outcomes from a multicenter review. *Neurosurgery* 43:405–413, 1998.

80. Ono Y, Ueki K, Joseph JT, Louis DN. Homozygous deletions of the CDKN2/p16 gene in dural hemangiopericytomas. *Acta Neuropathol (Berl)* 91(3):221–225, 1996.

81. Richard S, Campello C, Taillandier L, et al. Haemangioblastoma of the central nervous system in von Hippel-Lindau disease. French VHL Study Group. *J Intern Med* 243:547–553, 1998.

82. Chang SD, Meisel JA, Hancock SL, et al. Treatment of hemangioblastomas in von Hippel-Lindau disease with linear accelerator-based radiosurgery. *Neurosurgery* 43:28–34, 1998.

83. DeAngelis LM. Current management of primary central nervous system lymphoma. *Oncology (Huntingt)* 9:63–71, 1995.

84. Nassar SI, Haddad FS, Abdo A. Epidermoid tumors of the fourth ventricle. *Surg Neurol* 43:246–251, 1995.

85. Kallmes DF, Provenzale JM, Cloft HJ, et al. Typical and atypical MR imaging features of intracranial epidermoid tumors. *AJR Am J Roentgenol* 169:883–887, 1997.

86. Nagele T, Klose U, Grodd W, et al. Three-dimensional chemical shift-selective MRI of a ruptured intracranial dermoid cyst. *Neuroradiology* 38:572–574, 1996.

87. Mathiesen T, Grane P, Lindgren L, et al. Third ventricle colloid cysts: a consecutive 12-year series. *J Neurosurg* 86:5–12, 1997.

88. Shemie S, Jay V, Rutka J, et al. Acute obstructive hydrocephalus and sudden death in children. *Ann Emerg Med* 29:524–528, 1997.

89. Bunin GR, Surawicz TS, Witman PA, et al. The descriptive epidemiology of craniopharyngioma. *J Neurosurg* 89:547–551, 1998.

90. Breteau N, Demasure M, Lescrainier J, et al. Sacrococcygeal chordomas: potential role of high LET therapy. *Recent Results Cancer Res* 150:148–155, 1998.

91. Buatti JM, Marcus RB. Pituitary adenomas: current methods of diagnosis and treatment. *Oncology* 11:791–803, 1997.

92. Teramoto A, Hirakawa K, Sanno N, et al. Incidental pituitary lesions in 1000 unselected autopsy specimens. *Radiology* 193:161–164, 1994.

93. Sano T, Kovacs KT, Scheithauer BW, et al. Aging and the human pituitary gland. *Mayo Clin Proc* 68:971–977, 1993.

94. Kovacs K, Scheithauer BW, Horvath E, et al. The World Health Organization classification of adenohypophysial neoplasms. *Cancer* 78:502–510, 1996.

95. Blevins LS. Aggressive pituitary tumors. *Oncology* 12:1307–1316, 1998.

96. Shimon I, Melmed S. Genetic basis of endocrine disease: pituitary tumor pathogenesis. *J Clin Endocrinol Metab* 82:1675–1681, 1997.

97. Guru SC, Manickam P, Crabtree JS, et al. Identification and characterization of the multiple endocrine neoplasia type 1 (MEN1) gene. *J Intern Med* 243:433–439, 1998.

98. Shimon I, Melmed S. Genetic basis of endocrine disease: pituitary tumor pathogenesis. *J Clin Endocrinol Metab* 82:1675–1681, 1997.

99. Lamberts SW, De Herder WW, Van der Lely AJ. Pituitary insufficiency. *Lancet* 352:127–134, 1998.

100. Wiren L, Bengtsson BA, Johannsson G. Beneficial effects of long-term GH replacement therapy on quality of life in adults with GH deficiency. *Clin Endocrinol (Oxf)* 48:613–620, 1998.

101. Rolih CA, Ober KP. Pituitary apoplexy. *Endocrinol Metab Clin North Am* 22:291–302, 1993.

102. Nakasu Y, Itoh R, Nakasu S, et al. Postoperative sella: evaluation with fast spin echo T$_2$-weighted high-resolution imaging. *Neurosurgery* 43:440–446, 1998.

103. Morita A, Meyer FB, Laws ER Jr. Symptomatic pituitary metastases. *J Neurosurg* 89:69–73, 1998.

104. Honegger J, Fahlbusch R, Bornemann A, et al. Lymphocytic and granulomatous hypophysitis: experience with nine cases. *Neurosurgery* 40:713–722, 1997.

105. Thodou E, Asa SL, Kontogeorgos G, et al. Clinical case seminar: lymphocytic hypophysitis: clinicopathological findings. *J Clin Endocrinol Metab* 80:2302–2311, 1995.

106. Webster J, Piscitelli G, Polli A, et al. A comparison of cabergoline and bromocriptine in the treatment of hyper-

prolactinemic amenorrhea. *N Engl J Med* 331:904–909, 1994.

107. Newman CB, Melmed S, George A, et al. Octreotide as primary therapy for acromegaly. *J Clin Endocrinol Metab* 83:3034–3040, 1998.

108. Simmons NE, Laws ER Jr. Glioma occurrence after sellar irradiation: case report and review. *Neurosurgery* 42:172–178, 1998.

109. Lillehei KO, Kirschman DL, Kleinschmidt-DeMasters BK, et al. Reassessment of the role of radiation therapy in the treatment of endocrine-inactive pituitary macroadenomas. *Neurosurgery* 43:432–438, 1998.

110. Yoon SC, Suh TS, Jang HS, et al. Clinical results of 24 pituitary macroadenomas with linac-based stereotactic radiosurgery. *Int J Radiat Oncol Biol Phys* 41:849–853, 1998.

111. Muratori M, Arosio M, Gambino G, et al. Use of cabergoline in the long-term treatment of hyperprolactinemic and acromegalic patients. *J Endocrinol Invest* 20:537–546, 1997.

112. Colao A, Di Sarno A, Landi ML, et al. Long-term and low-dose treatment with cabergoline induces macroprolactinoma shrinkage. *J Clin Endocrinol Metab* 82:3574–3579, 1997.

113. Bevan JS, Adams CBT, Burke CW, et al. Factors in the outcome of transsphenoidal surgery for prolactinoma and non-functioning pituitary tumour, including pre-operative bromocriptine therapy. *Clin Endocrinol (Oxf)* 26:541–556, 1997.

114. Freda PU, Wardlaw SL, Post K. Long-term endocrinological follow-up evaluation in 115 patients who underwent transsphenoidal surgery for acromegaly. *J Neurosurg* 89:353–358, 1998.

115. Estrada J, Boronat M, Mielgo M, et al. The long-term outcome of pituitary irradiation after unsuccessful transsphenoidal surgery in Cushing's disease. *N Engl J Med* 336:172–177, 1997.

116. Young Jr WF, Scheithauer BW, Kovacs KT, et al. Gonadotroph adenoma of the pituitary gland: a clinicaopathologic analysis of 100 cases. *Mayo Clin Proc* 71:649–656, 1996.

117. Gittoes NJ, Bates AS, Tse W, et al. Radiotherapy for non-function pituitary tumours. *Clin Endocrinol (Oxf)* 48:331–337, 1998.

118. Tsang RW, Brierley JD, Panzarella T, et al. Radiation therapy for pituitary adenoma: treatment outcome and prognostic factors. *Int J Radiat Oncol Biol Phys* 30:557–565, 1994.

119. Cheung AYC, Sligh T, Bauserman S, et al. Evaluation of modern pathologic nomenclature, tumor imaging and treatment of pituitary adenomas in a recent surgical series. *J Neurooncol* 37:145–153, 1998.

120. Byrne TN, Waxman SG. *Spinal Cord Compression. Diagnosis and Principles of Management.* Philadelphia: Davis, 1990.

121. Boriani S, Weinstein JN, Biagini R. Primary bone tumors of the spine. Terminology and surgical staging. *Spine* 22:1036–1044, 1997.

122. Muthukumar N, Kondziolka D, Lunsford LD, et al. Stereotactic radiosurgery for chordoma and chondrosarcoma: further experiences. *Int J Radiat Oncol Biol Phys* 41:387–392, 1998.

123. Breteau N, Demasure M, Lescrainier J, et al. Sacrococcygeal chordomas: potential role of high LET therapy. *Recent Results Cancer Res* 150:148–155, 1998.

124. Seppala MT, Sainio MA, Haltia MJ, et al. Multiple schwannomas: schwannomatosis or neurofibromatosis type 2? *J Neurosurg* 89:36–41, 1998.

125. Moran CA, Rush W, Mena H. Primary spinal paragangliomas: a clinicopathological and immunohistochemical study of 30 cases. *Histopathology* 31:167–173, 1997.

126. Patchell RA, Tibbs PA, Walsh JW. A randomized trial of surgery in the treatment of single metastases to the brain. *N Engl J Med* 322:494–500, 1990.

127. Patchell RA, Tibbs PA, Regine WF, et al. Postoperative radiotherapy in the treatment of single metastases to the brain: a randomized trial. *JAMA* 280(17):1485–1489, 1998.

128. Seung SK, Sneed PK, McDermott MW, et al. Gamma knife radiosurgery for malignant melanoma brain metastases. *Cancer J Sci Am* 4(2):103–109, 1998.

129. Flickinger JC, Kondziolka D, Lunsford LD, et al. A multi-institutional experience with stereotactic radiosurgery for solitary brain metastasis. *Int J Radiat Oncol Biol Phys* 28:797–802, 1994.

130. Bindal AK, Bindal RK, Hess KR, et al. Surgery versus radiosurgery in the treatment of brain metastasis. *J Neurosurg* 84:748–754, 1996.

131. Schiff D, Shaw EG, Cascino TL. Outcome after spinal re-irradiation for malignant epidural spinal cord compression. *Ann Neurol* 37:583–589, 1995.

29

Malignant Tumors of the Eye

■ ■ ■

John E. Lahaniatis

Luther W. Brady

Jorge E. Freire

Jerry A. Shields

Carol L. Shields

Theodore E. Yaeger

THE AMERICAN CANCER SOCIETY ESTIMATES that in 2000, 2,200 new malignant tumors will involve the structures of the eye. Of these tumors, 75% will be choroidal melanomas, 20% will be retinoblastomas, and the remainder will be other tumors involving the orbit. However, the most common malignant tumor involving the eye is a metastasis: As patients are living longer because of more appropriate and proper systemic management, more patients are developing metastases to the orbit or to the choroid of the eye.

In general, radiotherapy is an extremely effective means for managing tumors involving the eye. Although surgery plays an important role in managing ocular tumors, numerous tumor sites also respond well to radiotherapy (e.g., choroidal melanomas).

OCULAR MALIGNANCIES
Eyelid Carcinomas

Basal cell and squamous cell carcinomas of the eyelid are managed effectively by surgical excision as first-line therapy or by radiotherapy, with an acceptable cosmesis as a consequence of treatment [1]. In radiotherapy, overall cure rates of 90% or better are achieved by using 45 to 60 Gy with electron beams or low-energy x-ray beams. This modality necessitates appropriate shielding to protect the underlying lens and other orbital structures [2]. Surgical excision gives similar cure rates but may produce more cosmetic defects. Cryotherapy is used in certain circumstances.

Meibomian Gland Carcinoma

Meibomian gland carcinomas are sebaceous gland carcinomas that may be multicentric and frequently recur after primary management. Surgery is considered first-line treatment in such management, with cryotherapy often used as a second-line alternative to surgery. Radiotherapy provides acceptable cosmesis both for primary treatment and for treatment of recurrent disease. Somewhat higher irradiation dosages in the range of 60 to 65 Gy in six to seven weeks are recommended, and the control rates are in the range of 80% to 90% or better.

UVEAL TUMORS

Metastatic Tumors of the Posterior Uvea

Carcinoma that metastasizes to the eye is the most common malignant disease involving the eye. Metastatic uveal lesions account for 15% of such cases, and the most common primary sites are breast or lung in women and lung or gastrointestinal tract in men. Most frequently, uveal metastases are unifocal, although multifocal disease within the same eye is fairly common. Metastatic uveal tumors can cause visual symptoms that necessitate treatment; hence, the aim of that therapy should be control of the tumor with return of visual function to affected patients. An important factor in the treatment decision is to differentiate among single metastatic tumors of the posterior uvea with no evidence of systemic disease; single lesions with active systemic disease; and multiple lesions with active systemic disease or no active systemic disease. In more favorable circumstances (i.e., inactive or no systemic disease), the treatment decision should be more aggressive in character as opposed to that for patients with active systemic disease calling for a more conservative course of treatment. In most instances, metastatic lesions to the posterior uvea are not treated as effectively by systemic chemotherapy alone; therefore, radiotherapy should be a part of this general management [2].

For those with active systemic disease, the recommended treatment is palliative irradiation in the range of 30 to 35 Gy over a three-week period to the entire ocular structure. However, in the absence of active systemic disease and in patients with anticipated long-term survival, the more aggressive approach of delivering 45 to 50 Gy in 4.5 to 5.5 weeks in 1.8 to 2.0 Gy per fraction is required. This treatment program can be delivered to include all the tumor, as determined using contrast-enhanced computed tomography or contrast-enhanced magnetic resonance imaging and shielding the normal structures to the greatest degree possible. Long-term control can be achieved using this approach to the prob-

lem. The efficacy of chemotherapy for metastatic neoplasms involving the uvea is largely unknown. Many patients receiving chemotherapy for metastatic disease may have clinically undetected uveal metastases that respond to chemotherapy.

Malignant Melanoma of the Posterior Uvea

Malignant melanomas of the posterior uvea represent 75% of primary malignant tumors involving the eye. Usually, melanoma involving the anterior uvea is detected earlier than melanomas involving the posterior uvea. Anterior uveal melanomas may be removed by iridectomy or iridocyclectomy.

Traditionally, posterior uveal melanomas have been treated by enucleation of the affected eye. Some investigators have raised questions as to the role for this treatment technique because it may promote seeding of tumor cells, thereby affecting affected patients' prognosis. Brachytherapy techniques using such varied radioactive sources as ^{60}Co, ^{125}I, ^{192}Ir, ^{198}Au seeds, and ^{109}Ru have been used, producing effective and positive results in the treatment of malignant melanomas of the posterior uvea [1–7]. In general, radioactive plaque radiotherapy should be used to treat (1) selected medium-sized melanomas that are growing, with an emphasis on the potential for preservation of vision, (2) medium-sized choroidal and ciliary body melanomas, and (3) an actively growing tumor in an affected patient's only useful eye. Transpupillary thermotherapy is an alternative modality for treating small choroidal melanomas.

For tumors that exceed 15 mm in diameter and 10 mm in thickness, enucleation with or without preoperative radiotherapy is preferred. However, some evidence suggests that preoperative irradiation is not helpful.

The ultimate visual outcome of treatment with radiotherapy depends on tumor size and the location relative to the fovea or the optic disk. Large tumors or those in the proximity to the fovea or optic disk place patients at high risk of radiation retinopathy and papillopathy after treatment. Radiation doses higher than 50 Gy delivered to the fovea or the optic disk present an increased risk of visual loss [5]. More recently, combined plaque irradiation and laser photocoagulation have been used to increase local control, particularly in those circumstances in which the tumors are close to the optic disk. (For a discussion of radiotherapeutic techniques, see Chapter 8.)

Large ocular melanomas or tumors with extrascleral

extension at diagnosis preferably are treated by exenteration of the orbit, as opposed to radiotherapy or simple enucleation [2].

Shields et al. [8] reported local control rates of 93% in patients with nonresectable, diffuse iris melanoma treated with custom-designed ^{125}I plaques. Similar overall local control rates have been reported in treating malignant melanomas of the posterior uvea in other locations.

RETINAL TUMORS

Retinoblastoma is the most common intraocular malignancy in children and constitutes approximately 20% to 25% of all primary malignant tumors of the eye. Some 600 new cases were recorded in 1999, according to data from the American Cancer Society. Retinoblastomas are bilateral in one-third of affected patients and are unilateral in two-thirds of patients. These tumors are hereditary in approximately 40% of diagnosed cases and are transmitted as an autosomal dominant trait (i.e., the "two-hit" hypothesis) [6]. The genetic abnormality involves deletion or mutation of the tumor suppressor gene *RB*, on the long arm of chromosome 13.

In general, the hereditary form is diagnosed earlier than is the nonhereditary form of the disease. Most patients with the hereditary form have bilateral disease. In most affected children, this tumor is diagnosed before the age of three to four years, presenting with leukokoria (white papillary reflex), strabismus, and a mass in the fundus. In general, these findings are noted as early as 6 to 24 months of age. Diagnostic workup should be complete, including recording of a history, physical examination and complete ophthalmologic examination with retinal drawings and photographs, ultrasonography for documentation of the tumor location and size, and cranial contrast-enhanced computed tomography. Routine cerebrospinal fluid study and bone marrow examination are not recommended except in the presence of signs and symptoms suggesting extraocular extension.

Factors that carry a poor prognosis include invasion of the choroid, involvement of the optic nerve, involvement of the scleral emissary veins and episcleral tissues, and central nervous system dissemination. The grouping system used most widely for retinoblastoma is that described by Reese and Ellsworth (see Chapter 25, under "Retinoblastoma") [9].

The primary goals for therapy are both cure and preservation of vision. In large measure, past treatment regimens have relied on enucleation in the unilateral eye when the eye is blind or enucleation of the more severely affected eye in bilateral disease. However, more emphasis recently is being placed on radiotherapeutic techniques for early disease, and chemotherapy prior to radiotherapy for late disease. Still, indications for enucleation include glaucoma after rubeosis iridis, with visual loss and tumor recurrence not amenable to more conservative therapy.

When the eye contains group I or group II tumors, external-beam radiotherapy using meticulous lens-sparing technology can preserve vision with minimal complications in almost all cases. In more advanced tumors, preservation of vision with external-beam radiotherapy drops to 79% in group III, 70% in group IV, and 29% in group V [6].

Radioactive plaque therapy offers a viable option for local treatment of retinoblastoma. Various sources have been used, including ^{60}Co, ^{125}I, ^{192}Ir, and [109]Ru. The advantages of ^{125}I plaque therapy are its physical properties of low energy, adequate dose distribution, and ease of shielding, which contributes to a decreased radiation dose to the opposite eye, to personnel, and to the surrounding orbital structures. Recommended dosages are 45 to 50 Gy to the tumor apex and 35 to 40 Gy if radiotherapy is combined with chemotherapy. In a series reporting 91 cases of recurrent or residual retinoblastoma, Shields et al. [10] reported a tumor control and salvage rate of 89% with ^{125}I plaque therapy involving a mean dose of 41 Gy to the apex of the tumor and a mean follow-up of 52 months. Recent investigations have shown encouraging results with multidrug chemotherapy in conjunction with local therapy, such as irradiation, radioactive plaque placement, and laser photocoagulation. The potential problem of second neoplasms after chemoirradiation remains open, as the risk of second malignancy is increased.

OPTIC NERVE GLIOMA

Optic nerve glioma is more common in children younger than 15 years and accounts for approximately 1% of all central nervous system tumors. More than 50% of the cases involve the optic chiasm. These tumors grow slowly and can cause visual defects, proptosis, optic atrophy, and nystagmus. Completeness of surgical excision correlates with survival, but intracranial surgery alone produces very low survival rates and major losses of vision.

Radiotherapy is indicated when intracranial or progressive symptoms are present. With careful treatment-planning techniques, dosages of 50 Gy in 5 to 5.5 weeks with 1.8 to 2.0 Gy per fraction can be delivered in adults, and 45 Gy in 4.5 to 5 weeks with 1.8 to 2.0 Gy per fraction can be delivered to children younger than 15; such treatment produces excellent preservation of vision and excellent control of tumors. Such tumors are indolent in character, and long-term survival ranging from 80% to 100% is achieved with radiotherapy. Complications related to calcification, necrosis, and chiasmal damage are rare. However, endocrine disorders in children are frequent. Chemotherapy does not play an established role in treatment of this disorder.

ORBITAL TUMORS
Rhabdomyosarcoma

Most often, rhabdomyosarcoma of the orbit is seen in young children, having a rapid onset with marked proptosis and swelling of the adnexal tissue. In the past, orbital exenteration was the recommended treatment, as many ophthalmologists thought that the tumor was not radioresponsive. However, this tumor has proved to be very radioresponsive, and currently the recommendation for management is combined-modality treatment consisting of radiotherapy and chemotherapy initially. Surgical intervention is limited to biopsy or local excision. Radiotherapy alone can result in local tumor control rates of approximately 90% and, when combined with chemotherapy, can produce five-year disease-free survivals of 90% or better. Thus, such combination therapy is preferred.

Malignant Orbital Lymphoma

Orbital lymphoma may be the only manifestation of lymphoma or may be a part of a generalized systemic disease process. The staging workup should be the same as that used for any patient with non-Hodgkin's lymphoma at other sites. Radiotherapy alone results in excellent local tumor control [4]. When the disease process is part of a generalized disease process, radiotherapy should be combined with chemotherapy. Radiotherapy doses in the range of 30 to 45 Gy administered in conventional fractionation are recommended for treatment of localized orbital lymphoma.

Lacrimal Gland Tumors

Lacrimal gland tumors tend to invade the surrounding orbital bone, rendering surgical resections difficult. The mortality associated with these tumors highlights radiotherapy as an important part of the treatment program to reduce postoperative recurrences. Tumor doses of 50 to 60 Gy are necessary, depending on the size of the lesion. When tumors have been excised completely, with all margins clear of tumor, no further treatment is indicated beyond case follow-up.

SEQUELAE OF TREATMENT

Skin changes resulting from radiotherapy include erythema, depigmentation, atrophy, and telangiectasia. Loss of eyebrows or eyelashes may or may not ensue, depending on whether they are included in the treatment field. Scalp hair loss may occur at the exit area of the external-beam portal, but this loss generally is transient and is followed by hair regrowth. Direct corneal injury may occur with irradiation doses of 48 Gy or higher. Reversible epithelial changes with minimal stromal damage can occur at doses of less than 48 Gy but are uncommon.

Radiation-induced cataract is of significant concern in radiotherapy treatment of the eye. A single dose of 2 Gy or a fractionated dose of 8 Gy at the level of the lens can significantly increase the risk of cataract formation. At higher doses, the risk is approximately 100%, but the onset of the cataract may be protracted. Treatment is the same as for non-irradiation-caused cataracts: surgical cataract extraction and insertion of a lens [11].

Radiation-induced retinopathy and retinal atrophy can result in gradual visual loss. Significant retinal damage will not occur at doses below 50 Gy, but the risk of radiation retinopathy is increased in patients with diabetes. Optic nerve damage may result either from ischemic injury due to small vessel changes or from retrobulbar optic neuropathy due to proximal nerve injury. Doses of 60 Gy or higher are associated with increased risk of optic nerve atrophy, particularly when the fraction sizes are larger than 1.9 Gy [12]. Cranial irradiation in children with optic glioma (particularly involving high radiation doses) can result in dysfunction of the hypothalamus or pituitary gland. Growth hormone deficiency and precocious puberty may result at doses in excess of 45 to 55 Gy.

SUMMARY

Over the last 25 years, a major and dramatic change has taken place in the programs of treatment for malignant tumors of the eye. The major shift has been from primary emphasis on surgery toward radiotherapy, with surgery being used for biopsy, and chemotherapy serving as an adjuvant mode of treatment of certain tumor types. Clearly, the major emphasis has been on preservation of the intact eye and preservation of vision without compromise in long-term outcome.

REFERENCES

1. Fitzpatrick PJ. Organ and functional preservation in the management of cancers of the eye and eyelid. *Cancer Invest* 13:66–74, 1995.
2. Freire JE, Brady LW, DePotter P, et al. Eye. In Perez CA, Brady LW (eds), *Principles and Practice of Radiation Oncology* (3rd ed). Philadelphia: Lippincott-Raven, 1998:867–888.
3. Bosworth JL, Packer S, Rotman M, et al. Choroidal melanoma: I-125 plaque therapy. *Radiology* 169:249–251, 1988.
4. Chao CKS, Lin H-S, Devineni VR, et al. Radiation therapy for primary orbital lymphoma. *Int J Radiat Oncol Biol Phys* 31:929–934, 1995.
5. Cruess AF, Augsburger JJ, Shields JA, et al. Visual results following cobalt plaque radiotherapy for posterior uveal melanoma. *Ophthalmology* 91:131–136, 1984.
6. Halperin EC. *Retinoblastoma: genetics, diagnosis, treatment and sequelae.* Presented at the thirty-ninth annual meeting of American Society for Therapeutic Radiology and Oncology (ASTRO), Orlando, FL, October 19–22, 1997.
7. Karlsson UL, Augsburger JJ, Shields JA, et al. Recurrence of posterior uveal melanoma after ^{60}Co episcleral plaque therapy. *Ophthalmology* 96:382–388, 1989.
8. Shields CL, Shields JA, DePotter P, et al. Treatment of nonresectable malignant iris tumors with designed plaque radiotherapy. *Br J Ophthalmol* 79:306–312, 1995.
9. Reese AB, Ellsworth RM. The evaluation and current concept of retinoblastoma therapy. *Trans Am Acad Ophthalmol Otolaryngol* 67:164–172, 1963.
10. Shields CL, Shields JA, DePotter P, et al. Plaque radiotherapy for residual or recurrent retinoblastoma in 91 cases. *J Pediatr Ophthalmol Strabismus* 31:242–245, 1994.
11. Merriam GR, Focht E. A clinical study of radiation cataracts and their relationship to dose. *Am J Roentgenol Radium Ther Nucl Med* 77:759, 1957.
12. Parsons JT, Bova FJ, Fitzgerald CR, et al. Radiation optic nerve neuropathy after megavoltage external-beam irradiation: analysis of time-dose factors. *Int J Radiat Oncol Biol Phys* 30:755–763, 1994.

30

Metastatic Cancer from an Unknown Primary Site

■ ■ ■

SRIDHAR RAMASWAMY
ROBERT T. OSTEEN
LAWRENCE N. SHULMAN

GENERAL CONSIDERATIONS

Metastatic cancer from an unknown primary site (MCUP) represents approximately 5% of new cancer diagnoses in the United States. One useful working definition of this entity is histologically confirmed metastatic cancer in patients in whom a complete medical history, careful physical examination, basic blood tests, selected radiologic examination, and sophisticated histopathologic studies fail to reveal the origin of the tumor.

Indeed, most practicing physicians can recall having seen such cases, which usually are memorable because of the attendant diagnostic uncertainty, the urgent concern and confusion of patients and their families, and the potentially time-consuming and frustrating search for the primary lesion. Often, this search involves a multitude of tests, at great expense, that may not shed any light on the problem at hand but might entail significant discomfort or risk for an affected patient without altering prognosis or therapy. Furthermore, the therapeutic goals for such patients are not uniform and may range from potential cure in a small number of patients with specific histologic and clinical features to palliation of symptoms for the majority of the remaining patients.

A great deal of pessimism persists concerning the treatment of such lesions and the prognosis for such patients. Generally, the patient with MCUP is thought to be elderly and debilitated with comorbid disease and to have multiple visceral metastases that respond poorly to chemotherapy. However, patients with MCUP represent a heterogeneous mix, with a wide range in clinical presentation, natural history, and response to therapy. Increasingly clear is that subsets of patients with MCUP can be treated using chemotherapy, radiotherapy, and surgery, with a small number of patients experiencing long-term survival after therapy. As such, the overriding goals for the clinician should be the systematic identification of treatable subsets of patients and the offer of therapy that can be useful and potentially lifesaving [1, 2].

DIAGNOSTIC EVALUATION

The typical patient with MCUP develops symptoms referable to the metastatic site, but a routine history, physical examination, chest radiograph, and laboratory studies fail to reveal a primary site. Further tests, including appropriate noninvasive and invasive studies, eventually may identify a primary tumor. Nevertheless, the primary site is identified in only approximately 20% of patients with MCUP, either at the time of presentation or later in their illness. An additional 50% to 60% of primary tumors may be identified at autopsy. However, even at autopsy, up to 16% of patients will not have an identifiable primary lesion [3]. The most common primary tumors ultimately identified in patients with MCUP are pancreatic and lung cancers, followed by certain other gastrointestinal tumors (hepatocellular, colorectal, gastric) and renal cell carcinoma [4].

Clinicians have attempted to determine positive and negative prognostic factors for patients with MCUP. Negative factors that seem to affect overall survival include a diagnosis of adenocarcinoma, solid-organ involvement (including hepatic, pulmonary, and osseous metastases), and more than three sites of disease [5].

Certainly, as medical imaging becomes ever more sophisticated, a greater number of tumors are being identified at an earlier stage. However, the impact of this information on survival is not yet clear [6]. Thus, patients with MCUP should undergo a systematic diagnostic evaluation (guided by the principles outlined next) to avoid needless, expensive, and potentially dangerous testing. The major focus of the clinician should be on identifying those subsets of patients who might respond to therapy (Table 30.1).

History, Physical Examination, and Selected Laboratory Studies

Most patients with MCUP seek medical attention because of signs or symptoms referable to sites of metastatic disease. Common locations for such metastases include the liver, lungs, bones, and lymph nodes. Such constitutional symptoms as weight loss, anorexia, and fatigue also may be prominent. In most cases, symptoms begin to appear shortly before presentation, a finding that might reflect the often rapid growth of such tumors.

A thorough history always should be obtained and may provide insight into the origin of a tumor. Any prior surgical procedures and biopsy specimens should be reviewed in detail to exclude a previous history of malignancy, and information about a patient's family history, social habits, and occupational exposure should be obtained. Occasionally, an adenocarcinoma from an unknown primary site may present with pulmonary embolism, deep venous thrombosis, or migratory thrombophlebitis (Trousseau's syndrome) in the absence of other causes of hypercoagulability (e.g., deficiencies of antithrombin III, protein C, or protein S; activated protein C resistance).

The physical evaluation must include a careful examination of the skin, thyroid, lymph nodes, breast, pelvis, testicles, prostate, and rectum. Occasionally, primary melanomas that have regressed can be identified with the help of a Wood's lamp examination. Occult head and neck cancer should be suspected in patients who present with cervical adenopathy in the upper or middle cervical region. Most of these malignancies will be squamous cell carcinomas. For patients with supraclavicular lymphadenopathy, the most likely sites of the primary tumor are the lungs or gastrointestinal organs. Enlarged inguinal lymph nodes may contain squamous cell carcinoma. Often, the primary tumor is located in the skin or in the genital or anal regions. These sites must be examined carefully, and both colposcopy and anoscopy should be considered.

Routine laboratory studies include a complete blood cell count, a chemistry panel (including liver function tests), urinalysis and microscopy, and studies for occult blood in the stool. In general, checking a battery of serum tumor markers is unrevealing because many tumors will produce multiple markers. In addition, elevated tumor markers may be more indicative of parenchymal invasion by tumor rather than the actual origin of the cancer [7, 8]. For example, both alpha-fetoprotein (AFP) and serum lactate dehydrogenase levels may be raised in the setting of liver metastases. However, selected studies guided by other clinical findings might be very useful. For example, a serum prostate-specific antigen (PSA) may point to prostatic adenocarcinoma in a 70-year-old man with MCUP. Further, although beta–human chorionic gonadotropin (β-HCG) or AFP levels or both can be elevated modestly in the setting of many tumors, a primary germ-cell tumor should be suspected in younger patients with markedly elevated levels of these tumor markers.

Though anemia often accompanies systemic cancer, bone marrow involvement should be suspected when other blood cell lines are affected or when leukoerythroblastic changes are evident in the peripheral blood smear. Bone marrow aspiration and biopsy may be used

Table 30.1   Evaluation of Patients with Carcinoma from an Unknown Primary Site, to Identify Those Whose Tumors May Be Treatable

Carcinoma	Clinical Evaluation	Pathologic Studies	Special Subgroups	Therapy	Prognosis
Adenocarcinoma (well-differentiated or moderately well-differentiated)	Abdominal CT; serum PSA in men, mammography in women	PSA stain in men; status of ERs and PRs in women	Women with axillary node involvement	Treat as primary breast cancer	Poor for entire group (median survival, 4 mo): better for subgroups
				Women with peritoneal carcinomatosis	Surgical cytoreduction + chemotherapy effective in ovarian cancer
				Men with blastic bone metastases, high serum PSA, or PSA tumor staining	Hormonal therapy for prostate cancer
				Patient with single peripheral nodal site of involvement	Lymph node dissection ± radiotherapy
Squamous carcinoma	Panendoscopy for cervical node presentation; pelvic + rectal examination; anoscopy for inguinal presentation	None	Cervical adenopathy	Radiotherapy ± neck dissection	5-yr survival, 25–50%
			Inguinal adenopathy	Inguinal node dissection + radiotherapy	Potential long-term survival
Poorly differentiated carcinoma or adenocarcinoma	Chest, abdominal CT; serum HCG, AFP	Immunoperoxidase staining (see Table 31.2), electron microscopy, chromosomal analysis	Atypical germ-cell tumors (identified by chromosomal abnormalities only)	Treatment for germ-cell tumor	Treatment results similar to those for extragonadal germ-cell tumor
			Neuroendocrine tumors	Cisplatin-based therapy	10–20% cured with therapy: high overall response rate
			Predominant tumor location in retroperitoneum, peripheral nodes	Cisplatin, etoposide, and bleomycin	

CT = computed tomography; PSA = prostate-specific antigen; ER = estrogen receptor; PR = progesterone receptor; HCG = human chorionic gonadotropin; AFP = alpha-fetoprotein.
Source: Reprinted with permission from JD Hainsworth, FA Greco, Treatment of patients with cancer of an unknown primary site. *N Engl J Med* 329:257–263, 1993. Copyright © 1993, Massachusetts Medical Society. All rights reserved.

in this setting to detect bone marrow metastases, which develop most commonly from primary tumors of the breast, lung, gastrointestinal tract, pancreas, and prostate gland.

Radiographic Studies

Good-quality posteroanterior and lateral chest radiographs should be obtained. Although chest radiographic findings may be nonspecific, solitary lesions, hilar masses, and pleural effusions may reflect a primary lung cancer or metastatic disease from another site. Multiple nodules are more indicative of metastatic disease. Abnormalities on chest radiography should be followed up with chest computed tomographic (CT) scanning with intravenous contrast. Bronchoscopy may be indicated in those patients with a smoking history, supraclavicular lymphadenopathy, and a suspicious chest radiograph or CT scan. A chest CT scan should be obtained in patients with isolated brain metastases, because lung primaries frequently are the source and can be missed with a routine chest radiograph [9].

CT scanning of the abdomen and pelvis with intravenous and oral contrast should be performed in all patients with MCUP. This noninvasive technique may reveal the primary site, may help to define the extent of metastatic disease, and may provide clues about possible complications, including biliary obstruction or hydronephrosis. In one older study, CT scanning identified the primary site in 35% of cases involving a metastatic adenocarcinoma from an unknown primary site [10]. In this series, pancreatic cancer was the tumor found most commonly. However, it is noteworthy that abdominal or pelvic CT scanning may yield a significant percentage of false-negative results. For example, CT scanning was normal in up to 30% of cases in which pancreatic cancer ultimately was found. As a result of improvements in the quality of CT scans over the last decade, an ever-increasing number of primary tumors probably are being discovered by radiographic means.

A bilateral mammogram should be obtained for women with MCUP. The yield of mammography may be higher either in women with metastatic adenocarcinoma or in women with axillary lymph node involvement at the time of initial presentation. However, in women with widely metastatic breast cancer, a palpable axillary mass usually is present at the time of presentation. Gadolinium-enhanced breast magnetic resonance imaging (MRI) may be more sensitive than routine mammography for identifying small breast lesions, although the lack of large, prospective studies of this imaging modality and the cost and availability of MRI still limit its broad use.

Other radiographic studies may be useful, depending on initial clinical findings. For example, young patients with rapidly enlarging retroperitoneal masses, mediastinal disease, or significant peripheral lymphadenopathy should be evaluated for the possibility of germ-cell tumors or lymphoma. Occult gonadal primary tumors in men may be revealed by testicular ultrasonography [11].

Patients who present with signs or symptoms that suggest an intracranial mass should be evaluated with either CT scanning or MRI to search for cerebral metastases. Primary tumors associated with intracranial metastases include lung cancer and malignant melanoma. Cancers of the breast, kidney, and gastrointestinal tract, lymphoma, and germ-cell tumors (especially choriocarcinoma) are less common but not infrequent sources. An intracranial mass should undergo biopsy if no other sites of disease are evident. Complete excision should be considered if the intracranial disease is confined to a single site and surgical removal is feasible. In general, postoperative whole-brain irradiation is administered to such patients [12].

In patients with isolated cervical adenopathy, CT scanning of the head and neck may reveal an occult primary tumor and can help to define the extent of lymphadenopathy. In such cases, a careful fiberoptic evaluation of the nasopharynx, larynx, base of tongue, and hypopharynx is essential, and biopsy specimens should be obtained from any suspicious areas. Many clinicians also recommend fiberoptically guided biopsies of normal-appearing oropharyngeal tissue in patients with MCUP and isolated cervical adenopathy, because of the high incidence of occult disease. In one study, this strategy revealed occult carcinoma in approximately 17% of cases [13].

Bone pain may be the first manifestation of MCUP. When bone metastases are suspected, plain films and bone scans should be obtained to identify the location and extent of metastatic disease. Areas that may be at risk for fracture should be assessed, and such prophylactic therapy as stabilization or radiotherapy should be considered. In addition, patients presenting with back pain in the setting of MCUP should be examined immediately to exclude the possibility of spinal cord compression. Spinal CT scanning or MRI may be particularly helpful in this setting. In asymptomatic patients with MCUP, bone scanning might be considered when one suspects a primary tumor with a propensity to form bony metastases, such as prostate cancer.

Considerable interest has been generated in the use of newer imaging modalities, such as positron emission tomography scanning, for evaluating patients with MCUP. However, the role and value of such studies remain to be defined.

Pathologic Studies

Pathologists play a crucial role in evaluating patients with MCUP [14]. Cooperation among the primary-care physician, medical oncologist, surgeon, and pathologist will ensure that adequate tissue samples are obtained and processed appropriately to provide as much information as possible. With the currently available variety of techniques and special studies for determining tumor types, the biopsy sample must be of sufficient size and must be handled with care. The site of the metastasis will dictate the type of specimen obtained but, when possible, the specimen should be divided into at least three portions. One part should be placed in formalin for routine histologic evaluation, another should be snap-frozen for immunocytochemical analysis, and the remaining portion should be placed in glutaraldehyde for possible electron microscopy. Immunoperoxidase assays also may be performed on tissue embedded in paraffin. Finally, additional fresh tissue may be needed for cytogenetic studies. Noteworthy, however, is that sensitive genetic techniques involving the polymerase chain reaction often can be used to obtain cytogenetic information from fixed tissue samples.

In numerous studies of patients with MCUP that span two decades, investigators have identified four major diagnostic categories based on light-microscopical evaluation: well- and moderately well-differentiated adenocarcinomas (60% of patients), poorly differentiated adenocarcinomas (30%), poorly differentiated neoplasms (5%), and squamous cell carcinomas (5%) [4, 15–17]. Patients who have a poorly differentiated carcinoma or adenocarcinoma are, on average, younger than are patients with well-differentiated or moderately differentiated adenocarcinoma and more often present with rapidly progressive tumors. In addition, involvement of the lymph nodes, mediastinum, and retroperitoneum is more common for patients with poorly differentiated histologic findings, whereas metastases to the liver, lungs, or bone are seen more often in patients with well-differentiated tumors [4].

Although adenocarcinomas and squamous cell carcinomas have characteristic histologic features that are identified readily, generally these features are not specific enough to permit identification of the site of origin. On occasion, however, some features may provide clues to the location of the primary malignancy. For example,

papillary features may suggest a thyroid or ovarian tumor, whereas signet cells may suggest a gastrointestinal or breast primary.

IMMUNOPEROXIDASE STUDIES

Immunoperoxidase staining, electron microscopy, and cytogenetic studies may provide useful pathologic information (Table 30.2). Immunoperoxidase studies may be directed against cellular enzymes (e.g., prostatic acid phosphatase, PSA, and neuron-specific enolase); structural components (e.g., cytokeratin, desmin, and vimentin); cell-specific components (e.g., leukocyte common antigen [LCA], epithelial membrane antigen, chromogranin, and S-100 protein); hormones (e.g., human chorionic gonadotropin, calcitonin, and thyroglobulin); hormone receptors (e.g., estrogen and progesterone receptors); and oncofetal antigens (e.g., carcinoembryonic antigen and AFP). Special attention should be paid to those studies that could direct the diagnosis toward more treatable tumors.

Staining for LCA is essential in evaluating poorly differentiated tumors. Non-Hodgkin's lymphoma, which is characteristically LCA-positive, may be detected in 35% to 60% of cases, and such patients can be cured with combination chemotherapy. After standard therapy was given to patients with anaplastic tumors identified as large-cell lymphomas on the basis of positive LCA staining, 45% were found to be free from disease progres-

Table 30.2 Immunoperoxidase Staining for the Differential Diagnosis of Poorly Differentiated Tumors

Tumor	Component Detectable by Immunostaining
Lymphoma	Leukocyte common antigen
Carcinoma	Cytokeratin
Specific carcinomas	
Prostate	Prostate-specific antigen
Follicular thyroid	Thyroglobulin
Medullary thyroid	Calcitonin
Neuroendocrine	Neuron-specific enolase, chromogranin
Germ cell tumors	Human chorionic gonadotropin, alpha-vimentin
Melanoma	S-100 protein, HMB-45 antigen, vimentin
Special sarcomas	
Rhabdomyosarcoma	Desmin
Angiosarcoma	Factor VIII antigen

Source: Reprinted with permission from JD Hainsworth, FA Greco, Treatment of patients with cancer of an unknown primary site. *N Engl J Med* 329:257–263, 1993. Copyright © 1993, Massachusetts Medical Society. All rights reserved.

sion at 30 months [18]. This outcome is similar to that seen among patients with diffuse large-cell lymphoma diagnosed and treated in a standard fashion.

A positive result on staining for cytokeratin and epithelial membrane antigen suggests carcinoma. This result is not completely specific, however, as other tumor types, such as sarcomas and germ-cell tumors, occasionally may be cytokeratin-positive. A mucin-positive stain in a poorly differentiated cancer is consistent with adenocarcinoma. In addition, the presence of PSA is indicative of prostate cancer, whereas the presence of thyroglobulin and calcitonin is consistent with medullary and thyroid cancers, respectively. An adenocarcinoma that stains positively for estrogen and progesterone receptors certainly suggests breast cancer. Although germ-cell tumors may be identified by positive staining for human chorionic gonadotropin and AFP, hepatocellular carcinoma also may be AFP-positive. A positive result on staining for S-100 protein and human melanoma black–45 is suggestive of melanoma. Similarly, rhabdomyosarcoma and angiosarcoma are suggested by positive stains for desmin and factor VIII antigen, respectively.

Despite its benefits, the use of immunocytochemistry has several potential drawbacks. As with any specialized technique, a pathologist with special skills is required to interpret the results accurately. In addition, appropriate positive and negative controls must be used.

ELECTRON MICROSCOPY

Electron microscopy may yield valuable information when routine histologic evaluation and immunocytochemical analysis are unrevealing. Certain cell features are diagnostic of specific cancers, including premelanosomes (melanoma), myofibrils (sarcoma), desmosomes (squamous cell cancer), microvilli (adenocarcinoma), and neurosecretory granules (neuroendocrine tumors).

CYTOGENETIC STUDIES

Newer cytogenetic techniques have made possible the identification of cancers that are associated with chromosomal abnormalities [19, 20]. For example, some lymphomas are characterized by immunoglobulin or T-cell receptor gene rearrangements (e.g., the association between Burkitt's lymphoma and the t(8;14) chromosomal translocation). Recent studies have demonstrated a link between specific chromosomal abnormalities and certain solid tumors. For example, abnormalities of chromosome 12 have been found in some testicular and extragonadal germ-cell tumors, whereas the t(11;22)

translocation has been associated with Ewing's sarcoma and peripheral neuroepithelioma.

THERAPY FOR METASTATIC CANCER FROM AN UNKNOWN PRIMARY SITE

Because patients with MCUP are a heterogeneous group, treatment may cover a broad range, including aggressive chemotherapy given with curative intent, palliative hormonal therapy or radiotherapy, or supportive care only. Attention should focus on both treatment of lymph node metastases as local disease and treatment of systemic disease. Physicians, patients, and affected families must frankly review the goals of treatment so that informed decisions can be made about the appropriateness of particular therapeutic interventions.

If the diagnostic evaluation strongly suggests a tumor for which effective, disease-specific therapy exists, this option should be discussed, provided that affected patients' general medical condition qualifies them as appropriate candidates for such treatment. Patients with lymphoma or germ-cell tumors possibly can be cured with combination chemotherapy, even when disseminated disease is present. In addition, as outlined later, patients who present with certain other clinical or histologic features may benefit from treatment.

Poorly Differentiated Carcinoma, Adenocarcinoma, and Neoplasms

Early studies seemed to indicate the chemoresponsiveness of patients with poorly differentiated carcinoma or poorly differentiated adenocarcinoma to cisplatin-based regimens. In one study, complete responses occurred in 26% of 220 patients treated, and the actuarial 10-year disease-free survival rate was 16% [16]. However, more recent studies have not confirmed these findings. A retrospective review of 1,400 patients with poorly differentiated carcinoma and adenocarcinoma seen at a large cancer referral center indicated the poor prognosis and poor response to chemotherapy of the majority of such patients. The authors of that review pointed out that the increasing sophistication of immunohistochemistry in their series might have resulted in more accurate identification of treatable tumors [21, 22]. Thus, this series probably is more indicative of the natural history of treated, poorly differentiated carcinoma and adenocarcinoma.

Cisplatin-based chemotherapy programs appear to

be useful for treating patients with features of neuroendocrine tumors, as evidenced by immunocytochemistry (positive staining for neuron-specific enolase or chromogranin) or electron microscopy (presence of neurosecretory granules). When cisplatin-based chemotherapy was used to treat 19 patients with poorly differentiated neuroendocrine tumors from an unknown primary site, researchers noted complete remissions in 6 of the 19 patients, and 3 of the 6 remained disease-free at 19, 20, and 100 months, respectively, after completing therapy. In addition, local modalities (excision with or without radiotherapy) were used to treat four patients with disease limited to a single site, and all four remained disease-free for the duration of the study [23].

Well-Differentiated or Moderately Differentiated Adenocarcinoma

Most patients with well-differentiated or moderately differentiated adenocarcinoma fare poorly; they are, on average, older and more debilitated and have a poorer performance status relative to patients with poorly differentiated tumors. Whether treatment has a significant effect on the overall survival of such patients is not yet clear. Although responders have been found to live longer, this outcome may indicate merely a more indolent tumor rather than reflecting treatment success. Nevertheless, some patients with well-differentiated or moderately differentiated adenocarcinoma of an unknown primary site have exhibited clear benefits as a result of treatment, and a minority of these patients are potentially curable [24].

Women who present with adenocarcinoma in the axillary lymph nodes, even those with normal breast examinations and mammograms, should be treated presumptively for breast cancer if clinical and radiographic evaluation fail to reveal another primary lesion. Assays for estrogen and progesterone receptors should be performed on the lymph node specimen, with a positive result considered presumptive evidence for a diagnosis of primary breast cancer. However, because negative results on these assays do not rule out breast cancer, receptor status should not affect the treatment approach. Women with isolated axillary involvement are potentially curable, and treatment outcomes are similar to those of women who have stage II breast cancer with an obvious primary tumor [25]. Traditionally, mastectomy has been recommended for women with axillary involvement and an unknown primary tumor; occult primary breast cancer may be found in approxi-

mately 50% to 70% of specimens from such patients. Some investigators have advocated the combined use of breast irradiation and axillary node dissection [26]. Adjuvant systemic treatment with chemotherapy or hormonal therapy (or both) is indicated in women with no additional systemic metastases. Chemotherapy or hormonal treatment appropriate for breast cancer can provide significant palliation for women with widely disseminated disease.

Women who present with peritoneal carcinomatosis from an adenocarcinoma of an unknown primary site form another distinct clinical group [27]. Although diffuse abdominal involvement sometimes is seen in breast or gastrointestinal cancer, this pattern is much more common in ovarian cancer. In particular, the entity of extraovarian peritoneal serous papillary carcinoma is well described and has a similar natural history in those patients presumptively treated as having ovarian cancer [28]. Consequently, a woman with peritoneal carcinomatosis from an unknown primary tumor should be treated presumptively for ovarian cancer, even if she has had a previous oophorectomy or if the ovaries appear normal on pathologic study. Women who are medically fit should be offered aggressive cytoreductive surgery followed by cisplatin-based chemotherapy. In several series, this approach yielded meaningful clinical responses in approximately one-third of the women treated, and some remained disease-free after more than 4 years of follow-up. Indeed, the prognosis in women with peritoneal carcinomatosis from an unknown primary site is identical to that for women with known ovarian cancer, as compared by stage of disease [26].

Men who present with adenocarcinoma and skeletal metastases may have prostate cancer and may benefit from empiric hormonal therapy. Hormonal interventions also should be considered in men with elevated serum levels of PSA or with tumors that stain positively for prostate markers, even when visceral metastases are present. Significant palliation may be achieved in this setting.

When one fails to identify a likely primary site in patients with well-differentiated or moderately differentiated adenocarcinoma, empiric chemotherapy should be considered for those symptomatic patients who have a good performance status. The drugs that are most effective in this setting have not been identified definitively. The earliest clinical studies suggested that regimens containing doxorubicin were promising, with associated response rates ranging from 7% to 37% and median survival ranging from 5 to 15 months. Although a number of recent trials have sought to improve on these results by adding cisplatin, results often have been contradictory, and these newer regimens generally have offered no significant survival advantage. For example, in one trial, the median survival times were 18 and 25 weeks, respectively, for a regimen involving doxorubicin plus mitomycin C and another involving cisplatin, vinblastine, and bleomycin [29]. In a separate study, the addition of cisplatin to a regimen of mitomycin C and doxorubicin actually reduced the median survival from 5.5 to 4.6 months [30]. A third trial found no apparent advantage when cisplatin and etoposide were added to a regimen consisting of vincristine, doxorubicin, and cyclophosphamide [31]. The possible role of 5-fluorouracil (5-FU) and leucovorin in this setting has not yet been determined in a large number of patients. However, because the value of 5-FU and leucovorin has been documented in metastatic gastrointestinal cancers [32], this regimen should be considered in patients with well-differentiated or moderately differentiated adenocarcinoma from an unknown primary site. More recently, some investigators have explored the use of paclitaxel for the treatment of MCUP, on the basis of its activity against a wide variety of cancers. Given the small numbers of patients reported thus far, the role of this drug in the treatment of MCUP remains to be defined in a randomized fashion, although increasing evidence suggests that this agent may induce clinical responses in some patients [33]. Before embarking on any empiric treatment program, clinicians must provide their patients with detailed information about the potential toxicities associated with the particular chemotherapy regimen.

Squamous Cell Carcinoma

Local treatment modalities, including radical neck dissection, high-dose irradiation, or both, have the potential to cure squamous cell carcinoma in the cervical lymph nodes in patients presenting with this disease. In general, 30% to 50% of patients or more remain disease-free after 5 years. However, because patients treated with surgery alone have a higher risk of developing a primary lesion in the head and neck (approximately 20–40%), usually the recommended treatment is radiotherapy, either alone or combined with surgery. The role of chemotherapy in this setting has not been defined fully. In one retrospective review, investigators compared the results obtained in patients treated with local modalities alone or in combination with cisplatin chemotherapy (with or without 5-FU) [33]. Although patients receiving the combined-modality therapy tended to have more locally advanced disease (N3), they

achieved a higher complete response rate (81% versus 28%) and had a longer median survival (37 months versus 24 months) than did patients treated with surgery or radiotherapy without chemotherapy [34].

In patients who present with squamous cell carcinoma in the inguinal nodes from an unknown primary site, disease-free survival may be prolonged by local therapy. In one retrospective review, 38% of patients with tumor localized to the inguinal or inguinal plus iliac regions were alive 5 years after treatment. Most of these patients were treated with excisional biopsy followed by radiotherapy or lymph node dissection [35]. Table 30.1 summarizes current approaches for the evaluation and treatment of patients with treatable subsets of MCUP; the table also includes information on prognosis.

Supportive Care

The vast majority of patients who present with MCUP can benefit from supportive care at some point during the course of their illness. For example, appropriate radiotherapy may provide significant palliation of neurologic symptoms caused by painful bony lesions or metastases. Aggressive pain control and treatment of metabolic or paraneoplastic complications also may improve the quality of life for this patient population. As with all patients with advanced cancer, issues surrounding end-of-life care, including hospice care, should be discussed in a proactive and open manner.

REFERENCES

1. Osteen RT, Kopf G, Wilson RE. In pursuit of the unknown primary. *Am J Surg* 135:494–498, 1978.
2. Leonard RJ, Nystrom JS. Diagnostic evaluation of patients with carcinoma of unknown primary tumor site. *Semin Oncol* 20:244–250, 1993.
3. Le Chevalier T, Cvitkovic E, Caille P, et al. Early metastatic cancer of unknown primary origin at presentation: a clinical study of 302 consecutive autopsied patients. *Arch Intern Med* 148:2035–2039, 1988.
4. Hainsworth JD, Greco FA. Treatment of patients with cancer of an unknown primary site. *N Engl J Med* 329:257–263, 1993.
5. Van der Gaast A, Verweij J, Planting AST, et al. Simple prognostic model to predict survival in patients with undifferentiated carcinoma of unknown primary site. *J Clin Oncol* 13:1720–1725, 1995.
6. Kagan AR, Steckel RJ. The limited role of radiologic imaging in patients with unknown tumor primary. *Semin Oncol* 18:170–173, 1991.

7. Briasoulis E, Pavlidis N. Cancer of unknown primary origin. *Oncologist* 2:142–152, 1997.

8. Ruddon RW, Norton SE. Use of biological markers in the diagnosis of cancers of unknown primary tumor. *Semin Oncol* 20:251–260, 1993.

9. Latief KH, White CS, Protopapas Z, et al. Search for a primary lung neoplasm in patients with brain metastases: is the chest radiograph sufficient? *Am J Roentgenol* 168:1339–1344, 1997.

10. McMillan H, Levine E, Stephans RH. Computed tomography in the evaluation of metastatic adenocarcinoma from an unknown primary site. *Radiology* 143:143–146, 1982.

11. Comiter CV, Benson CJ, Capeluoto CC, et al. Nonpalpable intratesticular masses detected sonographically. *J Urol* 154:1367–1369, 1995.

12. Patchell RA, Tibbs PA, Walsh JW, et al. Randomized trial of surgery in the treatment of single metastases to the brain. *N Engl J Med* 322:494–500, 1990.

13. Lee DJ, Rostock RA, Harris A, et al. Clinical evaluation of patients with metastatic squamous carcinoma of the neck with occult primary tumor. *South Med J* 79:979–983, 1986.

14. Mackay B, Ordonez NG. Pathological evaluation of neoplasms with unknown primary tumor site. *Semin Oncol* 20:206–228, 1993.

15. Hainsworth JD, Greco JA. Poorly differentiated carcinoma and poorly differentiated adenocarcinoma of unknown primary tumor site. *Semin Oncol* 20:279–286, 1993.

16. Hainsworth JD, Johnson DH, Greco FA. Cisplatin-based combination chemotherapy in the treatment of poorly differentiated carcinoma and poorly differentiated adenocarcinoma of unknown primary site: results of a 12-year experience. *J Clin Oncol* 10:912–922, 1992.

17. Hainsworth JD, Wright EP, Johnson DH, et al. Poorly differentiated carcinoma of unknown primary site: clinical usefulness of immunoperoxidase staining. *J Clin Oncol* 9:1931–1938, 1991.

18. Horning SJ, Carrier EK, Rouse RV, et al. Lymphoma presenting as histologically unclassified neoplasms: characteristics and response to treatment. *J Clin Oncol* 7:1281–1287, 1989.

19. Bell CW, Pathak S, Frost P. Unknown primary tumors. Establishment of cell lines, identification of chromosomal abnormalities, and implications for a second type of tumor progression. *Cancer Res* 49:4311–4315, 1989.

20. Ilson DH, Motzer RJ, Rodriguez E, et al. Genetic analysis in the diagnosis of neoplasms of unknown primary tumor site. *Semin Oncol* 20:229–237, 1993.

21. Abbruzzese JL, Abbruzzese MC, Hess KR, et al. Unknown primary carcinoma: natural history and prognostic factors in 657 consecutive patients. *J Clin Oncol* 12:1272–1280, 1994.

22. Lenzi R, Hess KR, Abbruzzese MC, et al. Poorly differentiated carcinoma and poorly differentiated adenocarcinoma of unknown origin: favorable subsets of patients with unknown primary carcinoma. *J Clin Oncol* 15:2056–2066, 1997.

23. Garrow GC, Greco FA, Hainsworth JD. Poorly differentiated neuroendocrine carcinoma of unknown primary tumor site. *Semin Oncol* 20:287–291, 1993.

24. Sporn JR, Greenberg BR. Empiric chemotherapy for adenocarcinoma of unknown primary tumor site. *Semin Oncol* 20:261–267, 1993.

25. Ellerbroek N, Holmes F, Singletary E, et al. Treatment of patients with isolated axillary nodal metastases from an occult primary carcinoma consistent with breast origin. *Cancer* 66:1461–1467, 1990.

26. Baron PL, Moore MP, Kinne DW, et al. Occult breast cancer presenting with axillary metastases: updated management. *Arch Surg* 125:210–215, 1990.

27. Muggia FM, Baranda J. Management of peritoneal carcinomatosis of unknown primary tumor site. *Semin Oncol* 20:268–272, 1993.

28. Dalrymple JC, Bannatyne P, Russell P, et al. Extraovarian peritoneal serous papillary carcinoma: a clinicopathologic study of 31 cases. *Cancer* 64:110–115, 1989.

29. Milliken ST, Tattersall MHN, Woods RL, et al. Metastatic adenocarcinoma of unknown primary site. A randomized study of two combination chemotherapy regimens. *Eur J Cancer Clin Oncol* 23:1645–1648, 1987.

30. Eagan RT, Themeau TM, Rubin J, et al. Lack of value for cisplatin added to mitomycin-doxorubicin combination chemotherapy for carcinoma of unknown primary site. *Am J Clin Oncol* 10:82–85, 1987.

31. de Campos ED, Menasce LP, Radford J, et al. Metastatic carcinoma of uncertain primary site: a retrospective review of 57 patients treated with vincristine, doxorubicin, cyclophosphamide (VAC) or VAC alternating with cisplatin and etoposide (VAC/PE). *Cancer* 73:470–475, 1994.

32. Bruchner HW, Crown J, McKenna A, et al. Leucovorin and 5-fluorouracil as a treatment for disseminated cancer of the pancreas and unknown primary tumors. *Cancer Res* 48:5570–5572, 1988.

33. Hainsworth JD, Erland JB, Kalman LA, et al. Carcinoma of unknown primary site: treatment with 1-hour paclitaxel, carboplatin, and extended-schedule etoposide. *J Clin Oncol* 15:2385–2393, 1997.

34. de Braud F, Al-Sarraf M. Diagnosis and management of squamous cell carcinoma of unknown primary tumor site of the neck. *Semin Oncol* 20:273–278, 1993.

35. Guarischi A, Keane TJ, Elhakim T. Metastatic inguinal nodes from an unknown primary neoplasm: a review of 56 cases. *Cancer* 59:572–577, 1987.

31

Paraneoplastic and Endocrine Syndromes

■ ■ ■

Paul E. Rosenthal

OVERVIEW

Tumors produce signs and symptoms by two major mechanisms. One involves dysfunction of normal tissues owing to invasion, compression, or destruction by a primary tumor or its metastases. The other involves distant or "remote" effects of the malignancy owing to the elaboration of biologically active substances that enter the circulation and cause physiologic changes. These remote effects are known collectively as *paraneoplastic syndromes.*

A paraneoplastic syndrome may precede the diagnosis of an underlying malignancy by months to years, may occur as the presenting symptom, or may develop during the course of the illness [1]. Up to 50% of patients with cancer will be affected by at least one paraneoplastic syndrome at some time during their illness. Prompt recognition that a given symptom complex is a remote effect of cancer may allow an occult tumor to be detected early. Sometimes, these syndromes can be treated successfully even when an underlying malignancy cannot be controlled. If effective treatment is available for the underlying malignancy, assessing the clinical syndrome or, preferably, measuring the specific substance that produces the syndrome may be useful in monitoring the response to treatment.

Several of the best-characterized paraneoplastic syndromes appear to be related to a tumor's elaboration of humoral substances that are comparable or identical to naturally occurring hormones, such as antidiuretic hormone, adrenocorticotropic hormone (ACTH), or insulin-like growth factor (Table 31.1). Other syndromes (cachexia, hypertrophic pulmonary osteoarthropathy) are presumed to be caused by a biologically active substance not yet completely understood. The effects of a tumor on a patient's immune function (autoimmunity, immune complex dysfunction, and immunosuppression) contribute to several other paraneoplastic phenomena.

Table 31.1   Common Paraneoplastic Syndromes

Type of Syndrome	Proposed Mechanism	Associated Tumor Type
Endocrinologic		
SIADH	Production and release of antidiuretic hormone by tumor cells	Small-cell lung cancer, many others
Cushing's syndrome	Production and release of ACTH by tumor cells	Small-cell lung cancer, bronchial carcinoid tumors
Hypercalcemia	Production and release of a polypeptide (possibly a growth factor with partial homology to parathormone) by tumor cells	Squamous cell lung cancer, squamous cell cancer of the head and neck, ovarian cancer
Musculoskeletal		
Dermatomyositis	Unknown (possibly an autoimmune reaction)	Visceral adenocarcinomas of lung, breast, colon, and other sites
Hypertrophic pulmonary osteoarthropathy	Unknown	Lung carcinoma, particularly adenocarcinoma and large-cell cancer
Dermatologic (various)	Possibly caused by production of a growth factor (e.g., transforming growth factor α, insulin-like growth factor, epidermal growth factor) by tumor cells	Gastric carcinoma, melanoma
Neurologic		
Eaton-Lambert syndrome	Autoimmune production of IgG reactive with motor end plate (possibly with calcium channels)	Small-cell cancer
Subacute cerebellar degeneration	Possible autoimmune reaction to cerebellar Purkinje cells	Small-cell cancer, ovarian cancer, lymphoma

SIADH = syndrome of inappropriate antidiuretic hormone; ACTH = adrenocorticotropic hormone.

Tumors of endocrine tissues can be functional. The excessive secretion of a tissue's normal physiologic products (polypeptides, catecholamines, or corticosteroids) may give rise to dramatic clinical syndromes. For example, overproduction of erythropoietin by a renal cell carcinoma may be an exaggeration of a normal physiologic phenomenon. As a result, the systemic effects of the tumor product may be greater than the local effects of tumor growth.

A hormone produced by a tumor-involving tissue that normally does not elaborate that hormone is said to be *ectopic*, whereas the normal hormones produced by endocrine tumors are termed *eutopic*. At one time considered a rare occurrence, ectopic hormone production by a tumor now is recognized as a common clinical phenomenon, and various mechanisms have been proposed to account for it.

One such mechanism is the so-called APUD (*a*mine *p*recursor *u*ptake and *d*ecarboxylation) concept, a term that refers to a widely distributed system of neuroendocrine cells. These cells are morphologically and biochemically distinct and are characterized by their capac-

ity for APUD. Melanocytes, thyroid C cells, pancreatic islet cells, and certain specialized epithelial cells in the respiratory, gastrointestinal (GI), and genitourinary systems are part of the APUD system. Some of these cells are believed to have a common embryologic origin (arising from the neural crest) and to be related embryologically to precursors of normal endocrine tissue. Thus, tumors resulting from the neoplastic proliferation of APUD cells in various locations could give rise to diverse hormonal syndromes. If the APUD concept is valid, it would explain why anatomically diverse tumors produce similar types of hormones. However, this theory may not explain all cases of ectopic hormone production because a wide variety of morphologic cell types may produce ectopic hormones [2].

Another proposed mechanism for paraneoplastic phenomena is *gene activation* in malignant or transformed cells. Although each cell contains the entire human genome, the genome is not expressed in its entirety. When cancer develops, specific genes are activated, leading to decreased control of transcription in parts of the genome that normally are inactive. The resultant gene products range from oncofetal antigens to complex polypeptide hormones. Several of these polypeptides may function as growth factors that stimulate tumor growth [3]. Exaggerated production of biologically active polypeptides may be a universal concomitant of neoplastic transformation and could lead to clinical paraneoplastic syndromes.

As a result of improved techniques for detecting substances secreted by tumors, even in the absence of an associated syndrome, some of these substances now can be used as clinical tumor markers. Ectopic or eutopic hormones may indicate a tumor, and their measurement may be useful in monitoring tumor recurrence or progression. In this regard, radioimmunoassays for human chorionic gonadotropin have proved invaluable in managing gestational choriocarcinoma and testicular cancer, and the oncofetal proteins carcinoembryonic antigen and alpha-fetoprotein are now measured as a means of monitoring treatment response in a number of malignancies. In the future, more precise determinations of these and other ectopically secreted hormones and related polypeptides may be of value in cancer diagnosis and treatment.

The presence of a clinical syndrome in a cancer patient does not necessarily indicate that the syndrome represents a remote effect of that cancer. Clinicians should be aware that frequent concomitants of malignancy (e.g., infection, nutritional deficiencies, or drug toxicity) may produce effects similar to those seen in paraneoplastic syndromes but may be much more amenable to treatment.

Corollaries of Koch's postulates have been proposed to judge whether a tumor is producing a hormone ectopically. These corollaries include (1) finding hormone concentrations in the tumor higher than those in surrounding normal tissue; (2) documenting that hormone concentrations in venous blood flowing from the tumor are greater than those in arterial blood flowing to the tumor; (3) observing that hormone levels have fallen or that clinical manifestations have reversed after successful tumor treatment; and, most conclusively, (4) demonstrating that ectopic hormone is produced by tumor cells in culture or tumor xenografts in animal models. New techniques of DNA and RNA analysis have confirmed that gene expression and the production of mRNA for the ectopic hormone occur directly within the tumor cells [4].

The foregoing criteria for ectopic polypeptide production have been met most often in syndromes related to overproduction of well-characterized hormones. Evidence of a paraneoplastic origin for other conditions, especially neurologic and musculoskeletal syndromes, is based on the clinical association of these syndromes with various malignancies; although clinical evidence suggests a humoral basis, the exact pathogenesis for these syndromes requires further definition.

GENERAL SYNDROMES
Fever

Fever not associated with infection may be a systemic manifestation of malignant disease. Most often, it occurs with renal cell carcinoma, lymphoma (especially Hodgkin's disease), and hepatic metastases from GI adenocarcinomas. Responsible mechanisms may include direct lymphokine production by tumor cells or reactive macrophages. Up to 20% of patients presenting with fever of unknown origin eventually will be found to have a malignancy, usually a lymphoma. Although some investigators have reported that certain patterns of temperature elevation, such as Pel-Epstein fever, suggest an underlying malignancy, such patterns rarely are seen. In patients with a documented malignancy, fever most often is due to an infection. Fever directly related to the malignancy can be treated according to the symptoms with antipyretics or nonsteroidal antiinflammatory agents. Tumor-related fever disappears when the underlying malignancy is treated successfully [5].

Cachexia

Most commonly, cachexia is associated with lung and GI carcinoma and is somewhat less common in lymphoma and breast cancer. However, it is found almost universally in patients with advanced cancer, and the chronic protein-calorie malnutrition associated with cancer cachexia often contributes to the death of such patients. Experimental and clinical data indicate that cachexia may be related to a tumor's production of humoral substances. Cachectin, a substance produced by monocytes and related closely to human tumor necrosis factor, also may be involved. A proteoglycan may be the putative "wasting factor" [6].

Usually, cancer cachexia is associated with pronounced anorexia and early satiety. Patients lose interest in food, describe food as tasteless, and are able to consume only a small amount at meals. Taste abnormalities are common, and food aversions, especially to meats, may be pronounced. In some cases, the sight of large portions of food or the aroma of food cooking may cause affected patients to feel nauseated. Physical examination reveals diffuse wasting of muscle and adipose tissue, and the classic "hippocratic facies of malignancy" is seen in advanced cases. Still not clear is whether cachexia is caused primarily by anorexia alone or by a catabolic effect associated with the malignancy.

Management of cancer cachexia can be difficult for affected patients, their families, and their physicians. Although successful eradication of the tumor will reverse the syndrome, such a solution rarely is possible, because cachexia usually is associated with advanced malignancy. Occasionally, small frequent feedings and protein-calorie supplements are beneficial. Corticosteroids, anabolic steroids, and progestins have been used but often are ineffective, and their side effects usually outweigh their potential benefits. Enteral and parenteral hyperalimentation may slow or even reverse the syndrome in some cases, but the use of intensive nutritional support should be limited to selected patients in appropriate clinical settings [7]. Research to improve our understanding of cancer cachexia and better methods of treatment could add to such patients' quality of life and might increase rates of survival (see Chapter 35).

ENDOCRINE SYNDROMES

Clinical syndromes produced by hormonally active substances are among the most common and best-characterized paraneoplastic syndromes. Polypeptides appear to be the only hormones that tumors produce ectopically; ectopic production of catecholamines or steroid hormones has not been described. In fact, every known polypeptide hormone normally secreted by endocrine tissue has been shown to be produced ectopically by various tumors of nonendocrine origin.

Although the ectopic hormone often appears identical or nearly identical to the native bioactive hormone, tumor cells may synthesize polypeptide hormones in an uncoordinated manner. Normally, in an orderly cycle termed the *peptide cascade*, polypeptide hormones undergo biochemical evolution during synthesis, storage, secretion, and catabolism. This sequential evolution may not occur in ectopic hormone production, a situation that gives rise to different molecules of varying size and biological activity in the plasma. Similarly, appropriate sugars may not be added after the synthesis of glycoprotein hormones (e.g., human chorionic gonadotropin), and this defect will change their chemical and biological characteristics. In hormones composed of two polypeptide subunits, gene activation may be markedly unbalanced, resulting in excesses of one of the subunits. These molecules may cross-react to varying degrees with the biologically active hormone in the radioimmunoassay being used to quantify circulating hormone levels but may exhibit little or no biological activity in the hormone's target tissues. Perhaps for this reason, patients with immunologic evidence of ectopic hormone production often have no clinical evidence of excess hormone.

Syndrome of Inappropriate Antidiuretic Hormone Secretion

The syndrome of inappropriate antidiuretic hormone secretion (SIADH) first was described more than 40 years ago in a patient with lung cancer. Currently, it is one of the ectopic hormone syndromes that is best characterized and encountered most frequently. SIADH is associated with a variety of malignancies, including lung cancer, thymoma, pancreatic cancer, and several others. However, it is encountered most often in small-cell lung cancer. Up to 10% of patients with that disorder have evidence of SIADH during the clinical course of the disease; up to 70% may demonstrate abnormalities of water metabolism during provocative water-loading tests [1]. Not uncommonly, SIADH will be the presenting symptom in small-cell lung cancer, and resolution of the syndrome indicates that the tumor is responding to therapy.

The clinical presentation in SIADH is determined by the degree of rapidity of onset of the associated hyponatremia. Typically, patients with mild hyponatremia complain of weakness and lethargy, whereas those with severe hyponatremia (serum sodium levels < 115 mEq/liter) may present with frank coma and generalized seizures. In addition to hyponatremia, the diagnostic criteria for SIADH include hyposmolality of extracellular fluids, urine that is less than maximally dilute, absence of volume depletion, sustained, appreciable renal excretion of sodium, and normal renal and adrenal function.

Because the basic pathophysiologic abnormality in SIADH is excessive retention of free water, mild cases may be managed by fluid restriction (intake < 1 liter/day). More severe disease (especially that involving seizures) may require saline infusions together with furosemide diuresis to prevent further volume overload. Successful control of the underlying malignancy with surgery, irradiation, or chemotherapy leads to prompt resolution of the syndrome, and such treatment should play an important role in management whenever appropriate.

Ectopic ACTH Syndrome

Ectopic production of the ACTH syndrome or of related polypeptides has been described in a variety of malignancies, including small-cell lung cancer, bronchial carcinoid, islet-cell tumors of the pancreas, medullary carcinoma, pheochromocytoma, and arrhenoblastoma of the ovary. Such production occurs when normal adrenal tissue produces excessive amounts of adrenocortical hormones in response to sustained stimulation by the ectopic polypeptide. Slow-growing tumors associated with this syndrome may produce the classic stigmata of *Cushing's syndrome*, which include truncal obesity, striae, and a "buffalo hump." However, the symptoms associated with the more common small-cell lung cancer do not resemble classic Cushing's syndrome. In such cases, the syndrome is characterized instead by severe muscle weakness, fatigue, weight loss, and pronounced metabolic abnormalities, including hypokalemia and metabolic alkalosis. Glucose intolerance and mild hypertension also may be present. Usually, these tumors are autonomous and rarely are suppressed with dexamethasone. Because ACTH is homologous to melanocyte-stimulating hormone, hyperpigmentation also is seen commonly in these patients. Treatment consists of judicious potassium replacement and management of the underlying malignancy. Occasionally, inhibitors of adrenal hormone synthesis (e.g., metyrapone, aminoglutethimide, and ketoconazole) will provide palliation [7].

Hypercalcemia

Hypercalcemia is relatively common among cancer patients. They may present with fatigue, weakness, anorexia, vomiting, abdominal pain, or coma. Most often, breast cancer is associated with this electrolyte abnormality, with 10% to 25% of affected patients being hypercalcemic at some time during the course of the disease. Usually, metastasis to bone is a prerequisite for hypercalcemia; in such cases, the underlying mechanism may be rapid turnover of bone as a direct result of metastatic activity. However, hypercalcemia sometimes appears as a true paraneoplastic effect (i.e., mediated directly by a humoral agent).

Commonly, hypercalcemia that is *not* associated with metastatic bone disease is found in cancer of the lung (especially of the squamous cell type); in cancer of the head and neck, kidney, ovary, cervix, and pancreas; and in hepatoma. In such cases, multiple *humoral mechanisms* appear to be involved. Humoral inducement of hypercalcemia of malignancy may be related to the production by different tumor tissues of a variety of hormones: parathormone-like substances, prostaglandins, or other as-yet unidentified materials. Members of this hormone family include tumor growth factor, interleukin-6, and tumor necrosis factor [8]. Apparently, some tumors elaborate a polypeptide that is biologically similar to parathormone. For example, a human lung cancer line has been found to produce a protein that has a molecular weight of 16,000 kD (approximately twice that of parathormone) and that is in many ways homologous to native parathormone. This finding may explain why protein derived from the tumor interacts with the parathormone receptor and, in turn, why clinical hypercalcemia develops [8].

A number of other substances may be associated with the hypercalcemia of malignancy, including prostaglandins, which induce bone resorption through osteoclastic stimulation. Increased prostaglandin synthesis has been reported in patients with renal cell carcinoma, squamous cell carcinoma of the lung, and other tumors. Although hypercalcemia may respond to inhibitors of prostaglandin synthesis (e.g., aspirin or indomethacin), such responses are rare. Reports indicate that a family of cytokinins—the osteoclast-activating factors—can be produced by myeloma cells, lymphoma cells, and peripheral blood lymphocytes and may play a role in the hypercalcemia associated with the hematologic malignancies.

Humoral hypercalcemia of malignancy is characterized by elevated blood calcium, variable blood levels of phosphorus, and increased urinary excretion of calcium, phosphorus, and cyclic adenosine monophosphate. However, the serum bicarbonate level usually is elevated, resulting in a metabolic alkalosis rather than in the metabolic acidosis typical of primary hyperparathyroidism. Moreover, the clinical course of cancer-related hypercalcemia is much more rapid than that seen in primary hyperparathyroidism. Because breast carcinoma rarely is associated with ectopic production of parathormone-like substances, the occurrence of hypercalcemia in patients with breast cancer but no bone metastases should prompt a search for primary hyperparathyroidism.

Hypoglycemia

Humoral hypoglycemia is rare, the exception being hypoglycemia characteristic of insulinoma of the pancreas. Presenting symptoms include confusion, lethargy, irritability, and coma, and laboratory assessment will reveal fasting hypoglycemia. Most cases of tumor-related hypoglycemia have been associated with hepatomas or massive mesenchymal tumors of the abdomen and retroperitoneum (e.g., fibrosarcomas, mesotheliomas, or liposarcomas).

Although the pathogenesis of paraneoplastic hypoglycemia is not understood well, in some instances the tumor appears to produce a substance having biological activity similar to that of insulin. A case report identified a leiomyosarcoma that produced ectopic insulin-like growth factor II [9]. Surgical removal of the tumor relieved the hypoglycemia, but the condition returned on relapse of the cancer. The tumor cells contained high levels of the growth factor and gene and mRNA coding for the factor. Other possible mechanisms for tumor-associated hypoglycemia include inappropriately high glucose use by the tumor itself and production by the tumor of specific inhibitors of hepatic gluconeogenesis. Often, hypoglycemia arises in the terminal stages of a malignancy, and palliation may be difficult. Glucose infusions, glucocorticoids, growth hormone, and the antihypertensive agent diazoxide have been used with varying degrees of success.

Excess Secretion of Human Chorionic Gonadotropin

Two clinical syndromes have been associated with excess secretion of human chorionic gonadotropin (HCG), a hormone normally secreted by the placenta. One is a rare syndrome of *precocious puberty* that affects prepubertal boys and has been associated with hepatoblastoma. The other is characterized by the appearance of *gynecomastia* in adult men with lung or testicular cancer. Biochemical evidence of excess HCG secretion without a clinical syndrome has been documented in lung, ovarian, and GI cancer (especially involving the stomach) and in melanoma [7].

Erythrocytosis

Erythrocytosis is defined as an absolute increase in the red blood cell mass to levels exceeding 30 ml/kg of body weight in men and exceeding 25 ml/kg of body weight in women. It has been associated with renal cell carcinoma, Wilms' tumor, sarcoma, hepatoma, cerebellar hemangioblastoma, uterine leiomyoma, ovarian carcinoma, pheochromocytoma and, in rare instances, thymoma and hepatic angiosarcoma. Patients with erythrocytosis may be asymptomatic or may complain of headache, dizziness, tinnitus, decreased exercise toler-

ance, or thrombotic phenomena. Incidence depends on the tumor cell type and varies from 1% to 5% in renal cell carcinoma, 5% to 10% in hepatoma, and up to 25% to 30% in cerebellar hemangioblastoma.

Several different mechanisms may produce erythrocytosis, including production of erythropoietin or erythropoietin-like material by the tumor; stimulation of erythropoietin secretion by renal tissue, either through humoral factors produced by prostaglandins or through a mass effect; enhancement of erythropoietin activity; or non-erythropoietin-mediated stimulation of erythropoiesis. Usually, erythrocytosis resolves after the responsible tumor has been treated successfully, and recurrence of the hematologic disorder may herald a cancer relapse.

If the hematocrit exceeds 54% in a man or 47% in a woman, the cause should be determined. Erythropoietin measurements obtained by radioimmunoassay may help to discriminate between polycythemia vera and secondary polycythemia. The majority of patients with polycythemia vera had erythropoietin concentrations well below 30 mU/ml. Usually, leukocyte and platelet counts are normal in secondary polycythemia but are increased in polycythemia vera. Occasionally, patients with cancer have leukocytosis from other causes. Leukocyte alkaline phosphatase levels will be elevated in polycythemia vera but usually are normal in cancer patients unless an intercurrent infection is present.

In some patients with untreatable tumors, phlebotomy will provide symptomatic relief. If elective surgery is planned, the hematocrit should be reduced preoperatively to near 46% to maintain normal cerebral flood flow, because flow is reduced when hematocrit values are elevated [10].

Thyrotoxicosis

Such trophoblastic tumors as hydatidiform moles and choriocarcinomas reportedly elaborate a thyroid-stimulating substance distinct from both pituitary thyroid-stimulating hormone and the long-acting thyroid stimulator of Graves' disease. Paraneoplastic thyrotoxicosis is characterized by mild hyperthyroidism with eyelid lag, tachycardia, weakness, hyperactive reflexes, and goiter, but it lacks the exophthalmos characteristic of Graves' disease. This thyroid-stimulating activity may stem from HCG, which is produced in large quantities by trophoblastic tumors but is a relatively weak thyroid stimulator. Thyroid storm is unusual in patients with paraneoplastic thyrotoxicosis. Laboratory studies show elevated triiodothyronine (T_3) and thyroxine (T_4) levels, whereas thyroid scans indicate that the gland is diffusely active. This condition is treated by surgical removal of the primary tumor or by chemotherapy.

GASTROINTESTINAL HORMONE SYNDROMES

The excess production of naturally occurring GI hormones by specific tumors has been associated with several dramatic clinical syndromes. Most of the disorders' symptoms result from the physiologic or endocrinologic effects of the tumor rather than from its size or replacement of normal tissue.

Zollinger-Ellison Syndrome

Zollinger-Ellison syndrome consists of severe peptic ulceration of the stomach, duodenum, and jejunum in association with pancreatic islet-cell tumors. Gastric acid secretion is excessive, and the ulcers tend to be highly resistant to treatment. Diarrhea and steatorrhea are common features. Zollinger-Ellison syndrome, which is caused by the tumor's excessive, sustained secretion of gastrin, usually can be controlled with histamine H_2-receptor blockers (e.g., cimetidine, ranitidine). In some cases, the tumor can be identified and resected. In patients with malignant gastrinomas and metastases, the antineoplastic agent streptozocin may be helpful [7].

Insulinoma

Pancreatic islet-cell tumors that arise from β cells and produce insulin are relatively rare. Approximately 90% of such tumors are benign, and they are distributed equally in the head, body, and tail of the pancreas; the 10% that are malignant tend to metastasize to the liver and regional lymph nodes. The clinical presentation may be subtle and may consist primarily of such neuropsychiatric symptoms as aberrant behavior and disorders of consciousness. Although it suggests the diagnosis, the finding of Whipple's triad—hypoglycemia induced by fasting or exercise and relieved by oral glucose with central nervous system and vasomotor system symptoms—is not specific. Laboratory tests reveal elevations in insulin or related polypeptides and an abnormal insulin-glucose ratio.

Definitive therapy requires surgical resection of the tumor. If the tumor is inoperable or metastatic disease

is present, streptozocin may provide palliation. Diazoxide, a nondiuretic thiazide, may help to raise plasma glucose levels.

Glucagonoma

Glucagonoma is a rare syndrome characterized by a distinctive skin rash (necrolytic, migratory erythema), glucose intolerance, and weight loss and by markedly elevated plasma glucagon levels. This syndrome is associated with pancreatic islet-cell tumors of the alpha cell type. Surgical removal of the tumor will lead to remission.

Verner-Morrison Syndrome

The Verner-Morrison syndrome, also known as *pancreatic cholera,* is characterized by severe, voluminous watery diarrhea. Dehydration, hypokalemia, and hypochlorhydria are common, and hypercalcemia also may be present. The syndrome appears to be related to the excess production of vasoactive intestinal peptide by a tumor, most commonly an islet-cell tumor or pheochromocytoma and, rarely, lung cancer.

Occasionally, prednisone or a somatostatin analog will help to relieve diarrheal symptoms. Definitive treatment requires surgical resection of the tumor. Again, streptozocin may be helpful if the syndrome occurs secondary to an unresectable islet-cell tumor.

Carcinoid Syndrome

The clinical manifestations of this dramatic syndrome may vary considerably, depending on the location of the associated carcinoid tumor and the extent of tumor growth. Most often, the classic syndrome is seen, with ileal carcinoid tumors and hepatic metastases. Carcinoid tumors secrete a variety of substances, including serotonin, kinin, histamine, and prostaglandins. The clinical syndrome consists of palpitations, facial flushing, diarrhea, abdominal cramps, and wheezing. Endocardial fibrosis may occur, with associated abnormalities of the tricuspid and pulmonic valves. Although the syndrome is distinctive, it does not always develop fully, rendering diagnosis difficult. Excessive excretion of the serotonin metabolite 5-hydroxyindolacetic acid remains the most useful marker of a carcinoid tumor.

Because the appearance of the syndrome usually reflects hepatic metastases, treatment of the underlying malignancy often is ineffective. Such antiserotonin drugs as methysergide and cyproheptadine may alleviate abdominal cramping. Attempts to control this syndrome with chemotherapy involving a variety of drugs, including streptozocin for underlying metastatic disease, have met with limited success. Finally, a recently introduced somatostatin analog, octreotide, may have an important role in the treatment of patients with malignant carcinoid syndrome [11, 12].

HEMATOLOGIC SYNDROMES
Red Blood Cell Disorders

Increased red blood cell production was discussed earlier (see under Erythrocytosis). A more common finding in patients with cancer is mild to moderate anemia, particularly the anemia of chronic disease and myelophthisic anemia. Usually, *anemia of chronic disease* is normochromic and normocytic, although hypochromia is seen occasionally with a concomitant decrease in serum iron and iron-binding capacity and an increase in serum ferritin. Examination of the bone marrow reveals increased hemosiderin within macrophages. The precise cause of this chronic anemia is not yet known, but it appears to be related to multiple factors, including decreased red blood cell survival, an impaired bone marrow response to anemia, and impaired release of iron by macrophages.

The *myelophthisic anemia of cancer* is caused by direct tumor cell invasion of the bone marrow. An important note is that tumor cells may not always be evident on bone marrow biopsy; conversely, bone marrow metastases may not result in a leukoerythroblastic peripheral blood smear.

Deficiencies of iron or other nutrients may exacerbate and modify the morphology of both these types of anemia. Exogenous administration of erythropoietin can reverse these anemias and can improve the quality of life for affected patients [13].

Sometimes, another red blood cell disorder, *antibody-mediated hemolytic anemia,* may be seen in patients with lymphoma or chronic lymphocytic leukemia. Rarely, it is seen with solid tumors (particularly those affecting the ovary) and with metastatic gastric carcinoma [14].

White Blood Cell Disorders

Patients with cancer may develop a *leukemoid blood reaction* with a marked increase in the total white blood cell count, usually neutrophilia. Occasionally, the number of immature myeloid cells increases to such an extent that the condition resembles a leukemic process. Although leukemoid reactions have been described for a variety of malignancies, they are most common in retroperitoneal sarcomas and in breast, gastric, and lung carcinomas. The underlying mechanism is the tumor's elaboration of a factor similar in activity to colony-stimulating factor. Morphologic markers specific for such acute leukemia as Auer bodies should be absent in a paraneoplastic leukemoid reaction.

Although eosinophilia has been described in many malignant diseases, it is seen most commonly in Hodgkin's disease and lung cancer (in < 1% of patients with cancer). This condition may be related to tumor necrosis, but its precise pathogenesis and prognostic significance have not yet been determined. *Monocytosis* has been observed in many malignancies, particularly in gastric, breast, and ovarian carcinomas and in malignant melanoma.

Platelet Disorders

Thrombocytosis, defined as an increase in the platelet count to greater than 400,000/mm^3, is seen in a variety of malignancies, especially lung cancer, Hodgkin's disease, and myeloproliferative disorders. It occurs without tumor invasion of the bone marrow, and the platelet count usually returns to normal once the tumor has been eradicated successfully. Treatment-related changes in platelet count are especially common in patients with Hodgkin's disease; in such cases, absolute platelet count may be a sensitive indicator of disease activity. An elevated platelet count does not seem to contribute to the frequent thrombotic events seen in patients with cancer, and specific attempts to lower the count usually are not warranted. *Thrombocytopenia* also is common in patients with cancer, but usually it occurs secondary to a complication of the cancer itself (e.g., disseminated intravascular coagulation or bone marrow invasion) or to its treatment.

Coagulation Disorders

Clinical and laboratory evidence of coagulation abnormalities is extremely common among patients with cancer. These disorders range from thrombotic phenomena to frank hemorrhage associated with a consumption coagulopathy. Perhaps the most graphic example of a cancer-associated hypercoagulable state is migratory superficial thrombophlebitis (Trousseau's syndrome) associated with pancreatic cancer. However, a tendency toward venous and arterial thrombosis has been associated with a great variety of malignancies, especially visceral adenocarcinomas. Sometimes, unexplained thrombophlebitis or even pulmonary embolism is the first indication of an undiagnosed malignancy [15]. Nonbacterial thrombotic endocarditis may be seen, or excessive fibrinolysis and hemorrhage may dominate the clinical picture.

The precise relationship between coagulation disorders and cancer still is unknown. Several malignancies, especially mucin-producing adenocarcinomas, release thromboplastic materials that may activate the clotting system. In addition, tumor cell extracts contain proteases capable of activating factor X. An abnormal tumor microvasculature might lead to factor XII activation and thus could initiate the entire coagulation cascade. Activation of fibrinolytic enzymes by tumors also has been well described.

Chronic subclinical disseminated intravascular coagulation is extremely common in cancer patients, especially those with metastatic disease. However, this condition rarely requires treatment because affected patients are asymptomatic. Usually, symptomatic thrombotic complications require heparin anticoagulation and the use of warfarin to achieve lasting control. Generally, *acute hemorrhagic* disseminated intravascular coagulation requires clotting-factor replacement, either alone or in combination with heparin, and management may be difficult. Finally, when it is possible, control of the underlying malignancy can play an important role in the management of paraneoplastic coagulation disorders.

SKIN AND CONNECTIVE TISSUE SYNDROMES

Acanthosis Nigricans

The term *acanthosis nigricans* refers to pigmented hyperkeratosis, consisting of verrucous and papillary lesions that occur in the skin flexures, particularly in the axillary and perineal areas. Usually, these lesions are symmetric and may be accompanied by pruritus. Acanthosis nigricans has been associated with visceral adenocarcinomas, particularly of the stomach. Its appearance usually precedes or coincides with the diagnosis of the malignancy and may, therefore, signify internal malignancy. Successful treatment of the associated cancer may lead to complete regression of these skin changes.

Ichthyosis

The term *ichthyosis* refers to a generalized dryness and scaling of the skin that may have a variety of causes, including hereditary syndromes. When ichthyosis develops late in life, it may be associated with lymphoma, particularly Hodgkin's disease.

Malignant Down

Hypertrichosis lanuginosa acquisita, or malignant down, is rare. It is a dramatic paraneoplastic syndrome characterized by excessive growth of the fine lanugo hair.

Leser-Trélat Sign

The Leser-Trélat sign is the sudden appearance and growth of multiple seborrheic keratoses. It occurs in association with an underlying visceral cancer.

Sweet's Syndrome

Sweet's syndrome is an acute febrile neutrophilic dermatosis. Approximately 20% of patients with Sweet's syndrome have an associated cancer (e.g., leukemia, lymphoma, or a solid tumor). The skin lesions and fever characteristic of this condition respond dramatically to corticosteroid treatment, regardless of whether the associated neoplasm responds to antitumor therapy.

Hyperpigmentation

Generalized hyperpigmentation has been observed with various neoplasms, including lung, liver, and pancreatic carcinomas. This syndrome is characterized by diffuse darkening of the exposed areas of the body (e.g., the face, neck, and dorsum of the hands) and of the axillae, palmar creases, and buccal mucosa. Almost always, paraneoplastic hyperpigmentation occurs in patients with the aforementioned ectopic ACTH syndrome. Substances that stimulate melanocyte production in humans arise from a large precursor molecule that also contains the polypeptide sequence for ACTH. Ongoing research seeks to determine whether the hyperpigmentation seen in these patients arises from extremely high ACTH levels or from the tumor's simultaneous release of ACTH and melanocyte-stimulating hormone. In rare instances, successful treatment of the tumor has led to a reversal of the hyperpigmentation.

Dermatomyositis

Dermatomyositis is characterized by polymyositis with proximal muscle weakness and a violaceous erythema on exposed parts of the body, especially the malar area and the eyelids. A muscle disorder with or without weakness may occur and progress over a period of weeks to months, with spontaneous remissions and exacerbations. Patients may complain of muscle pain, tenderness, and swelling. Dysphagia is common, and respiratory muscles may become weak. Laboratory findings may include elevated serum muscle enzymes (creatinine phosphokinase, aldolase, and transaminase) and elevated urinary creatinine.

Electromyography reveals evidence of primary muscle degeneration with spontaneous fibrillation. A muscle biopsy will document focal or diffuse necrosis of muscle fibers, regenerative activity evidenced by basophilia of the same fibers, and an inflammatory reaction consisting of interstitial and perivascular infiltration by lymphocytes and plasma cells. Although the relationship between dermatomyositis and visceral malignancy recently was questioned, studies of men older than 40 years show a clear-cut association between dermatomyositis and the subsequent neoplasia. The malignancies associated most commonly with this disease are visceral adenocarcinomas, usually arising in the stomach, breast, ovary, or lung.

Like the foregoing cutaneous disorders, the onset of dermatomyositis usually precedes the diagnosis of malignancy, sometimes by several years. Most patients appear to benefit at least temporarily from corticosteroids. Successful treatment of the associated malignancy may improve the muscle disorder, but the two diseases occasionally follow separate courses.

Hypertrophic Pulmonary Osteoarthropathy

Patients with hypertrophic pulmonary osteoarthropathy may have a variety of abnormalities that range from asymptomatic clubbing to a severe periostitis and polyarticular arthritis. Commonly, this syndrome is associated with intrathoracic malignancy, particularly lung carcinoma. Although clubbing of the fingers and toes alone may be associated with a variety of conditions unrelated to cancer (including cystic fibrosis, biliary cirrhosis, cyanotic congenital heart disease, and bacterial

endocarditis), the full-blown syndrome—arthritis, clubbing, and periosteal proliferation—usually is associated with malignancy. The articular symptoms may precede the periosteal changes and clubbing, and the joints involved most often are the knees, ankles, elbows, wrists, and metacarpophalangeal joints. Patients may complain of joint or leg pain. Periosteal thickening can be demonstrated radiographically, especially when it involves the tarsal and carpal bones and the long bones of the forearms and legs. Usually, joint involvement is symmetric. Serum alkaline phosphatase levels are normal, but a bone scan may be positive in areas of new bone formation.

The pathogenesis of hypertrophic pulmonary osteoarthropathy is unknown. This syndrome may regress promptly after successful tumor resection. Occasionally, treatment with salicylates or glucocorticoids can offer palliation [7].

NEUROLOGIC SYNDROMES

The remote effects of tumors on the nervous system can lead to a wide range of neurologic syndromes. The causes of these disorders are not completely understood, but evidence suggests a humoral or cellular autoimmune pathogenesis for most.

Subacute Cerebellar Degeneration

Patients with the dramatic subacute cerebellar degeneration syndrome present with evidence of cerebellar ataxia, dysarthria, dysphagia and, occasionally, dementia. The cerebrospinal fluid may show pleocytosis and slightly increased protein levels; however, these findings are not diagnostic. Pathologic assessment reveals diffuse cortical degeneration from the cerebellum, with panhemispheric loss of Purkinje cells. Although the cause of this syndrome is unknown, some investigators believe that an autoimmune process may be involved; antibodies to neuronal cells and some types of receptors have been demonstrated in serum. Most commonly, subacute cerebellar degeneration is associated with lung cancer, particularly of the small-cell type, and with ovarian and breast carcinoma and lymphoma [16].

Eaton-Lambert Syndrome

Frequently, classic myasthenia gravis is associated with a benign or malignant thymoma and rarely is seen in other malignancies. However, a variant known as *facilitating myasthenia* or *reverse myasthenia*, or *Eaton-Lambert syndrome*, occurs almost exclusively in patients with small-cell lung cancer. This syndrome differs from classic myasthenia gravis in several important ways.

Myasthenia gravis occurs primarily in young women, whereas Eaton-Lambert syndrome generally affects men older than 40 years. In classic myasthenia, the bulbar and ocular muscles tend to be involved initially. In contrast, the initial symptom of Eaton-Lambert syndrome usually is proximal muscle weakness related to impaired release of acetylcholine from the motor nerve terminal. Electromyography will reveal a striking finding in patients with Eaton-Lambert syndrome: Repeated stimuli produce impulse facilitation rather than the fatigue seen in classic myasthenia. High serum levels of IgG autoantibodies that block the voltage-dependent calcium channels are believed to be responsible for the presynaptic impairment discovered in patients with this syndrome. Occasionally, patients with Eaton-Lambert syndrome respond to guanidine; the anticholinesterases used to treat myasthenia gravis are ineffective. In several instances, successful antitumor treatment has reversed this syndrome.

Retinal Degeneration

A syndrome of progressive blindness secondary to retinal degeneration may occur in association with malignancy, particularly small-cell lung cancer. Serum IgG from several patients with paraneoplastic retinopathy has been found to react with both retinal ganglion cells and tumor cells, a finding consistent with an autoimmune phenomenon.

Carcinomatous Neuropathies

Probably, motor, sensory, and mixed neuropathies are the most common neurologic abnormalities seen in patients with cancer. Most often, the syndrome encountered is a mild, symmetric, sensory peripheral neuropathy that occurs with advanced malignancies. Further research is needed to determine whether this syndrome results from the general debility and poor nutritional status characteristic of patients with advanced cancer or whether it represents a distinct paraneoplastic effect of the neoplasm.

Other Neurologic Syndromes

Many neurologic disorders affecting virtually all levels of the nervous system and the muscles and neuromuscular junctions have been described in cancer patients. Their pathogenesis and the nature of their association with malignancy, if any, require further study [17].

RENAL SYNDROMES

The remote effects of a malignancy can produce renal dysfunction through a variety of mechanisms. Such cancer-related metabolic abnormalities as hypercalcemia or hyperuricemia may damage the kidney. Patients with multiple myeloma and Bence Jones proteinuria are at high risk for renal dysfunction and may incur damage secondary to renal amyloidosis. Glomerular injury may develop with extensive proteinuria in a variety of malignancies, including breast, colon, and lung cancers. In some instances, the complete nephrotic syndrome may be present. Often, pathologic examination demonstrates a membranous or membranoproliferative glomerulopathy, which appears to be related to the deposition of immune complexes on the glomerular membrane. These immune complexes appear secondary to circulating antigen-antibody complexes. In several cases, these antigens have been shown to be tumor-related (e.g., carcinoembryonic antigen).

Generally, the prognosis for patients with membranous or membranoproliferative glomerulopathies is poor, and remission of the renal lesion rarely has been noted, even when the tumor is treated successfully. In contrast, patients with nephrotic syndrome associated with Hodgkin's disease and other lymphomas ordinarily demonstrate minimal glomerular changes on renal biopsy, without evidence of immune complex formation. Successful treatment of the underlying lymphoma leads to prompt remission of the renal disease in such patients [7].

SUMMARY

The paraneoplastic syndromes offer an opportunity to increase understanding of malignancy from the standpoint of both basic biological research and clinical practice. The study of these syndromes may provide insight into the fundamental nature of neoplastic transformation. Some researchers have suggested that the hormones and other polypeptides or growth factors released by tumors may be required for tumor growth;

alternatively, these substances may confer a selective advantage favoring the growth of tumor cells over normal cells. With new information about these phenomena, approaches to cancer therapy may be improved. Techniques for precise identification of minute amounts of polypeptides may allow the early diagnosis of curable malignancies in asymptomatic individuals. Finally, if tumor-associated substances can be identified on cancer cell membranes, current approaches to cancer therapy may become more selective.

REFERENCES

1. Barri Y, Knochel J. Hypercalcemia and electrolyte disturbances in malignancy. *Hematol Oncol Clin North Am* 10: 775–790, 1996.
2. Moffat F, Ketcham A. Metastatic proclivity and patterns among APUD cell neoplasms. *Semin Surg Oncol* 9:443–452, 1993.
3. Yu H, Spitz M, Mistry J, et al. Plasma levels of insulin-like growth factor-I and lung cancer risk: a case-control analysis. *J Natl Cancer Inst* 91:151–156, 1999.
4. Kaffer J. Endocrinopathy and ectopic hormones in malignancy. *Hematol Oncol Clin North Am* 10:811–823, 1996.
5. Gelfand J, Dinarello C, Wolff S. Alterations in body temperature. In Isselbacher K, Braunwald E, Wilson J, et al. (eds), *Harrison's Principles of Internal Medicine* (13th ed). New York: McGraw-Hill, 1994:81–90.
6. Tisdale M. Biology of cachexia. *J Natl Cancer Inst* 89:1763–1773, 1997.
7. John W, Foon K, Patchell R. Paraneoplastic syndromes. In DeVita VT Jr, Hellman S, Rosenberg SA (eds), *Cancer: Principles and Practice of Oncology* (5th ed). Philadelphia: Lippincott-Raven, 1997:2397–2422.
8. Warnell R. Metabolic emergencies. In DeVita VT Jr, Hellman S, Rosenberg SA (eds), *Cancer: Principles and Practice of Oncology* (5th ed). Philadelphia: Lippincott-Raven, 1997:2486–2500.
9. Daughaday WH, Imanuele MA, Brooks MH, et al. Synthesis and secretion of insulin-like growth factor II by a leiomyosarcoma with associated hypoglycemia. *N Engl J Med* 319:1434–1440, 1988.
10. France-Saenz R. Hypercalcemia syndrome of inappropriate ADH and other endocrine syndromes. In Skeel RT, Lachant NA (eds), *Handbook of Cancer Chemotherapy.* Boston: Little, Brown, 1995:590–613.
11. Kvols L, Moertel C, O'Connell M, et al. Treatment of the malignant carcinoid syndrome. *N Engl J Med* 315:663–666, 1986.
12. Otte A, Muellar-Brand J, Dellas S, et al. Yttrium-90 labeled somatostatin analogue for cancer treatment. *Lancet* 351:417–418, 1998.
13. Spivak J. Recombinant human erythropoietin and the anemia of cancer. *Blood* 84:997–1004, 1994.
14. Antman KH, Skarin AT, Mayer RJ, et al. Microangiopathic hemolytic anemia and cancer: a review. *Medicine* 58:277–384, 1979.
15. Sorensen H, Mellamkjaer L, Steffansen F. The risk of a diagnosis of cancer after primary deep venous thrombosis or pulmonary embolism. *N Engl J Med* 338:1169–1173, 1998.
16. Sillevis Smitt P, Kinoshita A, De Leeuw B, et al. Paraneoplastic cerebellar ataxia due to autoantibodies against a glutamate receptor. *N Engl J Med* 342:21–27, 2000.
17. Hinton R. Paraneoplastic neurologic syndromes. *Hematol Oncol Clin North Am* 10:909–925, 1996.

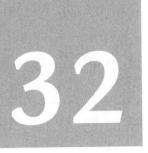

32

Cancer-Related Emergencies

■ ■ ■

Angela DeMichele
John H. Glick

OVERVIEW OF DIAGNOSIS AND MANAGEMENT OF ONCOLOGIC EMERGENCIES

Advances in radiotherapy, chemotherapy, and supportive care have increased the incidence of oncologic emergencies as survival of cancer patients improves. Before initiating treatment, several important management factors must be considered in evaluating and treating an oncologic emergency. Aggressive treatment is often indicated when a histologic diagnosis of malignancy is suspected, but has not been established, as well as in patients with an established diagnosis of cancer who have an excellent long-term prognosis. In advanced malignancies, the primary goal is often palliation and relief of symptoms, even if the patient has a limited life expectancy.

Frequently, restoring functional status leads to improved quality of life. However, a strong chance for cure or prolonged palliation with preservation of quality of life may warrant more aggressive measures, designed to support a patient through the acute manifestations of a treatable illness. If the oncologic emergency is directly due to the malignant process, the general approach is to treat the underlying malignancy if effective therapy is available and to initiate treatment promptly to prevent complications and permanent disability. However, for terminal cancer patients, foregoing treatment and controlling pain may be the most appropriate steps. Figure 32.1 illustrates the general approach to the evaluation and treatment of an oncologic emergency.

CARDIOPULMONARY EMERGENCIES
Pericardial Effusion and Neoplastic Cardiac Tamponade

At autopsy, up to 20% of cancer patients have cardiac or pericardial metastases [1]. Cancers of the lung or

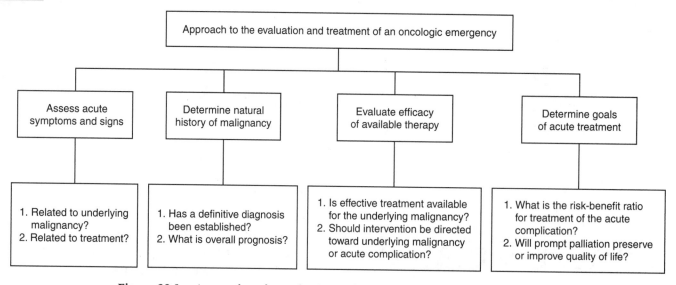

Figure 32.1. Approach to the evaluation and treatment of an oncologic emergency.

esophagus can grow by direct extension into the pericardium, while distant primary malignancies may metastasize to the pericardium hematogenously. Lung and breast carcinomas, lymphoma, leukemia, melanoma, gastrointestinal primaries, and sarcomas are the most common primary cancers associated with malignant pericardial effusions [1].

PATHOPHYSIOLOGIC FEATURES

Tamponade usually occurs because of cardiac compression from large malignant pericardial effusions, although, in some cases, encasement of the heart by tumor or postirradiation pericarditis can mimic tamponade as well [2]. With cardiac tamponade, signs of circulatory collapse appear suddenly, even though the effusion or constriction may have developed gradually. The severity of tamponade depends on the rate of pericardial fluid formation and the volume of fluid accumulated. Slow pericardial fluid accumulation may stretch the pericardium and cardiac contractility may not be greatly impaired. However, if the pericardium is surrounded by tumor or radiation fibrosis, even a small effusion may produce significant cardiac compression and hemodynamic compromise. Elevated pericardial pressures reduce ventricular expansion and diastolic filling. As stroke volume decreases, hypotension, compensatory tachycardia, and equalization and elevation of the mean left atrial, pulmonary arterial and venous, right atrial, and vena caval pressures occur. Tachycardia and peripheral vasoconstriction develop in an attempt to maintain arterial pressure, increase blood volume, and improve venous return.

CLINICAL PRESENTATION

In a large autopsy series, fewer than 30% of patients with malignant pericardial effusions had symptoms of pericarditis [3]. In most patients, the diagnosis of pericardial tumor is not detected prior to acute hemodynamic compromise or death. With tamponade or pericardial constriction, patients may complain of dyspnea, cough, and retrosternal chest pain relieved by leaning forward. When cardiac output falls, decreased cerebral blood flow, peripheral cyanosis, decreased systolic and pulse pressures, and pulsus paradoxus occur. Occasionally patients with large effusions develop hoarseness, hiccups, nausea, vomiting, or epigastric pain. Physical examination may reveal engorged neck veins, distant heart sounds, edema, ascites, hepatosplenomegaly, or hepatojugular reflux [1].

DIAGNOSTIC EVALUATION

More than half the patients with pericardial effusions have cardiac enlargement, mediastinal widening, or hilar adenopathy that can be seen on a chest x-ray. As the fluid increases, the mediastinum shortens and widens, the normal arcuate borders are lost, and the cardiac silhouette becomes globular [4]. Electrocardiographic abnormalities are often nonspecific. With pericarditis, the electrocardiogram may have low QRS voltage in the limb leads, sinus tachycardia, ST elevations, and T wave changes; with tamponade, electrical alternans may occur. Echocardiography is the most specific and sensitive noninvasive test for the presence of pericardial effusion or right ventricular collapse, suggesting tamponade. An echocardiogram should therefore be performed immediately if the diagnosis of percardial effusion or tamponade is suspected. With posterior effusions, two distinct echoes are seen: one from the effusion and the other from the posterior heart border. The space between these echoes indicates the size of the effusion or thickness of the pericardium [5, 6]. More recently, magnetic resonance imaging (MRI) has been advocated as a diagnostic tool in this setting because of its excellent resolution [7, 8]. Inconclusive physical examination and noninvasive studies require that a right heart catheterization be performed to diagnose pericardial tamponade or constriction [9].

Pericardiocentesis should be performed for both diagnostic and therapeutic purposes. The fluid is analyzed for cell count, cytology, and appropriate cultures [10]. The cytology is usually positive in patients with metastatic carcinoma, but is frequently inconclusive with lymphoma and mesothelioma. If a histologic diagnosis is important and pericardial fluid cytologies are negative, a pericardial biopsy should be performed either under local anesthesia with a subxiphoid approach or under general anesthesia with an anterior thoracotomy. The latter procedure is more sensitive because more tissue can be obtained, but has a higher attendant morbidity and mortality [11].

THERAPY

A clinically significant decrease in cardiac output is an indication for emergency pericardiocentesis before initiating definitive local therapy to prevent recurrent tamponade. Emergency pericardiocentesis should be considered if the patient develops (1) cyanosis, dyspnea, shock, or impaired consciousness; (2) a pulsus paradoxus greater than 50% of the pulse pressure; (3) a decrease of more than 20 mm of Hg in pulse pressure; or (4) peripheral venous pressures greater than 13 mm of Hg [9]. Oxygen should be administered, but positive pressure ventilation is contraindicated due to the potential for worsening venous return from increased intrapericardial and intrapleural pressures.

Tamponade will generally recur after an initial tap unless the patient receives prompt treatment to prevent pericardial fluid reaccumulation. Therapeutic options depend on the primary tumor's sensitivity to systematic chemotherapy, hormonal therapy, or local radiotherapy; prior treatment; and life expectancy. Pericardial windows, sclerosing agents, radiotherapy, effective systemic antineoplastic drugs, and pericardectomy have all produced excellent, long-term palliation in selected series [11–14]. These treatments are difficult to compare because responses are not based on objective criteria. Duration of response and survival are influenced by the extent of metastatic disease, and the chance of response to concurrent systemic hormonal therapy or chemotherapy [13, 15]

Tamponade can often be controlled for some time by pericardial catheter drainage and sclerosis. An indwelling pericardial catheter is left in place until pericardial drainage stops. Minocycline (10 mg/kg) or tetracycline (500–1,000 mg) is then instilled through the pericardial cannula and flushed with normal saline [14, 16]. The procedure is repeated every two to three days until there is no fluid drainage in the preceding 24 hours. The inflammatory response and fibrosis from intrapericardial tetracycline obliterates the space between the parietal and visceral pericardium and prevents fluid reaccumulation.

Effective pericardial sclerosis can also be achieved with 1–2 installations of bleomycin (20 mg) through the catheter [17]. Bleomycin is instilled after all the pericardial fluid has been evacuated for 24 hours, then the tube is clamped for 10 minutes and then withdrawn. In one series, no major side effects were noted, except for one transient elevation in temperature that resolved in less than 12 hours. Severe fibrosis was not reported after local installation, nor was fibrous thickening of the pericardium found at autopsy. None of the patients in the study died from pericardial tamponade. Bleomycin may have certain advantages over tetracycline, including fewer side effects (especially less pain). One recent study comparing doxycycline and bleomycin showed no difference in efficacy between the two agents, with bleomycin requiring a shorter duration of catheterization and fewer inpatient hospital days [18].

Palliation may also be obtained with pleural-pericardial windows. Under local anesthesia, inferior pericardiotomy provides immediate relief of cardiac compression and tissue for histologic diagnosis with complication rates less than 2% [13]. Tamponade symptoms reoccur in less than 5% of patients. Previously, thoracotomy was required if the heart is encased with tumor, or if additional tissue was required for a diagnostic purpose; now a less invasive laparoscopic technique can be used [19]. An even less invasive approach to recurrent large pericardial effusions involves the use of balloon pericardiotomy. This is a treatment in which a non-surgical pericardial window is created via the percutaneous subxiphoid route using a balloon dilating catheter. Recent reports have demonstrated that this procedure can be performed safely and effectively in patients with malignant pericardial effusions [20].

Pericardiectomy (or pericardial "stripping") may be necessary if radiation-induced pericardial disease is not controlled with conservative medical management, but it should not be performed when there is extensive pericardial tumor. With extensive pericardial metastases, life expectancy is short and surgical morbidity and mortality rates with pericardiectomy are high [13].

An alternative approach to the management of malignant pericardial effusions involves the use of local chemotherapy or radiation. Colleoni et al recently reported the direct installation of cytotoxic chemotherapy into the pericardial space [21]. Patients with malignant pericardial effusions were treated with intracavitary thiotepa (15 mg on days 1, 3, and 5) through an indwelling pericardial cannula after extraction of as much pericardial fluid as possible on day 0. Responses were assessed by clinical examination, computed tomographic (CT) scan, and echocardiography before treatment, one month after treatment, and every two months thereafter. Nineteen of the 23 patients studied (83%) responded to treatment with a rapid improvement of symptoms. The median time to pericardial effusion progression was nine months. No significant side effects were registered, except one patient who had transient grade III thrombocytopenia and leukopenia and one patient who had grade I leukopenia. Intracavitary platinum has also been used successfully in patients with recurrent tamponade due to lung cancer [22]. Cisplatin (10 mg in 20 ml of normal saline) was instilled over a five-minute period on five consecutive days (maximal total cisplatin dose in single course = 50 mg) directly into the pericardial space, with approximately 80% of patients obtaining relief for at least one month post-treatment. Although radiotherapy has been reported to control more than 50% of malignant pericardial effusions, the radiosensitivity of the tumor will determine the response and duration of palliation. Radiation doses are given in 1.5 Gy to 2.0 Gy fractions to a total dose of 25–30 Gy. Patients with lymphoma or leukemia may respond to lower doses (e.g., 15–20 Gy over a two-week period).

Once the patient is clinically stable, systemic therapy should be administered if effective treatment is available. If a rapid chemotherapeutic response can be obtained (e.g., in lymphoma or small-cell lung cancer), the patient may be treated with pericardial drainage and systemic chemotherapy. Recent data suggests that systemic cytotoxic therapy may be effective in chemotherapy-sensitive tumors such as lymphoma, leukemia, and breast cancer [23]. Patients with lymphoma who have not received first-line therapy have an excellent re-

sponse rate to combination chemotherapy for their pericardial effusions. In one series of three patients with malignant pericardial effusions due to breast cancer [23], control of effusion was achieved with single pericardiocentesis followed by systemic chemotherapy. No other local therapy was necessary. Similar results have also been observed in patients with effusions due to acute leukemia [24].

Superior Vena Cava Syndrome

ETIOLOGIC FACTORS AND PATHOPHYSIOLOGIC FEATURES

The superior vena cava (SVC) is easily compressed by adjacent, expanding masses. When obstructed, venous blockage produces pleural effusions and facial, arm, and tracheal edema. With severe SVC obstruction, brain edema and impaired cardiac filling may produce altered consciousness and focal neurologic signs. Symptoms depend on the extent and rapidity of SVC compression. If the SVC is gradually compressed and collateral circulation develops, symptoms may be indolent and subtle. The presence of SVC syndrome associated with malignancy is a poor prognostic factor, with average survival from time of diagnosis measured in months [25–27].

Most cases of SVC syndrome are caused by malignant, mediastinal tumors [27]. More than 75% of malignant SVC obstructions are secondary to advanced lung cancers. From 10% to 15% of neoplastic SVC syndromes are secondary to mediastinal lymphomas, most often diffuse large-cell subtypes [28]. Less than 15% are secondary to benign etiologies such as tuberculosis, aneurysms, and thrombus. The most common nonmalignant cause of SVC obstruction is thrombus in central venous catheters [29].

CLINICAL PRESENTATION AND DIAGNOSTIC EVALUATION

Diagnosis of severe SVC obstruction is suggested if facial edema, venous engorgement, and impaired consciousness are present. However, in its early stages, the presentation is often much more subtle, and may include facial plethora, upper extremity edema, neck vein distention, tachypnea, hoarseness (due to vocal cord paralysis), or onset of Horner's syndrome [30]. Chest computerized tomography (CT) scan with intravenous contrast or chest MRI scans are currently the preferred diagnostic tools [31]. MRI scans are often done prior to any intervention to provide excellent anatomic detail and help to define radiation portals. However, if SVC obstruction develops slowly, venography or radionuclide scans may be necessary to confirm the diagnosis. Angiographic or radionuclide studies also help to localize the site of obstruction, plan radiation portals, or guide interventional radiologic procedures [32].

Many patients with SVC syndrome do not present with a histologic diagnosis of malignancy. In such situations, the least invasive technique should be used to establish the diagnosis by biopsy or cytology. Sputum cytology, bronchoscopy with brushings and washings, or biopsy of palpable adenopathy provide the correct diagnosis in 70% of cases [30]. However, because of elevated venous pressures, these procedures are associated with a risk of post-operative bleeding and possible airway compromise that may necessitate rigid bronchoscopy and endotracheal balloon tamponade. If small-cell lung cancer or lymphoma is suspected, bone marrow aspiration or biopsies may confirm the diagnosis, abrogating the need for a pulmonary procedure. If necessary, invasive diagnostic procedures (e.g., thoracotomy or mediastinoscopy) can be performed safely if the trachea is not obstructed [33]. In the past, invasive procedures were postponed a few days until radiotherapy was begun to prevent complications from bleeding or airway compromise. However, delaying diagnostic procedures several days after radiotherapy may yield only necrotic tissue, preventing the establishment of a definitive diagnosis.

THERAPY

Only a small percentage of patients with rapid onset of SVC obstruction are at risk for life-threatening complications [34]. Emergency treatment is indicated when there is brain edema with marked mental status changes, decreased cardiac output with hemodynamic compromise or upper-airway edema with impending loss of airway. In such circumstances, intraluminal stent placement may effectively restore blood flow immediately and is often used prior to, or in conjunction with, radiotherapy [35]. This approach uses a combination of thrombolysis, angioplasty, and intravascular stents. Short-term results are excellent, with rapid patient recovery.

Most patients with non-life threatening malignant SVC obstruction are treated with radiotherapy with or without stent placement. Radiotherapy has traditionally been given in high daily fractions (4.0 Gy for three days), followed by 1.5–2.0 Gy per day to a total dose of 30–50 Gy. The radiation dose depends on tumor size, radioresponsiveness, and probability of achieving a response with systemic therapy [36, 37]. In a recent review of 46 patients with SVC syndrome due to malignancies, even higher initial doses of radiation treatment (8 Gy a day, three weekly fractions) were used. With this approach, complete responses were seen in 56% of patients, while 96% of patients had a partial response [38]. Patients with locally advanced non-small cell lung cancer without distant metastases should have the mediastinal, hilar, and supraclavicular lymph nodes and any adjacent parenchymal lesions irradiated. During radiation, patients improve clinically before objective signs of tumor shrinkage are evident on chest x-rays. Radiation palliates SVC obstruction in greater than 70% of patients with lung carcinoma and more than 95% with lymphoma [37]. The addition of chemotherapy to radiotherapy does not appear to improve response rate overall. Corticosteroids may decrease edema associated with inflammatory reactions following tumor necrosis from irradiation. If clinical signs of venous obstruction progress shortly after radiotherapy is initiated, steroids are administered until the signs and symptoms of inflammation are under control. Thus, radiation therapy is very effective for most cases of SVC syndrome due to malignancy, with resolution commonly occurring within approximately four weeks of diagnosis [31].

Chemotherapy alone may be preferable to radiation for patients with disseminated or highly chemosensitive disease if a prompt response is anticipated. For example, small-cell anaplastic carcinoma and lymphoma will respond to radiation; however, these malignancies may respond more rapidly to systemic chemotherapy or multimodality approaches [39].

The role of anticoagulation in the management of SVC syndrome remains controversial [40]. Anticoagulation may help relieve venous obstruction by preventing thrombus formation. Although anticoagulated patients improve more rapidly and have shorter hospitalizations, there is no difference in overall survival. Generally, the risks of hemorrhage associated with antithrombotic therapy outweigh the temporary benefit if the venous obstruction is due to tumor rather than clot. When SVC obstruction is due to thrombus around a central venous catheter, patients may be treated with fibrinolytics, anticoagulants or a superior vena cava filter [41], with or without catheter removal.

Finally, surgical approaches have been used to bypass the occluded SVC [42]. Doty et al reported 10 patients who had surgical intervention for SVC syndrome. Four patients had fibrosing mediastinitis and six had bronchogenic carcinoma. A composite spiral vein graft was placed between the left jugular-subclavian vein and the right atrium of each patient to bypass the completely occluded SVC. The graft was constructed from the patient's own saphenous vein, which was split longitudinally and wrapped around a stent in spiral fashion. The edges of the vein were sutured together to form a large autogenous conduit. All patients were immediately relieved of SVC obstructive symptoms and signs. Graft patency ranged from 7 days to 18 months, as determined by radionuclide venography or contrast-enhanced CT scanning. Patients with SVC obstruction resulting from cancer survived up to 21 months (mean = 10.7 months) postoperatively. Thus, in some cancer patients with a reasonable life-expectancy, spiral vein bypass graft may provide effective palliation for SVC obstruction with immediate relief of symptoms.

Airway Obstruction

ETIOLOGIC FACTORS AND PATHOPHYSIOLOGIC FEATURES

Airway obstruction due to malignancy must be treated promptly to prevent postobstructive pneumonia, respiratory distress, and/or irreversible lung collapse. Airway obstruction is usually caused by endobronchial or endotracheal malignancies, but may also be due to extraluminal compression secondary to parenchymal tumor or enlarged lymph nodes [43]. Endotracheal obstruction is typically caused by primary tumors of the head and neck, but can also be secondary to benign etiologies such as tracheal stenosis, tracheomalacia, or edema from infections or recent irradiation. Lung cancer is the primary cause of endobronchial obstruction. At diagnosis, partial or complete bronchial obstruction is present on chest x-rays in 53% of patients with squamous cell carcinoma; 25% with adenocarcinoma; 33% with large-cell anaplastic carcinomas; and 38% with small-cell carcinoma. Endobronchial tumor is seen in 70% of lung cancer patients at thoracotomy. Endobronchial lesions are found in the main stem and lobular bronchi in approximately 20% and 50% of cases, respectively [44].

In contrast to primary bronchogenic carcinomas, significant endobronchial metastatic lesions are rare [45]. Only 2% of cancer patients have significant endobronchial metastases. However, if patients with microscopic endobronchial disease are included, the incidence of endobronchial metastases ranges from 25% to 50%. The most common malignancies that metastasize to the bronchial tree are carcinomas of the breast, colon and kidney; sarcomas; melanomas; and ovarian cancer.

CLINICAL PRESENTATION

Bronchial and tracheal obstruction are often difficult to differentiate on physical examination. Presenting symptoms include dyspnea, orthopnea, cough, wheezing, stridor, hoarseness, and hemoptysis. Symptoms of bacterial postobstructive pneumonia may be found with complete obstruction of a bronchus. High-pitched breathing or inspiratory stridor are usually associated with laryngeal or tracheal obstruction. Wheezing and rhonchi may be audible or palpable over a partially obstructed airway. If the bronchus is significantly obstructed, the trachea will deviate toward the obstructed side.

DIAGNOSTIC EVALUATION

Lateral neck radiographs with soft tissue technique may provide a view of the upper one-third of the trachea. Chest roentgenographs may reveal atelectasis or segmental consolidation, but tracheal narrowing may not be seen on routine chest x-rays or bilateral oblique views. CT scanning of the neck and upper airways is often indicated to make the diagnosis of tracheal or bronchial obstruction by tumor [45]. In the acute setting, upper-airway obstruction can also be confirmed at the bedside with flow-volume loops using an 80% helium and 20% oxygen mixture (Heliox) [46]. Fiberoptic bronchoscopy is indicated in any patient with suspected airway compromise regardless of radiographic findings as a substantial number of clinically significant cases of tracheal obstruction may be radiographically undetectable [47]. Directed biopsies are usually needed to obtain a definitive histologic diagnosis. Cultures should be obtained if fever or other signs of postobstructive pneumonitis are present. However, these procedures can result in post-biopsy edema of the bronchial mucosa that can compound airway obstruction, sometimes necessitating endotrachial intubation.

THERAPY

Significant upper-airway obstruction requires immediate treatment to prevent respiratory failure and death. A low tracheostomy is most commonly performed if the obstruction is in the hypopharnyx, larynx, or upper one-third of the trachea. In highly selected patients, endoscopic laser treatment of malignant central airway obstructions can also be performed successfully [48]. In one recent preoperative series, 304 patients underwent 449 operative rigid bronchoscopies for airway obstructions, most involving the use of a neodymium:yttrium-aluminum-garnet laser [49]. The total resection rate was 9.5% (5% for squamous cell carcinoma, 75% for low-grade malignant bronchial tumors, and 75% for papillary thyroid cancer). The median period between operative rigid bronchoscopy and operation was 18 days. No complications were observed after endoscopic treatment and no anastomotic complications were observed in the subsequent tracheobronchoplastic procedures. Endobronchial stents have also been used to maintain airway patency [50]. Various stent models have been developed for the treatment of inoperable airway stenoses. They consist mainly of two types: metal and silicone devices, or combinations of both (hybrid models) [51]. The choice of a specific stent depends on the nature of the airway obstruction, the preference of the endoscopist, and the overall costs of the procedure.

Once the airway is secured, most patients are treated with emergency radiotherapy. External beam as well as high dose rate endobronchial irradiation have been successful in palliating symptomatic airway obstruction [52, 53]. Often high doses of corticosteroids (dexamethasone, 10 to 16 mg a day) are administered to decrease edema during the initial days of radiation. When curative radiotherapy is used for obstructing non-small cell lung cancer, it can initially be difficult to plan radiation portals because of obstructing pneumonitis. As atelectasis resolves, the portal can often be reduced. Patients with endobronchial obstruction from small-cell lung cancer may respond promptly to either combination chemotherapy or radiotherapy. If an endobronchial lesion regrows in the irradiated field, the patient may be palliated with laser therapy, iridium seed implantation, or cryosurgery [54]. Palliative airway stenting has met with limited success in patients who are not surgical candidates [55].

Patients with neoplasms that are very sensitive to chemotherapy, such as small cell lung cancer or lymphoma, may have a prompter response with combination chemotherapy [56]. Some have advocated the use of intratumoral cytotoxic chemotherapy. Recently, Celikoglu et al reported their experience with this procedure [57]. A total of 93 patients with nearly complete extrinsic obstruction of at least one major airway were treated by injection of anti-cancer drugs directly into the endobronchial tumors or infiltrated bronchial mucosa through a flexible fiber-optic bronchoscope. At every session of treatment 1–3 ml each of 50 mg/ml of 5-fluorouracil, 1 mg/ml of mitomycin, 5 mg/ml of methotrexate, 10 mg/ml of bleomycin, and 2 mg/ml of mitoxantrone were injected separately at different sites without pre-mixing. Local intratumoral chemotherapy relieved the obstruction in 81 of the 93 patients. Endoscopically visible tumors were reduced in size, and infiltrative changes were also improved. Obstruction was not relieved in 12 patients. The therapy was well tolerated and had no systemic side effects, and no serious complications.

CENTRAL NERVOUS SYSTEM EMERGENCIES

Spinal Cord Compression

ETIOLOGIC FACTORS AND PATHOPHYSIOLOGIC FEATURES

Spinal cord compression is always an emergency, especially when neurologic deterioration is rapid. Once the patient becomes paraplegic, there is little chance of regaining lost motor function. The most common tumors associated with spinal cord compression are carcinomas of the breast, lung, and prostate; multiple myeloma; and lymphoma [58, 59]. At autopsy, more than 5% of patients with metastatic disease have epidural tumors, which generally arise from within the vertebral body and grow along the epidural space anterior to the spinal cord. Patients with paraspinal tumors (e.g., lymphoma) may develop epidural metastases when the neoplasm grows through the intervertebral foramina from adjacent nodes. Spinal cord and nerve root compression may occur secondary to epidural tumor or vertebral collapse from destructive osseous metastases. Permanent neurologic dysfunction also may occur if vascular compromise produces prolonged ischemia or hemorrhage.

Spinal cord compression may also be due to a number of nonmechanical causes including paraneoplastic syndromes, carcinomatous myopathy or myelopathy, radiation myelopathy, herpes zoster, subacute myelopathy, pain from pelvic or long-bone metastases, anterior spinal artery occlusion, retroperitoneal tumor, or toxicity of cytotoxic drugs. Nonmalignant conditions such as herniated disks, osteoporotic vertebral fractures, and intraspinal abscess can also cause cord compression in the cancer patient.

CLINICAL PRESENTATION

More than 95% of patients with spinal cord compression complain of progressive central or radicular back pain. The pain is often aggravated by recumbency, weight bearing, coughing, sneezing, or the valsalva maneuver, and is relieved by sitting [58]. The earliest neurologic symptoms are sensory changes, including numbness, paresthesias, and coldness. The incidence of permanent motor dysfunction has significantly decreased in the last two decades due to earlier diagnosis and treatment [60]. Although bladder and bowel dysfunction are rarely the first objective signs of cord compression, metastases to the cauda equina typically produce impaired urethral, vaginal, and rectal sensation, bladder dysfunction, saddle anesthesia, and decreased sensation in the lumbosacral dermatomes. The level of cord compression can be determined by pain elicited by straight leg raising, neck flexion, or vertebral percussion. The upper limit of the sensory level is often one or two vertebral bodies below the site of compression. Decreased rectal tone and perineal sensation are often observed when there is automatic dysfunction. Deep tendon reflexes may be brisk with cord compression and diminished with nerve root compression [60].

DIAGNOSTIC EVALUATION

Neurologic signs and symptoms suggesting spinal cord compression are generally evaluated by plain films, myelography, MRI, or CT scan. The majority of patients with solid tumors presenting with spinal cord compression have x-ray abnormalities on plain films, but in the past, myelography was essential in radiotherapeutic management [61]. Solid tumors have a much higher incidence of bony involvement than do hematologic malignancies. Because abnormal bone radiographs are seen in only about one-third of patients with non-Hodgkin's lymphoma, Hodgkin's disease, or myeloma, there is a stronger role for alternative imaging strategies in patients with these malignancies [62].

Over the past decade, MRI has largely replaced myelography as the gold standard in diagnosing the presence and extent of spinal cord compression [63–65]. The accuracy of MRI in detecting metastatic compression of the spinal cord or cauda equina has been compared to findings at myelography, surgery, clinical follow-up, and autopsy results. Magnetic resonance imaging has been shown to have a sensitivity of 93%, a specificity of 97%, and an overall accuracy of 95%. It also has a distinct advantage over myelography because no contrast injections are required. Patients with a complete or partial block of the spinal canal from an epidural metastasis may also have additional epidural deposits at other levels and MRI may show these multiple sites, which may not be obvious on the initial myelogram unless special attention is given to these areas

[66]. However, the detection of cord displacement becomes less certain and more subjective when the spine is scoliotic. The use of surface coil may improve image detail. The disadvantage of MRI is the necessity for the patient to lie still in one position, which many patients with severe central back pain cannot maintain for long periods of time.

THERAPY

Corticosteroids may promptly reduce peritumoral edema and improve neurologic function [67]. Prior to emergency diagnostic procedures, patients with neurologic symptoms from possible cord compression should receive dexamethasone (10 mg). Generally, dexamethasone (4–10 mg every six hours) is continued during radiation therapy, then tapered. Steroids initially improve neurologic function, but it is not clear whether they affect the ultimate outcome following definitive therapy. The side effects of high-dose corticosteroids (listed in Table 32.1) must be considered when drug doses are prescribed.

Suspected spinal cord compression requires immediate consultation of the radiation oncologist and the neurosurgeon. Treatment decisions must be based on the tumor's radiosensitivity, clinical expertise with surgical decompression, the level of cord compression, rate of neurologic deterioration, and prior radiotherapy.

Radiotherapy is the primary treatment for most patients with epidural metastases and once the diagnosis of cord compression is confirmed, emergency radiotherapy should be given [68, 69]. Radiation portals include the entire area of block and two vertebral bodies above or below it. Radiation doses range from 30 Gy to 40 Gy given over a two to three-week period. Radioresponsive tumors (e.g., lymphoma and multiple myeloma) have

Table 32.1 Side Effects of Corticosteroids

Serious/Potentially Life Threatening	Bothersome/ Non-Life Threatening	Rare Side Effects
Diabetes mellitus	Weight gain	Hiccups
Adrenal insufficiency	Striae	Pseudorheumatoid arthritis
Susceptibility to infection	Moon facies	
Fluid retention	Acne	
Peptic ulcer disease	Insomnia	
Psychosis	Proximal muscle weakness	

higher response rates to radiotherapy than do radioresistant tumors (e.g., melanoma) [69]. More than half the patients with rapid neurologic deterioration improve with radiotherapy; however, the prognosis for patients with autonomic dysfunction or paraplegia is poor despite surgery or radiotherapy [70, 71]. In one recent series of 56 breast cancer patients with spinal cord metastases, 89% of patients with back pain prior to radiotherapy had the pain improve or disappear completely. Four of six cases (67%) with urinary dysfunction responded to radiation therapy. Of 35 cases with motor dysfunction at the time of diagnosis, 21 (60%) regained the ability to walk and another five (14%) who were able to walk with support at diagnosis did not deteriorate. All 21 cases without motor deficits before treatment maintained good motor performance after radiation therapy. Response to therapy was better in pretreatment walking than in nonwalking patients (97% versus 69%; $p < 0.02$). Probability of duration of response at one year was 59% and 10% for posttreatment walking and nonwalking patients, respectively ($p < 0.0001$). One-year survival probability was 66% for posttreatment walking and 10% for posttreatment nonwalking patients, respectively ($p < 0.0001$). Pretreatment and posttreatment ambulatory status were the most important prognostic factors [70]. Some patients who recur in the spine following radiotherapy for cord compression may be able to gain relief of symptoms through reirradiation, with minimal risk of severe myelopathy [72].

In patients who are not candidates for radiotherapy, surgical laminectomy can provide prompt decompression of the spinal cord and nerve roots. Anterior laminectomy is technically challenging, but more often successful in completely removing the tumor, since most epidural metastases arise in the vertebral bodies anterior to the spinal cord [73]. When epidural tumor is not entirely removed surgically, postoperative radiotherapy is given to decrease residual tumor, relieve pain, and improve functional status. Most ambulatory patients have improved neurologic function following surgical decompression, but those with severe preoperative neurologic deficits rarely benefit from surgery. Surgery is generally contraindicated when there are multiple areas of cord compression.

A recent review suggests that patients with vertebral collapse rarely benefit form surgical laminectomy due to a higher incidence of neurologic complications [74]. The data suggest that laminectomy in the presence of vertebral body collapse has a higher risk of major deterioration by at least one grade (50% compared with 24% in patients without vertebral collapse). This is probably caused by the presence of a destructive lesion in the anterior spinal column, which results in further instability with posterior laminectomy. In most cases, laminectomy is contraindicated in the presence of a collapsed vertebral body, and alternate methods of treatment should be applied. Although radiation therapy should not affect spinal stability, there is no evidence that radiation therapy improves neurologic results. The most logical approach may be to use an anterior surgical approach to the spine (i.e., transthoracic) and early mobilization [75].

In cases where there is no prior histologic diagnosis of malignancy or if infection or epidural hematoma must be ruled out, a laminectomy is required for both diagnosis and treatment. High cervical cord lesions can cause death from respiratory paralysis unless surgical decompression is accomplished. If surgery is not possible, the patient's neck should be stabilized in a halo. When neurologic signs progress over a 48–72-hour period despite high-dose steroids and radiotherapy, emergency decompression should be attempted although operative results are generally poor when there is rapid neurologic progression. If there is a long interval following radiotherapy for spinal cord compression, surgery may be beneficial when the epidural tumor recurs.

Chemotherapy rarely has a major therapeutic role in spinal cord compression but if the malignancy is sensitive to chemotherapy, the drug regimen can be administered concurrently or soon after radiotherapy or surgery is complete. Although the management of spinal cord compression due to multiple myeloma usually involves radiation, with or without decompressive surgery, chemotherapy may play a role in patients who have had prior radiation if they have a chance of response [76]. Spinal cord compression due to Hodgkin's disease, non-Hodgkin's lymphoma or neuroblastoma may also be responsive to chemotherapy in addition to radiotherapy [77, 78]. Neurologic recovery in patients with lymphoma and cord compression has been observed with single-agent chemotherapy. Paraplegia due to prostate cancer has been found to respond to hormonal manipulation without radiation treatment [79].

Carcinomatous Meningitis

ETIOLOGIC FACTORS AND CLINICAL PRESENTATION

Carcinomatous meningitis is increasing in frequency because of improved survival with systemic antineoplastic therapies and increased awareness of this problem among oncologists [80]. At autopsy, 4% of patients have leptomeningeal spread, most commonly associated with lymphoma, leukemia, cancers of the breast and lung, and melanoma [81]. Because most chemotherapy drugs fail to penetrate the blood-brain barrier, carcinomatous meningitis develops frequently in patients without signs of progressive systemic disease outside the central nervous system (CNS). At autopsy, the brain and spinal cord may be covered by a sheet of malignant cells, or areas of the spinal cord and cranial nerve roots may have multifocal metastases. The malignant cells tend to settle in the basal cisterns where they interfere with cerebrospinal fluid (CSF) flow and absorption, which may lead to obstructive hydrocephalus [80].

Carcinomatous meningitis should be suspected when neurologic signs indicate that more than one structural area of the nervous system is affected. Clinical symptoms depend on the extent of tumor involving the brain, cranial nerves, or spinal cord. Occasionally, neurologic symptoms may be subtle and exist for several weeks prior to diagnosis. Headache may be accompanied by nausea and vomiting, and mental status changes, lethargy, and decreased memory are frequent. The most common cranial nerve deficits result in diplopia, visual blurring, hearing loss, and facial numbness. More than 70% of patients have neurologic signs due to spinal cord or nerve root involvement and may have symptoms of spinal cord compression [59].

DIAGNOSTIC EVALUATION

The diagnosis of carcinomatous meningitis is established by cytologic examination of CSF. At least 5 ml of CSF should be sent for cytology, although the initial fluid analysis may not be diagnostic. Repeated lumbar punctures increase diagnostic yield, and are often required to confirm the diagnosis [82]. In a retrospective series of carcinomatous meningitis, malignant cells were seen cumulatively within the first, second, and third CSF samples in 42%, 66%, and 87% of patients, respectively, demonstrating that patients may have repeatedly negative lumbar CSF cytologies. More than half of the patients with carcinomatous meningitis have one or more of the following CSF abnormalities: an opening pressure greater than 160 mm of water, an increased white blood cell count, a reactive lymphocytosis, an elevated level of CSF protein, or a decreased level of glucose.

CT or MRI scans may reveal contrast enhancement in the meninges and periventricular area, hydrocepha-

lus, or brain metastases; concurrent brain metastases are present in 20% of patients [83] Emergency myelograms or MRI scans of the spine should be performed in patients with symptoms or signs due to metastases to the spinal cord or cauda equina.

THERAPY

Treatment for carcinomatous meningitis generally consists of intrathecal chemotherapy with or without radiation therapy to the areas of the neuroaxis responsible for the neurologic deficits. Without treatment, patients will die within four to six weeks. Even in those patients who respond to treatment, survival may only be extended by 6–10 months [80]. Treatment-related toxicity includes aseptic meningitis, thrombocytopenia, and neutropenia. In a recent series of 32 women with carcinomatous meningitis due to metastatic breast cancer treated with combined modality therapy, median survival was 7.5 months (range = 1.5–16 months) [80]. Eighteen women died of progressive carcinomatous meningitis or combined meningitis and systemic disease progression. Women with persistent interruption of CSF flow (due to extensive CNS disease) fared worse than women with normal CSF flow (median survival = 3 months versus 10 months; $p < 0.0001$).

Therapeutic drug levels are not generally achieved in the CSF with parenteral chemotherapy, and thus intrathecal administration is necessary. Intraventricular chemotherapy via an Ommaya reservoir generally is preferable to lumbar injections. With lumbar puncture, the drug may reach only the epidural or subdural spaces. Even when the chemotherapeutic drug reaches the subarachnoid space, therapeutic drug levels are rarely reached in the ventricles. Intraventricular injections via the Ommaya are also less painful than lumbar punctures and allow drug concentrations to follow the normal pathways for CSF flow [84]. When compared with retrospective series in which drugs were given by lumbar puncture, it appears that response rates are higher and longer in duration with intraventricular therapy and radiation therapy. In the series of Wasserstrom et al, more than 60% of patients with leptomeningeal metastases from breast cancer, 100% with lymphoma, 50% with lung cancer, and 40% with melanoma improved or stabilized with therapy. In this series, the median survival was 5.8 months with a range from one to 29 months [83]. Ommaya reservoirs can be placed with less than 2% morbidity and no mortality. If intracranial pressure is increased, an Ommaya reservoir can be placed and connected to a ventricular peritoneal shunt. The shunt has an on-off valve that allows it to be closed off for about four hours after intraventricular drug administration.

The most frequently used intrathecal drugs are methotrexate, thiotepa, and cytosine arabinoside. Leucovorin (10 mg orally every six hours for six doses) will decrease the systemic side effects of methotrexate. Since leukovorin does not cross the blood-brain barrier, the antitumor efficacy of methotrexate in the CSF will not be effected. Methotrexate and thiotepa are usually administered for solid tumors associated with carcinomatous meningitis. Cytosine arabinoside alone or with methotrexate is used in leukemic and lymphomatous meningitis. Intrathecal therapy is given twice a week until symptoms improve or stabilize and the cytology becomes negative. Intrathecal therapy may then be given weekly, and gradually spaced out to monthly injections if the cytologies are persistently negative [80, 83].

Whole-brain and brain-stem irradiation are used when there are cerebral or cranial nerve abnormalities. When spinal cord or nerve root signs are present, myelograms or MRI scans of the spine are required to plan radiation portals. Doses are usually 30 Gy over a two-week period.

Lymphomatous and leukemic meningitis are more responsive to intrathecal therapy and may also respond to high-dose systemic methotrexate with leucovorin rescue. Because of the high incidence of leptomeningeal involvement, patients with acute lymphocytic leukemia, acute lymphoblastic lymphoma, and Burkitt's lymphoma receive prophylactic intrathecal chemotherapy via lumbar puncture and whole-brain irradiation after a complete remission is obtained [85–87].

GASTROINTESTINAL AND INFECTION-RELATED EMERGENCIES

Acute Diarrheal Syndrome

PATHOPHYSIOLOGIC FEATURES

Cancer patients commonly develop diarrhea. The primary causes of diarrhea in this population can be grouped according to those that are tumor-related, those that are treatment-related and those due to infectious etiologies [88]. Tumor-related diarrhea can be either exudative or secretory, with the latter including tumor-related hypersecretory states as seen with endocrine tumors such as vasoactive intestinal polypeptide (VIP)omas, gastrinomas, other amine precursor uptake and decarboxylation cell (APUD)omas, and the carcinoid syndrome. In these patients, the tumor produces one or more substances that result in the secretion of fluid into the intestinal lumen, as a result of disturbances in the transport of water and electrolytes. Treatment-related diarrhea may be due to surgical morbidity or may stem from the toxic effects of chemotherapy or radiotherapy. Bowel resection, particularly right hemicolectomy, may lead to increased delivery of luminal fluid to the colon, overwhelming the reabsorption capacity of the colonic surface. Other mechanical abnormalities of motility can result from surgical resection, or the presence of tumor within the gastrointestinal tract.

Radiotherapy to either the large or small bowel is frequently associated with the development of diarrhea, as the intestinal lumen becomes atrophied leading to increased bowel transit times and decreased resorptive capacity. Chemotherapeutic agents that are most commonly associated with the development of severe diarrhea include 5-flourouracil and CPT-11, although many other agents can also contribute to diarrhea, including methotrexate, actinomycin D, leucovorin, mesna, doxorubicin, daunorubicin, topotecan, and streptozocin. Finally, infectious etiologies are important contributors to cancer-related diarrhea. Oncologic patients are often immunosuppressed, and this, combined with the decreased barrier to infection associated with bowel toxicity may lead to the development of infectious diarrhea due to common microorganisms. Agents such as *Shigella, Escherichia coli,* and *Salmonella* can cause illness by directly invading the bowel mucosa, while *Clostridium difficile* and some *E. coli* produce enterotoxins that result in secretory diarrhea. Finally, in transplant patients, graft-versus-host disease can involve the gastrointestinal tract, leading to severe diarrhea, which may be the first clinical manifestation of this potentially life-threatening condition.

CLINICAL PRESENTATION AND DIAGNOSTIC EVALUATION

Diarrhea in cancer patients can rapidly result in severe dehydration, electrolyte abnormalities, and other life-threatening consequences. Thus, early recognition and intervention are critical. Identification of patients at high risk for the development of severe diarrhea and its complications are important. Patients who have had abdominal surgery may be at risk due to the development of adhesions that may limit bowel motility, or due to limitations in bowel blood supply. Other at-risk patients include those with comorbid medical conditions such as diabetes mellitus, collagen vascular diseases, or inflammatory bowel disease [89]. Finally, patients receiving abdomino-pelvic radiotherapy or chemoradiotherapy, particularly with the use of 5-fluorouracil-based regimens, are vulnerable.

To provide a frame of reference, patients must be asked routinely about their baseline bowel habits to provide a frame of reference, as there is great variation in the "normal" number of daily bowel movements. The most commonly used tool to evaluate diarrhea in cancer patients is the National Cancer Institute-Common Toxicity Criteria (NCI-CTC) [90]. However, this tool evaluates only the number of bowel movements per day. Patients must also be instructed to take note of the volume and character of their bowel movements, and to report any change from baseline. Patients often present with frequent (hourly), large volume, watery bowel movements, or nocturnal incontinence. Tenesmus and hematochezia may be present, particularly in radiation enteritis and infectious etiologies. Diarrhea may or may not be accompanied by abdominal pain, nausea, or vomiting. Abdominal rebound and guarding are rarely present.

A careful history and physical examination are paramount. Patients should be questioned regarding recent antibiotic use, travel, or exposure to ill family members. A dietary history should be obtained, to rule out the possibility of food poisoning, as well as to document the patient's ability to maintain adequate intake of fluids in the face of severe gastrointestinal fluid losses. The presence of abdominal pain, constitutional symptoms, fever, nausea, or emesis may help narrow the differential diagnosis.

Laboratory evaluation includes serum chemistries (blood urea nitrogen [BUN], bicarbonate), complete blood count with an absolute neutrophil count, and liver function tests. Stool culture and examination for white blood cells should be performed before antimotility agents are instituted. However, the absence of white blood cells in the neutropenic patient does not eliminate the possibility of an infectious etiology. Further evaluation should be based on the clinical scenario. Radiologic studies (abdominal X-rays or CT scan) should be used in cases of high suspicion of mechanical obstruction. When graft-versus-host disease is suspected, the diagnosis may require endoscopy and biopsy.

THERAPY

Treatment for cancer-associated diarrhea should be determined both by etiology and symptomatology. For example, patients with mild chemotherapy-induced diarrhea may need only over-the-counter antidiarrheals, while those with diarrhea caused by *C. difficile* will need to be treated with antibiotics as well. Patients with severe diarrhea from any cause need aggressive supportive care, which often requires inpatient or home administration of intravenous fluids, careful monitoring and supplementation of electrolytes, and pharmacologic intervention. High volume fluid loss can rapidly become life-threatening in patients debilitated by cancer, in whom baseline reserve is limited. Furthermore, mild symptoms can progress within hours to become so severe that the patient can no longer compensate by increasing oral intake.

The approach to chemotherapy-induced diarrhea (CID) has recently been reviewed and published by an expert consensus panel convened in June 1997 [91]. This group, consisting of physicians specializing in medical oncology, bone marrow transplantation, radiation oncology, and gastroenterology, addressed the stepwise approach to the patient with CID. Initial management is nonpharmacologic, including avoidance of foods and medicines that can aggravate CID. Withdrawal of mild and milk products, as well as other foods that are high in fat, is recommended. Caffeine and alcohol should be limited or avoided, and patients should discontinue use of bulk laxatives, stool softeners, and promotility agents that are often used in conjunction with opoids for pain control.

Pharmacologic intervention typically begins with the opioids diphenoxylate and loperamide. These agents reduce diarrhea by decreasing peristalsis in the small and large intestines. Efficacy data from double-blind, crossover studies comparing these agents have suggested that loperamide is generally the more effective antidiarrheal agent [92–95] when used at a dose of 2 mg every 4 hours. High-dose loperamide has been shown to be effective for CPT-11-induced diarrhea, when given on an intensive schedule (2 mg every 2 hours) [96].

Octreotide (Sandostatin®) is a synthetic analog of somatostatin, a hormone that is produced throughout the gastrointestinal tract. This agent acts directly on epithelial cells to reduce the secretion of a number of pancreatic and gastrointestinal hormones, including VIP, gastrin, insulin, and serotonin [97]. The natural substance has a very short half-life, which allows it to tightly regulate bowel function. The synthetic analogs, including octreotide, have a longer duration of action (6–8 hours), but are limited in that they can only be administered by subcutaneous injection because oral bioavailability is poor. Octreotide has been used in a variety of diarrheal states, including radiation enteritis, chemotherapy-induced diarrhea [98], acquired immunodeficiency syndrome (AIDS) [99], graft-versus-host disease [100, 101], treatment-associated diarrhea [91, 97, 98, 102], and tumor-associated diarrhea [88] including the carcinoid syndrome. In early studies of diarrhea associated with the administration of fluoropyrimidines, symptoms have been amiliorated in approximately 90% of patients within three days of instituting therapy [103, 104]. The efficacy of octreotide is clearly dose-dependent, with data suggesting that higher doses are more effective than lower doses, without a substantial increase in toxicity. In phase I studies, the maximally tolerated dose was 2,000 μg, three times a day for five days, with dose-limiting toxicity above that level consisting of hypersensitivity reactions at the injection site and asymptomatic hypoglycemia [97]. Multiple studies have shown octreotide to be superior to loperamide in chemotherapy-induced diarrhea [98, 105], and in refractory diarrhea associated with bone marrow transplantation [102]. Thus, use of octreotide therapy is recommended for patients with persistent diarrhea of any severity who are refractory to high-dose loperamide therapy [91]. A starting dose of 100–150 μg should be administered subcutaneously until diarrhea resolves, with dose escalation by 50 μg increments up to a maximum dose of 2,000 μg three times a day for up to five days. The optimal dosage and schedule of octreotide in cancer-associated diarrhea is currently being evaluated in an NCI-sponsored, intergroup, randomized clinical trial.

Neutropenic Enterocolitis

PATHOPHYSIOLOGIC FEATURES

Neutropenic enterocolitis, also known as typhlitis, is a severe, often life-threatening complication of prolonged neutropenia. It is often diagnosed only at autopsy, with its true incidence unknown. It typically occurs in patients who have been neutropenic for at least 5–7 days, after recent treatment with chemotherapy, who have been on broad-spectrum antibiotics [106]. It is most commonly described in patients with acute leukemia. The presence of typhlitis was confirmed pathologically in approximately 25% of autopsies in patients with leukemia at the Texas Children's Hospital of Baylor College of Medicine [107]. However, it can also can occur in patients with solid tumors [108], AIDS, organ transplants, or cyclic neutropenia [106].

The cecum is primary anatomic site of involvement, although other segments of bowel can also be involved [109]. Typically, hemorrhage, edema, and fibrinous ex-

udate are seen on pathologic examination [110]. The cecum is thought to be at greatest risk due to its poor vascular supply and high volume of colonic bacteria. The cecum is further compromised by breakdown of the normal colonic surface due to the absence of neutrophils, the direct toxic effects of chemotherapy and the production of exotoxins by *Clostridia* and other bacteria [111]. When the cecum is not involved, the clinicopathologic picture is most commonly associated with chemotherapy-induced *C. difficile* colitis complicated by toxic megacolon [112].

Agents most commonly isolated in the stool and/or blood of patients with neutropenic enterocolitis include gram negative bacteria, especially *Pseudomonas aeruginosa*; and anaerobes, typically *C. septicum* and *C. difficile*. There have been other organisms infrequently reported, including one reported case of *Citrobacter freundii* [108].

CLINICAL PRESENTATION AND DIAGNOSTIC EVALUATION

Classically, neutropenic enterocolitis begins as a very nonspecific illness in a neutropenic patient, characterized by abdominal pain, nausea, bloating, fever, and diarrhea (with or without blood). Only one-third of patients have vomiting or bloody stool. The abdominal discomfort then may become more localized to the right lower quadrant, with 13% of patients having right-sided symptoms at some point in the course of the disease [109]. The evolution from non-specific to localized symptoms can occur over hours to days. The diagnosis is suspected by finding bowel wall thickening on abdominal ultrasound, X-ray, or CAT scan, in the setting of abdominal pain and an examination indicative of an acute abdomen. Endoscopic procedures are usually avoided because of the high risk of perforation. Serial abdominal examinations are typically undertaken, with monitoring of patient progression most commonly by this mechanism.

THERAPY

Historically, neutropenic enterocolitis has been associated with a mortality reaching 30–50% even when aggressive therapy such as surgery was performed, although more recent reports have described improved outcomes with early recognition and aggressive medical management alone [113]. This includes supportive care, consisting of aggressive hydration, bowel rest, and nasogastric suction, as well as antimicrobial therapy to cover resistant anaerobic and resistant gram-negative organisms. Despite these measures, however, a substantial proportion of patients will continue to progress, developing hemodynamic instability and frank sepsis which is almost universally fatal. In such cases, surgical resection of affected bowel has been undertaken, although its role in the salvage of patients with this disease remains controversial. Indications for surgical resection included gastrointestinal bleeding despite resolution of hematologic abnormalities, intraperitoneal bowel perforation, or clinical deterioration secondary to uncontrolled sepsis [114]. Surgical procedures typically used include right hemicolectomy, ileostomy, and mucous fistula [113]. Divided ileostomy for less severe cases may be useful. Despite this aggressive intervention, fulminant neutropenic enterocolitis remains a highly fatal condition. It remains unclear if early intervention or prophylactic bowel rest after chemotherapy will influence outcome; further studies are needed to clarify the optimal management strategy in this condition.

Neutropenic Fever and Sepsis

ETIOLOGIC FACTORS AND PATHOPHYSIOLOGIC FEATURES

Fever is a common occurrence in patients with cancer, particularly among those with decreased host defenses due to cancer treatment. However, when fever occurs in a patient who has deficient circulating neutrophils due to underlying disease or its treatment, overwhelming and life-threatening infection may quickly ensue, with devastating consequences. Historical series in the era prior to the use of prophylactic antibiotics document upwards of 95% mortality rates in febrile neutropenic episodes. Thus, febrile neutropenia is one of the most serious of the oncologic emergencies. It is critically important for the clinician to quickly and accurately diagnose febrile neutropenia, recognize signs and symptoms of infection in the neutropenic patient, and provide appropriate and timely management of this condition, since infections in these patients can be rapidly progressive resulting in a major source of morbidity and mortality.

Although fever in cancer patients is most often a result of infection, other noninfectious causes must also be considered. Pyrogenic medications (particularly cytotoxic agents such as bleomycin and cytosine arabinoside), blood products, allergic reactions, and the malignant process itself are potential sources of a febrile response [115]. Between 48% and 60% of neutropenic patients who become febrile have an established or occult infection [116]. However, no reliable criteria exist to allow the clinician to safely predict which episodes of febrile neutropenia are due to an infectious etiology. In examining this issue, Pizzo et al published a prospective study of 140 febrile neutropenic patients at the NCI [115]. Their study showed that it was not possible to distinguish patients with active infection from those with non-infectious causes by age, sex, underlying malignancy, or types of therapeutic modalities. Thus, it has become standard of care to treat empirically every patient with febrile neutropenia until an etiology has been established, or the episode has resolved.

While definitions of "febrile neutropenia" may vary slightly from institution to institution, the inverse relationship between host neutrophil count and infection has been well established. In the 1960s, Bodey et al [117] determined that when the neutrophil count decreased to < 1,000 cells/mm^3, increased susceptibility to infection can be expected, with the highest risk in patients with absolute neutrophil counts < 100 cell/mm^3. Other factors impacting the incidence of infection in neutropenic patients included the rate of decline in the count to low levels, the duration of the neutropenic period [116], phagocytic function (which may be impaired by the underlying disease or cytotoxic therapy), the status of the patient's immune system, alterations of physical defense barriers (as occurs with severe mucositis), and the patient's exposure to infectious agents (through either endogenous colonization or exposure to the hospital environment) [118].

A limited spectrum of bacterial, viral, fungal, and yeast organisms is responsible for the vast majority of documented infections in the neutropenic host. In the 1960s and 1970s, when the high risk of infection in neutropenic patients was first identified, the vast majority (71%) of documented infections was due to gram-negative organisms [119]. This proportion decreased to 31% during the 1980s, largely due to a decrease in the incidence of *P. aeruginosa* [119]. Aerobic gram-positive cocci (including coagulase-negative staphylococci, *viridans* streptococci, and *Staphylococcus aureus*) and aerobic gram-negative bacilli (including *E. coli*, *Klebsiella pneumoniae*, and *P. aeruginosa*) are now the most commonly identified bacterial pathogens [120]. Gram-positive organisms currently account for 60–70% of microbiologically documented infections. While many of these organisms are indolent, organisms that are methicillin-resistant (e.g., *S. aureus*, *viridans* streptococci, and pneumococci) may cause fulminant infections that can result in death if not treated promptly. Fungal infections tend to occur secondarily among patients who have received prolonged courses of broad-spectrum antibiotics, but these can also be a source of primary infection. Systemic fungal infections, especially candidiasis and aspergillosis, often occur during the course of prolonged antimicrobial therapy.

CLINICAL PRESENTATION AND DIAGNOSTIC EVALUATION

The definition of fever varies from institution to institution, but generally, a temperature clearly above the normal temperature for the patient constitutes a febrile state. A "fever" is typically defined as a single oral temperature $\geq 38.3°C$ (101°F) in the absence of obvious environmental causes [116]. However, in the case of the neutropenic patient, the consensus guidelines of the Immunocompromised Host Society define febrile neutropenia as a single temperature $\geq 38.5°C$, or the occurrence of three temperatures $\geq 38°C$ within a 24-hour period, taken at least four hours apart [121].

Likewise, the clinical definition of neutropenia is non-uniform. However, because of the high risk of life-threatening bacterial infections, the Infectious Disease Society of America (IDSA) defines neutropenia as "all patients with neutrophil counts of not more than 500/mm³ or those with counts of 500–1,000/mm³ in whom a further decrease can be anticipated" [116].

Anatomic sites for the development of infection in neutropenic cancer patients are limited and specific, differing from those of patients with chronic hereditary neutropenia who tend to have upper respiratory tract infections as the most common site. Neutropenic cancer patients most commonly have involvement of the alimentary tract, due primarily to damage by cytotoxic chemotherapy, or the integument, due to invasive procedures like central venous catheters [122]. Patients with low neutrophil counts tend to have a diminution in the inflammatory response, often leading to a lack of the typical signs and symptoms that indicate an infectious source. The physician should ascertain if the patient is receiving drugs that mask a febrile response (e.g., steroids, antipyretic-containing analgesics). Special attention must be paid to the specific areas that are most likely to be involved, including periodontium, pharynx, lower esophagus, lung, perineum (including perianal region), skin lesions, (including bone marrow aspiration sites and vascular catheter access sites), the eye (fungus), and the tissue surrounding nails.

Patients with febrile neutropenia should have a baseline chest x-ray, urinalysis, two sets of blood cultures, and cultures from any clinically suspicious and accessible anatomic site prior to the institution of therapy.

Patients with multilumen indwelling catheters should have one set of blood cultures from each port, as well as one set obtained from a peripheral vein. Studies examining the value of c-reactive protein, fever severity, or level of monocytopenia as predictors of bacteremia have found these indicators to be unreliable [121].

THERAPY

Antibiotic initiation, modification, and termination are the critical (and often controversial) decisions to be made in the febrile neutropenic patient. In 1997, the IDSA published practice guidelines for febrile neutropenia, a set of evidence-based recommendations to guide physicians caring for these patients [116]. The IDSA practice guidelines recommend the initiation of antibiotic therapy in all febrile patients with neutrophil counts $\leq 500/mm³$ or those with counts between 100/mm³ and 500/mm³ in whom a further decrease is anticipated. The regimen selected should be broad in its antimicrobial coverage, and should be administered by an intravenous route.

The approach to selecting agents for empiric antibiotic therapy depends upon the nature of the neutropenic host, characteristics of the clinical presentation, and the expected duration of neutropenia. Antibiotic selection should be guided by local epidemiologic patterns, taking into account antibiotic susceptibility patterns of recently isolated blood-borne pathogens [116, 123], as well as cost. The empirical regimen must be broad, achieve high bactericidal levels, and be as nontoxic and as simple to administer as possible. This has traditionally necessitated the combination of two or more antibiotics. Several regimens have been used, generally consisting of a cephalosporin or an extended-spectrum penicillin plus an aminoglycoside. No one regimen has been found to be superior to all others in clinical trials. Vancomycin may also be appropriate as part of the initial regimen.

Duration of treatment is also a complex issue. Few trials have addressed this issue, and the heterogeneity of the patient population requires that decisions be individualized. However, general guidelines published by IDSA [116] have included the following general principles. If fever resolves within first three days of treatment and no etiology is found through Gram stain or culture, low-risk neutropenic patients may be changed to an oral antibiotic; high-risk patients are recommended to remain on intravenous antibiotic therapy. If, however, an etiology is identified, the patient should be treated with a full course of antimicrobial therapy for that source.

The decision regarding duration of antibiotic therapy becomes complicated when either fever or neutropenia persist beyond the initial 72 hours after presentation. Patients recovering with an absolute neutrophil count (ANC) > 500 by day 7, with no source identified, may discontinue antibiotics at that time. High-risk patients with an ANC ≤ 500 on day 7 should be continued on antibiotics; discontinuation of antibiotics can be considered in persistently neutropenic, low-risk patients when afebrile for 5–7 days. Persistent fever during first three days of treatment should prompt reassessment, at which time the physician should consider a change in antibiotic regimen. At this time, it may also be reasonable to discontinue treatment with vancomycin. Fever persisting beyond days 5–7 should prompt the physician to consider adding amphotericin B, with or without antibiotic changes. In the patient who rapidly recovers with an ANC > 500, antibiotic therapy can be discontinued after 4–5 days if no source is identified. If the patient's ANC remains < 500, antibiotic therapy should continue for two weeks, at which time it may be discontinued, based upon the patients overall condition.

When used prophylactically, granulocyte-colony-stimulating factors (GM-CSF, G-CSF) can reduce the duration of neutropenia. However, the four studies that have looked at the initiation of colony-stimulating factors at the time of admission for febrile neutropenia have shown that use of growth factors decreases duration of hospitalization by 1–2 days, but has no effect upon number of documented infections or survival [124–126]. Therefore, because of their high cost and lack of effect upon mortality, colony-stimulating factors are not currently recommended at the time of presentation of all febrile neutropenic episodes. In rare instances, these agents may be indicated prophylactically, for example, in patients undergoing allogeneic or autologous bone marrow/stem cell transplants and in some heavily-pretreated patients with lymphoreticular malignancies.

UROLOGIC EMERGENCIES
Obstructive Uropathy
ETIOLOGIC FACTORS

Obstructive uropathy is frequently associated with intra-abdominal, retroperitoneal, and pelvic malignancies. The diagnostic procedures and therapeutic approach depend on whether the site of obstruction is in the bladder neck or ureter. Bladder outlet obstruction is often secondary to cancer of the prostate, cervix, or bladder, or to benign prostatic hypertrophy. Ureteral blockage is more often due to para-aortic malignancies such as lymphomas, sarcomas, and nodal metastases from carcinomas of the cervix, bladder, prostate, rectum, or ovary.

Most cancer patients have obstructive nephropathy due to tumor, but benign conditions must be considered in the differential diagnosis. Chronic hypercalcemia, hyperuricemia, or urinary tract infection predisposes patients to renal calculi. Ureteral strictures may be a delayed complication of both surgery and radiotherapy. Following retroperitoneal surgery, abscesses or hematomas can cause ureteral obstruction. Although the primary cause of acute hyperuricemic nephropathy is uric acid deposition in the renal tubules, ureteral obstruction from uric acid calculi has also been reported, particularly in association with myeloproliferative disorders. Bladder outlet obstruction may be secondary to clots, urethral strictures from radiation fibrosis, or cyclophosphamide-induced cystitis. Patients with locally advanced bladder cancer or with metastases in the brain, spinal cord, or sacral roots may have impaired bladder emptying secondary to neurologic dysfunction. Voiding problems may be secondary to medications that alter the central or autonomic nervous system. Regardless of the etiology of obstruction, uncorrected pathologic changes in the dilated structures proximal to the site may ultimately culminate in renal failure and death. Thus, the initial staging evaluation for patients with locally advanced pelvic or retroperitoneal malignancies should include studies to assure patency of the urinary tract.

CLINICAL PRESENTATION

Obstruction should be suspected when patients complain of urinary retention, flank pain, hematuria, or persistent urinary tract infections [127]. Unfortunately, ureteral obstruction often is not diagnosed until renal failure results in obtundation, seizures, volume overload, or anuria. Impaired bladder emptying can cause symptoms of hesitancy, urgency, nocturia, frequency, and decreased force of the urinary stream. Partial kidney obstruction should be suspected when polyuria alternates with oliguria. Physical examination may reveal enlargement of the prostate or bladder, or a pelvic, flank, or renal mass. Decreased anal sphincter tone or diminished bulbocavernosus reflexes suggest the presence of a neurogenic bladder [127].

DIAGNOSTIC EVALUATION

The diagnosis of obstructive uropathy can be made readily with intravenous pyelography, renal ultrasound, renal radionuclide scans, or CT. The bladder must be catheterized to exclude urethral obstruction. Routine serum chemistries, including creatinine, electrolytes, BUN, calcium, phosphorus, uric acid, and hematologic profiles should be monitored frequently. Pyuria and bacteriuria suggest infection behind an obstruction that requires immediate drainage and parenteral antibiotics.

The obstruction site must be determined prior to planning appropriate therapy. Hydronephrosis is most often initially confirmed by renal ultrasonography, since the risks of contrast-induced nephrotoxicity are high. Renal ultrasound can demonstrate pelvic or retroperitoneal masses, ureteral dilation, calculi, and the residual normal renal cortex [128]. Intravenous urograms will define the site of blockage in up to 80% of cases of acute urinary obstruction, but with the risk of worsening renal dysfunction due to the contrast dye used in these studies. CT is more expensive and less specific, but it can help differentiate hydronephrosis from renal cysts and identify obstructing masses. More recently, MRI has become the favored approach [129, 130]. MR urography is highly sensitive in diagnosing urinary tract obstruction and also suggests the underlying pathology in many cases. In nondilated systems it is not possible to get good images because MR urography only depicts fluid in the urinary tract. However, MR urography can provide a reliable alternative to other more invasive modalities, such as retrograde or antegrade urography, and is without the risk of contrast media and radiation exposure.

Percutaneous antegrade pyelography has the advantage of often both diagnosing and relieving obstruction obstructions without the risks of anesthesia [128]. Under ultrasound guidance, a catheter is inserted in the dilated renal pelvis. Urine is aspirated and sent for analysis and culture. To localize the site of obstruction, contrast is injected through the catheter. Once the site it determined, an attempt is made to advance the catheter through the obstruction to restore internal ureteral drainage. If the internal drainage is ineffective, external drainage can be done through the percutaneous catheter until indwelling ureteral stents are placed with cystoscopy and retrograde pyelography if possible [131]. Urodynamic and urethrocystography are helpful in differentiating bladder dysfunction secondary to neuromuscular or mechanical causes. Generally, transurethral or suprapubic cystoscopy is required to determine the cause of bladder output obstruction. The ureteral orifices must be visualized and urinary flow confirmed from each orifice. Appropriate biopsies and cytologies should be obtained [127].

THERAPY

Lower urinary tract obstruction can be temporarily relieved by an indwelling urethral catheter or suprapubic cystostomy. If bladder outlet obstruction cannot be promptly corrected, suprapubic cystostomy is preferable to an indwelling urethral catheter. Suprapubic cystostomies are more comfortable, carry a lower risk of infections, and avoid prostatic swelling [132]. For partially denervated bladders, parasympathomimetic drugs (e.g., bethanechol) can improve bladder contraction and prevent overflow incontinence. Low-pressure incontinence can be treated with adrenergic agonists (e.g., ephedrine). Anticholinergics (e.g., Pro-banthine®) are prescribed for patients with uninhibited or reflex neurogenic bladders [127]. Generally, prostatic obstruction is corrected by transurethral resection. Infection, hyperkalemia, and acidosis must be treated promptly. Unless obstruction is removed promptly, permanent renal damage will result.

Obstructive symptoms from advanced prostate cancer may also be improved by treatment of the primary tumor, including orchiectomy, hormonal therapy, chemotherapy or radiation [133]. However, temporary urinary diversion is still typically required because maximal benefit these treatments is often delayed for several weeks [132]. Appropriate dose adjustments must be made for renal insufficiency; nephrotoxic drugs (e.g., cisplatin and methotrexate) should be completely avoided. Cyclophosphamide and ifosfamide should not be given because severe damage to the uroepithelium occurs after prolonged exposure to the active urinary metabolites of these drugs. After the obstruction is relieved, appropriate intravenous or oral fluids are needed for a few days to compensate for any postobstructive diuresis.

The decision to relieve an obstructing lesion must be carefully considered in terminally ill patients, where patient comfort is paramount. Patients with severe pain or discomfort due to bladder distention may be appropriate candidates for interventions; however, those with asymptomatic obstruction may not.

Hemorrhagic Cystitis

ETIOLOGIC FACTORS AND PATHOPHYSIOLOGIC FAETURES

Hemorrhagic cystitis is an inflammation of the lining of the bladder that can be a severe complication of cancer or its treatment. This condition is most commonly due to intravesicular effects of toxic metabolites of chemotherapy, bladder irradiation, or viral infection. Oxazophosphorine-based alkylating agents, such as cyclophosphamide and ifosfamide, are the most commonly associated cytotoxic agents associated with this disorder. In early studies, hemorrhagic cystitis occurred in 40–70% of patients treated with cyclophosphamide [134, 135]. Both agents are metabolized by the hepatic microsomal enzyme system, to form phosphoramide mustard and acrolein. In 1979, Cox identified acrolein as the toxic metabolite of cyclophosphamide responsible for development of hemorrhagic cystitis [136]. Chloroacetaldehyde, another metabolite of ifosfamide, also appears to be toxic to the bladder endothelium, and is likely responsible for the greater incidence of hemorrhagic cystitis observed with ifosfamide compared with cyclophosphamide [137]. The exact mechanisms by which these substances damage the bladder wall are unknown.

Furthermore, up to 20% of patients receiving radiation for genitourinary cancers develop hemorrhagic cystitis [138]. Small vessel injury caused by radiation can lead to interstitial bladder wall fibrosis, reduced bladder capacity, and the formation of friable, telangiectatic blood vessels that can spontaneously rupture, leading to massive hemorrhage [139].

Finally, in patients receiving bone marrow transplants, hemorrhagic cystitis can be caused by reactivation of BK virus, a human polyoma virus. In a series of 53 patients reported by Arthur et al [140], 47% of transplant recipients excreted BK virus, and in all cases this was the result of the reactivation of latent virus. Hemorrhagic cystitis of long duration (greater than or equal to 7 days) was associated with BK viruria. The disease was four times more likely in patients who excreted BK virus than in those who did not, and the virus was identified in 55% of the urine specimens collected during episodes of cystitis compared with 8–11% of the specimens collected during cystitis-free periods. BK viruria often temporally preceded or coincided with the onset of the disease. Among 19 patients with BK viruria lasting seven days or longer, hemorrhagic cystitis occurred in 15. Occurrence of the disease was related to the source of bone marrow. The disease oc-

curred in 50% of 38 recipients of allogeneic marrow and in 7% of 15 recipients of syngeneic or autologous marrow. Among recipients of allogeneic marrow, the disease was observed in 71% of the 21 patients excreting BK virus and in 24% of the 17 not excreting the virus, suggesting that that reactivation of BK virus may account for a substantial proportion of late-onset, long-lasting hemorrhagic cystitis in recipients of bone marrow transplants.

CLINICAL PRESENTATION AND DIAGNOSTIC EVALUATION

In a series of 100 patients from the Mayo Clinic with hemorrhagic cystitis induced by cyclophosphamide, major symptoms were gross hematuria (78%) and irritative voiding symptoms (45%) [141]. Microhematuria developed in 93% of patients. Hemorrhagic cystitis developed at significantly lower doses and shorter durations of therapy in patients treated with cyclophosphamide intravenously than in patients treated orally. Twenty percent had bleeding severe enough to require transfusion. Cystectomy was required in nine patients and bladder cancer developed in five [141]. There are no clinical predictors to indicate which patients will experience this complication. Acute hemorrhage usually occurs during or shortly after treatment, whereas delayed hemorrhage is most common in patients who take oral cyclophosphamide long term [139].

THERAPY

The approach to hemorrhagic cystitis in cancer patients involves both prevention and early intervention with aggressive supportive measures. Mesna (sodium-2-mercapto-ethane sulfate) has been developed as the specific chemoprotective agent against acrolein-induced bladder toxicity. It inactivates alkylating metabolites in the bladder to form an inert thioether [142]. When administered orally or intravenously, mesna is converted to an inactive disulfide form, which is renally excreted and then converted back to the active parent form by glutathione reductase in the bladder. The efficacy of mesna in preventing ifosfamide-induced hemorrhagic cystitis has been demonstrated in a placebo-controlled double-blind comparative study. Ifosfamide was administered by intravenous drip infusion at a daily dose of 2 g/m^2 for five consecutive days, and mesna was intravenously administered at 20% of the ifosfamide dose, three times a day for five consecutive days. Of the 101 patients studied, the mesna group had significantly less dysuria, hematuria, and feeling of incomplete bladder emptying [143].

A decrease in chemotherapeutic efficacy with the addition of mesna to the regimen has never been documented. Because the half-life of mesna is only one hour, it must be administered beyond the completion of ifosfamide. Mesna appears to be safe, with minimal side effects that include diarrhea, headache, and limb pain [144]. A rare hypersensitivity reaction to mesna has been described, characterized by fever, myalgia, arthralgia, and skin lesions mimicking a vasculitis. Oral mesna has been evaluated; it is well-absorbed, but its use is limited by nausea and vomiting associated with its sulfurous taste, as well as the risk of poor patient adherence, particularly in the setting of concomitant emetogenic chemotherapy.

In addition to metabolite-neutralizing agents such as mesna, the patient at risk for hemorrhagic cystitis should be supported with aggressive pretreatment and intratreatment hydration, and close monitoring to assure adequate diuresis to dilute urinary acrolein. In a randomized trial comparing intravenous hydration with mesna to intravenous hydration with a three-way Foley catheter and continuous bladder irrigation with saline, Vose et al reported no difference in episodes of severe hemorrhagic cystitis between the groups, but patients treated with continuous bladder irrigation had a significantly greater incidence of urinary tract infections (27% versus 14%) and bladder spasms or pain (84% versus 2%) [145]. These data suggest that the combination of intravenous hydration and continuous infusion mesna is the most effective means of preventing chemotherapy-induced hemorrhagic cystitis. Other agents studied as uroprotectants include N-acetyl cysteine [146–148], intravesicular formalin [149], prostaglandins [150–153], and pentosanpolysulfate [154–156], with varying degrees of success.

Once the clinical manifestations of hemorrhagic cystitis have occurred, the treatment options are largely supportive. These include stopping or reducing the offending drug, increasing hydration with alkaline fluid, and pharmacologic induction of diuresis with agents such as furosemide. If these measures are unsuccessful, bladder irrigation and/or mesna can be added to further neutralize the toxic metabolites. Most cases will resolve within days of discontinuing the offending agent; however, occasionally prolonged, chronic symptoms may develop.

METABOLIC EMERGENCIES

Hypercalcemia

ETIOLOGIC FACTORS

The most frequent metabolic emergency in oncology is hypercalcemia, which develops when the rate of calcium mobilization from bone exceeds the renal threshold for calcium excretion. Neoplastic disease is the leading cause of hypercalcemia among inpatients [157]. The most common malignancies associated with hypercalcemia are carcinomas of the breast and lung, hypernephroma, and multiple myeloma, squamous cell carcinoma of the head and neck and esophagus, and thyroid cancer. Parathyroid carcinoma is a rare malignancy associated with intractable hypercalcemia due to elevated parathyroid hormone (PTH) levels.

Although more than 80% of patients with hypercalcemia have osseous metastases, the extent of bony disease does not correlate with the level of hypercalcemia. During the course of their disease, approximately 40–50% of patients with breast carcinoma metastatic to the bones will develop hypercalcemia. In most settings hypercalcemia suggests disease progression, but patients with metastatic breast cancer involving bone may develop hypercalcemia when they are placed on hormonal therapy. Estrogen and antiestrogens stimulate breast cancer cells to produce osteolytic prostaglandins and to increase bone resorption [158]. Within several days of initiating hormonal therapy for metastatic breast cancer, the calcium level may rise and the bone pain increase. This tumor flare, in response to hormonal therapy, usually implies that the patient will subsequently have an excellent antitumor response to hormonal treatment. However, if hypercalcemia is severe, the hormonal therapy must be temporarily held and the hypercalcemia corrected before the drug is reinstituted.

PATHOPHYSIOLOGIC FEATURES

In the past, cancer-related hypercalcemia was classified by the presence or absence of bone involvement. Hypercalcemia in the former group was believed to be associated with direct bony destruction by cancer cells (so-called local osteolytic hypercalcemia), and the second group was characterized by various "humorally mediated" mechanisms. Evidence now supports the notion that hypercalcemia—even in patients with extensive bone involvement by tumor—is mediated by a variety of mechanisms, including factors released by malignant calls that ultimately act to resorb calcium from bone [159]. Some of these factors also stimulate calcium reabsorption from the renal tubule, but this effect is secondary in importance to accelerated osteoclastic bone resorption. Bone metastases or the indirect effects of ectopic humoral substances directly stimulate osteoclast activity and proliferation. *In vitro* studies have shown that selected cancer cell lines are capable of reabsorbing bone without increasing osteoclast activity [158].

Patients with squamous cell carcinomas of the head and neck, and adenocarcinomas of the lung, breast, and esophagus may develop a clinical syndrome suggestive of hyperparathyroidism owing to ectopic secretion of parathyroid hormone or parathyroid hormone-related protein (PTH-RP) [160, 161]. Most cases of hypercalcemia, which were presumed to be secondary to ectopic PTH production, are now felt to be due to ectopic secretion of PTH-RP, which binds to the parathyroid receptor [162]. In contrast to hypercalcemia due to hyperparathyroidism, these patients have impaired production of 1,25-dihydroxy vitamin D and no evidence of renal bicarbonate wasting [163]. In association with hypercalcemia, patients develop hypophosphatemia, increased urinary cyclic AMP, and elevations in levels of bone alkaline phosphatase [163]. The presence of PTH-RP at the diagnosis of hypercalcemia has been associated with a reduced hypocalcemic response to bisphosphonates, a more advanced tumor state and, therefore, an extremely poor prognosis [164]. Recent work has also demonstrated the importance of PTH-RP as a tumor-produced factor in the pathogenesis of bone metastasis. Besides these cancer-related functions, work in the past decade has clearly established that parathyroid hormone-related peptide has many important functions in normal physiology related to growth and development, reproductive function and smooth muscle relaxation [165].

Osteolytic prostaglandins have been detected in hypercalcemic patients with carcinomas of the lung, kidney, and ovary [166]. Animal studies have shown that inhibitors of prostaglandin synthesis (such as aspirin, indomethacin, and other nonsteroidal anti-inflammatory drugs, as well as corticosteroids) are successful therapies, but these agents are less effective in clinical practice.

A variety of other "osteoclast activating substances" have been identified, and likely play a less important role in the development of malignancy-induced hypercalcemia. These include the transforming growth factors (TGFs), and interleukin-6 (IL-6) among others. Most osteotrophic tumors, such as breast and prostate cancer, appear to require proximity to bone to effect bone resorption, possibly via release of TGFs, PTH-RP, or prostaglandins [166]. The extensive osteolysis observed in multiple myeloma may be due to focally increased production of IL-6 and TGF-β that accelerates bone resorption by normal osteoclasts. A large number of patients with cancer have lytic bone disease, but only a small proportion develop hypercalcemia; thus, interaction of these factors and amplification of the pathophysiology by the kidney must also occur [167].

CLINICAL PRESENTATION AND DIAGNOSTIC EVALUATION

Hypercalcemia is rarely a presenting sign of malignancy, except in patients with parathyroid carcinoma, human T-cell lymphotropic virus type-1 lymphoma, or multiple myeloma. Most hypercalcemic patients present with nonspecific symptoms of fatigue, anorexia, nausea, polyuria, polydipsia, and constipation. Neurologic symptoms from hypercalcemia begin with vague muscle weakness, lethargy, apathy, and hyporeflexia. Without treatment, symptoms progress to profound alterations in mental status, psychotic behavior, seizures, coma, and ultimately death. Patients with prolonged hypercalcemia eventually develop permanent renal tubular abnormalities with renal tubular acidosis, glucosuria, aminoaciduria, and hyperphosphaturia [168]. Sudden death from cardiac arrhythmias may occur when the serum calcium rises acutely. Except for those with parathyroid cancer, hypercalcemic patients rarely live long enough to develop signs of chronic hypercalcemia.

All hypercalcemic patients should have serial levels of serum calcium phosphate, alkaline phosphatase, electrolytes, BUN, and creatinine measured. Elevated immunoreactive PTH levels in association with hypophosphatemia may suggest ectopic hormone production. In malnourished patients with low albumin levels, the ionized calcium value may be helpful in deciding on therapy, since hypercalcemic symptoms correlate with elevation in ionized rather than protein-bound calcium. Patients with multiple myeloma may have elevated serum calcium secondary to abnormal calcium binding to paraproteins without an elevation in ionized calcium, while malnourished patients with hypoalbuminemia may have symptoms of hypercalcemia with normal serum calcium levels. The electrocardiogram often reveals shortening of the QT interval, widening of the T wave, bradycardia, and PR prolongation [168].

THERAPY

The cause of hypercalcemia, severity of associated clinical signs, and chance of response to effective antitumor therapy must be considered in choosing the most appropriate therapy. Mild hypercalcemia is frequently corrected with intravenous hydration alone. If effective antitumor therapy is available, the serum calcium will gradually decline as the tumor regresses. However, most hypercalcemic cancer patients require additional hypocalcemic therapy until an antitumor response is obtained. Calcium balance can be corrected by directly decreasing bone reabsorption, promoting urinary calcium excretion, and decreasing oral calcium intake. Patients should be mobilized to avoid osteolysis. Constipation should be corrected, and medications (such as thiazide diuretics and vitamins A and D) that may elevate calcium levels should never be used.

Corticosteroids, which block bone reabsorption due to osteoclast-activating factor (OAF), were used widely for this condition prior to the development of newer calcium-lowering agents [169]. Corticosteroids have been effective in multiple myeloma, lymphoma, breast cancer, and leukemia. Corticosteroids block bone reabsorption due to OAF. High-dose steroids may also have hypocalcemic effects by increasing urinary calcium excretion, inhibiting vitamin D metabolism, decreasing calcium absorption, and after long-term use by producing negative calcium balance in bone. High doses of corticosteroids are generally required for several days before an effective hypocalcemic response is seen; most patients require 40–100 mg of prednisone a day [170].

In the past, the majority of hypercalcemic patients were treated with Mithracin (plicamycin), a chemotherapeutic agent that decreases bone reabsorption by reducing osteoclast number and activity [171]. Mithracin is effective in patients with hypercalcemia from either bone metastases or from bone reabsorption from ectopic humoral substances. The drug is a sclerosing agent and must be given as a bolus through a freshly started intravenous line. If extravasation occurs, patients will develop ulceration and ultimately fibrosis of the underlying tissues. Hypercalcemic patients will often require one or two injections of Mithracin (15–20 µg/kg) per week, unless effective antitumor therapy is initiated. The serum calcium level will begin to decrease within six to 48 hours. If no response occurs within the first two days, a second dose can be administered. Only low doses of Mithracin are typically necessary to control hypercalcemia and the majority of patients do not develop side effects (e.g., thrombocytopenia, coagulopathy, hypertension, liver function abnormalities, or nephrotoxicity) generally seen with high doses.

Also used infrequently in the treatment of hypercalcemia of malignancy is calcitonin. Calcitonin promptly inhibits bone reabsorption causing a decrease in serum calcium levels within hours of administration [171]. Although a prompt hypocalcemic response is obtained, tachyphylaxis develops unless glucocorticoid therapy is given with calcitonin. For unclear reasons, if the serum calcium levels begin to increase with calcitonin, the drug may be temporarily held and then reinstituted; occasionally a secondary response will occur within 48 hours. Calcitonin is given in daily doses (3–6 Medical Research Council [MRC] units/kg) intravenously or twice a day intramuscularly or subcutaneously (100–400 MRC units/kg) [171].

More recently, hydration and administration of bisphosphonates are the mainstays of acute therapy for malignancy-associated hypercalcemia [168]. All hypercalcemic patients are dehydrated because of polyuria from renal tubular dysfunction. Intravenous hydration with normal saline will increase urinary calcium excretion because the urinary clearance rates for calcium parallel sodium excretion. The development of bisphosphonates has revolutionized treatment of malignancy-induced hypercalcemia. These compounds, pyrophosphate analogs with a phosphate-calcium-phosphate backbone, which binds tightly to calcified bone matrix, include etidronate, clodronate, and pamidronate [172]. All three are useful for the treatment of hypercalcemia, but pamidronate seems to be the most effective. Randomized trials of pamidronate versus standard treatment with hydration, steroids and mithramycin have established the superiority of pamidronate in effectively lowering serum calcium, with few side effects [173]. Subsequent studies have defined the optimal dosing and administration of pamidronate for this indication [174, 175]. A four-hour infusion of pamidronate disodium (60 mg) was as safe and effective as a 24-hour infusion, and both were superior to saline alone in lowering corrected serum calcium concentrations in patients with cancer-associated hypercalcemia. In addition, pamidronate appears to have antitumor activity in several cell types [176], and has been shown to decrease pain and fractures associated with bone metastases in patients with breast cancer [177]

Hyponatremia

ETIOLOGIC FACTORS

Only 1–2% of patients with malignancy develop the syndrome of inappropriate antidiuretic hormone secretion (SIADH) [178]. Despite a low plasma osmolality, the urine is inappropriately concentrated with a high sodium level. This situation can also occur in renal disease, hypothyroidism, and adrenal insufficiency and these diseases must be excluded to confirm the diagnosis of SIADH. The majority of patients are asymptomatic unless the serum sodium concentration falls abruptly.

Ectopic antidiuretic hormone secretion has been confirmed in patients with bronchogenic carcinoma. Small-cell anaplastic carcinoma of the lung is the most common malignancy associated with SIADH [179]. At presentation, more than 50% of patients with small-cell lung cancer may develop hyponatremia following a water load, but fewer than 15% of patients will develop clinically significant hyponatremia [180]. Case reports of SIADH have also been published in patients with cancers of the prostate, adrenal cortex, esophagus, pancreas, colon, and head and neck; carcinoid; thymoma; lymphoma; and mesothelioma [178].

Because ectopic antidiuretic hormone production is rarely seen except in patients with small-cell carcinoma, SIADH is more frequently associated with pulmonary or CNS metastases. Inappropriate antidiuretic hormone secretion can also occur with medications including morphine, vincristine, and cyclophosphamide [181]. With advanced malignancy, patients may also develop hyponatremia due to a "reset osmostat" in which the serum sodium is usually mildly depressed and may be corrected to normal levels with effective antitumor therapy. Kerne et al [182] reported that SIADH secretion can occur with pituitary prolactinomas. These tumors may produce SIADH without detectable arginine vasopressin levels. In this setting, bromocriptine induces both tumor regression and correction of hyponatremia.

Adrenal insufficiency resulting from withdrawal of corticosteroids or metastases to the adrenal or pituitary glands may cause mild hyponatremia. In the setting of severe liver disease, heart failure, or acute renal insufficiency, patients may develop dilutional hyponatremia. Vomiting, diarrhea, ascites, or diuretics may precipitate hyponatremia. Patients with plasma cell dyscrasias may have artifactual hyponatremia. Electrolytes should be followed when patients are treated with high-dose cisplatin with mannitol diuresis.

PATHOPHYSIOLOGIC FEATURES

With increased ADH secretion, excessive water is reabsorbed in the collecting ducts [178]. This leads to increased distal sodium delivery by producing a mild increase in intravascular volume. Volume expansion also increases renal perfusion, decreases proximal tubular reabsorption of sodium, and decreases aldosterone ef-

fect. Ectopic ADH secretion has been measured in patients with small-cell lung carcinoma [183]. In other conditions associated with increased ADH secretion, there is excessive production of ADH by the posterior pituitary [184].

Dilutional hyponatremia occurs in volume overloaded states secondary to cardiac, hepatic, or renal dysfunction. Although the total body sodium and water content are increased, the circulating plasma volume is reduced. With impaired renal perfusion, there is greater reabsorption of water in the collecting duct and increased ADH secretion, resulting in a dilutional hyponatremic state. With dehydration, total body salt and water content are generally decreased, which results in decreased renal perfusion and increased ADH secretion. Diuretics, interstitial renal disease, and mineralocorticoid deficiency are also associated with excessive renal sodium losses. Pseudohyponatremia is associated with elevated parathyroid levels in patients with plasma cell dyscrasias. Since the plasma sodium concentration is measured as the sodium concentration per unit of plasma, with elevated paraprotein levels, the percentage of water in plasma is decreased. With mannitol infusion or hyperglycemia, an osmotic gradient produces increased water movement into the extravascular spaces resulting in hyponatremia.

CLINICAL PRESENTATION AND DIAGNOSTIC EVALUATION

With mild hyponatremia, patients may complain of anorexia, nausea, myalgias, and subtle neurologic symptoms. When hyponatremia develops rapidly or the sodium level decreases below 115 mg/dL, patients frequently have alterations in mental status ranging from lethargy to confusion and coma. Seizures and psychotic behavior have also been reported. With profound hyponatremia, alterations in mental status, pathologic reflexes, papilledema, and rarely, focal neurologic signs may be found on physical examination [179]. The cause of hyponatremia must be determined before appropriate therapy can be initiated. If pseudohyponatremia due to hyperproteinemia, hyperlipidemia, or hyperglycemia is suspected, serum protein electrophoresis should be done and levels of lipids and glucose should be checked. Medication records should be reviewed since chemotherapeutic agents (e.g., vincristine or cyclophosphamide), mannitol, morphine, diuretics, and abrupt steroid withdrawal may contribute to hyponatremia.

A careful history, physical examination, and review

of the patient's intake and output will help to determine whether the patient is volume expanded, dehydrated, or euvolemic. Serum and urine electrolytes, osmolality, and creatinine should be measured. With SIADH, there is inappropriate sodium concentration in the urine for the level of hyponatremia [184]. The urine osmolality is greater than plasma osmolality, but it is never maximally dilute. With SIADH, the BUN is usually low from volume expansion. Hypouricemia and hypophosphatemia may result from decreased proximal tubular reabsorption of these ions. Thyroid and adrenal dysfunction should be ruled out if laboratory studies suggest SIADH. Chest x-ray and CT scans of the brain may reveal pulmonary or neurologic disorders that may cause excessive ADH production.

THERAPY

Ideally, treatment should be given to correct the cause of the hyponatremia; SIADH will resolve when the underlying cause of excessive antidiuretic hormone production is removed. Following effective combination chemotherapy for a small-cell lung cancer, the sodium will rise to normal levels. Corticosteroids and radiotherapy may alleviate SIADH due to brain metastasis. If drug-induced SIADH occurs, the serum sodium will correct once the offending agent is discontinued. If the etiology of excessive ADH secretion cannot be corrected, the initial therapy is water restriction [178]. If free water intake is restricted to 500–1,000 cc per day, the negative free water balance will correct the hyponatremia within 7–10 days. If the serum sodium does not correct with water restriction, demeclocycline may correct the hyponatremia by decreasing the stimulus of ADH for free water reabsorption in the collecting ducts [180].

Demeclocycline produces a dose-dependent, reversible nephrogenic diabetes insipidus [185]. With demeclocycline, despite liberal fluid intake, the average pretreatment serum sodium (121 mEq/L) increased above 130 mEq/L within three to four days of initiating treatment. The only side effect of demeclocycline is reversible nephrotoxicity [186]. Renal dysfunction develops in fewer than half of the patients and is generally mild. The majority of patients who experienced nephrotoxicity were either receiving other nephrotoxic drugs or higher doses of demeclocycline. Demeclocycline is excreted in the urine and bile; patients with renal or hepatic dysfunction should either avoid this drug or have reduced doses administered. The initial daily demeclocycline dose is 600 mg, unless the patient has liver or kidney dysfunction or is receiving other nephrotoxic drugs. Doses may be increased up to 1,200 mg a day if hyponatremia persists. The total drug dose is divided and given two or three times a day.

Hypoglycemia

ETIOLOGIC FACTORS AND PATHOPHYSIOLOGIC FEATURES

Fasting hypoglycemia occurs with insulinomas and rarely, with other islet cell tumors of the pancreas [187]. Other tumors associated with hypoglycemia usually are large, bulky, slow-growing mesenchymal malignancies, including fibrosarcomas, mesotheliomas, and spindle-cell sarcomas [188].

Glucose homeostasis is normally maintained by appropriate hormonal regulation of gluconeogenesis and glycogenolysis in patients with adequate caloric intake. Tumor-induced hypoglycemia may be caused by secretion of insulin or an insulin-like substance, increased glucose utilization by the tumor, or alterations in the regulatory mechanisms for glucose homeostasis. Although insulin levels are elevated in hypoglycemia from islet cell cancers, increased insulin secretion has not been observed with other neoplasms [189]. Using bioassays, increased levels of substances with insulin-like activity have been measured in serum samples from patients with hypoglycemia and non-islet-cell malignancies. These substances are now referred to as non-suppressible insulin-like activity (NSILA) [190]. Only 5–10% of their insulin-like activity can be neutralized with antibodies to insulin. NSILA appears to be a combination of somatomedins A and C, high molecular weight glycoproteins, and low molecule weight growth factors. These substances have both the growth-promoting and metabolic effects of insulin. However, the growth-promoting effects of the low-molecular-weight substances are 54% greater than the effects of insulin, while their metabolic effects are only 1–2% as potent. The high molecular weight substances have minimal growth-promoting capabilities but maintain their metabolic effects.

Elevated levels of low molecular weight NSILA have been demonstrated in patients with non-islet-cell tumors causing hypoglycemia by both radioreceptor and bioassay techniques. Elevated levels of these substances have been demonstrated in patients with hemangiopericytomas, hepatomas, pheochromocytomas, adrenocortical carcinomas, and large mesenchymal tumors.

Low to normal levels of NSILA have been measured in patients with hypoglycemia in association of leukemia, lymphoma, or gastrointestinal primaries [189]. When there is a rapid reduction in glucose levels in the normal patient, counterregulatory mechanisms should increase secretion of adrenocorticotropic hormone (ACTH), glucocorticoids, growth hormone, and glucagon. However, in patients with tumor-induced hypoglycemia, the decrease in glucose is usually not rapid enough to increase these hormone levels.

Cancer patients have reduced rates of hepatic gluconeogenesis-reduced glycogen breakdown following epinephrine or glucagon, and decreased hepatic glycogen stores [191]. These data suggest that impaired glucose homeostasis may contribute to tumor-induced hypoglycemia. In the past, increased use of glucose by the tumor was thought to be one of the causes of hypoglycemia. However, increased glycogen breakdown and gluconeogenesis should compensate for increased glycolysis. Before assuming that the metabolic abnormality is caused by the malignancy, the more common causes of hypoglycemia (i.e., exogenous insulin use, oral diabetic agents, adrenal failure, pituitary insufficiency, alcohol abuse, or malnutrition) should be excluded.

CLINICAL PRESENTATION AND DIAGNOSTIC EVALUATION

Most patients will complain of excessive fatigue, weakness, dizziness, and confusion. Patients will rarely have symptoms to suggest reactive hypoglycemia. Symptoms tend to occur after fasting in the early morning or late afternoon. If the blood glucose level remains depressed below 40 mg/dL, seizures may result. Symptoms may be more nonspecific in the elderly, who can present with weight loss or change in mental status [192].

Fasting and late-afternoon glucose levels are most helpful in making the diagnosis. Patients with insulinomas will have increased insulin levels with fasting glucose levels less than 50 mg/dL, while patients with nonislet-cell tumors will have normal to low insulin levels during the periods of hypoglycemia [189]. Leukemic patients with high leukocyte counts may have artifactual hypoglycemia when blood remains in collection tubes for prolonged periods.

Insulinomas produce large amounts of proinsulin and have elevated proinsulin-to-insulin ratios. Higher proinsulin levels are seen with malignant insulinomas. If technically feasible, insulin-like plasma factors should be measured by bioassay or radioreceptor technique [193].

THERAPY

Hypoglycemia is corrected rapidly with intravenous injections of 50% dextrose, which should be followed by a continuous infusion of 10% dextrose. Insulinomas are frequently cured by surgery, while the rare patient with the inoperable insulinoma can be managed with chemotherapy or diazoxide.

If effective antitumor therapy is available for nonislet-cell tumors associated with hypoglycemia, the metabolic abnormalities should resolve with tumor regression. Following surgical resection of fibrosarcomas, hypoglycemia will resolve. Effective chemotherapy regimens for mesotheliomas have also corrected hypoglycemia [189]. To prevent nocturnal hypoglycemia, patients should be awakened from sleep for meals and have frequent between-meal and bedtime snacks. Occasionally, corticosteroids may provide temporary relief. Patients have also benefited from intermittent subcutaneous or long-acting, intramuscular, glucagon injections [194].

Tumor Lysis Syndrome

ETIOLOGIC FACTORS AND PATHOPHYSIOLOGIC FEATURES

Tumor lysis syndrome is usually associated with malignancies that have an increased rate of cell turnover, or that are highly sensitive to anti-tumor therapies. Although it can occur spontaneously, the condition most frequently is reported as a complication following cytotoxic therapy that produces a rapid antitumor response [195]. Rapid cell death increases uric acid production and results in hyperuricemia and uric acid crystal deposition in the urinary tract [196]. The most common tumors associated with tumor lysis syndrome are leukemia and lymphoma, but this condition has also been reported among patients with solid tumors, including lung cancer [197, 198], breast cancer [195], small cell tumors [196], multiple myeloma, and squamous-cell carcinomas of the head and neck. In addition, certain cytotoxic treatments may be associated with the disorder. Reports have linked CPT-11 in colorectal cancer [199] and fludarabine [200] with this disorder.

Hyperuricemia and associated renal uric acid deposition can lead to uric acid nephropathy. Most episodes of uric acid nephropathy are associated with effective cytotoxic chemotherapy or radiation therapy, but spontaneous hyperuricemic nephropathy in hematologic malignancies has been occasionally reported in lymphoma and leukemia patients, particularly with high tumor burden [201]. The incidence and severity of hyperuricemic nephropathy have decreased with prophylactic treatment with allopurinol, vigorous hydration, and alkalinization of the urine. In previous studies, mortality rates from hyperuricemic nephropathy ranged from 47% to 100%. However, with current aggressive medical therapy, the majority of patients regain normal renal function within a few days of treatment [201].

CLINICAL PRESENTATION AND DIAGNOSTIC EVALUATION

Tumor lysis syndrome occurs as a result of rapid release of intracellular contents into the bloodstream, which then increase to life-threatening concentrations. The syndrome is characterized by hyperuricemia, hyperkalemia, hyperphosphatemia, and hypocalcemia [201]. Serial blood studies for electrolytes, BUN, creatinine, calcium, phosphorus, and uric acid must be obtained. Lethal cardiac arrhythmias are the most serious consequences of hyperkalemia. Hyperphosphatemia may result in acute renal failure [202]. Hypocalcemia (a result of hyperphosphatemia) can cause muscle cramps, cardiac arrhythmias, and tetany.

Renal involvement commonly presents with signs and symptoms of uremia, including nausea, vomiting, lethargy, and oliguria [201]. Early treatment provides an excellent chance of rapidly reversing renal dysfunction. It can be difficult to differentiate acute uric acid nephropathy from other causes of renal failure with secondary hyperuricemia. If flank pain or gross hematuria occurs, a renal ultrasound should be performed to exclude ureteral obstruction. Hyperuricemia increases the incidence of dye-induced renal dysfunction, so intravenous contrast should be avoided. In the tumor lysis syndrome, hyperphosphatemia and hypocalcemia often occur out of proportion to the degree of renal insufficiency. The urinalysis will be helpful if uric acid crystals are seen, but their absence does not exclude the diagnosis since crystalluria and hematuria occur only in the acute phase [196]. Kelton et al have demonstrated that a urinary uric acid-to-creatinine ratio > 1 is relatively specific for hyperuricemia nephropathy [203].

THERAPY

The primary goal of therapy should be the prevention of hyperuricemia and other associated metabolic derangements. Patients at high risk should be treated with allopurinol, vigorous hydration, and urinary alkalinization for at least 48 hours prior to cytotoxic therapy. Drugs that block tubular reabsorption of uric acid (such as aspirin, radiographic contrast, probenecid, and thiazide diuretics) should be avoided. Serum electrolytes, uric acid, phosphorus, calcium and creatinine should be checked every few hours for three to four days after initiating cytotoxic treatment. The frequency of monitoring should depend on the clinical condition of the patient. If significant hyperkalemia or hypocalcemia become evident, an electrocardiogram should be obtained and the cardiac rhythm should be monitored while these abnormalities are corrected.

Prior to chemotherapy, the serum uric acid level should be normal, the urine pH > 7, and intravenous hydration should be given to ensure a high urine volume [204]. To alkalinize the urine, intravenous sodium bicarbonate (100 mEq/m²) should be given daily. When the urinary pH is > 7.5, uric acid solubility is maximal and it is not necessary to produce significant metabolic alkalosis, which may complicate the clinical situation. Serum potassium and magnesium levels should be followed closely and allopurinol administered in doses ranging from 300 mg/day to 800 mg/day to decrease uric acid production by competitively inhibiting xanthine oxidase. Although high xanthine levels might precipitate xanthine stones, this has not been reported in patients treated for hyperuricemic nephropathy. Prophylactic colchicine is not required when allopurinol is administered because patients rarely develop acute gouty arthritis.

If oliguria or anuria develops, ureteral obstruction must be excluded by renal ultrasound or antegrade or retrograde pyelography; nephrotoxic contrast must be avoided. Once ureteral obstruction is excluded, mannitol or high-dose furosemide should be given in an attempt to restore urine flow. A Foley catheter should be inserted to accurately measure urine output. If a prompt diuresis does not occur within a few hours, emergency hemodialysis may be necessary to reverse uric acid obstruction of the urinary tubules [205].

A hollow-fiber kidney apparatus will decrease serum uric acid levels more rapidly than either peritoneal or coil dialysis [206]. Patients with hypotension may not be able to tolerate standard hemodialysis, however. In such patients, continuous arteriovenous hemofiltration (CAVH) and conventional continuous arteriovenous hemodialysis (CAVHD) may be effective [205]. Patients may require multiple days of dialysis before hyperuricemia resolves and renal function returns to baseline normal values [207]. Fortunately, with early recognition and aggressive measures for prevention and treatment, acute uric acid nephropathy now has an extremely low morbidity and mortality rate [201].

Adrenal Gland Failure

ETIOLOGIC FACTORS AND PATHOPHYSIOLOGIC FEATURES

Adrenal gland insufficiency in cancer patients may result from progression of the disease process or as a side effect of treatment. The adrenal gland may be a site of primary tumor development, or, more commonly, a site of metastasis [208–210]. Metastases to the adrenal gland due to breast, lung, or colon cancer, which are being discovered more frequently as CT and MRI imaging improve, only rarely cause adrenal gland insufficiency; most are asymptomatic. Iatrogenic causes include surgery (adrenalectomy) or treatment with agents that are either directly toxic (suramin, mitotane) or that inhibit steroid synthesis, such as aminoglutethamide [211], megestrol [212], or corticosteroids [213]. A series reported by the Massachusetts General Hospital in 1984 found that 19% of patients with metastatic cancer and adrenal enlargement by CT developed symptoms of adrenal gland insufficiency [214].

CLINICAL PRESENTATION AND DIAGNOSTIC EVALUATION

Classic signs and symptoms of adrenal insufficiency include weakness, weight loss, anorexia, hyperpigmentation, and postural hypotension. Development of this condition is typically insidious rather than abrupt, with circulatory collapse or shock uncommon [215, 216]. The diagnostic study of choice is the ACTH-stimulation test. Patients are given Cosyntropin, 0.25 mg intravenously, and serum cortisol is monitored at baseline, at 30 minutes, and at 60 minutes. Adrenal insufficiency is defined as a failure to increase serum cortisol by at least 5 micrograms/100 ml to a minimum of 15 micrograms/100 ml at either 30 or 60 minutes postcosyntropin [215]. However, if the diagnosis is strongly suspected on clinical grounds, steroids and supportive care should be started immediately, and subsequent treatment can be modified when test results become available [217].

THERAPY

Physiologic glucocorticoid replacement is attained by administration of cortisone acetate (25 mg in the morning and 12.5 mg in the early evening). During periods of stress (e.g., operative procedures or infection), these doses may need to be doubled or tripled. Occasionally, mineralocorticoid replacement with 0.05–0.1 mg of fludrocortisone is required in addition to cortisone acetate. In patients with no adrenocortical function whatsoever, maintenance doses of dexamethasone or prednisone do not provide adequate mineralocorticoid coverage and fludrocortisone must be given. Pharmacologic doses of parenteral glucocorticoids are required in the setting of acute adrenal failure and circulatory collapse. Typically, water-soluble forms of hydrocortisone (e.g., sodium succinate salt), 100 mg intravenously every eight hours, are required. Thereafter, the patient should be monitored for evidence of hyperglycemia, hypokalemia, or hypernatremia [144].

SUMMARY

The diagnosis of malignancy is frequently complicated by the development of cancer-related emergencies. These conditions, which involve a variety of organ systems, may be sudden, severe and/or potentially life-threatening. Many develop as the first indicator of the presence of malignancy, and thus alert the physician to the presence of an underlying diagnosis. Others develop as the malignancy progresses, or as a result of cytotoxic therapy. As antitumor therapy becomes more effective and less toxic, it is imperative to recognize potentially life-threatening or permanently disabling complications that may be prevented or reversed by prompt action. Accurate diagnosis and treatment of oncologic emergencies can improve quality of life and prolong survival, allowing more patients to receive an adequate trial of definitive therapy designed to eradicate or effectively palliate their malignant disease.

REFERENCES

1. McAllister HA Jr, Hall RJ, Cooley DA. Tumors of the heart and pericardium. *Curr Probl Cardiol* 24:57–116, 1999.
2. DeCamp MM Jr, Mentzer SJ, Swanson SJ, Sugarbaker DJ. Malignant effusive disease of the pleura and pericardium. *Chest* 112(suppl 4):291S–295S, 1997.
3. Habboush HW, Dhundee J, Okati DA, Davies AG. Constrictive pericarditis in B cell chronic lymphatic leukaemia. *Clin Lab Haematol* 18:117–119, 1996.
4. Woodring JH. The lateral chest radiograph in the detection of pericardial effusion: a reevaluation. *J KY Med Assoc* 96:218–224, 1998.

5. Hancock E. Constrictive pericarditis: clinical clues to diagnosis. *JAMA* 232:176–177, 1975.

6. Millman A, Meller J, Motro M. Pericardial tumor or fibrosis mimicking pericardial effusion by echocardiography. *Ann Intern Med* 86:434–436, 1977.

7. Hudson R. *Diseases of the Pericardium.* New York: McGraw-Hill, 1998.

8. White CS. MR evaluation of the pericardium and cardiac malignancies. *Magn Reson Imaging Clin North Am* 4:237–251, 1996.

9. Mader MT, Poulton TB, White RD. Malignant tumors of the heart and great vessels: MR imaging appearance. *Radiographics* 17:145–153, 1997.

10. Bardales RH, Stanley MW, Schaefer RF, et al. Secondary pericardial malignancies: a critical appraisal of the role of cytology, pericardial biopsy, and DNA ploidy analysis. *Am J Clin Pathol* 106:29–34, 1996.

11. Figueroa W, Alankar S, Pai N, Dave M. Subxiphoid pericardial window for pericardial effusion in end-stage renal disease. *Am J Kidney Dis* 27:664–667, 1996.

12. Laham RJ, Cohen DJ, Kuntz RE, et al. Pericardial effusion in patients with cancer: outcome with contemporary management strategies. *Heart* 75:67–71, 1996.

13. Shepherd FA. Malignant pericardial effusion (see comments). *Curr Opin Oncol* 9:170–174, 1997.

14. Maher EA, Shepherd FA, Todd TJ. Pericardial sclerosis as the primary management of malignant pericardial effusion and cardiac tamponade. *J Thorac Cardiovasc Surg* 112:637–643, 1996.

15. Fiocco M, Krasna MJ. The management of malignant pleural and pericardial effusions. *Hematol Oncol Clin North Am* 11:253–265, 1997.

16. Lashevsky I, Ben Yosef R, Rinkevich D, et al. Intrapericardial minocycline sclerosis for malignant pericardial effusion (see comments). *Chest* 109:1452–1454, 1996.

17. van Belle SJ, Volckaert A, Taeymans Y, et al. Treatment of malignant pericardial tamponade with sclerosis induced by instillation of bleomycin. *Int J Cardiol* 16:155–160, 1987.

18. Liu G, Crump M, Goss PE, et al. Prospective comparison of the sclerosing agents doxycycline and bleomycin for the primary management of malignant pericardial effusion and cardiac tamponade. *J Clin Oncol* 14:3141–3147, 1996.

19. Rodriguez MI, Ash K, Foley RW, Liston W. Pericardioperitoneal window: laparoscopic approach. *Surg Endosc* 13:409–411, 1999.

20. Law DA, Haque R, Jain A. Percutaneous balloon pericardiotomy: non-surgical treatment for patients with cardiac tamponade. *WV Med J* 93:310–312, 1997.

21. Colleoni M, Martinelli G, Beretta F, et al. Intracavitary chemotherapy with thiotepa in malignant pericardial effusions: an active and well-tolerated regimen. *J Clin Oncol* 16:2371–2376, 1998.

22. Tomkowski WZ, Filipecki S. Intrapericardial cisplatin for the management of patients with large malignant pericardial effusion in the course of the lung cancer. *Lung Cancer* 16:215–222, 1997.

23. Buzaid AC, Garewal HS, Greenberg BR. Managing malignant pericardial effusion. *West J Med* 150:174–179, 1989.

24. Handa R, Bhatia S, Wali JP, et al. Acute leukemia presenting as pericardial effusion—a case report. *Singapore Med J* 38:491–492, 1997.

25. Furuta M, Hayakawa K, Saito Y, et al. Clinical implication of symptoms in patients with non-small-cell lung cancer treated with definitive radiation therapy. *Lung Cancer* 13:275–283, 1995.

26. Urban T, Lebeau B, Chastang C, et al. Superior vena cava syndrome in small-cell lung cancer. *Arch Intern Med* 153:384–387, 1993.

27. Chen YM, Yang S, Perng RP, Tsai CM. Superior vena cava syndrome revisited. *Jpn J Clin Oncol* 25:32–36, 1995.

28. Markman M. Common complications and emergencies associated with cancer and its therapy. *Cleve Clin J Med* 61:105–114, 1994.

29. Puel V, Caudry M, Le Metayer P, et al. Superior vena cava thrombosis related to catheter malposition in cancer chemotherapy given through implanted ports. *Cancer* 72:2248–2252, 1993.

30. Perez CA, Presant CA, van Amburg ALD. Management of superior vena cava syndrome. *Semin Oncol* 5:123–134, 1978.

31. Chen JC, Bongard F, Klein SR. A contemporary perspective on superior vena cava syndrome. *Am J Surg* 160:207–211, 1990.

32. Sharma RP, Keller CE, Shetty PC, Burke MW. Superior vena cava obstruction: evaluation with digital subtraction angiography. *Radiology* 160:845, 1986.

33. Mineo TC, Ambrogi V, Nofroni I, Pistolese C. Mediastinoscopy in superior vena cava obstruction: analysis of 80 consecutive patients. *Ann Thorac Surg* 68:223–226, 1999.

34. Baker GL, Barnes HJ. Superior vena cava syndrome: etiology, diagnosis, and treatment. *Am J Crit Care* 1:54–64, 1992.

35. Schindler N, Vogelzang RL. Superior vena cava syndrome. Experience with endovascular stents and surgical therapy. *Surg Clin North Am* 79:683–694, 1999.

36. Egelmeers A, Goor C, van Meerbeeck J, et al. Palliative effectiveness of radiation therapy in the treatment of superior vena cava syndrome. *Bull Cancer Radiother* 83:153–157, 1996.

37. Hoegler D. Radiotherapy for palliation of symptoms in incurable cancer. *Curr Probl Cancer* 21:129–183, 1997.

38. Rodrigues CI, Njo KH, Karim AB. Hypofractionated radiation therapy in the treatment of superior vena cava syndrome. *Lung Cancer* 10:221–228, 1993.

39. Chan RH, Dar AR, Yu E, et al. Superior vena cava obstruction in small-cell lung cancer. *Int J Radiat Oncol Biol Phys* 38:513–520, 1997.

40. Nomori H, Nara S, Morinaga S, Soejima K. Primary malignant lymphoma of superior vena cava. *Ann Thorac Surg* 66:1423–1424, 1998.

41. Adelstein DJ, Hines JD, Carter SG, Sacco D. Thromboembolic events in patients with malignant superior vena cava syndrome and the role of anticoagulation. *Cancer* 62:2258–2262, 1988.

42. Doty DB. Bypass of superior vena cava: six years' experience with spiral vein graft for obstruction of superior vena cava due to benign and malignant disease. *J Thorac Cardiovasc Surg* 83:326–338, 1982.

43. Shepherd FA. Intrathoracic complications of malignancy and its treatment (see comments). *Curr Opin Oncol* 7:150–157, 1995.

44. Nally AT. Critical care of the patient with lung cancer. *AACN Clin Issues* 7:79–94, 1996.

45. Taichman DB, Tino G, Aronchick J, et al. Diffuse airway narrowing from carcinoma metastatic to the bronchial submucosa: identification by chest CT. *Chest* 114:1217–1220, 1998.

46. Lunn WW, Sheller JR. Flow volume loops in the evaluation of upper airway obstruction. *Otolaryngol Clin North Am* 28:721–729, 1995.

47. Shure D. Radiographically occult endobronchial obstruction in bronchogenic carcinoma. *Am J Med* 91:19–22. 1991.

48. Ramser ER, Beamis JF Jr. Laser bronchoscopy. *Clin Chest Med* 16:415–426, 1995.

49. Daddi G, Puma F, Avenia N, et al. Resection with curative intent after endoscopic treatment of airway obstruction. *Ann Thorac Surg* 65:203–207, 1998.

50. Stohr S, Bolliger CT. Stents in the management of malignant airway obstruction. *Monaldi Arch Chest Dis* 54:264–268, 1999.

51. Tojo T, Iioka S, Kitamura S, et al. Management of malignant tracheobronchial stenosis with metal stents and Dumon stents. *Ann Thorac Surg* 61:1074–1078, 1996.

52. Chang LF, Horvath J, Peyton W, Ling SS. High dose rate afterloading intraluminal brachytherapy in malignant airway obstruction of lung cancer (see comments). *Int J Radiat Oncol Biol Phys* 28:589–596. 1994.

53. Pisch J, Villamena PC, Harvey JC, et al. High dose-rate endobronchial irradiation in malignant airway obstruction. *Chest* 104:721–725, 1993.

54. Sheski FD, Mathur PN. Cryotherapy, electrocautery, and brachytherapy. *Clin Chest Med* 20:123–138, 1999.

55. Zwischenberger JB, Wittich GR, van Sonnenberg E, et al. Airway simulation to guide stent placement for tracheobronchial obstruction in lung cancer. *Ann Thorac Surg* 64:1619–1625, 1997.

56. Tanaka H, Nakahara K, Sakai S, et al. [A case of Hodgkin's disease with endotracheal tumor presenting with severe airflow obstruction.] *(Nihon Kyobu Shikkan Gakkai Zasshi) Jpn J Thorac Dis* 30:1732–1737, 1992.

57. Celikoglu SI, Karayel T, Demirci S, et al. Direct injection of anti-cancer drugs into endobronchial tumours for palliation of major airway obstruction. *Postgrad Med J* 73:159–162, 1997.

58. Schiff D, Batchelor T, Wen PY. Neurologic emergencies in cancer patients. *Neurol Clin* 16:449–483, 1998.

59. Posner JB. Management of central nervous system metastases. *Semin Oncol* 4:81–91, 1977.

60. Pedersen AG, Bach F, Melgaard B. Frequency, diagnosis, and prognosis of spinal cord compression in small cell bronchogenic carcinoma. A review of 817 consecutive patients. *Cancer* 55:1818–1822, 1985.

61. Calkins AR, Olson MA, Ellis JH. Impact of myelography on the radiotherapeutic management of malignant spinal cord compression. *Neurosurgery* 19:614–616, 1986.

62. Lim CC, Chong BK. Spinal epidural non-Hodgkin's lymphoma: case reports of three patients presenting with spinal cord compression. *Singapore Med J* 37:497–500, 1996.

63. Fujii Y, Higashi Y, Owada F, et al. Magnetic resonance imaging for the diagnosis of prostate cancer metastatic to bone. *Br J Urol* 75:54–58, 1995.

64. Berman CG, Clark RA. Diagnostic imaging in cancer. *Prim Care* 19:677–713, 1992.

65. Tryciecky EW, Gottschalk A, Ludema K. Oncologic imaging: interactions of nuclear medicine with CT and MRI using the bone scan as a model. *Semin Nucl Med* 27:142–151, 1997.

66. Heldmann U, Myschetzky PS, Thomsen HS. Frequency of unexpected multifocal metastasis in patients with acute spinal cord compression. Evaluation by low-field MR imaging in cancer patients. *Acta Radiol* 38:372–375, 1997.

67. Koehler PJ. Use of corticosteroids in neuro-oncology. *Anticancer Drugs* 6:19–33, 1995.

68. Latini P, Maranzano E, Ricci S, et al. Role of radiotherapy in metastatic spinal cord compression: preliminary results from a prospective trial. *Radiother Oncol* 15:227–233, 1989.

69. Janjan NA. Radiotherapeutic management of spinal metastases. *J Pain Symptom Manage* 11:47–56, 1996.

70. Maranzano E, Latini P, Checcaglini F, et al. Radiation therapy of spinal cord compression caused by breast cancer: report of a prospective trial. *Int J Radiat Oncol Biol Phys* 24:301–306, 1992.

71. Huddart RA, Rajan B, Law M, et al. Spinal cord compression in prostate cancer: treatment outcome and prognostic factors. *Radiother Oncol* 44:229–236, 1997.

72. Schiff D, Shaw EG, Cascino TL. Outcome after spinal re-irradiation for malignant epidural spinal cord compression. *Ann Neurol* 37:583–589, 1995.

73. Sucher E, Margulies JY, Floman Y, Robin GC. Prognostic factors in anterior decompression for metastatic cord compression. An analysis of results. *Eur Spine J* 3:70–75, 1994.

74. Findlay GF. The role of vertebral body collapse in the management of malignant spinal cord compression. *J Neurol Neurosurg Psychiatry* 50:151–154, 1987.

75. Findlay GF. Adverse effects of the management of malignant spinal cord compression. *J Neurol Neurosurg Psychiatry* 47:761–768, 1984.

76. Burch PA, Grossman SA. Treatment of epidural cord compressions from Hodgkin's disease with chemotherapy. A report of two cases and a review of the literature. *Am J Med* 84:555–558, 1988.

77. Katagiri H, Takahashi M, Inagaki J, et al. Clinical results of nonsurgical treatment for spinal metastases. *Int J Radiat Oncol Biol Phys* 42:1127–1132, 1998.

78. Higgins SA, Peschel RE. Hodgkin's disease with spinal cord compression. A case report and a review of the literature. *Cancer* 75:94–98, 1995.

79. Osborn JL, Getzenberg RH, Trump DL. Spinal cord compression in prostate cancer. *J Neurooncol* 23:135–147, 1995.

80. Chamberlain MC, Kormanik PR. Carcinomatous meningitis secondary to breast cancer: predictors of response to

combined modality therapy. *J Neurooncol* 35:55–64, 1997.

81. Zachariah B, Zachariah SB, Varghese R, Balducci L. Carcinomatous meningitis: clinical manifestations and management. *Int J Clin Pharmacol Ther* 33:7–12, 1995.

82. Chamberlain MC. Cytologically negative carcinomatous meningitis: usefulness of CSF biochemical markers. *Neurology* 50:1173–1175, 1998.

83. Wasserstrom WR, Glass JP, Posner JB. Diagnosis and treatment of leptomeningeal metastases from solid tumors: experience with 90 patients. *Cancer* 49:759–772, 1982.

84. Obbens EA, Leavens ME, Beal JW, Lee YY. Ommaya reservoirs in 387 cancer patients: a 15-year experience. *Neurology* 35:1274–1278, 1985.

85. Preti A, Kantarjian HM. Management of adult acute lymphocytic leukemia: present issues and key challenges. *J Clin Oncol* 12:1312–1322, 1994.

86. van Besien K, Forman A, Champlin R. Central nervous system relapse of lymphoid malignancies in adults: the role of high-dose chemotherapy. *Ann Oncol* 8:515–524, 1997.

87. Horak ID, Kremer AB, Magrath IT. Management of histologically aggressive lymphomas with a high risk of CNS disease. *Baillieres Clin Haematol* 9:707–726, 1996.

88. Cascinu S. Management of diarrhea induced by tumors or cancer therapy. *Curr Opin Oncol* 7:325–329, 1995.

89. Baillie-Johnson HR. Octreotide in the management of treatment-related diarrhoea. *Anticancer Drugs* 7(suppl 1):11–15, 1996.

90. US Department of Health and Human Services, National Institutes of Health, National Cancer Institute. *Investigator's Handbook: A Manual for Participants in Clinical Trials of Investigational Agents.* Bethesda, MD: National Cancer Institute, 1993.

91. Wadler S, Benson 3rd AB, Engelking C, et al. Recommended guidelines for the treatment of chemotherapy-induced diarrhea. *J Clin Oncol* 16:3169–3178, 1998.

92. Bergman L, Djarv L. A comparative study of loperamide and diphenoxylate in the treatment of chronic diarrhoea caused by intestinal resection. *Ann Clin Res* 13:402–405, 1981.

93. Palmer KR, Corbett CL, Holdsworth CD. Double-blind cross-over study comparing loperamide, codeine and diphenoxylate in the treatment of chronic diarrhea. *Gastroenterology* 79:1272–1275, 1980.

94. Pelemans W, Vantrappen F. A double blind crossover comparison of loperamide with diphenoxylate in the symptomatic treatment of chronic diarrhea. *Gastroenterology* 70:1030–1034, 1976.

95. Jaffe G. A comparison of lomotil and imodium in acute non-specific diarrhoea. *J Int Med Res* 5:195–198, 1977.

96. Abigerges D, Armand JP, Chabot GG, et al. Irinotecan (CPT-11) high-dose escalation using intensive high-dose loperamide to control diarrhea. *J Natl Cancer Inst* 86:446–449, 1994.

97. Wadler S, Haynes H, Wiernik PH. Phase I trial of the somatostatin analog octreotide acetate in the treatment of fluoropyrimidine-induced diarrhea. *J Clin Oncol* 13:222–226, 1995.

98. Cascinu S, Fedeli A, Fedeli SL, Catalano G. Octreotide versus loperamide in the treatment of fluorouracil-induced diarrhea: a randomized trial. *J Clin Oncol* 11:148–151, 1993.

99. Farthing MJ. The role of somatostatin analogues in the treatment of refractory diarrhoea. *Digestion* 57 (suppl 1):107–113, 1996.

100. Crouch MA, Restino MS, Cruz JM, et al. Octreotide acetate in refractory bone marrow transplant-associated diarrhea. *Ann Pharmacother* 30:331–336, 1996.

101. Morton AJ, Durrant ST. Efficacy of octreotide in controlling refractory diarrhea following bone marrow transplantation. *Clin Transplant* 9:205–208, 1995.

102. Geller RB, Gilmore CE, Dix SP, et al. Randomized trial of loperamide versus dose escalation of octreotide acetate for chemotherapy-induced diarrhea in bone marrow transplant and leukemia patients. *Am J Hematol* 50:167–172, 1995.

103. Cascinu S, Fedeli A, Fedeli SL, Catalano G. Control of chemotherapy-induced diarrhea with octreotide. A randomized trial with placebo in patients receiving cisplatin. *Oncology* 51:70–73, 1994.

104. Petrelli NJ, Rodriguez-Bigas M, Rustum Y, et al. Bowel rest, intravenous hydration, and continuous high-dose infusion of octreotide acetate for the treatment of chemotherapy-induced diarrhea in patients with colorectal carcinoma. *Cancer* 72:1543–1546, 1993.

105. Gebbia V, Carreca I, Testa A, et al. Subcutaneous octreotide versus oral loperamide in the treatment of diarrhea following chemotherapy. *Anticancer Drugs* 4:443–445, 1993.

106. Case records of the Massachusetts General Hospital. Weekly clinicopathological exercises. Case 3–1997. A 39-year-old man with diarrhea and abdominal pain after chemotherapy for acute leukemia (clinical conference). *N Engl J Med* 336:277–284, 1997.

107. Katz JA, Wagner ML, Gresik MV, et al. Typhlitis. An 18-year experience and postmortem review. *Cancer* 65:1041–1047, 1990.

108. Clemons MJ, Valle JW, Harris M, et al. *Citrobacter freundii* and fatal neutropenic enterocolitis following adjuvant chemotherapy for breast cancer. *Clini Oncol (R Coll Radiol)* 9:172–175, 1997.

109. Weinberger M, Hollingsworth H, Feuerstein IM, et al. Successful surgical management of neutropenic enterocolitis in two patients with severe aplastic anemia. Case reports and review of the literature. *Arch Intern Med* 153:107–113, 1993.

110. Anonymous. *Clostridium septicum* and neutropenic enterocolitis (editorial). *Lancet* 2:608, 1987.

111. Hopkins DG, Kushner JP. Clostridial species in the pathogenesis of necrotizing enterocolitis in patients with neutropenia. *Am J Hematol* 14:289–295, 1983.

112. Anand A, Glatt AE. *Clostridium difficile* infection associated with antineoplastic chemotherapy: a review. *Clin Infect Dis* 17:109–113, 1993.

113. Moir CR, Scudamore CH, Benny WB. Typhlitis: selective surgical management. *Am J Surg* 151:563–566, 1986.

114. Shamberger RC, Weinstein HJ, Delorey MJ, Levey RH. The medical and surgical management of typhlitis in

children with acute nonlymphocytic (myelogenous) leukemia. *Cancer* 57:603–609, 1986.

115. Pizzo PA, Robichaud KJ, Wesley R, Commers JA. Fever in the pediatric and young adult patient with cancer: a prospective study of 1001 episodes. *Medicine* 61:153–165, 1982.

116. Hughes WT, Armstrong D, Bodey GP, et al. Infectious Diseases Society of America 1997 guidelines for the use of antimicrobial agents in neutropenic patients with unexplained fever. *Clin Infect Dis* 25:551–573, 1997.

117. Bodey GP, Buckley M, Sathe YS, Freireich EJ. Quantitative relationships between circulating leukocytes and infection in patients with acute leukemia. *Ann Intern Med* 64:328–340, 1966.

118. Paschal BR, Gradon JD, Rolston KVI, et al. Fever in patients with neutropenia. *N Engl J Med* 329:1279–1280, 1993.

119. Freifeld AG, Pizzo PA. The outpatient management of febrile neutropenia in cancer patients. *Oncology* 10:599–612, 1996.

120. Bochud PY, Eggiman P, Calandra T, et al. Bacteremia due to viridans streptococcus in neutropenic patients with cancer: clinical spectrum and risk factors (see comments). *Clin Infect Dis* 18:25–31, 1994.

121. Freifeld AG WT, Pizzo PA. Infections in the cancer patient. In DeVita VT, Hellman S, Rosenberg SA (eds), *Cancer: Principles and Practice of Oncology* (5th ed). Philadelphia: Lippincott-Raven, 1997:2659–2704.

122. Dale DC, Guerry DT, Wewerka JR, et al. Chronic neutropenia. *Medicine* 58:128–144, 1979.

123. Pizzo PA. Drug therapy: Management of fever in patients with cancer and treatment-induced neutropenia. *N Engl J Med* 328:1323–1332, 1993.

124. Mitchell PL, Morland B, Stevens MC, et al. Granulocyte colony-stimulating factor in established febrile neutropenia: a randomized study of pediatric patients. *J Clin Oncol* 15:1163–1170, 1997.

125. Anaissie EJ, Vartivarian S, Bodey GP, et al. Randomized comparison between antibiotics alone and antibiotics plus granulocyte-macrophage colony-stimulating factor (*Escherichia coli*-derived) in cancer patients with fever and neutropenia (see comments). *Am J Med* 100:17–23, 1996.

126. Maher DW, Lieschke GJ, Green M, et al. Filgrastim in patients with chemotherapy-induced febrile neutropenia. A double-blind, placebo-controlled trial (see comments). *Ann Intern Med* 121:492–501, 1994.

127. Herwig KR. Management of urinary incontinence and retention in the patient with advanced cancer. *JAMA* 244:2203–2204, 1980.

128. Platt JF. Urinary obstruction. *Radiol Clin North Am* 34:1113–1129, 1996.

129. Louca G, Liberopoulos K, Fidas A, et al. MR urography in the diagnosis of urinary tract obstruction. *Eur Urol* 35:102–108, 1999.

130. Hussain S, O'Malley M, Jara H, et al. MR urography. *Magn Reson Imaging Clin North Am* 5:95–106, 1997.

131. Bordinazzo R, Benecchi L, Cazzaniga A, et al. Ureteral obstruction associated with prostate cancer: the outcome after ultrasonographic percutaneous nephrostomy. *Arch Ital Urol Androl* 66(suppl 4):101–106, 1994.

132. Hollander JB, Diokno AC. Urinary diversion and reconstruction in the patient with spinal cord injury. *Urol Clin North Am* 20:465–474, 1993.

133. Schellhammer PF, Whitmore RBD, Kuban DA, et al. Morbidity and mortality of local failure after definitive therapy for prostate cancer. *J Urol* 141:567–571, 1989.

134. Costanzi JJ, Gagliano R, Loukas D, et al. Ifosfamide in the treatment of recurrent or disseminated lung cancer: a phase II study of two dose schedules. *Cancer* 41:1715–1719, 1978.

135. Ershler WB, Gilchrist KW, Citrin DL. Adriamycin enhancement of cyclophosphamide-induced bladder injury. *J Urol* 123:121–122, 1980.

136. Cox PJ. Cyclophosphamide cystitis—identification of acrolein as the causative agent. *Biochem Pharmacol* 28:2045–2049, 1979.

137. Brade WP, Herdrich K, Varini M. Ifosfamide—pharmacology, safety and therapeutic potential. *Cancer Treat Rev* 12:1–47, 1985.

138. Dean RJ, Lytton B. Urologic complications of pelvic irradiation. *J Urol* 119:64–67, 1978.

139. de Vries CR, Freiha FS. Hemorrhagic cystitis: a review. *J Urol* 143:1–9, 1990.

140. Arthur RR, Shah KV, Baust SJ, et al. Association of BK viruria with hemorrhagic cystitis in recipients of bone marrow transplants. *N Engl J Med* 315:230–234, 1986.

141. Stillwell TJ, Benson RC Jr. Cyclophosphamide-induced hemorrhagic cystitis. A review of 100 patients. *Cancer* 61:451–457, 1988.

142. Lewis C. A review of the use of chemoprotectants in cancer chemotherapy. *Drug Saf* 11:153–162, 1994.

143. Fukuoka M, Negoro S, Masuda N, et al. Placebo-controlled double-blind comparative study on the preventive efficacy of mesna against ifosfamide-induced urinary disorders. *J Cancer Res Clin Oncol* 117:473–478, 1991.

144. Warrell RPJ. Oncologic emergencies. In DeVita VT, Hellman S, Rosenberg SA (eds), *Cancer: Principles and Practice of Oncology* (5th ed). Philadelphia: Lippincott-Raven, 1997:2469–2522.

145. Vose JM, Reed EC, Pippert GC, et al. Mesna compared with continuous bladder irrigation as uroprotection during high-dose chemotherapy and transplantation: a randomized trial. *J Clin Oncol* 11:1306–1310, 1993.

146. de Flora S, Cesarone CF, Balansky RM, et al. Chemopreventive properties and mechanisms of *N*-acetylcysteine. The experimental background. *J Cellular Biochem Suppl* 22:33–41, 1995.

147. Dorr RT. Chemoprotectants for cancer chemotherapy. *Semin Oncol* 18(suppl 2):48–58, 1991.

148. Palma PC, Villaca CJ Jr, Netto NR Jr. *N*-acetylcysteine in the prevention of cyclophosphamide induced haemorrhagic cystitis. *Int Surg* 71:36–37, 1986.

149. Donahue LA, Frank IN. Intravesical formalin for hemorrhagic cystitis: analysis of therapy. *J Urol* 141:809–812, 1989.

150. Kelly JD, Young MR, Johnston SR, Keane PF. Clinical response to an oral prostaglandin analogue in patients with interstitial cystitis. *Eur Urol* 34:53–56, 1998.

151. Miller LJ, Chandler SW, Ippoliti CM. Treatment of cyclo-

phosphamide-induced hemorrhagic cystitis with prostaglandins. *Ann Pharmacother* 28:590–594, 1994.

152. Levine LA, Kranc DM. Evaluation of carboprost tromethamine in the treatment of cyclophosphamide-induced hemorrhagic cystitis. *Cancer* 66:242–245, 1990.

153. Hemal AK, Praveen BV, Sankaranarayanan A, Vaidyanathan S. Control of persistent vesical bleeding due to radiation cystitis by intravesical application of 15 (S) 15-methyl prostaglandin F2-alpha. *Indian J Cancer* 26:99–101, 1989.

154. Jepsen JV, Sall M, Rhodes PR, et al. Long-term experience with pentosanpolysulfate in interstitial cystitis. *Urology* 51:381–387, 1998.

155. Hwang P, Auclair B, Beechinor D, et al. Efficacy of pentosan polysulfate in the treatment of interstitial cystitis: a meta-analysis. *Urology* 50:39–43, 1997.

156. Parsons CL, Mulholland SG. Successful therapy of interstitial cystitis with pentosanpolysulfate. *J Urol* 138:513–516, 1987.

157. Kelly PJ, Eisman JA. Hypercalcaemia of malignancy. *Cancer Metastasis Rev* 8:23–52, 1989.

158. Mundy GR. Malignancy and the skeleton. *Horm Metab Res* 29:120–127, 1997.

159. Kaplan M. Hypercalcemia of malignancy: a review of advances in pathophysiology. *Oncol Nurs Forum* 21:1039–1046, 1994.

160. Moseley JM, Kubota M, Diefenbach-Jagger H, et al. Parathyroid hormone-related protein purified from a human lung cancer cell line. *Proc Natl Acad Sci USA* 84:5048–5052, 1987.

161. Broadus AE, Mangin M, Ikeda K, et al. Humoral hypercalcemia of cancer. Identification of a novel parathyroid hormone-like peptide. *N Engl J Med* 319:556–563, 1988.

162. Abou-Samra AB, Juppner H, Force T, et al. Expression cloning of a common receptor for parathyroid hormone and parathyroid hormone-related peptide from rat osteoblast-like cells: a single receptor stimulates intracellular accumulation of both cAMP and inositol trisphosphates and increases intracellular free calcium. *Proc Natl Acad Sci USA* 89:2732–2736, 1992.

163. Mundy GR. Pathophysiology of cancer-associated hypercalcemia. *Semin Oncol* 17(suppl 5):10–15, 1990.

164. Pecherstorfer M, Schilling T, Blind E, et al. Parathyroid hormone-related protein and life expectancy in hypercalcemic cancer patients. *J Clin Endocrinol Metab* 78:1268–1270, 1994.

165. Guise TA, Mundy GR. Physiological and pathological roles of parathyroid hormone-related peptide. *Curr Opin Nephrol Hypertens* 5:307–315, 1996.

166. Ikeda K, Ogata E. Humoral hypercalcemia of malignancy: some enigmas on the clinical features. *J Cell Biochem* 57:384–391, 1995.

167. Warrell RP Jr. Etiology and current management of cancer-related hypercalcemia. *Oncology* 6:37–43, 1992.

168. Edelson GW, Kleerekoper M. Hypercalcemic crisis. *Med Clin North Am* 79:79–92, 1995.

169. Ashkar FS, Miller R, Katims RB. Effect of corticosteroids on hypercalcaemia of malignant disease. *Lancet* 1:41, 1971.

170. Bockman RS. Hypercalcaemia in malignancy. *Clin Endocrinol Metab* 9:317–333, 1980.

171. Chisholm MA, Mulloy AL, Taylor AT. Acute management of cancer-related hypercalcemia. *Ann Pharmacother* 30:507–513, 1996.

172. Coleman RE. Bisphosphonate treatment of bone metastases and hypercalcemia of malignancy. *Oncology* 5:55–62, 1991.

173. Ostenstad B, Andersen OK. Disodium pamidronate versus mithramycin in the management of tumour-associated hypercalcemia. *Acta Oncol* 31:861–864, 1992.

174. Gucalp R, Theriault R, Gill I, et al. Treatment of cancer-associated hypercalcemia. Double-blind comparison of rapid and slow intravenous infusion regimens of pamidronate disodium and saline alone (see comments). *Arch Intern Med* 154:1935–1944, 1994.

175. Gallacher SJ, Ralston SH, Fraser WD, et al. A comparison of low versus high dose pamidronate in cancer-associated hypercalcaemia. *Bone Mineral* 15:249–256, 1991.

176. Fitton A, McTavish D. Pamidronate. A review of its pharmacological properties and therapeutic efficacy in resorptive bone disease. *Drugs* 41:289–318, 1991. (Published erratum appears in *Drugs* 43:145, 1992.)

177. Hortobagyi GN, Theriault RL, Lipton A, et al. Long-term prevention of skeletal complications of metastatic breast cancer with pamidronate. Protocol 19 Aredia Breast Cancer Study Group. *J Clin Oncol* 16:2038–2044, 1998.

178. Keenan AM. Syndrome of inappropriate secretion of antidiuretic hormone in malignancy. *Semin Oncol Nurs* 15:160–167, 1999.

179. Shapiro J, Richardson GE. Hyponatremia of malignancy. *Crit Rev Oncol Hematol* 18:129–135, 1995.

180. Lockton JA, Thatcher N. A retrospective study of thirty-two patients with small-cell bronchogenic carcinoma and inappropriate secretion of antidiuretic hormone. *Clin Radiol* 37:47–50, 1986.

181. Goldberg M. Hyponatremia. *Med Clin North Am* 65:251–269, 1981.

182. Kern PA, Robbins RJ, Bichet D, et al. Syndrome of inappropriate antidiuresis in the absence of arginine vasopressin. *J Clin Endocrinol Metab* 62:148–152, 1986.

183. Spencer HW, Yarger WE, Robinson RR. Alterations of renal function during dietary-induced hyperuricemia in the rat. *Kidney Int* 9:489–500, 1976.

184. Kovacs L, Robertson GL. Syndrome of inappropriate antidiuresis. *Endocrinol Metab Clin North Am* 21:859–875, 1992.

185. Kinzie BJ. Management of the syndrome of inappropriate secretion of antidiuretic hormone. *Clin Pharm* 6:625–633, 1987.

186. Trump DL. Serious hyponatremia in patients with cancer: management with demeclocycline. *Cancer* 47:2908–2912, 1981.

187. Soga J, Yakuwa Y, Osaka M. Insulinoma/hypoglycemic syndrome: a statistical evaluation of 1085 reported cases of a Japanese series. *J Exp Clin Cancer Res* 17:379–388, 1998.

188. Anderson N, Lokich JJ. Mesenchymal tumors associated with hypoglycemia: case report and review of the literature. *Cancer* 44:785–790, 1979.

189. Kahn CR. The riddle of tumour hypoglycaemia revisited. *Clin Endocrinol Metab* 9:335–360, 1980.

190. Zapf J, Rinderknecht E, Humbel RE, Froesch ER. Non-suppressible insulin-like activity (NSILA) from human serum: recent accomplishments and their physiologic implications. *Metabolism* 272:1803–1828, 1978.

191. Pisters PW, Cersosimo E, Rogatko A, Brennan MF. Insulin action on glucose and branched-chain amino acid metabolism in cancer cachexia: differential effects of insulin. *Surgery* 111:301–310, 1992.

192. Shilo S, Berezovsky S, Friedlander Y, Sonnenblick M. Hypoglycemia in hospitalized nondiabetic older patients. *J Am Geriatr Soc* 46:978–982, 1998.

193. LeRoith D, Clemmons D, Nissley P, Rechler MM. NIH conference. Insulin-like growth factors in health and disease (see comments). *Ann Intern Med* 116:854–862, 1992.

194. Mullans EA, Cohen PR. Iatrogenic necrolytic migratory erythema: a case report and review of nonglucagonoma-associated necrolytic migratory erythema. *J Am Acad Dermatol* 38:866–873, 1998.

195. Drakos P, Bar-Ziv J, Catane R. Tumor lysis syndrome in nonhematologic malignancies. Report of a case and review of the literature. *Am J Clin Oncol* 17:502–505, 1994.

196. Kalemkerian GP, Darwish B, Varterasian ML. Tumor lysis syndrome in small cell carcinoma and other solid tumors. *Am J Med* 103:363–367, 1997.

197. Hussein AM, Feun LG. Tumor lysis syndrome after induction chemotherapy in small-cell lung carcinoma. *Am J Clin Oncol* 13:10–13, 1990.

198. Persons DA, Garst J, Vollmer R, Crawford J. Tumor lysis syndrome and acute renal failure after treatment of non-small-cell lung carcinoma with combination irinotecan and cisplatin. *Am J Clin Oncol* 21:426–429, 1998.

199. Boisseau M, Bugat R, Mahjoubi M. Rapid tumour lysis syndrome in a metastatic colorectal cancer increased by treatment (CPT-11) (letter). *Eur J Cancer* 32A:737–738, 1996.

200. Cheson BD, Frame JN, Vena D, et al. Tumor lysis syndrome: an uncommon complication of fludarabine therapy of chronic lymphocytic leukemia. *J Clin Oncol* 16:2313–2320, 1998.

201. Arrambide K, Toto RD. Tumor lysis syndrome. *Semin Nephrol* 13:273–280, 1993.

202. Schilsky RL. Renal and metabolic toxicities of cancer chemotherapy. *Semin Oncol* 9:75–83, 1982.

203. Kelton J, Kelley WN, Holmes EW. A rapid method for the diagnosis of acute uric acid nephropathy. *Arch Intern Med* 138:612–615, 1978.

204. Cunningham SG. Fluid and electrolyte disturbances associated with cancer and its treatment. *Nurs Clin North Am* 17:579–593, 1982.

205. Schelling JR, Ghandour FZ, Strickland TJ, Sedor JR. Management of tumor lysis syndrome with standard continuous arteriovenous hemodialysis: case report and a review of the literature. *Ren Fail* 20:635–644, 1998.

206. Pichette V, Leblanc M, Bonnardeaux A, et al. High dialysate flow rate continuous arteriovenous hemodialysis: a new approach for the treatment of acute renal failure and tumor lysis syndrome. *Am J Kidney Dis* 23:591–596, 1994.

207. Jeffrey RF, Khan AA, Prabhu P, et al. A comparison of molecular clearance rates during continuous hemofiltration and hemodialysis with a novel volumetric continuous renal replacement system. *Artif Organs* 18:425–428, 1994.

208. Davi MV, Francia G, Brazzarola P, et al. An unusual case of adrenal failure due to isolated metastases of breast cancer. *J Endocrinol Invest* 19:488–489, 1996.

209. Black RM, Daniels GH, Coggins CH, et al. Adrenal insufficiency from metastatic colonic carcinoma masquerading as isolated aldosterone deficiency. Report of a case and review of the literature. *Acta Endocrinol* 98:586–591, 1981.

210. Payne DK, Levine SN, Franco DP, Giyanani VL. Adrenal insufficiency due to metastatic lung carcinoma and shown by abdominal CT scan. *South Med J* 77:1592–1593, 1984.

211. Hoffken K, Kempf H, Miller AA, et al. Aminoglutethimide without hydrocortisone in the treatment of postmenopausal patients with advanced breast cancer. *Cancer Treat Rep* 70:1153–1157, 1986.

212. Subramanian S, Goker H, Kanji A, Sweeney H. Clinical adrenal insufficiency in patients receiving megestrol therapy. *Arch Intern Med* 157:1008–1011, 1997.

213. Spiegel RJ, Vigersky RA, Oliff AI, et al. Adrenal suppression after short-term corticosteroid therapy. *Lancet* 1:630–633, 1979.

214. Seidenwurm DJ, Elmer EB, Kaplan LM, et al. Metastases to the adrenal glands and the development of Addison's disease. *Cancer* 54:552–557, 1984.

215. Redman BG, Pazdur R, Zingas AP, Loredo R. Prospective evaluation of adrenal insufficiency in patients with adrenal metastasis. *Cancer* 60:103–107, 1987.

216. Lawton JM. Acute adrenal insufficiency: hemodynamic and echocardiographic characteristics. *Wisc Med J* 91:214–216, 1992.

217. Hockings GI, Strakosch CR, Jackson RV. Secondary adrenocortical insufficiency: avoiding potentially fatal pitfalls in diagnosis and treatment (editorial). *Med J Aust* 166:400–401, 1997.

33

Effective Pain Treatment in Cancer Patients

■ ■ ■

C. Stratton Hill, Jr.
Charles S. Cleeland
Howard B. Gutstein

In a significant percentage of cancer patients, the inadequate treatment of pain causes needless suffering [1–4]. This problem is not new. Knowledge about all aspects of pain and its treatment has increased over the last two decades. In addition, the number of organizations dedicated to disseminating this knowledge has increased significantly. Despite these efforts, progress in improving pain treatment has been inordinately slow.

Providing adequate pain relief for cancer patients is a complex issue. Merely giving health care providers modern information about drugs and interventional pain-relieving techniques is not adequate to effect improvement in the treatment of patients' pain. The problem is multifactorial and involves barriers related to health care providers, the health care system, and patients and their families [4, 5]. In addition to exhibiting major knowledge deficits about pain management, health care professionals fear disciplinary action by state health-care licensing boards and state and federal drug enforcement agencies relating to the appropriate and adequate use of opioids (narcotics) [6]. Society has become increasingly concerned about inadequate pain relief and its contribution to a poor quality of life [7]. Incumbent on all health care professionals is the provision of the best possible pain relief to cancer patients in pain.

This chapter relates barriers to the delivery of good pain management to recommendations about the assessment and treatment process. Specific barriers that prevent effective pain relief are discussed at points at which they usually arise in patient evaluation and are reviewed in toto at the end of the chapter.

A goal of this chapter is to provide to every physician caring for cancer patients in pain the tools for becoming a "pain treatment expert," using modalities available to all physicians. The chapter emphasizes the proper use of analgesic drugs. Most patients do not require sophisticated pain treatment modalities [5]. Because of the multitude of factors contributing to the experience of chronic pain, support from other health care personnel is desirable. In most communities, some type of team, such as a combination of nurses, pharmacists, social workers, and clergy, can be assembled to address some or all the factors involved in patients' pain.

PREVALENCE, SEVERITY, AND RISK FOR PAIN

Between 60% and 80% of cancer patients with terminal disease will require pain management. Often, pain occurs much earlier than in the terminal stage and occurs intermittently throughout the course of the disease. Many patients with months or years to live will be compromised by poorly controlled pain. Among patients with metastatic cancer, the percentage of patients in pain increases dramatically. In the United States, even with the availability of a full range of analgesics and other pain treatments, more than half of all outpatients with metastatic disease will have cancer-related pain, and one-third report pain so severe that it significantly impairs their quality of life. Multicenter studies indicate that approximately 40% of patients with cancer pain do not receive prescriptions for analgesics potent enough to manage their pain and that others do not receive sufficient dosing of the prescribed analgesic [4].

As a result of the prescribing of inadequate-strength analgesics, patients in minority treatment settings, female patients, and older patients are at greater risk for poorly controlled pain. In urban clinics treating underserved patients, two-thirds receive prescriptions for analgesic drugs of inadequate strength and, for many patients, no analgesic is prescribed [4]. Additional groups at high risk for poor pain management include children, cognitively impaired adults, and other vulnerable members of society.

CAUSES OF PAIN

Direct tumor involvement is the most common cause of pain, present in approximately two-thirds of those with pain from metastatic cancer. Tumor invasion of bone is the physical basis of pain in approximately one-half of those experiencing tumor-related pain. In the remaining patients, this pain is brought on by nerve compression or infiltration or by involvement of the gastro-intestinal (GI) tract or soft tissue. Persistent posttherapy pain from long-term effects of surgery, radiotherapy, and chemotherapy accounts for an additional 20% of all who report pain from metastatic cancer; a small residual group experiences pain from non-cancer-related conditions.

The majority of patients with advanced cancer have pain that occurs at multiple sites and is caused by multiple mechanisms. A new complaint of pain in patients with metastatic cancer should first be considered to be disease-related, but other causes always should be considered and ruled out.

Mechanisms of Pain Generation

Pain sensation is generated either by stimulation of peripheral pain receptors or by damage to the peripheral nervous system or the central nervous system (CNS). Peripheral pain receptors can be stimulated by pressure, compression, and traction, and by disease-related chemical changes. Pain due to stimulation of these pain receptors is called *nociceptive* pain. Damage to visceral or somatic nerves or to autonomic nerve trunks and to CNS nerve structures produces what is termed *neuropathic* pain. Neuropathic pain may be caused by spontaneous activity in nerves damaged by disease or treatment. Often, cancer patients have both nociceptive and neuropathic pain. Neuropathic pain is less responsive to opioid analgesics and requires the use of other drugs.

Pain in cancer patients can be attributed to the following causes: (1) tumor impingement on, or invasion of, pain-sensitive structures; (2) any type of treatment for the tumor, specifically treatments that damage the nervous system; (3) body structure changes from tumor effects that cause muscle imbalance or other changes resulting in painful mechanical skeletal stresses; and (4) acute or chronic painful medical conditions (or both) and acute surgical conditions unrelated to the malignant disease.

Usually, nociceptive pain is associated with overt tissue damage and is the type of pain commonly encountered by cancer patients. A common example of nociceptive pain is acute postoperative pain and that associated with trauma. Nociceptive pain may be defined as a state of continuous stimulation of pain receptors, called *nociceptors*, by a noxious stimulus. Usually, nociceptive pain is relieved effectively by removal of the stimulus or by treatment with pharmacologic agents or interventional techniques. Distinguishing nociceptive from neuropathic pain is increasingly important be-

Table 33.1   Clinical Features of Neuropathic Pain

Delay in onset of pain, ranging from days to weeks to months after the event that produced nerve damage (e.g., surgery, irradiation, chemotherapy, biological therapy, or combinations thereof)

Failure of examination of painful area to reveal an ongoing tissue-damaging process that would be considered painful (e.g., pain in a mastectomy site that appears to be healed)

Sensations that an affected patient considers painful but describes as abnormal, unfamiliar, unpleasant, "strange," or "weird," possibly causing the physician to consider the patient histrionic

Sensations seem strange and unfamiliar to the patient and are often described as burning, pressure, twisting, or torque-like sensations; stabbing, knife-like sensations; and shooting, electrical sensations

Paroxysmal sensations of varied duration, possibly alternating from place to place in the same general area

Pain in the affected area produced by stimuli that usually are not painful (e.g., touch)

Pronounced summation and after-reaction with repetitive stimuli

Pain in an area of numbness

Less effective relief (generally) with nonopioid and opioid analgesics as compared to the relief achieved with these agents in nociceptive pain; pain effectiveness synergistically improved by use of coanalgesics

---

cause of treatment implications and the apparent increase in the incidence of neuropathic pain in cancer patients.

Neuropathic Pain

Cancer patients may experience pain due to nerve damage caused directly by a tumor or its treatment. A common site for nerve-related or neuropathic pain is tumor involvement of the brachial and lumbar plexuses. Aggressive cancer treatment with cytotoxic drugs and other modalities is occurring more frequently and accounts for the apparent increase in the incidence of neuropathic pain. These treatments may injure the peripheral nervous system. Injury to a peripheral nerve can occur simply by cutting it, as in surgery; likewise, injury to nerves can occur with external-beam or other types of irradiation, neurotoxic chemotherapy, and biological therapy. Therefore, injury occurs in the course of necessary treatment and does not imply negligence. Why neuropathic pain occurs in only a small percentage of identically treated patients is not understood.

Neuropathic pain can occur in any part of the body. Several recognizable neuropathic pain syndromes occur. Two associated with surgery are postmastectomy and postthoracotomy syndromes. Peripheral neuropathies are the most frequent postchemotherapy syndromes. Any nerve can be affected, but the sensory cutaneous nerves of the soles of the feet frequently are involved, causing a persistent, burning pain.

Often, patients experiencing the strange painful sensations associated with neuropathic pain are reluctant to reveal them for fear that they will be considered "crazy" or histrionic, a factor adding to their psychological distress. These feelings are compounded when af-

fected patients obtain only partial pain relief with commonly prescribed analgesics, including strong opioids. Patients may encounter skepticism by health care providers who may be unfamiliar with this type of pain and openly may express surprise and doubt about the report of only partial pain relief with strong opioids.

Neuropathic pain is characterized by some or all of the features listed in Table 33.1. Two very important diagnostic features of neuropathic pain derived from patients' history and physical examination are the delay in pain onset after damage to the nervous system and the absence of an obvious ongoing cause for the pain. A classic example of these two features is the postmastectomy syndrome. A patient may have a mastectomy and can suffer postoperative (nociceptive) pain but may recover and return to activities of daily living and even return to work. After a variable period, many of the features described in Table 33.1 occur. On physical examination, nothing but the mastectomy scar is visible, essentially leaving no evidence for an obvious pain-producing process.

Various terms (*neurogenic, deafferentation,* etc.) have been applied to this type of pain. However, Fields [8] suggested the term *neuropathic pain* as the most appropriate because it implies only that the pain is due to functional abnormalities of the nervous system. Treatment of neuropathic pain is problematic. In probably no other painful experience is the actual participation of physicians and their staff essential in obtaining an acceptable level of pain control. The first tasks are to assure affected patients that their reports of symptoms (e.g., the strangeness of the pain they are experiencing) are believed and to help them to develop a realistic set of expectations about results. Patients must be aware that treatment results often will not be dramatic: *Patience* is the watchword. In addition to analgesics, medi-

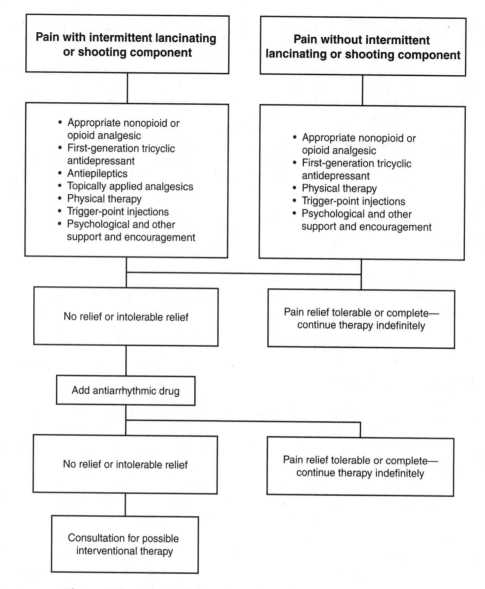

Figure 33.1 Suggested algorithm for treatment of neuropathic pain.

cations recommended for treatment of this type of pain include antidepressants, antiepileptics, antiarrhythmics, and steroid drugs, and they must be taken continuously despite the facts that little immediate relief of pain is evident and that undesirable side effects occur. A schema for treatment is presented in Figure 33.1.

Analgesic drugs are very effective in relieving nociceptive pain. In contrast, neuropathic pain is not relieved as effectively by the commonly used nonopioid or weak or strong opioid analgesics. Because most patients with pain of all types are treated with opioids given orally, the failure of patients with neuropathic pain to experience relief often is attributed to the oral route of administration. However, changing the route of

drug administration to other sites, including the spinal route, fails to improve responsiveness to opioids [9, 10].

Pain Associated with Tumor Impingement or Invasion

Most often, pain in cancer patients is caused by the effects of the tumor itself. When pain occurs, meticulous initial and ongoing efforts to demonstrate tumor presence are imperative. Early detection of recurrent tumor offers the best opportunity for effective treatment of both the pain and the tumor. An appropriate investigation always should be performed, keeping in mind that pain often precedes examiners' ability to demonstrate the tumor's presence objectively by either physical examination or sophisticated imaging techniques. Treatment decisions based on an erroneous assumption about etiology are likely to be ineffective and can be detrimental to affected patients. Though efforts to demonstrate the presence of a tumor or other causes of pain are continuing, symptomatic treatment of the pain should be started with analgesics that are strong enough and are appropriate for the specific cause of the pain.

Characteristically, some tumors metastasize to certain areas of the body (e.g., breast and prostate cancers metastasizing to bone); however, pain in any area of the body of a cancer patient should be investigated to rule out metastasis. Pain in the head and neck requires the early use of sophisticated imaging techniques, because plain radiography of this area may not detect tumor invasion or bone destruction (or both). Computed tomography (CT) and magnetic resonance imaging (MRI) are the procedures of choice for demonstrating lesions in this area.

Back pain commonly is observed in cancer patients because many tumors metastasize to vertebral bodies and other spinal structures. Two conditions warrant special mention: epidural metastatic disease and spasm of paravertebral and other back muscles. If epidural metastatic disease goes undetected, most likely it ultimately will cause paralysis from spinal cord compression. Epidural spinal cord compression should be considered in the differential diagnosis in all cases of back pain in cancer patients and should be treated as a medical emergency. Early diagnosis and prompt treatment can prevent paralysis in the majority of cases. Vertebral body metastases, with or without subsequent partial or complete collapse of the vertebrae, are a frequent cause of spasm of the paravertebral muscles and cause moderate to severe pain. Pain caused by vertebral body invasion, in the absence of vertebral collapse and muscle imbalance and associated muscle spasm, is a nociceptive pain and is more likely to be controlled by an analgesic than is pain caused by muscle spasm. Usually, muscle spasm pain is controlled more effectively by physical therapy modalities. A common cause of failure to control back pain caused by muscle spasm is an overreliance on analgesic and muscle relaxant drugs in lieu of physical therapy modalities. Often, superficial and deep heat (ultrasonography) are contraindicated in treating muscle spasm because of a belief that these approaches will accelerate tumor growth. The data to support this belief are questionable.

Invasion of individual nerves or plexuses and inva-sion of pain-sensitive structures in soft tissues are other common causes of pain related to direct tumor involvement. The character of the pain will vary, depending on the structure involved. Invasion of nerves with subsequent nerve damage produces neuropathic pain. Damage to axons and myelin sheaths has been suggested as a mechanism for this type of pain [11]. Another characteristic of tumor involvement of these structures is motor weakness.

Abdominal visceral pain is caused by tumor obstruction of hollow organs, tumor invasion of pain-sensitive soft tissues, and peritoneal irritation. Tumor obstruction of hollow organs can be partial or complete; either condition may require surgical intervention. Characteristically, visceral pain caused by tumor invasion of pain-sensitive soft tissue and peritoneum is diffuse and poorly localized.

Pain Associated with Cancer Treatment

Patients expect pain, discomfort, and other distressing symptoms during active cancer treatment and for a variable period after treatment, regardless of treatment modality. Most patients, however, expect these symptoms to diminish gradually during healing until they eventually disappear. In the majority of cases, that progression takes place but, in a minority of patients, pain either may persist or may develop after a pain-free interval of varying length, despite apparent healing of the damaged tissue. This minority is the subpopulation of pain patients who are suffering from neuropathic pain. However, in all situations in which pain is thought to be due to treatment, the possibility of recurrent tumor still must be ruled out as a cause of pain.

Pain Associated with Structural Body Changes

Tumor invasion of vertebral bodies may cause pain in two ways. First, the direct involvement of a vertebra activates nociceptors located there; second, collapse of the vertebra as a result of tumor invasion often causes changes in body structure, particularly muscle imbalance, which causes paravertebral and other muscle spasms. Sustained spasm causes pain in the muscle involved and secondary tenderness in the surrounding muscles (secondary hyperalgesia).

Scoliosis after thoracic surgery for thoracic tumors causes muscle imbalance and can be painful. Usually, such pain occurs only in the upright position (i.e., incident pain—that occurring only when this position is assumed) and, for that reason, treating it is difficult. Frequently, doses of opioids sufficient to relieve pain when affected patients are upright are excessive when such patients lie down. Exercises designed to strengthen compensatory muscles may be helpful in controlling this type of pain.

Pain from Other Causes

Cancer patients may suffer from chronic painful medical illnesses acquired either before or after the diagnosis of cancer. Treatment for these conditions is the same as it would be had the patient never had cancer, unless such treatment causes complications or interferes with cancer therapy. Acute painful surgical conditions that occur in cancer patients can be unrelated to their cancer or may be a complication of tumor progression or its treatment. A list of common causes of pain and specific pain syndromes in cancer patients is presented in Table 33.2.

ASSESSING PATIENT PAIN

Proper pain management requires a clear understanding of the characteristics of a given pain and its physical basis. The changing expression of cancer pain demands repeated assessment, as new causes for pain can emerge rapidly. In advanced cancer cases, pain from multiple etiologies is the rule, not the exception.

Assessment of pain includes three components: (1) the initial assessment, (2) persistent, frequent reassessments as long as the pain persists, and (3) routine assessment for the occurrence of new pain. It is achieved primarily by recording a thorough pain history. However, certain tools are available to assess some of the pain parameters (e.g., scales to measure intensity). These scales can be used also in reassessment (Fig. 33.2) [12]. A careful pain history includes questions concerning the location, severity, and quality of the pain and the impact of the pain on an affected patient's life.

Initial Assessment

Pain severity always is the initial determination, as often it will drive the major treatment decisions that must be made. The initial assessment additionally determines

Table 33.2   Common Causes of Pain and Specific Pain Syndromes in Cancer Patients

Pain syndromes associated with direct tumor involvement
　Tumor infiltration of bone
　　Base-of-skull syndromes
　　　Jugular foramen metastases
　　　Clivus metastases
　　　Sphenoid sinus metastases
　　Vertebral body syndromes
　　　C2 metastases
　　　C7–T1 metastases
　　　L1 metastases
　　Sacral syndromes
　Tumor infiltration of nerve
　　Peripheral nerve (peripheral neuropathy)
　　Plexus
　　　Brachial plexopathy
　　　Lumbar plexopathy
　　　Sacral plexopathy
　　Root (leptomeningeal metastases)
　　Spinal cord (epidural spinal cord compression)

Pain syndromes associated with cancer therapy
　Postoperative syndromes
　　Postthoracotomy syndrome
　　Postmastectomy syndrome
　　Post–radical neck syndrome
　　Phantom limb syndrome
　Postchemotherapy syndromes
　　Peripheral neuropathy
　　Aseptic necrosis of the femoral head
　　Steroid pseudorheumatism
　　Postherpetic neuralgia
　Postirradiation syndromes
　　Radiation fibrosis of the brachial and lumbar plexus
　　Radiation myelopathy
　　Radiation-induced second primary tumors
　　Radiation-induced necrosis of bone

Pain syndromes not associated with cancer or cancer therapy
　Cervical and lumbar osteoarthritis
　Thoracic and abdominal aneurysms
　Diabetic neuropathy

the pain's location, onset, and characteristics (e.g., quality, possible radiation); clues to its etiology, intensity, dynamics (e.g., static, progressive), and influence on patients' psychosocial function and activities of daily living; the influence of previous therapy on etiology and the kind and effectiveness of previous pain treatment; whether patients have discovered methods to modulate the pain (e.g., lying down, standing up); whether pain is *incident* (i.e., pain associated with a specific incident, such as weight bearing or movement); and whether *breakthrough* pain is present.

Visual Analog Scale

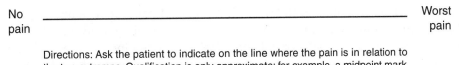

No pain ———————————————————————————— Worst pain

Directions: Ask the patient to indicate on the line where the pain is in relation to the two extremes. Qualification is only approximate; for example, a midpoint mark would indicate that the pain is approximately half of the worst possible pain.

Graphic Rating Scale

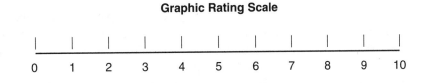

0   1   2   3   4   5   6   7   8   9   10

Verbal Rating Scale

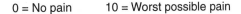

0 = No pain   10 = Worst possible pain

Pain Faces Scale

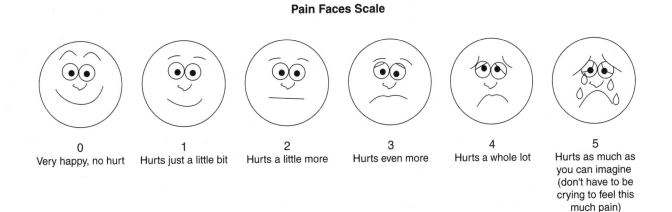

0	1	2	3	4	5
Very happy, no hurt	Hurts just a little bit	Hurts a little more	Hurts even more	Hurts a whole lot	Hurts as much as you can imagine (don't have to be crying to feel this much pain)

Figure 33.2 Representative samples of pain intensity rating scales. (Reprinted with permission of Mosby, St. Louis, MO, from DL Wong, M Hockenberry-Eaton, D Wilson, ML Winkelstein, E Ahmann, PA DeVito-Thomas, *Whaley and Wong's Nursing Care of Infants and Children* (6th ed), 1999: 1153. © by Mosby-Year Book, Inc.)

Occasionally, during the initial assessment of a pain report, cancer is found in patients who appear healthy and are not suspected of having the disease. Unless the pain in such patients is proved unequivocally to result from the cancer, investigation of the pain complaint should not stop with diagnosing either primary or metastatic cancer, because many cancers in their early stages are not painful. The pain may have another cause. Patients with pain unrelated to their cancer should have treatment appropriate for the specific cause of the pain.

SEVERITY

Inadequate pain assessment and poor physician-patient communication about pain are major barriers to good pain care [13]. Frequently, intensity is the only characteristic of pain assessed by health care providers, but assessment should go beyond this. Physicians and nurses tend to underestimate pain intensity, especially when it is severe. Patients whose doctors underestimate their pain are at high risk for poor pain management and compromised function. A small minority of cancer patients may complain of pain in a dramatic fashion, but many more patients underreport the severity of their pain and the lack of adequate pain relief. This reluctance to report pain arises from patients' unwillingness to acknowledge that their disease is progressing, to divert a physician's attention from treating the disease, and to indicate to the physician that the prescribed treatment plan is not working. Patients may not want to be treated with opioid analgesics because of their misconception about addiction, because they fear psychoactive components of opioids, because they are concerned that using opioids "too early" will preclude pain relief when and if pain becomes more severe, or because they fear that being placed on opioids signals that death is near [14]. Presenting information that addresses these concerns in a straightforward manner will allay most of these fears and should be considered an essential step in providing pain control. Most important is that patients understand that they will function better if their pain is controlled.

Communication about pain is aided greatly by having affected patients use a scale to report pain. A simple rating scale ranges from 0 to 10 (0, "no pain;" 10, pain "as bad as you can imagine"). Used properly, pain severity scales can be invaluable in titrating analgesics and in monitoring for increased pain with progressive disease. Though pain scales are the most useful instruments for assessing the intensity of pain, such scales are useful only in following the course of pain in the *same* individual; they are not valid for comparing one patient's pain to another patient's [4]. Nonetheless, changes in intensity of pain are meaningful. Most often, inexorable progression of intensity signals progression of a cancer, whereas lessening of intensity means either control of the cancer or adequate pain relief. Pain intensity may start as mild and can progress in crescendo fashion to severe; alternately, it may be severe at onset. Accurate evaluation of pain intensity is important because pain treatment should be tailored to address the intensity of pain at presentation (i.e., strong opioids for severe pain at onset and nonopioids or weak opioids for mild pain at onset).

Often, mild pain is well tolerated and has minimal impact on affected patients' activities. However, beyond a certain threshold, pain is especially disruptive. Usually, this threshold is the point at which patients rate the severity of their pain at 5 or greater on a 0-to-10 scale. When it is too great (usually 7 or more on this scale, which is severe pain that must be addressed aggressively), pain becomes the primary focus of attention and prohibits most activity not related directly to pain (Fig. 33.3) [15]. Though total elimination of pain may not be possible, reducing its severity by several numbers on the severity scale ought to be a minimum standard of pain therapy.

In addition to determining pain severity, assessment should contain, at a minimum, the following information, though each interview must be tailored to individual clinical situations.

LOCATION

Identifying the location of pain will help to determine whether it is related to a primary tumor or its metastases, whether it is referred or is of radicular or musculoskeletal origin, and whether it is unrelated to a cancer. Having affected patients draw the location of pain on both front and back poses of a figure of the human body (see Fig. 33.3) is very helpful in determining location. The examiner should bear in mind that a person can experience pain in several locations simultaneously.

ONSET

Determining the onset of pain will help to identify whether the pain is cancer-related (the presenting symptom of cancer that prompted an affected patient to seek medical advice) or whether it was an unrelated, preexisting pain. If it is the former, subsequent episodes of pain almost invariably will be interpreted by affected patients as tumor recurrence or progression. However, subsequent pain experienced by a cancer patient cannot be assumed to be caused inevitably by a cancer.

Because of its prevalence in the general population, preexisting back pain is common in patients who subsequently develop cancer. If a successful program for treatment of this pain exists, it should be continued. However, such patients also may develop back pain or pain in other parts of the body owing to their cancer. Separate treatments for preexisting pain and pain due to cancer are necessary for optimum pain relief.

CHARACTERISTICS

Descriptors are important in determining the type of pain experienced by affected patients. Some descriptors for neuropathic pain are fairly distinct from descriptors for nociceptive pain. Examples of descriptors are shown in Figure 33.4 [16]. The two types of pain may coexist; thus, descriptors for both types of pain may be used by affected patients. Because treatment is different for each pain type, being alert to descriptors that identify each type is important.

SPECIAL ETIOLOGIC CLUES

Obviously, pain in the region of a primary tumor or metastatic lesion is considered prima facie to be due to the presence of the tumor. Other etiologic clues from an affected patient's health history include tumor treatment—surgery, radiotherapy, chemotherapy, and biological response modifiers—that may cause nerve damage and, therefore, neuropathic pain. Thus, all previous cancer treatments are potential chronic pain producers. Evidence of other medical conditions that produce pain (e.g., various arthritides, diabetic neuropathy, herpes zoster) will help to establish a differential pain diagnosis.

PSYCHOLOGICAL ISSUES

Teaching specific pain management skills can be helpful to a majority of affected patients, especially those who face pain for months to years. Often, evaluation and prescription of the specific skills most beneficial to affected individuals can be obtained through consultation with a behavioral psychologist, a psychiatrist, or a pain nurse specialist. (Note, however, that such techniques never should be used as a substitute for appropriate analgesia.) Skills include relaxation, self-hypnosis, and other distraction and cognitive control techniques. These measures can affect the sensation of pain by reducing muscle tension on pain-generating lesions and

by maximizing patients' ability to cope with pain and to remain as active as their disease permits.

Invariably, myriad psychological issues are associated with cancer patients who experience chronic pain. Such issues include the effect of pain on patients and the psychosocial consequences to them, their families, and their friends. Health care providers must recognize these issues and either address them or consult with appropriate professionals to ensure that they are addressed. Optimum pain relief is unlikely if psychological issues are not resolved.

The psychological issues depend, to a large degree, on affected patients' perceived responsibility to their families in meeting financial, interpersonal, advisory, supportive, intercessory, and other needs. The hope is that ensuring fulfillment of these needs will render patients and their families more functional and will allow for optimum well-being of family members during the illness.

IMPACT ON PSYCHOSOCIAL FUNCTION AND DAILY LIVING

Data support the negative impact of moderate to severe pain on affected patients' quality of life, and the elements of this impact must be evaluated [17]. Prominent among the factors affecting the quality of life are sleep disturbance, tension-producing anxiety, and clinical depression. Patients who report that the number of hours they sleep now is fewer than that of the last pain-free interval and who experience difficulties with sleep onset, frequent interruptions of sleep, and early-morning awakening suggest the need for pharmacologic intervention, often consisting of the addition of a low-dose antidepressant or sedative drug at bedtime. Just as affected patients hesitate to report severe pain, they may hesitate to report symptoms indicative of depression and anxiety. Helping such patients to recognize depression or anxiety and to report it in a quasi-quantitative manner (e.g., using a scale of 0 to 10, on which 10 is as bad as the patient can imagine) may help to overcome some of this reluctance. Significant depression and anxiety should be treated with appropriate medications, if practitioners feel competent in this area, or through psychiatric or psychological consultation, especially if such depression and anxiety persist in the face of adequate pain relief.

A very small percentage of cancer patients in severe psychosocial distress will express many of their psychological losses and concerns (inability to perform in their roles as breadwinner, monetary provider, etc.) as physical pain. An important aspect of treatment is to recog-

STUDY ID#__________ HOSPITAL#__________

DO NOT WRITE ABOVE THIS LINE

Brief Pain Inventory (Short Form)

Date: _____/_____/_____ Time:_____

Name: __________ (Last) __________ (First) __________ (Middle Initial)

1. Throughout our lives, most of us have had pain from time to time (such as minor headaches, sprains, and toothaches). Have you had pain other than these everyday kinds of pain today?

1. Yes 2. No

2. On the diagram, shade in the areas where you feel pain. Put an X on the area that hurts the most.

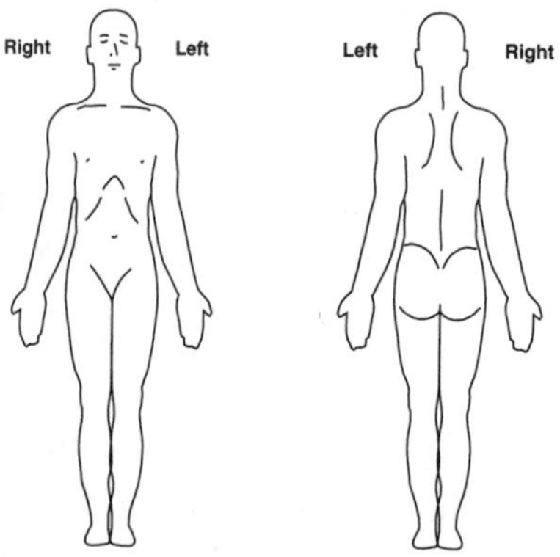

3. Please rate your pain by circling the one number that best describes your pain at its *worst* in the last 24 hours.

0	1	2	3	4	5	6	7	8	9	10
No pain										Pain as bad as you can imagine

4. Please rate your pain by circling the one number that best describes your pain at its *least* in the last 24 hours.

0	1	2	3	4	5	6	7	8	9	10
No pain										Pain as bad as you can imagine

5. Please rate your pain by circling the one number that best describes your pain on the *average*.

0	1	2	3	4	5	6	7	8	9	10
No pain										Pain as bad as you can imagine

6. Please rate your pain by circling the one number that tells how much pain you have *right now*.

0	1	2	3	4	5	6	7	8	9	10
No pain										Pain as bad as you can imagine

Figure 33.3 Brief pain inventory. (Reprinted from *Advances in Pain Research and Therapy,* vol 12. Courtesy of the Pain Research Group, University of Texas, MD Anderson Cancer Center, Houston, TX.)

7. **What treatments or medications are you receiving for your pain?**

_____

_____

8. **In the last 24 hours, how much relief have pain treatments or medications provided? Please circle the one percentage that most shows how much relief you have received.**

0%	10%	20%	30%	40%	50%	60%	70%	80%	90%	100%
No relief										Complete relief

9. **Circle the one number that describes how, during the past 24 hours, pain has interfered with your:**

A. General activity

0   1   2   3   4   5   6   7   8   9   10
Does not interfere   Completely interferes

B. Mood

0   1   2   3   4   5   6   7   8   9   10
Does not interfere   Completely interferes

C. Walking ability

0   1   2   3   4   5   6   7   8   9   10
Does not interfere   Completely interferes

D. Normal work (includes both work outside the home and housework)

0   1   2   3   4   5   6   7   8   9   10
Does not interfere   Completely interferes

E. Relations with other people

0   1   2   3   4   5   6   7   8   9   10
Does not interfere   Completely interferes

F. Sleep

0   1   2   3   4   5   6   7   8   9   10
Does not interfere   Completely interferes

G. Enjoyment of life

0   1   2   3   4   5   6   7   8   9   10
Does not interfere   Completely interferes

MD Anderson Cancer Center Pain Intensity Scale

Rate your pain at the times listed below. Mark a ✓ at the place in the line that best describes your pain at the time.

Date _____ Patient _____ # _____

Time	No pain at all	Just noticeable	Mild	Not something I could tolerate all the time	Severe	So bad I almost pass out	Worst pain I can imagine	Medication/ comments
_____								_____
_____								_____
_____								_____
_____								_____
_____								_____
_____								_____
_____								_____
_____								_____
_____								_____
_____								_____

MDACC Pain Intensity Tracking Tool

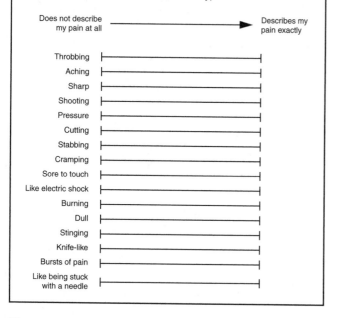

Pain Characteristics

For each word or phrase below, mark a ✓ on the corresponding line at the place that best shows how well that word or phrase describes your pain. Please make a mark on the line for each word or phrase indicating the degree to which it describes your pain (i.e., not at all, somewhat, or exactly).

Does not describe my pain at all → Describes my pain exactly

Throbbing
Aching
Sharp
Shooting
Pressure
Cutting
Stabbing
Cramping
Sore to touch
Like electric shock
Burning
Dull
Stinging
Knife-like
Bursts of pain
Like being stuck with a needle

Pain Disruptiveness

For each phrase listed below, mark a ✓ at the place on the corresponding line that best shows how well that phrase describes the effects of your pain on your daily activities. Be sure to make a mark for each phrase indicating the degree to which it describes your pain (i.e., not at all, somewhat, or exactly).

Does not describe my pain at all → Describes my pain exactly

Makes me want to give up
My pain is all I can think about
All I can do is lie in bed
Can't do the things I feel I need to
Can't go out
Makes me irritable
Can't do what I enjoy
Keeps me awake
Unable to eat
Makes me tired
Annoys me, but I can distract myself and go on

Figure 33.4 Descriptors of pain. MDACC = *M.D.* Anderson Cancer Center. (Adapted from SR Nemni, *A psychophysical methodology for the development of measurement scales: the quantification of the qualities of cancer pain.* Unpublished doctoral dissertation, Texas Christian University, Fort Worth, TX, December 1988.)

nize somatization and to deal with this problem or to provide such patients with psychological or psychiatric referral or counseling. However, physicians more often misdiagnose true pain as depression or anxiety. Assessment of patients who are cognitively impaired, particularly those experiencing agitation, may be extremely difficult. In such patients, the differentiation between agitated delirium and pain may be especially difficult. Patients in whom pain was well controlled before the development of delirium are unlikely to be agitated because of uncontrolled pain. Frequent discussions between various health care professionals and patients' families will be required.

Some patients who are experiencing pain and have a recent history of alcoholism or drug addiction may request analgesics for their psychological effects rather than for their analgesic effect. However, this reaction is unlikely in patients without a clear history of severe addictive behavior. On the other hand, treating patients who are recovering alcoholics or drug abusers may be difficult because of their resistance to analgesics for fear of a relapse of their former abuse problem. Although their care is more complex, patients with drug or alcohol addiction never should be denied appropriate pain medications. If the purpose of pain-relieving drugs is suspected to be solely that of maintaining an abuse problem, affected patients should be confronted with this behavior, and an agreement should be reached regarding the use of opioids for the management of pain rather than for producing mood alterations. For patients in this group, oral medication with long-acting opioids is preferable to short-acting opioids. Prescriptions by a single physician would simplify the negotiation process with such patients.

Frequently, chronic pain spawns a variety of negative emotions that culminate in clinical depression and other psychological conditions. These conditions can produce profound changes in interpersonal relationships. When present, these effects of chronic pain must be recognized and treated appropriately if the desired outcome of adequate pain relief and return to normal, or near-normal, lifestyle is to be achieved.

EFFECT OF PREVIOUS TREATMENT

It is important that the physician know what role previous treatment for a tumor (or another medical condition) might be playing in causing pain. For example, neurotoxic chemotherapeutic agents can cause severe peripheral neuropathy and consequent neuropathic pain. Equally important is knowing what prior pain treatments have been used and whether they were effective. Failure of previous analgesics to relieve pain may have resulted from use of an analgesic insufficiently potent to match the intensity of pain or from prescription of an insufficient dose; it may also be attributable to a nontolerated dose or, possibly, the patient suffers from neuropathic pain. Most likely, neuropathic pain will require the use of coanalgesics combined with the appropriate analgesic drug.

PATIENT CAPACITY TO MODULATE PAIN

Patients can, on occasion, modulate pain by using such techniques as biofeedback, guided imagery, relaxation, and self-hypnosis as primary or adjuvant treatment modalities. Use of these methods should be judged on their effectiveness (i.e., pain relief or enhancement of relief). Learning specific skills for managing pain is helpful for most patients, especially those who will have to deal with pain for months to years. These skills can be categorized as educational preparation for managing pain and as specific behavioral skills that will work synergistically with analgesics and adjuvant drugs to reduce pain or pain perception. All patients need educational preparation for systematically reporting their pain, for identifying and managing side effects, and for appropriate use of scheduled and breakthrough analgesics. Patients also need to be disabused of unnecessary concern about addiction or nonexistent side effects, such as loss of social control or excessive euphoria.

Many patients derive substantial benefit from specific behavioral training in self-hypnosis, relaxation, distraction, and cognitive control or restructuring. Often, evaluation and prescription of the specific skills most beneficial to affected individuals can be obtained through consultation with behavioral psychologists, psychiatrists, or pain nurse specialists. These measures can affect the sensation of pain by reducing muscle tension on pain-generating lesions and by maximizing patients' ability to cope with the pain and remain as active as their disease permits. Recent research with such neuroimaging techniques as positron emission tomography and functional MRI have shown that these behavioral measures can alter the activation of deep brain structures known to be critical to the appreciation of pain [18].

INCIDENT AND BREAKTHROUGH PAIN

Incident and breakthrough pain deserve special mention because of the treatment implications involved.

Breakthrough pain may be defined as a transient flare in pain intensity during the course of an otherwise successful treatment of a persistent pain [19]. It can be idiopathic or spontaneous (or both) and can result from an end-of-dose failure (i.e., failure of a dose of a controlled-release analgesic to control the pain for the period during which it is supposed to be effective). Usually, end-of-dose failure is caused by an insufficient dose of the controlled-release analgesic.

Incident pain may be considered a specific type of breakthrough pain if a persistent pain successfully controlled in the absence of an incident is not controlled when such an incident occurs. Controlling this type of breakthrough pain is more difficult than controlling idiopathic, spontaneous and end-of-dose breakthrough pains. The dose necessary to control incident pain may be excessive for treating the underlying persistent pain, causing such undesirable side effects as drowsiness, sedation, or mental confusion (or all these effects).

The most effective treatment of incident pain is to administer the breakthrough medication sufficiently in advance of an anticipated incident. An effective breakthrough analgesic is a short-acting analgesic with a rapid onset, having minimal or no side effects, and preferably being noninvasive. The breakthrough dose with a short-acting opioid analgesic should be approximately one-sixth of the total daily dose of the controlled-release opioid analgesic.

RELIABILITY OF PAIN REPORTING

Cognitive problems, especially loss of memory, are a serious problem in evaluating the effect of pain treatment from one day to the next. Usually, remembering the intensity or other characteristics of pain from the previous day is impossible for patients with defective memory. Confusion based on organic or metabolic impediments should be recognized so that it is not attributed to patient manipulation to obtain drugs for mood-altering purposes or to temporary confusion resulting from opioid administration. Patients providing inconsistent answers about their pain experience and those having apparent trouble with memory should undergo a neuropsychological mental status examination. Metabolic encephalopathies caused by such conditions as electrolyte derangement and reversible liver and kidney failure may be temporary and can disappear with the correction of the metabolic problem.

Reassessment

All the components of an initial assessment are likely to function in a reassessment as well. Pain is a dynamic process, and treatment must be evaluated constantly to determine its effectiveness. Constant surveillance and decision making are required. The frequency of reassessment varies from hourly to only those times at which a change in affected patients' symptoms occurs. Nurses and other health care providers, family members, and friends are important allies in reassessing effectiveness of treatment and thereby helping physicians to make treatment decisions.

INTERPRETING ASSESSMENT

After an affected patient's report of pain is considered in light of knowledge of all of the causes of pain, likely a reasonable preliminary diagnosis about its etiology and a tentative treatment plan can be made. Meticulously obtained health histories provide physicians with sufficient information about the characteristics and causes of pain and how it affects patients to enable them better to focus on specific elements of the physical examination and to select appropriate laboratory and imaging studies. Physical examinations should elaborate and expand on information gained from integrating knowledge of the causes of pain with the patient's report of pain.

Physical Examination

Quality medical practice requires that all patients undergo a thorough physical examination. (The reader is referred to Table 33.3 for a glossary of terms used in the physical examination and care of patients with pain.) Besides performing a standard complete physical examination, physicians should use information gained from the historical assessment as a guide to focus on the local examination of the painful area, skin, and musculoskeletal and nervous systems. Maneuvers that stress the area under examination and reproduce the pain also are important in identifying the pain source.

Each painful area should be examined carefully for physical changes, such as swelling and inflammation, that contribute to the pain experience. Muscle tenderness and spasm may account for pain. If the etiology of these findings is not apparent from the physical examination, appropriate diagnostic studies should be or-

Table 33.3 Glossary of Terms Used in the Assessment and Management of Cancer Patients with Pain

Term	Definition
Allodynia	Pain caused by a stimulus that ordinarily does not cause pain (e.g., touch, pressure from clothes, cold air blowing on the skin). Commonly, patients perceive this sensation when the skin is stimulated.
Breakthrough pain	A transient flare in pain intensity during the course of otherwise successful treatment of a persistent pain. It may be idiopathic or spontaneous (or both) or it may be an end-of-dose failure (i.e., the dose of controlled-release analgesic fails to maintain pain control for its expected period).
Ceiling effect	The dose level of a drug beyond which increasing the dose does not produce increased effect of the drug. Increasing the dose after its maximum desired effect is likely to produce intolerable side effects or drug toxicity.
Central pain	Pain associated with a lesion of the central nervous system.
Coanalgesic	A drug whose action serves primarily for conditions other than pain relief but that, under special conditions, relieves pain (e.g., antidepressants, antiepileptics, and corticosteroids). They have their greatest utility in the treatment of neuropathic pain.
Dysesthesia	An unpleasant abnormal sensation, whether spontaneous or evoked by normal stimuli.
Hypalgesia	Diminished sensitivity to noxious stimulation.
Hyperalgesia, primary	A state of increased pain sensation caused by a stimulus that ordinarily produces a pain of lesser degree and occurs at the site of injury.
Hyperalgesia, secondary	A state of increased pain sensation (as described for *primary hyperalgesia*) but occurring in apparently unaffected tissue, usually immediately surrounding a site of injury.
Incident pain	Pain occurring with movement, position, or other "incident," regardless of what the pain-producing incident is. Patient may be entirely free of pain when the incident is not happening, or the incident may serve to exacerbate a constant pain. Incident pain is a form of breakthrough pain.
Neuropathic pain	Pain that occurs as a result of nerve damage, or pain due to functional abnormalities of the nervous system. Nerves may be damaged by a variety of circumstances (e.g., cutting, as in surgery, irradiation, chemotherapy, and biological therapy).
Nociceptive pain	Pain caused by activation of nociceptors. Usually, activation is by overt tissue damage. This is the pain most commonly experienced by patients and is represented by any condition that causes tissue damage.
Nociceptor	A peripheral nervous system receptor that is preferentially sensitive to a noxious stimulus.
Noxious stimulus	Any stimulus that elicits the sensation of pain.
Pain	An unpleasant sensory experience perceived as arising from a specific body region and often associated with actual or potential tissue damage, or described in terms of such damage. Evokes various negative emotions, especially when chronic.
Paraneoplastic syndrome	Painful syndromes occurring in the presence of malignancy but apparently not directly caused by it. Usually, these syndromes affect the muscles, joints, bones, or a combination thereof.
Paresthesia	Morbid or perverted sensation, whether spontaneous or evoked, and contrasted with dysesthesia (an unpleasant, abnormal sensation brought on by normal stimuli).
Postmastectomy syndrome	Pain occurring in a mastectomy site (usually the inner aspect of an extremity on the mastectomy side) having characteristics of neuropathic pain (see Table 33.1).
Postthoracotomy syndrome	Pain occurring on the hemithorax of the thoracotomy site and having characteristics of neuropathic pain (see Table 33.1).
Trigger point	A circumscribed point of increased painful sensitivity on the skin and underlying muscular structures. It is detected by direct palpation and reproduces the pain of which the patient complains.

dered. Pain may vary with positional changes; for example, pain may be present when a patient is sitting but may disappear completely with reclining, or vice versa.

ABDOMEN

Because, during the course of a patient's illness, the abdomen frequently is the site of intermittent, acute painful disorders secondary to obstruction by either tumor or adhesions from previous surgery or radiotherapy, pain in the abdomen should be evaluated carefully. Neuropathic pain secondary to previous therapy of all types also may be located in the abdomen. Because outward or ongoing evidence of a pain-producing process frequently is absent, patients complaining of neuropathic abdominal pain often have difficulty in convincing physicians that such pain actually exists. Bladder, bowel, rectal, and vaginal spasms and a distressful bearing-down sensation deep in the pelvis and rectal area are frequent sequelae of radiotherapy for pelvic lesions; they are visceral forms of neuropathic pain. Because these symptoms frequently are episodic or may be constant with periodic exacerbation, achieving complete pain control is difficult.

SKIN

In examining the skin, examiners may find allodynia, hyperalgesia, dysesthesia, hypalgesia, numbness, cellulitis, neuritis, neuropathy, edema, heat, ulceration, direct tumor invasion, trophic changes, and various dermatologic eruptions. Some of these findings provide support for the diagnosis of neuropathic pain. They also help to determine a complete treatment plan (e.g., antibiotic therapy to relieve the pain of cellulitis and local treatment with salves and ointments to relieve pain of skin ulceration, in addition to systemic analgesic drugs).

MUSCULOSKELETAL SYSTEM

Examination may reveal both joint and muscle signs and symptoms, and changes in these structures may affect overall skeletal structural integrity. Function of major muscle groups should be tested. Muscle spasm, atrophy, tenderness (perhaps secondary hyperalgesia), a hypersensitive focal area or site in muscle or connective tissue (trigger point), and muscle imbalance secondary to previous surgery may be present. Joint swelling and tenderness may indicate an acute or chronic process, possibly related to the malignant process. Frequently, paraneoplastic syndromes involve the nervous and musculoskeletal systems. Limited motion in a joint (e.g., the shoulder) may cause a painful adhesive capsulitis (frozen shoulder) not infrequently seen in patients with limited motion in the shoulder after breast and thoracic surgery. Often, physical therapy modalities are more effective than is drug treatment for long-term improvement. However, analgesics and muscle relaxants may be necessary to facilitate physical therapy.

PERIPHERAL AND CENTRAL NERVOUS SYSTEMS

The nervous system probably is the system affected most frequently by cancer and its treatment. Particular attention should be paid to examination of this system. At a minimum, all sensory and motor deficits should be identified. Knowledge of specific neurologic deficits can help to locate obscure metastatic deposits in difficult-to-identify locations. As mentioned, special attention should be given to back pain in identifying leptomeningeal disease and the possibility of spinal cord compression. Preventing spinal cord compression, with its subsequent likelihood of paralysis, can enhance significantly the quality of affected patients' remaining period of life. Spinal cord compression requires immediate treatment with corticosteroids; they reduce swelling, thus relieving pain, and may provide interim protection against permanent damage to neurologic structures until application of definitive measures (e.g., irradiation or surgery or both). Differentiation between peripheral and central causes of pain can be achieved by careful neurologic examination. This determination is important in directing application of treatment.

Laboratory and Imaging Studies

Perhaps the two most important diagnostic tests for patients with pain are CT and MRI. Both are noninvasive and give relatively detailed images of normal and abnormal anatomic structures. Nervous system structures are visualized better with MRI, and this modality is particularly useful for detecting early spinal cord compression. Positron emission tomography has the potential to demonstrate specific metabolic and functional CNS changes, but it still is an investigational tool.

Testing of muscle and peripheral nerves by electromyography and nerve conduction studies is useful in selected cases. Electroencephalography is beneficial for evaluating patients with suspected seizure disorders and metabolic derangements of the brain. Psychological testing may be helpful in identifying brain metastases and in assessing higher integrative functioning; it is useful also in evaluating the validity of patients' responses to questions and the state of their memory and can provide a clue to their ability to comply with instructions.

Blood chemistry tests that reflect the functioning capacity of the major organ systems are important for determining how affected organs are likely to metabolize analgesics and other drugs used to treat pain and other distressing symptoms. Proper dosing with analgesics will depend on this information. The kidney and liver are the two most important systems involved in analgesic metabolism and functional derangements, and failure of either or both will require adjusting the dose of analgesic administered.

DEVELOPMENT OF A TREATMENT PLAN

Knowledge of the causes of pain and information obtained from assessment of the pain report by the patient, from the physical examination, and from appropriate laboratory studies permit development of a treatment plan. For patients who have pain because of a primary or metastatic tumor, the first treatment consideration for both tumor control and pain relief is that directed at the neoplastic process. Treatments designed to remove or otherwise ablate a tumor—surgery, radiotherapy, chemotherapy, and biological response modifiers—should be selected on the basis of their effectiveness alone or in combination. However, providing pain relief with appropriate analgesics (be they nonopioids or strong opioids) is necessary during treatment for the tumor and until treatment relieves the pain.

The pain treatment emphasis in this chapter, however, is on patients in whom the cause of pain cannot be removed or who cannot be treated effectively by pain pathway blockade (nerve blocks), neurosurgical techniques, or other treatment modalities and who must be treated with systemic analgesics, including potent opioids. From 60% to 90% of cancer patients will experience diffuse pain that is so intense that systemic, potent opioids will be required [20]. Reliance on potent opioids renders this group of patients the most likely to experience inadequate pain relief. They fall into the following categories [6]:

- Patients whose pain treatment requires opioids in "unusual" doses (doses considered high) over protracted periods
- Patients who have predominantly neuropathic pain or pain only partially responsive to opioids and who are treated with opioids only
- Patients whose pain can be relieved by opioids but, because no anatomic, physiologic, or pathologic cause for pain can be demonstrated by either physical examination or diagnostic techniques, are denied access to opioids
- Patients who have cancer pain and concomitantly abuse drugs, those who previously abused drugs, and those who fit the presumed profile of a drug abuser.

Most pain in cancer patients is of nociceptive origin and can be relieved adequately by the means readily available to most physicians and other health care providers. Specialized pain-relieving techniques will continue to be carried out in hospitals and pain treatment centers. However, this type of service is needed only in a select, relatively small percentage of patients in pain [5].

Guidelines

All health care professionals who treat cancer patients should be familiar with the guidelines, "Management of Cancer Pain," published in 1994 by the Agency for Health Care Policy and Research [5]. The guidelines do not include some newer analgesic preparations and de-

livery systems but present a review of evidence-based approaches to cancer pain management. Newer guidelines and critical pathways for cancer pain treatment have been developed by the American Pain Society [21] and the National Comprehensive Cancer Network [22] and should be consulted for the latest in recommendations for adequate pain treatment. Evidence suggests that following such guidelines improves cancer pain management.

Frequently, the prompt relief of pain from cancer involves the use of simultaneously (rather than serially) administered combinations of drug and nondrug therapies. Identification of a treatable neoplasm as a factor in pain production calls for appropriate radiotherapy or radionuclide and bisphosphonate compounds (e.g., to bone metastases), chemotherapy or, in some instances, surgical debulking. Until such treatment can be effective (possibly taking days to weeks), affected patients' pain must be managed with analgesics. In many instances, these agents are the only pain treatment available because of the patients' condition, the physical basis of the pain, or limited treatment options.

Analgesic Ladder

The World Health Organization (WHO) recommends an "analgesic ladder" approach (Fig. 33.5) to pain treatment: patients whose pain begins as mild and progresses to severe are treated in a stepwise fashion using increasingly stronger analgesics, which may or may not be combined with a nonsteroidal antiinflammatory drug (NSAID) or various adjuvant or coanalgesic drugs [23]. For mild pain, a nonopioid analgesic (e.g., acetaminophen, aspirin, another NSAID) can be used with such adjuvant drugs as antidepressants, antiepileptics, or other coanalgesics. For moderate pain, a weak opioid alone or in combination with acetaminophen, aspirin, or another NSAID is recommended, again adding the aforementioned adjuvant drugs; this combined regimen used in conjunction with a strong opioid will serve for severe pain. The minimum dose of opioid employed for any degree of pain should be that adequate to relieve the pain. The so-called usual or recommended doses found in pharmacology texts or other standard references are merely recommended starting doses; frequently, they will be inadequate and must be exceeded to provide optimum relief.

What must be kept in mind is that the analgesic ladder can be accessed initially on any "rung." Pain may not progress in a crescendo fashion: At the onset, it may be severe and may require starting treatment at the top

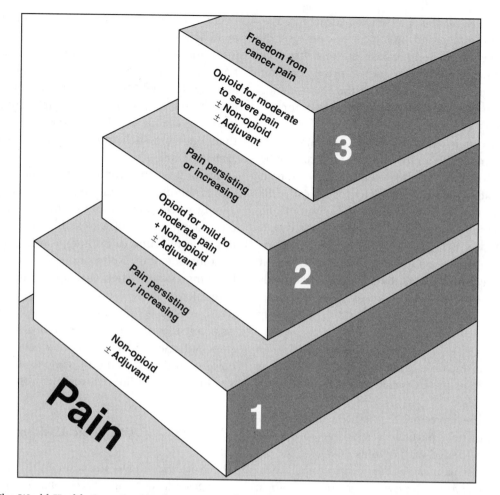

Figure 33.5   The World Health Organization three-step analgesic ladder for cancer pain relief. (Reprinted with permission of the World Health Organization from Cancer pain relief and palliative care. Report of a WHO expert committee. *World Health Organ Tech Rep Ser* 804: 1990.)

rung of the ladder using a strong opioid. Assessing the intensity of the pain as described by an affected patient is essential to selecting at pain onset the proper analgesic to achieve optimum relief.

Special Patient Populations

Certain populations of patients in pain require special consideration: children, minorities, underserved groups, vulnerable members of our society (e.g., individuals with criminal records; present and past substance abusers; patients with painful conditions from such sexually transmitted diseases as the acquired immunodeficiency syndrome [AIDS], the cognitively impaired; and persons currently in prison.)

Patients in such populations should not be denied adequate pain relief on the basis of nonmedical factors. Anecdotal case reports from such populations reveal

that any report of pain is considered automatically as overstated or as a manipulative maneuver. Caregivers may be judgmental and might consider such individuals as deserving of what is happening to them. Caregivers should guard against adopting such attitudes in dealing with these populations. The scope of this chapter prohibits addressing each of these groups in detail. Nonetheless, we believe that treatment of pain in children warrants special attention.

PAIN TREATMENT IN CHILDREN

Though cancer is a rare disease in children, affecting only 0.2% of the general population, pain is common in pediatric cancer. Two-thirds of children with cancer present with pain symptoms. Neither the causes nor the treatment of cancer pain in children are as well studied or characterized as they are for adults. In addition, lack of training of primary caregivers has limited the use of strong analgesics in children. However, advances in education and therapy have improved this situation markedly in recent years [24].

Pain experienced by children with cancer is different from that felt by adults. The main reason for this difference is the variation in malignancies that present in different age groups. The most common types of childhood malignancy are hematologic; in adults, carcinomas and sarcomas (solid tumors) are more common. Often, pain secondary to hematologic cancer is not as severe or localized, yet is intense enough to be the presenting symptom for the majority of children with cancer.

Many types of childhood malignancies respond well to multimodal therapy. Therapy itself is also a major source of pain, but pain secondary to treatment often is very predictable and well treated by conventional means. Often, the natural history of childhood cancer consists of long disease-free intervals. Thus, children experience less of the chronic, debilitating types of pain so characteristic of adult cancers.

Etiologic Features of Pain in Children

The causes of cancer-related pain in children also are unique. In general, cancer causes pain in four ways: by inducing secretion of pain-causing cytokines, by invasion of surrounding soft tissues and other pain-sensitive structures, by compression of nerves, and by obstruction of hollow organs. Whether the patient is a child or an adult, all these factors should be considered in evaluating pain, especially in patients with solid-tumor malignancies. However, because solid tumors are rare in childhood, more pain may be caused by therapy than by the tumor itself. Up to 80% of children report pain from therapy, with pain from diagnostic procedures playing a significant role.

The etiology of pain may be mixed. The location of pain in children also may be more generalized than that in adults, owing to the nature of the disease. Because pain complaints may be vague, localization may be difficult. The keeping of a pain diary is useful to characterize the temporal pattern of pain; such a diary may be kept by affected children or by their parents or by both.

Pain not caused directly by disease or treatment also can be prominent. Generalized debilitation can lead to painful bedsores and muscle cramping. Research suggests that children with preexisting cancer pain may be more sensitive to other, superimposed pain [25]. Finally, psychosocial and perceptual factors can play an important role in the perception of pain and must not

be overlooked. Both social and financial family stresses brought on by cancer may have an adverse impact on affected children, depending on their age. Some children may experience guilt because of their perception of having caused such family problems.

The stress of coping with a potentially fatal disease and with the resulting physical debilitation also can be significant for affected children. Again, such children's sense of time and their understanding of the natural history of their disease vary with their age, leading to differing impacts of these factors. Children will experience varying degrees of difficulty in coping with the physical changes induced by cancer or its treatment (e.g., baldness, indwelling catheters, cachexia). The interplay of school and socialization problems (e.g., taunting by classmates, rapid tiring, falling behind with schoolwork, isolation due to missed school attendance) may alter pain perception. Detecting or diagnosing depression can be difficult in such children. Masked depression can be reported as pain and should be considered in every child with cancer.

Pain Assessment

Evaluation of cancer pain in children always should follow a well-organized structure. Factors to be considered include etiology, location, temporal pattern, intensity, quality of pain, and the effectiveness of previous interventions. These criteria are similar to those used in the evaluation of adult cancer pain; however, visually observed cues and reports from affected children's parents will play an important role in the evaluation, as will a direct, age-appropriate discussion with such children.

The intensity of pain in younger children can be evaluated accurately using validated modifications of a visual analog scale, such as the faces scale (see Fig. 33.2). Often, older children and adolescents can use the standard visual analog scale. However, some older children may be unable to communicate pain because of coexisting conditions (e.g., developmental delay, communication disorder, inability to speak because of endotracheal intubation). The ability of such patients to communicate their distress accurately and appropriately will vary widely. With developmental delay, behaviors appropriate to earlier stages of development may be seen. Practitioners should be sensitive to these issues. Consulting professionals with requisite expertise may be necessary in dealing with children who have communication problems.

Assessment of pain in preverbal children presents a unique challenge. Because such children cannot communicate the location or intensity of their pain, these qualities must be inferred from changes in behaviors and from physiologic signs. Physiologic parameters include heart and respiratory rates and palm sweating. Stress hormone responses have been profiled as a measure of pain, but the practicality of this approach is questionable. However, none of these responses is specific for noxious stimulation, and pain behaviors themselves cannot be used as a quantitative assessment of pain. Such responses are modified by learning and the emotional state of the child and must be interpreted in that context [25]. Another important factor is realizing that pain behaviors change as children develop. For example, an infant may respond to pain with generalized movements, changes in facial expression, and crying patterns, whereas toddlers may be capable of more localized reactions to pain.

Pain quality and characteristics can be represented using standard descriptors, reported by either child or parent. These descriptors will provide additional information about the etiology of pain and can help to suggest effective treatment. The outcome of any previous interventions for pain also should be noted. Awareness of doses and effectiveness of administered drugs will help to improve further treatments. Children who develop symptoms of tolerance to the effects of opioid and sedative drugs should also be assessed for signs of physical and psychological dependence.

Devising a General Treatment Plan

Treatment of cancer pain in children involves many of the same concepts used in the treatment of adult pain, with some minor variations. The first factor to consider is the venue for initiating treatment. Adequate pain management can be initiated on either an inpatient or outpatient basis, depending on the severity of pain, its anticipated progression, and psychosocial factors. Caregivers, patients' families, and insurance companies should be apprised that valid indications for hospitalization include pain or symptom control and patient and family education that can be carried out best in the hospital. Often, even relatively brief hospital stays are sufficient to familiarize patients and their families with their pain treatment modalities and can help to avert serious discomfort or emergency admissions in the future. These principles are valid both for such technologically "advanced" forms of analgesic management as patient-controlled analgesia (PCA) and for more routine oral medication management.

The presumed natural history of the pain will help

to determine the nature of the treatment. For example, continuous pain from mucositis may require continuous administration of analgesic agents, whereas intermittent pains may require an entirely different strategy. The routes of analgesic administration normally available to adults may not be usable in children. For example, regional analgesia often is not a reasonable option in children because of the diffuse nature of the pain they experience and the pancytopenia that accompanies cancer treatment. Oral administration of analgesics may not be effective, owing to lack of compliance in young children and the presence of oral mucositis in some children undergoing chemotherapy. As a result, such alternative routes as opioid patches, iontophoresis, and rectal or transmucosal administration (fentanyl) must be considered.

All analgesic medications that are useful in adults work well in children. Analgesics that interact adversely with other medicines in affected children's therapeutic regimens should be avoided. Determining potential adverse reactions requires exactitude and close collaboration with children's primary caregivers.

The WHO analgesic ladder can be applied to treatment of children as well as adults. Experience will dictate where on the ladder treatment should be initiated for children with specific conditions. Generally, intermittent dosing of analgesics is satisfactory for outpatients. In most cases, weak and potent opioids can be combined with other adjuvant agents to produce adequate pain relief. However, some types of constant pain are managed better by continuous opioid infusion, even in outpatients. This modality requires a minor operative procedure for insertion of either a long-term indwelling central venous catheter or a long line, often threaded centrally from an antecubital vein. Then infusions can be maintained using one of several available types of infusion pumps specifically designed for this purpose. All doses used in children are calculated on a milligram-per-kilogram basis, and commonly employed intravenous doses of narcotics are listed on a sample inpatient PCA order sheet (Fig. 33.6).

Anecdotal reports indicate that PCA is employed safely in children as young as eight years, and some caregivers have reported unassisted use of PCA (with appropriate training) in children as young as four years. Parents can help by pushing the PCA button for small children who can communicate their discomfort but who are not yet capable of associating pushing the button with pain relief. Managing infants and preverbal toddlers via parent-assisted PCA is much more difficult: Though many experienced clinicians, using multiple clinical cues, excel at distinguishing pain from other

UNIVERSITY OF MICHIGAN
HOSPITALS AND HEALTH CENTERS
PEDIATRIC ANALGESIA ORDER SHEET

BIRTHDATE

NAME

CPI No.

SEX: M F   VISIT NO. ____ ____ ____ ____

AGE	WEIGHT

1. No other narcotics or sedatives to be administered while on PCA unless Pain Service has ordered them or been notified. Consult Pain Service before discontinuing PCA. **(Page 1534)**

2. **Mode:**   ☐ PCA ONLY   ☐ PCA + CONTINUOUS   ☐ NURSE CONTROLLED   ☐ CONTINUOUS

3. **Drug Selection and Pump settings:**

Drug Selection (choose one)	Loading Dose	Continuous Infusion Rate	PCA Dose	4 Hour Limit
☐ Morphine 1 mg/ml	_____ mg 0.05–0.10 mg/kg	_____ mg/hr 0.01–0.02 mg/kg/hr	_____ mg 0.02–0.03 mg/kg	_____ mg 0.25–0.3 mg/kg
☐ Morphine 100 µg/ml (3 mg/30 cc) use for pts < 15 kg	_____ µg 50–100 µg/kg	_____ µg/hr 10–20 µg/kg	_____ µg 20–30 µg/kg	_____ µg 250–300 µg/kg
☐ Hydromorphone 1 mg/ml	_____ mg 0.005–0.010 mg/kg	_____ mg/hr 0.002–0.004 mg/kg	_____ mg 0.002–0.004 mg/kg	_____ mg 0.02–0.04 mg/kg
☐ Hydromorphone 100 µg/ml (3 mg/30 cc) use for pts < 40 kg	_____ µg 5–10 µg/kg	_____ µg/hr 2–4 µg/kg	_____ µg 2–4 µg/kg	_____ µg 20–40 µg/kg
☐ Meperidine 10 mg/ml	_____ mg 0.5–1.0 mg/kg		_____ mg 0.2–0.3 mg/kg	_____ mg 2.5–3.0 mg/kg
☐ Other _____	_____	_____ /hr	_____	_____

Lockout interval _____ minutes (8–15 min)

4. **Monitoring:**   Respiratory rate and sedation level
  Neonates and infants to 1 yr = q1h × 8 hr and then q2h
  Children 1 yr and older = q2h × 8 hr and then q4h
  Pain scores q2h × 8 hr and then q4–8h. If pain not controlled after 1 hr, page 2522 or 1534

5. **Treatment of side effects:**
  a. **Nausea and vomiting:**

  ☐ Metoclopramide (Reglan) _____ mg IV q6h prn (0.15 mg/kg/dose)
  ☐ Droperidol _____ µg IV q4h prn (20–25 µg/kg/dose, max of 1250 µg/dose)
  ☐ Per Primary service
  ☐ Other: _____

  b. **Pruritus** ☐ Diphenhydramine (Benadryl) _____ mg IV over 15 min q6h prn (0.5 mg/kg/dose)

  c. **Excessive sedation** (score > 2) or respiratory rate < _____ discontinue PCA and page 1534 or 2522.

  d. **Critical sedation** (score = 4) or respiratory rate < _____ discontinue PCA and **page 1534 Pain Service and Primary Service STAT,** and give Naloxone _____ mg IV (0.01 mg/kg/dose, max of 0.1 mg/dose) may repeat q2min × 2

6. Acute Pain Service staff may change PCA orders by increasing or decreasing pump settings by 20%.

7. **Additional orders**

DOCTOR'S SIGNATURE	DR. NO.	DATE	TIME	CLERK'S INIT.	UNIT	DATE	TIME
			AM PM				AM PM

DO-2060305/DS   Rev.12/98   **MEDICAL RECORD ORIG.**   University of Michigan Health System   PEDIATRIC ANALGESIA ORDER SHEET

A

Figure 33.6 (A) Sample pediatric analgesia order sheet. (B) Sample pediatric epidural analgesia order. (C) Sample pediatric patient-controlled analgesia (*PCA*) dosage table. (Reprinted courtesy of Sandra Merkel, RN, Director, the University of Michigan Medical School, Department of Anesthesiology, Pediatric Pain Service, Ann Arbor, MI.)

UNIVERSITY OF MICHIGAN HOSPITALS AND HEALTH CENTERS
PEDIATRIC EPIDURAL ANALGESIA ORDERS

BIRTHDATE

NAME

CPI No.

SEX: M F   VISIT NO. ____ ____ ____ ____

AGE	WEIGHT

1. No other opioids or sedatives are to be administered while receiving epidural analgesia unless Pediatric Pain Service has ordered them or been notified. Consult Pain Service before discontinuing epidural. **(Page 1534)**

2. Epidural medication must be preservative-free, in sodium chloride 0.9%, 250 ml exact volume

Epidural Drug Section:

☐ Fentanyl 2 µg/ml   ☐ Bupivacaine 0.0625%
☐ _____   ☐ Bupivacaine 0.1%
Rate: 0.1–0.4 ml/kg/hr

☐ Duramorph (pts<15 kg) _____ mg in 250 ml
   ($2 \times$ wt [kg] $\times 250$ = µg per 250 ml; divide by 1000 for mg). 1 ml/hr = 2 µg/kg/hr.
☐ Duramorph (pts>15 kg) _____ mg in 250 ml
   (wt [kg] $\times 250$ = µg per 250 ml; divide by 1000 for mg). 1 ml/hr = 1 µg/kg/hr.
Rate: 3–5 µg/kg/hr

3. **Pump Setting:**   LL1 - Prescribed rate: Infusion _____ ml/hr
                        LL0 - Maximum setting: Infusion _____ ml/hr

Adolescents only: >12 years	Bolus Dose _____ ml Time Interval _____ min Dose/hr_____

4. **Epidural catheter and dressing:**   Epidural tubing must be clearly labeled "Epidural"
                                           Epidural dressing to be changed only by the Pain Service

5. **Monitoring:**   Resp Rate q1h (pts<12 mos must be on CR monitor)
   Duramorph epidural = continuous pulse oximetry until 24 hr after infusion stopped
   Temperature, sensory level, and check epidural site q8h
   Pain score, sedation, heart rate, BP q4h
   Maintain IV access for 8 hr after fentanyl epidural infusion and at least 18 hr after
        duramorph epidural infusion are discontinued
   All assessment continues until 8 hr after epidural infusion is stopped

6. **Activity:**   Out-of-bed activity must be supervised.

7. **Treatment of side effects:**

   Pruritus   ☐ Diphenhydramine (Benadryl) _____ mg IV over 15 min q6h prn (0.5 mg/kg)
                   ☐ Naloxone (Narcan) _____ IV q1–2h prn (1–2 µg/kg)
   Nausea   ☐ Metoclopramide (Reglan) _____mg IV q6h prn (0.15 mg/kg)
                   ☐ Other _____

8. **Page Pain Service:**   Resp Rate < _____ Heart Rate < _____ Systolic BP < _____
   (1534 or 2522)   Sedation scores > 2 (asleep, difficult to arouse)
                         Unrelieved pain and uncontrolled pruritus or nausea
                         Temp over 101˚, urinary retention (notify primary service as well)
                         No movement of feet or toes
                         Bleeding, leakage, tenderness at epidural site

9. **Excessive and Critical Sedation**
   Resp Rate < _____ Systolic BP < _____: **stop infusion and page Pain Service 1534**
   Cyanotic, unresponsive, resp rate < _____, or apnea: **apply oxygen, stimulate patient,**
        turn off infusion, page 1534 Pain Service and Primary Service STAT and give
        Naloxone _____mg IV (0.01 mg/kg/dose, max of 0.1 mg/dose) may repeat q2min x 2

DOCTOR'S SIGNATURE	DR. NO.	DATE	TIME	CLERK'S INIT.	UNIT	DATE	TIME
			AM PM				AM PM

DO-2048273/DS   Rev.12/98   **MEDICAL RECORD ORIG.**   M⚕ University of Michigan Health System   PEDIATRIC EPIDURAL ANALGESIA ORDERS

B

Figure 33.6   continued

Pediatric PCA Dosage Table

	Morphine[1]	Meperidine	Hydromorphone[2] (Dilaudid)	Fentanyl[3]
Loading dose	0.05–0.15 mg/kg	0.5–1.5 mg/kg	5–10 µg/kg	1–2 µg/kg
Infusion	0.01–0.02 mg/kg/hr	0.1–0.2 mg/kg/hr	2–3 µg/kg/hr	0.1–0.5 µg/kg/hr
Demand dose	0.02–0.04 mg/kg	0.2–0.4 mg/kg	2–4 µg/kg	0.2–0.5 µg/kg
4-Hr limit	0.25–0.30 mg/kg	2.5 mg/kg	20–40 µg/kg	2–4 µg/kg
Lockout time	8–15 min	8–15 min	8–15 min	8–15 min

The PCA pump has preset concentrations, but the pump can also be programmed in micrograms or milligrams for a specific concentration.

1. For children weighing < 15 kg, use a morphine concentration of 100 µg/ml.

2. Hydromorphone dose is calculated as 10 times as potent as morphine. Literature indicates equivalent doses ranging from 7–10 times as potent as morphine. Hydromorphone via PCA can be written in two concentrations:
   a. *For patients weighing < 40 kg* = 100 µg/ml (3.0 mg in 30 ml); write all PCA parameters in micrograms.
   b. *For patients weighing > 40 kg* = 1 mg/ml (30.0 mg in 30 ml); write all PCA parameters in milligrams.

3. Not recommended for routine PCA use. Pruritus is a problem when total dose = 1 µg/kg/hr.

C

Figure 33.6   continued

causes of distress, affected young children's parents often find this process very difficult. For this reason, a better approach is to implement continuous infusion therapy alone or to employ nurse-controlled analgesia.

Nonpharmacologic adjunctive measures that have proved useful in adults can be altered appropriately to provide relief for children. Such measures include biofeedback, relaxation therapy, operant conditioning, distraction, desensitization, hypnosis, and psychological counseling for both affected children and their families. Though such measures have a success rate lower than that of conventional pharmacologic therapy, they often provide or improve pain and symptom relief where other methods have failed. Adjuncts also can minimize side effects by reducing drug doses required to achieve and maintain effective analgesia. The diverse nature of these interventions again highlights the need for a multidisciplinary team approach in evaluating children's pain. This approach is more time-consuming and expensive than are less complex strategies but is well worth the investment for the improved quality of life it provides.

Managing Procedural Pain

A key issue in treating children is the management of procedural pain. This problem is very serious for children who often are not taken seriously or who are treated inadequately. Procedural pain management has an impact on children undergoing cancer care because often they endure multiple procedures during the course of their illness.

Issues other than pain also must be addressed. Often, the fear of a strange, threatening environment can be overwhelming to children. Fear of the unknown, accentuated by inadequate or inappropriate explanation of necessary procedures, can create great difficulty in managing a child. A frightened child might not understand the need for immobility during procedures. This lack of understanding can result in the appearance of inability to cooperate, thus prolonging what might have been an otherwise brief procedure.

Some practitioners doubt that "conscious sedation" is an effective and safe technique for the management of procedural pain in children. Great effort is required to find a plane of analgesia that will produce comfort, relaxation, and immobility in affected children without adversely affecting the maintenance and protection of the airway (as, to a lesser extent, in adults). With the advent of less restrictive fasting guidelines for general anesthetics (allowable administration approximately three hours after clear liquid ingestion), the use of ultra-short-acting general anesthetics is a simple and less disruptive alternative to conscious sedation and other forms of sedation for invasive procedures. The new inhaled anesthetic sevoflurane or such intravenous agents as propofol and remifentanil are especially well suited for this purpose [26]. This approach is especially advantageous for frequent procedures, such as radiotherapy, requiring scheduling of several weeks of daily procedures. Such procedures can be performed early in the day, and rapid recovery causes less disruption to affected children's daily routine.

Regular use of inhaled anesthetics also can avoid the need for disfiguring and potentially infectious chronic indwelling venous catheters placed only for the purpose of sedative administration. This approach does require the presence of an anesthesiologist. However, the increase in cost can be offset by the decrease in disruption of daily family routine. With careful coordination among anesthesiologists, oncologists, and third-party payers, this arrangement can be mutually beneficial to all concerned.

Sedation with less potent but longer-acting drugs (e.g., pentobarbital) poses its own set of problems. Though sedation using these compounds often is carried out by standard protocols using non–anesthesiology specialists, any cost savings is negated by the longer recovery times needed for procedures that often are extremely brief and by the undesirable side effects of prolonged drug action. The advantages of routine use of inhaled anesthetics is a strong argument for substituting them for longer-acting drugs.

Adjunctive measures should be employed in the management of procedural pain. Psychological interventions can impart a sense of control and can help to minimize the emotional stress associated with procedures. For example, whenever possible, procedures should be performed in an environment familiar to affected patients: either at the bedside or in a room specially designed and decorated for this purpose. When appropriate, parents can be permitted to stay while their children fall asleep. Children can be allowed to administer their own medications (hold the face mask, inject needleless syringes). EMLA® cream (*e*utectic *m*ixture of *l*ocal *a*nesthetics) or iontophoretic administration of local anesthetic can be used at procedural sites to help to minimize analgesic requirements. These adjuncts are appropriate for such relatively minor procedures as in-travenous insertion or blood drawing and can render much more tolerable the most feared part of cancer for many children.

Summary of Considerations in Managing Childhood Cancer Pain

In sum, the management of cancer pain in children employs many of the same principles used in adults. Age- or size-appropriate adjustments in drug dosages and alteration of administration routes based on the nature of disease and developmental considerations are necessary, of course. In addition, the developmental immaturity of children mandates that adjunctive and age-appropriate psychological measures receive an increasingly important role in the management of pain and other symptoms in children. A multidisciplinary approach is preferable to address these issues. Appropriate, rather than cost-effective, care for affected children should be the goal of treatment. Pain and other symptom management should occupy an equal position with cancer treatment programs and should be as routine as checking vital signs.

SELECTION OF A PHARMACOLOGIC REGIMEN

Appropriate pain control can be achieved in most patients using various nonopioids, opioids, adjuvant drugs, coanalgesics, and combinations thereof. The immediate challenge facing physicians treating chronic pain patients is determining whether a pharmacologic approach is appropriate and, if so, which drugs to use, singly or in combination, to achieve optimum pain relief. Adequate pain control can be achieved in the majority of patients using relatively simple techniques.

Nonopioid Analgesics

The major group of nonopioid analgesics is the NSAIDs. Acetaminophen, although not technically an NSAID, often is included in this group because of its analgesic properties. These analgesics relieve pain using a mechanism different from that operating in opioid analgesics. Analgesia is related strongly to the ability of NSAIDs to inhibit the action of the enzyme cyclooxygenase (COX), an enzyme that releases inflammatory mediators (predominantly prostaglandins) known to sensitize or activate peripheral nociceptors in producing pain [27].

These inhibitors block the production of prostaglandin endoperoxides by the COX enzyme. The therapeutic efficacy of NSAIDs largely parallels their potency to inhibit this enzyme [27]. COX exists in two isoforms known as COX-1, the constitutive form, and COX-2, the inducible form. COX-1 activates the production of prostacyclin that, when released by the endothelium, is antithrombogenic and when released by the gastric mucosa is cytoprotective. COX-2 is induced by inflammatory stimuli and cytokines in migratory and other cells. Therefore, antiinflammatory actions of NSAIDs are postulated to be due to inhibition of COX-2, and the unwanted side effects (e.g., irritation of the stomach lining) are due to inhibition of COX-1.

Typical NSAIDs inhibit both isoforms. A significant advancement in NSAID therapy has been achieved with the identification of selective COX enzyme inhibitors (i.e., inhibitors for a specific isoform). Two new drugs, celecoxib (Celebrex) and rofecoxib (Vioxx), are the first drugs developed to target the COX-2 enzyme alone. Studies have shown that these drugs will relieve arthritis pain and inflammation effectively by blocking the inflammation-producing effect of the COX-2 enzyme while potentially causing fewer side effects, most notably in the GI tract, by not blocking the COX-1 gastric cytoprotective effect. As a general precaution, however, both physician and patient should be on constant alert for GI tract bleeding. Also, studies in laboratory animals show severe disruptions in renal function, suggesting that affected patients should be monitored for evidence of renal impairment, especially if doses exceeding those recommended or usual are contemplated. Interestingly, COX-2 inhibition may play a role also in the chemoprevention of colon cancer in genetically susceptible populations and may reduce the incidence of Alzheimer's disease [28, 29].

A useful treatment strategy is to administer opioids and nonopioids simultaneously to affected patients. This approach takes advantage of each drug's mode of action and potentiates analgesic synergy.

INDICATIONS

A specific indication for the use of NSAIDs in treating cancer patients is pain associated with an inflammatory reaction (not necessarily infectious in origin) surrounding a tumor. Such a reaction is most obvious in cutaneous metastatic nodules or infiltration. A second specific indication is pain associated with bone metastases [30]. A body of anecdotal evidence indicates that NSAIDs provide additional relief of bone pain when used in combination with opioids. The synergism of NSAIDs with opioids is another indication for their use, because a reduction in the dose of opioid may be possible in patients suffering from the undesirable side effects of oversedation and mental cloudiness. This reduction may eliminate the side effects without sacrificing pain control.

DOSING AND ROUTES OF ADMINISTRATION

Most studies of dosing with NSAIDs have been conducted with patients having chronic, nonmalignant painful medical conditions, yet dosages derived from these studies are recommended for treatment of pain in cancer patients. Therefore, careful thought must precede using these dosages in cancer patients; usually, cancer patients are older, may have single or multiple organ compromise or failure, and may be receiving cytotoxic or other drugs with effects uncomplementary to those of NSAIDs. Under these circumstances, dosages may have to be lower than those recommended. Conversely, higher dosages may be needed if the desired effect is not achieved and no contraindications caution against increasing the dose.

However, the cardinal pharmacologic principle regulating dosing with NSAIDs is the "ceiling effect," whereby increasing the dose of a drug above a certain level will fail to provide additional pain relief but may indeed produce adverse effects. In general, NSAIDs produce analgesic effects at lower doses and produce antiinflammatory effects at higher doses [31]. Dose ranges for selected NSAIDs are given in Table 33.4.

Three routes of administration are available for NSAIDs. The majority must be given orally. Indomethacin is available also in rectal suppository form, and ketorolac, a potent NSAID popular for postoperative pain, is available for intramuscular and intravenous administration [32]. The physical status of affected patients will help to determine which of these routes of administration is most appropriate.

SIDE EFFECTS

The major toxic effects of NSAIDs on organ systems occur in the kidney and GI tract; however, adverse effects may occur in any organ system and have been reported in the CNS, lung, and liver [33]. Patients who have impaired renal function should be given NSAIDs cautiously. Patients who have a history of GI bleeding or current dyspepsia either should be treated with a selective COX enzyme inhibitor or should not be treated with NSAIDs. Patients with a remote history of GI bleeding or a vague history of peptic disease should be

Table 33.4　Commonly Used Nonsteroidal Antiinflammatory Drugs

Generic Name and Class	Trade Name	Approx. Half-Life (hr)	Dosing Schedule	Recommended Starting Dose (mg/day)	Maximum Recommended Dose (mg/day)
Salicylates					
Acetylsalicylic acid	Aspirin, etc.	3–12	q4–6h	2,600	6,000
Choline magnesium trisalicylate*	Trilisate	8–12	q8–12h	1,500 × 1, then 500 q12h	4,000
Salsalate	Disalcid	8–12	q8–12h	1,500 × 1, then 500 q12h	4,000
Diflunisal	Dolobid, Dolobis	8–12	q12h	1,000 × 1, then 500 q12h	1,500
Acetic acid derivatives					
Indomethacin	Indocin, Indocid, Indomethine	4–5	q8–12h	75	200
Sulindac	Clinoril, Arthorobid	14	q12h	300	400
Tolmetin	Tolectin	1	q6–8h	600	2,000
Ketorolac	Toradol	4–7	q4–6h	120	240
Suprofen	—	2–4	q6h	600	800
Fenamates					
Mefenamic acid	Ponstel, Ponstan, Ponstil, Namphen	2	q6h	4	1,000
Meclofenamate sodium	Meclomen	2–4	q6–8h	150	400
Propionic acid derivatives					
Ibuprofen	Motrin, Advil, Nuprin, Rifen	3–4	q4–8h	1,200	4,200
Naproxen	Naprosyn, Naprosine, Proxen	13	q12h	500	1,000
Fenoprofen	Nalfon, Fenopran, Nalgesic, Progesic	2–3	q6h	800	3,200
Ketoprofen	Orudis, Alrheumat	2–3	q6–8h	150	300
Flurbiprofen	Ansaid	5–6	q8–12h	100	300
Diclofenac	Voltaren	2	q6h	75	200
Oxaprozin	Daypro	50–60	q24h	1,200	1,800
Oxicams					
Piroxicam	Feldene	45	q24h	20	40
Pyranocarboxylic acids					
Etodolac	Lodine	7.3	q6–8h	800	1,200
Naphthylalkanones					
Nabumetone	Relafen	22–30	q12–24h	1,000	4,000
Selective COX-2[†] inhibitors					
Celecoxib	Celebrex	11.2	q12h	100–200	400
Rofecoxib*	Vioxx	17	Daily	12.5–25.0	25

*Available in liquid form.
[†]COX = cyclooxygenase.

given cytoprotective and antiulcer therapy on a prophylactic basis if conventional NSAIDs are used, or they should be treated with a selective COX enzyme–inhibitor NSAID.

Treatment with a drug having the potential to cause bleeding is of particularly concern in cancer patients because frequently these patients have compromised platelet levels and poorly functioning platelets secondary to use of chemotherapeutic agents or other anticancer drugs. Choline magnesium trisalicylate, salsalate, and diflunisal (all nonacetylated salicylates) are the NSAIDs of choice for treating patients with platelet abnormalities if NSAIDs must be used in this circumstance. Choline magnesium trisalicylate is available in liquid form, rendering its administration possible in patients unable to swallow pills.

SPECIFIC NSAIDS

A wide variety of NSAIDs are available for use (see Table 33.4). Generally, studies are inconclusive as to whether one drug is superior to another in antiinflammatory effect, pain-relieving qualities, or side effects. Clinical experience has shown that none are consistently reliable for pain relief in all patients. Except for indications cited earlier, selection is empiric: If one drug fails to provide the desired effect, trying another is appropriate. Each drug should be administered for an interval long enough to allow an adequate trial (generally, one week).

Distinctions among NSAIDs are based on differences in their pharmacologic characteristics rather than in their therapeutic efficacy. For example, piroxicam has a long half-life and can be given only once daily. This dosing is convenient for patients and encourages better compliance. A specific NSAID also might be chosen because of its lack of inhibition of platelet function. Nonacetylated NSAIDs possess this property, in contrast to all the others. Consequently, they are the NSAID of choice in patients at risk for bleeding disorders and in patients who are receiving chemotherapy and whose platelet count may be in jeopardy.

The discovery of COX-inhibiting NSAIDs tempts physicians to treat all patients requiring an NSAID with these drugs, owing to their more favorable side effect profile. At the time of this writing, these drugs are considerably more expensive than are conventional, nonselective COX-inhibiting NSAIDs. Certainly, treating all patients with the selective COX enzyme–inhibiting NSAIDs is not necessary. Patients who were previously treated with NSAIDs that caused peptic distress or GI bleeding definitely should be treated with the selective

agents. Other patients who have no previous experience with NSAIDs and no contraindications to their use can be given a trial with a conventional NSAID and can be monitored carefully for all adverse side effects. If none develop, such patients can continue use of such agents with instructions for continued monitoring. Where cost is a major factor, this approach to NSAID use is reasonable.

Opioid Analgesics

CLASSIFICATION

One useful classification of opioids divides them into three categories on the basis of their predominant pharmacologic action (Table 33.5): pure agonists, mixed agonist-antagonists, and partial agonists. The prototypical agonist opioid is morphine. The prototypical antagonist is naloxone, a drug that will reverse analgesia and all other pharmacologic actions of opioids and, in opioid-dependent patients, can cause the withdrawal syndrome. The predominant action of mixed agonist-antagonists and partial agonists is agonist, but these agents also have a potentially significant antagonist action.

The practical significance of this classification system relates to switching affected patients' medication from one category to another. Patients who have been treated with pure agonists should not be switched to either mixed agonist-antagonists or partial agonists because the antagonist component of the drug may pre-

Table 33.5 Pharmacologic Classification of Opioids

Classification	Opioid
Pure agonists	Propoxyphene
	Codeine
	Dihydrocodeine
	Oxycodone
	Hydrocodone
	Morphine
	Hydromorphone
	Methadone
	Levorphanol
	Meperidine
Mixed agonist-antagonists	Pentazocine
	Butorphanol
	Nalbuphine
	Dezocine
Partial agonists	Buprenorphine

Table 33.6 Classification of Opioids Based on Analgesic Potency

Classification	Opioid
Weak opioids	Propoxyphene
	Codeine
	Hydrocodone
Potent opioids	Morphine
	Hydromorphone
	Oxycodone
	Fentanyl
	Methadone
	Levorphanol
	Meperidine

cipitate a withdrawal reaction. However, patients who have been treated with mixed agonist-antagonists or partial agonists may be switched to pure agonists with impunity because doing so presents no potential for a withdrawal reaction.

Another practical classification of opioids separates them as either *weak* or *potent* on the basis of their capacity to relieve mild, moderate, or severe pain (Table 33.6). Perhaps any narcotic could relieve any pain, but the side effects accompanying the necessary dosage render impractical the use of weaker narcotics for severe pain.

PRACTICAL PHARMACOLOGIC FEATURES

As with all drugs, the two pharmacologic features—pharmacokinetic and pharmacodynamic—have practical therapeutic importance for opioids. *Pharmacokinetics* is a term that refers to the body's effect on the drug before it reaches binding sites; the term *pharmacodynamics* refers to the drug's effect on the body after it reaches the binding site in the CNS. Morphine serves as a representative of these characteristics for this category of opioids.

Pharmacokinetics

Morphine is absorbed readily from the GI tract and is metabolized to morphine-3-glucuronide and morphine-6-glucuronide. Morphine-6-glucuronide is a potent analgesic, but morphine-3-glucuronide may antagonize its analgesic effect [34].

Through a first-pass effect (biotransformation), metabolism in the liver inactivates approximately two-thirds of an orally administered dose. Parenterally administered doses are not affected by this first-pass effect because they reach binding sites before the liver reduces their effectiveness; consequently, clinicians often perceive parenterally administered opioids to be more effective than those administered orally. To overcome the first-pass effect with oral opioids, the dose administered must be adjusted upward. Adherence to this principle can ensure success in oral administration of opioids in the vast majority of patients.

Pharmacodynamics

Morphine affects primarily the CNS and the bowel. The CNS effects in individuals who are experiencing pain differ from those in individuals who are not [35]. Pain antagonizes the analgesic effects of opioids; therefore, patients in severe pain will require a dose of opioid higher than that usually recommended in standard pharmacology textbooks or other references. Respiratory depression also is antagonized by pain [35]. As long as a dose is not increased excessively beyond that necessary to control the pain, respiratory depression is exceedingly unlikely. Often, confusion about these points has resulted in the administration of inadequate doses of morphine or other opioids to patients in pain. However, if the source of pain is removed suddenly, excessive sedation and respiratory depression may occur.

Morphine's effects on the CNS are diverse and include analgesia, drowsiness, changes in mood, decrease in mental acuity, nausea, vomiting, and alterations in the endocrine and autonomic nervous systems. Incremental increases in doses can be expected to produce additional analgesia in patients whose pain is nociceptive. The pharmacologic principle of "dosing to effect"—that is, increasing the dose either until the desired effect is achieved or until undesirable side effects prevent further escalation—always should be followed in using morphine. In general, side effects are encountered only with the onset of therapy, and they are transient. Occasionally, pain less responsive to morphine can be managed effectively by using another potent opioid (e.g., hydromorphone or fentanyl).

Effects on the small and large intestines are a marked decrease or halting of propulsive contractions and peristaltic waves. Tolerance to effects on the bowel seldom occurs; therefore, instituting a bowel-cleaning program is essential in administering long-term morphine. Morphine also may affect urinary bladder function, causing both urgency and urinary retention because of increased sphincter tone. Blood pressure may drop, owing to peripheral arteriolar and venous dilation.

The pharmacodynamics of other opioids are essentially the same as for morphine. Significant clinical differences are discussed with the specific opioids.

Table 33.7 Oral-to-Parenteral Dose Ratios of Weak and Potent Opioids for Treatment of Moderate to Severe Pain

	Route	Equianalgesic Dose[a,b] (mg)	Duration (hr)	Plasma Half-Life (hr)
Narcotic agonists				
Morphine	P	10	4–6	2.0–3.5
	PO	30	4–7	
Codeine	P	130	4–6	3
	PO	200	4–6	
Oxycodone	P	NA		–
	PO	15–20	3–5	
Levorphanol	P	2	4–6	12–16
(Levo-dromoran)	PO	4	4–7	
Hydromorphone	P	1.5	4–5	2–3
(Dilaudid)	PO	7.5	4–6	
Oxymorphone	P	1	4–6	2–3
(Numorphan)	PR	10	4–6	
Meperidine	P	75	4–5	3–4
(Demerol)	PO	300	4–6	12–16
Methadone	P	10		15–30
(Dolophine)	PO	20		
Fentanyl	TD, TM	100 μg/hr[c]	1–3	3.5
(Duragesic, Actiq)				
Tramadol (Ultram)	PO	50–100	3–7	6
Mixed agonist-antagonists				
Pentazocine	P	60	4–6	2–3
(Talwin)	PO	180	4–7	
Nalbuphine	P	10	4–6	5
(Nubain)	PO	–		
Butorphanol	P	2	4–6	2.5–3.5
(Stadol)	PO	–		
Partial agonists				
Buprenorphine	P	0.4	4–6	7
(Temgesic)	SL	0.8	5–6	

P = parenteral; PO = per os (orally); NA = not available; PR = per rectum; TD = transdermal; TM = transmucosal; SL = sublingual.
[a]For these equianalgesic doses, the time of peak analgesia ranges from 1.5 to 2.0 hours and the duration ranges from 4 to 6 hours.
[b]These are recommended starting doses from which the optimal dose for each patient is determined by titration and the maximal dose is limited only by adverse effects.
[c]Note that dose is expressed as micrograms/hour.

MECHANISM OF ACTION

Exogenous opioids act as ligands that bind to opioid receptors in the CNS and other tissues (e.g., the large bowel) [36]. These receptors also function in endogenous analgesic systems. Reasonably firm evidence identifies three major categories of CNS receptors: mu, kappa, and delta. These receptors are believed to mediate the various effects of the opioids. The affinity with which an opioid binds to one or more of these receptors may account for its characteristic action. For example, dysphoria and psychotomimetic effects are associated with opioids that have a stronger affinity for kappa receptors. Most clinically used analgesics are mu receptor agonists. Because clinically used opioids act by binding to mu receptors, combining them in the treatment of pain seldom is advantageous. For example, simultaneous use of morphine, hydromorphone, and meperidine to treat a patient provides no therapeutic benefit over an adequate dose of only one of these drugs. Such polypharmacy is practiced commonly, probably because of a reluctance simply to increase the dose of a single opioid to an effective level, albeit one that may exceed the usual or recommended dose. However, this untested practice has become traditional most likely because of fear of sanction by state and federal regulatory agencies for prescribing one drug outside the usual or recommended dosage range. From a patient's perspective, use of an adequate dose of a single agent is less confusing, and the results are the same.

Combining drugs that have similar mechanisms of action is appropriate when the objective is to take advantage of a specific pharmacologic characteristic of each drug. For example, use of methadone, a drug with a long half-life and a possible dosing interval of six hours, requires concomitant prescription of a complementary short-acting drug, such as morphine or hydromorphone, for breakthrough pain that may occur before the end of six hours. Taking advantage of synergistic interactions between opioids and various nonopioid analgesics also is an appropriate therapeutic maneuver and may limit undesirable side effects associated with either category of analgesic.

DOSING

Probably the most common error in using opioids is underdosing [3]. Usually, the dose of morphine recommended for the treatment of severe pain is 10 mg intramuscularly. This dose was determined by single-dose studies of postoperative patients [37]. However, pain associated with cancer and pain from many chronic benign conditions frequently is much more severe than is postoperative pain and will require doses higher than 10 mg. A maxim about the proper dose of morphine is "whatever it takes to relieve the pain." A 10-mg intramuscular dose or an equianalgesic oral dose may be a reasonable starting dose, but the pain relief achieved by this dose should be evaluated within 30 to 60 minutes after administration; if pain has not been relieved, the dose should be titrated upward until it is. The use of intravenous PCA renders titration easier and faster.

Titration upward can be achieved by either oral or intravenous administration of additional doses. Rapid upward titration is possible because of the antagonistic effect of pain on the respiratory depressant effect of opioids. As long as an affected patient is experiencing pain, the possible complication of respiratory depression should not be a deterrent to administering a dose adequate to relieve pain.

To titrate upward by the oral route, affected patients are instructed to take a "breakthrough" dose of immediate-release morphine between the scheduled doses of this agent whenever the pain returns. The duration of action of immediate-release morphine is ap-

proximately four hours. Therefore, the breakthrough dose will be taken anytime during the four-hour interval of the scheduled dose. If the combination of scheduled and breakthrough doses is inadequate to control pain, the combined dose for the 24-hour period is used as a new scheduled dose in divided doses every four hours, and a new breakthrough dose is used (50% higher than the previous breakthrough dose).

To titrate upward by the intravenous route, morphine is administered intravenously until pain is relieved or until intolerable side effects appear or until it is determined that a patient has pain that is only partially responsive to opioids (i.e., neuropathic pain). Incremental doses for titrating upward (either bolus or rapid infusions) range from 5 to 15 mg; choice of the appropriate dose is determined by the assessment of the severity of pain. Patients whose dose is titrated by this method and whose pain is relieved immediately do not experience unnecessary delayed titration intervals that occur with the oral titration method.

In a multicenter study, dosages of morphine to relieve cancer pain adequately varied from 60 to 3,000 mg orally every 24 hours in divided doses [38]. These figures, however, should not be considered upper or lower limits but merely as an illustration of the wide range necessary to individualize adequate dosing. As regards nociceptive pain, anecdotal reports cite patients who received 36 to 50 g morphine every 24 hours and were alert and able to function satisfactorily. Undertreatment of pain will occur if dosing intervals exceed four hours when immediate-release morphine is used. To obviate this problem, morphine now is available in a controlled-release form that extends its effectiveness to 12 hours or longer. Combining this form of morphine with immediate-release morphine can provide nearly constant pain control. A method of pain control using combined immediate-release and controlled-release morphine is described and illustrated later.

Table 33.7 shows the oral-to-parenteral dose ratios and the equianalgesic doses for commonly used opioids. This table can be used to convert the dose of one opioid into that of another and to convert one route of administration to another. The reference standard is 10 mg of morphine given intramuscularly for treatment of severe pain. Table 33.8 lists the oral analgesics used commonly for mild to moderate pain.

SIDE EFFECTS

Side effects are simply manifestations of the pharmacodynamics of opioids in organ systems other than the

Table 33.8   Oral Analgesics Used Commonly for Mild to Moderate Pain

Drug	Dose* (mg)	Dose Range (mg)	Comments	Precautions
Non-narcotics				
Aspirin	325–650	1,950–3,900	Often used in combination with opioid-type analgesics	Renal dysfunction; Avoid in hematologic disorders and in combination with steroids
Choline magnesium trisalicylate	6,500	1,500–3,000	Longer duration of action than aspirin	Minimal GI side effects; no effect on platelets
Acetaminophen	325–650	1,950–3,900	No significant antiinflammatory effects	Minimal GI side effects; no effect on platelets
Ibuprofen (Motrin)	400–800	2,400–4,800	Antiinflammatory and analgesic effects	
Diflunisal (Dolobid)	500–1,000	1,000–2,000	Longer duration of action than ibuprofen; higher analgesic potential than aspirin	Like aspirin
Naproxen (Naprosyn)	250–500	1,500–3,000		
Celecoxib (Celebrex)	200	200–400	Selective COX-2 enzyme inhibitor	
Refecoxib (Vioxx)	12.5	12.5–25.0	Selective COX-2 enzyme inhibitor; may require only a single daily dose	
Morphine-like agonists				
Codeine	15–60	90–360	Often used in combination with nonopioid analgesics; biotransformed in part to morphine	Impaired ventilation; bronchial asthma; increased intracranial pressure
Meperidine (Demerol)	150–300	900–1,800	Shorter-acting; biotransformed to normeperidine, a potentially toxic metabolite. Not recommended for treatment of chronic pain.	Normeperidine accumulates with repetitive dosing, causing CNS excitation; not for patients with impaired renal function or receiving monoamine oxidase inhibitors
Propoxyphene HCl (Darvon)	65–130	390–780	"Weak" narcotic; often used in combination with nonopioid analgesics; longer half-life; biotransformed to a potentially toxic metabolite (norpropoxyphene)	Propoxyphene and metabolite accumulate with repetitive dosing; overdose complicated by convulsions. Not recommended for treatment of chronic pain
Mixed agonist-antagonists				
Pentazocine (Talwin)	50–100	300–600	In combination with nonopioids; in combination with naloxone to discourage parenteral abuse	May cause psychotomimetic effects; may precipitate withdrawal in opioid-dependent patients; not recommended for chronic pain

GI = gastrointestinal; COX = cyclooxygenase; CNS = central nervous system.
*These are recommended starting doses from which the optimal dose for each patient is determined by titration and the maximal dose is limited only by adverse effects.
Note: For these analgesics (see also Comments), the time of peak analgesia ranges from 1.5 to 2.0 hours and the duration ranges from 4 to 6 hours.

CNS. In most situations, side effects are considered undesirable; however, certain effects may be desirable (e.g., in controlling diarrhea secondary to tumor of the GI tract or in controlling persistent cough secondary to lung cancer).

The pharmacodynamics of other opioid drugs are similar to those of morphine, although individuals may experience more or fewer side effects with other drugs, and the same drug may cause different side effects in different patients. For example, morphine may cause nausea and vomiting in one patient but not in another. These side effects may occur with any of the opioids, and changing from one to another may be necessary for specific patients. Also, pharmacologic differences are found among the clinically used opioids; these are discussed in the sections describing specific opioids.

Side effects may be transient or persistent. Side effects that usually are transient and associated with initiation of opioid therapy are sedation, mental clouding (including transient hallucinations), dizziness, urinary retention, nausea, vomiting, and itching. These side effects should be evaluated carefully before concluding that opioids in general or a particular opioid and route of administration must be abandoned. Multiple causes can underlie symptoms and, for an opioid to be implicated, a definite causal relationship should be established.

Administering antiemetics with an opioid controls nausea and vomiting. Often, after a week or two, the antiemetics can be discontinued, and affected patients can continue to take an oral narcotic without experiencing nausea and vomiting. Patients who have persistent problems urinating can be taught to catheterize themselves; after several days, urination may occur normally. Many of these transient side effects are dose-dependent, and once the dose is adjusted properly, the side effects are minimized or disappear.

Persistent side effects should be treated vigorously. Sedation can be treated with CNS stimulants (e.g., dextroamphetamine sulfate or methylphenidate). Dextroamphetamine sulfate is known to have a synergistic action with opioids and not only may correct the sedation but may enhance pain relief [39].

Patients who have experienced unrelieved pain for a significant period may be sleep-deprived from inability to sleep for much of that period. With adequate pain relief, they may be able to sleep and may do so for an extended period simply to "catch up." However, this method of recovering from sleep deprivation should not be confused with sedation.

The most consistent and persistent side effect of opioids is constipation. It occurs with all (even weak) opioids and with all routes of administration. Thus, a bowel-cleaning program should be instituted immediately with the prescription of opioids, especially when chronic administration is anticipated. Because propulsion is the action blocked by opioids, administering stool softeners alone is not sufficient to alleviate this side effect; softeners should be combined with a mild laxative for effective relief. Failure to control constipation may cause nausea and vomiting. Frequently, patients who suffer this side effect are labeled as allergic when, in fact, they simply are not moving their bowels as they should.

The intrinsic attributes of opioids may be confused with side effects. Tolerance is thought to occur in anyone on long-term administration of opioids. In cancer patients, clinical tolerance seldom is observed. If dose escalation is required, the need more often results from progression of disease than from development of tolerance. Physical dependence occurs but is of no consequence, because it does not cause symptoms or undesirable effects until the opioid no longer is needed and a patient abruptly discontinues it. Abrupt discontinuation will produce the distressful symptoms of an abstinence or withdrawal reaction. This can be avoided by reducing the opioid dose gradually. Cancer patients taking opioids for pain relief welcome the discontinuation of these drugs when pain abates, and ample evidence suggests that patients taking such opioids do not develop psychological dependence on them [40, 41]. Addiction to a drug has been shown to involve factors more complex than the mere exposure to it. The likelihood that cancer patients who take opioids for pain will become drug abusers or typical street drug addicts is remote [41].

Most patients can be treated with oral opioids, even for the severest pain, if adequate attention is paid to treatment of side effects. Patience in overcoming side effects, on the part of both physicians and patients, can pay big dividends in optimum pain relief and cost containment. Frequently, side effects that occur, regardless of route of administration, are misinterpreted as an allergy to the opioid. However, true allergies to opioids are extremely rare. True allergic signs (e.g., skin eruptions, urticaria) should be present before a diagnosis of allergy is reached.

ROUTES OF ADMINISTRATION

Oral Route

Opioids are effective pain relievers when given by mouth, and patients prefer this route of administration to all others because of its effectiveness and convenience. Recognition and application of basic pharmacokinetic principles in treating pain with orally administered opioids will demonstrate achievement of pain control like that of any other route of administration. Infrequently, the route of administration may cause transient, undesirable side effects that may occur with initiation of opioid treatment, but the route should not be abandoned simply because of this reaction. Every effort should be made to treat side effects aggressively and to ensure the success of oral administration, because other routes of administration are more cumbersome, potentially more dangerous, and often more expensive.

Frequently, lack of effect with oral opioids is given as a reason to change routes of administration. Such a conclusion requires careful pharmacodynamic analysis [42]. Reaching such a conclusion as lack of effect seems unlikely. In the case of opioids, dose titration upward should be continued until one of two results occur: Pain relief is achieved with no intolerable or untreatable side effects *or* intolerable or untreatable side effects prevent further dose escalation. An oral dose of opioid that is perceived to be unusually high and produces neither pain relief nor side effects cannot be considered dosing to effect. Therefore, the oral route cannot be ruled ineffective in the absence of one or the other results cited.

Administration via Rectum and Other Body Orifices

Most analgesics administered via the rectum and other body orifices are effective, but patients generally have an aversion to them, especially if the dose requires insertion of multiple suppositories or if treatment extends over a long interval. However, such routes are particularly useful if nausea and vomiting of short duration precludes oral administration.

Rectal administration is the route used most commonly; however, it is contraindicated in patients with low platelet counts. Drugs are absorbed readily via the vagina, and this route should be considered as an alternative to rectal administration in selected circumstances.

Parenteral Route

Parenteral routes include intramuscular, intravenous, subcutaneous, and intraspinal administration. Once again, use of these routes is governed by pharmacokinetic principles; in this regard, intramuscular, intravenous, and subcutaneous routes are similar, whereas the intraspinal route is different. Claims that the parenteral route is superior to other routes are anecdotal. Usually, the parenteral route is chosen simply because of various other practical dosing considerations. The traditional intramuscular route of parenteral administration is becoming less popular because it is traumatic for affected patients and produces less consistent results. The most common reason for parenteral administration is unavailability of the oral route: Persistent nausea and vomiting, difficulty in or defective swallowing (e.g., tracheoesophageal fistula), mental cloudiness or obtundation, and intestinal obstruction are common conditions precluding medication by this route. Another indication for parenteral administration is increased pain intensity requiring an unusually large dose (i.e., to avoid the

impracticality of swallowing large numbers of tablets). Because the requisite equianalgesic parenteral dose is smaller, administering the drug by this route may be more practical.

Transdermal or Iontophoretic Administration

Transdermal administration of fentanyl ("patches") has been approved for use for moderate to severe pain. Fentanyl is an extremely potent and short-acting opioid that, when used transdermally, is appropriate for the ambulatory treatment of chronic cancer pain. The traditional intravenous route would be impractical for administration of fentanyl to outpatients. With the transdermal system, fentanyl permeates the skin, and a "depot" is established in the stratum corneum layer. Anatomic position of the patch does not effect absorption. However, fever can lead to increased absorption and potential overdose.

This modality is well suited for use in patients with cancer pain because of its ease of use, prolonged duration of action, and stable blood levels. It takes up to 12 hours to detect significant analgesia and up to 16 hours to observe full clinical effects. Plasma levels plateau after two sequential patch applications, and fentanyl kinetics do not appear to change with repeated applications. Dermatologic side effects from the patch (e.g., rash, pruritus) seldom occur and are mild. In the unlikely event that excessive sedation or respiratory depression should occur, treatment with naloxone (Narcan®) should be instituted and maintained for an appropriate interval after patch removal, owing to the depot effect (slow release) from the subcutaneous fat. Multiple doses of naloxone may be necessary because of its relatively short half-life. The transdermal route is an attractive choice when the oral route is unavailable, because it is noninvasive and use is easy.

Transmucosal Route

Opiates administered through the oral mucosa can be absorbed more quickly than are those given through the stomach. Bioavailability of oral transmucosal fentanyl citrate (OTFC) is 52%, as compared with 32% for orally administered fentanyl, owing to avoidance of the liver's first-pass effect. In adults using OTFC, significant analgesia has been demonstrated to develop within 15 minutes and to last for two hours. Dose-dependent sedation with an onset of 20 to 60 minutes also was observed. Respiratory depression occurred only with higher doses, primarily in opioid-naive individuals.

This method has proved effective also as an outpatient treatment for breakthrough pain. In this setting, OTFC provided pain relief within 15 minutes, and patients were able to titrate the appropriate dose easily [43].

Inhalation

Studies have demonstrated that opioid analgesics can be delivered by nebulizer. However, development of this route of administration awaits further refinement to render it practical as an alternative to other routes of administration for use by non-pain specialists.

Intranasal Route

Intranasal drug delivery has the advantage of rapid absorption. Therefore, therapeutic blood levels are achieved rapidly second only to intravenous administration. Intranasal fentanyl has been found effective for postoperative analgesia and surgical premedication in adults. However, evaluation of the effectiveness of this method of delivery has not been sufficient. Further studies of this route for breakthrough pain are warranted. The only product currently available for intranasal instillation is butorphanol (Stadol), but this agonist-antagonist is not recommended for chronic pain.

Invasive Routes Requiring Specially Trained Experts

Generally, invasive routes of opioid administration are employed for reasons of practicality and convenience rather than because they offer superior methods of pain relief. Affected patients may be unable to receive a drug in a simpler manner, or administering the required dose may be easier by an invasive technique rather than noninvasively. Devices for administering drugs by such routes range in sophistication from a simple syringe-driver administering a drug subcutaneously to a totally implanted, computer-programmable infusion pump system administering a drug via an intraspinal catheter. However, controlled studies of indications for use of these sophisticated techniques are not available, and pain control experts do not agree as to when a specific technique is indicated. An important consideration in the use of these techniques is that as the degree of sophistication increases, so does the level of expertise required of the caregiver and the support staff responsible for administering and supervising the technique. Invasive techniques have been demonstrated to be appropriate for only 20% of cancer patients with pain [5].

ADVANCING ANALGESIC THERAPY WITH POTENT OPIOIDS

When pain intensity increases and pain diffuses throughout the body, only the most potent opioids can control the pain. The decision to advance pain therapy by switching to a more potent opioid and thereby escalating the dose as necessary is associated with a feeling of trepidation on the part of most physicians. The most likely reasons for this trepidation are concern about side effects, about patients' development of tolerance, about creation of an "addict," and about sanctions by regulatory authorities, as well as a misconception about a ceiling effect. This trepidation has led physicians to delay or reserve the use of potent and effective opioids until the terminal phase of patients' illness [44]. Obviously, pain of such severity that it can be relieved only by opioids is an indication for their use regardless of whether the pain occurs in the early (or localized) stage of the disease or in its advanced stage. Frequently, polypharmacologic prescription of analgesic drugs using weak opioids singly or in combination with nonopioid analgesics is practiced far beyond the point of the drugs' usefulness. An additional consideration is the inconvenience and unpleasantness of taking a large number of pills rather than only a few pills. Thus, physicians should set aside their fears and prescribe opioids whenever they are needed for adequate alleviation of pain.

The decision to initiate opioid therapy for pain should be made in either of two circumstances: The intensity of initial pain obviously calls for potent opioids to relieve it, or nonopioid and less potent opioid analgesics no longer are capable of relieving pain intensity as it increases during disease progression. In the first circumstance, the decision to initiate opioid analgesics should be made easily because of the obvious intensity of the pain and the imperative to relieve it. In the second circumstance, the decision is less obvious because of the evolving and sometimes subtle nature of pain increase.

A maxim of pain treatment with opioids is to begin with the weakest opioid having analgesic properties sufficient to relieve pain, thereby minimizing the possibility of undesirable side effects. Ongoing reassessment of pain relief is the most reliable procedure for determining when an opioid should be started. A weak opioid, as defined in Table 33.6, may be used alone or in combination with a nonopioid analgesic. Again, ongoing reassessment will indicate when the drug no longer is effective. A clue that pain intensity is increasing or that tolerance is developing is a decrease in the effectiveness interval of a single dose of a medication. Most opioids are effective for 3 to 4 hours. If pain is controlled for only 2 to 2.5 hours, an increased dose or a change to a more potent opioid is indicated.

Often, reluctance to begin prescribing potent opioids results in increasing the number of dose-units of a weak opioid or nonopioid analgesic combination. The limiting factor in increasing an opioid dose in a combination opioid and nonopioid analgesic (usually acetaminophen or an NSAID) is the amount of nonopioid present. Increasing the number of dose-units to increase the dosage of the opioid eventually will increase the nonopioid portion to toxic levels. Potent opioids alone should be started long before toxic levels of the nonopioid are reached.

Frequently, opioid therapy is delayed for patients with a possible long-term painful prognosis because of concerns about tolerance and physical and psychological dependency (addiction). Prognosis and survival time should not be determining factors for initiating opioid therapy. Similarly, tolerance and physical dependence should not be deterrents to possible long-term use. Clinical experience with cancer patients indicates that tolerance may not occur or can be managed simply by increasing the opioid dose. Physical dependence on opioids is a normal and expected pharmacologic phenomenon with a sole consequence of withdrawal reaction if opioids are discontinued abruptly—a process that can be avoided simply by decreasing the dosage gradually as pain intensity decreases. Psychological dependency seldom occurs when opioids are used for legitimate medical purposes [45]. Therefore, the possibility of opioid addiction in cancer patients is remote. No logical reason supports the postponement of opioid use because of the fear of tolerance, physical dependency, and psychological dependency.

SPECIFIC OPIOIDS

Once the decision has been made to use an opioid, the appropriate agent must be chosen. That selection depends on pain intensity. Mild to moderate pain requires only weak opioids, whereas severe pain requires potent opioids.

Weak Opioids
Propoxyphene
Propoxyphene is one of the four stereoisomers of methadone and the only one that has analgesic activity. Given orally, its analgesic potency is approximately half to two-thirds that of codeine. Studies are in conflict as to whether this drug is more effective than appropriate doses of aspirin, other NSAIDs, or acetaminophen. Nonetheless, trying propoxyphene in patients with mild pain is useful. However, it should not necessarily be considered a step up the analgesic ladder for those patients whose pain no longer is relieved by aspirin or acetaminophen, notwithstanding the fact that technically it is an opioid.

Codeine
Codeine, the opioid probably used most widely for treating cancer pain, is effective in controlling mild pain. Frequently, it is combined with either aspirin or acetaminophen, a combination that produces a synergistic analgesic effect. Continuing the use of codeine, either alone or in combination, after it no longer is adequate to relieve pain is a common practice because of reluctance to prescribe a more potent opioid.

Hydrocodone
Hydrocodone is used extensively in antitussive compounds. It is used also in fixed combination with acetaminophen and NSAIDs for the treatment of mild to moderate pain; it is not available as a separate analgesic. No studies are available comparing hydrocodone's potency with that of other analgesics. Generally, it is considered weaker than the combination oxycodone products. A particular precaution for fixed-combination hydrocodone products is that some of them contain as much as 650 to 750 mg of acetaminophen (Anexsia 7.5/650; Vicodin ES®) in a single tablet, and toxic doses of acetaminophen will be reached more quickly if the number of tablets is increased or the interval of administration is decreased to avoid use of a more potent opioid.

Potent Opioids
Morphine
Morphine is the prototype for potent opioids because it is the opioid used most widely worldwide and it has been studied more extensively than any other opioid. Consequently, more clinical experience and more investigational data are available for this agent than for other opioids. However, despite this wealth of experience and data, probably more myths and misconceptions circulate about morphine than about any other opioid [46].

Hydromorphone
Hydromorphone is absorbed readily from the GI tract and will control severe pain when given orally. It is more potent by weight than is morphine, with 1.3 mg of hydromorphone being equianalgesic to 10 mg of morphine given intramuscularly. Because of biotransformation in the liver (first-pass effect), the oral dose of hydromorphone must be four to five times the parenteral dose to produce an equianalgesic effect (see Table 33.7) When given orally, hydromorphone reaches its peak effect slightly more rapidly than does morphine and also has a slightly shorter duration of action. Ad-

ministration of hydromorphone at 3-hour intervals may be necessary.

Oxycodone

Until recently, oxycodone was not available in the United States except in combination with either aspirin or acetaminophen (Percodan®, Percocet®, Tylox®). Oxycodone is now available separately as a 5-mg tablet, as a liquid (1 mg/ml and 20 mg/ml), and as a controlled-release product of 10, 20, 40, and 80 mg. It is useful for moderate to severe pain and for alleviating concerns about reaching toxic levels of nonnarcotics with escalating doses of combination products.

Initially, oxycodone was classified as a weak opioid. However, more recent evidence suggests a potency similar to that of morphine, probably on the basis of the increased bioavailability of oxycodone as compared to morphine [47]. The equianalgesic dose is 15 to 20 mg of oral oxycodone to 30 mg of morphine (see Table 33.7). Controlled-release oxycodone preparations are as efficacious as similar formulations of morphine in the treatment of chronic pain of both malignant and nonmalignant origin. Patient compliance also is improved with the controlled-release product, because frequent dosing is obviated.

Fentanyl

Fentanyl is a potent agonist opioid. It is approximately 100 times more potent than morphine by weight. Recently, it was introduced as an analgesic for the treatment of chronic pain. Previously, its major use was as a general anesthetic agent. Since its introduction as a treatment of chronic pain, considerable experience has accumulated for its use.

Some pharmacologic characteristics of the drug shed light on its usefulness for relieving chronic pain. In single intravenous doses, its duration of analgesia is 30 to 60 minutes. However, because its use for chronic pain control is confined to transdermal administration, this pharmacodynamic information is irrelevant; the transdermal system delivers the drug continuously until the system is exhausted. The transdermal route is analogous to an intravenous infusion. In the majority of patients, the system is effective for 72 hours but, in some, it is effective for only 48 hours.

With the transdermal system, the prescribed concentration of fentanyl in the blood is not reached for 12 or more hours after initiation of therapy. Therefore, doses of a rapidly acting opioid agonist must be given, whether transmucosally, orally, rectally, or parenterally, during the first 12 or more hours so as to provide adequate pain control while fentanyl reaches its prescribed concentration. If affected patients experience an adverse drug effect during the course of treatment and the drug is discontinued, they must be monitored for up to 24 hours after discontinuation of fentanyl, because the drug is stored in subcutaneous fat and a 50% decline in the serum concentration of fentanyl may take 17 or more hours.

It is preferable to initiate chronic pain treatment with a short-acting agonist until a dose of that agent is established that controls the pain, then to convert from that drug to an equianalgesic dose of transdermal fentanyl. Initiating and titrating with transdermal fentanyl may be difficult because of the duration of delivery by the system.

Methadone

Methadone is as potent an analgesic as is morphine in comparable doses when administered intramuscularly. However, because of its favorable oral-to-parenteral ratio of 2:1 (a slighter first-pass effect), the equianalgesic oral dose must be only twice the parenteral dose. The most important clinical consideration in the use of methadone is its long half-life. Although the duration of analgesic effectiveness of single oral doses is approximately four hours, the drug's terminal elimination half-life varies from 13 to 51 hours. When repeated doses are given every four hours, the drug accumulates, and the blood concentration may reach toxic levels. Initial dosing must be administered carefully to avoid this complication. After the first three to four days, the interval of administration can be extended, effectively reducing the total 24-hour dosage while maintaining the same analgesic level. Methadone may be effective when administered every 6 to 12 hours.

Controlling pain with methadone may be difficult in older patients and in cancer patients whose disease is progressing rapidly and who experience frequent changes in pain level. Also, some patients associate methadone with the treatment of heroin (or other) drug addiction and fear that taking methadone will stigmatize them as being drug addicts.

Levorphanol

Levorphanol can be used orally to control severe pain. It is absorbed readily from the GI tract and has a favorable oral-to-parenteral ratio of approximately 1:1. The drug has a half-life of approximately 11 hours; therefore, some accumulation occurs, and dosing intervals of longer than 4 hours may be possible.

Meperidine

Although used extensively for postoperative pain, meperidine is not recommended for the treatment of chronic pain. It is absorbed readily from the GI tract, but it has an unfavorable oral-to-parenteral ratio of 4:1. A 75- to 100-mg dose of meperidine is equianalgesic to a 10-mg dose of morphine when given intramuscularly. When given orally, 300 mg is equianalgesic to 30 mg of morphine. Meperidine's duration of action is three hours or less, rendering frequent dosing necessary.

The most serious drawback to the chronic administration of meperidine is the accumulation of the metabolite normeperidine. Its half-life is longer than that of the parent meperidine. Normeperidine is a CNS stimulant and may cause tremors, muscle twitches, and seizures. Toxicity is more likely to occur in the presence of renal failure.

MIXED AGONISTS-ANTAGONISTS AND PARTIAL AGONISTS

Opioids with mixed agonist-antagonist activity and partial agonists are not recommended for the treatment of chronic cancer pain. The incidence of psychotomimetic reactions is higher than with the pure agonists [48], and only pentazocine is available for oral administration in the United States. Additionally, patients should not be switched abruptly from or tapered off a pure agonist to an agonist-antagonist or a partial agonist because of the potential for precipitating a withdrawal reaction. The partial agonist buprenorphine also will precipitate a withdrawal reaction in patients who are tolerant to morphinelike agonists, and the respiratory depression caused by this drug is not reversed easily by naloxone [49].

Newer Analgesics with Varying Modes of Action

TRAMADOL

Tramadol (Ultram®) is a relatively new analgesic with a complex mode of action. It has weak opioid activity at the mu opioid receptor, and it also activates alpha$_2$ receptors. Analgesic activity stems from its antidepressant-like ability to inhibit serotonin and norepinephrine reuptake at the synaptic level. It appears to have very little tolerance or dependency liability. Currently, tramadol is available only in oral form in the United States. The side effect profile includes seizures (especially in patients concomitantly treated with antidepressants), dizziness, dry mouth, sedation, nausea, and vomiting.

Tramadol for relief of cancer pain was found in studies to be as effective as morphine in the treatment of mild to moderate pain. However, tramadol does not appear to be very effective in the treatment of pain of neuropathic origin. For that reason, tramadol appears to have a limited place in the routine treatment of cancer pain. A specialized application would serve for those patients who have moderate pain but in whom conventional opioids are not tolerated well.

TOPICAL CAPSAICIN ANALOGS

Topical capsaicin analog compounds have been used for centuries to relieve pain. Capsaicin is the active ingredient in a variety of peppers or paprika. It acts on specific nociceptive neurons, expressing the recently cloned capsaicin receptor. Initially causing pain owing to the enhanced release of substance P from the neuron, repetitive use of the compound depletes sensory neurons of substance P, providing useful analgesia. Normal sensory thresholds do not appear to be altered with chronic use. This compound has been effective in postherpetic neuralgia, diabetic neuropathy, postmastectomy pain, and even cluster headaches [50, 51]. Better characterization of the structural and functional characteristics of the capsaicin receptor undoubtedly will lead to an increase in currently available treatment options.

N-METHYL-D-ASPARTATE RECEPTOR ANTAGONISTS

Strong evidence indicates that the strange, painful sensations associated with neuropathic pain originate in damaged somatosensory afferent axons. A nerve can be damaged by any trauma (e.g., cutting, as in surgery, and injury from irradiation, chemotherapy, or other therapy). Nerve damage does not imply negligence on the part of health care providers. All damaged afferent axons begin to discharge spontaneously—that is, no external stimulus is required to activate them. This discharge gives rise to abnormal, spontaneous sensations experienced by affected patients. In response to this action, C fibers in the nerve (C-fiber nociceptors) release glutamate, an amino acid that sensitizes the postsynaptic cell to respond more strongly to all its inputs [52]. The glutamate effects this change by binding to N-methyl-D-aspartate (NMDA) receptors. NMDA antagonists can prevent this reaction, thus preventing the occurrence of pain by this mechanism.

Clinically, the NMDA antagonists ketamine and dextromethorphan have been used to treat chronic pain. Ketamine's effectiveness has been limited by psychotomimetic side effects, whereas dextromethorphan has limited efficacy as an NMDA receptor antagonist. One possible strategy for the use of ketamine is in extremely low dose infusions (1–3 mg/kg/day). This use may limit psychiatric side effects and may permit some adjuvant function. Notably, NMDA receptor antagonists have been shown also to inhibit the development of opioid tolerance and dependence [52]. Thus, these compounds could have value both as adjuvant analgesics and as compounds that prolong the analgesic effectiveness of opioids in patients with cancer pain. The development and application of NMDA antagonists with improved potency and fewer side effects (e.g., memantine) eventually should enable us to realize the full potential of this class of adjuvants.

ALPHA₂-RECEPTOR AGONISTS

A particularly exciting area of adjuvant pain control has been the clinical development of alpha₂-receptor agonists. These compounds work synergistically with opioids to provide pain relief. Alpha₂ agonists produce analgesia by actions at presynaptic (and possibly postsynaptic) spinal sites and have other central modes of action. Clonidine is the alpha₂ agonist used most commonly. It has been administered intrathecally and epidurally and now is available for transdermal patch administration. Clonidine has been shown to provide satisfactory analgesia for extended periods in cancer patients tolerant to opioids. However, animal studies suggest that the possibility for cross-tolerance between opioids and alpha₂ agonists does exist. Commonly observed side effects of clonidine therapy are hypotension, bradycardia, and sedation. More selective and potent alpha₂ drugs are being tested in the hope of diminishing these side effects. In patients who can tolerate the side effects, an alpha₂ agonist should be considered in the course of treating refractory chronic pain.

Adjuvant Drugs and Coanalgesics

Adjuvant drugs and coanalgesics are those agents that exhibit a primary pharmacologic action other than analgesia but that, in special situations, also have analgesic properties, enhance the pain-relieving properties of primary analgesics, or indirectly contribute to the overall relief of pain. This definition is broad and might be considered so broad as to include almost all categories of drugs. The terms *adjuvant* and *coanalgesic* are arbitrary when used in this context. Although reports of beneficial use of these drugs often are provocative [41], the specific indications for their use can be confusing. Practitioners treating pain patients recognize that drugs other than primary analgesics are useful in treating pain, and they use them empirically. For practical purposes, the categories of drugs that fit the definition provided and that seem to produce the most useful results are antidepressants, antiepileptics, oral local anesthetics, corticosteroids, and CNS stimulants.

ANTIDEPRESSANTS

Tricyclic Antidepressants

Tricyclic antidepressants are reported to be useful in a variety of neuropathic painful conditions of both malignant and nonmalignant origin [53, 54]. Because pain associated with cancer frequently includes pain secondary to nerve damage (neuropathic pain), treatment of pain of any origin using these drugs as adjuvants with either nonopioid or opioid analgesics is justified, as long as their use is not contraindicated. The group of first-generation antidepressant agents has been demonstrated to be more effective in treating neuropathic pain than are later generations of these drugs [54].

The dose required for treatment of neuropathic pain is much lower than that required for the treatment of depression. Initiating therapy with a small dose is advisable. For example, in patients younger than age 40, a single, daily dose of 25 mg of amitriptyline given close to 9:00 PM usually is tolerated. For patients older than 40, the advisable single daily dose is 10 mg given at the same time of day. Once this dose is determined to be tolerated, incremental increases in the dose—usually every other day—can be made. Should unacceptable side effects be experienced with the increased dose, it should be scaled back to the previous dose. If one tricyclic antidepressant is not tolerated, another drug in this class should be tried.

A favorable side effect of these drugs is their sedative action secondary to improvement in the sleep pattern. Usually, patients experience this benefit immediately, whereas the beneficial effect on the pain may be delayed by a variable period after onset of therapy. However, the beneficial effect of these drugs on neuropathic pain usually occurs prior to the time required for them to influence depression. The watchword for use of these drugs in patients with neuropathic pain is *patience*.

Selective Serotonin Reuptake Inhibitors

The new class of antidepressants known as *selective serotonin reuptake inhibitors* (SSRIs) initially held the promise of providing analgesia similar to that seen with tricyclic antidepressants, though with a much reduced incidence of side effects. However, results using these compounds have been mixed. Adequate analgesia has been reported in cases of mixed chronic pain syndromes and rheumatoid disease. However, results in the treatment of headache, diabetic neuropathy, and fibromyalgia have been disappointing. In some circumstances, SSRIs may be effective, but the reduced cost, wider efficacy, and greater clinical experience with the tricyclic agents still support use of the latter in chronic pain states.

ANTIEPILEPTICS

Antiepileptic drugs have proved useful in treating patients with neuropathic pain, especially those who experience a sharp, shooting, or lancinating pain component. However, the drugs may be effective also in treating patients who have neuropathic pain without this characteristic. These agents' effectiveness has been demonstrated in a wide variety of clinical pain states, and empiric trials with them are justified for all patients who experience neuropathic pain [55]. As with the use of antidepressants, antiepileptics should be given at a low starting dosage and gradually should be increased to the therapeutic ranges used in treatment of convulsive disorders. Carbamazepine, phenytoin, valproate, and clonazepam are antiepileptics currently used for treating this type of pain. Blood levels of carbamazepine and phenytoin should be monitored at regular intervals to prevent toxicity from these drugs.

Recently, gabapentin (Neurontin®) was approved and released as an antiepileptic compound. As have other antiepileptics, it has demonstrated usefulness in the management of chronic pain, especially neuropathic pain. Gabapentin may act by regulating postsynaptic glutamate receptors or by augmenting gamma-aminobutyric acid function indirectly. Studies have demonstrated the efficacy of gabapentin in treating neuropathic pain of peripheral origin, although results in treating central pain syndromes are controversial [56]. The advantage of gabapentin lies in its more favorable side effect profile as compared to that of tricyclic antidepressants or other antiepileptic medications. This drug should be considered early in the course of cancer pain treatment, after conventional opioid ladder therapy has failed to produce optimum pain relief, or in cases in which a significant neuropathic component is suspected. Gabapentin should also be used in patients who may not tolerate the side effects of conventional antidepressants or antiepileptics.

ORAL LOCAL ANESTHETICS

Mexiletine, an orally active antiarrhythmic agent structurally similar to lidocaine, has been effective in the treatment of neuropathic pain in certain patients. Its use should be considered only after adequate trials with combined antidepressant and antiepileptic drugs have failed to produce the desired results. Clinically, mexiletine usually is not considered an agent to supplant the aforementioned two categories of drugs but instead usually is given in addition to them.

CORTICOSTEROIDS

Clinical experience with corticosteroids has proved them to be useful in treating the pain associated with bone metastasis and tumor infiltration of neural structures. When corticosteroids are effective, pain relief usually is dramatic. Any corticosteroid may be used, but dexamethasone is the common choice because of its minimal effect on electrolytes and other metabolic functions. Usually, a dose of 16 mg/day given in divided oral doses is effective. Short-term use is preferable because of the potential metabolic side effects but, in some patients, long-term use with vigorous treatment of the side effects may be necessary. Other side effects of corticosteroids that may occur but are beneficial to the patient are increased appetite and an improved sense of well-being.

CNS STIMULANTS

Low-dose dextroamphetamine and methylphenidate are useful in counteracting the sedative effects of opioids and other CNS depressants used to treat pain and other distressing symptoms of advanced cancer. These drugs should be administered in the early morning and again around noon only if necessary. Administering them after noon may interfere with a patient's sleeping at night. Alleviating sedation may allow the opioid dose to be increased, thereby alleviating more pain.

METHOTRIMEPRAZINE

Methotrimeprazine is the only phenothiazine that has demonstrated analgesic properties. Originally, it was useful in patients who had pain and suffered anxiety and agitation. It no longer is available in the United States.

USEFUL PAIN MANAGEMENT STRATEGIES

Avoiding Unnecessary Polypharmacy

Prescribing multiple opioids with identical mechanisms of action and choosing multiple opioids with no discernible pharmacokinetic or pharmacodynamic rationale have become traditions for physicians using potent opioids. This unfocused and unnecessary use of multiple opioids for pain treatment serves no useful purpose and is confusing to affected patients. However, if opioids are combined to take advantage of pharmacologic differences in specific agents (e.g., differences in duration of effect), such combination is justified and desirable.

An example of needless polypharmacy is combining opioids having a similar duration of action (e.g., morphine and hydromorphone)—and even additional similar opioids—in their usual or recommended doses to control increasingly intense pain, in lieu of escalating the dose of a single drug as necessary. Strategies of this type probably developed because of physicians' fear of sanction by government disciplinary and regulatory agencies. Physicians should resist this fear and prescribe opioids (preferably a single drug in an appropriate dose) in a simple manner that is not confusing to their patients.

Justified Opioid Combination

Combining opioids can be useful, and indeed desirable, if doing so is based on sound principles of these agents' use (e.g., combining opioids with long and short half-lives). Opioids with long half-lives are desirable because they can be administered at longer intervals (e.g., every six hours), thus requiring fewer doses during a 24-hour interval. This approach is a convenience to affected patients and has a positive psychological effect because patients are less frequently reminded of their infirmity. However, additional pain that may occur during the interval between doses of the agent may require supplemental opioid. A short-acting drug can fill this need. In this way, consistent pain relief is achieved by combining two opioids.

However, managing a therapeutic regimen of opioids with long half-lives is difficult in patients whose pain intensity changes frequently, because of the lag in achieving pain relief after a dose is changed. If such a regimen is inadequately managed, the long half-life of the prescribed drug eventually causes oversedation. This problem is especially prevalent in the elderly. Development of controlled-release morphine and oxycodone obviated problems associated with combining drugs having long and short half-lives. Prolonged effectiveness of controlled-release products is a result of the slow release of the drug over a 12- to 24-hour period, rather than a result of the drug's long half-life. Frequently, adequate pain control can be achieved using the controlled-release regimen alone. Should breakthrough pain occur during the expected control interval, it can be treated with an immediate-release opioid. Use of a combination of controlled- and immediate-release opioids can permit a treatment regimen analogous to that used in treating an insulin-dependent diabetic with long- and short-acting insulin.

The first consideration in devising such a treatment regimen is to determine the amount of immediate-release opioid necessary to control the patient's pain over a 24-hour period. This 24-hour dosage is determined by multiplying (1) the single dose of an immediate-release opioid necessary to maintain pain control for a specified time period by (2) the total number of doses required to maintain a pain-free state during a 24-hour period. For example, if a patient requires 60 mg of immediate-release opioid to relieve pain effectively for 4 hours, the dosage for a 24-hour period would be $6 \times 60 = 360$ mg. This 24-hour dosage will be the amount of controlled-release opioid that will be administered in once- or twice-daily doses. In the example cited, 180 mg is administered every 12 hours or 360 mg is administered every 24 hours. If pain is controlled with the controlled-release opioid, no additional pain medication will be required. However, immediate-release opioids always are prescribed with controlled-release opioids, for use as needed should breakthrough pain occur during the specified interval (i.e., pain not alleviated by the controlled-release opioid). The breakthrough dose for adequate pain relief should be approximately one-sixth of the total daily dose of the controlled-release opioid analgesic, but it should be titrated, not determined arbitrarily.

After an affected patient begins taking a controlled-release opioid, the number of doses required to maintain pain control serves as a marker for determining when the dose should be increased. For example, for 12-hour drugs, when the number of breakthrough doses exceeds two during the daytime 12-hour interval and exceeds one during the nighttime 12-hour interval, the dosage should be increased. The dose of controlled-release opioid is increased by the amount of immediate-release opioid required to alleviate breakthrough pain. This total dose is divided into two 12-hour-interval doses. For 24-hour drugs, the dose of controlled-release agent should be increased if three breakthrough doses are necessary to maintain 24-hour control.

Any immediate-release, short-acting opioid can be used in conjunction with a controlled-release opioid (e.g., morphine) for treating breakthrough pain. Using immediate-release morphine obviates converting a breakthrough nonmorphine opioid dosage to a morphine dosage when the controlled-release morphine dose must be increased. Also, the medication process is simplified by keeping to a minimum the number of different medications given to affected patients.

The combination regimen has many advantages. First, it is convenient: Ambulatory patients can carry their medication in inconspicuous containers. Second, frequent dosing is unnecessary; therefore, patients are not obvious when taking medication. Third, pain is controlled throughout the night; thus, neither pain nor the need to take medicine interferes with sleep. Similar advantages can be achieved for 48 to 72 hours using a transdermal fentanyl system. These advantages support consideration of a combination regimen of pain management for all patients with persistent pain (Fig. 33.7).

USE OF CONSULTANTS

Frequently, patients who do not respond to simple pain control measures are considered for some type of special technique. Most often, such a technique employs a novel route of opioid administration, alone or in combination with a local anesthetic, or some type of neurostimulatory or neuroablative invasive procedure. These procedures necessitate the involvement of specially trained physicians. The criteria for using these procedures is not well established. Frequently absent is evidence that patients are unresponsive to adequate simple pain treatment. Most invasive techniques alter the pharmacokinetics of opioids, and comparison of equianalgesic doses in treatment methods is difficult. In addition, deafferentation procedures may provide temporary relief but, in the long run, more severe pain may ensue. Treatment of the late-appearing pain may be even more difficult than that for the original pain, with a significantly decreased quality of life for affected patients.

In consulting with experts, physicians responsible for long-term management of patient pain and other distressing symptoms should discuss what the outcome is likely to be and what the medical, nursing, and supportive requirements are for maintaining the contemplated system. The discussion also should include associated complications and the likelihood of repeating the procedure to correct any malfunction. An additional factor in contemplating invasive and ablative procedures is patient longevity, as some ablative procedures are effective for only a few months. If patients' expected survival is shorter than the expected effectiveness of a procedure, the procedure is indicated; however, if anticipated survival exceeds such effectiveness, undertaking the procedure is problematic, because the plasticity of the nervous system probably will cause the emergence of pain more severe than the original.

BARRIERS TO ADEQUATE PAIN CONTROL

Despite efforts to provide adequate information about specific methods of pain control, pain in cancer patients continues to be treated inadequately. As most cancer patients are likely to require opioid analgesics, the barriers to pain control relate to adequate and appropriate opioid use. Both medical and extramedical factors must be recognized and corrected if adequate pain relief is to be a reality for cancer patients.

Cultural and Societal Barriers

Prejudicial attitudes and misconceptions about the pharmacologic properties of opioids and confusion about the legitimate and illegitimate use of these drugs are thoroughly ingrained in our culture. Changing culturally rooted societal behavior, including that of health care professionals, is difficult. It is no less difficult in the case both of health care providers' behavior regarding the prescription, dispensing, and administration of opioids and, in many instances, patients' willingness to accept them. Behavior validated by a culture becomes instinctive, and deviating from it through a volitional decision can produce anxiety and perhaps a sense of betrayal of the culture in those who decide to do so. The undertreatment of pain with opioids seems to have attained this position.

Unquestionably, the intent and desire of the majority of health care professionals is to relieve pain in their patients. A resolve to do so necessitates departing from certain instinctive behaviors and making a volitional, reasoned decision to prescribe opioids on the basis of

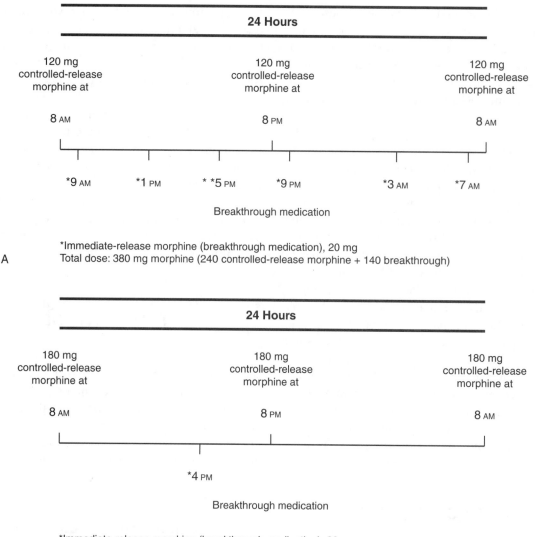

Figure 33.7 Illustration of treatment program using a combination of controlled-release and immediate-release morphine. (A) Patient in this model is receiving inadequate doses of controlled-release morphine and so requires multiple doses of breakthrough medication over 24 hours. (B) Patient in this model is receiving an adequate dose of controlled-release morphine and so requires only an occasional dose of breakthrough medication over 24 hours. This patient can sleep through the night without interruption because of pain.

scientific principles. Emphasis must be placed on outcome, not process.

Emphasis on process focuses on the treatment modality used by health care professionals (fairly frequently, on the provider's training). For example, an interventionist trained in nerve blocks will tend to persist in using that method regardless of whether it provides adequate pain relief for a significant period. A behaviorist likewise uses certain techniques specific to behavioral science, techniques that may or may not be effective. If treatment methods fail, patients sometimes are blamed

for the failure, accused of not being diligent in applying the techniques. In some cases, practitioners are evangelical about their methods and emotionally denounce other methods of treatment. This attitude is especially true for those with a bias against opioids (termed *opiophobia* by Morgan [57]). Emphasis on outcome focuses on pain relief as the end result. The process of achieving it is not paramount, provided safety standards are maintained, side effects are acceptable, and function and quality of life are improved.

Cultural and societal barriers are found also in affected patients, their families, and their friends. These barriers stem primarily from their confusion about opioids: a failure to understand the difference between *patients* taking opioids for a legitimate medical purpose and *individuals* abusing them for nonmedical purposes. Health care providers should work with patients to ensure their understanding of this distinction so that they no longer are confused but feel comfortable taking opioids for relief.

The demonstrated slow pace in improving pain relief may require educating affected patients, their families, and their friends to demand better pain relief. These individuals should be empowered to know that poor pain relief is unacceptable and that they can demand that it be adequate [58].

Knowledge Deficits

Persistent knowledge deficits among health care providers result from a prevailing unawareness of new knowledge of opioid pharmacology gleaned from studies of pain treatment with long-term opioids in cancer patients. Information about dosing with opioids, initially incorporated in most pharmacology textbooks, was obtained in early, single-dose studies that used as the pain model patients with postoperative pain [39]. In general, postoperative pain is less severe than is the chronic pain of cancer and other medical conditions. Recent studies of cancer patients treated with long-term opioids has provided a new body of knowledge of opioid use for pain relief. Studies of other pharmacodynamic effects of opioids (e.g., tolerance and respiratory depression) were performed with volunteers having no symptoms. These individuals were opioid-naive and, in the absence of symptoms, the pharmacodynamics were fairly different from those in symptomatic patients.

Now that modern treatment has extended cancer patients' lives, many patients experience chronic pain of varying severity and duration; thus, they serve as a new model for studying opioid pharmacology. Several salient facts have emerged:

- Pain is a natural "antagonist" to the analgesic effects of opioids; therefore, adequate doses (in many cases seemingly high) must be used to overcome this effect.
- Pain similarly "antagonizes" respiratory depression; therefore, respiratory depression is not a deterrent to choosing an adequate dose of opioid to relieve pain.

- Psychological dependence (addiction) on opioids seldom occurs in patients taking opioids for their legitimate pain-relieving qualities.
- No ceiling effect limits dosing with opioids for patients with nociceptive pain. Each incremental dose increase triggers an appropriate increase in pain relief.

This knowledge provides a scientific basis for prescribing opioids.

Regulatory Barriers

State licensing and disciplinary boards and state and federal drug enforcement agencies continue practices that deter physicians—and pharmacists—from prescribing opioids adequately. Therefore, physicians, pharmacists, health care professionals, and government officials should work to establish proper guidelines to govern opioid use, so that all involved clearly understand what the standard of practice is. The goals should be availability of adequate opioids for patients who legitimately need them and prevention of illegal use.

Over the last five years, significant progress has been made in removing real or perceived regulatory barriers and setting a clear standard of practice for opioid use. This progress includes intractable-pain treatment acts and rules that govern the use of opioids for treating pain from both malignant and nonmalignant origins. However, because health care professionals still are largely unaware of these efforts and remain skeptical about their protection from sanctions, an improved feeling of trust must be developed among all concerned.

REFERENCES

1. Edwards WT. Optimizing opioid treatment of postoperative pain. *J Pain Symptom Manage* 5:S24–S36, 1990.
2. Foley KM. Advances in cancer pain. *Arch Neurol* 56:413–417, 1999.
3. Marks RE, Sachar EJ. Undertreatment of medical inpatients with narcotic analgesics. *Ann Intern Med* 78:173–181, 1973.
4. Cleeland CS, Gorin R, Hatfield AK, et al. Pain and its treatment in outpatients with metastatic cancer. *N Engl J Med* 330:592–596, 1994.
5. Jacox A, Carr DB, Payne R, et al. *Management of Cancer Pain: Clinical Practice Guideline No. 9.* [AHCPR Pub. No. 94–0592.] Rockville, MD: Agency for Health Care Policy and Research, US Department of Health and Human Services, Public Health Service, 1994.

6. Hill CS Jr. Relationship among cultural, educational, and regulatory agency influences on optimum cancer pain treatment. *J Pain Symptom Manage* 5:S37–S45, 1990.

7. Ferrell BR. The impact of pain on quality of life. *Nurs Clin North Am* 30:609–624, 1995.

8. Fields HL. *Pain.* New York: McGraw-Hill, 1987:133–169.

9. Arner S, Arner B. Differential effects of epidural morphine in the treatment of cancer related pain. *Acta Anaesthesiol Scand* 29:32–36, 1985.

10. Arner S, Meyerson BA. Lack of analgesic effect of opioids on neuropathic and idiopathic forms of pain. *Pain* 33:11–23, 1988.

11. Foley KM. Pain syndromes in patients with cancer. *Med Clin North Am* 71:169–184, 1987.

12. Wong D, Whaley LF. *Clinical Handbook of Pediatric Nursing.* St Louis: Mosby, 1986.

13. Von Roenn JH, Cleeland CS, Gonin R, et al. Physician attitudes and practice in cancer pain management. A survey from the Eastern Cooperative Oncology Group. *Ann Intern Med* 119:121–126, 1993.

14. Hodes RL. Cancer patients' needs and concerns when using narcotic analgesics. In Hill CS Jr, Fields WS (eds), *Advances in Pain Research and Therapy,* vol 11. New York: Raven Press, 1989:91–99.

15. Cleeland CS. Measurement of pain by subjective report. In Chapman CR, Loeser JD (eds), *Advances in Pain Research and Therapy,* vol 12. New York: Raven Press, 1989: 391–403.

16. Nemni SR. *A psychophysical methodology for the development of measurement scales: the quantification of the qualities of cancer pain.* Unpublished doctoral dissertation, Texas Christian University, Fort Worth, TX, December 1988.

17. Serlin RC, Mendoza TR, Nakamura Y, et al. When is cancer pain mild, moderate, or severe? Grading pain severity by its interference with function. *Pain* 61:277–284, 1995.

18. Rainville P, Duncan GH, Price DD, et al. Pain affect encoded in human anterior cingulate but not somatosensory cortex. *Science* 277:968–971, 1997.

19. Portenoy RK, Payne D, Jacobsen P. Breakthrough pain: characteristics and impact in patients with cancer pain. *Pain* 81:129–134, 1999.

20. World Health Organization. *Cancer Pain Relief and Palliative Care: Report of a WHO Expert Committee.* (WHO Technical Report Series No. 804.) Geneva: World Health Organization, 1990.

21. Max MB, Payne R (eds). *Principles of Analgesic Use in the Treatment of Acute Pain and Cancer Pain* (4th ed). Glenview, IL: American Pain Society, 1999.

22. Grossman SA, Benedetti C, Payne R, Syrjala K. NCCN practice guidelines for cancer pain. *Oncology* 13:33–44, 1999.

23. World Health Organization. Cancer pain relief and palliative care. Report of a WHO expert committee. *World Health Organ Tech Rep Ser* 804: 1990.

24. Schechter NL, Berde CB, Yaster M (eds). *Pain in Infants, Children, and Adolescents.* Baltimore: Williams & Wilkins, 1993.

25. McGrath PA. *Pain in Children: Nature, Assessment, and Treatment.* New York: Guilford Press, 1990.

26. Tyler DC, Krane ES (eds). *Advances in Pain Research and Therapy,* vol 15. New York: Raven Press, 1990.

27. Vane JR, Botting RM. Mechanism of action of nonsteroidal anti-inflammatory drugs. *Am J Med* 104(3A):2S–8S, 1998.

28. Sheehan KM, Sheahan K, O'Donoghue DP, et al. The relationship between cyclooxygenase-2 and colorectal cancer. *JAMA* 282:254–257, 1999.

29. Vane JR, Bakhle YS, Botting RM. Cyclooxygenases 1 and 2. *Annu Rev Pharmacol Toxicol* 38:97–120, 1998.

30. Janjan NA, Payne R, Gillis T, et al. Presenting symptoms in patients referred to a multidisciplinary clinic for bone metastases. *J Pain Symptom Manage* 16:171–178, 1998.

31. Waldman SD, Kilbride MJ. The nonsteroidal anti-inflammatory drugs: current concepts. *Pain Digest* 2:289–294, 1992.

32. Miller LJ, Kramer MA. Pain management with intravenous ketorolac. *Ann Pharmacother* 27:307–308, 1993.

33. Stambaugh JE Jr. Role of nonsteroidal anti-inflammatory drugs. In Patt RB (ed), *Cancer Pain.* Philadelphia: Lippincott, 1993:111–114.

34. Smith MT, Watt JA, Cramond T. Morphine-3-glucuronide, a potent antagonist of morphine analgesia. *Life Sci* 47:579–585, 1990.

35. Hanks GW, Twycross RG, Lloyd JW. Unexpected complication of successful nerve block. *Anaesthesia* 36:37–39, 1981.

36. Snyder SH. Drug and neurotransmitter receptors in the brain. *Science* 224:22–31, 1984.

37. Twycross RG. The management of pain in cancer: a guide to drugs and dosages. *Oncology (Huntingt)* 2:35–44, 1988.

38. Kaiko RF, Grandy RP, Oshlack B, et al. The United States experience with oral controlled-release morphine (MS Contin Tablets). *Cancer* 63(suppl 11):2348–2354, 1989.

39. Bruera E, Ripamonti C. Adjuvants to opioid analgesics. In Patt RB (ed), *Cancer Pain.* Philadelphia: Lippincott, 1993: 143–159.

40. Perry S, Heidrich G. Management of pain during débridement: a survey of U.S. burn units. *Pain* 13:267–280, 1982.

41. Ingham JM, Foley KM. Pain and the barriers to its relief at the end of life: a lesson for improving end of life health care. *Hospice J* 13:89–100, 1998.

42. Portenoy RK, Foley KM, Inturrisi CE. The nature of opioid responsiveness and its implications for neuropathic pain: new hypotheses derived from studies of opioid infusions. *Pain* 43:273–286, 1990.

43. Portenoy RK, Payne R, Coluzzi P, et al. Oral transmucosal fentanyl citrate (OTFC) for the treatment of breakthrough pain in cancer patients: a controlled dose titration study. *Pain* 79:303–312, 1999.

44. Cleeland CS. Pain control: public and physicians' attitudes. In Hill CS, Fields WS (eds), *Advances in Pain Research and Therapy,* vol 11. New York: Raven Press, 1989:81–89.

45. Porter J, Jick H. Addiction rare in patients treated with narcotics (letter). *N Engl J Med* 302:123, 1980.

46. Twycross RG, Lack SA. *Symptom Control in Far Advanced Cancer: Pain Relief.* London: Pitman Publishing, 1983.

47. Reder RF, Oshlack B, Miotto JB, et al. Steady-state bioavailability of controlled-release oxycodone in normal subjects. *Clin Ther* 18:95–105, 1996.

48. Houde RW. Analgesic effectiveness of the narcotic agonist/antagonists. *Br J Clin Pharmacol* 1(suppl 3):297s–308s, 1979.

49. Inturrisi CE. Management of cancer pain: pharmacology and principles of management. *Cancer* 63(suppl 11):2308–2320, 1989.

50. Alaberca R, Ochoa JJ. Cluster tic syndrome. *Neurology* 44:996–999, 1994.

51. Bernstein JE, Bickers DR, Dahl MV, et al. Treatment of chronic postherpetic neuralgia with topical capsaicin. *J Am Acad Dermatol* 17:93–96, 1987.

52. Mayer DJ, Mao J, Holt J, Price DD. Cellular mechanisms of neuropathic pain, morphine tolerance, and their interactions. *Proc Natl Acad Sci USA* 96:7731–7736, 1999.

53. Max MB. Treatment of post-herpetic neuralgia: antidepressants. *Ann Neurol* 35(suppl):S50–S53, 1994.

54. McQuay HJ. Pharmacological treatment of neuralgic and neuropathic pain. *Cancer Surv* 7:141–159, 1988.

55. McQuay H, Carrol LD, Jadad AR, et al. Anticonvulsant drugs for management of pain: a systemic review. *BMJ* 311:1047–1052, 1995.

56. Rowbotham M, Harden N, Stacey B, et al. Gabapentin for the treatment of postherpetic neuralgia: a randomized controlled trial. *JAMA* 280:1837–1842, 1998.

57. Morgan JP. American opiophobia: customary underutilization of opioid analgesics. In Hill CS Jr, Fields WS (eds), *Advances in Pain Research and Therapy,* vol 11. New York: Raven Press, 1989.

58. Hill CS Jr. When will adequate pain treatment be the norm? (editorial). *JAMA* 274:1881–1882, 1995.

34

Nutrition and the Cancer Patient

■ ■ ■

Marvin J. Lopez
Hassan Y. Tehrani

FREQUENTLY, MALNUTRITION AND WEIGHT LOSS accompany a new diagnosis of cancer. Despite the current multidisciplinary approach to cancer and advances in multimodality therapies, protein-calorie malnutrition remains the second most frequent diagnosis in cancer patients. Malnutrition has an impact not only on morbidity and median survival but on patients' tolerance of and response to antineoplastic therapy [1].

This chapter outlines the mechanisms and effects of cancer cachexia. It describes the methods of nutritional assessment of cancer patients and the current options available for providing optimal nutritional support.

CANCER CACHEXIA

Cancer cachexia is a syndrome characterized by anorexia, early satiety, progressive weight loss, and asthenia accompanied by depletion of adipose tissue and skeletal muscle and resulting in visceral organ atrophy [2–4]. In a study of more than 3,000 patients by DeWys et al. [1], the frequency of weight loss ranged between 31% and 87% in patients with newly diagnosed cancer prior to the initiation of chemotherapy. In addition, this study demonstrated that weight loss was associated with a decreased median survival in this group of patients, as compared with those whose weight remained stable. The consequences of cachexia in the host can be summarized as follows:

- Immunosuppression with increased susceptibility to infections
- Reduced responsiveness and tolerance to chemotherapy

We thank Sarah Boardman, BA, Valerie Goldman, MS, RD, and Karen Klein, RD, for their assistance in preparing this chapter.

- Increased incidence of perioperative complications (prolonged ileus, sepsis, poor wound healing)
- Less tolerance to radiotherapy regimens

The exact etiology of cancer cachexia has yet to be elucidated fully. It appears to be related to a combination of diminished nutrient intake and alterations in host substrate metabolism, with tumor-host competition for nutrients. Furthermore, antineoplastic modalities (e.g., chemotherapy, radiotherapy, and surgery), with their inherent side effects and complications, only add to cancer patients' malnourished state.

Diminished Nutrient Intake

Anorexia may be defined as the spontaneous, unintended decline in food intake. It is a common symptom of malignancy, occurring in 15% to 40% of patients at initial presentation. However, anorexia alone cannot account for the weight loss seen with cancer cachexia. The reasons are threefold: Measured food intake fails to correspond to the degree of weight loss, weight loss precedes the decline in food intake, and attempts to reverse cachexia by dietary counseling and increasing food intake have been unsuccessful [3–5].

Anorexia probably is due to the action of centrally mediated biochemical tumor factors and psychological factors acting in combination to reduce appetite. The biochemical factors that have been implicated include increasing circulating levels of interleukin-1 (IL-1), increased central serotoninergic activity, production of satietins, and alterations in hypothalamic neuropeptide Y receptors [6–9].

The psychological factors of anorexia involve the interplay of behavioral, emotional, and perceptual responses. The behavioral consequences include learned food aversions, changes in food preferences, and anticipatory nausea and vomiting. Emotional responses manifest as fear, depression, and anxiety, which typically are associated with a diagnosis of cancer. The perceptual responses include the presence of food, the timing of meals, self-assessment of intake, palatability of foods, and beliefs about food. The palatability of food is cognition-dependent, with multiple studies demonstrating alterations in taste sensations in cancer patients [10–12].

The primary tumor or its metastases may cause localized effects on the gastrointestinal tract. Mass effects may be intraluminal or extraluminal. Oropharyngeal and esophageal tumors may cause dysphagia or odynophagia. Compression of the stomach or duodenum may

Table 34.1 Complications of Antineoplastic Therapies Affecting the Nutritional Status of the Host

Therapy	Complications
Chemotherapy	Anorexia, nausea, vomiting, diarrhea, mucositis, hepatitis, pancreatitis
Radiotherapy	Anorexia, nausea, vomiting, diarrhea, mucositis, xerostomia, dysphagia, odynophagia, malabsorption, gastrointestinal stricture, obstruction, fistulas
Surgery	Prolonged starvation, malabsorption, complications resulting in gastrointestinal stricture, obstruction, and fistulas, fluid and electrolyte imbalances

result in nausea, early satiety, or obstruction. In the intestines, a tumor mass may cause either partial or complete obstruction. Fistulas, which may be internal or external, may arise at any point along the gastrointestinal tract as a result of local tumor effects or of antineoplastic therapies. Gastrointestinal fistulas cause diminished nutrient intake as a result of the bypassing of functional segments of bowel. Significant fluid and electrolyte imbalances may occur, particularly in high-output fistulas [13]. Tumors of the biliary tree or pancreas may diminish nutrient intake as a consequence of malabsorption due to alterations in the bile salt pool or decreased pancreatic exocrine secretions. The effects of antineoplastic therapies on nutrient intake are summarized in Table 34.1.

Altered Host Metabolism

Cancer patients experience changes in carbohydrate, lipid, and protein metabolism. In addition, they undergo alterations in fluid and electrolyte composition and in metabolic rate [14]. The complex interrelated metabolic alterations in cancer patients can be summarized as follows:

- Increased total body water, electrolyte, and mineral enzymatic alterations
- Marked gluconeogenesis, insulin resistance, glucose intolerance
- Mobilization of adipose stores, increased fatty acid oxidation
- Diminished protein synthesis, increased proteolysis, increased use of protein as substrate, tumor-host competition for amino acids, negative nitrogen balance

It is hypothesized that two pathways constitute the mechanisms by which metabolism is altered. The first pathway is mediated by tumor-produced catabolic factors (e.g., neurotensin, bombesin, and toxohormone-L). The second is mediated by the cytokine network. Among the cytokines implicated are IL-1, IL-6, interferon gamma, tumor necrosis factor–alpha (TNF-α), and leukemia inhibitory factor [14–17].

In the chronic fasting state, adipose tissue becomes the body's primary fuel source, with released free fatty acids being converted for use as ketone bodies. This process results in conservation of muscle mass. In this state, basal energy expenditures (BEEs) are reduced [4]. However, in the cancer patient, loss of adipose tissue and muscle mass occurs in equal amounts. Cancer patients may have reduced, normal, or increased resting metabolic rates. Changes in metabolic rates are highly variable. They depend not only on tumor type (with solid gastrointestinal tumors tending toward higher metabolic rates) but on the tumor stage along the time continuum and, finally, on the therapeutic approaches applied against it. Interestingly, tumor burden or evidence of spread does not appear to be a factor in metabolic rate change [14, 18–20].

CARBOHYDRATE METABOLISM

In cancer patients, the changes seen in carbohydrate metabolism are an increase in glucose production and development of insulin resistance. Combined, they tend toward a state of glucose intolerance [21, 22]. Tumor cells may act as a glucose drain; they are able to metabolize glucose at high rates and are critically dependent on glycolytic pathways for more than 50% of their energy requirements. Particularly important in this process is the mitochondria-based hexokinase type II enzyme, which has been shown to be expressed in higher levels in tumor cells versus normal cells [23]. Other significant pathways for glucose production are an increase in Cori cycle activity and an increase in hepatic glucose production, mediated by lipid-mobilizing factor, which acts to stimulate adenylate cyclase in a guanosine triphosphate–dependent manner [24].

LIPID METABOLISM

Cancer patients manifest the changes in lipid metabolism by mobilization of adipose stores, with a concomitant increase in fatty acid oxidation [25]. The presence of lipolysis-promoting activity factors has been demonstrated in the sera of cancer-bearing patients. These factors induce lipolysis by the activation of protein kinase, which in turn converts hormone-sensitive lipase from its inactive to its active form via phosphorylation. The tumor itself may be the ultimate benefactor of free fatty acids: They may act as a substrate for augmenting tumor growth, increasing the cells' mitotic rate by inhibiting guanosine triphosphatase–activating protein [26, 27].

PROTEIN METABOLISM

In uncomplicated starvation, adipose tissue predominates as the fuel source, resulting in sparing of muscle protein. Cancer patients, however, experience a proportionately greater use of protein as substrate, with tumor-host competition for amino acids. Cancer-bearing hosts demonstrate a decrease in skeletal muscle protein synthesis and an increase in proteolysis, leading to a net negative nitrogen balance [28]. Evidence implicating IL-1, IL-6, and TNF-α as signals for proteolysis, either singly or in combination, remains controversial [29]. Animal studies, however, have demonstrated that protein degradation is associated with significant elevations in prostaglandin E_2 production. Other demonstrated mechanisms of proteolysis are extralysosomal adenosine triphosphate and ubiquitin-dependent proteases [30, 31].

Pharmacologic Treatment of Cancer Cachexia

The pharmacologic agents available to treat cancer cachexia can be divided into three different classes, according to their mechanisms of action. The first group includes megestrol acetate and medroxyprogesterone acetate. These agents are synthetic derivatives of the naturally occurring hormone progesterone. Both have appetite-stimulating properties and anabolic effects. The weight gain seen in cancer patients is due primarily to an increase in adipose tissue, with a lesser amount of weight gain accruing from an increase in body fluid but no gain in lean muscle mass. Traditionally, megestrol acetate has been used in the treatment of advanced breast and endometrial cancers. An observed side effect seen in patients with these disorders was an improvement in appetite and weight gain. Subsequent trials in nonhormonally sensitive cancer patients have demonstrated the effectiveness of this agent, starting at 160 mg/day in divided doses. Most responses occur within 2 weeks. Higher doses may be needed in initial nonresponders: One study found the optimal dose to be 800 mg/day [32, 33]. Side effects are infrequent and dose-dependent and include deep venous thrombosis, diarrhea, rash, and impotence. Traditionally, medroxy-progesterone acetate has been used also in the treatment of advanced breast and uterine cancers. The effective dose that has been shown to improve appetite and to increase weight gain is 1,000 mg/day in divided doses [34, 35]. Side effects include deep venous thrombosis, rash, and changes in menstrual flow.

In the second group is delta-9-tetrahydrocannabinol, a naturally occurring extract from *Cannabis sativa* (marijuana), commercially known as Dronabinol. This acts to increase appetite and also decreases nausea and vomiting associated with cancer chemotherapy [36]. Doses range from 2.5 to 20 mg/day. Initial starting doses are 2.5 mg administered orally twice daily (before lunch and dinner). Predictable side effects are central nervous system–related, including euphoria, dizziness, and confusion.

The third group of agents, still experimental, are those that act directly to oppose the cachexia-promoting effects of tumors. Two of these agents are eicosapentaenoic acid (EPA) and lentinan. EPA is a polyunsaturated fatty acid found in fish oil. In multiple animal studies, a diet supplemented with EPA has been found to reverse cachexia, an outcome demonstrated also in a small human trial in patients with advanced pancreatic cancer. The mechanism of action of EPA is believed to be inhibition of cyclic adenosine monophosphate elevation in adipocytes in response to lipid-mobilizing factor and inhibition of a rise in muscle protein prostaglandin E_2, preventing protein degradation [37–39]. Lentinan is a β-glucan derived from the mushroom *Lentinus edodes*. Although no human trials exist, Tamura et al. [40] have produced promising results in the reversal of cancer-induced cachexia in rats, thought to be mediated by the anti-TNF actions of lentinan.

In summary, the exact pathways by which cancer patients become cachectic remain to be defined. However, on the basis of the foregoing discussion, several metabolic mechanisms have been clarified. Although medications for controlling the symptoms of cancer-related anorexia are in widespread use, the development of agents designed specifically to block the cachexia pathways still is in its infancy.

NUTRITIONAL ASSESSMENT

Nutritional assessment of cancer patients includes the evaluation of their medical history, physical examination, anthropometric measurements, and laboratory data. The goal of assessment is to formulate a strategy so that any necessary, appropriate nutritional intervention can be implemented. The history should detail weight loss, food intake patterns, symptomatology, medical and surgical history, current medications, and psychosocial factors. Physical examination includes the accurate measurement of height and weight, assessment of fat and muscle wasting, assessment of skin integrity, and elucidation of signs of specific nutrient deficiency (e.g., syndromes of vitamin and trace element deficits) [41].

The anthropometric measurements of triceps and subscapular skin-fold thickness provide a measure of body fat. Muscle mass can be determined by midarm muscle circumference. Standard tables are based on data from studies by Jelliffe [42] and Frisancho [43]. However, these standards suffer from various limitations, including select population subsets, inconsistencies between observers, and changes in hydration status affecting those measurements [44, 45].

Detsky et al. [46] and others have proposed subjective global assessment (SGA) as a way of assessing nutritional status (Fig. 34.1). In the SGA, the history features five areas: weight loss, food intake patterns, gastrointestinal symptoms, functional capacity, and primary diagnosis. The physical examination also focuses on five areas: assessment of subcutaneous fat and muscle wasting and the presence or absence of ankle edema, sacral edema, or ascites. Assessment areas are graded as normal (0) or as affected by mild (1+), moderate (2+), or severe (3+) changes. On the basis of the combined history and physical examination, an SGA rank is assigned: *A* indicates well-nourished; *B*, moderate or suspected malnutrition; or *C*, severe malnutrition. Derivation of an SGA rank is not based on numeric weighting of any individual area but rather on subjective weighting by the observer. In addition, SGA has been shown to have a greater than 90% reproducibility between observers and can be taught easily to a variety of medical and paramedical staff [46–48].

The traditional laboratory assessments of nutritional status have included serum albumin, prealbumin, and transferrin. Albumin, the most abundant plasma protein, functions to maintain plasma oncotic pressure and to transport a variety of molecules and drugs. The concentration of serum albumin depends on its synthesis, degradation, gastrointestinal and renal losses, exchange between bodily compartments, and volume of distribution. Because inflammatory processes, gastrointestinal and renal disease states, and hydration status affect its serum concentration, albumin is not an accurate measure of nutritional status. However, it does have prognostic value, with low serum concentrations (< 3.4 g/dl) being associated with increased morbidity and mortality in hospitalized patients [44, 49].

Patient History

Weight change and height

Current height: _____ cm   weight: _____ kg

Overall weight loss in last 6 months: _____ kg

Change in last 2 weeks:
☐ decreased   ☐ not changed   ☐ increased

Food intake over past month

☐ less than usual   ☐ unchanged   ☐ more than usual

Current intake: ☐ suboptimal solid diet
                   ☐ full liquids
                   ☐ hypocaloric liquids
                   ☐ starvation

Gastrointestinal symptoms (persisting > 2 weeks)

☐ none ☐ nausea ☐ vomiting ☐ diarrhea ☐ anorexia

Functional capacity

☐ no dysfunction   ☐ dysfunction: duration _____ weeks

Type of dysfunction:
☐ working suboptimally   ☐ ambulatory   ☐ bedridden

Disease and its relation to nutritional requirements

Primary diagnosis _____

Metabolic demand:
☐ no stress ☐ low stress ☐ moderate stress ☐ high stress

Physical status (for each trait specify: 0 = normal,
1 = mild, 2 = moderate, 3 = severe)

_____ loss of subcutaneous fat (triceps, chest)
_____ muscle wasting (quadriceps, deltoids)
_____ ankle edema
_____ sacral edema
_____ ascites

SGA rating: ☐ A = well-nourished
                 ☐ B = moderately (or suspected of being)
                     malnourished
                 ☐ C = severely malnourished

Figure 34.1 Features of subjective global assessment (*SGA*). (Reprinted with permission from AS Detsky, JR McLaughlin, JP Baker, et al., What is subjective global assessment of nutritional status? *JPEN J Parenter Enteral Nutr* 11[1]:8–13, 1987.)

Serum prealbumin is a transport protein for thyroid hormones. It has a much shorter half-life as compared to albumin (2–3 days versus 17–20 days). Serum prealbumin has been proposed as the laboratory measure of choice for assessing visceral protein and for monitoring nutritional status and the impact of nutritional therapy.

Serum levels of thyroxine-binding prealbumin below 150 mg/liter suggest an at-risk patient who should be monitored carefully. Thyroxine-binding prealbumin levels below 110 mg/liter are an indication for aggressive nutritional intervention. Serum transferrin has been used also as a marker of nutritional status. However, its half-life of 8 days and interference by iron metabolism offer little advantage over albumin [50].

The use of immune competence to assess nutritional status, as measured by delayed-type hypersensitivity to common recall antigens, remains controversial. Sepsis, steroids, surgery, and chemotherapy nonspecifically alter the presence or absence of anergy. Therefore, immunity is not a specific indicator of malnutrition but has been found to be a useful prognostic marker [2, 44, 51].

Accurate assessment of the nutritional status of cancer patients should entail a focused history and physical examination along with careful evaluation of biochemical data. In addition, this process should be dynamic so as to monitor not only the effect of the tumor on the host but the effectiveness of nutritional therapy.

NUTRITIONAL REQUIREMENTS

Before nutritional therapy can be instituted, patient-specific daily requirements of calories, protein, vitamins, and minerals have to be considered. Daily caloric needs may be calculated using predictive equations or by measurements using indirect calorimetry. Typically, the caloric needs for nonmetabolically stressed hospitalized patients are met by supplying 25 to 35 kcal/kg body wt/day. The Harris-Benedict equations provide a convenient method for calculating BEE on the basis of height, weight, age, and gender. However, these equations have been shown systematically to overestimate BEE by approximately 5% [52]. Others have modified the equations to include allowances for metabolic stress and activity, thereby permitting calculation of total energy expenditure (Table 34.2) [53]. Indirect calorimetry provides an accurate measurement of BEE. This method involves the use of a metabolic cart to measure total body oxygen consumption and carbon dioxide production, providing measurements from which energy expenditure can be calculated. Although they have been found to be useful in intensive care unit settings, these methods entail equipment costs and complexity that limit their value for routine inpatient or outpatient use.

Typically, the amount of lipids and carbohydrates supplied as the nonprotein portion of calories should be in a ratio of no more than 30% lipid to 70% carbohydrate. It is essential that sufficient nonprotein calories

Table 34.2   Determining Energy Requirements

Basal energy expenditure (BEE); Harris-Benedict equation
  For men: BEE (kcal/d) = 66 + 13.7W + 5H − 6.8A
  For women: BEE (kcal/d) = 655 + 9.6W + 1.7H − 4.7A

Stress factors
  Starvation   0.85
  Minor surgery   1.0–1.2
  Sepsis   1.4–1.8
  Cancer   1.1–1.45

Activity factor
  Bedbound   1.2
  Ambulatory   1.3

Total energy expenditure = BEE × stress factor × activity factor

W = weight in kilograms; H = height in centimeters; A = age in years.
Source: Adapted from LK Shanbhogue, WJ Chwals, M Weintraub, et al., Parenteral nutrition in the surgical patient. *Br J Surg* 74(3): 172–180, 1987.

Table 34.3   Recommended Daily Requirements of Vitamins and Trace Elements

Vitamin or Element	Enteral Dose	Parenteral Dose
Vitamin		
Vitamin A	1,000 µg	3,300 IU
Vitamin B$_{12}$	3 µg	5 µg
Vitamin C	60 mg	100 mg
Vitamin D	5 µg	200 IU
Vitamin E	10 mg	10 IU
Vitamin K	100 µg	10 mg
Thiamine (B$_1$)	2 mg	3 mg
Riboflavin (B$_2$)	2 mg	4 mg
Pyridoxine (B$_6$)	2 mg	4 mg
Pantothenic acid	6 mg	15 mg
Biotin	150 µg	60 µg
Folate	400 µg	400 µg
Trace element		
Chromium	200 µg	15 µg
Copper	3 mg	1.5 mg
Iodine	150 µg	150 µg
Iron	10 mg	2.5 mg
Manganese	5 mg	100 µg
Selenium	200 µg	70 µg
Zinc	15 mg	4 mg

Source: Adapted with permission from PL Marino, *The ICU Book* (2nd ed). Baltimore: Williams & Wilkins, 1997:721–736.

be provided so as to avoid degradation of administered protein for energy use. Under normal circumstances, protein intake requirements may be met by supplying 0.8 to 1.0 g/kg/day, though this figure may rise to 1.2 to 1.6 g/kg/day in metabolically stressed cancer patients. The total body nitrogen balance may be determined by measuring daily protein intake and 24-hour urinary urea nitrogen excretion (UUN; in grams):

$$\text{Nitrogen balance} = \text{Protein intake (in grams)}/6.25 - (\text{UUN} + 4)$$

The goal is to maintain a positive nitrogen balance of 4 to 6 g/day. The nitrogen balance can be determined on a weekly basis to follow trends and to allow for adjustments in nutritional intervention [54].

Twelve vitamins and seven trace elements are essential to the daily diet and must be administered to avoid deficiency syndromes. They are listed in Table 34.3 with their respective enteral and parenteral doses [54]. The amount of free water that meets requirements for homeostasis is in the range of 30 to 35 ml/kg/day. Appropriate adjustments must be made for those patients with comorbidities of cardiac, hepatic, or renal disease.

NUTRITIONAL THERAPY

Four levels of nutritional intervention may be applied to cancer patients: dietary counseling, supplemental oral feeding, enteral support, and total parenteral nutrition. These interventions are hierarchic with respect to

expertise needed for their application, invasiveness, associated potential complications, and costs. The level of support needed is highly variable and depends on a patient's nutritional status, the disease process, and the antineoplastic therapy directed against the process. Although survival itself may not be improved by improving the nutritional status of cancer patients with specific support, such support allows for improved tolerance and response to antineoplastic treatment. In addition, it can enhance such patients' quality of life and sense of well-being.

Dietary Counseling

The interplay of behavioral, emotional, and perceptual responses of cancer patients to their disease process and its treatment may contribute to diminished nutrient intake. Patients should be educated about their disease process and the importance of nutrition in the overall management plan. Advice should be given concerning those foods that are nutritious and provide a healthy, well-balanced diet for particular patients. Numerous simple measures can facilitate an increase in oral intake. In the hospital setting, creating a clean and pleasant eating environment may be helpful. Unnecessary tests or procedures should not disrupt mealtimes. Certain diagnostic tests and procedures necessitate a fasting status, but this status should be kept to a minimum. Patients with anorexia benefit from frequent small meals that are high in calories and protein. Early satiety may be prevented by minimizing fluid intake with meals. For those patients suffering from nausea, excessively greasy or sweet foods should be avoided, and antiemetics or promotility agents should be considered. Alterations in taste sensations may inhibit patients from taking their usual foods, and attempts should be made to accommodate different preferences. Relatives and friends should be encouraged to bring home-cooked foods if patients desire them. Furthermore, the preparation and presentation of food always should render it appealing and inviting.

Patients with head and neck cancers have unique problems. Ablative neck resections may leave such patients with a lesser ability to chew and swallow food. In such instances, a softer diet may be helpful. Those suffering from dysphagia or odynophagia also may benefit from a softer or a liquid diet. In addition, these diets are beneficial to patients with mucositis secondary to chemotherapy or radiotherapy. Xerostomia secondary to head and neck irradiation can be particularly distressing and can be treated with artificial saliva and frequent rinses with soda water or citrus juice, all of which stimulate saliva production. Dietitians must be involved in assessing and counseling patients as early as possible, preferably before antineoplastic therapy is instituted [2, 10].

Patients with treatment-induced diarrhea may benefit from low-fat diets and dietary supplements that contain water-soluble fiber in conjunction with antidiarrheal agents. If a lactase deficiency is suspected, milk products should be eliminated from the diet, or commercial Lactaid products can be used. Patients with short-bowel syndrome may require predigested or elemental preparations to maintain an adequate postoperative nutritional state. Pancreatic insufficiency can be treated orally with pancreatic enzymes. Diarrhea-causing opportunistic infections, such as those due to *Clostridium difficile*, must be recognized and treated appropriately [2].

Supplemental Oral Feeding

Most cancer patients are able to tolerate an oral diet, though not in volumes large enough to support an adequate caloric intake. For such patients, a large number of available commercially prepared solid and liquid supplements may be used alone or in combination with regular diets to increase protein-calorie intake. The typical liquid preparations contain 1 to 2 kcal/ml. Polymeric formulations that contain intact carbohydrate, fat, and protein are preferred because of their palatability, cost, and ability to stimulate normal digestion. Many of these preparations are available also in the form of nutrition bars that may be preferred by some patients. Special formulations do exist for patients with comorbidities of diabetes (those lower in carbohydrate content), renal disease (those with modified protein, sodium, and potassium levels), and hepatic disease (those low in aromatic amino acids). Elemental formulas (oligomeric or monomeric) consisting of free amino acids or dipeptides or tripeptides are available for those with digestive or absorptive abnormalities. Modular preparations consist of the individual nutrients of carbohydrates, lipids, or protein. Such preparations may be combined to create a custom formula or may be added to an existing formula to increase the delivery of that particular nutrient. The composition of these formulas varies widely with respect to water and electrolyte content and thus osmolarity, and they should, therefore, be prescribed with care. The polymeric formulations are the mainstay of supplemental feeds. The nonpolymeric and special feeds do have a place in certain circumstances but are limited for oral use because of their lack of palatability and, therefore, are used mostly for feeding by one of several alternative methods [54].

Enteral Support

The enteral route of nutrition always is preferable to the parenteral. The provision of enteral nutrients not only maintains the functional morphology of intestinal mucosa but supports host defenses against septic sequelae resulting from bacterial translocation [55]. In addition, enteral feeding is less expensive and carries less morbidity as compared with parenteral feeding. The enteral route of feeding using a tube should be considered when patients have a functional gastrointestinal tract but cannot or will not eat. Access may be obtained by either nasoenteric tubes or by tube gastrostomy or jejunostomy.

Nasoenteric feeding tubes are appropriate when their anticipated period of use is less than 4 weeks. The distal tip of the tube may be positioned in the stomach, duodenum, or jejunum, either by using bedside techniques (e.g., positioning in the right lateral decubitus position) or by radiographic guidance. In addition, such promotility agents as metoclopramide or erythromycin can be administered to facilitate placement of tubes beyond the pylorus. Typically, tube sizes for adults range from No. 8 Fr. to No. 12 Fr. , with or without a weighted tip. Smaller sizes are more comfortable for patients but have the drawback of being more prone to clogging. Although nasoduodenal or nasojejunal feeding demonstrates no nutritional benefit over nasogastric feeding, tubes positioned in the distal duodenum or beyond are associated with a lesser risk of aspiration. Other potential complications of nasoenteric tubes include clogging, diarrhea, pulmonary intubation, gastrointestinal perforation, sinusitis, and tube dislodgment [56].

If the need for enteral support is anticipated for longer than 4 weeks, percutaneous enteric tube support should be considered. Available options include percutaneous endoscopic gastrostomy (PEG), percutaneous endoscopic gastrojejunostomy, and surgical gastrostomy or jejunostomy with or without laparoscopic assistance. Each technique has its advantages and disadvantages. Placement of PEG tubes technically is easier and less expensive. However, for patients with a history of aspiration, reflux esophagitis, or gastroparesis or when early postoperative feeding after major surgery is indicated, jejunostomy tubes are preferred. Complications associated with these tubes include aspiration, clogging, diarrhea, wound infections, and peritubal leakage [57].

For the majority of patients, nutritional needs can be met with standard isotonic polymeric formulas. Other patients (as discussed) may benefit from special formulas or elemental or modular diets. Patients with gastrostomy tubes are maintained on a feeding regimen with intermittent boluses every 3 to 6 hours. Volumes can start at 50 ml per bolus and can be increased incrementally until predetermined goals are met. Typically, bolus volumes should not exceed 400 ml to avoid gastric distention. Residual volumes can be checked periodically before the next bolus to ensure that they are being tolerated. Patients with jejunostomy tubes should receive continuous feeding only using a pump. Typically, feeding starts at 20 ml/hr and can be increased by 10 ml every 8 hours until the goal rate is met. Residual volumes for jejunostomy tubes cannot be checked as they can be for gastrostomy tubes. Instead, patients are followed clinically: Complaints of nausea, distention, or diarrhea suggest that the feeds are not being tolerated. Diarrhea is not unusual when jejunostomy feeds are started, particularly when hypertonic formulas are used. This side effect may be minimized (as suggested) by starting at a low feeding rate and increasing the rate slowly. If diarrhea is persistent, a change to an isotonic or elemental formula should be considered, or antiperistaltic agents should be administered. Jejunostomy

feeds may be cycled conveniently at night for those outpatients motivated to be ambulatory and independent during daytime hours. In addition, all tubes should be flushed every 6 to 8 hours with 20 to 30 ml of normal saline to minimize clogging [54, 56].

Total Parenteral Nutrition

Total parenteral nutrition (TPN) should be considered in cancer patients only when the enteral route is not feasible. However, in those terminally ill patients with advanced stages of disease, TPN is not indicated. Typically, TPN is administered through a centrally placed catheter lying in either the internal jugular or subclavian veins, but another convenient route is a peripherally inserted central catheter using the antecubital veins for access.

TPN formulations are prepared from standard concentrations of dextrose, amino acids, and lipids. Additives include vitamins and minerals to meet recommended daily requirements, heparin to maintain catheter patency and, if necessary, insulin and H_2 blockers. The formulas are prepared in laminar flow cabinets using strict aseptic technique. Local policy guidelines should be followed regarding handling of the TPN bag, intravenous tubing, and catheter to minimize contamination. In-line micropore filters should be used as part of the administration set to help decrease the chance of

Table 34.4   Complications of Total Parenteral Nutrition

Catheter-related
   Pneumothorax
   Great-vessel injury
   Air embolism
   Venous thrombosis
   Malposition
   Catheter blockage
   Catheter fracture

Metabolism-related
   Hyperglycemia, hypoglycemia
   Hypokalemia
   Hypermagnesemia, hypomagnesemia
   Hyperphosphatemia, hypophosphatemia
   Fatty liver
   Vitamin deficiency
   Trace element deficiency
   Refeeding syndrome
   Essential fatty acid deficiency

Sepsis-related
   Line sepsis
   TPN solution contamination

TPN = total parenteral nutrition.

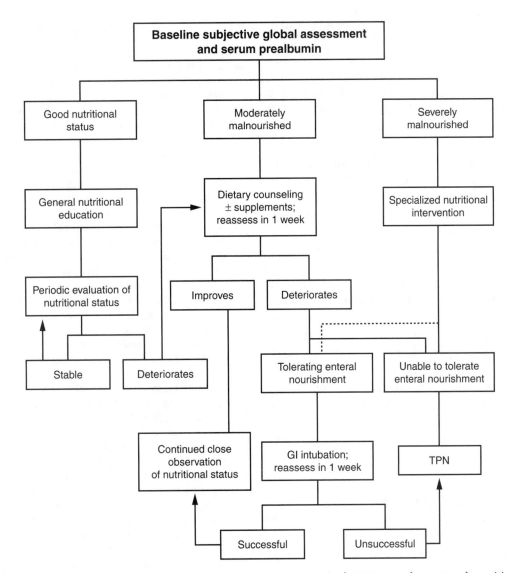

Figure 34.2   A nutritional support pathway. *GI* = gastrointestinal; *TPN* = total parenteral nutrition.

infusing contaminants and precipitants. As for enteral support, the provision of calories should be maintained in a ratio of 70% to 85% to 15% to 25% for carbohydrates to lipids, with administration of enough protein to maintain a positive nitrogen balance. Using standard formulations satisfies most patients' requirements, though some may need customized preparations.

The oxidation of intravenous glucose provides 3.4 kcal/g. Glucose use is optimal when given at rates of 4 to 5 mg/kg/min. Infusion at rates above 7 mg/kg/min does not increase oxidation rates. Standard TPN includes dextrose in a 50% solution, rendering it hyperosmolar (2,525 mOsm/liter). Concentrations of up to 70% are available to supply adequate calories in a lesser volume in those patients whose fluid intake is restricted.

Intravenous lipids have a caloric value of 10 kcal/g. Lipid emulsions consist of polyunsaturated long-chain triglycerides derived from sunflower or soybean oils, rich in linoleic acid. The emulsions are isotonic and are available in strengths of 10% (1.1 kcal/ml) or 20% (2.2 kcal/ml). Linoleic acid is the only essential lipid. Its deficiency can be prevented by supplying it in a concentration of at least 0.5% fatty acids delivered.

Standard amino acid formulas consist of 50% essential and 50% nonessential amino acids, typically in a 7% strength, with a caloric value of 4 kcal/g. Glutamine is the primary fuel source of the enterocyte. Enrichment of TPN formulas with glutamine has been shown to reduce intestinal cell atrophy during periods of bowel rest and thus may be beneficial in maintaining bowel integrity against bacterial translocation. Commercially available preparations of electrolytes, vitamins, and minerals are available and can be added directly to the mixtures to complete patients' requirements [53, 58–60].

Monitoring of patients should begin prior to initiation of TPN, with a complete blood cell count; a full assessment of electrolytes, blood urea nitrogen, creatinine, glucose, and prealbumin; liver function tests; and a lipid profile. During the first week of TPN, the serum electrolytes, blood urea nitrogen, and creatinine should be checked daily and then twice weekly if they are stable. Triglycerides and liver function tests should be checked weekly. Lipids should not be administered if triglycerides rise more than 500 mg/dl. Blood glucose values should be obtained every 6 hours until stable. Appropriate insulin coverage should be ordered for patients with glucose intolerance or diabetes. Measurements of the complete blood cell count, prealbumin, and weight, and a calculation of nitrogen balance should be performed on a weekly basis. Most patients can be started on a volume of 1,000 ml/day, which can be increased incrementally on a daily basis to meet their requirements. Once the enteral route is functional, however, TPN patients should be weaned rapidly. TPN is associated with some potentially serious or fatal complications. These complications fall into the categories of catheter-related, metabolism-related, and sepsis-related (Table 34.4).

CONCLUSION

Cachexia is a prevalent finding among cancer patients. The precise final pathways have yet to be elucidated fully. A few available agents may block its effects partially and may produce weight gain. Nutritional assessment of cancer patients should be a dynamic process throughout the disease process. Intervention should be multidisciplinary, the team consisting of physicians, nurses, dietitians, and social workers.

Nutritional therapy must be highly individualized and hierarchic, with an intervention being instituted only when the next simplest option is not applicable to a patient (Fig. 34.2). TPN is invasive and costly and carries with it a risk of potentially serious complications. It is indicated in only a small subset of the cancer population, and its liberal use in the presence of a functioning gastrointestinal tract should be condemned. Finally, no firm evidence substantiates that aggressive nutritional intervention promotes tumor growth. Therefore, no justification can be presented for withdrawing appropriate nutritional support from cancer patients for whom available curative or palliative therapy exists.

REFERENCES

1. De Wys WD, Begg C, Lavin PT, et al. Prognostic effect of weight loss prior to chemotherapy in cancer patients. *Am J Med* 69:491–497, 1980.
2. Lopez MJ, Dwyer JT, Frank JL. Nutrition and the cancer patient. In Osteen R (ed), *Cancer Manual* (9th ed). Boston: American Cancer Society, Massachusetts Division, 1996:201–209.
3. Albrecht JT, Canada TW. Cachexia and anorexia in malignancy. *Hematol Oncol Clin North Am* 10(4):791–800, 1996.
4. Tisdale MJ. Biology of cachexia. *J Natl Cancer Inst* 89(23):1763–1773, 1997.
5. Ovesen L, Allingstrup L, Hannibal J, et al. Effect of dietary counseling on food intake, body weight, response rate, survival and quality of life in cancer patients undergoing chemotherapy: a prospective randomized study. *J Clin Oncol* 11:2043–2049, 1993.
6. Laviano A, Renvyle T, Meguid MM, et al. Relationship between interleukin-1 and cancer anorexia. *Nutrition* 11:680s–683s, 1995.
7. Chance WT, Balasubramaniam A, Fischer JE. Neuropeptide Y and the development of cancer anorexia. *Ann Surg* 221:579–587, 1995.
8. Knoll J. Endogenous anorectic agents—satietins. *Annu Rev Pharmacol Toxicol* 28:247–268, 1988.
9. Cangiano C, Testa U, Muscaritoli M, et al. Cytokines, tryptophan and anorexia in cancer patients before and after surgical tumor ablation. *Anticancer Res* 14:1451–1455, 1994.
10. Padilla GV. Psychological aspects of nutrition and cancer. *Surg Clin North Am* 66:1121–1135, 1986.
11. De Wys WD, Walters K. Abnormalities of taste sensation in cancer patients. *Cancer* 36:1888–1896, 1975.
12. Berstein IL. Physiological and psychological mechanisms of cancer anorexia. *Cancer Res* 42:7152s–7172s, 1982.
13. Moser AJ, Roslyn JJ. Enterocutaneous fistula. In Cameron JL (ed), *Current Surgical Therapy* (6th ed). St Louis: Mosby, 1998:155–159.
14. Giacosa A, Frascio F, Sukkar SG, Roncella S. Food intake and body composition in cancer cachexia. *Nutrition* 12:s20–s23, 1996.
15. Cederholm T, Wretlind B, Hellstrom K, et al. Enhanced generation of interleukins 1 beta and 6 may contribute to the cachexia of chronic disease. *Am J Clin Nutr* 65:876–882, 1997.
16. Todorov P, Cariuk P, McDevitt T, et al. Characterization of a cancer cachectic factor. *Nature* 379:739–742, 1996.
17. Moldawer LL, Copeland EM. Proinflammatory cytokines, nutritional support, and the cachexia syndrome: interactions and therapeutic options. *Cancer* 79:1828–1839, 1997.
18. Staal van den Brekel AJ, Dentener MA, Schols AM, et al. Increased resting energy expenditure and weight loss are related to a systemic inflammatory response in lung cancer patients. *J Clin Oncol* 13:2600–2605, 1995.
19. Fredrix EW, Soeters PB, Wouters EF, et al. Effect of different tumor types on resting energy expenditure. *Cancer Res* 15:6138–6141, 1991.

20. Falconer JS, Fearon KC, Plester CE, et al. Cytokines, the acute phase response, and resting energy expenditure in cachectic patients with pancreatic cancer. *Ann Surg* 219:325–331, 1994.

21. Tayek JA, Manglik S, Abemayor E. Insulin secretion, glucose production, and insulin sensitivity in underweight and normal-weight cancer patients: a Clinical Research Center study. *Metabolism* 46:140–145, 1997.

22. Tayek JA. A review of cancer cachexia and abnormal glucose metabolism in humans with cancer. *J Am Coll Nutr* 11:445–456, 1992.

23. Mathupala SJ, Rempel A, Pederson PL. Glucose catabolism in cancer cells. *J Biol Chem* 270:16918–16925, 1995.

24. Hirai K, Ishiko O, Tisdale M. Mechanisms of depletion of liver glycogen in cancer cachexia. *Biochem Biophys Res Commun* 241:49–52, 1997.

25. Mulligan HD, Beck SA, Tisdale MJ. Lipid metabolism in cancer cachexia. *Br J Cancer* 66:57–61, 1992.

26. Taylor GC, Doering DL, Kraemer FB, Taylor DD. Aberrations in normal systemic lipid metabolism in ovarian cancer patients. *Gynecol Oncol* 60:35–41, 1996.

27. Toomey D, Redmond P, Hayes DB. Mechanisms mediating cancer cachexia. *Cancer* 76:2418–2426, 1995.

28. Dworzak F, Ferrari P, Gavazzi C, et al. Effects of cachexia due to cancer on whole body and skeletal muscle protein turnover. *Cancer* 82:42–48, 1998.

29. Lorite MJ, Cariuk P, Tisdale MJ. Induction of muscle protein degradation by a tumor factor. *Br J Cancer* 76:1035–1040, 1997.

30. Cariuk P, Lorite MJ, Todorov PT, et al. Induction of cachexia in mice by a product isolated from the urine of cachectic cancer patients. *Br J Cancer* 76:603–613, 1997.

31. Llovera M, Martinez CG, Agell N, et al. Muscle wasting associated with cancer cachexia is linked to an important activation of the ATP-dependent ubiquitin-mediated proteolysis. *Int J Cancer* 61:138–141, 1995.

32. Gebbia V, Testa A, Gebbia N. Prospective randomised trial of two doses of megestrol acetate in the management of anorexia-cachexia syndrome in patients with metastatic cancer. *Br J Cancer* 73:1576–1580, 1996.

33. Loprinzi CL, Michalak JC, Schaid DJ, et al. Phase III evaluation of four doses of megestrol acetate as therapy for patients with cancer anorexia and/or cachexia. *J Clin Oncol* 11:762–767, 1993.

34. Simons JP, Schols AM, Hoefnagels JM, et al. Effects of medroxyprogesterone acetate on food intake, body composition, and resting energy expenditure in patients with advanced, nonhormone-sensitive cancer: a randomized, placebo-controlled trial. *Cancer* 82:553–560, 1998.

35. Neri B, Garosi VL, Intini C. Effect of medroxyprogesterone acetate on the quality of life of the oncologic patient: a multicentric cooperative study. *Anticancer Drugs* 8:459–465, 1997.

36. Nelson K, Walsh D, Deeter P, Sheehan F. A phase II study of delta-9-tetrahydrocannabinol for appetite stimulation in cancer associated anorexia. *J Palliat Care* 10:14–18, 1994.

37. Tisdale MJ. Inhibition of lipolysis and muscle protein degradation by EPA in cancer cachexia. *Nutrition* 12:s31–s33, 1996.

38. Ohira T, Nishio K, Ohe Y, et al. Improvement by eicosanoids in cancer cachexia induced by LLC-IL6 transplantation. *J Cancer Res Clin Oncol* 122:711–715, 1996.

39. Wigmore SJ, Ross JA, Falconer JS, et al. The effect of polyunsaturated fatty acids on the progress of cachexia in patients with pancreatic cancer. *Nutrition* 12:s27–s30, 1996.

40. Tamura R, Tanebe K, Kawanishi C, et al. Effects of lentinan on abnormal ingestive behaviors induced by tumor necrosis factor. *Physiol Behav* 61:399–410, 1997.

41. Council on Practice Quality Management Committee. ADA's definition for nutrition screening and assessment. *J Am Diet Assoc* 94:838–839, 1994.

42. Jelliffe DB. *The Assessment of the Nutritional Status of the Community: With Special Reference to Field Surveys in Developing Regions of the World* [monograph]. Geneva: World Health Organization, 1966.

43. Frisancho AR. New norms of upper limb fat and muscle areas for assessment of nutritional status. *Am J Clin Nutr* 34:2540–2545, 1981.

44. Jeejeebhoy KN. Nutritional assessment. *Gastroenterol Clin North Am* 27:347–369, 1998.

45. Thuluvath PJ, Triger DR. How valid are our reference standards of nutrition? *Nutrition* 11:731–733, 1995.

46. Detsky AS, McLaughlin JR, Baker JP, et al. What is subjective global assessment of nutritional status? *JPEN J Parenter Enteral Nutr* 11:8–13, 1987.

47. Hirsch S, de Obaldia N, Petermann M, et al. Subjective global assessment of nutritional status: further validation. *Nutrition* 7:35–37, 1991.

48. Ottery FD. Definition of standardized nutritional assessment and interventional pathways in oncology. *Nutrition* 12:s15–s19, 1996.

49. Gray GE, Meguid MM. The myth of serum albumin as a measure of nutritional status. *Gastroenterology* 99:1845–1851, 1990.

50. Prealbumin in Nutritional Care Consensus Group. Measurement of visceral protein status in assessing protein and energy malnutrition: standard of care. *Nutrition* 11:169–171, 1995.

51. Lopez MJ, Robinson P, Madden T, Highbarger T. Nutritional support and prognosis in patients with head and neck cancer. *J Surg Oncol* 55:33–36, 1994.

52. Frankenfield DC, Muth ER, Rowe WA. The Harris-Benedict studies of human basal metabolism: history and limitations. *J Am Diet Assoc* 98:439–445, 1998.

53. Shanbhogue LK, Chwals WJ, Weintraub M, et al. Parenteral nutrition in the surgical patient. *Br J Surg* 74:172–180, 1987.

54. Marino PL. Nutrient and energy requirements. In Marino PL (ed), *The ICU Book* (2nd ed). Baltimore: Williams & Wilkins, 1997:721–736.

55. Unno N, Fink MP. Intestinal epithelial hyperpermeability. Mechanisms and relevance to disease. *Gastroenterol Clin North Am* 27:289–307, 1998.

56. Rodman DP, Gaskins SE. Optimizing enteral nutrition. *Am Fam Physician* 53:2535–2542, 1996.

57. American Gastroenterological Association Patient Care Committee. American Gastroenterological Association technical review on tube feeding for enteral nutrition. *Gastroenterology* 108:1282–1301, 1995.

58. National Advisory Group on Standards and Practice Guidelines for Parenteral Nutrition. Safe practices for parenteral nutrition formulations. *JPEN J Parenter Enteral Nutr* 22:49–66, 1998.

59. Fish J, Sporay G, Beyer K, et al. A prospective randomized study of glutamine-enriched parenteral compared with enteral feeding in postoperative patients. *Am J Clin Nutr* 65:977–983, 1997.

60. Buchman AL, Moukarzel AA, Bhuta S, et al. Parenteral nutrition is associated with intestinal morphological changes in humans. *JPEN J Parenter Enteral Nutr* 19:453–460, 1995.

35

Rehabilitation and Survivorship

■ ■ ■

CLAUDETTE G. VARRICCHIO
NOREEN AZIZ

SURVIVORSHIP AND REHABILITATION ARE closely interwoven concepts when applied to the cancer experience. Planning for both should begin when a diagnosis of cancer and a treatment plan are made. The increasing ability to treat cancer successfully and to aid in the maintenance of productive lives for those people who are living with cancer requires addressing the issues related to rehabilitation and survivorship simultaneously with early detection, diagnosis, and treatment of cancer. Both medical and psychological problems have been reported consistently by cancer survivors, and any comprehensive model of disease management carries with it the essential aspect of preventing or effectively treating such sequelae. Thus, both rehabilitation and management of survivorship are integral aspects of optimal, comprehensive cancer care [1].

In the United States, more than 1.2 million persons will be diagnosed each year with cancer. Nearly 60% will be alive in five years. There are currently approximately 8.4 million cancer survivors in the United States [2]. This trend to prolonged survival shows an even greater increase when adjusted by the primary cancer site. Data from 1974 to 1976 and from 1981 to 1987 reported by a Surveillance, Epidemiology, and End Results survey [3] demonstrated significant improvements in the five-year relative survival rates for melanoma; for breast, uterine, prostate, testicular, and bladder cancer; and for Hodgkin's disease and non-Hodgkin's lymphoma. A continuous and sustained decline in cancer mortality has occurred in the United States from 1990 to 1995 [4].

Almost all persons in whom cancer has been diagnosed and treated need some form of rehabilitation and preemptive medical and psychosocial management of the physiologic, psychological, social, and economic sequelae of survivorship from this disease. Problems facing cancer survivors are unique and multifaceted [5]. They include physical, emotional, and social stresses arising as a result of the effects of treatment, changes in lifestyle, disruption of home and family roles, and the fear of recurrence. Physical, psychological, and social morbidity are issues for cancer survivors [6]. Such persons live with compromise and uncertainty and face numerous challenges that arise as a result of changes in their strength, endurance, reproductive capacity, sexuality, and body image [7].

Each person with cancer has unique needs based on the extent of the disease, effects of treatment, prior health, functional level, coping skills, support systems, and many other influences. This complexity requires an interdisciplinary approach by all health professionals. Cancer rehabilitation and survivorship services should represent an organized, systematic approach geared toward the provision of quality interdisciplinary care. This approach helps cancer patients to adapt to their situation regardless of whether the deficits and changes are temporary or permanent [8].

Frequently, cancer and cancer treatment result in disabilities that warrant the same consideration given to disabilities arising from other causes. The inclusion of cancer in the language of the Americans with Disabilities Act attests to this. Common problems that are found in persons treated for cancer and that require rehabilitation include paralysis, paresis, intellectual-perceptual deficits, communication impairments, contractures, pressure sores, ambulation or transfer difficulties, self-care deficits, fractures, and lymphedema (by no means an exhaustive list). Additionally, the concept of cancer survivorship encompasses a multitude of medical and psychosocial disease and treatment sequelae that have been reported widely in cancer patients [9]. Areas of overlap exist. Many patients who have physical disabilities also experience psychological problems. Cancer survivors without physical problems may evince an increased incidence of psychological problems [8, 10].

The relevance of cancer rehabilitation and survivorship to oncologic clinical practice has increased as cancer therapy has improved. A sign of success is the significant number of cancer survivors who require some level of rehabilitation services. Clinical practice in this area is empirically based, because little research-derived evidence is available to guide decision making.

DEFINITIONS
Survivorship

Cancer survivorship first was described as a concept by Fitzhugh Mullan, a physician who had been given a diagnosis of cancer [11]. His definition coincides with that widely accepted today: "Everyone diagnosed as having cancer, beginning from the point of diagnosis to the end of life, is a cancer survivor." Mullan also described the survivorship experience and equated it with the climatic seasons of the year. He recognized three phases of survival: (1) acute survival (extending from diagnosis to the completion of initial treatment; issues dominated by treatment and its side effects); (2) extended survival (beginning with the completion of initial treatment for the primary disease or remission of disease [or both] and dominated by watchful waiting, regular follow-up examinations, and intermittent therapy); and, (3) permanent survival (not a single moment in time, evolving from extended disease-free survival when the likelihood of recurrence is sufficiently low).

Owing to the tremendous strides in disease treatment, cancer survivors are living for extended periods beyond their initial diagnosis—hence the need for recognition and definition of long-term survivors. Generally, long-term cancer survivors are defined as being 5, 10, 15, or 20 years beyond the diagnosis of their primary disease, and they embody the concept of permanent survival as defined by Mullan.

Because cancer is a disease with both physical and psychosocial sequelae, it is important to note that the issues facing cancer survivors are *not* extensions of the issues and concerns of cancer patients in treatment. The qualitative difference [12] lies in the diversity of the sequelae, encompassing physical and physiologic sequelae that require medical management, prevention, and treatment on the one hand, and the less medically oriented trend away from illness-related problems and toward societal and interpersonal issues on the other [13].

Rehabilitation

"Cancer rehabilitation is a concept struggling for definition, recognition, and direction . . . Rehabilitation should constitute an umbrella concept in cancer care" [14]. This statement, made in 1990 by Watson, remains true today. The concept of adaptive cancer rehabilitation, as introduced by Dietz [1, 15], consisted of four categories: prevention, restoration, support, and palliation. Preventive rehabilitation includes interventions designed to improve physical functioning and to reduce morbidity and disability. Restorative rehabilitation has as goals the control, circumvention, or elimination of residual cancer disability. Supportive rehabilitation is intended to lessen disability and other associated problems. Palliative rehabilitation is used in advanced and active disease to attenuate the disability.

In further defining rehabilitation, other authors use such words as *adaptation, readaptation, physical functioning, quality of life,* and *maximal levels of functioning* within the limits imposed by the disease [16]. More recent attempts to define cancer rehabilitation have proposed these definitions: "Cancer rehabilitation is a process by which individuals within their environments are assisted to achieve optimal functioning within the limits imposed by cancer" [10]. "Cancer rehabilitation is a dynamic, health-oriented process designed to promote maximum levels of functioning in individuals with cancer-related health problems" [1]. Cancer rehabilitation has been defined also as "a team approach to helping both the patient and family remain as independent as possible within the limitations of the disease, functionally, emotionally, spiritually, and socially, throughout the continuum of care" [17].

CLINICAL IMPLICATIONS

Questions of particular importance to cancer survivors include the risk of recurrence; surveillance for the adverse sequelae of treatment and the development of new cancers; effects on reproduction and offspring; and issues of quality of life and psychosocial adjustment beyond the acute treatment period. These questions not only occupy a central core of importance; they have the potential to influence such infrastructural systems as databases, follow-up requirements for clinical trials, new therapeutic approaches, dosages of chemotherapeutic drugs, surveillance recommendations, and the cancer research agenda itself [5, 6, 8].

Decisions concerning specific requirements of follow-up care benefit from information derived from studies of the medical and psychological outcomes of both the cancer experience and therapy. Providing information, education, and other forms of intervention during active cancer treatment and beyond may have implications for the prevention of future illness and for the overall quality of life [18]. Cancer survivors also are a rich source of information for the study of other conditions (e.g., second cancers and potential comorbidities) arising as a consequence of the cancer diagnosis and treatment.

Though research directed toward cancer biology, risk prevention, diagnosis, detection, and treatment of cancer is extensive, relatively modest research efforts address cancer survivors in general and long-term survivors (defined as living 5, 10, 15, or 20 years beyond the diagnosis of their primary disease) in particular. Priority areas for cancer survivorship research [19] include certain essential issues. One is quality of life (e.g., prevalence and longitudinal incidence studies of changes in quality of life over time). Another is physiologic outcomes. Similarly structured studies would address physiologic late effects (e.g., cardiac toxicities and events; pulmonary compromise; late effects of limb-sparing and reconstructive surgery; ovarian failure; renal failure; and diminished cognitive function and mentation).

Another fruitful area for research is reproduction and sexuality. Studies could target offspring of cancer survivors, evaluating birth defects, delayed developmental milestones, and malformation rates. Second cancers also are a concern; both prevalence and incidence should be investigated. Still another area is economic outcomes. Often, survivors and their families encounter job and insurance discrimination [20]; such individuals would profit from exploration of the impact of survivorship relative to such discrimination [21]. Studies should encompass the economic impact of follow-up medical monitoring; outcomes of follow-up that affect costs; comparisons of how follow-up care is delivered; relative cost of specialty-based follow-up care as compared to primary-physician-based care; and evaluation of effectiveness and cost of psychosocial and other interventions that will affect outcomes [22].

Frequently, education and communication needs arise in the lives of cancer survivors. Such demanding areas should be researched for their impact on these individuals. Also in need of further research are preventive interventions. These must be evaluated to prevent both the physiologic and the psychological sequelae of survivorship. Such preventive measures include the use of cardioprotective agents, modification of diet and lifestyle or administration of agents to reduce the risk of second cancers, maintenance of fertility, and early interventions during treatment to diminish the negative impact of potential side effects.

As regards data resources, development of the Surveillance, Epidemiology, and End Results registry and other established registries could yield information about survivors and could help in the formation of cohorts of cancer survivors. Surveillance research studies should evaluate trends in expected cancer survival time, attributable medical care costs, impact of an intervention on survival time in a cohort of cancer survivors, and the delineation of factors relevant to the successful tracing of cohorts of cancer survivors.

Additionally, certain areas exhibit a dearth of both exploratory and validation studies [19]. Research is needed to address the development and testing of diverse methodologic approaches specific to cancer survivors. Also needed are pilot studies of preliminary basic science analyses to explore mechanisms of action; epidemiologic hypothesis-generating studies; and population-based studies of incidence and prevalence of cancer outcomes and sequelae.

Physiologic Sequelae

The physiologic sequelae of cancer and its treatment incorporate two related areas. *Long-term* physiologic effects are chronic physiologic side effects persisting beyond the acute cancer treatment phase. *Late* effects are delayed physiologic health effects occurring months to years after treatment. Physiologic sequelae can be classified further. System-specific sequelae include such effects as organ damage, failure, or premature aging; immunosuppression or compromised immune systems; and endocrine damage. Development of second malignant neoplasms comprises increased risk of recurrent malignancy, increased risk of a certain cancer associated with the primary malignancy, or increased risk of secondary malignancies associated with cytotoxic or radiologic cancer therapies. Functional changes include lymphedema, incontinence, pain syndromes, neuropathies, and fatigue. They also are seen in such cosmetic changes as amputations, ostomies, and skin and hair alterations and frequently surface as associated comorbidities (e.g., osteoporosis, arthritis, scleroderma, and hypertension).

Psychosocial and Quality-of-Life Sequelae

The psychosocial and quality-of-life sequelae incorporate aspects of survivorship relating to two areas. One involves patients' adaptation to the personal consequences of cancer diagnosis and treatment, seen in issues of self-concept, body image, personal autonomy, coping strategies, intimacy, interpersonal and family interactions, and living with uncertainty. A second area encompasses adjustment to the social consequences of cancer, exemplified in societal or familial perceptions and expectations; survivors' adjustment to altered interpersonal relationships, family roles, and functions; and issues of financial stability, job security, health insurance, job lock, or discrimination.

Economic Sequelae

Economic sequelae include such issues as job security, job discrimination, and job lock (inability to change jobs because of fear of losing insurance coverage), which have an economic impact on the patient and the patient's family, patterns of care, and cancer control practices in health maintenance organizations or other service delivery settings. Other issues include costs of cancer care by disease site or stage; costs of standard and experimental therapies for cancer; factors that influence treatment-related decision making by providers or patients; and decision-making issues and outcomes associated with genetic testing of survivors or their families. Economic sequelae are interwoven closely with both physiologic and psychosocial health outcomes.

IMPACT ON THE FAMILY

Only recently has cancer been recognized as a family disease [23]. Both stress and depression have been noted to increase in patients and their family members as a result of concerns regarding recurrence. Annual follow-up visits and physical loss of a body part serve as reminders about the chronic nature of the disease for both survivors and their families [24]. Parents of childhood cancer survivors report personal levels of post-traumatic stress symptoms significantly higher than those of the actual survivors themselves [25]. Additionally, some preliminary studies have shown that family members, particularly adolescent daughters of women with breast cancer and spouses of patients with lung cancer, are at increased risk of depressive or stress-related clinical symptomatology. Clearly, this area of clinical impact is underrepresented, and studies are needed to delineate both the prevalence of such symptomatology and any interventions geared toward preventing or minimizing the deleterious impact of the cancer diagnosis on families.

PREVENTION AND EARLY DETECTION

A challenge is inherent in conducting survivorship research and in successfully introducing appropriate interventions that could effect improvements in the care and management of cancer survivors, which in turn could lead to better quality of life and a favorable long-term survival. Inherent in that challenge is recognizing the importance both of preventing premature mortality from the disease or its treatment and of preventing or detecting early both the physiologic and psychological sources of morbidity. Prevention of second cancers and recurrences of the primary disease require watchful follow-up and optimal use of such early-detection screening techniques as mammograms. Methodological challenges continue to loom; still unresolved are the questions of optimal long-term follow-up guidelines, the method of delivery of medical, psychosocial, and follow-up care to cancer survivors, and the prevention of further morbidity in long-term survivors of cancer.

TREATMENT AND INTERVENTIONS

Physical symptom management is as important in survivorship and rehabilitation as it is during treatment. The persistence of symptoms long past the end of treatment is well documented. Pain, fatigue, neuropathies, and other functional limitations (e.g., lymphedema and problems in swallowing, speech, ambulation, and body image) present long-range management problems.

Effective symptom management during treatment may prevent or decrease lasting effects. Attention to psychosocial problems and problems of coping and adjustment during treatment provides the foundation of preventive interventions to promote more satisfactory quality of life after cancer.

No consensus has been reached regarding the recommendations for routine follow-up after cancer therapy. Some groups are preparing guidelines and decision trees for regular monitoring of health status after cancer treatment [26, 27]. Regular follow-up (1) permits the timely diagnosis and treatment of long-term complications of cancer treatment; (2) provides the opportunity to institute such preventive strategies as diet modification, tobacco cessation, and other lifestyle changes; (3) facilitates screening and the early detection of a second cancer; (4) results in timely diagnosis and treatment of recurrent cancer; and (5) leads to the detection of functional or physical or psychological disability [28].

Cognitive Deficits

The survival of children with diagnosed and treated cancer is one of the successes in cancer care. Often, this survival improvement comes at a cost to the quality of life. Reports in the literature indicate that children receiving cranial irradiation and chemotherapy perform less well on intellectual and educational tests than do those in nonirradiated groups, verbal and attentional deficits being most pronounced. Children receiving chemotherapy alone performed at levels similar to those of controls, suggesting that such treatment is not associated with adverse neurobehavioral sequelae (i.e., registration of information and psychomotor speed) [29]. These findings suggest a need to investigate treatment delivery modifications that would diminish such cognitive deficits without sacrificing therapeutic effectiveness. They also point out a need for cognitive rehabilitation for children who have undergone cranial irradiation or intrathecal therapy.

Long-term cognitive impairment can arise also as a side effect of chemotherapy. Months or years after completion of treatment, neuropsychological symptoms, particularly memory and concentration problems, frequently have been reported by cancer patients treated with chemotherapy [30]. Another recent study has reported that breast cancer patients treated with adjuvant chemotherapy combining cyclophosphamide, methotrexate, and 5-fluorouracil are at a significantly higher risk for late cognitive impairment as compared to breast cancer patients not treated with chemotherapy (odds ratio = 6.4). This cognitive impairment was unaffected by anxiety, depression, fatigue, and time elapsed since treatment. It also was unrelated to self-reported complaints of cognitive dysfunction [31].

Future clinical trials and studies should recognize the importance of evaluating impaired cognition as a side effect of chemotherapy. This information should form the basis for preventive or remedial interventions in clinical practice.

Fatigue

Fatigue is receiving increasing attention as one of the most prevalent and distressing symptoms experienced by persons who have been treated for cancer. Fatigue has been described as "the missing link to quality of life" [32]. It is the most frequently reported symptom related to cancer and cancer treatment [33]. Fatigue can influence all aspects of quality of life, and it persists as a limiting factor long after treatment has been completed. Health care providers assume that they understand acute fatigue because they have experienced it themselves. However, cancer treatment–related fatigue is chronic and is not relieved by rest. Existing research suggests that fatigue or a sense of low energy persists after treatment, and persistent fatigue will result in a decrease in activity. Emerging literature also describes such chronic fatigue after cancer treatment. Thus far, little available evidence identifies the cause of this chronic fatigue, and few evidence-based interventions are available to reduce treatment-related fatigue or to reestablish pretreatment levels of energy [34].

Nutrition

Nutritional guidance is a part of successful rehabilitation and survivorship. Knowledge of good nutrition to maintain strength is essential. Cancer survivors must have knowledge of what comprises a healthy diet and lifestyle comparable to that advocated for the prevention of primary cancer. Because the prevention of recurring or second primary cancer is of great concern to survivors, they want all the information and guidance possible regarding how to stay healthy and to avoid cancer-related illness or other comorbidities. In view of what is known about the effect of certain dietary elements on cancer risk and protection, research is necessary to delineate the impact of nutritional interventions on cancer risk reduction or modulation. Some studies are under way, but their findings have not yet been defined. Owing to this lack of specific evidence for nutritional guidelines, the recommendations could be to follow the same nutritional advice given for risk reduction in persons who do not have diagnosed cancer.

Communication

Often, cancer and its treatment cause major changes in functioning, thereby creating a variety of psychological problems and problems in managing daily life. Limitations in function and mobility affect work and family roles. The need for emotional and social support may increase. Persons with cancer may experience fear, uncertainty about their future, loss of self-esteem, high levels of stress, and distress from persistent physical symptoms. The ability to communicate these concerns to physicians, caregivers, and families is necessary for obtaining supportive care and education for the management and resolution of these stressors. Physicians, caregivers, and families must be able to hear and observe what affected patients are trying to communicate. Good communication helps to reduce fear and anxiety, to counter feelings of isolation, to correct misconceptions, and to obtain appropriate symptom relief. If good communication is established between affected patients and all care providers, it will help to maintain trust and hope and to improve the quality of life through improving symptom management [1].

Because cancer patients and their families consider health care providers to be a primary, trusted source of information, patient education is the responsibility of all such providers [35]. Each has an area of expertise from which to provide guidance to promote comfort and adaptation. Such guidance can help affected patients to reach what will be an optimum level of wellness and functioning, both physical and psychological, within the context of the disease and treatment effects.

A person with cancer should be told—realistically but optimistically—the truth about his or her condition [1]. Most patients actively seek knowledge about their cancer and about the treatment they will receive. If they do not obtain satisfaction and a perception of openness in information from their caregivers, they will seek alternative sources of information, sources that may be less than accurate.

However, providing information alone, regardless of the format, is insufficient. Patients' understanding of such information must be assessed, as should their preferred mode of information access: by reading, by listening, by observing demonstration, or by a combination of these. Caregivers must determine patients' reading comprehension levels and the language they prefer for communicating and receiving information.

A growing body of research suggests that a diagnosis of cancer affects the entire family. Most studies show that psychological distress is experienced by family members at the time of diagnosis, during treatment, and in the early bereavement phase after death of the patient. As an increasing number of persons become survivors of cancer, their experience and that of family members more closely resembles that of living with a chronic disease [36]. Care should be taken to provide affected families with current and relevant information about the disease and its treatment. Caregivers should ensure that patients' family members also have an understanding of the effect of such patients' diagnosis on their risk profile. The time during which patients are being treated for cancer may present an opportunity to provide their families with information about cancer prevention, lifestyle changes, risk, and screening.

Psychological Support

Persons who have cancer experience the impact of the disease in many different ways and at different times. Common concerns involve such factors as the threatened loss of life; of independence, a job, and relationships; and of body integrity and function. These fears have an effect on perceived quality of life and contribute to the meaning of cancer for affected patients. Patient age and the degree to which the disease and treatment effects threaten life goals and activities modify the meaning of cancer for such individuals. At any age, even temporary disruption of function becomes disturbing if it involves valued life activities or forces a change in goals [1].

For most people, cancer is a new experience. Most people know little about cancer treatment, be it surgery, chemotherapy, irradiation, or biological therapies. If they have any opinion, they are likely to have strong preconceived notions about the negative side effects of these therapies. These notions are likely to engender fear and psychological distress. Plans and procedures should be explained as often as necessary. Health care providers should reinforce educational efforts daily. Psychological support is necessary throughout the course of treatment and often into the survivorship stage to control side effects, to prevent long-term and late psychological effects, and to maintain hope [1]. All persons with cancer should be treated in an emotionally supportive manner by all health professionals with whom they interact. Providing information and support continuously throughout the course of the disease may go a long way toward preventing the development of adjustment disorders or major depression. If such conditions develop, a relatively short term of psychotherapy should prove effective in most cases [1].

Support groups may be a helpful and practical approach to providing psychological support. Support group leaders should be knowledgeable about cancer care, the natural history of the disease, and psychology and the group process [37]. Recent research shows that most people cope well with cancer and may need formal counseling and support only in times of crisis or when their usual coping mechanisms are ineffective [38].

Certain strong myths relate to cancer and depression. A prevalent misconception is that all cancer patients are depressed. Many studies have demonstrated evidence to the contrary and have cited those who exhibit widely varying degrees of depression. A second myth is that persons with cancer *should* be depressed and that, therefore, treatment is unnecessary [1]. Depression involves feelings of sadness, grief, hopelessness, and helplessness. Some level of sadness and grief is a normal response to the diagnosis of cancer and its treatment. The degree of these feelings and their manifestations distinguishes between normal responses and depression. This continuum ranges from sadness to depressed mood [1]. The current general assumption is that at least 25% of all persons with cancer will meet the criteria for adjustment disorder, with depressed mood or major depression [39]. Studies have shown that cancer patients are no more likely to suffer from depression than are other equally seriously ill medical patients [40].

Sexuality

Usually, a patient's sexuality is markedly affected by the diagnosis and treatment of cancer. Estimates of the prevalence of sexual dysfunction in cancer patients range from 20% to 90%. The main concept that must be conveyed by the health care provider is that sexual feelings and function can resume after treatment. Sometimes, these feelings and functions return in different behavioral patterns, and often barriers must be removed to allow this area of human nature to be expressed [1].

Cancer treatment can alter sexual function directly when a tumor involves the sexual or reproductive organs. In men, tumor sites associated with sexual dysfunction include prostate cancer, penile cancer, and testicular cancer. Without rehabilitation, approximately 85% to 90% of men with prostate cancer suffer erectile dysfunction and impotence secondary to surgery or irradiation [1, 41]. Impaired sexual response for a large number of breast cancer patients occurs several months postoperatively rather than at the time of surgery [42].

Often, patients receiving chemotherapy suffer from malaise, fatigue, and nausea, all of which can reduce libido. In addition, such treatment-induced conditions as alopecia can cause affected patients to feel less attractive and can diminish sexual desire. Certain chemotherapeutic regimens, particularly those involving alkylating agents, may suppress gonadal functions. For example, women may experience ovarian failure, with associated dyspareunia and decrease in vaginal lubrication. When not contraindicated, hormone replacement can help to reverse these symptoms for women. However, these same agents may impair fertility in men [43].

Cancer can have indirect but dramatic effects on sexual function secondary to affected patients' emotional response to diagnosis or treatment. Such bodily changes as creation of a stoma or removal of a breast can limit patients' interest in sex and can interfere with sexual arousal and satisfaction. Distracted by pain or preoccupied with bodily function, affected patients may be unable to relax and enjoy sex. Others may see themselves as diseased and contagious and may withdraw both socially and sexually. By learning what cancer means to such patients, clinicians can correct misinformation and thereby facilitate patients' adjustment to the illness [36]. Medications also might affect sexual function or responsiveness. The most common offenders are anti-hypertensive and anticholinergic agents [36].

The sequelae of malignancy affect not only patients themselves but their sexual partners. A partner's response to a particular sexual change can be either similar to or much different from that of a patient. Regardless of the role of sexuality within the relationship and the changes that occur, couples who are able to communicate their needs and feelings have the best chance of adjusting successfully to change. The way in which clinicians address sexual issues with both patients and their partners can facilitate this adjustment [36].

In 1995, a survey [44] of various aspects of quality of life for 191 women at five years or more from diagnosis found that the women reported good psychological states and relative satisfaction with their sexual lives. Women who had experienced a recurrence of their cancer, were longer-term survivors, or suffered from breast cancer all reported higher levels of somatic concerns.

Reluctance to discuss sexual problems with health care providers is an issue in sexual rehabilitation. It is the responsibility of health care providers to ask about sexual functioning after treatment (Table 35.1).

Maintenance of Fertility Options

Remarkable advances have been made in the treatment of cancers that affect persons of reproductive age. Many survivors now must face effects on gonadal function, and such persons have concerns about reproductive capacity. Increasingly, assisted reproductive technologies and ways of preserving the ability to have children are the targets of cancer care professionals [45]. Health care providers are shifting the focus of oncologic care toward improving the quality of life, particularly with regard to fertility.

Cancer therapy either temporarily or permanently can damage sperm and ova production, resulting in infertility. Alternative treatment regimens can preserve reproductive function while maintaining high therapeutic efficacy [46]. The cryopreservation of ovarian tissue is a promising new method for conserving the fertility of young women being treated for cancer [47]. Sperm banking long has been an option for men. Now researchers are exploring ways to stimulate the recovery of spermatogenesis after chemotherapy and radiotherapy [48]. Most men of reproductive age will survive the treatment of their cancer, but reproductive function is a concern of such men.

The maintenance of fertility after cancer therapy brings with it a concern about effects on the offspring

Table 35.1   Physician Guidelines for Addressing Sexual Rehabilitation After Cancer Treatment

Record a sexual history, including the quality of patients' sexual activity.
Include patients' partners when applicable.
Convey a positive message: Some form of sexual expression always is possible.
Perform a thorough medical workup to diagnose any associated medical or treatment-related conditions impeding sexual functioning.
Counsel with simple direct suggestions.
Refer patients to a sex therapist for persistent sexual problems.

Source: Adapted from RJ McKenna, D Wellisch, F Fawsy, Rehabilitation and supportive care of the cancer patient. In GP Murphy, W Lawrence Jr, RE Lenhard Jr (eds), *American Cancer Society Textbook of Clinical Oncology* (2nd ed). Atlanta: American Cancer Society, 1995:635–654.

of cancer survivors. A recent study of the risk of cancer among 5,847 offspring of 14,652 survivors of childhood cancer diagnosed since the 1940s and 1950s in Scandinavia and Iceland showed no evidence of a significantly increased risk of nonhereditary cancer among the offspring of survivors of childhood cancer [49].

Quality of Life

Quality-of-life evaluation tools may be used during treatment to assess the impact of the disease and treatment and to predict survival of persons with cancer. Quality-of-life scores have prognostic value independent of other factors [50]. Attention to factors that influence quality of life during treatment will have an impact on the quality of survival. Attention to minimizing treatment-related sequelae and to the effects of persistent long-term symptoms of treatment toxicity should be a standard of care and a focus of research.

The long-term survival of persons with diagnosed cancer has risen dramatically during the last few decades. Very little is known about the quality of life experienced by such survivors [49]. Many assumptions have been made, but little systematic investigation has addressed the reality of survival. A review of 34 articles published from January 1, 1980, through February 12, 1998, by Gotay and Muraoka [51] revealed that many survivors continue to experience negative effects of cancer or treatment (or both) well beyond the completion of therapy. Several of the reviewed reports documented positive coping strategies and enhanced quality of life in long-term survivors of cancer. These findings support the need to assess positive as well as negative effects of cancer and its treatment. Other studies are beginning to support the observation that as survival extends, the reported quality of life is closer to that of healthy persons who have not had cancer [52, 53]. Additional information from well-designed studies is needed to increase understanding of the needs of long-term survivors, especially of those who are not represented in published quality-of-life studies.

The well-documented improvements in survival from childhood cancer raise questions about the physical and psychological aspects of quality of life in survivors. These questions have brought about the evaluation of physical, hormonal, and endocrine function on the one hand and cognitive and behavioral outcomes on the other. Far less attention is paid to the consequences for social and emotional adjustment. However, recent work is showing that these developmental aspects may be compromised in survivors of childhood cancer [54].

REHABILITATION

Rehabilitation is a largely overlooked aspect of cancer care. As the goals of reduction of cancer mortality are achieved, cancer rehabilitation must be a major focus of cancer care and cannot be divorced from cancer treatment. Cancer survivor rehabilitation can reduce the negative impact of cancer and its treatment on individuals, families, and communities. However, such rehabilitation rarely is mentioned in the "war on cancer," the "march to end cancer," or cancer prevention efforts and other cancer control programs.

Treatment approaches that include surgery, radiotherapy, and chemotherapy can have sequelae that affect cancer patients' quality of life and functional status. Health care providers must focus not only on the control or eradication of disease but on restoration of function and maintenance of psychological well-being. In the words of one author addressing cancer survivorship, "Cancer care is incomplete unless rehabilitation is addressed" (Table 35.2) [55].

Physical Rehabilitation

Those in the field of cancer rehabilitation are beginning to recognize the need for physical rehabilitation programs similar to those in cardiac rehabilitation. Exercise programs are being developed as interventions to improve physical functioning of persons with mobility

problems resulting from therapy. They also are being evaluated for use in weight control during maintenance therapy in breast cancer and as an intervention to lessen the effects of chronic fatigue. General physical therapy programs for reeducation after amputations have been a staple in cancer survivor rehabilitation programs.

Psychosocial Rehabilitation

The diagnosis of cancer in one member of a family or social system can have a significant impact on all family members. Cancer is a family disease, and all affected individuals should be the focus of supportive and adaptive interventions. The primary emphasis in research into the psychosocial aspects of cancer has been individual patients' responses to cancer and its treatment. Family members can play a significant role in how affected patients cope with and adjust to the illness and in the quality of survival [56].

The emotional support offered by specialized groups can be especially helpful to cancer patients and their families. The many different types of available support groups propose diverse goals: to decrease the sense of alienation by talking with others in a similar situation; to reduce anxiety about treatments and their effects; to

Table 35.2 Cancer Rehabilitation–Related Services

Cancer-specific rehabilitative services (e.g., related to ostomy care, continence, mobility)
Counseling services
Enterostomal therapy
Exercise classes
Family support services
Formal counseling
Information and education
Lymphedema management
Music and art therapy
Nutritional consultation
Occupational therapy
Physical therapy
Recreational therapy
Relaxation and yoga classes
Social services
Speech-language pathology
Spiritual care
Stress management
Support and education groups
Survivorship services

Note: This list represents expertise that should be available in the cancer center or by referral.
Source: Adapted from SL Frymark, Sexuality and body image in younger women with breast cancer. *Cancer Manage* Jan–Feb:8–13, 1998.

assist in clarifying misperceptions and misinformation; and to diminish feelings of isolation, helplessness, hopelessness, and neglect by others. The most common group approaches are education, behavioral training, problem-solving and coping skills, and psychological support. Professionally led and peer-led self-help groups have expanded in recent decades [1, 57].

Some of the more visible groups on a national level are I Can Cope, Y Me, Reach to Recovery, and Us Too. In addition, many diverse services are sponsored and provided by local groups. Some research has shown that these behavioral-educational interventions enhance the quality of life and, in some cases, prolong survival for cancer patients [40, 58].

RISK REDUCTION

Health-related beliefs and behaviors of long-term survivors of childhood cancer are important because of their vulnerability to adverse late effects of their cancer and its treatment. Areas of concern to be targeted for educational interventions and other appropriate monitoring include alcohol and tobacco use, diet, exercise, sleep, dental habits, and other lifestyle influences on health status and cancer risk. A study of health-related behaviors of survivors of childhood cancer showed that more than 80% of parents and 60% of young adult survivors believed that remaining healthy was more important for cancer survivors than for most other people [59]. However, this shared belief in increased vulnerability was expressed inconsistently in the survivors' health behaviors (i.e., smoking and other activities carrying a high risk for carcinogenesis).

AMERICANS WITH DISABILITIES ACT

Cancer survivors have experienced discrimination in the workplace because cancer often is perceived as a fatal disease. Employers also are reluctant to "take a chance" on cancer survivors because of preconceived notions that cancer survivors will be unable to do their jobs and because of the increasing costs of fringe benefits, including health insurance. Though employment discrimination continues to exist, it is less frequent now than in the past, primarily owing to public education in that regard [1].

Approximately 25% of the more than seven million cancer survivors experience unequal treatment in the workplace solely because of their history of cancer [21]. Many employers do not realize that in the United States more than half the persons with diagnosed cancer will overcome their disease and will have productivity rates relatively equal to those of other workers who have not had cancer.

For employment befitting their skills, training, and experience, cancer patients should have the same opportunity as those without a cancer history. Hiring, promotion, and treatment in the workplace should depend on ability and qualifications and should not be affected by a history of cancer. Sections 503 and 504 of the Federal Rehabilitation Act of 1973 provide that employment discrimination is illegal, but many workers are not covered by this act [60].

Now cancer patients can rely on the Americans with Disabilities Act (ADA) to overcome employment discrimination (Table 35.3). The ADA, which became effective on July 26, 1992, expands the protection of sections 503 and 504 of the Federal Rehabilitation Act by including employers with 25 or more employees. As of July 1994, businesses with 15 to 24 employees must follow the employment provisions specified in the ADA. Under provisions of the ADA, all cancer survivors are considered legally disabled. The ADA is a federal civil rights law requiring that disabled people be given the same opportunities as the able-bodied. The law provides

Table 35.3 Provisions of the Americans with Disabilities Act

Cancer survivors are considered legally disabled.
Disabled people must be given chances and opportunities equal to those given to the able-bodied.
Employers cannot discriminate in any phase of employment.
The act is not an affirmative-action statute.
Provisions apply to all qualified individuals who have a disability but can perform the essential functions of the job, regardless of whether a reasonable accommodation from the employer is needed.
The act protects individuals with a record of impairment. A provision protects cancer survivors for the remainder of their lives.
The act protects cancer survivors whose disease is cured, controlled, or in remission.
Cancer patients cannot be asked about, and do not have to disclose, any disability that would affect job performance.
The act does not require an explanation of gaps in employment history.

Source: Adapted from RJ McKenna, D Wellisch, F Fawzy, Rehabilitation and supportive care of the cancer patient. In GP Murphy, W Lawrence Jr, RE Lenhard Jr (eds), *American Cancer Society Textbook of Clinical Oncology* (2nd ed). Atlanta: American Cancer Society, 1995:635–654.

that employers cannot discriminate against persons with a disability in any phase of employment: hiring, training, job assignment, classification, promotion, transfer, benefits, leave of absence, layoff, or termination. The ADA is not an affirmative-action statute; it contains no quotas or goals for hiring the disabled [1]. Decisions that deny employment opportunities to cancer survivors and are based on misconceptions about cancer, rather than on individual ability to perform the work, may violate survivors' legal rights. Such discrimination may violate most federal and state laws that prohibit employment discrimination on the basis of actual or perceived disabilities [21].

RELAPSE AND PALLIATION

Many persons with cancer live in fear of recurrence, a normal anxiety about having had cancer. Those who cope best are those with realistic expectations. A perfectly reasonable reaction is for patients to ask their physician to gauge the risks of recurrence. Health care providers should be honest when responding to this question.

Recurrence of cancer, whether it occurs soon after treatment cessation or many years later, is a shattering experience. A diagnosis of recurrent, metastatic, or advanced disease can be even more traumatic than the original diagnosis. Often, patients interpret a diagnosis of recurrent disease as a death sentence. Emotions are likely to be more intense as such patients relive the trauma experienced at the original diagnosis. Open communication with affected health care providers and patients' families should be encouraged at all times. Support is required because making and facing treatment decisions may be more difficult for such patients at this stage. Most patients are less anxious if they know that their wishes will be honored and that they will have the information needed to make decisions even if their families are reluctant to address their concerns.

Depression and anticipatory grief also are normal reactions. Health care providers must be prepared to be supportive and to provide services and referrals needed by patients and families at the time of recurrence or at diagnosis of metastatic or advanced disease. Often, as with many aspects of cancer care and treatment decisions, what matters most is not what has happened but what can be done about it. Information about treatment options and other matters that will assist in decision making is as important at this stage of the disease as it is at initial diagnosis.

Symptom Management at the End of Life

Palliative care programs are based on the principle that care should be directed to cancer-affected families as a unit. Knowledge of family functioning can give health care providers insight into and understanding of why providing optimal care to some patients is more difficult than providing it for others. Health care providers should adjust their care according to affected families' level of functioning; they must appreciate that working with some families may be more demanding and that the outcomes may be less satisfactory. Families exhibiting consensus about problems, open and direct communication, and flexibility in adapting to change can be approached as a cohesive unit. In those families demonstrating indirect communication, little agreement about the nature of their problems, and rigidly entrenched roles, care must be tailored to their level of functioning. Families do not come to health care providers for help in changing their family systems; they come for help in dealing with the impending death of a family member [61].

Pain is a common distressing symptom experienced by cancer patients in the period close to the end of life. It affects physical functioning, social interaction, psychological status, and quality of life. Often, pain remains treated at a less-than-optimal level despite the extensive available body of knowledge regarding cancer pain assessment and management (see Chapter 33). [62]

When cure is not possible, the goals of care change to the prolongation of life and the palliation of symptoms. Palliative care is concerned mainly with managing side effects, controlling symptoms, and supporting overall quality of life [63, 64]. Assessment of quality of life at the end of life is an integral part of competent care. Early studies equated quality of life with functional status and usually measured it by the Karnofsky Performance Status Scale [65], the Zubrod Scale [66], the Eastern Cooperative Oncology Group scale, or other performance scales that provide an assessment of ambulatory and functional status. Studies of functional status and health-related quality of life have shown weak correlations and suggest that though functional status and quality of life are related, the concept of quality of life is broader than its component domains: physical symptoms and psychosocial, family, and spiritual elements. Measures of quality of life should be multidimensional, subjective, useful in a given setting, valid, and reliable [67]. Caregivers have been found to be consistently poor surrogate reporters of a patient's quality of life.

Supportive Care: Hospice

Hospice is an integral part of the broad spectrum of cancer care. It is defined as an integrated program of appropriate hospital and home care for cancer patients with a limited life expectancy. The usual goal is to help such patients live as fully as possible for whatever time remains but not to perform heroic, uncomfortable, or meaningless treatments or procedures. Hospice is not necessary for every dying person, but it is an option [1]. Timely referral to hospice is essential if the benefits of hospice care are to be experienced by affected patients and their families.

Hospice programs can provide improved outcomes of better pain control, better psychological support for patients and their families, and improved nursing and supportive services. Hospice can give affected families a respite from direct care and can provide a setting to support such families in their attempts to provide physical and psychological care for related patients. Hospice can provide support and rehabilitation for surviving families.

Data from the National Hospice Study [68] indicate that as patients approach death, their Quality of Life Index scores decreased. This finding was supported by other studies. The Hospice Quality of Life Index [69] has been developed to assess the overall quality of life of hospice patients. Four major categories are assessed: physical-functional, psychological, social-spiritual, and financial. It is the only tool designed specifically for use in palliative care settings. Other quality-of-life assessment tools were designed and validated for use with patients undergoing active treatment with curative intent. Such tools may be useful in palliative care settings, but additional validity and reliability data are required to ascertain their appropriateness and accuracy with patients who are receiving palliative care [70].

REFERENCES

1. McKenna RJ, Wellisch D, Fawsy F. Rehabilitation and supportive care of the cancer patient. In Murphy GP, Lawrence W Jr, Lenhard RE Jr, (eds), *American Cancer Society Textbook of Clinical Oncology* (2nd ed). Atlanta: American Cancer Society, 1995:635–654.
2. Greenlee RT, Murray T, Bolden S, Wingo PA. Cancer statistics, 2000. *CA Cancer J Clin* 50:7–33, 2000.
3. National Cancer Institute, Division of Cancer Prevention and Control, Surveillance Program. *Cancer Statistics Review, 1973–1988.* [NIH Pub. No. 91–279.] Washington, DC: US Department of Health and Human Services, 1991.
4. Cole P, Rodu B. Declining cancer mortality in the United States. *Cancer* 78:2045–2058, 1996.
5. Smith K, Lesko LM. Psychosocial problems in cancer survivors. *Oncology* 2:33–40, 1988.
6. Ellman R, Thomas BA. Is psychological well-being impaired in long-term survivors of breast cancer. *J Med Screen* 2:5–9, 1995.
7. Schover LR. Sexuality and body image in younger women with breast cancer. *Monogr J Natl Cancer Inst* 16:177–182, 1994.
8. Frymark SL. Providing cancer rehabilitation services. *Cancer Manage* Jan–Feb:8–13, 1998.
9. Harpham WS. Long-term survivorship. Late effects. In Berger A, et al. (eds), *Principles and Practices of Supportive Oncology.* Philadelphia: Lippincott-Raven, 1998:889–907.
10. Lehmann JF, DeLisa JA, Warren CG. Cancer rehabilitation: assessment of need development and evaluation of a model of care. *Arch Phys Med Rehab* 89:1281–1284, 1998.
11. Mullan F. Seasons of survival: reflections of a physician with cancer. *N Engl J Med* 313:270–273, 1985.
12. Broder S. The human costs of cancer and the response of the National Cancer Program. *Cancer* 67:1716–1717, 1985.
13. Clark EJ, Stovall EL, Leigh S, et al. *Imperatives for Quality Care: Access, Advocacy, Action and Accountability.* Silver Spring, MD: National Coalition for Cancer Survivorship, 1996.
14. Watson PG. Cancer rehabilitation. The evolution of a concept. *Cancer Nurs* 13:2–12, 1990.
15. Dietz JH. Rehabilitation of the cancer patient. *Med Clin North Am* 53:1066–1069, 1969.
16. Dudas S, Carlson C. Cancer rehabilitation. *Oncol Nurs Forum* 15:183–188, 1988.
17. Mayer C, O'Connor L. Rehabilitation of persons with cancer: an ONS Position Statement. *Oncol Nurs Forum* 16:424–427, 1989.
18. Ganz PA, Hirji K, Sim MS, et al. Predicting psychosocial risk in patients with breast cancer. *Med Care* 31:419–431, 1993.
19. Meadows A. *Meeting Summary and Recommendations: Unresolved Issues in Cancer Survivorship.* Bethesda, MD: National Cancer Institute, Office of Cancer Survivorship, 1996.
20. Berry DL, Catanzaro M. Persons with cancer and their return to the workplace. *Cancer Nurs* 15:40–46, 1992.
21. Hoffman B. Employment discrimination: another hurdle for cancer survivors. *Cancer Invest* 9:589–598, 1991.
22. Weeks J. Taking quality of life into account in health economic analysis. *Monogr J Natl Cancer Inst* 20:23–27, 1996.
23. Veach TA, Nicholas DR. Understanding families of adults with cancer: combining the clinical course and cancer stages of family development. *J Counsel Dev* 76:144–155, 1998.
24. Zabora J, Smith E. Family dysfunction and the cancer patient: early recognition and intervention. *Oncology (Huntingt)* 4:31–41, 1991.
25. Barakat LP, Kazak AE, Meadows AT, et al. Families surviving childhood cancer: a comparison of posttraumatic stress symptoms with families of healthy children. *J Pediatr Psychol* 6:843–859, 1997.
26. National Comprehensive Cancer Network. NCCN proceedings: oncology practice guidelines. *Oncology (Huntingt)* 12:11A, 1998.
27. National Comprehensive Cancer Network. NCCN proceedings. *Oncology (Huntingt)* 13:51, 1999.

28. Lenhard RE Jr, Lawrence W Jr, McKenna RJ. General approach to the patient. In Murphy GP, Lawrence W Jr, Lenhard RE Jr, (eds), *American Cancer Society Textbook of Clinical Oncology* (2nd ed). Atlanta: American Cancer Society, 1995:64–74.

29. Anderson V, Smibert E, Ekert H, et al. Intellectual, educational and behavioural sequelae after irradiation and chemotherapy. *Arch Dis Child* 70:476–483, 1994.

30. Wieneke MH, Dienst ER. Neuropsychologic assessment of cognitive functioning following chemotherapy for breast cancer. *Psychooncology* 4:61–66, 1995.

31. Schagen SB, Frits van Dam SAM, Muller MJ, et al. Cognitive deficits after postoperative adjuvant chemotherapy for breast carcinoma. *Cancer* 85:640–650, 1999.

32. Winningham ML. Fatigue: the missing link to quality of life. *Fatigue* 4:2–7, 1995.

33. Piper BF. Fatigue. In Carrierie-Kohlman V, Lindsey A, West C (eds), *Pathophysiological Phenomena in Nursing. Human Responses to Illness* (2nd ed). Philadelphia: Saunders, 1993:279–301.

34. Nail LM, Jones LS. Fatigue as a side effect of cancer treatment: impact on quality of life. *Fatigue* 4:8–13, 1995.

35. Harris KA. The informational needs of patients with cancer and their families. *Cancer Pract* 6:39–46, 1988.

36. Ell K, Nishimoto R, Mantell J, Hamovitch M. Longitudinal analysis of psychological adaptation among family members of patients with cancer. *J Psychom Res* 32:429–438, 1988.

37. Kriss A. Psychosocial/psychotherapeutic interventions in cancer patients: consensus statement. *Support Care Cancer* 3:270–271, 1995.

38. Cunningham AJ. Group psychological therapy for cancer patients. *Support Care Cancer* 3:244–247, 1995.

39. Massie MJ, Holland JC. Depression and the American cancer patients. *J Clin Psychiatr* 51:252–256, 1995.

40. Spiegel D. Essentials of psychotherapeutic interventions for cancer patients. *Support Care Cancer* 3:252–256, 1995.

41. Stroudmire A, Techman T, Graham S. Sexual assessment of the urologic oncology patient. *Psychosomatics* 26:405–410, 1985.

42. Maguire G, Lee G, Bevington C, et al. Psychiatric problems in the first year after mastectomy. *Br Med J* 1:963–965, 1978.

43. Halfin VP, Morgentaler A, Barton Burke M, Goldstein I. Sexuality and cancer. In Osteen R (ed), *Cancer Manual* (9th ed). Framingham MA: American Cancer Society, Massachusetts Division, 1996:222–236.

44. Kurtz ME, Wyatt G, Kurtz JC. Psychological and sexual well-being, philosophical/spiritual views, and health habits of long-term cancer survivors. *Health Care Women Int* 16:253–262, 1995.

45. Shahin MS, Puscheck E. Reproductive sequelae of cancer treatment. *Obstet Gynecol Clin North Am* 25:423–433, 1998.

46. Costabile RA, Spevak M. Cancer and male factor infertility. *Oncology* 12:557–562, 1998.

47. Newton H. The cryopreservation of ovarian tissue as a strategy for preserving the fertility of cancer patients. *Human Reprod Update* 4:237–247, 1998.

48. Meistrich ML. Hormonal stimulation of the recovery of spermatogenesis following chemo- or radiotherapy. *APMIS* 106:37–45, 1998.

49. Sankila R, Olsen JH, Anderson H, et al. Risk of cancer among offspring of childhood-cancer survivors. Association of the Nordic Cancer Registries and the Nordic Society of Paediatric Haematology and Oncology. *N Engl J Med* 338:1339–1344, 1998.

50. Coates A, Porzsolt F, Osoba D. Quality of life in oncology practice: prognostic value of EORTC QLQ-C30 scores in patients with advanced malignancy. *Eur J Cancer* 33:1025–1030, 1997.

51. Gotay CC, Muraoka MY. Quality of life in long-term survivors of adult-onset cancers. *J Natl Cancer Inst* 9:656–667, 1998.

52. Dorval M, Maunsell E, Deschenes L, et al. Long-term quality of life after breast cancer: comparison of 8-year survivors with population controls. *J Clin Oncol* 16:487–494, 1998.

53. Olweny CLM, Juttner CA, Rolfe P, et al. Long-term effects of cancer treatment and consequences of cure: cancer survivors enjoy quality of life similar to their neighbours. *Eur J Cancer* 29A:826–830, 1993.

54. Eiser C, Havermans T. Long term social adjustment after treatment for childhood cancer. *Arch Dis Child* 70:66–70, 1994.

55. Clarke LK. Rehabilitation of the head and neck cancer patient. *Oncology* 12:81–89, 1998.

56. Manne S. Cancer in the marital context: a review of the literature. *Cancer Invest* 16:188–202, 1998.

57. Meyer TJ, Mark MM. Effects of psychosocial interventions with adult cancer patients: a meta-analysis of randomized experiments. *Health Psychol* 2:101–108, 1995.

58. Fawsz IF. A short-term psychoeducational intervention for patients newly diagnosed with cancer. *Support Care Cancer* 3:235–238, 1995.

59. Mulhern RK, Tyc VL, Phipps S, et al. Health-related behaviors of survivors of childhood cancer. *Med Pediatr Oncol* 25:159–165, 1996.

60. McKenna RJ, Toghia N. Maximizing the productive activities of the cancer patient: policy issues in work and illness. In Barofsky I (ed), *The Cancer Patient*. New York: Praeger, 1989.

61. Davis B, Reimer JC, Martens N. Family functioning and its implications for palliative care. *J Palliat Care* 10:29–36, 1994.

62. Committee on Care at the End of Life. *Approaching Death: Improving Care at the End of Life*. Washington, DC: National Academy Press, 1997.

63. Ingham JM, Foley KM. Pain and the barriers to its relief at the end of life: a lesson for improving end of life health care. *Hosp J* 13:89–100, 1998.

64. Cella DF. Measuring quality of life in palliative care. *Semin Oncol Suppl* 3:73–81, 1995.

65. Karnofsky DA, Abelmann WH, Craver LF, et al. The use of nitrogen mustards in the palliative treatment of carcinoma. *Cancer* 1:634–656, 1948.

66. Zubrod CG, Schneiderman M, Frei E, et al. Appraisal of methods for the study of chemotherapy of cancer in man: comparative therapeutic trial of nitrogen mustard and triethylene thiophosphoramide. *J Chron Dis* 11:703, 1960.

67. Padilla GV, Frank-Stromborg M. Single instruments for measuring quality of life. In Frank-Stromborg M, Olsen

SJ (eds), *Instruments for Clinical Health-Care Research* (2nd ed). Boston: Jones & Bartlett, 1997:114–134.

68. Kane RL, Klein SJ, Bernstein L, et al. Hospice role in alleviating the emotional stress of terminal patients and their families. *Med Care* 23:189–197, 1985.

69. McMillan SC, Mahon M. Measuring quality of life in hospice patients using a newly developed Hospice Quality of Life Index. *Qual Life Res* 2:437–447, 1994.

70. McMillan SC. Quality of Life Assessment in Palliative Care, 1999. <http://www.moffitt.usf.edu/providers/ccj/v3n3/article4.html>

36

Psychiatric Complications in Cancer Patients

∎ ∎ ∎

ANDREW J. ROTH
MARY JANE MASSIE

CANCER IS COMPOSED OF A GROUP OF DIS-eases that for centuries has struck fear in the hearts of people. Its previously certain fatal outcome, absence of known cause or cure, and association with suffering, pain, and disfigurement made it particularly frightening. Physicians long avoided telling patients that they had cancer, believing that the diagnosis would be too painful to hear. The press avoided printing the word, and affected families colluded with physicians to keep the diagnosis a secret from afflicted patients.

Multiple factors have contributed to attitude changes in the United States. Founded in 1913, the American Cancer Society began to educate the public about the importance of early cancer diagnosis and treatment. In the 1950s and the 1960s, physicians and patients became less pessimistic about cancer, as radiotherapy and chemotherapy altered the pattern of outcome for several neoplasms in children and young adults. The hospice movement in Europe and the pioneering work of Dr. Elisabeth Kübler-Ross in the United States led to improvement in care for dying patients by focusing attention on pain and symptom control. In the 1960s and 1970s, after clinical studies demonstrated that compassionate honesty is helpful, not damaging, for both adult and pediatric patients, clinicians began discussing more openly all aspects of the illness with patients and families. These types of discussions may have been encouraged also by consumer advocacy and the need for informed consent. Patients who wished to discuss their fears of advanced cancer and death could do so because the situation's reality could be acknowledged.

Cancer's transition from a group of neglected and hopeless diseases to one of potential cures, increased

The authors gratefully acknowledge assistance by Theresa Carpenter, Kathleen Zoe McClear, and Alex Pisani in the preparation of this manuscript. This work was supported in part by William E. Pelton, Sylvia Rosenberg, and Margaret and R. Peter Sullivan III.

treatment efforts, and extensive research generated more interest in the disease's psychosocial aspects. The field of psycho-oncology pioneered by Morton Bard, Arthur Sutherland, Avery Weisman, Jimmie Holland, and others was developed to deal with the human dimensions of cancer and its impact on the psychological and social functioning of patients, their families, and treating staff [1].

PSYCHOLOGICAL IMPACT OF CANCER

Persons who receive diagnoses of cancer exhibit characteristic normal responses. A period of initial disbelief, denial, or despair is common and generally lasts for 2 to 5 days. Patients often state "This just can't be happening to me," or "Pathology must have mixed up my slides," or "There is no reason to take treatment; it won't work." The second phase, characterized by dysphoric mood, lasts from 1 to 2 weeks. Often, patients report having anxiety symptoms, depressed mood, anorexia, insomnia, or irritability. The ability to concentrate and to carry out usual daily activities is impaired, and intrusive thoughts of the illness and uncertainty about the future are present. Usually, adaptation begins after several weeks and continues for months as patients integrate new information, confront reality issues, find reasons for optimism, and resume activities [2].

Patients' perceptions of the disease, its manifestations, and the stigma commonly attached to cancer contribute to these responses. For adults, fear of a painful death is a primary concern. All patients fear the potential for disability, dependency on family and health care providers, altered appearance, and changed body function. The new role of being sick or different involves a change in nearly every aspect of adults' or children's lives. The fear of being separated from or abandoned by family, friends, and colleagues is common.

Although such concerns are pervasive, the initial level of psychological distress is highly variable and relates to three factors: (1) medical (cancer type and site; stage at diagnosis; such symptoms as pain; treatments required; rehabilitation available; clinical course of illness; caregiver attitudes; and associated medical and psychiatric conditions); (2) patient-related (level of cognitive and psychological development; ability to cope with stressful events; emotional maturity; ability to accept altered life goals; prior experiences with cancer; concurrent life losses and stresses; emotional and economic support by family and others); and (3) societal and cultural (attitudes toward cancer and treatment; stigma associated with diagnoses; health care policies) [3]. Consideration of these factors enables physicians to evaluate the patient better.

Cancer treatment, often lengthy and arduous, necessitates flexibility in patterns of emotional adaptation. Beyond the initial adjustment, the possibility of cure changes the threat of death to a focus on uncertainty and management of treatment side effects. Simultaneously, patients must meet normal school, work, and family obligations, must maintain a sense of control and confidence in the outcome, and must manage financial burdens.

PEDIATRIC AND FAMILY ISSUES

Discussing the cancer diagnosis with sick children is as routine in pediatric care as in the care of adult patients. The diagnosis and prognosis, including the issue of death, are discussed in a developmentally appropriate manner on several occasions with participation of the family [4]. Efforts to reduce "keeping secrets" will diminish the possibility of pathologic communication patterns in affected families. Compliance is enhanced by a child's sense of involvement in the treatment.

The effects of cancer on affected families include reactions of disbelief, anger, grief, hostility, guilt, and mourning for possible loss [5]. For most parents, the diagnosis of cancer in their child means "death," despite recent changes in the prognosis for many neoplasms. An intellectual understanding that many medical advances have occurred does little to decrease family members' distress and fears: They must accept the rigors of treatment without any guarantee of success. The illness alters all aspects of family life. The parents' goals, wishes, and expectations for the ill child are changed forever. The diagnosis of cancer in children or adults most likely will aggravate existing family problems. However, contrary to popular belief, the likelihood of divorce is not increased, nor are couples generally brought closer together [6].

The devotion of parents' time to affected children's clinic visits and hospitalizations may occasion inadvertent parental neglect of the siblings. Many concerns of siblings are strikingly similar to those of sick children: symptoms of anxiety, social isolation, decreased self-esteem, and a sense of vulnerability to illness and injury. Numerous behavioral and school problems have been documented; thus, communication with teachers about the cancer issues facing an affected family may be helpful [7].

PREVALENCE OF PSYCHIATRIC DISORDERS IN CANCER PATIENTS

The many myths about psychological problems in cancer patients vary from expressing a universal need for help to outright denial. One of the first efforts in psycho-oncology was to obtain objective data on the type and frequency of emotional problems in cancer patients. Using criteria from the *Diagnostic and Statistical Manual of Mental Disorders* classification of psychiatric disorders, the Psychosocial Collaborative Oncology Group at three cancer centers determined the prevalence of psychiatric disorders in 215 randomly assessed hospitalized and ambulatory adult patients with cancer (Fig. 36.1) [1]. Slightly more than one-half (53%) were adjusting normally to the crisis of illness. The remainder (47%) had sufficient distress to receive a diagnosis of a psychiatric disorder. Adjustment disorder with depressed or anxious mood (or both) was by far the most common diagnosis (68%). Major depressive disorder was next (13%), followed by organic mental disorder (delirium; 8%), personality disorder (7%), and preexisting anxiety disorder (4%). Nearly 90% of the psychiatric disorders—adjustment disorders, organic mental disorders (delirium), and major depression—were related to responses to disease or treatment. Only 11% represented psychiatric problems that antedated the cancer diagnosis (e.g., personality and anxiety disorders). Comparable research in children is lacking, but clinical data appear to reflect a similar spectrum of problems. Physicians who treat cancer patients can expect to find, for the most part, a group of psychologically healthy individuals who are responding to significant stresses posed by cancer and its treatment.

DISORDERS IN CANCER PATIENTS WITH PAIN

In the Psychosocial Collaborative Oncology Group Study, 39% of those who received a psychiatric diagnosis experienced significant pain. In contrast, only 19% of patients who did not receive a psychiatric diagnosis had significant pain. The psychiatric diagnosis of the patients was predominantly adjustment disorder with depressed or mixed mood (69%) but, notably, 15% of patients with significant pain had symptoms of a major depression.

Both data and clinical observation show that the psychiatric symptoms of patients who are in pain must be considered initially to be a consequence of uncontrolled

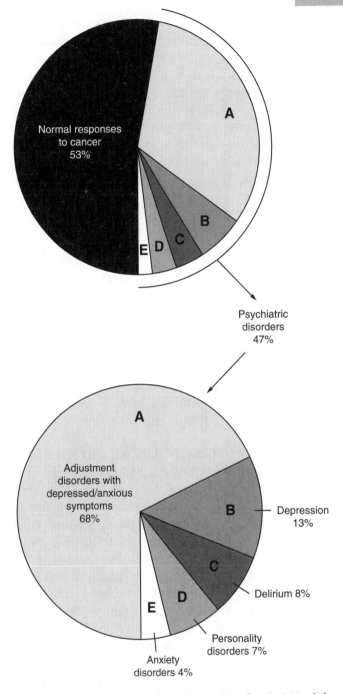

Figure 36.1 Prevalence of psychiatric disorders in 215 adult cancer patients indicated that slightly more than half were adjusting normally to the crisis of illness. Adjustment disorder with depressed or anxious mood (or both) was the most common psychiatric disorder diagnosed. (© 1983, Reprinted with permission of the American Medical Association from LR Derogatis, GR Morrow, J Fetting, et al., Prevalence of psychiatric disorders among cancer patients. *JAMA* 249:751–757, 1983.)

pain. Acute anxiety, depression with despair (especially when adult patients believe that the pain means disease progression), agitation, irritability, lack of cooperation, anger, and insomnia may be the emotional or behavioral concomitants of pain. In physically ill children, chronic pain may present with symptoms of apathy, withdrawal, and clinging behaviors. These symptoms are not labeled as a psychiatric disorder unless they persist after pain is controlled adequately.

Clinicians first should assist in pain control and then should reassess patients' mental state after pain is controlled, to determine whether such patients have a psychiatric disorder. Undertreatment of pain is a major problem in both adult and pediatric settings [8]. Aggressive pain management strategies, including narcotics, are essential to the emotional care of physically ill children and adults (see Chapter 33). Long-term psychiatric sequelae are less likely in children whose pain is well treated. No evidence substantiates increased risk of subsequent drug abuse in either children or adults receiving narcotic analgesia. In fact, patients associate the narcotic effects with the unpleasant aspects of the illness and seek to avoid them during the recovery phase.

SPECIFIC PSYCHOLOGICAL PROBLEMS AND THEIR MEDICAL MANAGEMENT

Though most adults and children adjust well to the stress of cancer, a persistent, severe, or intolerable level of emotional distress that prohibits such patients' usual functioning is not normal and requires evaluation, diagnosis, and management by a mental health professional. Seven psychiatric disorders occur frequently enough in cancer to warrant a description of their clinical picture. Three are direct responses to illness: adjustment disorders with anxiety or depression (or both), major depressive disorder, and delirium. The remaining four—primary anxiety disorders, personality disorders, schizophrenia, and bipolar disorders—are preexisting conditions that often are exacerbated by illness.

Adjustment Disorders

The most common psychiatric disorder diagnosed in adults and children with cancer is an adjustment disorder in reaction to the stress of illness. The characteristic symptoms are those of anxiety and depression. The key features of adjustment disorders are the unusual persistence of symptoms and undue interference with occupational, social, or school functioning. When symptoms are severe, differentiating adjustment disorders from major depression or generalized anxiety disorders is difficult. Regular patient follow-up usually clarifies such diagnostic questions.

Interventions are directed at helping the patient to adapt to the stresses of cancer and to resume successful coping. Individual psychotherapy focuses on clarifying the medical situation and the meaning of illness and on reinforcing successful coping strategies. A helpful technique is to include a spouse, partner, or family member in some sessions to enhance support at home. Often, group therapy is helpful, as are such behavioral methods as relaxation and hypnosis. The decision to prescribe psychotropic medication is based on the presence of a high level of distress or an inability to carry out daily activities. A therapeutic trial of a benzodiazepine (e.g., lorazepam, 0.5 mg orally bid or tid; alprazolam, 0.25 mg orally tid) may control symptoms effectively and can facilitate other therapeutic interventions. Although the common fear of inciting drug addiction in both adult and pediatric cancer patients is unfounded, benzodiazepines are remarkably underprescribed. Consequently, patients experience distress that could be controlled easily by judicious use of medication.

Depressive Disorders

The overlap of physical illness and symptoms of depression is recognized widely. Diagnosis of depression in physically healthy adults and children requires the presence of somatic complaints—insomnia, anorexia, fatigue, and weight loss—in addition to depressed mood and cognitive symptoms. These symptoms, however, are common to both cancer and depression. In cancer patients, the diagnosis of depression must depend on cognitive symptoms: dysphoric mood, apathy, crying, anhedonia, feelings of helplessness, decreased self-esteem, guilt, social withdrawal, and thoughts of "wishing for death" or suicide.

Depression in both adult and pediatric cancer patients has been studied using a range of assessment methods [9–11]. In general, the more narrowly the term *depression* is defined, the lower the prevalence of depression that is reported. Several studies using patient self-report and observer ratings found major depression in approximately one-fourth of hospitalized adult cancer patients [9, 10]. This prevalence is similar to that seen in patients with other serious medical illnesses, suggesting that the level of illness, not the specific diagnosis, is the primary determinant [12, 13]. Factors associated with a higher prevalence of depression in cancer patients are a greater level of physical impairment, advanced stages of illness, inadequately controlled pain, prior history of depression, and the presence of other significant life stresses or losses [11].

The clinical evaluation of affected patients includes a careful assessment of both symptoms and history, particularly previous depressive episodes, family history of depression or suicide, concurrent life stresses, and level of social support. Exploring the patient's understanding of the medical situation and the meaning of illness is essential. The contribution of pain to depressive symptoms must be determined because no psychiatric disorder can be diagnosed with certainty until pain is controlled [14].

Symptoms of depression can be produced by numerous commonly prescribed medications, including methyldopa, reserpine, barbiturates, diazepam, and propranolol. Of the hundreds of cancer chemotherapeutic agents, depressive symptoms are produced by relatively few: prednisone, dexamethasone, vincristine, vinblastine, procarbazine, asparaginase, amphotericin B, tamoxifen, interferon, and interleukin-2. Many metabolic, nutritional, endocrine, and neurologic disorders produce depressive symptoms [15]. Adult cancer patients with abnormal levels of potassium, sodium, or calcium may become depressed, as can patients with a variety of nutritional deficiencies (folate, vitamin B_{12}). Hypothyroidism or hyperthyroidism and adrenal insufficiency also can produce depressive symptoms.

Suicidal ideation requires careful assessment to determine whether it reflects depressive illness or expresses a wish to have ultimate control over intolerable symptoms. Adult cancer patients who are at higher risk are those with poor prognosis, advanced stages of illness, a psychiatric history or history of substance abuse, previous suicide attempts, or a family history of suicide. A recent death of a friend or partner, few social supports, depression with extreme hopelessness, poorly controlled pain, delirium, and recent information of a grave prognosis are significant risk factors [16].

TREATMENT OF DEPRESSIVE DISORDERS

Usually, prolonged and severe depression requires treatment that combines psychotherapy with medication or, rarely, with electroconvulsive therapy. Pharmacologic treatments appropriate for use in adult cancer patients are the newer agents, including selective serotonin reuptake inhibitors (SSRIs), the tricyclic antidepressants (TCAs), psychostimulants, mood stabilizers, and monoamine oxidase inhibitors (MAOIs; Table 36.1) [17, 18].

New Antidepressant Agents

The SSRIs fluoxetine, sertraline, and paroxetine are the antidepressants prescribed first in cancer settings because they have fewer sedative and autonomic effects than do the TCAs. The most common side effects are mild nausea, gastrointestinal disturbance, headache, somnolence or insomnia, and a brief period of increased anxiety; hyponatremia is an uncommon adverse effect. These drugs may cause appetite suppression that usually lasts several weeks. Some cancer patients experience transient weight loss; however, weight usually returns to baseline level, and the anorectic properties of these drugs have not been a limiting factor in cancer patients already struggling with anorexia. Paroxetine has no active metabolites, and sertraline has fewer active metabolites than does fluoxetine; both paroxetine and sertraline have a short half-life, a characteristic important in efforts to avoid accumulation of the drug and to allow for more precise titration. All SSRIs can cause sexual dysfunction in both men and women, a side effect that often leads to cessation of use of the drug. Citalopram, the newest SSRI, is reportedly easier for patients to tolerate. Dosages for fluoxetine and paroxetine start at 5 or 10 mg/day and can be increased to 20 mg/day. Sertraline is started at 25 mg/day and is titrated slowly to an effective dose (50–150 mg/day). Citalopram can be started at 10 to 20 mg/day and increased to 20 to 40 mg/day.

Bupropion and trazodone are prescribed less frequently than are the SSRIs for individuals with cancer. Buproprion is considered if patients have a poor response to a reasonable trial of other antidepressants. Its activating profile makes it useful in lethargic medically ill patients; it should be avoided in patients with a history of seizure disorder or brain tumor and in those who are malnourished. Slow-release bupropion may be helpful for patients wanting to discontinue tobacco smoking (i.e., those with lung cancer, head and neck cancer, etc.). Trazodone is strongly sedating and, in low doses (50–100 mg at bedtime), is helpful in the treatment of depressed cancer patients with insomnia. Often, effective antidepressant doses are greater than 300 mg/day. Trazodone has been associated with priapism and should, therefore, be used with caution in male patients. Venlafaxine, nefazodone, and mirtazapine are the newest antidepressant medications available; little information is available thus far regarding their use in cancer patients. Venlafaxine affects both norepinephrine and serotonin neurotransmitter systems, but it does not produce the same uncomfortable antimuscarinic and antiadrenergic side effects as do the TCAs. Hypertensive side effects at higher doses can be problematic

Table 36.1 Antidepressant Medications Used in Cancer Patients

Drug	Starting Daily Dosage (mg PO)	Therapeutic Daily Dosage (mg PO)
Newer agents		
Serotonin reuptake inhibitors		
Fluoxetine	10	20–60
Sertraline	25	50–200
Paroxetine	10	10–40
Citalopram	20	20–40
Others		
Trazodone	50	150–300
Bupropion	75	200–300
Venlafaxine	18.75	75–225
Nefazodone	50–100	300–600
Mirtazapine	15	15–45
Tricyclic antidepressants		
Amitriptyline	25	50–150
Doxepin	25	50–200
Desipramine	25	50–200
Nortriptyline	25	50–150
Psychostimulants		
Dextroamphetamine	2.5 at 8:00 AM and noon	5–30
Methylphenidate	2.5 at 8:00 AM and noon	5–30
Pemoline	18.75 in morning and at noon	37.5–150
Monoamine oxidase inhibitors		
Isocarboxazid	10	20–40
Phenelzine	15	30–60
Tranylcypromine	10	20–40
Lithium carbonate	300	600–1,200

PO = per os (orally).

in medically ill patients. Nefazodone also affects serotonin and norepinephrine systems. It is useful in patients with agitated depression and insomnia. Mirtazapine, another sedating antidepressant, is efficacious for agitated depressions. It has fewer gastrointestinal side effects than do the other antidepressants and can be less sedating at higher dosages. Bupropion, nefazodone, and mirtazapine are less likely to cause sexual dysfunction than are the SSRIs and venlafaxine.

Tricyclic Antidepressants

TCAs (amitriptyline, imipramine, desipramine, doxepin, nortriptyline, etc.) still are used in the oncology setting for both adults and children with cancer [19]. For cancer patients, nortriptyline and desipramine have the most favorable side-effect profiles in this class of antidepressants. Dosing is initiated at 10 to 25 mg at bedtime, especially in debilitated patients, and the dose is increased by 25 mg every 1 to 2 days until a beneficial effect is achieved. For reasons that are unclear, depressed cancer patients often show a therapeutic response to a TCA at much lower doses (75–125 mg/day) than usually are required in physically healthy, depressed patients (150–300 mg/day). Serum levels of the medications can be helpful in titrating dosages (especially with nortriptyline) and in monitoring toxicity and compliance. Frequently, the effects on appetite and sleep are immediate; the effects on mood may be delayed.

Psychostimulants

In cancer patients, low doses of a psychostimulant (i.e., dextroamphetamine, methylphenidate, and pemoline) promote a sense of well-being, decrease fatigue, and stimulate appetite. An advantage of these drugs is a rapid onset of antidepressant action as compared with other antidepressants. Psychostimulants also can potentiate the analgesic effects of opioid analgesics and are used commonly to counteract opioid-induced sedation.

Side effects at low doses include insomnia, tachycardia, euphoria, and mood lability. High doses and long-term use may produce nightmares, insomnia, and paranoia. Patients should be cardiologically and neurologically stable before starting on a stimulant. Usually, treatment with dextroamphetamine and methylphenidate is initiated at a dose of 2.5 mg at 8 AM and at noon. Pemoline, a chewable and gentler psychostimulant, usually is initiated at a dose of 18.75 mg at 8 AM and is the drug of choice for frail, debilitated patients or for those who cannot swallow pills. Pemoline should be used with caution in patients with renal impairment; liver and renal function tests should be monitored periodically with longer-term treatment.

Typically, patients are maintained on a psychostimulant for 1 to 2 months, after which time approximately two-thirds will be able to be withdrawn without a recurrence of depressive symptoms. Those who develop recurrence of depressive symptoms can be maintained for long periods (e.g., up to 1 year). Tapering of the psychostimulant may be aided by concurrent use of another antidepressant.

Mood Stabilizers

Patients who have been receiving lithium carbonate for bipolar affective disorder prior to developing cancer should be maintained on the agent throughout cancer treatment, although close monitoring is necessary when the intake of fluids and electrolytes is restricted, such as during preoperative and postoperative periods. The maintenance dose of lithium may have to be reduced in seriously ill patients. Lithium should be prescribed with caution in patients receiving cisplatin or other potentially nephrotoxic drugs.

Use of carbamazepine as a mood stabilizer can be problematic in cancer patients because of its bone marrow–suppressing properties. Although use of valproic acid and gabapentin in this population has not been studied, these drugs appear to be tolerated better.

Monoamine Oxidase Inhibitors

If patients have responded well to an MAOI for depression prior to treatment for cancer, its continued use is warranted. Most psychiatrists, however, are reluctant to start depressed cancer patients on MAOIs because the need for dietary restriction is received poorly by patients who already have dietary limitations and nutritional deficiencies secondary to cancer illness and treatment. MAOIs should be prescribed cautiously in patients receiving the antineoplastic agent procarbazine, because it has some monoamine oxidase inhibitory activity. The opioid meperidine should not be prescribed for patients taking MAOIs, as hypertensive crisis and death can result.

Electroconvulsive Therapy

Occasionally, electroconvulsive therapy must be considered for adult cancer patients whose depression is resistant to other interventions and in whom it represents a life-threatening complication of cancer. When prominent psychotic features are present or treatment with antidepressants poses unacceptable side effects, electroconvulsive therapy should be considered.

CHOICE OF ANTIDEPRESSANTS

The choice of antidepressant depends on the nature of the depressive symptoms, the medical problems present, and the side effects of the specific drug to be exploited or avoided. Depressed patients who are agitated and have insomnia will benefit from the use of an antidepressant that has sedating effects, such as amitriptyline, doxepin, trazodone, nefazodone, and mirtazapine. Patients with psychomotor slowing will benefit from the use of compounds with the least sedating effects, such as protriptyline, desipramine, fluoxetine, and bupropion. Patients who have stomatitis secondary to chemotherapy or radiotherapy or who have slowed intestinal motility or urinary retention should receive an antidepressant with the least anticholinergic effects, such as desipramine, nortriptyline, or one of the newer serotonin-based drugs. Low doses of antidepressants (i.e., amitriptyline or nortriptyline, 10–50 mg) can be especially useful as adjuvant pain medications in those patients with neuropathic pain syndromes.

Patients who are unable to swallow pills may be able to take an antidepressant in an elixir form (amitriptyline, nortriptyline, fluoxetine, paroxetine) or in an intramuscular form (amitriptyline or imipramine). Hospital pharmacies can prepare some TCAs (e.g., amitriptyline) in rectal suppository form, but absorption by this route has not been studied in cancer patients. Parenteral administration of the TCAs may be considered for cancer patients who are unable to tolerate oral administration because of the absence of a swallowing reflex, the presence of gastric or jejunal drainage tubes, or obstruction. Although three TCAs (amitriptyline, imipramine, and clomipramine) are available in injectable form, the US Food and Drug Administration has approved imipramine and amitriptyline for oral and muscular administration and clomipramine for oral use only. Cardiac monitoring is suggested for this type of administration. The psychostimulant pemoline may be absorbed through the buccal mucosa and obviates the need for swallowing.

Delirium

Delirium, the second most common psychiatric diagnosis among cancer patients, is due both to the direct effects of cancer on the central nervous system (CNS) and the indirect CNS complications of the disease and treatment. Posner [20] has reported that 15% to 20% of hospitalized cancer patients have cognitive function abnormalities unrelated to structural disease. Approximately one-fifth of psychiatric consultations are for assistance in the diagnosis and management of delirium [2]. Usually, delirium is due to one or more causes: medications, electrolyte imbalance, nutritional deficiencies, metabolic abnormalities, infections, hematologic abnormalities, hormone-producing tumors, or paraneoplastic syndromes [21].

Often, early symptoms of delirium are unrecognized in both adults and children and, hence, are undertreated. Any adult who shows acute onset of agitation, behavioral changes, impaired cognitive function, altered attention span, or a fluctuating level of consciousness should be evaluated for presence of delirium. Children may exhibit symptoms of agitation, confusion, and fear. Predominant causes include the cumulative sedative effects of antihistamines, benzodiazepines, and analgesics. Treatment strategies include reevaluation of the necessity of all sedating drugs, verbal reassurance by a consistent companion, and low-dose neuroleptic treatment (e.g., haloperidol).

Many drugs can cause acute confusional states. Confusion is a common adverse effect of opioids. Delirium has been associated with methotrexate (by intrathecal or intravenous administration), fluorouracil, vincristine, vinblastine, bleomycin, carmustine (BCNU), cisplatin, asparaginase, procarbazine, cytosine arabinoside, ifosfamide, and corticosteroids (among the more than 300 chemotherapeutic agents now available for cancer treatment). Other medications that are prescribed commonly for cancer patients and can cause confusional states are interleukin-2, amphotericin, and acyclovir.

Steroid compounds (prednisone, dexamethasone) are a frequent cause of delirium. Psychiatric disturbances range from minor mood disturbances to psychosis [22]. Characteristic symptoms include affective changes (emotional lability, euphoria, depressed mood), anxiety, fears, paranoid interpretation of events, suspiciousness, delusions, and hallucinations. More severe symptoms develop within four to five days of high-dose

steroid treatment or with rapidly tapered doses, but psychiatric symptoms also can develop while patients are on a maintenance dose or from doses commonly prescribed for antiemetic therapy. No relationship has been shown between the development of steroid-induced mental status changes and premorbid personality or psychiatric history [23].

Management of delirium requires corrective medical interventions, but interim symptomatic treatment may be necessary. General care should include sensory stimulation to avoid deprivation effects, provision of such familiar stimuli as family, use of companions to ensure safety, and frequent monitoring by staff members.

Delirious adult and pediatric patients with psychotic symptoms or agitation respond to neuroleptic medication. Haloperidol is the medication prescribed most commonly because of its excellent safety record, producing little effect on heart rate, blood pressure, respiration, or cardiac output. It can be given orally in tablet or concentrate form or can be administered parenterally (intramuscularly or intravenously). Peak plasma concentrations are achieved in 2 to 4 hours after an oral dose, and measurable plasma concentrations occur in 15 to 30 minutes after parenteral administration.

The initial dose of haloperidol for both adult and pediatric cancer patients is low (0.5–1.0 mg administered orally or 0.25–0.5 mg parenterally). The dose can be repeated at 30-minute intervals until symptoms are controlled. If psychotic symptoms are reduced but agitation remains, low-dose benzodiazepines can be added.

Anxiety Disorders

The types of anxiety encountered in the oncology setting are (1) episodes of acute anxiety related to the stress of cancer and its treatment, (2) anxiety resulting from medical illness and treatments, and (3) chronic anxiety disorders that antedate the cancer diagnosis and are exacerbated during treatment [24]. Situational anxiety is common: Most patients are anxious while waiting to hear their diagnosis; before stressful or painful procedures (bone marrow aspiration, chemotherapy administration, radiotherapy, wound débridement); prior to surgery; and while awaiting test results. Anxiety is expected at these times, and most patients manage with the reassurance and support from their physicians.

At times, further treatment is necessary. Extreme fearfulness, inability to cooperate or understand procedures, a prior history of panic attacks, needle phobia, or claustrophobia may require an anxiolytic medication (e.g., lorazepam, 0.5 mg orally tid; alprazolam, 0.25–0.5 mg orally tid; clonazepam, 0.5 mg orally bid) to reduce symptoms to a manageable level. Hypnotics (e.g., triazolam, 0.125–0.25 mg orally) are particularly useful during the perioperative period.

The differential diagnosis of anxiety in cancer patients can be complex. Patients in severe pain may appear anxious or agitated and usually respond to adequate pain control with analgesics. The anxiety that accompanies respiratory distress (e.g., pulmonary embolus), though eventually relieved by medical intervention, often requires use of an anxiolytic. Many patients on steroids experience insomnia and anxiety, which is treated with benzodiazepines. Patients developing metabolic encephalopathy (delirium) can appear restless or anxious, and treatment with neuroleptics often is required as determination and correction (if possible) of the cause is begun. Anxiety symptoms also are features of withdrawal from narcotics, benzodiazepines, and barbiturates. Because patients who abuse alcohol or drugs commonly underreport substance intake prior to admission, physicians need to consider alcohol or drug withdrawal in all patients who develop otherwise unexplained anxiety symptoms during the first week of hospitalization. Other medical conditions in which anxiety is prominent or is the presenting symptom are hyperthyroidism, hypoglycemia, hypocalcemia, and hormone-secreting tumors.

Anxiety disorders that antedate the onset of cancer can compromise medical treatment. Phobias and panic disorder are the most common types. Occasionally, patients have their first episode of panic while being treated in a medical setting. Psychiatric evaluation prior to undertaking cancer treatment is essential in patients with a history of panic disorder or phobia. Patients with claustrophobia may have extreme anxiety in the confined spaces of diagnostic scanning devices or radiotherapy treatment rooms. Patients with needle phobias report having avoided medical evaluations for years because of their fears. Often, patients with agoraphobia are unable to tolerate hospitalization unless accompanied by a family member.

Phobias related to medical procedures are common in children with cancer. Though careful attention to preparation of children (e.g., role playing) in advance of painful procedures may limit the incidence of anxiety, specific behavioral interventions, including relaxation training and distraction, may be indicated for specific symptoms [25]. Self-hypnosis is an effective treatment for both generalized anxiety and specific phobias in children, adolescents, and adults.

Posttraumatic stress disorder (PTSD) is a specific type of anxiety disorder due to the effects of traumatic experiences, including military combat, natural catastrophes, assault, rape, accidents, and life-threatening illness. Recall of prior painful or frightening treatments are common causes of PTSD in cancer patients, especially children. Illness also can exacerbate feelings about earlier traumas, noted particularly in cancer patients who are holocaust survivors. In both adult and pediatric cancer patients, symptoms can develop at various stages of illness but are frequent at the time of diagnosis. Important variables in the disorder's development are patients' personality traits, patients' biological vulnerability to stressful events, and the severity of the stressor. In general, pediatric and geriatric populations have more difficulty in coping with stressful events and are at risk for PTSD. The underdeveloped emotional state of children prevents them from using various adaptive strategies, and the elderly are likely to have fixed coping mechanisms that minimize their flexibility in dealing with trauma.

The reported prevalence of PTSD in cancer survivors ranges from 4% to 25% [26, 27]. Newer research using more stringent diagnostic criteria is providing clinicians a more accurate understanding of the magnitude of the problem in patients, survivors, and parents of children.

In adults, the typical presenting symptoms include periods of intrusive repetition of the stressful event (nightmares, flashbacks, and intrusive thoughts) along with denial, emotional numbness, and depression. A syndrome of recurrent nightmares, separation anxiety, and emotional blunting consistent with the diagnosis of PTSD has been reported in children being treated for cancer [28]. In both adults and children, use of denial is prominent and minimizes the painful event. Distinguishing the diagnosis from a generalized anxiety disorder, depression, or panic disorder is rendered difficult by the nonspecific emotional symptoms. Questions about intrusive phenomena help to determine the specific diagnosis.

Many patients with intermittent anxiety, simple phobias, or PTSD find relaxation therapy and distraction techniques helpful. Generally, play therapy is indicated for children with PTSD. When the need for a diagnostic procedure or treatment is urgent, benzodiazepines should be used (e.g., prior to venipuncture, intravenous chemotherapy administration, a scanning procedure, or radiotherapy treatment).

Benzodiazepines are the drugs of choice for both acute and chronic anxiety states. The most common side effects—sedation and confusion—occur more frequently in older patients and in those with impaired liver function. Short-acting benzodiazepines, such as

Table 36.2 Commonly Prescribed Benzodiazepines in Cancer Patients

Drug Name (by Class)	Approximate Dose Equivalent	Initial Dosage (mg PO)	Elimination Half-Life Drug Metabolites (hr)	Active Metabolite
Short-acting				
Alprazolam	0.5	0.25–0.5 tid	10–15	Yes
Oxazepam	10.0	10–15 tid	5–15	No
Lorazepam	1.0	0.5–2.0 tid	10–20	No
Temazepam*	15.0	15–30 qhs	10–15	No
Triazolam*	0.25	0.125–0.25 qhs	1–5	No
Intermediate-acting				
Chlordiazepoxide	10.0	10–25 tid	10–40	Yes
Long-acting				
Diazepam	5.0	5–10 bid	20–100	Yes
Clorazepate	7.5	7.5–15 bid	30–200	Yes
Clonazepam	0.5	0.25–1 bid	18–50	No

PO = per os (orally); tid = three times day; bid = twice a day; qhs = daily at bedtime.
*Hypnotic agent.

alprazolam, lorazepam, and oxazepam, often are prescribed. Oxazepam and lorazepam are metabolized by conjugation and are excreted by the kidney and, hence, are better tolerated by patients with impaired hepatic function and by those taking other medications with sedative effects (e.g., analgesics). Both lorazepam and alprazolam reduce vomiting in cancer patients receiving emetogenic cancer chemotherapeutic agents. Clonazepam, a longer-acting benzodiazepine, is useful for individuals who have end-of-dose failure with recurrence of anxiety symptoms from short-acting benzodiazepines.

Table 36.2 lists the usual initial dose of benzodiazepines, approximate dose equivalent, half-life, and presence or absence of active metabolites. The dose schedule depends on patients' tolerance and the anxiolytic's duration of action. When a long-acting benzodiazepine is used in patients with chronic anxiety, the dose usually does not exceed twice per day. The shorter-acting benzodiazepines are given three to four times per day. Increasing the dose is preferred to switching to another agent in patients with persistent symptoms.

Patients who experience severe anticipatory anxiety (i.e., anxiety before chemotherapy administration) are given an anxiolytic (e.g., lorazepam) both the night before and immediately prior to the treatment. Patients with chronic anxiety states require anxiolytics daily or intermittently for months or years. Cancer patients, even those with chronic anxiety, usually do not take more medication than they absolutely require and ea-gerly discontinue medications as soon as their symptoms remit.

The most common side effects of the benzodiazepines are dose-dependent and include drowsiness, confusion, and motor incoordination. When the dose is lowered, uncomfortable sedation often disappears, while the antianxiety effects continue. Sedation is most common and most severe in patients with impaired liver function. With medications that have CNS-depressant properties, such as narcotics, physicians should be aware of the synergistic effects of the benzodiazepines.

Low-dose neuroleptics are effective in patients with severe anxiety that is not controlled with maximal therapeutic doses of benzodiazepines or for those patients who cannot tolerate side effects of benzodiazepines, such as sedation or respiratory depression. The low efficacy of the antihistamines for anxiety limits their general usefulness, although they are prescribed for control of anxiety in patients with respiratory impairment or other conditions where benzodiazepines are contraindicated. Antidepressants and buspirone are non-benzodiazepine alternatives to the treatment of anxiety symptoms for patients who cannot tolerate or do not respond to benzodiazepines.

Often, PTSD is treated with antidepressants that reduce both panic and depressive symptoms in most adult patients. In children, benzodiazepines are useful because of their effect on the often-noted anxiety and restlessness.

Personality Disorders

Patients (or families) with "difficult" personalities frustrate and anger those who treat them. The stress of cancer exaggerates these patients' maladaptive coping strategies, and often they become even more difficult than usual. Personality disorders are identified by the exaggeration of common characteristics: the paranoid person who is suspicious and threatens litigation; the obsessive person whose excessive attention to details of care is accompanied by repeated criticism; the dependent person who demands care far beyond objective needs and who may be dependent on alcohol or drugs; the patient who has borderline disorder and is unable to conform to rules, manipulates and divides, and may disturb staff and other patients; the narcissistic person who, with airs of grandiosity and arrogance and with the need to be admired, feels entitled to special care and flies into a rage at the slightest sense that these needs are not met; and the histrionic person who dramatizes symptoms and distress. Because personality disorders are not perceived by patients to be a problem, effective management depends on staff members' ability to understand a patient's maladaptive pattern and to manage that patient's behavior. Many of these patients benefit from consistent limit setting, applied in a quiet, firm, but kindly manner [29].

ADDITIONAL INDICATIONS FOR PSYCHIATRIC CONSULTATION

Many mild to moderately severe psychiatric disorders are managed successfully by oncologists and a sensitive support staff. However, cancer patients clearly experience a significant number of psychiatric disorders requiring accurate diagnosis by a mental health professional for precise and effective treatment. Once treatment is outlined, management often may be carried out by oncologists with help of nurses and social workers. The more severe psychiatric problems, such as schizophrenia and bipolar disorders, require close collaboration between oncologists and psychiatrists.

Disorders directly related to illness, preexisting psychiatric disorders exacerbated by illness, and major mental disorders have been described. Four additional indications also warrant discussion.

Capacity to Consent to or Refuse Treatment

A psychiatric consultation is requested when a patient refuses a procedure critical to survival or when the capacity to give informed consent is in question. Occasionally, legal advice or a judge's decision is necessary for emergency treatment. However, when elective treatment is planned for a mentally impaired patient with no family, court direction may be needed. An increasingly common concern are patients who refuse a clearly life-sustaining treatment, such as dialysis, as part of a decision to forgo all further treatment. Often, oncologists and nurses are not certain whether such patients truly are capable of assessing all their options. The presence of acute depression, delirium, or dementia, which dulls mental processes and strongly biases decisions, poses a difficult and sometimes urgent reason for psychiatric consultation [1, 29].

Leaving Against Medical Advice

Requests to leave the hospital against advice are due most commonly to the presence of a confusional state secondary to illness or medication and, as such, often represent an acute danger to self, allowing for brief restraint and treatment after psychiatric evaluation. An acutely psychotic state or an exacerbated prior psychiatric disorder also may result in poor judgment. The cause of the behavior must be determined, and a decision must be made as to whether affected patients can be managed safely at home or whether they must remain in the hospital with a relative or companion. Often, the severity of such patients' cancer illness prevents safe transfer to a medical psychiatric unit, but improvement occurs rapidly with care by familiar medical staff members, with one-to-one observation and low doses of a neuroleptic drug, such as haloperidol.

Sexual Dysfunction

Often, infertility and sexual dysfunction are unavoidable consequences of irradiation, surgery, and chemotherapy [30]. In men, the opportunity for sperm banking before treatment can both arouse and assuage concerns about infertility. Information given to men with newly diagnosed prostate cancer about the likelihood of sexual dysfunction with different treatment options can aid treatment decisions. In women, a very useful approach in diminishing the inevitable adverse reactions is found in psychological preparation for the premature menopause and sterility associated with chemotherapy or the altered sexual function that results from gynecologic surgery. Psycho-oncologists should initiate discussions of sex early on during their interactions with patients, in an attempt to establish a sexual interest and performance baseline. Although many patients on active cancer treatment report little interest in sex or inability to engage in sex because of nausea, fatigue, and other treatment side effects, most are reassured to learn that the sexual consequences of cancer treatment are important to their treating physicians and will be monitored by their doctors during and after cancer treatment. Psycho-oncologists can be particularly helpful members of the cancer treatment team by reinforcing the teams' interest in helping affected patients to maintain a sex life during cancer treatment (if possible) and in restoring a healthy and "normal" sex life after the cessation of treatment.

Significant Distress from Conflict with Family or Staff

Sometimes, care for a patient becomes imbued with persistent conflict. This condition may stem from a patient's personality, but often it involves an affected family's problems or, less often, staff members' inadvertent mishandling. A psychiatric consultation can provide an objective assessment that identifies and confronts the sources of the problematic behavior. Family meetings, possibly with the patient and selected staff members present, often help to ease family distress. Similarly, multidisciplinary staff conferences encourage a more concerted and effective approach to both family and patient [1].

PSYCHOLOGICAL INTERVENTIONS FOR CANCER PATIENTS

The types of interventions used most commonly by health professionals working with cancer patients include education, behavioral training, group interventions, and individual psychotherapy [31]. The cornerstone of psychological interventions in cancer is emotional support [32]. Psychoeducational counseling focusing on advice and information about illness can be helpful to both patients and family members and can be carried out by different members of the treatment team. Religious or spiritual counseling is meaningful for many patients during the existential crisis created by cancer. Often, a visit by a "veteran" patient who has successfully negotiated the same cancer treatment can help.

Usually, psychotherapy provided by a mental health professional consists of short-term, crisis-oriented supportive therapy to assist affected patients to strengthen adaptive defenses and to cope better with the problems of illness. Group therapy, led either by professionals or cancer survivors, is useful in several ways. First, groups have an educational function in orienting and teaching patients. Second, groups encourage emotional learning and can relieve anxiety by allowing individuals to share similar problems and solutions. Third, groups often become a voice for social awareness and change, giving participants a valuable sense of strength and providing doctors with new insights into patients' concerns.

Behavioral therapies emphasize self-regulatory interventions and are well received by many patients. Many learn relaxation exercises, visual imagery for distraction, and self-hypnotic suggestions. Although these techniques do not have antitumor effect, such techniques are particularly effective in reducing anticipatory nausea and vomiting in patients receiving chemotherapy.

LONG-TERM SURVIVORS AND CURED PATIENTS

Advances in cancer treatment have resulted in a rapidly growing population of more than 5 million long-term survivors, many of them children and young adults. Psychiatric sequelae of cancer in both children and adults include those related to the direct effects of the disease and those that are consequences of the treatments, of family factors, and of the individual psychology of the affected person. The long-term adjustment of survivors of childhood cancer appears largely unimpaired [33]. Cured cancer patients have special medical and psychiatric concerns, including fears of termination of treatment, preoccupation with disease recurrence, and minor physical problems; a sense of greater vulnerability to illness (the Damocles syndrome); pervasive awareness of mortality and difficulty with reentry into normal life (the Lazarus syndrome); persistent guilt (the survivor syndrome); difficult adjustment to physical losses and handicaps; a sense of physical inferiority; diminished self-esteem or confidence; perceived loss of job mobility; and fear of insurance discrimination. Concerns about infertility, often understandably submerged at the time of diagnosis and treatment, reappear when patients consider marrying.

Survivors' intellectual functioning is a major concern. Children and adults with brain tumors and those undergoing bone marrow transplantation are at risk from both their disease and treatment. Most have residual deficits with neuropsychological impairment, including compromised motor and cognitive test performance [34].

Many centers around the country are developing "survivor clinics" that incorporate a multidisciplinary approach to the cured child, adolescent, or adult. As the number of cancer survivors grows, more attention is being given to societal attitudes. The National Coalition of Cancer Survivorship is an outgrowth of survivors' need for and value of support. The issues surrounding health and life insurance policies are a prime example of an area in which research is needed to delineate problems and advocacy is needed to encourage solutions.

MANAGEMENT OF GRIEF

Frequently, grief is encountered in the oncology setting, and staff management can affect the nature of bereavement and influence the family's long-term adjustment. Once death has occurred, grieving has acute and chronic components [35]. Reminders of the deceased precipitate waves of an overwhelming sense of loss, crying, fatigue, and agitation. The intense distress of the first few months is characterized by social withdrawal, preoccupation with the deceased, diminished concentration, restlessness, depressed mood, anxiety, insomnia, or anorexia. The bereaved spouse or parent repeatedly recalls how the final days were handled, how the painful news of grave prognosis and death were conveyed, and how sensitively the final moments were managed. The surviving relatives may search for fault and tend to blame both themselves and staff members. Physicians must recognize that they have a special meaning to survivors and must understand survivors' reactions in this context. A meeting held 1 to 2 months after the death is a valuable setting wherein autopsy findings and any troubling questions can be discussed.

Over months, grief usually diminishes in intensity. The duration of normal grieving is much more variable than originally assumed and often extends well beyond a year. Often, parents and older spouses from a long union report that they are "never the same again;" some truly never recover [36]. Individual psychotherapy or group psychotherapy can assist family members in coping with loss and bereavement issues.

PSYCHOLOGICAL PROBLEMS IN HIGH-RISK INDIVIDUALS

The current explosion of information about genetic contribution to the development of cancer has brought into existence a new population: people whose family history is such that they are clearly at high risk for certain cancers. A psychologically useful approach is differentiating between people who are afraid they *might* be at risk and people who are afraid because they *know* they are at risk. Those in the first group benefit from being educated about what, if any, is their increased risk. Some will remain excessively anxious even in the absence of objective reason and may be said to suffer from cancerophobia; they benefit from psychological support and regular checkups with a trusted internist to prevent them from squandering time and resources consulting with numerous physicians.

Patients in the second group (those who are at an increased genetic risk) need detailed genetic and psychological counseling to help them in making difficult decisions regarding genetic testing, marriage, childbearing, prenatal testing, or risk-reducing surgeries (e.g., prophylactic mastectomy or oophorectomy). For high-risk individuals who have medicosurgical, genetic counseling, and psychiatric issues, surveillance programs provide clinical examination, diagnostic screenings, information, and support delivered by coordinated multidisciplinary team members.

STRESSES ON ONCOLOGY STAFF

Recent studies have helped to clarify the picture of emotional reactions of patients and their relatives to cancer; but few studies have addressed the stresses on oncologists and its effect on personal and professional life [37, 38]. Studies show that, despite recent criticism of medicine as uncaring, patients still accept treatment largely because they trust their doctors' recommendations. Overworked, stressed oncologists are compromised in their ability to give attention to the art of medicine, yet seldom is this human aspect of care more important than in oncology [1].

Generally, most physicians tolerate work stresses well and have personality characteristics that are known to buffer stress: a strong commitment to work, a sense of control of their work without letting the magnitude of the problems become overwhelming, and a view of daily problems as a challenge [39]. However, physicians also have the characteristics that predispose them to chronic stress. Many work long hours, are chronically fatigued, and seek little recreation; many have trouble in saying no to requests for additional work.

The practice of oncology carries specific additional strains: the uncertainty inherent in many treatment decisions and the repeated impact of patients' deaths. Some personal stress inevitably accompanies decisions about withholding or stopping life—sustaining treatment amid all the medical, social, and ethical ambiguities that abound in the current climate. Learning to discuss these issues with patients and families is difficult and painful.

Physicians with symptoms of emotional fatigue or burnout notice they have less zest and enthusiasm for work; depressed mood may ensue. They may begin to work longer hours and have a sense that no one but they can do the work correctly and that no one else works as hard as they do, when in fact they are less efficient and less effective. The need for a few drinks after work or experimenting with drugs to relax are ominous signs. On the physical side, insomnia is common. Appetite change may lead to weight gain or weight loss. Stressed physicians report feeling tired all the time. Headaches or somatic pains are indicators of distress. At this point, such physicians may tune out and feel detached from their patients. Detachment is an early sign of stress in house staff members, who say they feel less able to care and are more cynical and pessimistic about the meaning of their work.

Monitoring symptoms of emotional fatigue and acknowledging stress are important for anyone working in oncology. Survival tactics that must be instituted include recognizing limitations, developing a comfortable perspective on self and work, accepting personal and medical inadequacies, using gallows humor to lighten the meaning of painful events, working a normal workday, stopping when others do, taking a long weekend, and regular exercise. When symptoms do not remit, psychiatric consultation should be sought.

SUMMARY

The most common psychiatric complications in both adults and children with cancer are depression, anxiety, and delirium. Important factors for patient comfort and quality of life are evaluating and managing the psychological distress in patients with cancer. Psychotherapeutic, psychopharmacologic, and behavioral interventions can be tailored to very ill patients' needs. Clinical observation and research has furthered our understanding of the problems of long-term survivors, cured patients,

grieving families, individuals at high genetic risk of developing cancer, and oncology staff.

REFERENCES

1. Massie MJ, Spiegel L, Lederberg MS, Holland JC. Psychiatric complications in cancer patients. In Murphy GP, Lawrence Jr W, Lenhard Jr RE (eds), *American Cancer Society Textbook of Clinical Oncology* (2nd ed). Atlanta: American Cancer Society, 1995:685–698.
2. Massie MJ, Holland JC. Consultation and liaison issues in cancer care. *Psychiatr Med* 5:343–359, 1987.
3. Holland JC. Psychological aspects of cancer. In Holland JF, Frei E (eds), *Cancer Medicine* (2nd ed). Philadelphia: Lea & Febiger, 1982:1175–1203, 2325–2331.
4. Lewis M, Lewis DO, Schonfeld DJ. Dying and death in childhood and adolescence. In Lewis M (ed), *Child and Adolescent Psychiatry: A Comprehensive Textbook.* Baltimore: Williams & Williams, 1991:1051–1059.
5. Powazek M, Schijving J, Goff JR, et al. Psychosocial ramifications of childhood leukemia: one year post-diagnosis. In Schulman JL, Kupat MJ (eds), *The Child with Cancer.* Springfield, IL: Charles C. Thomas, 1980:143–155.
6. Lansky SB, Cairns NU, Hassannein R, et al. Childhood cancer: parent discord and divorce. *Pediatrics* 62:184–188, 1978.
7. Kagen-Goodheart L. Reentry: living with childhood cancer. *Am J Orthopsychiatry* 47:651–658, 1977.
8. Weisman S, Schechter N. The management of pain in children. *Pediatr Rev* 12:237–243, 1991.
9. Bukberg J, Penman D, Holland JC. Depression in hospitalized cancer patients. *Psychosom Med* 46:199–212, 1984.
10. DeFlorio ML, Massie MJ. Review of depression in cancer: gender differences. *Depression* 3:66–80, 1995.
11. Massie MJ, Popkin M. Depressive disorders. In Holland JC, (ed), *Psycho-oncology.* New York: Oxford University Press, 1998:518–540.
12. Moffic H, Paykel ES. Depression in medical inpatients. *Br J Psychiatry* 126:346–353, 1975.
13. Schwab JJ, Bialow M, Brown JM, Holzer CE. Diagnosing depression in medical inpatients. *Ann Intern Med* 67:695–707, 1967.
14. Massie MJ, Holland JC. The cancer patient with pain: psychiatric complications and their management. *Med Clin North Am* 71:243–258, 1987.
15. Hall RCW, Popkin MK, Devaul RA, et al. Physical illness presenting as psychiatric disease. *Arch Gen Psychiatry* 35:1315–1320, 1978.
16. Breitbart W. Suicide in cancer patients. In Holland JC, Rowland JH (eds), *Handbook of Psycho-oncology: Psychological Care of the Patient with Cancer.* New York: Oxford University Press, 1989:291–299.
17. Massie MJ, Holland JC. Psychiatric complications of cancer pain. *J Pain Symptom Manage* 7:99–109, 1992.
18. Roth AJ, McClear KZ, Massie MJ. Oncology. In Stoudemire A, Fogel B, Greenberg D (eds), *Psychiatric Care of the Medical Patient* (2nd ed). New York: Oxford University Press, 2000, 733–755.

19. Pfefferbaum-Levin B, Kumor K, Cangir A, et al. Tricyclic antidepressants for children with cancer. *Am J Psychiatry* 20:99–113, 1983.

20. Posner JB. Neurologic complications in systemic cancer. *Dis Mon* 2:7–60, 1978.

21. Lipowsky ZJ. *Delirium: Acute Brain Failure in Man*. Springfield, IL: Charles C Thomas, 1980.

22. Hall RCW, Popkin MK, Stickney SK, Gardner ER. Presentation of the steroid psychosis. *J Nerv Ment Dis* 167:229–236, 1979.

23. Stiefel FC, Breitbart WS, Holland JC. Corticosteroids in cancer: neuropsychiatric complications. *Cancer Invest* 7:479–491, 1989.

24. Noyes R, Holt CS, Massie MJ. Anxiety disorders. In Holland JC (ed), *Psychooncology*. New York: Oxford University Press, 1998:548–563.

25. Redd WH, Jacobsen PB, Die-Trill M, et al. Cognitive-attentional distraction in the control of conditioned nausea in pediatric cancer patients receiving chemotherapy. *J Consult Clin Psychol* 55:391–395, 1987.

26. Green BL, Rowland JH, Krupnick JL, et al. Prevalence of posttraumatic stress disorder in women with breast cancer. *Psychosomatics* 39:102–111, 1998.

27. Jacobsen PJ, Widows MR, Hann DM, et al. Posttraumatic stress disorder symptoms after bone marrow transplantation for breast cancer. *Psychosom Med* 60:366–371, 1998.

28. Nir Y. Post-traumatic stress disorder in children with cancer. In Pynoos RS, Eth S (eds), *Post-Traumatic Stress Disorder in Children*. Washington, DC: American Psychiatric Press, 1985:121–132.

29. Lederberg MS, Massie MJ. Psychosocial and ethical issues in the care of cancer patients. In DeVita VT, Hellman S, Rosenberg SA (eds), *Cancer: Principles and Practice of Oncology* (4th ed). Philadelphia: Lippincott, 1993:2448.

30. Schover LR. *Sexuality and Fertility After Cancer*. New York: Wiley, 1997.

31. Fawzy Fl, Fawzy NW, Arndt LA, Pasnau RO. Critical review of psycho-social interventions in cancer care. *Arch Gen Psychiatry* 52:100–113, 1995.

32. Sourkes B, Massie MJ, Holland JC. Psychotherapeutic issues. In Holland JC (ed), *Psycho-oncology*. New York: Oxford University Press, 1998:694–700.

33. Greenberg HS, Kazak AE, Meadows AT. Psychological function in 8- to 16-year-old cancer survivors and their parents. *J Pediatr* 114:488–493, 1989.

34. Andrykowski MA, Schmitt FA, Gregg ME, et al. Neuropsychological impairment in adult bone marrow transplant candidates. *Cancer* 70:2288–2297, 1992.

35. Osterweis M, Solomon F, Green M (eds). *Bereavement Reactions, Consequences and Care*. Washington, DC: National Academy Press, 1984.

36. Parkes CM, Wess R. *Recovery from Bereavement*. New York: Basic Books, 1983.

37. Kash K, Holland JC. Special problems of physicians and hose staff. In Holland JC, Rowland JH (eds), *Handbook of Psycho-Oncology: Psychological Care of the Patient with Cancer*. New York: Oxford University Press, 1989:647–657.

38. Lederberg MS. Psychological problems of staff and their management. In Holland JC, Rowland JH (eds), *Handbook of Psycho-Oncology: Psychological Care of the Patient with Cancer*. New York: Oxford University Press, 1989:631–646.

39. Kobasa SC, Pucceti MD. Personality and social resources in stress-resistance. *J Pers Soc Psychol* 45:839–850, 1983.

37

Fertility and Sexuality After Cancer Treatment

■ ■ ■

BARBARA L. ANDERSEN
DANIEL M. GREEN

FERTILITY AND SEXUAL OUTCOMES FOR CHILDHOOD AND ADOLESCENT CANCER SURVIVORS

Successful therapy for children and adolescents with cancer includes the use of ionizing irradiation or chemotherapeutic agents (or both). The use of such treatments has yielded survival improvements, as 70% of patients will survive for at least five years after diagnosis [1]; many live much longer. An issue of great concern to such survivors is the effect of their cancer and its treatment on their sexuality and fertility and on the health of their offspring. The treatments may produce DNA damage, with resultant gonadal sterilization or germ-cell DNA damage. Sterilization may be temporary or it may be premature, as in the case of premature menopause. DNA damage may be identified by an increased risk for chromosomal syndromes, single-gene defects, or major congenital malformations in the offspring of survivors.

Management of cancer in pediatric and adolescent patients must include recognition of these potential outcomes, provision of counseling regarding strategies for germ-cell preservation, and the addition of long-term follow-up of the offspring of cancer survivors to determine their increased risk, if any, for adverse pregnancy outcomes, genetic disease, and cancer.

Germ-Cell Survival

Ovarian damage can result in both sterilization and loss of hormone production, because ovarian hormonal production is related closely to the presence of ova and to maturation of primary follicles. These functions are not linked as closely in the testis. As a result, men may have normal androgen production in the presence of azoospermia. For these reasons, we review outcomes for both genders.

Ovarian Functioning for Female Survivors

Developmental changes occur in the number of oocytes in the ovary, with the most dramatic changes from fetal to childhood periods. The number of oocytes reaches a peak of 6.8×10^6 at five months of gestation; at birth, approximately 2×10^6 primordial follicles are present; at age six months, the number decreases to 0.7×10^6, and the number declines further to 0.3×10^6 by age 7 [2]. Thus, the nonrenewable nature of oocytes renders the ovary uniquely susceptible to damage by radiotherapy and chemotherapeutic agents.

IRRADIATION

Taken together, data indicate that the extent of germ-cell morbidity covaries with the dose and volume of radiotherapy and, for some, the timing of delivery, with higher dose volume and older age increasing the risk for morbidity. For example, all women who receive total-body irradiation prior to bone marrow transplantation develop amenorrhea, with only those younger than the mid-twenties apt to recover their ovarian function [3].

In the more common treatment circumstance, irradiation is delivered to the abdomen or pelvis when the ovaries are directly in the treatment field. Whole-abdomen irradiation (doses of 2,000 to 3,000 cGy) produces severe ovarian damage. In one series, 71% of affected women failed to enter puberty; of those who did, 26% had premature menopause [4, 5]. Data indicate that if treatment volume can be reduced, ovarian failure may be prevented [6–9]. For example, one study reported a 0% occurrence of ovarian failure in women who received abdominal irradiation to a volume that did not include both ovaries, a 14% occurrence in those whose ovaries were at the edge of the abdominal treatment volume, and a 68% occurrence in women whose ovaries were entirely within the treatment volume [10].

Ovarian failure is correlated also with the radiotherapy dose. Such failure occurred in 69%, 87%, 94%, and 100%, respectively, of women whose treatment doses increased from a low of 250 to 374 roentgens (R) to a maximum of 625 to 749 R to both ovaries [11]. Moreover, the frequency of ovarian failure was least among women who were younger than 40 years and had received radiotherapeutic doses of less than 624 R [11].

Surgical techniques have been developed to limit the ovarian dose. This can be accomplished in selected patients using midline oophoropexy [12, 13], lateral ovarian transposition [14], or heterotopic ovarian autotransplantation [15]. Data have indicated that with midline oophoropexy, for example, the ovarian doses received from pelvic irradiation can be limited to 220 to 550 cGy when the treatment dose is 4,400 cGy [12]. Thus, for women who are younger than 25 at the time of treatment, ovarian failure is infrequent (Table 37.1) [12, 16, 17]. Procedures such as these should be considered prior to pelvic irradiation of female children or adolescents.

CHEMOTHERAPY

Ovarian function has been evaluated in women after treatment with combination chemotherapy (Table 37.2) [18–21]. With combined regimens, if the data are separated by women's age at treatment, the sensitivity of older patients to the gonadal toxicity of such therapy can be illustrated (Table 37.3) [22–25]. Moreover, for individual regimens, the number of cycles also is important, as illustrated in Table 37.4 [26], which compares three versus six cycles. These data indicate that younger women and women receiving a lower radiation dosage had lower rates of amenorrhea morbidity after treatment.

At this time, only small sample studies report single-

Table 37.1 Relationship Between Ovarian Irradiation Dose and the Occurrence of Amenorrhea

Dose (cGy)	Amenorrhea Occurrence (no. of patients)
0–100	16% (1/6)
101–200	14% (1/7)
201–300	12% (1/8)
301–400	25% (1/4)
401–500	44% (4/9)
501–600	50% (3/6)
601–700	25% (1/4)

Table 37.2 Frequency of Amenorrhea After Treatment with Combination Chemotherapy

Patient Age	Regimen	Amenorrhea Frequency (no. of patients)
All ages	MVPP	63% (20/32)
All ages	MOPP	39% (17/44)
All ages	ChlVPP	19% (6/32)
All ages	ChlVPP/EVA	80% (16/20)

MVPP = nitrogen mustard, vinblastine, procarbazine, and prednisone; MOPP = nitrogen mustard, vincristine (Oncovin®), procarbazine, and prednisone; ChlVPP = chlorambucil, vinblastine, procarbazine, and prednisone; EVA = etoposide, vincristine, and doxorubicin (Adriamycin).

Table 37.3 Relationship Between Age at Treatment and Frequency of Amenorrhea After Treatment with Combination Chemotherapy

Patient Age (yr)	Regimen	Amenorrhea Frequency (no. of patients)
< 30	MVPP	52% (17/33)
30–51	MVPP	86% (31/36)
< 25	MOPP	20% (3/15)
> 25	MOPP	89% (8/9)
< 30	MOPP	0% (0/10)
30–40	MOPP	50% (5/10)

MVPP = nitrogen mustard, vinblastine, procarbazine, and prednisone; MOPP = nitrogen mustard, vincristine (Oncovin®), procarbazine, and prednisone.

Table 37.4 Relationship Among Age at Treatment, Number of Cycles, and Frequency of Amenorrhea After Treatment with Combination Chemotherapy (MOPP)

Patient Age (yr)	No. of Cycles	Amenorrhea Frequency (no. of patients)
16–30	3	3% (1/31)
	6	9% (1/11)
31–45	3	61% (11/18)
	6	62% (5/8)

MOPP = nitrogen mustard, vincristine (Oncovin®), procarbazine, and prednisone.

drug regimens. For example, one study reported that ovarian function was normal in all of six women treated for non-Hodgkin's lymphoma with a cyclophosphamide-containing drug combination [27]. Others reported that pubertal progression was affected adversely in 5.8% of 17 patients treated before puberty, as compared to 33.3% of 18 patients treated during puberty or after menarche [28]. Cisplatin administration resulted in amenorrhea in 14% of seven patients [29]. Chemotherapy with doxorubicin, cyclophosphamide, and high-dose methotrexate produced irregular menses in 20% of five women and resulted in persistent amenorrhea in 20% of five women treated for soft-tissue sarcomas [30]. Therapy with high-dose methotrexate (250 mg/kg/dose) with or without vincristine did not cause ovarian failure in any of four women evaluated after the completion of therapy [31]. Treatment with nitrosoureas with or without procarbazine produced ovarian damage in young women treated with craniospinal irradiation for malignant brain tumors [32].

Relevant data also come from studies of adult chemotherapy patients. For premenopausal women, recovery of ovarian function is unlikely if menstrual periods do not return within three months after cessation of treatment [24]. For postmenopausal women, reports cite significant changes in libido and sexual function in the period after chemotherapy [33]. Even in the presence of apparently "normal" ovarian function at the completion of chemotherapy, ovarian injury still may have occurred. Relevant data from childhood cancer survivors have documented premature menopause, especially in those individuals originally treated with both an alkylating agent and abdominal irradiation [34]. However, if the treatment can exclude both pelvic irradiation and combination chemotherapy, the incidence of premature menopause is reduced [35].

Testicular Functioning for Male Survivors

SURGICAL TREATMENT

Pelvic or genital surgery can produce considerable disruption of testicular function. For example, pelvic dissections as performed to remove a rhabdomyosarcoma of the prostate [36] can produce erectile difficulties. Even pelvic nodal dissection (e.g., bilateral retroperitoneal lymph node dissection [RPLND] for testicular tumors) can cause retrograde ejaculation [37, 38].

IRRADIATION

Early experimental evidence from human tests demonstrated the dose-response outcomes of recovery of spermatogenesis after irradiation. Inmate volunteers from the Oregon State Penitentiary were assigned to different irradiation dosages and then underwent vasectomy to document sperm counts. Recovery time was correlated with treatment dosage, such that complete recovery was observed 9 to 18 months after treatment in those given 100 cGy, after 30 months in those treated with 200 or 300 cGy, and only after 60 or more months in those treated with 400 or 600 cGy [39, 40].

Men in whom larger fields are treated (whole-abdomen irradiation) also may develop gonadal dysfunction. Five of 10 men were azoospermic, and two were severely oligospermic in posttreatment evaluations at ages 17 to 36. They had been treated for Wilms' tumors at ages 1 to 11 with whole-abdomen irradiation; however, the penis and scrotum either were excluded from the treatment volume or were shielded with 3 mm of lead [41]. The testicular irradiation doses varied from 796 to 983 cGy [41]. Others reported zoospermia in 100% of 10 men at 2 to 40 months after radiotherapeutic doses of 140 to 300 cGy to both testes [42]. Similarly, azoospermia was demonstrated in 100% of 10 men after testicular radiotherapeutic doses of 118 to 228 cGy. Recovery of spermatogenesis occurred after 44 to 77 weeks in 50% of the men, although three of the five with recovery had sperm counts below 20 × 10⁶/ml [43]. Oligospermia or azoospermia was reported in 33% of 18 men evaluated 6 to 70 months after receiving testicular irradiation doses of 28 to 135 cGy [44]. In another report, none of five men who received testicular irradiation doses of less than 20 cGy became azoospermic. By contrast, two who received testicular irradiation doses of 55 to 70 cGy developed temporary oligospermia, with recovery to sperm counts greater than 20 × 10⁶/ml at 18 to 24 months after treatment [45].

Administration of higher doses (e.g., 2,400 cGy, which is used for the treatment of testicular relapse of acute lymphoblastic leukemia) results in both sterilization and Leydig cell dysfunction [46]. Craniospinal irradiation produced primary germ-cell damage in 17% of 23 children with acute lymphoblastic leukemia [47] but in none of 4 children with medulloblastoma [48]. With adequate shielding, gonadal failure is infrequent after radiotherapy to a volume that does not include the testis [49].

CHEMOTHERAPY

Many studies have indicated that combination chemotherapy, including an alkylating agent and procarbazine, causes severe damage to the testicular germinal epithelium (Table 37.5) [19–21, 50–59]. Other data with nitrogen mustard, vinblastine, procarbazine, and prednisone (MVPP) chemotherapy indicate that azoospermia occurred as soon as after only two cycles. Even by three to four years after treatment, more than 80% of affected men did not recover spermatogenesis [54]. When the effects of two versus six cycles of nitrogen mustard, vincristine (Oncovin®), procarbazine, and prednisone (MOPP) were compared, azoospermia occurred less frequently after two treatment cycles (in 0 of 7 patients [0%]) than after six cycles (in 9 of 10 patients [90%]) [60]. Other data indicated that elevation of the basal follicle-stimulating hormone (FSH) level, reflecting impaired spermatogenesis, was less frequent among patients receiving two courses of vincristine, procarbazine, prednisone, and doxorubicin (Adriamycin) than among those who received two courses of this combination with two or more courses of cyclophosphamide, vincristine, procarbazine, and prednisone [61].

Many studies suggest that procarbazine contributes significantly to the testicular toxicity of combination

Table 37.5 Frequency of Azoospermia After Completion of Combination Chemotherapy

Treatment Regimen	Azoospermia Frequency (no. of patients)
MOPP	75% (42/56)
M(O/V)PP, COPP	87% (5/6)
MVPP	86% (132/154)
COPP	100% (106/106)
ChlVPP	100% (11/11)
ChlVPP/EVA	95% (21/22)
ABVD	0% (0/13)

MOPP = nitrogen mustard, vincristine (Oncovin®), procarbazine, prednisone; M(O/V)PP = nitrogen mustard, vincristine or vinblastine, procarbazine, prednisone; COPP = cyclophosphamide; vincristine (Oncovin®), procarbazine, prednisone; MVPP = nitrogen mustard, vinblastine, procarbazine, and prednisone; ChlVPP = chlorambucil, vinblastine, procarbazine, and prednisone; EVA = etoposide, vincristine, and doxorubicin (Adriamycin); ABVD = doxorubicin (Adriamycin), bleomycin, vinblastine, dimethyltriazeno-imidazole-carboxamide (DTIC).

chemotherapy regimens. The combination of doxorubicin, bleomycin, vinblastine, and dacarbazine (DTIC) produced oligospermia or azoospermia frequently during the course of treatment. However, recovery of spermatogenesis occurred after treatment was completed, in contrast to the experience reported after treatment with MOPP [56].

An early report suggested that prepubertal testes were less sensitive to damage by MOPP chemotherapy than were postpubertal testes [53]. Several groups of investigators reported that damage to prepubertal testes could not be identified until affected patients entered puberty, if the frequency of testicular damage was estimated by the presence of an elevated serum FSH level [50, 62–65]. None of these studies reported that prepubertal males were at lower risk for chemotherapy-induced testicular damage than were postpubertal patients.

Usually, treatment for nonseminomatous germ-cell tumors of the testis includes the combination of cisplatin, vinblastine, and bleomycin. Oligospermia or azoospermia was reported in most men after treatment with this chemotherapy regimen, and azoospermia still was present in 25% to 30% of men 24 to 94 months after treatment was complete [66–68]. Interpretation of these results and of those reported in men with Hodgkin's disease is complicated by the high frequency of oligospermia or azoospermia in such patients prior to initiation of treatment.

Testicular function was evaluated after treatment with combination chemotherapy in patients with acute lymphoblastic leukemia during childhood. Basal serum FSH and luteinizing hormone levels were normal in 32 prepubertal boys evaluated, whereas three (37.5%) of eight early-pubertal boys and two (50%) of four late-pubertal boys had raised basal serum FSH levels [69]. The factors that influenced the severity of testicular damage were the total dose of cyclophosphamide, administration of a cumulative dose of cytosine arabinoside exceeding 1 g/m², and the length of time between the cessation of treatment and testicular biopsy [70]. Blatt et al. [71] reported normal testicular function in 14 boys treated for acute lymphoid leukemia with therapy that did not include either cyclophosphamide or intravenous cytosine arabinoside, emphasizing the importance of the agents employed in determining the gonadal toxicity of a combination chemotherapy program.

Three of four men treated with high-dose methotrexate for osteosarcoma had normal sperm counts, whereas the fourth was severely oligospermic when first evaluated after cessation of treatment [31]. Treatment with doxorubicin, cyclophosphamide, and high-dose methotrexate for soft-tissue sarcoma produced azoospermia in eight (100%) of eight men after chemotherapy and proximal radiotherapy, in two (25%) of eight men after chemotherapy and distal radiotherapy, and in one (20%) of five men treated with chemotherapy only. Recovery of spermatogenesis was documented in men treated with chemotherapy only or with chemotherapy and distal irradiation, whereas azoospermia persisted in those men treated with chemotherapy and proximal radiotherapy [72]. Similar results have been reported in two studies: male non-Hodgkin's lymphoma survivors in whom pelvic radiotherapy and a cumulative cyclophosphamide dose greater than 9.5 g/m² were independent determinants of failure to recover spermatogenesis [73] and survivors of Ewing's and soft-tissue sarcoma in whom treatment with a cumulative cyclophosphamide dose greater than 7.5 g/m², correlated with persistent oligospermia or azoospermia [74].

Fertility

Treatment of childhood cancer results in impaired fertility for survivors. For example, the adjusted relative fertility of survivors as compared to that of their siblings was 0.85 (95% confidence interval [CI], 0.78–0.92). When male and female subjects are compared, the adjusted relative fertility of male survivors (0.76; 95% CI, 0.68–0.86) is slightly lower than that of female survivors (0.93; 95% CI, 0.83–1.04). The most impaired re-

sponse rates have been found in men who had been treated with alkylating agents with or without infradiaphragmatic irradiation [75].

Fertility may be impaired also by damage to the pelvic structures. For conception to occur, sperm must reach the uterine cervix, and conditions in the uterus must be appropriate for implantation. As noted, retrograde ejaculation occurs with significant frequency in men who undergo bilateral RPLND. Other studies have shown that uterine length is significantly shorter in women treated with whole-abdomen irradiation [76]. Related data indicate that endometrial thickness did not increase in response to hormone replacement therapy [76]. These data are important as the feasibility of assisted reproduction is considered for survivors.

Risks to the Offspring of Cancer Survivors

Most chemotherapeutic agents are mutagenic, with the potential to cause germ-cell chromosomal injury. Possible outcomes of such injury include an increase in the frequency of genetic diseases or congenital anomalies in the offspring. Early studies of affected offspring identified no apparent adverse effects [77–79]. However, data from offspring of patients treated for Wilms' tumor demonstrated that the birth weight of children born to women who had received abdominal irradiation was significantly lower than that of children born to women who had not received such irradiation [80], a finding that has been replicated [81–83]. The abnormalities of uterine structure and blood flow previously noted may be related to these clinical outcomes. Though the early studies were of small sample sizes of either patients or offspring, subsequent larger-scale efforts have not found an increased frequency of major congenital malformations [79, 84–90], genetic disease [79], or childhood cancer [90–92], even among the offspring of bone marrow transplantation patients [93]. Though these data are reassuring, the number of patients available for study is small, and length of follow-up with the offspring has been limited. These two circumstances preclude definitive statements regarding the risks to offspring of cancer survivors.

Patient Management

Patients who are to receive therapy that can put their fertility at risk need sensitive, informed management. Important elements of management can include considerations of gonadal protection, germ-cell storage, and assisted fertilization.

Protection of the ovary has been attempted with the use of oral contraceptive agents and luteinizing hormone–releasing hormone (LHRH) agonists, but the results are mixed. In one study in which women were treated with MVPP, permanent amenorrhea did not occur in six (ages 18–31 years) who received an oral contraceptive during chemotherapy treatment [94], yet these results were not confirmed in a similar study [18]. Initial amenorrhea occurred in all eight women (ages 17–34 years) treated with an LHRH agonist (Buserelin), and in three of 10 MVPP-treated female controls, but four of the Buserelin-treated women recovered their ovarian function [95].

A similar strategy has been used in treating male patients. In an evaluation of Buserelin, no protective effect, as estimated by posttherapy sperm count, was evident in 20 Buserelin-treated men compared with 10 untreated men [95]. Similarly, no protective effect on spermatogenesis was detected in the use of another LHRH agonist, D-Trp6-Pro9-N-ethylamide-LHRH (LHRHa), for six men receiving treatment with MOPP [96].

Frequently, the semen of men with previously untreated Hodgkin's disease and testicular carcinoma exhibits low numbers of inadequately mobile sperm [97–102]. Artificial insemination by husband has been successful when frozen semen specimens were used from patients whose pretreatment samples had adequate numbers ($> 20 \times 10^6$/ml) of mobile sperm [98, 99–101]. However, fertilization is possible also with lower sperm concentrations using gamete intrafallopian tube transfer or in vitro fertilization. Thus, sperm banking should be considered for any man who is not azoospermic prior to therapy and whose therapy may result in azoospermia [103].

Occasionally, retrograde ejaculation may be treated successfully with sympathomimetic agents [104]. Several reports published recently have detailed successful fertilization using spermatozoa recovered after sexual activity from urine of men with retrograde ejaculation [105–108].

Assisted reproductive technology has extended the possibility of pregnancy to women with treatment-induced ovarian failure. Frozen embryos have implanted successfully after transfer [109], although infrequently, and several reports have cited successful initiation and progression of pregnancy in postmenopausal women who were given exogenous hormone replacement and embryos produced from donor oocytes and their male partners' sperm [110–112].

Finally, recent laboratory investigations have demonstrated that spermatogenesis may be reconstituted in the mouse from frozen spermatogonial stem cells [113–115] and that fertility could be restored by implantation of frozen-thawed primordial follicles or ovarian cortical slices [116, 117]. These techniques may allow reconstitution of fertility in humans using the stored tissues of affected patients obtained prior to initiation of cancer treatment.

Summary

Gonadal damage is not infrequent in survivors of childhood and adolescent cancer. Surgical removal of the ovaries from radiotherapeutic treatment volumes should be performed when possible. Careful attention must be paid to radiotherapeutic technique, especially the use of effective shielding of the testes and ovaries from the irradiation beam, when such use will not have an adverse impact on the likelihood of local tumor control. Gamete banking offers the potential for later reproduction, using assisted reproductive technology when sterilization is an unavoidable sequela of successful treatment. Counseling of survivors should include discussions of the possibility of immediate sterilization or premature menopause as the result of treatment. Young women must assess the risk of premature menopause when contemplating postponement of pregnancy to allow completion of graduate education or career development. Adolescent and young adult survivors need to be aware that sterilization is not a generic outcome of cancer therapy and that precautions to prevent pregnancy still must be taken if pregnancy is not the desired outcome of sexual activity.

SEXUAL MORBIDITY
Overview

The sexual problems both of healthy individuals and of those with cancer exhibit many similarities, but we highlight some obvious differences. First, the sexual problems of adult cancer patients typically have an acute onset, appearing immediately after treatment. Prior to receiving their diagnosis, most cancer patients have had satisfactory sexual adjustment. The usual clinical pattern for the appearance of sexual problems after cancer treatment is that they begin as soon as intercourse is resumed. This suddenness and, for some, the severity of difficulty is distressing. Others may experience reductions in sexual desire, even if their functioning is not impaired. The distress of affected individuals may be heightened if they have not been forewarned by their health care providers about the likelihood or nature of these and related difficulties.

Second, sexual difficulties for cancer patients usually are pervasive, with major alterations in the frequency or range of sexual behavior and disruption of more than one phase of the sexual response cycle. Because of this, some patients may be concerned about maintaining any sexual activity. In contrast, the sexual difficulties of healthy individuals are more likely to be circumscribed, such as being most severe for one phase (e.g., orgasmic disruption) and displaying much less impairment of the other phases.

Third, maintaining sexual self-esteem or sexual activity may be difficult because of other disease and treatment side effects, the control of which is difficult. Fatigue or low energy and pain are two such disrupters. After treatment, many cancer patients report residual and activity-disrupting fatigue [118], factors that may, in turn, lead to lowered sexual desire. Also, genital or other pains are deterrents to desire for and arousal during sexual activity.

Fourth, data suggest that the response cycle disruptions for cancer patients differ from those of healthy individuals. Disruption of sexual desire may be a primary problem, with or without concomitant arousal deficits. Many cancer patients maintain their sexual desire, and some even continue sexual relations in the presence of significant deterrents, such as dyspareunia [119]. This latter scenario underscores the importance that many place on maintaining their sexual life after cancer. For cancer patients, difficulty with sexual excitement—both in terms of bodily response (erection or lubrication) and of subjective feelings of arousal—is a common problem. Orgasmic dysfunction is common, because of either lowered excitement or specific impairment, and the difficulty usually is pervasive rather than situational, as often is the case for healthy individuals. For example, women who were orgasmic during intercourse prior to surgery and irradiation treatments for cervical cancer might discover that they are nonorgasmic and further might feel insufficiently aroused even to approach orgasm. Similarly, men who are treated surgically for prostate cancer may be unable to achieve erection. Problematic resolution responses among cancer patients are varied. Often, those who experience pain during intercourse have residual discomfort. Those who are without pain but have disruptions of desire, excitement, or orgasm may feel sexual tension or disappointment or may fear that their sexual responsiveness is changed permanently.

Finally, the prognosis for sexual problems among healthy individuals is positive [120], whereas treatment of the sexual problems of cancer patients is likely to be difficult, and such problems may be refractory. Prevention through provision of the least disruptive but comparably curative cancer treatment is the single most important strategy. For example, research has demonstrated that breast-saving treatments as opposed to radical surgeries result in significantly better psychological and sexual adjustment [121]. Similar findings are emerging for treatment of in situ vulvar disease, prostate cancer, and disease at other sites. Interventions to reduce the incidence and severity of problems would be most effective if delivered during the diagnostic, treatment, and early posttreatment periods.

Interventions would have to be tailored to specific disease and treatment effects, and accurate and detailed explanations of the anticipated sexual disruptions would be central. The latter would enable patients to anticipate difficulties. Additional information might include specific strategies for managing their problems.

Sexual Schema and Other Psychological Contributors

Though medical factors contribute to morbidity, psychological-behavioral variables may be the most important. The model in Figure 37.1 begins with "baseline" psychological-behavioral factors, particularly age and sexual functioning (active or inactive and prior frequency of important sexual activities [e.g., intercourse]). These factors emerged as important predictors of sexual activity in the earliest research on sexuality [122] as well as in contemporary research [123]. These variables are important predictors in studies of healthy individuals, but their predictive utility is found also in studies of individuals with chronic conditions and illnesses [124, 125].

In the effort to identify a psychologically relevant variable, many investigators have tested the role of body image, because it has been hypothesized as relevant to sexuality for healthy women [126] and for women with cancer [127]. Descriptive findings of poor body concept among cancer patients have been reported, particularly in early studies of women with breast cancer [128]. However, often the measures of body image could not predict sexual outcomes among cancer patients for whom body image was thought to be important, such as breast cancer patients [129] or gynecologic cancer patients [130]. Instead, recent data indicate that rather than examination of a view of the

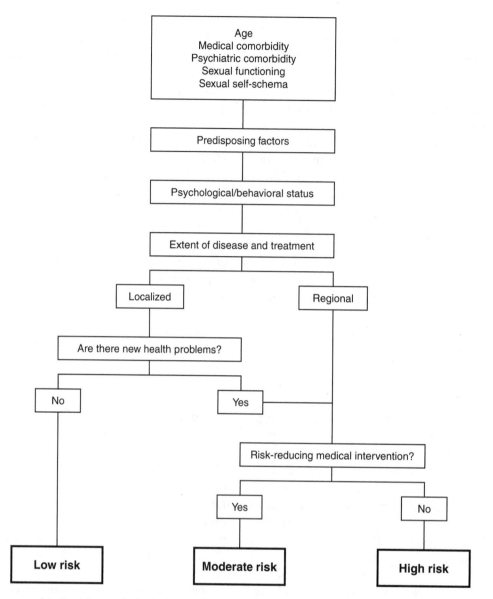

Figure 37.1 Demographic, health, psychological, sexual, and disease and treatment factors leading to low, moderate, and high levels of risk for sexual morbidity during the survivorship period.

body per se, a more central perspective of individuals' views of themselves as sexual persons—their sexual self-view or sexual self-schema—is an important predictor of sexual morbidity. Sexual self-schema (or sexual self-concept) is a cognitive view about sexual aspects of self; it is derived from sexual experiences, it affects current sexual experiences, and it guides men's and women's approaches to sexual situations with others [131, 132].

Research indicates that women's cognitive self-view of sexuality includes two positive aspects: an inclination to experience romantic or passionate emotions and a behavioral openness to sexual experiences or relation-

ships (or both). The other, negative aspect is that of embarrassment or conservatism (or both), which appears to be a deterrent to sexual expression [131]. Sexual schema predicts sexual behavior, attitudes, and responsiveness in healthy women, and it is an important, individual difference measure of female sexuality. In addition, it can predict risk for sexual morbidity after gynecologic cancer. Women who are "negative" in their sexual self-concept, in contrast to women with a "positive" sexual self-concept, are at greatest risk for sexual difficulty [125]. Women with a negative sexual self-view appear to have more difficulties because generally they are less romantic or passionate in their emotions,

Table 37.6 Sexual Morbidity Estimates for Men

Site and Subgroup	Method Rating*	Area of Sexual Functioning Difficulty			
		No Sexual Activity (%)	Desire (%)	Excitement (%)	Orgasm (%)
Colon-rectum					
Anterior resection	3	10–30	30–60	10–30	10–30
Abdominoperineal resection	3	60–100	30–60	50–90	70–100
Bladder	3	30–50	30–70	50–90	25–35
Prostate					
Retropubic	3	—	—	85	78
Perineal	3	—	—	88	100
Retropubic or perineal + hormone therapy	3	—	—	100	100
RT	3	—	—	37	—
Interstitial therapy + lymphadenectomy	4	—	—	15–25	30
Testicle					
Seminoma: Orch + RT	4	—	12	15	10
Nonseminoma: Orch + RL ± CTx	4	—	15–20	5–15	20–40
Nonseminoma: Orch + RL + RT ± CTx	4	—	50	24	55
Hodgkin's disease	2	—	—	20–30	—

RT = radiotherapy; Orch = orchiectomy; RL = radical lymphadenectomy; CTx = chemotherapy.
*Methodology rating scale for prior empirical literature: 2 = single-group longitudinal investigations with or without control(s); 3 = more than three retrospective studies; 4 = only one to two retrospective studies.

less open to sexual experiences, and more likely to have negative feelings about their sexuality. Thus, in the context of cancer, with disease or treatment factors causing direct changes to the body or sexual responses, women with negative sexual self-schemas are found to be at greater risk. Women with negative self-views of their sexuality also report that their sexual arousal level is lower, they are less apt to try new sexual activities as a way to cope with their sexual difficulties, and they have more negative cognitions or feelings (e.g., embarrassment) about any body changes.

Men's sexual self-views also consist of three primary components, although not completely parallel to those observed in women. All three male schema factors are positive traits: passionate or loving, powerful or independent, and open or liberal self-views [132]. Whereas women's sexual self-views may range from negative to positive, men's sexual self-views vary from "aschematic" to "schematic" (with schematic men holding highly positive views of the sexual self and aschematic men not viewing themselves as particularly sexual beings). Men who hold strong and well-developed sexual self-schemas tend to view themselves as romantic, powerful, and open individuals, whereas aschematic men do not view these traits as particularly self-descriptive.

Thus, men who score lowest on the sexual self-schema scale are not describing themselves in negative terms; they simply are not endorsing positive, sexually relevant modifiers as particularly self-descriptive.

Efforts to prevent sexual morbidity or to provide rehabilitation will be important for individuals with more negative (or aschematic) sexual self-concepts [133]. Such efforts could provide specific strategies for managing sexual difficulties, information to challenge affected women's typical self-view, and strategies for enhancing sexual self-schemas (e.g., ways to become more open to arousal and to sexual experiences and less inhibited or embarrassed).

Site-Specific Review of Sexual Outcomes

To summarize the incidence and types of sexual problems, Tables 37.6 and 37.7 (for men and women, respectively) provide estimates of behavioral and sexual response cycle disruptions. These data are composites from the available studies. The methodology rating in each table categorizes the types and number of studies that contributed to the estimate. As can be seen, the bulk of the research consists of retrospective studies of

Table 37.7   Sexual Morbidity Estimates for Women

Site and Subgroup	Method Rating*	Area of Sexual Functioning Difficulty				
		No Sexual Activity (%)	Desire (%)	Excitement (%)	Orgasm (%)	Dyspareunia (%)
Breast						
MRM	2	—	—	30–40	—	—
Lumpectomy + RT ± CTx	1	—	—	15–25	—	—
Colon-rectum						
Anterior resection	3	10–30	30–60	10–30	10–30	—
Abdominoperineal resection	3	60–100	30–60	50–90	70–100	—
Bladder	4	25	10	0	0	75
Cervix, endometrial	2	15	30–50	25–50	25–40	30–50
Surgery	2	—	30–40	25–35	25	30
RT	2	—	30–50	35–45	35	40–60
Surgery + RT	2	—	40–50	40–60	40	40–60
Vulva						
In situ	4	33	15	36	28	8
Invasive (vulvectomy)	3	50	15	40	30	20
Hodgkin's disease	2	20	32	—	—	—

MRM = modified radical mastectomy; RT = radiotherapy; CTx = chemotherapy.
*Methodology rating scale for prior empirical literature: 1 = randomized trials; 2 = single-group longitudinal investigations with or without control(s); 3 = more than three retrospective studies; 4 = only one to two retrospective studies.

limited patient samples, and the assessment of sexual outcomes usually were modest measures taken from interviews with patients. However, more recent data demonstrate that sexuality measures can be incorporated effectively into clinical trial investigations [134].

BREAST

In recent decades, considerable discussion and change have taken place in oncology regarding the appropriate standard surgical therapy for women with breast cancer. An impetus for clinical trials comparing the surgical therapies was to reduce morbidity (defined broadly but including quality of life) without sacrificing cure rate. Currently, the data suggest that conservative surgery (i.e., breast-conserving therapy [BCT]) with radiotherapy produces survival rates comparable to those achieved with modified radical mastectomy for women with early-stage disease [134]. However, not all women are eligible for BCT (because of size, location, or spread of the tumor), and they must undergo mastectomy. Still others, when given the choice, *elect* mastectomy. Subsequently, women are faced with the question of reconstruction: to proceed or not to proceed, and if so, when?

Data suggest that the sexuality pattern for women receiving reconstructive surgery (modified radical mastectomy with reconstruction [MRMR]) was significantly different—with lower rates of activity and fewer signs of sexual responsiveness—from that for women receiving either BCT or modified radical mastectomy (MRM) [135]. The behavioral disruption (failure to resume intercourse) can be particularly obvious. The finding of statistically equivalent sexual outcomes between BCT and MRM is consistent with the meta-analytical findings of Moyer [121]. That author reported extremely small (and nonsignificant [ns]) differences in effect size (ES) between BCT and MRM groups, considering both randomized (ES = 0.06; ns) and non-randomized (ES = 0.11; ns) investigations.

Comparison regarding dimensions of body-change stress reveals a consistent pattern of results for the three surgical groups but one that differs from the previously discussed sexual outcomes [135]. Specifically, significantly higher levels of traumatic stress and situational distress regarding the breast changes were reported by all women treated with mastectomy (i.e., both MRM and MRMR) in contrast to the levels in women treated with BCT. The pattern of less body-change stress accruing to women receiving BCT than to those receiving MRM is not surprising. Indeed, this effect is robust, is found in both randomized and nonrandomized investigations, and occurs regardless of whether the follow-up interval is short or long (i.e., less than or greater than 12 months postoperatively) [121]. Far fewer studies have included a sample of women who have undergone reconstruction. The finding of equivalent levels of distress for both the MRMR and MRM groups [135], however, is consistent with data from cross-sectional studies of heterogeneous samples of women assessed from two months to two years [136, 137] postoperatively and for longer than three years postoperatively [138]. Also, the data from the single study that randomly assigned women to either BCT or MRMR [139] found better outcomes for the women undergoing BCT and no apparent body image benefit for the women undergoing reconstruction.

In summary, women receiving MRMR find that their immediate postoperative sexual behavior and sexual responses are disrupted, significantly more so than are those in women receiving lesser surgery (BCT) or comparable breast surgery but no reconstruction (MRM). Moreover, the data suggest that the reconstruction achieves no reduction in body-change stress, at least when assessed during the early postoperative period: The reconstruction group reported levels of stress equivalent to those of the women receiving MRM only, and both mastectomy groups reported body-change stress significantly higher (in some cases, twice as high) as the responses of the women receiving BCT. Descriptive data from the few women who request bilateral mastectomy suggest that more radical surgical therapy does, indeed, result in greater psychological and behavioral morbidity [135].

COLON AND RECTUM

Treatment comparisons suggest consistently better sexual outcomes reported for those patients receiving an anterior resection rather than abdominoperineal resection (APR) of the rectum. For men, estimates of sexual dysfunction range between less than 50% for anterior resection and greater than 50% (and usually approaching 90–100%) for the abdominoperineal approach. These differences may be due to the effects of greater denervation of the sympathetic nerves with APR and to adjustment to having an abdominal stoma. These sexual data are consistent also with other data suggesting a more difficult adjustment in general after APR. Estimates for women come from much smaller

samples but, generally, studies report more positive outcomes than for men, regardless of the surgical approach.

BLADDER

Superficial bladder tumors are treated by transurethral resection and fulguration, and treatment may result in minimal sexual disruption; however, documenting data are not available. Men and women undergoing repeated cystoscopies have been noted to report reduced sexual desire and may have pain with intercourse, owing to urethral irritation [140]. As average bladder cancer patients are in their late sixties, lower frequencies of sexual activity and frequent lapses in functioning (e.g., erectile failure) would be expected. Historically, treatment for invasive bladder cancer has consisted of radical cystectomy with urinary diversion via an external conduit with ileal stoma. Of those men attempting to remain sexually active, inadequately rigid or only brief erections commonly occur. Orgasm, if experienced, is reported as less intense and occurs without ejaculate. Outcomes such as these have intensified efforts to modify surgical procedures and lower morbidity.

The sexual outcomes for women with bladder cancer have been studied on a very limited basis. In many respects, the outcomes are similar to those reported in women who have gynecologic cancer and are receiving an anterior pelvic exenteration, a procedure in which the vagina is narrowed instead of removed. Vaginal tightness and lack of lubrication appear to be the primary causes of the dyspareunia that often is reported.

The steps that have been taken to improve sexual outcomes have included nerve-sparing cystoprostatectomy with urethrectomy, continent diversions, and penile prosthesis surgery. Other related surgical procedures include intraabdominal reservoirs for urinary diversions, which patients are able to empty with self-catheterization. Mansson et al. [141] compared two patient groups, one whose members received the standard conduit diversion and the other whose members received the reservoir. Both groups had substantial sexual difficulties; however, those in the reservoir group had better overall adjustment. The latter finding was attributed to the absence of odor, leakage, and embarrassment, common problems for patients with urinary conduits. When total urethrectomy is necessary, the glans penis can collapse, causing difficulties with orgasm and appearance. Sexual outcome data suggest an improved outcome after less radical procedures or after aggressive reconstructive efforts (or both).

MALE GENITALIA

Prostate

Prostate treatments produce substantial sexual changes, and even a diagnostic biopsy may result in sexual difficulties. Many men report erectile failure and a complete loss (or at least a reduced amount) of seminal fluid ejaculated. Radical surgical prostatectomy for cancer is performed by the perineal, retropubic, or transpubic route. The rates of sexual dysfunction are three to four times higher than those for patients treated with less extensive surgery for benign prostate disease. If hormone therapy or orchiectomy is included, virtually all affected patients experience both erectile failure and ejaculation difficulty. Not surprisingly, therefore, some patients with local disease opt for supervoltage irradiation, which is used also in patients with regional disease. Again, the incidence of sexual difficulties is high, but it is less than half the estimates reported for radical surgery. Patients with metastatic disease or extensive regional spread are treated with such regimens as bilateral orchiectomy, estrogen administration, or both. The majority of patients who receive estrogen develop gynecomastia (the excessive development of male mammary glands), a troubling side effect.

Testicle

Cancer of the testicle accounts for only 1% of cancer in male individuals, but it is the most common site for disease among those aged 15 to 35 years. The surge of studies of sexual and reproductive outcomes for such persons is perhaps due to two factors. First, improvements in cure rates, particularly for disseminated tumors, have been achieved with chemotherapy. Second, the disease strikes men in the prime of their fatherhood and sexual-functioning years. As they become older and develop serious relationships, fertility status and sexuality will be a larger concern.

Testicular cancer is classified either as pure seminoma (accounting for roughly 40% of the cases) or nonseminoma. Treatment of the two differs and results in different sexual outcomes. Pure seminoma is radiosensitive; the usual treatment for it consists of radical orchiectomy of the testicle (occurrence of disease in both testicles being rare) followed by retroperitoneal nodal irradiation. Nonseminomas are treated with radical orchiectomy followed, for some, by chemotherapy. Data indicate that RPLND has a significantly negative impact on sexual functioning and fertility, owing to permanent difficulty with ejaculation. Of those men who receive orchiectomy and radiotherapy for seminoma,

10% to 20% report erectile or orgasmic dysfunction and low rates of sexual activity and desire. Reduced semen volume also can result, a side effect that has been hypothesized to occur from irradiation scatter to the prostate and seminal vesicles. Some studies indicate that higher irradiation dosages to the periaortic field is predictive of greater erectile and orgasmic difficulties.

In studies of nonseminoma patients, reduced ejaculate volume occurs in the majority of men. In fact, the data for both testicular cancer types suggest that RPLND likely reduces or eliminates semen outflow. Sexual outcomes for patients receiving orchiectomy and RPLND with or without chemotherapy appear similar. In contrast, if orchiectomy, RPLND, and radiotherapy are given with or without chemotherapy, sexual outcomes are worsened.

Penis

When cancer is confined to the penis, total penectomy leaves patients significantly impaired; however, stimulation of the remaining genital tissue, including the mons pubis, the perineum, and the scrotum, can produce orgasm for some [142]. Ejaculation can occur though the perineal urethrostomy and by the accompanying sensations of the bulbocavernosus and ischiocavernosus musculature. Patients who undergo partial excisions can remain capable of erection, orgasm, and ejaculation [143].

FEMALE GENITALIA

Cervix, Endometrium, and Ovary

The majority of the many retrospective studies that have been conducted with cervical cancer patients focus on the treatment alternatives of radical hysterectomy, radiotherapy, or combination treatment for those with early-stage disease. The widespread belief that radiotherapy is the most disruptive treatment comes from findings of poorly controlled studies. When they are compared in randomized studies [144], the outcomes for the two major treatment options appear similar; however, nonrandomized comparisons typically reveal more frequent and more problematic functioning for women treated with radiotherapy, either alone or in combination with surgery [145]. Other longitudinal research indicates that the primary sexual behavior disrupted by the disease and treatment process is the frequency of intercourse [119].

Regarding the sexual response cycle, the difficulty with sexual excitement is substantial. After treatment, women report lower arousal levels for sexual activities with their partners. A likely reason for the arousal deficits is the co-occurrence of significant disrupters (e.g., dyspareunia, due in part to irradiation effects or induced menopause or both) [146]. Promising intervention data suggest that severity of the latter difficulties can be reduced partly with psychological-behavioral interventions that provide information about the effects of cancer treatments and teach rehabilitation methods (e.g., using a vaginal dilator to reduce vaginal adhesions) [147].

Vulva

Typically, vulvar cancer occurs late in life; the average age of onset is 65 years. In contrast, the mean age for women with in situ disease is in the thirties and forties. Primary treatment for this disease has been radical vulvectomy. However, individualized and, consequently, more conservative approaches for treatment of vulvar cancer have been advocated, and studies indicate no differences in survival rates but significantly lower rates of morbidity (e.g., wound breakdown) [148]. Sexual disruption is substantial, even for women treated with wide local excision and related treatments for in situ disease. Overall, women appear more likely to be sexually inactive at follow-up [149]. A substantial number (30–50%) of women with invasive carcinoma treated with radical or modified radical vulvectomy (with or without groin dissection) cease all sexual activity; 60% to 70% of the women who remain sexually active report multiple sexual dysfunctions [150]. For women who become sexually inactive, many factors may be contributory. For some, the choice to be inactive is due to negative feelings (on the part of the women or their partners) about the physical changes to the body. For others, it may be due to severe dyspareunia, such as may occur with a narrowed introitus.

The single prospective study concerns the outcomes for 10 women treated for vulvar cancer [151]. A 77% participation rate was recorded; however, two-year follow-up data are available for only seven (70%) of the participants. In addition to the pretreatment assessment, follow-up assessments were conducted 6, 12, and 24 months after treatment. A comparison group of 24 healthy women was assessed on one occasion and demonstrated reductions in the frequency of sexual behavior and disruption of sexual desire and arousal at six months but with some improvement by 12 months; the gains remained stable during the next 12 months. All women remained sexually active despite a 50% increase in negative sensations during sexual arousal. These results are more favorable than are outcomes reported in the retrospective studies of vulvectomy patients and may be due to the selected samples participating in each (i.e., more dysfunctional patients in the retrospective studies and more "adjusted" patients continuing in this prospective report).

Hodgkin's Disease

Fertility and sexual morbidity associated with current therapies for Hodgkin's disease appear to be common. Also, decreased energy for and interest in sexual activity, with resultant lowered activity levels, may be problems for at least 25% of affected men and women. Specific sexual dysfunctions (e.g., erectile failure) have not been reported, but with treatment-induced ovarian failure, reports of dyspareunia would not be unexpected. Some data also suggest that Hodgkin's disease patients may be at greater risk for marital disruption, possibly owing to the extended strain on families during the lengthy treatment period and to the difficulties with impaired fertility [152].

ASSESSMENT OF SEXUAL FUNCTIONING

For cancer patients, the diagnostic period is a crisis [153]. Despite this reality, patients must process complex information and instructions as they undergo diagnostic studies and learn of treatment possibilities. Survival is a central concern. As this issue is clarified, concerns about impending treatments and their short- and long-term effects become paramount. In this context, assessment of affected patients' previous sexual functioning and explanation of any sexual morbidity from the disease and treatment become important. Assessment of patients' predisease sexual functioning will (1) enable health care providers to individualize the explanation of the anticipated sexual difficulties for affected patients (e.g., disruption in fertility as possibly important to a heterosexual man but not to a homosexual man); (2) provide important baseline information for understanding any posttreatment sexual problems; and (3) establish a context and precedent for patients to voice their sexual concerns.

Finally, a brief assessment of and information about probable sexual difficulties will prevent the occurrence of many sexual problems that may arise from lack of information or from confusion. Table 37.8 provides such an assessment model designed to evaluate both important

Table 37.8 ALARM Model for the Assessment of Sexual Functioning (Sample Questions)

Activity (frequency of such current sexual activities as intercourse, kissing, masturbation)
1. Prior to the appearance of any signs or symptoms of your illness, how frequently were you engaging in intercourse (specific weekly or monthly estimate)?
2. On occasions other than when having intercourse (or an equivalent intimate activity), do you share other forms of physical affection with your partner, such as kissing or hugging (or both) on a daily basis?
3. In the recent past (e.g., last 6 mo) have you masturbated? If so, estimate how often this has occurred (specific weekly or monthly estimate).

Libido-desire (desire for sexual activity and interest in initiating or responding to partner's initiations of sexual activity)
1. Prior to the appearance of your illness, would you have described yourself as generally interested in having sex?
2. Considering your current regular sexual relationship, who usually initiates sexual activity?
3. You indicated that your current frequency for intercourse is x times per week or month. Would you prefer to have intercourse more often, less often, or at the current frequency?

Arousal and orgasm (occurrence of erection-lubrication and ejaculation-vaginal contractions, accompanied by feelings of excitement)
For men
1. When you are interested in having sexual activity with your partner or alone, do you have any difficulty in achieving an erection? Do you feel emotionally aroused?
2. If you experience erectile difficulty, when did this problem start; how often does it occur; do certain particular circumstances trigger its occurrence (e.g., with partner only); and what do you understand to be the cause of the difficulty?
3. During sexual activity either alone or with a partner, do you have any difficulty with ejaculation (e.g., coming "too soon" or only after an extended period of time)?
4. If you experience premature or delayed ejaculation, how long would you estimate that it takes, on the average, to ejaculate after intensive stimulation begins?
For women
1. When you are interested in engaging in sexual activity, do you notice that your genitals become moist?
2. If you are postmenopausal, have you noticed any change in vaginal lubrication during sexual activity since the menopause, and are you currently taking hormonal replacement therapy?
3. If you experience arousal deficit, do you experience any pain with intercourse; how long have you had problems with becoming aroused during sexual activity; and do some circumstances cause you to feel more arousal than at other times?
4. During sexual activity either alone or with a partner, can you experience a climax or orgasm?
5. If orgasm does not occur, are you bothered at all by its absence?

Resolution (feelings of tension release after sexual activity and satisfaction with current sexual life)
1. After intercourse or masturbation, do you feel that sexual tension has been released?
2. On a scale from 1 (it could not be worse) to 10 (it could not be better), how would you rate your current sexual life?
3. Do you have any feelings of discomfort or pain immediately after sexual activity?
4. If you experience difficulty in resolution, what problems do you have after sexual activity; how long have they been occurring; and what is your understanding of their cause(s)?

Medical history relevant to sexuality
1. Current age and medical history: Have you had diabetes or hypertension?
2. Psychiatric history: In the past, have you had emotional difficulties for which you have sought treatment?
3. Substance use history: Do you consume alcohol or nonprescription drugs that may cause disruption of sexual activity or responses?

Note: ALARM refers to assessment of the following: sexual *a*ctivities, *l*ibido-desire, *a*rousal and orgasm, *r*esolution, and any *m*edical history relevant to sexual functioning. The examples used are for heterosexual individuals; some modification would be necessary for gay or lesbian individuals.

sexual behaviors (e.g., intercourse) and the sexual response cycle. Many relevant areas, such as marital adjustment, are omitted, but we assume assessment will be individualized within these central areas. Another strategy is to use very brief questionnaires [154].

Two important aspects of conducting brief assessments are understanding sexual behavior and functioning in healthy individuals and possessing the ability to discuss sexual functioning in a frank and nonjudgmental manner. To the extent that health care providers are informed, comfortable, and interested in addressing these concerns, cancer patients will begin to feel more hopeful and confident in coping with any sexual difficulties they may face.

REFERENCES

1. Kosary CL, Ries LAG, Miller BA, et al. (eds). *SEER Cancer Statistics Review, 1973–1992: Tables and Graphs.* [NIH Publication No. 96–2789.] Bethesda, MD: National Cancer Institute, 1995.
2. Baker TG. A quantitative and cytological study of germ cells in human ovaries. *Proc R Soc Lond B Biol Sci* 158:417–433, 1963.
3. Sanders JE, Buckner CD, Amos D, et al. Ovarian function following marrow transplantation for aplastic anemia or leukemia. *Blood* 6:813–818, 1988.
4. Wallace WHB, Shalet SM, Crowne EC, et al. Ovarian failure following abdominal irradiation in childhood: natural history and prognosis. *Clin Oncol* 1:75–79, 1989.
5. Scott JES. Pubertal development in children treated for nephroblastoma. *J Pediatr Surg* 16:122–125, 1981.
6. Hamre MR, Robison LL, Nesbit ME, et al. Effects of radiation on ovarian function in long-term survivors of childhood acute lymphoblastic leukemia: a report from the Children's Cancer Study Group. *J Clin Oncol* 5:1759–1765, 1987.
7. Wallace WHB, Shalet SM, Tetlow LJ, et al. Ovarian function following the treatment of childhood acute lymphoblastic leukemia. *Med Pediatr Oncol* 21:333–339, 1993.
8. Himelstein-Braw R, Peters H, Faber M. Influence of irradiation and chemotherapy on the ovaries of children with abdominal tumours. *Br J Cancer* 36:269–275, 1977.
9. Wallace WHB, Shalet SM, Hendry JH, et al. Ovarian failure following abdominal irradiation in childhood: the radiosensitivity of the human oocyte. *Br J Radiol* 62:995–998, 1989.
10. Stillman RJ, Schinfeld JS, Schiff I, et al. Ovarian failure in long-term survivors of childhood malignancy. *Am J Obstet Gynecol* 139:62–66, 1981.
11. Peck WS, McGreer JT, Kretzschmar NR, Brown WE. Castration of the female by irradiation. *Radiology* 34:176–186, 1940.
12. Sy Ortin TT, Shostak CA, Donaldson SS. Gonadal status and reproductive function following treatment for Hodgkin's disease in childhood: the Stanford experience. *Int J Rad Oncol Biol Phys* 19:873–880, 1990.
13. Horning SJ, Hoppe RT, Kaplan HS, et al. Female reproductive potential after treatment for Hodgkin's disease. *N Engl J Med* 304:1377–1382, 1981.
14. Husseinzadeh N, Nahhas WA, Velkley DE, et al. The preservation of ovarian function in young women undergoing pelvic radiation therapy. *Gynecol Oncol* 18:373–379, 1984.
15. Leporrier M, von Theobald P, Roffe J-L, et al. A new technique to protect ovarian function before pelvic irradiation. Heterotopic ovarian autotransplantation. *Cancer* 60:2201–2204, 1987.
16. Thomas PRM, Winstanly D, Peckham MJ, et al. Reproductive and endocrine function in patients with Hodgkin's disease: effects of oophoropexy and irradiation. *Br J Cancer* 33:226–231, 1976.
17. Ray GR, Trueblood HW, Enright LP, et al. Oophoropexy: a means of preserving ovarian function following pelvic megavoltage radiotherapy for Hodgkin's disease. *Radiology* 96:175–180, 1970.
18. Whitehead E, Shalet SM, Blackledge G, et al. The effect of combination chemotherapy on ovarian function in women treated for Hodgkin's disease. *Cancer* 52:988–993, 1983.
19. King DJ, Ratcliffe MA, Dawson AA, et al. Fertility in young men and women after treatment for lymphoma: a study of a population. *J Clin Pathol* 38:1247–1251, 1985.
20. Mackie EJ, Radford M, Shalet SM. Gonadal function following chemotherapy for childhood Hodgkin's disease. *Med Pediatr Oncol* 27:74–78, 1996.
21. Clark ST, Radford JA, Crowther D, et al. Gonadal function following chemotherapy for Hodgkin's disease: a comparative study of MVPP and a seven-drug hybrid regimen. *J Clin Oncol* 13:134–139, 1995.
22. Chapman RM, Sutcliffe SB, Malpas JS. Cytotoxic-induced ovarian failure in women with Hodgkin's disease: I. Hormone function. *JAMA* 242:1877–1881, 1979.
23. Schilsky RL, Sherins RJ, Hubbard SM, et al. Long-term follow-up of ovarian function in women treated with MOPP chemotherapy for Hodgkin's disease. *Am J Med* 71:552–556, 1981.
24. Waxman JHX, Terry YA, Wrigley PFM, et al. Gonadal function in Hodgkin's disease: long-term follow-up of chemotherapy. *Br Med J* 285:1612–1613, 1982.
25. Santoro A, Bonadonna G, Valagussa P, et al. Long-term results of combined chemotherapy-radiotherapy approach in Hodgkin's disease: superiority of ABVD plus radiotherapy versus MOPP plus radiotherapy. *J Clin Oncol* 5:27–37, 1987.
26. Andrieu JM, Ochoa-Molina ME. Menstrual cycle, pregnancies and offspring before and after MOPP therapy for Hodgkin's disease. *Cancer* 52:435–438, 1983.
27. Green DM, Yakar D, Brecher ML, et al. Ovarian function in adolescent women following successful treatment for non-Hodgkin's lymphoma. *Am J Pediatr Hematol Oncol* 5:27–31, 1983.
28. Siris ES, Leventhal BG, Vaitukaitis JL. Effects of childhood leukemia and chemotherapy on puberty and reproductive function in girls. *N Engl J Med* 294:1143–1146, 1976.
29. Wallace WHB, Shalet SM, Crowne EC, et al. Gonadal dysfunction due to *cis*-platinum. *Med Pediatr Oncol* 17:409–413, 1989.
30. Shamberger RC, Sherins RJ, Ziegler JL, et al. Effects of postoperative adjuvant chemotherapy and radiotherapy on ovarian function in women undergoing treatment for soft tissue sarcoma. *J Natl Cancer Inst* 67:1213–1218, 1981.
31. Shamberger RC, Rosenberg SA, Seipp CA, Sherins RJ. Effects of high-dose methotrexate and vincristine on ovarian and testicular function in patients undergoing postoperative adjuvant treatment of osteosarcoma. *Cancer Treat Res* 65:739–746, 1981.

32. Clayton PE, Shalet SM, Price DA, et al. Ovarian function following chemotherapy for childhood brain tumors. *Med Pediatr Oncol* 17:92–96, 1989.

33. Chapman RM, Sutcliffe SB, Malpas JS. Cytotoxic-induced ovarian failure in Hodgkin's disease: II. Effects on sexual function. *JAMA* 242:1882–1884, 1979.

34. Byrne J, Fears TR, Gail MH, Pee D, et al. Early menopause in long-term survivors of cancer during adolescence. *Am J Obstet Gynecol* 166:788–793, 1992.

35. Madsen BL, Giudice L, Donaldson SS. Radiation-induced premature menopause: a misconception. *Int J Radiat Oncol Biol Phys* 32:1461–1464, 1995.

36. Schlegel PN, Walsh PC. Neuroanatomical approach to radical cystoprostatectomy with preservation of sexual function. *J Urol* 138:1402–1406, 1987.

37. Narayan P, Lange PH, Fraley EE. Ejaculation and fertility after extended retroperitoneal lymph node dissection for testicular cancer. *J Urol* 127:685–688, 1982.

38. Nijman JM, Jager S, Boer PW, et al. The treatment of ejaculation disorders after retroperitoneal lymph node dissection. *Cancer* 50:2967–2971, 1982.

39. Rowley MJ, Leach DR, Warner GA, Heller CG. Effect of graded doses of ionizing radiation on the human testis. *Radiat Res* 59:665–678, 1974.

40. Heller CG, Wootton P, Rowley MJ, et al. Action of radiation upon human spermatogenesis. In Gual C (ed), *Proceedings of the Sixth Pan-American Congress of Endocrinology* (International Congress Series No. 112). Amsterdam: Excerpta Medica, 1966:408–410.

41. Shalet SM, Beardwell CG, Jacobs HS, et al. Testicular function following irradiation of the human prepubertal testis. *Clin Endocrinol* 9:483–490, 1978.

42. Speiser B, Rubin P, Casarett G. Aspermia following lower truncal irradiation in Hodgkin's disease. *Cancer* 32:692–698, 1973.

43. Hahn EW, Feingold SM, Nisce L. Aspermia and recovery of spermatogenesis in cancer patients following incidental gonadal irradiation during treatment: a progress report. *Radiology* 119:223–225, 1976.

44. Pedrick TJ, Hoppe RT. Recovery of spermatogenesis following pelvic irradiation for Hodgkin's disease. *Int J Radiat Oncol Biol Phys* 12:117–121, 1986.

45. Kinsella TJ, Trivette G, Rowland J, et al. Long-term follow-up of testicular function following radiation therapy for early-stage Hodgkin's disease. *J Clin Oncol* 7:718–724, 1989.

46. Blatt J, Sherins RJ, Niebrugge D, et al. Leydig cell function in boys following treatment for testicular relapse of acute lymphoblastic leukemia. *J Clin Oncol* 3:1227–1231, 1985.

47. Sklar CA, Robison LL, Nesbit ME, et al. Effects of radiation on testicular function in long-term survivors of childhood acute lymphoblastic leukemia: a report from the Children's Cancer Study Group. *J Clin Oncol* 8:1981–1987, 1990.

48. Ahmed SR, Shalet SM, Campbell RHA, et al. Primary gonadal damage following treatment of brain tumors in childhood. *J Pediatr* 103:562–565, 1983.

49. Fraass BA, Kinsella TJ, Harrington FS, et al. Peripheral dose to the testes: the design and clinical use of a practical and effective gonadal shield. *Int J Radiat Oncol Biol Phys* 11:609–615, 1985.

50. Shafford EA, Kingston JE, Malpas JS, et al. Testicular function following the treatment of Hodgkin's disease in childhood. *Br J Cancer* 68:1199–1204, 1993.

51. DeVita VT, Arseneau JC, Sherins RJ, et al. Intensive chemotherapy for Hodgkin's disease: Long-term complications. *Natl Cancer Inst Monogr* 36:447–454, 1973.

52. Asbjornsen G, Molne K, Klepp O, Aakvaag A. Testicular function after combination chemotherapy for Hodgkin's disease. *Scand J Haematol* 16:66–69, 1976.

53. Sherins RJ, Olweny CLM, Ziegler JL. Gynecomastia and gonadal dysfunction in adolescent boys treated with combination chemotherapy for Hodgkin's disease. *N Engl J Med* 299:12–16, 1978.

54. Chapman RM, Rees LH, Sutcliffe SB, et al. Cyclical combination chemotherapy and gonadal function. *Lancet* 1:285–289, 1979.

55. Chapman RM, Sutcliffe SB, Malpas JS. Male gonadal dysfunction in Hodgkin's disease. *JAMA* 245:1323–1328, 1981.

56. Viviani S, Santoro A, Ragni G, et al. Gonadal toxicity after combination chemotherapy for Hodgkin's disease. Comparative results of MOPP vs ABVD. *Eur J Cancer Clin Oncol* 21:601–605, 1985.

57. Charak BS, Gupta R, Mandrekar P, et al. Testicular dysfunction after cyclophosphamide-vincristine-procarbazine-prednisolone chemotherapy for advanced Hodgkin's disease. A long-term follow-up study. *Cancer* 65:1903–1906, 1990.

58. Dhabhar BN, Malhotra H, Joseph R, et al. Gonadal function in prepubertal boys following treatment for Hodgkin's disease. *Am J Pediatr Hematol Oncol* 15:306–310, 1993.

59. Heikens J, Behrendt H, Adriaansse R, Berghout A. Irreversible gonadal damage in male survivors of pediatric Hodgkin's disease. *Cancer* 78:2020–2024, 1996.

60. da Cunha MF, Meistrich ML, Fuller LM, et al. Recovery of spermatogenesis after treatment for Hodgkin's disease: limiting dose of MOPP chemotherapy. *J Clin Oncol* 2:571–577, 1984.

61. Braumswig JH, Heimes U, Heiermann E, et al. The effects of different cumulative doses of chemotherapy on testicular function. Results in 75 patients treated for Hodgkin's disease during childhood or adolescence. *Cancer* 65:1298–1302, 1990.

62. Green DM, Brecher ML, Lindsay AN, et al. Gonadal function in pediatric patients following treatment for Hodgkin's disease. *Med Pediatr Oncol* 9:235–244, 1981.

63. Whitehead E, Shalet SM, Morris-Jones PH, et al. Gonadal function after combination chemotherapy for Hodgkin's disease in childhood. *Arch Dis Child* 47:287–291, 1982.

64. Aubier F, Flamant F, Brauner R, et al. Male gonadal function after chemotherapy for solid tumors in childhood. *J Clin Oncol* 7:304–309, 1989.

65. Jaffe N, Sullivan MP, Ried H, et al. Male reproductive function in long-term survivors of childhood cancer. *Med Pediatr Oncol* 16:241–247, 1988.

66. Hansen SW, Berthelsen JG, Von Der Maase H. Long-term

fertility and Leydig cell function in patients treated for germ cell cancer with cisplatin, vinblastine, and bleomycin versus surveillance. *J Clin Oncol* 8:1695–1698, 1990.

67. Drasga RE, Einhorn LE, Williams SD, et al. Fertility after chemotherapy for testicular cancer. *J Clin Oncol* 1:179–183, 1983.

68. Johnson DH, Hainsworth JD, Linde RB, Greco FA. Testicular function following combination chemotherapy with *cis*-platin, vinblastine, and bleomycin. *Med Pediatr Oncol* 12:233–238, 1984.

69. Shalet SM, Hann IM, Lendon M, et al. Testicular function after combination chemotherapy for acute lymphoblastic leukemia. *Arch Dis Child* 56:275–278, 1981.

70. Lendon M, Palmer MK, Morris-Jones PH, et al. Testicular histology after combination chemotherapy in childhood for acute lymphoblastic leukaemia. *Lancet* 2:439–441, 1978.

71. Blatt J, Poplack DG, Sherins RJ. Testicular function in boys after chemotherapy for acute lymphoblastic leukemia. *N Engl J Med* 304:1121–1124, 1981.

72. Shamberger RC, Sherins RJ, Rosenberg SA. The effects of postoperative adjuvant chemotherapy and radiotherapy on testicular function in men undergoing treatment for soft tissue sarcoma. *Cancer* 47:2368–2374, 1981.

73. Pryzant RM, Meistrich ML, Wilson G, et al. Long-term reduction in sperm count after chemotherapy with and without radiation therapy for non-Hodgkin's lymphoma. *J Clin Oncol* 11:239–247, 1993.

74. Meistrich ML, Wilson G, Brown BW, et al. Impact of cyclophosphamide and long-term reduction in sperm count in men treated with combination chemotherapy for Ewing and soft tissue sarcomas. *Cancer* 70:2703–2712, 1992.

75. Byrne J, Mulvihill JJ, Myers MH, et al. Effects of treatment on fertility in long-term survivors of childhood or adolescent cancer. *N Engl J Med* 317:1315–1321, 1987.

76. Critchley HOD, Wallace WHB, Shalet SM, et al. Abdominal irradiation in childhood: the potential for pregnancy. *Br J Obstet Gynecol* 99:392–394, 1992.

77. Li FP, Fine W, Jaffe N, et al. Offspring of patients treated for cancer in childhood. *J Natl Cancer Inst* 62:1193–1197, 1979.

78. Hawkins MM, Smith RA, Curtice LJ. Childhood cancer survivors and their offspring studied through a postal survey of general practitioners: Preliminary results. *J R Coll Gen Pract* 38:102–105, 1988.

79. Mulvihill JJ, Byrne J, Steinhorn SA, et el. Genetic disease in offspring of survivors of cancer in the young (abstract). *Am J Hum Genet* 39:A7a, 1986.

80. Green DM, Fine WE, Li FP. Offspring of patients treated for unilateral Wilms' tumor in childhood. *Cancer* 49:2285–2288, 1982.

81. Byrne J, Mulvihill JJ, Connelly RR, et al. Reproductive problems and birth defects in survivors of Wilms' tumor and their relatives. *Med Pediatr Oncol* 16:233–240, 1988.

82. Li FP, Gimbrere K, Gelber RD, et al. Outcome of pregnancy in survivors of Wilms' tumor. *JAMA* 257:216–219, 1987.

83. Hawkins MM, Smith RA. Pregnancy outcomes in childhood cancer survivors: probable effects of abdominal irradiation. *Int J Cancer* 43:399–402, 1989.

84. Hawkins MM. Is there evidence of a therapy-related increase in germ cell mutation among childhood cancer survivors? *J Natl Cancer Inst* 83:1643–1650, 1991.

85. Green DM, Zevon MA, Lowrie G, et al. Pregnancy outcome following treatment with chemotherapy for cancer in childhood and adolescence. *N Engl J Med* 325:141–146, 1991.

86. Nygaard R, Clausen N, Siimes MA, et al. Reproduction following treatment for childhood leukemia: a population-based prospective cohort study of fertility and offspring. *Med Pediatr Oncol* 19:459–466, 1991.

87. Janov AJ, Anderson J, Cella DF, et al. Pregnancy outcome in survivors of advanced Hodgkin disease. *Cancer* 70:688–692, 1992.

88. Dodds I, Marrett LD, Tomkins DJ, et al. Case-control study of congenital anomalies in children of cancer patients. *Br Med J* 307:164–168, 1993.

89. Kenny LB, Nicholson HS, Brasseux C, et al. Birth defects in offspring of adult survivors of childhood acute lymphoblastic leukemia. *Cancer* 78:169–176, 1996.

90. Green DM, Fiorello A, Zevon MA, et al. Birth defects and childhood cancer in offspring of survivors of childhood cancer. *Arch Pediatr Adolesc Med* 151:379–383, 1997.

91. Mulvihill JJ, Myers MH, Connelly RR, et al. Cancer in offspring of long-term survivors of childhood and adolescent cancer. *Lancet* 2:813–817, 1987.

92. Hawkins JJ, Draper GJ, Smith RA. Cancer among 1,348 offspring of survivors of childhood cancer. *Int J Cancer* 43:975–978, 1989.

93. Sanders JE, Hawley J, Levy W, et al. Pregnancies following high-dose cyclophosphamide with or without high-dose busulfan or total-body irradiation and bone marrow transplantation. *Blood* 87:3045–3052, 1996.

94. Chapman RM, Sutcliffe SB. Protection of ovarian function by oral contraceptives in women receiving chemotherapy for Hodgkin's disease. *Blood* 58:849–851, 1981.

95. Waxman JH, Ahmed R, Smith D, et al. Failure to preserve fertility in patients with Hodgkin's disease. *Cancer Chemo Pharmacol* 19:159–162, 1987.

96. Johnson DH, Linde R, Hainsworth JD, et al. Effect of a luteinizing hormone–releasing hormone agonist given during combination chemotherapy on posttherapy fertility in male patients with lymphoma: preliminary observations. *Blood* 65:832–836, 1985.

97. Marmor D, Elefant E, Dauchez C, et al. Semen analysis in Hodgkin's disease before the onset of treatment. *Cancer* 57:1986–1987, 1986.

98. Reed E, Sanger WG, Armitage JO. Results of semen cryopreservation in young men with testicular carcinoma and lymphoma. *J Clin Oncol* 4:537–539, 1986.

99. Scammell GE, Stedronska J, Edmonds DK, et al. Cryopreservation of semen in men with testicular tumour or Hodgkin's disease: results of artificial insemination of their partners. *Lancet* 2:31–32, 1985.

100. Redman JR, Bajorunas DR, Goldstein MC, et al. Semen cryopreservation and artificial insemination for Hodgkin's disease. *J Clin Oncol* 5:233–238, 1987.

101. Hendry WF, Stedronska J, Jones CR, et al. Semen anal-

ysis in testicular cancer and Hodgkin's disease: pre- and post-treatment findings and implications for cryopreservation. *Br J Cancer* 55:769–773, 1983.

102. Hansen PV, Trykker H, Andersen J, et al. Germ cell function and hormonal status in patients with testicular cancer. *Cancer* 64:956–961, 1989.

103. Sigman M. Assisted reproductive techniques and male infertility. *Urol Clin North Am* 21:505–515, 1994.

104. Glezerman M, Lunenfeld B, Potashnik G, et al. Retrograde ejaculation: pathophysiologic aspects and report of two successfully treated cases. *Fertil Steril* 27:796–800, 1976.

105. Brassesco M, Viscasillas P, Burrel L et al. Sperm recuperation and cervical insemination in retrograde ejaculation. *Fertil Steril* 49:923–925, 1988.

106. Vernon M, Wilson E, Muse K et al. Successful pregnancies from men with retrograde ejaculation with the use of washed sperm and gamete intrafallopian tube transfer (GIFT). *Fertil Steril* 50:822–824, 1988.

107. Urry RL, Middleton RG, McGavin S. A simple and effective technique for increasing pregnancy rates in couples with retrograde ejaculation. *Fertil Steril* 46:1124–1127, 1986.

108. Van Der Linden PJ, Nan PM et al. Retrograde ejaculation: successful treatment with artificial insemination. *Obstet Gynecol* 79:126–128, 1992.

109. Levran D, Dor J, Rudak E, et al. Pregnancy potential of human oocytes—the effect of cryopreservation. *N Engl J Med* 323:1153–1156, 1990.

110. Borini A, Bafaro G, Violini F et al. Pregnancies in postmenopausal women over 50 years old in an oocyte donation program. *Fertil Steril* 63:258–261, 1995.

111. Sauer MV, Paulson RJ, Lobo RA. Pregnancy after age 50: application of oocyte donation to women after natural menopause. *Lancet* 341:321–323, 1993.

112. Sauer MV, Paulson RJ, Lobo RA. A preliminary report on oocyte donation extending reproductive potential to women over 50. *N Engl J Med* 323:1157–1160, 1990.

113. Avarbock MR, Brinster CJ, Brinster RL. Reconstitution of spermatogenesis from frozen spermatogonial stem cells. *Nature Med* 2:693–696, 1996.

114. Brinster RL, Zimmerman JW. Spermatogenesis following male germ-cell transplantation. *Proc Natl Acad Sci USA* 91:11298–11302, 1994.

115. Brinster RL, Avarbock MR. Germline transmission of donor haplotype following spermatogonial transplantation. *Proc Natl Acad Sci USA* 91:11303–11307, 1994.

116. Carroll J, Gosden RG. Transplantation of frozen-thawed mouse primordial follicles. *Hum Reprod* 8:1163–1167, 1993.

117. Gosden RG, Baird DT, Wade JC, et al. Restoration of fertility to oophorectomized sheep by ovarian autografts stored at -196°C. *Hum Reprod* 9:597–603, 1994.

118. Devlen J, Maguire P, Phillips P, et al. Psychological problems associated with diagnosis and treatment of lymphomas: II. Prospective study. *Br Med J* 295:955–957, 1987.

119. Andersen BL, Anderson B, Deprosse C. Controlled prospective longitudinal study of women with cancer: I. Sexual functioning outcomes. *J Consult Clin Psychol* 57:683–691, 1989.

120. Wincze JP, Carey MP. *Sexual Dysfunction: A Guide for Assessment and Treatment.* New York: Guilford Press, 1991.

121. Moyer A. Psychosocial outcomes of breast-conserving surgery versus mastectomy: a meta-analytic review. *Health Psychol* 16:284–298, 1997.

122. Kinsey A, Pomeroy WG, Martin EC, et al. *Sexual Behavior in the Human Female.* Philadelphia: Saunders, 1953.

123. Laumann EO, Gagnon JH, Michael RT, et al. *The Social Organization of Sexuality: Sexual Practices in the United States.* Chicago: University of Chicago Press, 1994.

124. Curry SL, Levine SB, Jones PK, et al. Medical and psychosocial predictors of sexual outcome among women with systemic lupus erythematosus. *Arthritis Care Res* 6:23–30, 1993.

125. Andersen BL, Woods X, Copeland LJ. Sexual self-schema and sexual morbidity among gynecologic cancer survivors. *J Consult Clin Psychol* 65:221–229, 1997.

126. Cash TF. *Body Image Therapy: A Program for Self-Directed Change.* New York: Guilford Publications, 1991.

127. Derogatis L. Breast and gynecologic cancers: their unique impact on body image and sexual identity in women. In Vaeth JM (ed), *Front Radiat Ther Oncol* 14:1–11, 1980.

128. de Haes JCC, Welvaart K. Quality of life after breast cancer surgery. *J Surg Oncol* 28:123–125, 1985.

129. Andersen BL, Jochimsen PR. Sexual functioning among breast cancer, gynecologic cancer, and healthy women. *J Consult Clin Psychol* 53:25–32, 1985.

130. Andersen BL, LeGrand J. Body image for women: conceptualization, assessment, and a test of its importance to sexual dysfunction and medical illness. *J Sex Res* 28:457–477, 1991.

131. Andersen BL, Cyranowski JM. Women's sexual self-schema. *J Pers Soc Psychol* 67:1079–1100, 1994.

132. Andersen BL, Cyranowski JM, Espindle D. Men's sexual self-schema. *J Pers Soc Psycol* 76:645–661, 1999.

133. Cyranowski JC, Aarestad SL, Andersen BL. The role of sexual self schemas in a diathesis-stress model of sexual dysfunction. *Appl Prevent Psychol* 8:217–228, 1999.

134. Stead ML, Crocombe WD, Fallowfield LJ, et al. Sexual activity questionnaires in clinical trials: acceptability to patients with gynaecological disorders. *Br J Obstet Gynaecol* 106:50–54, 1999.

135. Yurek D, Farrar W, Andersen BL. Breast cancer surgery: comparing surgical groups and determining individual differences in postoperative sexuality and body change stress. *J Consult Clin Psychol* 68: 697–709, 2000.

136. Mock V. Body image in women treated for breast cancer. *Nurs Res* 42:153–157, 1993.

137. Noguchi M, Saito Y, Nishijima H, et al. The psychological and cosmetic aspects of breast-conserving therapy compared with radical mastectomy. *Surg Today* 23:598–602, 1993.

138. Margolis GJ, Goodman RL, Rubin A. Psychological effects of breast-conserving cancer treatment and mastectomy. *Psychosomatics* 31:33–39, 1990.

139. Schain WS, d'Angelo TM, Dunhn ME, et al. Mastectomy versus conservative surgery and radiation therapy. *Cancer* 73:1221–1228, 1994.

140. Schover LR, Von Eschenbach AC, Smith DB, et al. Sexual rehabilitation of urologic cancer patients: a practical approach. *CA Cancer J Clin* 34:3–11, 1984.

141. Mansson A, Johnson G, Mansson W. Quality of life after cystectomy: comparison between patients with conduit and those with caeca reservoir diversion. *Br J Urol* 62:240–245, 1988.

142. Witkin MH, Kaplan HS. Sex therapy and penectomy. *J Sex Marital Ther* 8:209–221, 1989.

143. Bracken RB, Johnson DE. Sexual function and fecundity after treatment for testicular tumors. *Urology* 7:35–38, 1976.

144. Vincent CE, Vincent B, Greiss FC, et al. Some marital-sexual concomitants of carcinoma of the cervix. *South Med J* 68:551–558, 1975.

145. Yeo BKL, Perera I. Sexuality of women with carcinoma of the cervix. *Ann Acad Med Singapore* 24:676–678, 1995.

146. Bergmark K, Avall-Lundqvist E, Dickman, PW, et al. Vaginal changes and sexuality in women with a history of cervical cancer. *N Engl J Med* 340:1383–1389, 1999.

147. Robinson JW, Faris PD, Scott CB. Psychoeducational group increases vaginal dilation for younger women and reduces sexual fears for women of all ages with gynecological carcinoma treated with radiotherapy. *Int J Radiat Oncol Biol Phys* 44:497–506, 1999.

148. Rodriguez M, Sevin B-U, Averette HE, et al. Conservative trends in the surgical management of vulvar cancer: a University of Miami patient care evaluation study. *Int J Gynecol Cancer* 7:151–157, 1997.

149. Andersen BL, Turnquist D, LaPolla J, et al. Sexual functioning after treatment of in-situ vulvar cancer: preliminary report. *Obstet Gynecol* 71:15–19, 1988.

150. Andersen BL, Hacker NF. Psychosexual adjustment after vulvar surgery. *Obstet Gynecol* 62:457–462, 1983.

151. Weimar Schultz WCM, van de Wiel HBM, Bouma J, et al. Psychosexual functioning after treatment for cancer of the vulva: a longitudinal study. *Cancer* 66: 402–407, 1991.

152. Fobair P, Hoppe RT, Bloom J, et al. Psychosocial problems among survivors of Hodgkin's disease. *J Clin Oncol* 4:805–814, 1986.

153. Andersen BL, Anderson B, Deprosse C. Controlled prospective longitudinal study of women with cancer: II. Psychological outcomes. *J Consult Clin Psychol* 57:692–697, 1989.

154. McGahuey CA, Delgado PL, Gelenberg AJ. Assessment of sexual dysfunction using the Arizona Sexual Experiences Scale (ASEX) an implications for treatment of depression. *Psychiatr Ann* 29:39–45, 1999.

38

Complementary and Alternative Therapies

■ ■ ■

BARRIE R. CASSILETH

ALONG WITH MANAGED CARE, ADVANCES IN biotechnology, and other significant medical and societal events, acceptance of unconventional therapies contributed importantly to the major changes that marked health care in the 1990s. The popularity of complementary and alternative medicine (CAM) has affected every component of the health care system and all specialties of medicine, including oncology. It has left its mark on the thinking and practice of physicians and other health professionals and has broadened patients' involvement and influence in their own care. No longer a collection of covert practices, unconventional medicine today is highly visible, and information about it is widely available to the general public. It is a multibillion-dollar business in the United States and of equivalent impact and importance throughout the developed world.

Despite broad public acceptance of CAM in North America, the professional oncology community is hardly unanimous in its approval. To some extent, this dichotomy of opinion is attributable to problems of inconsistent terminology and definition (discussed later).

This chapter aims to accomplish three goals: to describe the current status of both unconventional medicine and specific alternative and complementary practices and their use and value; to delineate mainstream acceptance, concerns, and regulatory issues; and to discuss the implications of the deepening trend in health care represented by this growth industry. Resources for additional information also are provided.

DEFINITION OF CAM

The terminology associated with unconventional medicine continues to change over time. CAM may be defined as "diagnosis, treatment and/or prevention which complements mainstream medicine by contributing to a common whole, by satisfying a demand not met by orthodoxy or by diversifying the conceptual frameworks of medicine" [1]. This European definition addresses *complementary* medicine, the term commonly applied to CAM in Europe. It does not address *alternative* medicine, the umbrella term applied most often to CAM in the United States.

Nonetheless, this definition is more accurate than are recent previous efforts, which depended on distinctions between what is and is not taught in medical schools or what is and is not practiced in mainstream hospitals. Complementary therapies are found in many (if not most) hospitals today. *Complementary therapies* is also a more complete and accurate term and is less pejorative than such previous language as *unorthodox, unconventional, questionable,* or *unproved therapy,* or *quackery,* the 1914 epithet applied by the American Cancer Society.

An advantage of the phrase *complementary and alternative* is that it offers the opportunity to make important distinctions between the two. Alternatives are literally that; they are promoted for use *instead* of mainstream therapy. Complementary or adjunctive therapies are used for symptom management and to enhance quality of life *in concert* with mainstream care.

This distinction, however, is not universally applied: Often, *CAM, alternative,* and *complementary* are used indiscriminately as interchangeable umbrella terms for a host of disparate activities and products. In addition to naming unconventional therapies, the terms sometimes are used to include self-care, routine private responses to aches and pains, efforts to maintain fitness, and lifestyle activities. The tendency to "medicalize" social and personal activities [2] is prominent in this field. *Complementary* and *alternative* also may include nutritional cancer "cures;" energy healing and other unproved and sometimes harmful methods; and spiritual care and other support services that have been in mainstream use for decades.

Alternative therapies for cancer are promoted as independent treatments for use instead of surgery, chemotherapy, and irradiation. Typically, invasive and biologically active alternative regimens are unproved, expensive, and potentially harmful. They may harm directly through biological activity or indirectly when patients postpone receipt of mainstream care. Examples in cancer medicine include the metabolic therapies available in Tijuana, shark cartilage, and high-dose vitamins and other products sold over the counter in the United States.

Although research evidence is scanty [3], apparently 8% to 10% or so of patients with tissue biopsy–diagnosed cancer eschew mainstream therapy and immediately seek alternative care. The vast majority of CAM users seek complementary, not alternative, medicine. Specific CAM therapies are discussed later.

CAM USE AND USERS
Prevalence of and Preferred CAM Therapies

Worldwide, the use of CAM for cancer is widespread. A recent systematic review of relevant published data located 26 cancer patient surveys from 13 countries, including 5 from the United States [4]. The average prevalence across all studies was 31%. Therapies used most commonly around the world include dietary treatments, herbs, homeopathy, hypnotherapy, imagery and visualization, meditation, megavitamins, relaxation, and spiritual healing. New investigations substantiate these results [5–7].

All but one of the US surveys obtained information about specific therapies employed. Patients used Laetrile, metabolic therapies, diets, spiritual healing, megavitamins, imagery, and "immune system stimulants" [4]. Across samples, the prevalence of CAM use in the United States ranged from 7% to 50%.

Additional surveys (involving not cancer patients but members of the US general public) uncovered 1997 prevalence rates of 50% of 113 family-practice patients [8] and 42% of 1,500 members of the general populace [9]. An earlier telephone survey of a representative national sample of 1,539 adults found that one-third had used CAM [10].

Prevalence rates from all CAM studies, conducted in the United States and internationally, range from less than 10% to more than 50%. This broad range, with its apparent discrepancies, may be attributed primarily to differences in understanding and defining CAM. Often, surveys do not define CAM or define it extremely broadly, resulting in the inclusion of such lifestyle activities as weight-loss efforts and such support activities as group counseling.

Additional data emerge from studies that request and report information about specific therapies used. One of the large surveys of US adults [10] was conducted in 1991. Results showed that relaxation techniques (used by 13% of respondents), chiropractic (10%), and massage (7%) were sought most commonly. Herbal medicines were used by 3% of respondents. In contrast, the 1997 general public survey revealed the most common CAM therapies to be herbal remedies (used by 17% of respondents) and chiropractic (used by 16% of those surveyed) [9].

The profound influence of 1994 legislation allowing herbal medicines and other "food supplements" to be sold over the counter without US Food and Drug Administration (FDA) review is evident in the increased use of herbal remedies, from 3% in 1991 to 17% in 1997. Sales of dietary supplements are estimated to have doubled since passage of the 1994 law. Similarly, expanding insurance coverage of chiropractic care during that period may account for commensurate growth in use of this therapeutic modality (see later discussion). Homeopathy, acupuncture, folk remedies, and the like were used by a maximum of only 2% of respondents in both studies.

To date, almost all studies of cancer patients and of the international general public show that those who seek CAM therapies tend to be female, better-educated, of higher socioeconomic status, and younger than those who do not. The growth in CAM use by cancer patients in recent years is evident [4]; secondary analysis of nearly 3,000 cancer patients estimated a 64% increase in CAM use since 1997 [11].

CAM Use Among Pediatric Cancer Patients

The use of CAM methods among pediatric oncology patients represents a special and understudied issue. Surveys in Australia and Finland [4], in British Columbia [7], and in the Netherlands [12] indicate substantial interest in CAM, especially in more recent years, with 40% to 50% of pediatric oncology patients in those countries receiving alternative or complementary therapies.

In the only study of CAM use among US pediatric oncology patients published during the last 10 years, the authors found that 65% of 81 cancer patients used CAM, whereas 51% of 80 control-group children receiving routine checkups did so [13]. Of particular interest is the type of CAM received. Prayer, exercise, and spiritual healing accounted for more than 96% of CAM therapies used. However, excluded from this sample, by definition, are the pediatric patients brought for alternative treatment to clinics in the United States, Mexico, or elsewhere.

MAINSTREAM ACCEPTANCE OF CAM

In contrast to the situation 15 years ago, when even determining the whereabouts of CAM practitioners re-quired underground investigation, CAM today is very much a public issue. CAM is discussed widely in the electronic media, and information about it is found readily on the Internet. Magazines provide the general public with details about new CAM therapies. Typically, the *Yellow Pages* of telephone books in most cities and towns list various types of CAM practitioners.

Public Access to Information

Information available to the public varies widely in accuracy. Many World Wide Web sites and publications that appear to be objective actually are sponsored by commercial enterprises that promote and sell the products they report. (Reputable Web sites are listed at the end of this chapter.)

Often, distinguishing between reputable sources of information and those that present vested interests is difficult for patients. Some promotional material and books are written by medical doctors and appear to present legitimate information. An example is a magazine delivered unsolicited by mail and appearing to be a medical journal for the public. Called *M.D.'s Journal,* this quarterly, 61-page publication contains such article titles as "M.D. Cures Terminal Cancer" and "How to Make Yourself Almost Immune to Breast Cancer." Actually, the articles are advertisements for "free reports" that accompany a $79.90 subscription to a periodical [14]. This approach is not uncommon. The accompanying photograph of an apparently kindly, white-coated doctor, stethoscope around his neck, delivers a powerful message.

National Institutes of Health Activity

In addition to gaining acceptance by public sources of information, CAM also has entered mainstream medicine in an unprecedented fashion. An Office of Alternative Medicine (OAM) was established at the National Institutes of Health (NIH) by Congressional mandate in 1992, its stated purpose being to investigate unconventional medical practices [15]. In October 1998, Congress elevated the status of the Office of Alternative Medicine by designating it as the National Center for Complementary and Alternative Medicine (CCAM), appropriating $50 million for its support. Currently, the CCAM supports 14 CAM research centers. Most, including the Center for Alternative Medicine Research in Cancer at the University of Texas Health Science Center in Houston [16], are based at major universities. With the CCAM, the relevant NIH institute shares support of both basic science and clinical research within its purview.

Medical Schools and Medical Centers

Another marker of mainstream acceptance is the emergence of medical school courses in CAM. Elective courses in CAM and portions of required courses are taught in at least 75 medical schools in the United States [17]. In addition, numerous hospitals and medical centers have developed research and clinical service programs in CAM. Cancer programs and many comprehensive cancer centers have implemented or are creating CAM programs of varying complexity. Hospital programs differ by departmental base, types of clients served (inpatients, outpatients, community), access (physician or self-referral), administrative staff (physician, nurse, CAM expert), and services provided.

Services range from mind-body sessions only, to massage and exercise, to the provision of herbs and food supplements, to services even more removed from mainstream care, such as colonics and homeopathy. Some clinical programs designated as CAM are merely repackaged support services, previously available to patients as spiritual care, group and individual counseling, art therapy, nutritional guidance, and the like.

Recognition by Mainstream Journals and Physicians

A survey of 295 family physicians in the Maryland-Virginia region [18] revealed that up to 90% view such complementary therapies as diet and exercise, behavioral medicine, and hypnotherapy as legitimate medical practices. A majority of these physicians refer patients to nonphysicians for these therapies or provide the services themselves. In the same survey, homeopathy, Native American medicine, and traditional Oriental medicine were not seen as legitimate practices.

Two hundred Canadian general practitioners held similar views, noting their patients' interest especially in chiropractic. These physicians perceive chiropractic care, hypnosis, and acupuncture for chronic pain as the most effective CAM therapies and view homeopathy and reflexology as less efficacious [19]. A meta-analysis of 12 studies in Great Britain suggests that British physicians view complementary medicine as moderately effective [20], a level of enthusiasm that contrasts with

the fervent efforts of the British Royal Family to promote homeopathy and other complementary therapies and to merge them with mainstream care.

A survey of physicians in Massachusetts, Washington, New Mexico, and Israel showed that primary-care physicians are more likely than other specialists to use, and to refer patients for, alternative therapies [21]. An early survey revealed that mainstream physicians practicing alternative medicine almost exclusively tended to be family practitioners and psychiatrists [3].

In addition to the increasing coverage of CAM services by health insurers (discussed in "Mainstream Disapproval"), a final marker of mainstream acceptance noted here is the publication of CAM research articles in major mainstream medical journals. Articles about CAM in major journals throughout the 1970s shifted from expressing realistic concern about quackery [22–24] to surveys of patients' knowledge and use of unproved methods in the 1980s [25–27], to reports of actual research results starting primarily in the mid-1990s.

The *Journal of the American Medical Association*, the *New England Journal of Medicine*, the *Lancet*, the *British Medical Journal*, and such specialty journals as *Cancer* and the *Journal of Clinical Oncology* have published reports of CAM research in recent years. From 1996 through 1997, the National Library of Medicine added many new CAM search terms to its medical subject headings and began to cover for inclusion in Medline alternative medicine journals not reviewed previously.

Mainstream Disapproval

Not all mainstream physicians are pleased with CAM, with current efforts to integrate CAM and mainstream medicine, or with a separate NIH research entity for alternative medicine [28–30]. Vigorous opposition to CAM has been voiced, labeling it as pseudoscience based on absurd beliefs. CAM's deviation from basic scientific principles (e.g., implicit in homeopathy and therapeutic touch) is decried.

A 1997 letter to the US Senate Subcommittee on Public Health and Safety signed by prominent scientists, including four Nobel Laureates, deplored the lack of critical thinking and scientific rigor in OAM-supported research. Many claim that the very existence of the CCAM as an entity apart from existing NIH research institutes supports a separate, inferior level of research and an antiscience bias. Alternative medicine is a quintessential example of the sociopolitical force behind medical change.

CAM COSTS AND INSURANCE COVERAGE

Health insurance programs increasingly cover CAM services and providers. More than 30 major insurers, half of them Blues plans, cover more than one alternative method [31]. Some examples are given in Table 38.1.

Expanding insurance coverage of CAM therapies reflects consumer demand, but it also represents managed-care efforts to control costs. CAM therapies were covered on the assumption that alternative practitioners and products would be less expensive than those in the mainstream. Typically, most alternative practitioners do provide an opportunity for cost savings, and food supplements are less costly than are prescription pharmaceuticals if used instead of the latter.

However, practitioners of naturopathy; acupuncture; chiropractic; traditional Chinese, Native American, and Ayurvedic (Indian) medicine; and homeopathy and other alternative therapists rely heavily on so-called natural remedies for treating many problems. Such remedies include herbs and other botanical remedies, enzymes, amino acids, vitamins and minerals, and homeopathic products. Although formal analyses of the costs of these products to insurers are not available, unpublished data from the Blue Cross of Washington and the Alaska AlternaPath project have been reported. Analyzing their 1994 to 1995 costs, project coordinators determined that 39 cents of each benefit dollar was spent on natural products [32]. In 1994, the program took in $170,000 and paid out $650,000 [33]. It is believed that some of this cost overrun was due to subscribers stocking up on nutritional supplements [33]. Public interest and willingness to pay out-of-pocket expense is evident in the 73% growth of pharmacy sales of natural remedies and supplements from 1991 to 1995. Prescription drug sales during this same period rose 31% [34].

A similar unanticipated cost overrun occurred when Blue Cross of Arizona was required by 1983 legislation to cover chiropractic care. The assumption behind this mandate was that the competition would decrease health care costs. However, the average chiropractic case cost was $576, 8% higher than surgeons' costs and 352% higher than the cost of general-practice doctors [33]. The cost-effectiveness of chiropractic services remains a contentious and uncertain issue [35].

Naturopathic care is covered by approximately 100 insurance companies in the United States; most of these companies are concentrated in Alaska, Connecticut, and Washington [36]. Acupuncture, massage therapy,

Table 38.1 Examples of Managed-Care Coverage of Complementary and Alternative Medicine Services and Practitioners

Blue Cross of Washington and Alaska	AlternaPath program employs naturopaths and other alternative practitioners
American Western Life Insurance	Wellness Plan recognizes alternative providers; maintains 24-hour holistic hotline (hotline reduced physician visits by 29%); offers 123-page pamphlet describing natural remedies for common ailments; membership open to anyone; cost: $10 enrollment plus $8 per month
Oxford Health Plans (Connecticut)	Added thousands of alternative practitioners to its physician provider list
Griffin Health Services Corp. (Connecticut)	Combines primary care, wellness center, alternative practitioners
American Medical Security	Markets alternative-oriented health plans nationally
Prudential Insurance Company of America	Covers acupuncture for chronic pain and other alternative services
Mutual of Omaha	Sends heart patients to lifestyle centers
Boston's Harvard Community Health Plan	Offers course in relaxation and coping skills
Kaiser Permanente Alternative Medicine Clinic	Covers acupressure, acupuncture, herbal medications, relaxation training–stress reduction, yoga, nutritional counseling

and other CAM services are covered by many insurers [37]. Coverage most likely applies if patients have a physician's prescription for a given therapy.

CAM THERAPIES

Alternative therapies may be categorized in a variety of ways. The seven categories enumerated here are based on those developed by the OAM [38]: (1) diet and nutrition; (2) mind-body techniques; (3) bioelectromagnetics; (4) alternative medical systems; (5) pharmacologic and biological treatments; (6) manual healing methods; and (7) herbal medicine. Currently popular therapies within each of these categories are discussed later. Most of these approaches are unproved methods promoted as alternatives to mainstream cancer treatment.

Diet and Nutrition

Typically, today's proponents of dietary cancer treatments extrapolate the idea that food or vitamins can cure cancer from mainstream knowledge about the protective effects of fruits, vegetables, fiber, and avoidance of excessive dietary fat in reducing cancer risk. Proponents of this belief make their claims in books with such titles as *The Food Pharmacy: Dramatic New Evidence That Food Is Your Best Medicine; Prescription for Nutritional Healing;* and *New Choices in Natural Healing.* After criticizing chemotherapy, radiotherapy, and surgery as "highly invasive [methods] . . . [that] may shorten the patient's life," the chapter on cancer in a popular tome, *Alternative Medicine,* recommends that therapy instead address the entire body and employ a "non-toxic approach . . . incorporating treatments that rely on biopharmaceutical, immune enhancement, metabolic, nutritional, and herbal, non-toxic methods" [39].

METABOLIC THERAPIES AND DETOXIFICATION

Metabolic therapies continue to draw patients from North America to the many clinics in Tijuana, Mexico. One of the best-known clinics is the Gerson Clinic, where treatment is based on the belief that toxic products of cancer cells accumulate in the liver, leading to liver failure and death. The Gerson treatment aims to counteract liver damage with a low-salt, high-potassium diet, coffee enemas, and a gallon of fruit and vegetable juice daily. The clinic's use of liquefied raw calf-liver injections was suspended in 1997 after the outbreak of sepsis in a number of patients [40].

Other Tijuana clinics provide their own versions of metabolic therapy, each applying an individualized dietary and detoxification regimen. Additional components of treatment are included according to practitioners' preferences. (A rare example of a US oncologist practicing alternative medicine is Dr. Nicholas Gonzalez, who offers a version of metabolic therapy in New York.)

Metabolic regimens are based on belief in the importance of detoxification, which is considered necessary for the body to heal itself. Practitioners view cancer and other illnesses as symptoms of the accumulation of toxins. Neither the toxins nor the benefit of eliminating them has been documented. This is a nonphysiologic

but venerable concept that originated in ancient Egyptian, Ayurvedic, and other early efforts to understand illness and death, both of which were believed to be caused by the putrefaction of food in the colon. Decay and purging were major themes in early cultures' therapeutic regimens.

Contemporary detoxification with high colonics involves infusion into the colon of 20 or more gallons of water containing herbs, coffee, enzymes, or other substances believed useful by the practitioner. High colonics remain a central component of current Ayurvedic medicine and other current practices. In some cities, high-colonic detoxification is available independently from colonic practitioners and in storefront walk-in colonic clinics as a means of maintaining health. It has no known benefits and has been associated with serious clinical problems [40–42].

MEGAVITAMIN AND ORTHOMOLECULAR THERAPY

The popular use of nutritional supplements as treatment contrasts ironically with alternative medicine's simultaneous emphasis on "natural" foods and therapies. Some patients and alternative practitioners believe that large dosages of vitamins—typically hundreds of pills a day—or intravenous infusions of high-dose vitamin C can cure disease.

In 1968, Nobel Laureate Linus Pauling coined the term *orthomolecular* to describe the treatment of disease with large quantities of nutrients. His claims that massive doses of vitamin C could cure cancer were disproved in three clinical trials, but megavitamin and orthomolecular therapy (the latter adds minerals and other nutrients) remain popular among cancer patients. Perhaps the simplicity of this approach and the fact that patients can prescribe and provide their own over-the-counter therapy contribute to its appeal. No evidence supports megavitamin or orthomolecular therapy as effective in treating any disorder.

Some patients with treatable cancers turn to megavitamin therapy rather than to mainstream care. During last year, a major US television news program aired a segment about one of its own producers, a young woman who had recently diagnosed early-stage breast cancer and opted for hundreds of vitamin-and-mineral pills daily instead of surgery. As is typical of many media efforts, no follow-up report announced her death, leaving the public with the impression that alternatives to mainstream care—in this case, megavitamin therapy—are viable options for cancer patients.

THE MACROBIOTIC DIET

Although a relatively recent creation, the macrobiotic diet is rooted in the ancient yin-yang principle of balance. Yin and yang, the concept of opposite forces on which traditional Chinese medicine is based, are believed to describe all components of life and the universe. In macrobiotics, this world view of balance is embodied in diet, including the selection, preparation, and consumption of foods.

The macrobiotic diet was developed in the 1930s by George Ohsawa, a Japanese philosopher who sought to integrate traditional Oriental medicine, Christian teachings, and aspects of Western medicine [33]. The macrobiotic diet is embedded in a philosophy of living and a fully formed, fanciful concept of human physiology and disease that holds, for example, that blood cells are produced not in the bone marrow but in the stomach, where they are birthed by a "mother red blood cell" [43]. Macrobiotic diagnostic techniques, including iridology and pulse diagnosis, are similarly misguided.

Nonetheless, the diet as currently constructed is similar to recent US Department of Agriculture dietary pyramid recommendations for healthful eating. The macrobiotic diet derives 50% to 60% of its calories from whole grains, 25% to 30% from vegetables, and the remainder from beans, seaweed, and soups. The diet avoids meat, certain vegetables, and processed foods and promotes soybean consumption. Soups made with miso, a product of the fermentation of soybeans, remain an important dietary component.

Genistein, a substance in soybeans, may contribute to Asian women's lower rates of breast and other cancers. Soy versus animal protein significantly decreases total cholesterol, low-density lipoproteins, and triglycerides. Dietary soy products may contribute to reduced incidence of breast cancer [44]. However, no evidence substantiates that the macrobiotic diet is beneficial for patients with diagnosed cancer. Moreover, versions of this diet are nutritionally deficient and can cause weight loss in cancer patients.

Mind-Body Techniques

The potential to use our minds to influence our health is an extremely appealing concept in the United States. It affirms the power of the individual, a belief intrinsic to US culture. Not surprisingly, then, mind-body medicine is extremely popular in the United States.

Some mind-body interventions have moved from the category of alternative, unconventional therapies into mainstream medicine. Good documentation exists, for example, for the effectiveness of meditation, biofeedback, and yoga in stress reduction and in the control of particular physiologic reactions [45, 46].

Some proponents argue that patients can use mental attributes and mind-body work to prevent or cure cancer. This belief is attractive because it ascribes to patients almost complete control over the course of their illness [47]. Although they may involve small numbers of patients or remain nonreplicated, widely publicized studies suggest that mental factors or prayer influence the course of cancer. An example is a 1989 *Lancet* article suggesting that women who had breast cancer and attended weekly support-group sessions had double the survival time of women who did not attend [48]. Prospective versions of this study have not replicated the 1989 results.

Bernie Siegel, MD, former surgical oncologist and author of *Love, Medicine, and Miracles* [49] and other bestsellers, is a popular proponent of the active link between mind and cancer. Siegel developed groups of "exceptional cancer patients" (E-CaP), based on his observation that attitude appeared to influence survival time. In these groups, patients are encouraged to maintain positive attitudes and to assume responsibility for their own health. They are asked to consider why they might "need" their cancer. The premise is that cancer results from unhealthy emotional patterns, correction of which can cure cancer or prolong remission .

A study coauthored by Siegel, however, found no difference in length of survival between E-CaP and non-E-CaP patients who had completed standard mainstream therapy for breast cancer [50]. Had these results been positive, the study no doubt would have received publicity similar to that afforded Siegel's best-selling books. Because the results did not confirm more than 12 years of public statements, the article received scant, if any, media attention and even failed to alter proponents' claims.

Attending to the psychological health of cancer patients is a fundamental component of good cancer care. Support groups, good doctor-patient relationships, and the emotional and instrumental help of family and friends are vital. However, the idea that patients can influence the course of their disease through mental or emotional work is not substantiated and can evoke feelings of guilt and inadequacy when disease continues to advance despite patients' best spiritual or mental efforts [47].

Bioelectromagnetics

Bioelectromagnetics is the study of interactions between living organisms and their electromagnetic fields. According to proponents, magnetic fields penetrate the body and heal damaged tissues, including cancers [39]. No peer-reviewed publications could be located to substantiate this claim or any clinical cancer-related claims regarding bioelectromagnetics.

In 1993, the NIH OAM funded a pilot study of electrochemical treatment, which was conducted by the department of radiation research preclinical laboratory at the City of Hope Medical Center in Los Angeles. Treating mouse and rat fibrosarcomas with direct current produced long-term tumor-free animal survival. Cell culture studies demonstrated that electrochemical treatment inhibited cell proliferation and DNA synthesis. This preliminary effort was based on a technique widely used in China today to treat cancer in humans. Further research is under way at the City of Hope Medical Center [51].

Decades ago, on the basis of a belief that a large magnet placed at the foot of a patient's bed would pull cancer out of the body, magnets were sold as cancer cures. Today, simple magnets are sold to reduce pain. They can be purchased as arm, leg, or body bands, shoe inserts, or entire mattresses. These commercial efforts stem from anecdotal reports plus data from recent preliminary investigations demonstrating magnet-induced pain relief for pain from polio [52] and for pain originating from localized musculoskeletal injuries [53].

Alternative Medical Systems

The category of alternative medical systems includes ancient systems of healing typically based on concepts of human physiology that differ from those accepted by modern Western science. Two of the most popular healing systems are traditional Chinese medicine and India's Ayurvedic medicine, popularized by best-selling author Deepak Chopra, MD [54].

The term *Ayurveda* comes from the Sanskrit words *ayur* (life) and *veda* (knowledge). Ayurveda's 5,000-year-old healing techniques are based on the classification of people into one of three predominant body types. For each body type, the system delineates specific remedies for disease and regimens to promote health. Ayurveda has a strong mind-body component that stresses the need to keep consciousness in balance. To accomplish that balance, it uses such techniques as yoga and meditation. Ayurveda also emphasizes regular detoxification and cleansing through all bodily orifices.

Ten Ayurveda clinics are said to exist in North America, including one hospital-based clinic that has served 25,000 patients since 1985 [38]. The new Chopra Center for Well-Being in La Jolla, CA, offers a luxury spa setting for Ayurvedic treatments. The number of cancer patients who seek care at Ayurvedic clinics and spas is not documented.

Traditional Chinese medicine explains the body in terms of its relationship to the environment and the cosmos. Concepts of human physiology and disease are interwoven with geographic features of ancient China and with the forces of nature. Chi, the life force said to run through all of nature, flows in the human body through vertical energy channels known as *meridians*. The 12 main meridians, corresponding to the 12 main rivers of ancient China, are believed to be dotted with acupoints. Each of the original 365 acupoints corresponds to a specific body organ or system, so needling or pressing the acupoint can redress the life-force imbalance that is causing the problem in that particular organ.

To determine the source of the blockage, a practitioner relies on pulse diagnosis, a technique applied by doctors of traditional Chinese medicine today as it was millennia ago. It involves concentration on several body pulses by a practitioner for approximately 45 minutes.

In addition to acupuncture and acupressure, basic therapeutic tools include *qi gong* and *tai chi* to strengthen and balance chi. Traditional Chinese medicine also includes a full herbal pharmacopoeia with remedies for most ailments, including cancer [55]. Chinese herbal teas and relaxation techniques are soothing and appealing to many cancer patients, who use them as complementary therapies. The potential anticancer benefits of Chinese green tea and other herbal remedies are under investigation [56–58].

Pharmacologic and Biological Treatments

Alternative pharmacologic and biological treatments remain highly controversial. Probably the best-known and most popular pharmacologic therapy today is antineoplastons, developed by Stanislaw Burzynski, MD, and available in his clinic in Houston, TX [59]. Laboratory analysis conducted by a respected scientist concluded that antineoplastons did not normalize tumor cells [60]. However, preliminary clinical data encouraged a limited clinical trial for pediatric patients with brain tumors, but a joint research effort by the CCAM and the National Cancer Institute (NCI) failed to accrue patients.

Further research at the Burzynski Institute was permitted under an Investigational New Drug application, but preliminary data recently were criticized as uninterpretable, and the therapy was characterized as useless and toxic by respected mainstream scientists [61]. Burzynski and his patients continue the antineoplaston therapy and speak out in favor of its efficacy, disclaiming the critiques.

For the public, the effectiveness of this treatment remains unclear. Although the therapy is unproved and outside the realm of mainstream medicine, numerous patients report anecdotal success. Moreover, researchers at the NCI and elsewhere continue to investigate phenylacetate, a metabolite of the amino acid phenylalanine, which constitutes 80% of antineoplaston AS2–1. Recent results of a study conducted at the Memorial Sloan-Kettering Cancer Center indicate, "The safety profile and efficacy of phenylacetate make it an attractive agent for the treatment of pancreatic cancer" [62], and a Japanese investigation of three patients with advanced cancer concluded that "antineoplaston A10 and AS2–1 may be contributing to the rapid antitumor response" [63].

Immunoaugmentive therapy (IAT) was developed by the late Lawrence Burton, PhD, and is offered in his clinic in the Bahamas. Injected IAT is said to balance four protein components in the blood and to strengthen affected patients' immune system. According to proponent literature, Burton claimed that IAT was particularly effective in treating mesothelioma [64]. Documentation of IAT's efficacy remains anecdotal. The clinic has continued to operate since Burton's death, but its popularity seems to have waned [65].

Interest in shark cartilage as a cancer therapy was activated by a 1992 book by I. William Lane, PhD, *Sharks Don't Get Cancer,* and by a television special that displayed apparent remissions in patients treated with shark cartilage in Cuba. The televised outcome was disputed strongly by oncologists in the United States. Advocates base their therapy on its putative antiangiogenic properties [66], but the shark cartilage protein molecules are too large to be absorbed by the gastrointestinal tract and would be destroyed if absorbed. Actually, shark cartilage decomposes into inert ingredients and is excreted. A recent phase I–II trial of shark cartilage found no clinical benefit [67]. The dwindling commercial success of shark cartilage as a treatment for cancer

has led to its promotion for a different set of problems. Full-page color advertisements in alternative medicine journals read, "The most important joint decision you'll ever make. Your patients can now fight aging bone conditions. The secret is shark cartilage." Because the advertisements avoid specific indication that the therapy can cure an ailment, they fall within the guidelines of the 1994 Food Supplement Act. Thus, they are permitted even though no data address safety or efficacy for this product as a treatment for any condition.

Another well-known biological remedy, Cancell, appears to be especially popular in Florida and midwestern United States. Proponents claim that it returns cancer cells to a "primitive state" from which they can be digested and rendered inert. FDA laboratory studies that showed Cancell to be composed of common chemicals, including nitric acid, sodium sulfite, potassium hydroxide, sulfuric acid, and catechol, found no basis for proponents' claims of Cancell's effectiveness against cancer [68].

Manual Healing Methods

Manual healing includes a variety of touch and manipulation techniques. Osteopathic and chiropractic doctors were among the earliest groups to use manual methods. For its stress-reducing benefits, hands-on massage is a useful adjunctive technique for cancer patients and others. The value of chiropractic treatment of low back pain was supported by an NIH consensus conference [69], but its value is disputed widely by mainstream physicians [35].

One of the most popular manual healing methods is therapeutic touch (TT). Despite its name, it involves no direct contact. In TT, healers move their hands a few inches above a patient's body and sweep away "blockages" to the patient's energy field, although a study in the *Journal of the American Medical Association* showed that experienced TT practitioners were unable to detect the investigator's "energy field" [70]. Despite mainstream scientists' unwillingness to accept its fundamental premises, TT is taught in North American nursing schools and is practiced widely by nurses in the United States and other countries [71].

Skeptics' groups have offered $1 million, a sum that, with interest, now has grown to $1,100,000, to any TT practitioner able to demonstrate scientifically the existence of the human energy field. No one has applied. Debates between skeptics and TT believers enliven numerous Web sites [72].

Herbal Remedies for Cancer

Typically, herbal remedies are part of traditional and folk healing methods with long histories of use. Throughout history, some form of herbal medicine has been found is most areas of the world and across all cultures. Although many herbal remedies are claimed to have anticancer effects, only a few have gained substantial popularity as alternative cancer therapies.

Essiac is one of the most popular herbal cancer alternatives in North America. It was popularized by a Canadian nurse, Rene Caisse (*Essiac* is *Caisse* spelled backward) but was developed initially by a native Canadian healer. Essiac is composed of four herbs: burdock, Turkey rhubarb, sorrel, and slippery elm. Researchers at the NCI and elsewhere found that it has no anticancer effect. The sale of Essiac is illegal in Canada [38], but the product is widely available in US pharmacies and health food stores.

Iscador, a derivative of mistletoe, is a popular cancer remedy in Europe, where it is said to have been in continuous use as folk treatment since the time of the Druids. Iscador is available in many mainstream European cancer clinics. Although European governments have funded studies of iscador's effectiveness against cancer [38], definitive data have not emerged.

Pau d'arco tea is said to be an old Inca Indian remedy for many illnesses, including cancer. Made from the bark of an indigenous South American evergreen tree, its active ingredient, lapachol, has been isolated. Although lapachol showed antitumor activity in animal studies conducted in the 1970s, it does not appear to affect human malignancies. The tea does induce nausea and vomiting. Despite the absence of efficacy, *pau d'arco* tea is sold as a cancer remedy in health food stores, by mail, and on the Internet.

Other Herbal Medicines

Cancer patients use over-the-counter herbal products in addition to or instead of those promoted specifically as cancer treatments. An important precaution is to differentiate between herbal remedies that may help cancer patients and those that are toxic or that interact with other medications (Table 38.2). Because the FDA does not examine herbal remedies for safety and effectiveness, few products have been tested formally for side effects or quality control. However, information is beginning to emerge on the basis of public experience with over-the-counter supplements.

Recent reports in the literature describe severe liver

Table 38.2 Herbal Products with Serious Toxic Effects

Chaparral tea: promoted as an antioxidant, pain reliever, etc.; has caused liver failure requiring liver transplantation

Chaste tree berry: used for premenstrual syndrome; can interfere with dopamine-receptor antagonists

Chomper: "herbal laxative" and "cleansing" agent to be used as part of a diet regimen; contaminated with digitalis

Comfrey: ingested or used on bruises; can obstruct blood flow to the liver and possibly lead to death

Feverfew: used for migraines, premenstrual syndrome; can interact with anticoagulants and increase bleeding

Garlic: numerous preventive and therapeutic uses; can interact with anticoagulants and increase bleeding

Ginger: for nausea; can interact with anticoagulants and increase bleeding

Gingko: dilates arteries; can interact with anticoagulants and increase bleeding

Jin Bu Huan: sedative and analgesic containing morphinelike substances; can cause hepatitis

Laxatives: senna, cascara, aloe, and the like; can cause potassium loss when used over time; particularly dangerous when used with digitalis or prescription diuretics

Licorice: used to treat peptic ulcers and as expectorant; contraindicated with cardiac glycosides

Lobella: an emetic; may cause coma and death at high doses; such lesser effects as rapid heartbeat and breathing problems

Ma huang (ephedra): herbal form of the central nervous system stimulant commonly known as *speed;* sold with such names as *Herbal Ecstasy, Cloud 9,* and *Ultimate XPhoria*

Plantain leaves: cut or powdered; found in plantain extract, Nature Cleanse Tablets, BotaniCleanse brands, Blessed Herbs, and the like; contaminated with digitalis glycosides

"Siberian ginseng" capsules: may contain instead a weed composed of male hormonelike chemicals

Yohimbe: body builder; "enhances male performance;" has caused seizures, kidney failure, and death

and kidney damage from some herbal remedies (see Table 38.2). These reports underscore the fact that contrary to apparent consumer belief, "natural" products are not necessarily safe or harmless [57, 73–75]. Indeed, herbs are dilute natural drugs. They may contain hundreds of different chemicals, most of which have not been documented. Effects are not always predictable.

Regulatory and Safety Issues: Herbal Remedies and Other Food Supplements

Botanical remedies are sold in many forms, including capsules, liquids, and tea leaves. They may contain one or a collection of herbs and other ingredients, which typically are not described and often are unknown. No

COMPLEMENTARY AND ALTERNATIVE THERAPIES

legal standards govern the processing or packaging of herbs. According to research conducted by *Consumer Reports,* the content of herbal remedies often differs widely from one bottle to the next—even within the same brand—and from claims made on their labels.

St. John's Wort, a popular over-the-counter antidepressant, was analyzed by an independent laboratory in a recent study commissioned by the *Los Angeles Times.* This analysis revealed that 3 of 10 brands tested contained less than one-half the potency listed on the label [76]. The California Department of Health conducted an investigation of the ingredients in Asian patent medicines. Unsafe levels both of mercury and other toxic metals and of prescription drug compounds were discovered in more than one-third of products tested. The American Botanical Council found that some ginseng products contain no ginseng. A recent journal article reported heart problems resulting from digitalis-contaminated supplements [77].

Quality-control standards and reviews of such products are needed. Because they are not mandatory, however, few food supplement companies voluntarily self-impose quality evaluation and control. Consumer protection and enforcement agencies cannot provide protection against contaminated or falsely advertised products. Current federal regulations do not permit such oversight, and regulatory capability would prohibit full analysis and ongoing oversight of the estimated 20,000 food supplement items now sold over the counter.

Although store shelves contain harmful and worthless products, they also offer a wide range of genuinely useful remedies that can provide safe relief from a variety of ailments. The challenge is to avoid contaminated products and those that may interact with prescription pharmaceuticals. Dietitians and pharmacists and reputable books and Web sites (Table 38.3) can offer the necessary guidance.

Table 38.3 Reputable Sources of Complementary and Alternative Medicine Information

---

Cancer-specific sites
American Association for Cancer Research: http://www.aacr.org
American Cancer Society: www.cancer.org
Association of Community Cancer Centers: http://www.assoc-cancer-ctrs.org
CancerGuide by Steve Dunn: http://cancerguide.org
National Cancer Institute: www.cancernet.nci.nih.gov/
Office of Alternative Medicine: www.altmed.od.nih.gov
Oncolink (University of PA Cancer Center): http://www.oncolink.org
St. Jude Children's Research Hospital: http://www.stjude.org
Tufts University: http//www.altmedicine.com/
University of Texas Center for Alternative Medicine Research in Cancer: http://chprd.sph.uth.tmc.edu/utcam/

Herb and other food supplement sites
American Botanical Council: www.herbalgram.org
Medical Herbalism: A Journal for the Clinical Practitioner: www.medherb.com
Pharmaceutical Information Network: http://pharminfo.com
US Pharmacopoeia Consumer Information (Botanicals): http://www.usp.org/infofor/patient1htm

Regulatory and government agency sites
National Institutes of Health: www.nih.gov
NIH Medline Search: http://www.medscape.com
US Food and Drug Administration: www.fda.gov

Information about alternative and unproved methods
National Council Against Health Fraud: www.ncahf.org
Quackwatch: www.quackwatch.com

General complementary and alternative medicine information
Bibliographic summary of international complementary and alternative medicine information: http://cpmcnet.columbia.edu/dept/rosenthal/databases/AM_databases.html
HealthAtoZ: http://www.healthatoz.com
HealthTel Corp Links: www.medmatrix.org/index.asp
Natural Health Village: www.netvillage.com/
NIH Office of Alternative Medicine Citation Index: http://altmed.od.nih.gov/oam/resources/cam-ci/

CAM PRACTITIONERS AND PRACTICES

Major categories of CAM practitioners outside of mainstream medicine include chiropractors, naturopaths, and acupuncturists; the latter often practice a broader range of traditional Chinese medicine involving herbal therapeutics [78]. Chiropractic requires 4 years of training and prepares students to provide primary clinical services, including wellness maintenance, diagnosis of illness, and primary care in addition to musculoskeletal care. Fifteen percent of clinical training is devoted to organ systems other than the musculoskeletal system.

All 50 states plus the District of Columbia have licensure programs for chiropractors. The accrediting agency for chiropractic medicine was established in 1971, and a standardized national examination was created in 1982 [78, 79].

Naturopathic doctoral degrees are awarded after 4 years of postbaccalaureate training. Naturopathic education is designed to prepare primary-care providers. Training emphasizes health promotion, disease prevention, and the use of such natural remedies as botanicals. All 11 states that license naturopaths permit the designation of *N.D.* (doctor of naturopathic medicine) [80].

The accrediting agency for naturopathy was established in 1978, and standardized tests were first offered in 1986.

Practitioners of acupuncture and herbal medicine in the United States are trained for 3 years. They learn to diagnosis disease using pulse diagnosis and other traditional Chinese medicine techniques and to treat common problems with acupuncture and herbal remedies. Acupuncturists are recognized and licensed in 34 states, and three additional jurisdictions permit practice under M.D. supervision [81]. In 1982, acupuncturists were accredited, and their standardized national test was created.

CAM RESEARCH ISSUES

Numerous CAM journals have been established in the last 3 or 4 years. Most represent a second tier of publication, in which peer review often means evaluation by CAM proponents who have little training or experience in research. The validity and reliability of articles in these publications do not meet standards of mainstream peer-reviewed journals, and they should be read with caution and attention to methodology and the reliability of conclusions. Few articles in these journals stand the test of scientific scrutiny.

Very recently, three new journals that present scientific evaluations of CAM have appeared: *The Scientific Review of Alternative Medicine* (www.hutch.demon.co.uk/altmed/index.htm); *FACT* (*Focus on Alternative and Complementary Therapies*; www.fact@exeter.ac.com); and *Integrative Medicine*.

Identifying reliable journals and articles is particularly important with regard to CAM. Some CAM proponents have argued that research is not necessary to determine the effectiveness of alternative therapies for cancer; others claim that evaluating CAM is not possible because the therapies are too subtle or are too individualized to study with usual scientific methods [82]. Some say that clinical trials are unethical; others claim that alternative methodologies are required for alternative therapies.

In fact, *any* therapy can be evaluated properly [82–86]. Several CAM-interested scientists, including the current director of the OAM, mandate the importance of rigorous, scientific CAM evaluation and outline guidelines for its implementation [84–88]. The notion that proper evaluation is unnecessary or impossible for CAM is held by a minority of CAM proponents. The widely accepted view—articulated in the work of the Cochrane Collaboration on CAM and in such publications as those previously cited—is that CAM therapies require and warrant standard, scientifically accepted research methodologies.

REFERENCES

1. Ernst E, Resch KL, Mills S, et al. Complementary medicine—a definition. *Br J Gen Pract* 45:506, 1995.
2. Cassileth BR. This study "medicalizes" self-help activities by labeling them unconventional. *Advances* 9:12–13, 1993. (Invited comment on Eisenberg DM, Kessler RC, Foster C, et al. Unconventional medicine in the United States. *N Engl J Med* 328:246–252, 1993.)
3. Cassileth BR, Lusk EJ, Strouse TB, Bodenheimer BJ. Contemporary unorthodox treatments in cancer medicine: a study of patients, treatments and practitioners. *Ann Intern Med* 101:105–112, 1984.
4. Ernst E, Cassileth BR. The prevalence of complementary/alternative medicine in cancer: a systematic review. *Cancer* 83:777–782, 1998.
5. Miller M, Boyer MJ, Butow PN, et al. The use of unproven methods of treatment by cancer patients. Frequency, expectations and cost. *Support Care Cancer* 6:337–347, 1998.
6. Crocetti E, Crotti N, Feltrin A, et al. The use of complementary therapies by breast cancer patients attending conventional treatment. *Eur J Cancer* 34:324–328, 1998.
7. Fernandez CV, Stutzer CA, MacWilliam L, Fryer C. Alternative and complementary therapy use in pediatric oncology patients in British Columbia: prevalence and reasons for use and nonuse. *J Clin Oncol* 16:1279–1286, 1998.
8. Elder NC, Gillcrist A, Minz R. Use of alternative health care by family practice patients. *Arch Fam Med* 6:181–184, 1997.
9. The Landmark Report. November, 1997. <*http://www.landmarkhealthcare.com*>
10. Eisenberg DM, Kessler RC, Foster C, et al. Unconventional medicine in the United States. *N Engl J Med* 328:246–252, 1993.
11. Abu-Realh MH, Magwood G, Narayan MC, et al. The use of complementary therapies by cancer patients. *Nurs Connect* 9:3–12 1996.
12. Grootenhuis MA, Last BF, de Graff-Nijkerk JH, van der Wel M. Use of alternative treatment in pediatric oncology. *Cancer Nurs* 21:282–288, 1998.
13. Friedman T, Slayton WB, Allen LS, et al. Use of alternative therapies in children with cancer (electronic article). *Pediatrics* 100:1–6, 1998.
14. Whitaker Wellness Institute. *M.D.'s Journal.* Summer 1998.
15. Unconventional Medical Practices. Senate Appropriations Committee Report, 1992:141.
16. Center for Alternative Medicine Research in Cancer, Houston, TX. <http://www.sph.uth.tmc.edu/utcam/>
17. Wetzel MS, Eisenberg DM, Kaptchuk TJ. Courses involving complementary and alternative medicine at US medical schools. *JAMA* 280:784–778, 1998.
18. Berman BM, Singh BK, Lao L, et al. Physicians' attitudes toward complementary or alternative medicine: a regional survey. *J Am Board Fam Pract* 8:361–366, 1995.
19. Verhoef MJ, Sutherland LR. General practitioners' assess-

ment of and interest in alternative medicine in Canada. *Soc Sci Med* 41:511–515, 1995.

20. Ernst E, Resch K-L, White AR. Complementary medicine: what physicians think of it: a meta-analysis. *Arch Intern Med* 155:2405–2408, 1995.

21. Borkan J, Neher JO, Anson O, Smoker B. Referrals for alternative medicine. *J Fam Pract* 39:545–550, 1994.

22. Soffer A. Chihuahuas and laetrile, chelation therapy, and honey from Boulder, Colo. *Arch Intern Med* 136:865–866, 1976.

23. Jukes TH. Laetrile for cancer. *JAMA* 236:1284–1286, 1976.

24. Ingelfinger FJ. Quenchless quest for questionable cure. *N Engl J Med* 295:838–839, 1976.

25. Pendergrass TW, Davis S. Knowledge and use of "alternative" cancer therapies in children. *Am J Pediatr Hematol Oncol* 3:339–345, 1981.

26. Eidinger RN, Schapira DV. Cancer patients' insight into their treatment, prognosis, and unconventional therapies. *Cancer* 53:2736–2740, 1984.

27. Fulder SJ, Munro RE. Complementary medicine in the United Kingdom: patients, practitioners, and consultations. *Lancet* 2:542–545, 1985.

28. Park RL, Goodenough U. Buying snake oil with tax dollars. *New York Times,* January 3, 1996:A11.

29. Barrett S. Quackwatch: Your Guide to Health Fraud, Quackery, and Intelligent Decisions. <http://www.quackwatch.com>

30. Angell M, Kassirer JP. Alternative medicine—the risks of untested and unregulated remedies. *N Engl J Med* 339(12):839–841, 1998.

31. Kilgore C. Expanding coverage signals growing demand, acceptance for alternative care. *Med Health* 52(suppl)1–4, 1998.

32. Weeks J. The emerging role of alternative medicine in managed care. *Drug Benefit Trends* 9(4):14–16, 25–28, 1997.

33. Jarvis W. The idea vs the reality of "alternative" medicine. *NCAHF Newsletter* 20:1–3, 1997.

34. Finding a prescription for economic pain: pharmacies devote more space to alternative remedies. *Washington Post* January 16, 1997:E1, E4.

35. Shekelle PG. What role for chiropractic in health care? *N Engl J Med* 339:1074–1075, 1998.

36. Naturopathy—Health Insurance for N.D. Care. <http://homearts.com/hl/articles/68natu91.htm>

37. Moore NG. A review of reimbursement policies for alternative and complementary therapies. *Altern Ther Health Med* 3:26–29, 91–92, 1997.

38. Workshop on Alternative Medicine. Alternative medicine: expanding medical horizons. A report to the National Institutes of Health on alternative medical systems and practices in the United States. Washington, DC: US Government Printing Office, 1992.

39. Burton Goldberg Group. *Alternative Medicine: The Definitive Guide.* Puyallup, WA: Future Publishing, 1993:571.

40. Gerson Method. <www.quackwatch.com>

41. Eisele JW, Reay DT. Deaths related to coffee enemas. *JAMA* 244:1608–1609, 1980.

42. Istre GR, Kreiss K, Hopkins RS, et al. An outbreak of amebiasis spread by colonic irrigation at a chiropractic clinic. *N Engl J Med* 307:339–342, 1982.

43. Kushi M. *The Macrobiotic Approach to Cancer.* Wayne, NJ: Avery Publishing, 1982.

44. Anderson JW, Johnstone BM, Cook-Newell ME. Meta-analysis of the effects of soy protein intake on serum lipids. *N Engl J Med* 333:276–282, 1995.

45. NIH Technology Assessment Panel on Integration of Behavioral and Relaxation Approaches into the Treatment of Chronic Pain and Insomnia. Integration of behavioral and relaxation approaches into the treatment of chronic pain and insomnia. *JAMA* 276:313–318, 1996.

46. Sundar S, Agrawal SK, Singh VP, et al. Role of yoga in management of essential hypertension. *Acta Cardiol* 39:203–208, 1984.

47. Cassileth BR. The social implications of mind-body cancer research. *Cancer Invest* 7:361–3644, 1989.

48. Spiegel D, Bloom JR, Kraemer H, Gottheil E. Effect of psychosocial treatment on survival of patients with metastatic breast cancer. *Lancet* 2(8668):888–891, 1989.

49. Siegel BS. *Love, Medicine, and Miracles: Lessons Learned About Self-Healing from a Surgeon's Experience.* New York: Harper & Row, 1986.

50. Gellert GA, Maxwell RM, Siegel BS. Survival of breast cancer patients receiving adjunctive psychosocial support therapy: a 10-year follow-up study. *J Clin Oncol* 11:66–69, 1993.

51. <http://altmed.od.nih.gov/oam/resources/cam-ci/>

52. Vallbona C, Hazlewood CF, Jurida G. Response of pain to static magnetic fields in postpolio patients: a double-blind pilot study. *Arch Phys Med Rehabil* 78:1200–1203, 1997.

53. Pujol J, Pascual-Leone A, Dolz C, et al. The effect of repetitive magnetic stimulation on localized musculoskeletal pain. *Neuroreport* 9:1745–1748, 1998.

54. Chopra D. *Ageless Body, Timeless Mind.* New York: Harmony Books, 1993.

55. Hsu HY. *Treating Cancer with Chinese Herbs.* Los Angeles: Oriental Healing Arts Institute, 1982.

56. Bushman JL. Green tea and cancer in humans: a review of the literature. *Nutr Cancer* 31:151–159, 1998.

57. DiPaola RS, Zhang H, Lambert GH, et al. Clinical and biologic activity of an estrogenic herbal combination (PC-SPES) in prostate cancer. *N Engl J Med* 339:785–791, 1998.

58. Kurashige S, Jin R, Akuzawa Y, Endo F. Anticarcinogenic effects of shikaron, a preparation of eight Chinese herbs in mice treated with a carcinogen, *N*-butyl-*N*′-butanolnitrosoamine. *Cancer Invest* 16:166–169, 1998.

59. Burzynski S, Kubove E. Initial clinical study with antineoplaston A2 injections in cancer patients with five years' follow-up. *Drugs Exp Clin Res* 13S:1–11, 1987.

60. Green S. Antineoplastons: an unproved cancer therapy. *JAMA* 267:2924–2928, 1992.

61. Experts say interpretable results unlikely in Burzynski's antineoplastons studies. *Cancer Lett* 24:1–16, 1998.

62. Harrison LE, Wojciechowicz DC, Brennan MF, Paty PB. Phenylacetate inhibits isoprenoid biosynthesis and suppresses growth of human pancreatic carcinoma. *Surgery* 124:541–550, 1998.

63. Tsuda H, Sata M, Kumabe T, et al. Quick response of advanced cancer to chemoradiation therapy with antineoplastons. *Oncol Rep* 5:597–600, 1998.

64. Moss RW. *Cancer Therapy: The Independent Consumer's Guide.* New York: Equinox Press, 1992.

65. American Cancer Society. Immuno-augmentative therapy (IAT). *CA Cancer J Clin* 41:357–364, 1991.

66. American Cancer Society. *Shark Cartilage/Angiogenesis.* [Rep. no. 8100.] Atlanta: American Cancer Society, 1992.

67. Miller DR, Anderson GT, Stark JJ, et al. Phase I/II Trial of the safety and efficacy of shark cartilage in the treatment of advanced cancer. *J Clin Oncol* 16:3649–3655, 1998.

68. Butler K. *A Consumer's Guide to Alternative Medicine.* Buffalo, NY: Prometheus Books, 1992.

69. Lawrence DJ. Report from the Consensus Conference on the Validation of Chiropractic Methods. *J Manipulative Physiol Ther* 13:295–296, 1990.

70. Rosa L, Rosa E, Sarner L, et al. A close look at therapeutic touch. *JAMA* 279:1005–1010, 1998.

71. Jaroff L. A no-touch therapy. *Time,* November 21, 1994: 88–89.

72. Therapeutic Touch. <www.voicenet.com/~eric/tt/>

73. Drew AK, Myers SP. Safety issues in herbal medicine: implications for the health professions. *Med J Aust* 166:538–541 1997.

74. Vanherweghem JL, Depierreux M, Tielemans C, et al. Rapidly progressing interstitial renal fibrosis in young women: association with slimming regimen including Chinese herbs. *Lancet* 341:387–391, 1993.

75. Gordon DW, Rosenthal G, Hart J, et al. Chaparral ingestion: the broadening spectrum of liver injury caused by herbal medications. *JAMA* 273:489–490, 1995.

76. Monmaney T. Remedy's sales zoom, but quality control lags; St. John's Wort: regulatory vacuum leaves doubt about potency, effects of herb used for depression. *Los Angeles Times,* August 31, 1998:A-1.

77. Slifman NR, Obermeyer WR, Aloi BK, et al. Contamination of botanical dietary supplements by *Digitalis lanata. N Engl J Med* 339:806–811, 1998.

78. Cooper RA, Henderson T, Dietrich CL. Roles of nonphysician clinicians as autonomous providers of patient care. *JAMA* 280:795–802, 1998.

79. American Chiropractic Association. *Chiropractic: State of the Art.* Arlington, VA: American Chiropractic Association, 1994.

80. Council on Naturopathic Registration and Accreditation, Inc. <www.cnra.org>

81. Ergil KV. Acupuncture licensure, training and certification in the United States. In *NIH Consensus Development Conference on Acupuncture.* Bethesda, MD: National Institutes of Health, 1997:31–38.

82. Ernst E. Complementary medicine: common misperceptions. *J R Soc Med* 88:244–247, 1995.

83. Cassileth BR, Lusk EJ, Guerry D, et al. Survival and quality of life among patients on unproven versus conventional cancer therapy. *N Engl J Med* 324:1180–1185, 1991.

84. Vickers A. A proposal for teaching critical thinking to students and practitioners of complementary medicine. *Altern Ther Health Med* 3:57–62, 1997.

85. Vickers A, Cassileth BR, Ernst E, et al. How should we research unconventional therapies? *Int J Technol Assess* 13:111–121, 1997.

86. Cassidy C, Cassileth BR, Jonas W, et al. A guide for the alternative researcher [Appendix F]. In *Workshop on Alternative Medicine. Alternative Medicine: Expanding Medical Horizons. A Report to the National Institutes of Health on Alternative Medical Systems and Practices in the United States.* Washington, DC: US Government Printing Office, 1992.

87. Jonas W. Researching alternative medicine. *Nature Med* 3:824–827, 1997.

88. Cassileth BR. *The Alternative Medicine Handbook: The Complete Reference Guide to Alternative and Complementary Therapies.* New York: Norton, 1998.

SELECTED READINGS

Duke, James A. *The Green Pharmacy.* New York: Rodale Press, 1997.

Robbers JE, Tyler VE. *Tyler's Herbs of Choice: The Therapeutic Use of Phytomedicinals.* Binghamton, NY: Howarth Press, 1994.

Tyler VE. *The Honest Herbal: A Sensible Guide to the Use of Herbs and Related Remedies.* London: Pharmaceutical Press, 1993.

39

Clinical Trials

■ ■ ■

Leslie G. Ford
Rose Mary Padberg

ADVANCES IN CLINICAL CANCER RESEARCH have been made through the meticulous design and implementation of clinical trials. One example of this progress is that today newly diagnosed childhood cancers often are treated effectively and are cured. This improvement in response rate is due to the use of effective treatments that have been identified through the enrollment of numerous children in cancer clinical trials [1]. The findings of clinical trials can assure oncology professionals and their patients that the interventions identified for cancer prevention, early detection, and treatment are the best that science can offer.

Identifying successful treatment interventions is not accomplished easily, inexpensively, or quickly. Years of development, implementation, and monitoring of such interventions in specific groups of patients are required to prove that the intervention can be generalized to similar patients.

Multiple challenges are presented to the completion of a clinical trial. Frequently, investigators mention that the primary barrier is the time commitment required to recruit and retain patients in a clinical trial. This situation is especially true in the changing health care environment wherein professional staff members spend markedly less time with patients per visit than was true in the past.

Another barrier mentioned by investigators is the use of placebo-controlled studies. Though these studies offer scientific credibility, engaging interest in them by patients and physicians is difficult because of the preference for the "active agent." Often, patients misunderstand the concept of randomization and blinding, and they confer untested "benefit" to the active agent.

Slow accrual is a continual concern of study investigators. A scientific idea that is translated into a funded clinical trial can wait years for approval. Any innovative idea has a window of opportunity to be tested before other competing ideas are tested. Investigators must work diligently to develop a dedicated, educated staff that is able to recruit and retain study subjects through to completion. Obviously, study accrual is assisted by the involvement of multiple collaborating sites. However, this advantage is tempered with the requirement for additional funding for training and monitoring of the study staff to assure compliance to study guidelines.

DEFINITION OF CANCER CLINICAL TRIALS

Clinical trials comprise research that is designed and evaluated carefully so as to provide reliable information about interventions for preventing, detecting, or treating cancer or for improving quality of life for patients who have the disease. Studies should be conducted in a manner that will allow for generalization to populations of cancer patients who are being studied and will lead to a logical next step in a series of studies. Such studies are conducted in clinical settings (i.e., hospitals, medical centers, clinics, etc.), and they involve human subjects. Depending on their purpose, trials may recruit participants who have cancer or, in the case of prevention trials, who demonstrate a defined risk of developing the disease.

The various types of clinical trials differ with respect to their stated goals. These different types [2] of trials include the following:

1. Prevention trials designed to identify interventions that can prevent cancer
2. Prevention trials designed to retard the development of a second cancer in people who have had cancer
3. Early detection trials to identify methods to detect cancer early in its development
4. Treatment trials to identify interventions that are effective in reversing, stopping, or slowing the growth of cancer
5. Quality-of-life trials to identify strategies to improve the quality of patients' lives during and after treatment of cancer
6. Symptom management trials to identify interventions that alleviate the symptoms of both cancer and its treatment

The objective of a clinical trial is to determine the effectiveness of a proposed intervention in achieving its stated goal. People participating in clinical trials may benefit personally; however, they have no guarantee of direct therapeutic benefit. Furthermore, negative effects may be experienced. If the benefit of the intervention were assured, the study would not have to be conducted. In fact, the balance between the desirable effects and the negative effects actually determines whether an intervention tested in a clinical trial will be useful in preventing or treating cancer. This information about prevention and treatment ultimately benefits the public's health.

IMPORTANCE OF CLINICAL TRIALS

Seeking advances in medical knowledge through clinical trials is important in the study of any disease. This is especially true for cancer, for which both the morbidity and mortality are high. Nationally sponsored clinical cancer trials provide a valid scientific method of combining the data from multiple participating centers to identify promising interventions more quickly. Results of these studies are shared through scientific journals and presentations. Physicians draw on such published information to offer to their patients state-of-the-art therapies that they hope can replicate the successful outcomes achieved in the original studies [3].

METHODS OF CONDUCTING CLINICAL TRIALS

To protect clinical trials participants and to be more certain of the results, clinical trials follow rigorous scientific and ethical principles. Careful planning of a study is performed by physicians, statisticians, and other researchers to ensure that the methods used for conducting the study address the research questions in a manner that is both valid and reliable and that the study will provide sufficient data for appropriate statistical analysis. The research procedures also must ensure that standards for informed consent, confidentiality, and other ethical issues are addressed.

Around the world, clinical cancer trials are conducted by investigators in university hospitals, cancer centers, clinics, and doctor's offices. In the not-so-distant past, cancer patients had to travel to specialized research centers to participate in a clinical trial. Now, through national and international networks of cooperative groups, many of the studies can be found in the offices of community-based physicians active in clinical trial research. This availability is a great convenience for the patients and their families, who do not need to travel away from the comfort of home to obtain cancer therapy as part of a clinical trial.

CLINICAL TRIAL DESIGN
Protocol

Clinical trials are conducted according to (1) a set of standardized criteria for eligibility in the study, (2) a standardized diagnostic or therapeutic intervention, (3) standardized tests and measurements performed at specific intervals, and (4) statistical analysis. The protocol is the written, mutually accepted document followed by all investigators to ensure comparability of results. It is the investigators' guide to scientific rationale and background, to the specific intervention to be studied, and to the collection of data needed for statistical analysis. Every clinical investigator involved in the study follows the same protocol to ensure that patients receive identical interventions and that study results can be combined and compared.

Eligibility

A clinical trial participant needs to have specific attributes that are shared with other trial participants so that their information can be combined. Some of the elements that determine eligibility are age, gender, disease stage, laboratory test results, cancer risk status, and the like. Eligibility criteria identify specific personal characteristics that a potential participant must possess to qualify for participation.

Phases of Clinical Trials

Clinical trials embody three levels or phases; each phase represents a distinct level of knowledge about the potential value of an intervention. In phase I, an intervention is tested in people for the first time. These small studies seek to find and to document the optimum dose, its side effects, and most effective method of administration. Phase II seeks to determine whether the intervention is effective against a specific type of cancer or precancerous condition. Phase III studies are conducted with larger numbers of participants. They test a new research therapy against the standard treatment or prevention approach for a specific cancer. The goal of phase III studies is to determine whether the novel, experimental therapy is as good as or better than the standard therapy.

Randomization

Randomization is a scientific method that distributes clinical trial participants equally into intervention and control groups. Participants have a random chance of being placed in either group. Randomization uses computers algorithms to determine the group to which a prospective trial participant will be assigned. The purpose of this procedure is to reduce the potential bias due to preferential selection of a given participant for one or the other group.

If randomly assigned participants decide to leave the active study, they are urged strongly to allow the investigators to continue collecting follow-up data. This step ensures that their data are analyzed according to the group to which they were randomly assigned. This follow-up is called *intent-to-treat analysis* and it is used to reduce bias.

Blinding

Blinding occurs when two or more treatments are to be compared in a prospective study. To avoid bias in the evaluation of treatments, the pharmacy provides drugs in a packaging and formulation that do not allow either investigators or patients to recognize the treatment being given.

Informed Consent

The process of informed consent is the cornerstone of human clinical trials and is relatively new. The first efforts to protect human subjects in medical research were an outcome of the 1946 trial of 23 Nazi (German) doctors in Nuremberg. This trial resulted in the development of the Nuremberg Code, the first principle of which stresses the importance of obtaining informed consent from research subjects [4]. Today, three basic protections in place in federal regulation and policy protect human subjects participating in clinical research. The first protection is the institutional assurance. An assurance states that the institution will comply with the federal requirements to conduct properly reviewed and approved research. The second protection is an institutional review board composed of at least five local community members of varying backgrounds. An institutional review board reviews and approves all covered research. The last protection is the informed consent, a process that informs involved patients about the proposed research, from preenrollment through active study involvement and into the completion of the fol-low-up period.

To enable cancer patients to make an informed decision to participate or to decline participation in a study, the process of informed consent must provide a complete understanding of the rationale driving the study and of the study's goals, potential risks, and benefits. Participation in a clinical trial is voluntary, and participants are free to leave the study at any time. Participants should understand that any treatment being offered is research and is not a proved method. Although details of the proposed study are contained in the informed consent document, discussion with the health care team, supplemental reading materials, and computer-based programs often will enhance the potential study participant's understanding of the study. This flow of information to participants should continue throughout the study.

CHALLENGES

Increasing patient accrual, assuring insurance coverage for individuals participating in clinical trials, and increasing patient diversity are three of the challenges that clinical trial researchers experience. Increasing patient accrual is important for obtaining answers to a study question more quickly. According to the National Cancer Institute (NCI), approximately 3% of adult cancer patients enroll in clinical trials. The discovery of effective interventions for the cancer disease burden will take longer if participation in research studies continues to be limited to such a small subset of cancer patients. In the past, information about cancer clinical trials was provided to patients by physician referral, lectures, brochures, telephone information services, and videos. Now, a great deal of information about cancer clinical trials is available from national organizations on the World Wide Web. Fourteen years ago, the NCI developed the physician data query, a computerized clinical trial information service. However, only recently has the interest in and availability of Web sites grown to the point that significant numbers of people have access to this information.

Though low participation in clinical trials has many causes, exclusion of coverage by insurers is a major barrier. The penetration of managed-care plans has had an impact on cancer research sites across the country. Cancer care is expensive, and usually managed-care organizations focus on providing efficient care that often does not include research. This coverage by insurers varies from location to location, and potential participants are urged to talk with the clinical trial staff for better understanding of the insurance issues at their location. Discussion of reimbursement with insurers has been pursued actively for years by such organizations as the NCI and the National Coalition of Cancer Survivors.

Equal access and proportional representation of all racial and ethnic groups in cancer clinical trials is critical. Tejeda et al. [5] suggested that this goal is being realized in cancer treatment trials. However, this experience does not extend to cancer prevention trials [6]. Two of the large NCI chemoprevention trials in breast and prostate cancer were able to recruit only 3% to 4% minority participants, even after vigorous efforts were made to train site staff regarding cultural and racial barriers to clinical participation. Sites participating in clinical trials also should develop community affiliations (e.g., churches, community organizations) that engender on-going trusting and sharing rapport between the health care staff and the local residents.

CONCLUSION

Medical science advances through clinical trials. Physicians treating patients with such diseases as cancer, which still entails many unanswered questions about optimal prevention and treatment, should be aware of the availability of research studies not only to help their patients but to advance knowledge in the field. We are indebted to previous generations of research investigators for providing us with tools that have led to improved survival and quality of life for many cancer patients. We owe future generations the same legacy.

REFERENCES

1. MacArthur CA, Vietti T. The importance of phase I/II trials in pediatric oncology. *Invest New Drugs* 14:33–35, 1996.
2. National Cancer Institute. *Cancer Clinical Trials Education Program.* Bethesda, MD: National Cancer Institute, 1998.
3. Maxwell MB. Principles of treatment planning. In Groenwald SL, Frogge M, Goodman M, Henke Yarbro C (eds), *Cancer Nursing: Principles and Practice* (4th ed). Boston: Jones & Bartlett, 1997:225.
4. Katz J. The Nuremberg Code and the Nuremberg trial. A reappraisal. *JAMA* 276:1662–1665, 1996.
5. Tejeda HA, Green SB, Trimble EL, et al. Representation of African-Americans, Hispanics, and whites in NCI cancer treatment trials. *J Natl Cancer Inst* 88:812–816, 1996.
6. Fisher B, Costantino J, Wickerham D, et al. Tamoxifen for prevention of breast cancer: Report of the National Surgical Adjuvant Breast and Bowel Project P-1 study. *J Natl Cancer Inst* 90:1371–1388, 1998.

Index

Page numbers followed by "f" represent figures; those followed by "t" represent tables. Color plates are identified by the plate numbers, e.g., PL11.1.